The Routledge Handbook of Phonetics

The Routledge Handbook of Phonetics provides a comprehensive and up-to-date compilation of research, history, and techniques in phonetics. With contributions from 41 prominent authors from North America, Europe, Australia, and Japan, and including more than 130 figures to illustrate key points, this handbook covers all the most important areas in the field, including:

- the history and scope of techniques used, including speech synthesis, vocal tract imaging techniques, and obtaining information on under-researched languages from language archives;
- the physiological bases of speech and hearing, including auditory, articulatory, and neural explanations of hearing, speech, and language processes;
- theories and models of speech perception and production related to the processing of consonants, vowels, prosody, tone, and intonation;
- linguistic phonetics, with discussions of the phonetics-phonology interface, sound change, second language acquisition, sociophonetics, and second language teaching research;
- applications and extensions, including phonetics and gender, clinical phonetics, and forensic phonetics.

The Routledge Handbook of Phonetics will be indispensable reading for students and practitioners in the fields of speech, language, linguistics, and hearing sciences.

William F. Katz is Professor for the School of Behavioral and Brain Sciences at the University of Texas at Dallas, U.S.A.

Peter F. Assmann is Professor for the School of Behavioral and Brain Sciences at the University of Texas at Dallas, U.S.A.

Routledge Handbooks in Linguistics

Routledge Handbooks in Linguistics provide overviews of a whole subject area or sub-discipline in linguistics, and survey the state of the discipline including emerging and cutting edge areas. Edited by leading scholars, these volumes include contributions from key academics from around the world and are essential reading for both advanced undergraduate and postgraduate students.

The Routledge Handbook of Metaphor and Language
Edited by Elena Semino and Zsófia Demjén

The Routledge Handbook of Systemic Functional Linguistics
Edited by Tom Bartlett, Gerard O'Grady

The Routledge Handbook of Heritage Language Education
From Innovation to Program Building
Edited by Olga E. Kagan, Maria M. Carreira and Claire Hitchins Chik

The Routledge Handbook of Language and Humor
Edited by Salvatore Attardo

The Routledge Handbook of Language and Dialogue
Edited by Edda Weigand

The Routledge Handbook of Language and Politics
Edited by Ruth Wodak and Bernhard Forchtner

The Routledge Handbook of Language and Media
Edited by Daniel Perrin and Colleen Cotter

The Routledge Handbook of Ecolinguistics
Edited by Alwin F. Fill and Hermine Penz

The Routledge Handbook of Lexicography
Edited by Pedro A. Fuertes-Olivera

The Routledge Handbook of Discourse Processes, Second Edition
Edited by Michael F. Schober, David N. Rapp, and M. Anne Britt

The Routledge Handbook of Phonetics
Edited by William F. Katz and Peter F. Assmann

Further titles in this series can be found online at www.routledge.com/series/RHIL

The Routledge Handbook of Phonetics

Edited by William F. Katz and Peter F. Assmann

Routledge
Taylor & Francis Group
LONDON AND NEW YORK

First published 2019
by Routledge
2 Park Square, Milton Park, Abingdon, Oxon OX14 4RN

and by Routledge
52 Vanderbilt Avenue, New York, NY 10017

Routledge is an imprint of the Taylor & Francis Group, an informa business

British Library Cataloguing-in-Publication Data
A catalogue record for this book is available from the British Library

Library of Congress Cataloging-in-Publication Data
Names: Katz, William F., editor. | Assmann, Peter F., editor.
Title: The Routledge handbook of phonetics / edited by William F. Katz and Peter F. Assmann.
Description: Abingdon, Oxon ; New York, NY : Routledge, 2019. | Series: Routledge handbooks in linguistics | Includes bibliographical references and index.
Identifiers: LCCN 2018048253 | ISBN 9781138648333 (hardback) | ISBN 9780429056253 (e-book)
Subjects: LCSH: Phonetics.
Classification: LCC P221 .R75 2019 | DDC 414/.8—dc23
LC record available at https://lccn.loc.gov/2018048253

ISBN: 978-1-138-64833-3 (hbk)
ISBN: 978-0-429-05625-3 (ebk)

Typeset in Times New Roman
by Apex CoVantage, LLC

Contents

Illustrations

Figures

Tables

Abbreviations

aCGg	Anterior cingulate gyrus
aCO	Anterior central operculum
adSTs	Anterior dorsal superior temporal sulcus
AE	American English
aFO	Anterior frontal operculum
Ag	Angular gyrus
aINS	Anterior insula
ASHA	American Speech-Language-Hearing Association
aSMg	Anterior supramarginal gyrus
ASP	Automatic Selective Perception (theory)
aSTg	Anterior superior temporal gyrus
ASY	Articulatory synthesizer (Haskins Laboratories)
AV	Audio-visual
BA	Brodmann Area
Bark	Zwicker's auditory frequency scale
BOLD	Blood oxygenation level dependent
CAPT	Computer-assisted pronunciation teaching
CT	Computed tomography
CV	Consonant-vowel
dBA	Sound pressure level in decibels (A weighting)
dCMA	Dorsal cingulate motor area
dIFo	Dorsal inferior frontal gyrus, *pars opercularis*
DIVA	Directions into Velocities of Articulators (neurocomputational model)
dMC	Dorsal motor cortex
DNN	Deep neural network
DoF	Degrees of freedom
dSC	Dorsal somatosensory cortex
EEG	Electroencephalography
EMA	Electromagnetic articulography
EPG	Electropalatogram
ERB	Equivalent rectangular bandwidth
ERP	Event-related potential
f_0	Fundamental frequency
F_1	First formant (second formant F2, …)

fMRI	Functional magnetic resonance imaging
GABA	Gamma-Aminobutyric acid
GGA	Anterior Genioglossus
GGM	Middle Genioglossus
GGP	Posterior Genioglossus
GODIVA	Gradient Order DIVA (neurocomputational model)
GP	Globus pallidus
GUI	Graphical user interface
H1	First harmonic (second harmonic H2, …)
Hg	Heschl's gyrus
HNR	Harmonics-to-noise ratio
IFG	Inferior frontal gyrus
IFo	Inferior frontal gyrus, *pars opercularis*
IFS	Inferior frontal sulcus
IFt	Inferior frontal gyrus, *pars triangularis*
IL	Inferior Longitudinal
IPA	International Phonetic Alphabet (International Phonetic Association)
L1	First language
L2	Second language
Lg	Lingual gyrus
LPC	Linear predictive coding
LVP	Levator Veli Palatini
MEG	Magnetoencephalography
Mel	Stevens' pitch scale
MEN	Mentalis
MFCCs	Mel frequency cepstral coefficients
midMC	Middle motor cortex
midPMC	Middle premotor cortex
midSC	Middle somatosensory cortex
ML	Mylohyoid
MRI	Magnetic Resonance Imaging
MTG	Middle temporal gyrus
NLM	Native Language Magnet (theory)
NSF	National Science Foundation
OC	Occipital cortex
OO	Orbicularis Oris
OOp	Peripheral Orbicularis Oris
OPI	Oropharyngeal Isthmus
OT	Optimality theory
PAM	Perceptual assimilation model
PB	Peterson and Barney 1952 database
pCO	Posterior central operculum
pdPMC	Posterior dorsal premotor cortex
pdSTs	Posterior dorsal superior temporal sulcus
pdSTs	Posterior dorsal superior temporal sulcus
PET	Positron emission tomography
pFO	Posterior frontal operculum
pIFS	Posterior inferior frontal sulcus

pINS	Posterior insula
pMTg	Posterior middle temporal gyrus
PO	Parietal operculum
PP	Planum polare
preSMA	Pre-supplementary motor area
pSMg	Posterior supramarginal gyrus
pSTg	Posterior superior temporal gyrus
PT	Planum temporale
Put	Putamen
pvSTs	Posterior ventral superior temporal sulcus
RIS	Risorius
SL	Superior Longitudinal
SLM	Speech learning model
SLP	Speech language pathologist
SMA	Supplementary motor area
smCB	Superior medial cerebellum
SPL	Superior parietal lobule
Spt	Sylvian-parietal-temporal area
TIMIT	Phonetically balanced speech database, Texas Instruments and MIT
TMS	Transcranial magnetic stimulation
TOEFL	Test of English as a foreign language
UPSID	UCLA phonological segment inventory database
US	Ultrasound
VA	Ventral anterior nucleus of the thalamus
vCMA	Ventral cingulate motor area
vIFo	Ventral inferior frontal gyrus, *pars opercularis*
vIFt	Ventral inferior frontal gyrus, *pars triangularis*
VL	Ventrolateral thalamic nucleus
vMC	Ventral motor cortex
Vocoder	Voice coder
VOT	Voice onset time
vPMC	Ventral premotor cortex
VPP	Velopharyngeal Port
VRT	Verticalis
vSC	Ventral somatosensory cortex

Contributors

Takayuki Arai received his PhD from Sophia University in 1994. He was a visiting scientist at Oregon Graduate Institute (Portland, OR, U.S.A.) in 1992–1993 and 1995–1996, International Computer Science Institute (Berkeley, CA, U.S.A.) in 1997–1998, and Massachusetts Institute of Technology (Cambridge, MA, U.S.A.) in 2003–2004. He is currently Professor of the Department of Information and Communication Sciences, Sophia University.

Peter F. Assmann is a Professor in the School of Behavioral and Brain Sciences at the University of Texas at Dallas. His research interests focus on two overlapping problems in speech perception: How listeners cope with the enormous variability in the acoustic patterns of speech across talkers, and how speech communication is conducted with extraordinary resilience under adverse listening conditions.

Molly Babel is Associate Professor of Linguistics at the University of British Columbia. Her research focuses on the production and perception of phonetic variation, using theories and methods from Phonetics, Psycholinguistics, and Sociolinguistics. She is a member of the Royal Society of Canada's College of New Scholars, Artists, and Scientists.

Jason W. Bohland is Associate Director and Senior Research Scientist at the Boston University Cognitive Neuroimaging Center. His research focuses on understanding the functional architecture of neural systems in the human brain, with emphasis on those that support speech and language. This work utilizes computational, informatics, and neuroimaging methods to inform contemporary models of speech processing at multiple levels of organization.

Dani Byrd is Professor of Linguistics and former Executive Vice Dean at the University of Southern California. Her research focuses on the signatures of linguistic structure in articulatory timing. She has co-written the textbook *Discovering Speech, Words, and Mind* (Wiley-Blackwell, 2010), is a fellow of the Acoustical Society of America, and is on the editorial board of the *Journal of Phonetics*.

Charles B. Chang is Assistant Professor of Linguistics at Boston University, where he directs the Phonetics, Acquisition and Multilingualism Lab (PAMLab). His research concerns the processing, representation, and development of speech sounds in the context of multilingualism and language contact, as well as the cross-language interactions that occur during second-language learning and first-language attrition.

Tracey M. Derwing is Professor Emeritus of TESL at the University of Alberta, and an adjunct professor in Linguistics at Simon Fraser University. With Murray Munro, she has extensively researched L2 pronunciation and fluency; in 2015 they co-authored *Pronunciation Fundamentals: Evidence-based Perspectives for L2 Teaching and Research*, Amsterdam: John Benjamins. Tracey has also investigated interventions to enhance native speakers' comprehension of L2-accented speech.

Ewald Enzinger is a Research Engineer at Eduworks Corporation. He has previously held research appointments at the Acoustics Research Institute of the Austrian Academy of Sciences. He has contributed to analyses of forensic voice evidence for presentation in court in multiple cases and has collaborated with researchers and practitioners at law-enforcement agencies in Australia, Germany, and the Netherlands.

Marc Garellek is Associate Professor of Linguistics at University of California, San Diego. His research deals with the phonetics and linguistic functions of voice quality and other suprasegmental articulations such as stress, tone, and nasalization. He is currently an associate editor of *The Journal of the Acoustical Society of America-Express Letters*.

Bryan Gick is a Professor and Guggenheim fellow in the Department of Linguistics at the University of British Columbia, and a senior scientist at Haskins Laboratories. Gick's research develops an embodied approach to speech, deepening links between speech production and multimodal perception, biomechanics, motor control, the nervous system, and the development and learning of speech communication.

Louis Goldstein is Professor of Linguistics at the University of Southern California. His research focuses on the development of articulatory phonology, an approach that decomposes speech into units of articulatory coordination. He is a fellow of the Acoustical Society of America and the Linguistic Society of America, and is on the editorial board of *Phonetica*.

Frank H. Guenther is Professor of Speech Language, and Hearing Sciences and Biomedical Engineering at Boston University and a research affiliate at Massachusetts General Hospital and the Massachusetts Institute of Technology. His research combines theoretical modeling with behavioral and neuroimaging experiments to characterize the neural computations underlying speech. He also develops brain–machine interfaces to restore speech communication to severely paralyzed individuals.

Jonathan Harrington directs the Institute of Phonetics and Speech Processing at Ludwig-Maximilian University, Munich. His main research is in human speech processing and its relationship to sound change. He also has a long-standing interest in the development of tools for analyzing speech corpora and speech physiology research.

James M. Hillenbrand is Distinguished Faculty Scholar in the Department of Speech, Language, and Hearing Sciences at Western Michigan University. He held previous positions at Northwestern University and as director of research in the Intelligent Systems Division of RIT Research Corporation. His research focuses on the acoustics, perception, and synthesis of speech, the perception of vocal quality, and the modeling of auditory frequency analysis.

William F. Katz is a Professor at the University of Texas at Dallas, School of Behavioral and Brain Sciences, in the Department of Communication Disorders. His research concerns clinical phonetics, particularly speech production in adults with communication disorders resulting from brain injury.

Michael Kiefte is a Professor in the School of Communication Sciences and Disorders at Dalhousie University. His current research focus is on speech perception and production and with an emphasis on statistical modeling.

John Kingston is Professor of Linguistics at the University of Massachusetts, Amherst, where he has been since 1990. He previously taught at Cornell University (1986–1990) and the University of Texas, Austin (1984–1986). He received a PhD in Linguistics from the University of California, Berkeley in 1985. His research focuses principally on speech perception and its influence on phonology. He also does field work on Chinantecan and Chatino languages.

Felicitas Kleber is a Lecturer and Senior Researcher at the Institute of Phonetics and Speech Processing, Ludwig-Maximilian University, Munich. Her research interests are in prosody and intonation, sound change, German dialectology, and the acquisition of speech.

Joyce McDonough is a Phonetician and a Morphologist broadly interested in the structure encoded in the linguistic speech signal. She is especially interested in the phonetic patterns of morphological structure in complex morphologies and the coding of speech in the brain. One of her goals is to reintroduce phonetic methods and analyses into contemporary language documentation and description practices.

Geoffrey Stewart Morrison is Associate Professor of Forensic Speech Science, Aston University. His past appointments include Simons Foundation Visiting Fellow, Isaac Newton Institute for Mathematical Sciences; Scientific Counsel, Office of Legal Affairs, INTERPOL; and director of the Forensic Voice Comparison Laboratory, University of New South Wales. He has forensic casework experience in Australia, Canada, Northern Ireland, Sweden, and the United States.

Murray J. Munro is Professor of Linguistics at Simon Fraser University. His research – much of it carried out with Tracey M. Derwing – focuses on issues in applied phonetics and has appeared in a wide range of journals in the speech sciences and education. His most recent book, co-edited with John Levis, is *Pronunciation* (Routledge, 2017).

Benjamin Munson is a Professor in the Department of Speech-Language-Hearing Sciences at University of Minnesota. His research examines how lexical knowledge and sociolinguistic knowledge influence speech perception and speech production in children with typical and atypical language profiles.

Shrikanth Narayanan is Professor of Electrical Engineering, Computer Science, Linguistics, Psychology, Neuroscience and Pediatrics at the University of Southern California and directs the Signal Analysis and Interpretation Laboratory. He is a fellow of the IEEE, National Academy of Inventors, Acoustical Society of America, Association for Psychological Science, International Speech Communication Association, and the American Association for the Advancement of Science.

Terrance M. Nearey is Emeritus Professor of Linguistics at the University of Alberta. He continues to study speech perception and technical phonetics.

Jonathan E. Peelle is an Associate Professor in the Department of Otolaryngology at Washington University in Saint Louis. He obtained his PhD in Neuroscience from Brandeis University, and went on for postdoctoral training in Cognitive Neuroscience. His research investigates the neuroscience of speech comprehension, aging, and hearing impairment using a combination of behavioral and brain imaging methods.

Ulrich Reubold is a Senior Researcher at the Institute of Phonetics and Speech Processing, Ludwig-Maximilian University, Munich. His research interests are in laboratory phonology and sound change, concentrating on longitudinal change within the same person.

Murray Schellenberg works as a Researcher in the Interdisciplinary Speech Research Laboratory at the University of British Columbia. His research focuses on the intersection of language and music with a particular emphasis on issues of musical text-setting and the acoustics/articulation of singing performance.

Florian Schiel directs the Bavarian Archive for Speech Signals (BAS) at Ludwig-Maximilian University, Munich; BAS is located at the Institute of Phonetics and Speech Processing. His research interests include the analysis and modeling of user-specific states in large speech datasets, empirical speech analysis in general, speech corpus production and evaluation, speaker verification, forensic phonetics, and agent-based modeling.

Ian Stavness is Associate Professor of Computer Science at the University of Saskatchewan. He directs the Biological Imaging and Graphics lab, which is focused on three-dimensional computational modeling, image analysis, and deep learning for biological and biomedical applications. He has been recognized as an OpenSim fellow for his work on biomechanical modeling and its translation to rehabilitation medicine.

Mary Stevens is a Senior Researcher at the Institute of Phonetics and Speech Processing, Ludwig-Maximilian University, Munich. Her research interests include descriptive phonetics (including research on lesser documented languages and varieties of Italian), laboratory phonology, and sound change.

Christian E. Stilp is Associate Professor of Psychological and Brain Sciences at the University of Louisville. His research examines how perception of speech and other complex sounds is shaped by predictability and unpredictability in the acoustic environment. He is a member of the Acoustical Society of America.

Brad H. Story is Professor of Speech, Language, and Hearing Sciences at the University of Arizona. He also holds appointments in Biomedical Engineering, Cognitive Science, Second Language Acquisition, and Ethnomusicology. His research is concerned with the acoustics, mechanics, and physiology of human sound production, and understanding how listeners decode the information in the acoustic speech signal.

Marija Tabain is Associate Professor of Phonetics at La Trobe University. She is a member of the Permanent Council of the International Phonetic Association, and is on the editorial boards of the *Journal of Phonetics* and the *Journal of the International Phonetic Association*.

Ryan C. Taylor is a Postdoctoral Fellow in the Interdisciplinary Speech Research Laboratory at the University of British Columbia. He teaches in the Cognitive Systems Program and is a member of the Language Sciences Initiative. His research deals with the physiological and mental underpinnings of speech in communication, with emphasis on the phonetics and pragmatics of prosody.

Erik R. Thomas is a Professor in the English Department at North Carolina State University. His research deals with phonetic aspects of sociolinguistics, much of it focusing on minority dialects of English. He has written or edited six books, including *Sociophonetics: An Introduction* (Palgrave Macmillan, 2011) and *Mexican American English: Substrate Influence and the Birth of an Ethnolect* (Cambridge University Press, 2019).

Jason A. Tourville is a Research Assistant Professor in the Department of Speech, Language, and Hearing Sciences at Boston University. His research combines neuroimaging methods and computational modeling to study the neural mechanisms that underlie speech and speech disorders. He also uses an extensive background in human neuroanatomy to develop improved expert-guided semi-automated brain region labeling methods.

Asterios Toutios is Research Assistant Professor of Electrical Engineering at the University of Southern California. His research focuses on modeling human speech production based on direct observations of the vocal-tract dynamic configuration, with a view to helping assess speech disorders and enhance speech technologies like recognition and synthesis.

D. H. Whalen is the Founder and Chair of the Board of Directors of the Endangered Language Fund. He is also Distinguished Professor in the Speech-Language-Hearing Sciences program, Graduate Center, City University of New York (CUNY), as well as appointments in the linguistics departments of CUNY and Yale University. He is also Vice President of Research at Haskins Laboratories.

Matthew B. Winn is an Assistant Professor of Speech-Language-Hearing Sciences at the University of Minnesota. His research deals with the speech perception in people with hearing impairment, mainly focusing on phonetics and listening effort. He is also a clinically trained audiologist and a member of the Acoustical Society of America.

Yi Xu is Professor of Speech Sciences at University College London. He received his PhD in 1993 from the University of Connecticut. His research is primarily concerned with the basic mechanisms of speech production and perception in connected discourse, especially in terms of how multiple layers of communicative meanings are encoded through a common process of articulation.

Acknowledgments

The editors would like to thank the following copyright holders for permission to reproduce the following material:

Figure 4: De Cheveigné, A., and Kawahara, H., 1999. Missing-data model of vowel identification. *The Journal of the Acoustical Society of America*, 105(6), pp. 3497–3508.

Figure 5: Katz, W. F., and Mehta, S., 2015. Visual feedback of tongue movement for novel speech sound learning. *Frontiers in Human Neuroscience*, 9, p. 612.

Chapter 2, Figure 2.3 and Chapter 4, Figure 4.2: Morrison, G. S., and Assmann, P. F., eds. 2012. *Vowel inherent spectral change*. Springer Science and Business Media.

While the publishers have made every effort to contact copyright holders of material used in this volume, they would be grateful to hear from any they were unable to contact.

Editors' acknowledgments

This handbook, designed to provide a state-of-the-art view of modern phonetics, was made possible through the efforts of many talented individuals. Above all, we thank the authors, whose patience and perseverance in responding to deadlines and delays are greatly appreciated. We also thank the many researchers who provided thoughtful and constructive reviews of the chapters, including Martin J. Ball, Ryan Bennett, Suzanne Boyce, Lisa Davidson, Laura Dilley, John Esling, Sam Evans, Marc Garellek, Lisa Goffman, John Hansen, Allard Jongman, Lucie Menard, Patrick Reidy, Philip Rubin, Geoffrey Schwartz, Ron Thomson, Paschal Trembley, Siri Tuttle, and Melanie Weinrich.

Editors' introduction

A handbook of phonetics

William F. Katz and Peter F. Assmann

Overview

Phonetics, the branch of linguistics concerned with the production and perception of speech sounds, has experienced tremendous growth in recent years. As the chapters in this handbook indicate, phonetics is involved in speech technology and computing; social media and advertising; legal proceedings; second language instruction; and speech, hearing, and language pathology. As people increasingly communicate with "virtual assistants" and interact with personal devices that rely critically on speech and voice, basic research into the physical, social, and statistical aspects of speech plays a central role.

Phonetics has always had an important role as a bridging discipline: It shares common bonds with several other fields, including psychology, neuroscience, physics, and engineering. Phonetics links linguistics to the physical sciences through the study of speech acoustics and the mechanisms of speech production associated with phonation and articulation on the one hand, and the sensory and neural processing of speech on the other. As a result of expansive developments in each of these fields, phonetics continues to become a broader and deeper field.

As teachers of phonetics, we are struck by the tremendous growth of this field and note a need for integrative reviews to provide our students with important new lines of research and relate them to traditional issues. While one cannot begin to cover all the various new directions of phonetics within a single volume, we have tried to compile topics addressing both traditional themes and new directions, including a balance of empirical and theoretical work.

Themes and chapters

This handbook includes 21 chapters, from 39 authors, describing a wide range of languages and areas of research. The handbook is organized around five major themes. The first theme surveys a variety of techniques used in the field of phonetics, tracing their history and describing current and future developments.

Story (2019, Chapter 1, this volume) reviews the history of speech synthesis, a technology that is invaluable for phoneticians and links speech production and speech perception. Story traces the fascinating history of talking machines, from early resonating tube models through electronic circuits to modern digital synthesis. His chapter highlights the importance of models and physical representations in the development of speech synthesis and concludes with a discussion of the importance of uncovering the "rules" that govern the production of fluent speech, which in turn may be regarded as "synonymous with understanding many aspects of speech production and perception."

Toutios, Byrd, Goldstein, and Narayanan (2019, Chapter 2, this volume) present a survey of methods for visualizing the shapes and movements of the vocal tract during speech in real time. Focusing on dynamic real-time magnetic resonance imaging (rtMRI), they describe various attributes of segmental and suprasegmental production, including cross-linguistic differences in context dependence. In addition, they note how imaging data can inform current models of speech production. Examples are given concerning the development of rtMRI databases, and some remaining challenges are discussed.

Whalen and McDonough (2019, Chapter 3, this volume) describe the use of state-of-the art archival research methods to document the phonetic properties of endangered and under-researched languages. The authors note that adequate phonetic documentation has not been provided for many of the world's languages, and in the past, descriptions have often relied on small samples and impressionistic accounts. The chapter provides a survey of present-day language archives, from "A" (ANLC – Alaskan Native Language Center), to "U" (UCLA-University of California Los Angeles Phonetic Archive), and summarizes the phonetic analyses derived from them, along with recommendations for future archival phonetics research.

The second theme, covering the physiological basis of speech and hearing, includes five chapters. Garellek (2019, Chapter 4, this volume) examines the phonetics of voice, including the vibrations of the vocal folds and their acoustic and perceptual consequences, as well as the use of voice properties to form phonological and lexical contrasts. The chapter examines the complexities of vocal fold dynamics and their acoustic consequences, and considers how these properties are related to voice quality. It describes the current state of articulatory and psychoacoustic modeling to account for these interactions.

Gick, Schellenberg, Stavness and Taylor (2019, Chapter 5, this volume) detail the current state of articulatory phonetics, raising important questions concerning the basic components or "units" of articulation. Their aim is to encourage the reader to rethink the current mapping of descriptive terms onto specific groupings of nerves and muscles used to produce speech sounds. Drawing on examples from various languages, they demonstrate that a particular set of articulators such as the "lips" may be used differently across languages and indeed across phonemes within a language, causing one to consider whether a rather general designation such as "lips" is particularly helpful in the first place. Novel ways of viewing lingual behavior (including "bracing" for vowels) and uvular actions are discussed. This chapter also describes biomechanical simulations that tackle several timely issues in phonetics, including models of coarticulation and speech motor control.

Bohland, Tourville, and Guenther (2019, Chapter 6, this volume) delineate the neural systems and structures involved in the production of speech. Focusing primarily on data from functional magnetic resonance (fMRI) imaging, they review the neural systems active during speech, describing both healthy speech and patterns noted in speech and language disorders such as Parkinson's disease, ataxic dysarthria, and apraxia of speech. Brain imaging and behavioral data are related to the predictions made by neurocomputational models designed to simulate phonetic processing corresponding roughly to the level of phonemes or syllables ("DIVA" model) and, more recently, to multisyllabic words or phrases ("GODIVA" model). The potential of these models for achieving new insights and testing novel hypotheses concerning the neural control of speech is discussed.

The auditory and neural processing of speech is covered by Winn and Stilp (2019, Chapter 7, this volume). They provide examples to illustrate how the complex and nonlinear transformations in the auditory periphery affect the processing of speech, and show how a detailed knowledge of these mechanisms can inform phonetic analysis as well as theory. They note that auditory processing is especially sensitive to spectral change over time, providing a basis for contrast enhancement and a mechanism that contributes to well-documented spectral contrast effects in vowels and consonants.

Peelle (2019, Chapter 8, this volume) reviews the cortical structures that are enlisted during the auditory and audiovisual (AV) perception of speech. The chapter examines progressively larger linguistic units, ranging from isolated phonemes, individual words, and sentences in connected speech. Peelle considers how the different levels of speech processing interact with specific auditory and audiovisual neural processing networks. In addition to considering fMRI data, attention is paid to electrophysiological studies, including discussion of how oscillatory patterns noted in auditory cortex under different testing conditions suggest that the visual stream affects auditory processing during the AV perception of speech. The chapter concludes by considering how "real world" phonetic processing (i.e., in the noisy world outside of the phonetics lab!) can pose special challenges that need be considered in order to more fully understand the cognitive resources used in the processing of speech and language.

The third theme of the handbook addresses theories and models of speech perception and production. Hillenbrand (2019, Chapter 9, this volume) provides a systematic review of theories and mechanisms of vowel perception, with a primary focus on the vowels of North American English. Beginning with a review of the source-filter theory of vowel production and an acoustic characterization of vowel quality, the chapter reviews evidence related to the question of whether vowel perception is based on formants, spectral shape, or an alternative representation. It considers the role of vowel-inherent spectral change (VISC) in vowel identification and theories of talker normalization, the mechanism by which listeners accommodate to changes in the acoustic properties when the same vowel is spoken by different talkers.

Tabain (2019, Chapter 10, this volume) considers the phonetic properties of consonants, starting with an analysis of the descriptive framework of the phonetic features of voicing, place, and manner. The chapter emphasizes the complexity of the relationships between articulatory and acoustic properties and their encoding in (or omission from) the transcription system of the International Phonetic Alphabet (IPA). Using examples that include a number of Australian languages, the chapter provides a thorough examination of the relationships between acoustic, articulatory and perceptual properties of consonants.

Kiefte and Nearey (2019, Chapter 11, this volume) review theories and models of speech perception. Their main focus is on two questions: (a) What are the units of speech (from the combined perspectives of the listener and speaker) and (b) how do listeners map the acoustic signal to these units in perception? They evaluate two theoretical frameworks: *articulatory* and *gestural*, in which the listener is assumed to recover the linguistic units from the articulatory or gestural features involved in producing the signal; and *auditory*, whereby the linguistic units are recovered directly from the auditory representation of the signal. "Strong" forms of each of these approaches are rejected in favor of a "double-weak" framework, in which both gestural and auditory patterns are assumed to provide indirect links between acoustic properties and linguistic units.

Xu (2019, Chapter 12, this volume) covers prosody, tone, and intonation. The chapter begins with a review of the articulatory and aerodynamic properties underlying these three related domains and a discussion of how the associated perceptual properties of pitch, duration, and voice quality are transmitted in parallel to create segmental and suprasegmental contrasts. Several fascinating topics are included relating to context-dependent tonal alternations (e.g., pre-low raising and post-low bouncing), paralinguistic prosody, and the relation between boundary stress level and the rhythm class hypothesis that divides languages into categories such as "stress-timed," "syllable-timed," and "morae-timed." Many interesting comparisons between tonal languages (e.g., Mandarin) and non-tonal languages (e.g., English) are included.

The fourth theme of the book covers phonetics and linguistic variation. Kingston (2019, Chapter 13, this volume) discusses proposals for and against an "interface" between phonetics and phonology. The concept of such an interface is to provide a mechanism for translating between the phonological representation of speech, assumed to be composed of discrete linguistic categories, and the phonetic representation, which consists of continuous (acoustic and articulatory) measures. Arguments for and against a phonetics-phonology interface are carefully laid out, and Kingston identifies future steps that are needed to resolve these competing approaches.

Harrington, Kleber, Reubold, Schiel, and Stevens (2019, Chapter 14, this volume) review the nature of sound change, its origin, and its spread. They examine how ambiguities in the transmission of speech dynamics between the speaker and the hearer can lead to sound change. They consider in detail how hyper- and hypoarticulation contribute to sound change, and describe the steps involved in implementing agent-based models to explain how sound change develops and spreads in the population.

Chang (2019, Chapter 15, this volume) considers the mechanisms and processes involved in learning a second language (L2). The main focus of his chapter is a comparison and evaluation of current theories and models of L2 acquisition. Factors taken into account include the amount of L2 experience and the time course of learning, the acoustic-phonetic similarity of L1 and L2 sounds, and the relationship between perception and production.

Thomas (2019, Chapter 16, this volume) describes the recent history and developments in the new discipline of sociophonetics, which studies variation in the acoustic, articulatory and perceptual properties of speech, including regional variation (dialect) and social indexicality (gender, ethnicity, social class). Recent findings and developments in the field are highlighted, including descriptive studies of regional phonetic variation, sound mergers and the effects of language contact. A key development is that many studies have extended beyond the descriptive characterization of phonetic variation to develop and evaluate models of sound production and perception. The chapter concludes with a model of speech processing that combines episodic properties (associated with individual speakers) and abstract properties (related to the speaker's knowledge of phonological categories) to consider how these properties interact and shift over time.

Munro and Derwing (2019, Chapter 17, this volume) cover the principles and practices of second language teaching. Following a review of the history of phonetics and language pedagogy, they outline several principles to guide effective L2 instruction, emphasizing intelligibility over native-like pronunciation. They review recent findings on the effectiveness of pronunciation training, indicating the presence of individual differences in pronunciation learning success, and they show that accentedness, intelligibility and comprehensibility are at least partially independent factors. They conclude that evidence-based pronunciation instruction is both possible and necessary, and identify remaining pedagogical goals for intelligibility and comprehensibility to meet the needs of individual learners.

The final theme of the book covers applications and extensions. Munson and Babel (2019, Chapter 18, this volume) examine the impact of sex and gender in phonetics. They review the anatomical and physiological differences between male and female vocal tracts and the articulatory, acoustic, and perceptual differences between male and female speech. Clear evidence is presented that some of these differences cannot be explicitly assigned to physical properties of the articulators, but result as a consequence of learned social behaviors.

Katz (2019, Chapter 19, this volume) provides a summary and review of recent developments in the field of clinical phonetics. This chapter also surveys multisensory information in speech processing and argues that such information is critical for understanding the phonetics of disordered language acquisition and breakdown. Examples of audiovisual speech processing involving the head, face, lips, jaw, and tongue are provided for healthy individuals and clinical populations. A final section considers how studies of visual feedback depicting articulator movement are being applied to a number of issues in L2 acquisition and clinical phonetics.

Arai (2019, Chapter 20, this volume) considers how physical models of the vocal tract may be used to better understand the concepts and principles of sound production for the teaching of phonetics, as a research platform, and for practical applications such as training new sound contrasts in an unfamiliar language. Using examples from Japanese and English, evidence is provided concerning the usefulness of these physical models in describing concepts relevant to speech production and phonetics, including the relation between vocal tract configurations and vowel quality.

Morrison and Enzinger (2019, Chapter 21, this volume) review the field of forensic voice comparison, comparing auditory, spectrographic, acoustic-phonetic, and automatic approaches. A common scenario in forensic voice comparison involves determining whether the voices on two audio recordings represent the same person. The challenges faced in this area of research overlap with those experienced in other areas of phonetics, namely that there are sources of variability (e.g., background noise and reverberation, contextual differences) that complicate the decision process. The overall conclusion of the chapter is that automatic approaches perform better under forensically realistic conditions and require fewer resources. However, the authors find that automatic procedures depend critically on human supervision, and note there have been few attempts to evaluate acoustic-phonetic statistical approaches under forensically realistic conditions.

Taken together, these themes provide, we believe, a glimpse of the dynamic field of phonetics. Given the rapid growth of scientific knowledge, we are aware that much more data will be available by the time that the ink dries on this page. This, of course, is how it *should* be! In closing, it is our hope that this volume gives impetus for "newbies" to find novel areas to study, while providing more seasoned researchers with some details or viewpoints of which they may not have been aware. We certainly learned a great deal from working on this project and we hope this sentiment will also be shared by you, the reader.

References

Arai (2019, Chapter 20, this volume) Vocal tract models in phonetic teaching and research

Babel and Munson (2019, Chapter 18, this volume) Phonetics and gender

Bohland, Tourville and Guenther (2019, Chapter 6, this volume) Neural bases of speech production

Chang (2019, Chapter 15, this volume) Phonetics of second language acquisition

Garellek (2019, Chapter 4, this volume) The phonetics of voice

Gick, Schellenberg, Stavness and Taylor (2019, Chapter 5, this volume) Articulatory phonetics

Harrington, Kleber, Reubold, Schiel and Stevens (2019, Chapter 14, this volume) The phonetic basis of the origin and spread of sound change
Hillenbrand (2019, Chapter 9, this volume) The acoustics and perception of North American English vowels
Katz (2019, Chapter 19, this volume) New horizons in clinical phonetics
Kiefte and Nearey (2019, Chapter 11, this volume) Theories and models of speech perception
Kingston (2019, Chapter 13, this volume) Phonetics-phonology interface
Morrison and Enzinger (2019, Chapter 21, this volume) Forensic phonetics
Munro and Derwing (2019, Chapter 17, this volume) Phonetics and second language teaching research
Peelle (2019, Chapter 8, this volume) Neural bases of auditory and audiovisual speech perception
Story (2019, Chapter 1, this volume) History of speech synthesis
Tabain (2019, Chapter 10, this volume) Phonetic properties of the consonants
Thomas (2019, Chapter 16, this volume) Innovations in sociophonetics
Toutios, Byrd, Goldstein and Narayanan (2019, Chapter 2, this volume) Imaging and vocal tract development
Whalen and McDonough (2019, Chapter 3, this volume) Under-researched languages: Phonetic results from language archives
Winn and Stilp (2019, Chapter 7, this volume) Phonetics and the auditory system
Xu (2019, Chapter 12, this volume) Prosody, tone, and intonation

Part I

History, scope, and techniques

1
History of speech synthesis

Brad H. Story

Introduction

For the past two centuries or more, a variety of devices capable of generating artificial or synthetic speech have been developed and used to investigate phonetic phenomena. The aim of this chapter is to provide a brief history of synthetic speech systems, including mechanical, electrical, and digital types. The primary goal, however, is not to reiterate the details of constructing specific synthesizers but rather to focus on the motivations for developing various synthesis paradigms and illustrate how they have facilitated research in phonetics.

The mechanical and electro-mechanical era

On the morning of December 20, 1845, a prominent American scientist attended a private exhibition of what he would later refer to as a "wonderful invention." The scientist was Joseph Henry, an expert on electromagnetic induction and the first Secretary of the Smithsonian Institution. The "wonderful invention" was a *machine that could talk*, meticulously crafted by a disheveled 60-year-old tinkerer from Freiburg, Germany named Joseph Faber. Their unlikely meeting in Philadelphia, Pennsylvania, arranged by an acquaintance of Henry from the American Philosophical Society, might have occurred more than a year earlier had Faber not destroyed a previous version of his talking machine in a bout of depression and intoxication. Although he had spent some 20 years perfecting the first device, Faber was able to reconstruct a second version of equal quality in a year's time (Patterson, 1845).

The layout of the talking machine, described in a letter from Henry to his colleague H.M. Alexander, was like that of a small chamber organ whose keyboard was connected via strings and levers to mechanical constructions of the speech organs. A carved wooden face was fitted with a hinged jaw, and behind it was an ivory tongue that was moveable enough to modulate the shape of the cavity in which it was housed. A foot-operated bellows supplied air to a rubber glottis whose vibration provided the raw sound that could be shaped into speech by pressing various sequences or combinations of 16 keys available on a keyboard. Each key was marked with a symbol representing an "elementary" sound that, through its linkage to the artificial organs, imposed time-varying changes to the air cavity appropriate for generating apparently convincing renditions of connected speech. Several years earlier Henry had been shown a talking machine built by the English scientist Charles Wheatstone, but he noted that Faber's machine was far superior because instead of uttering just a few words, it was "capable of speaking whole sentences composed of any words what ever" (Rothenberg et al., 1992, p. 362).

In the same letter, Henry mused about the possibility of placing two or more of Faber's talking machines at various locations and connecting them via telegraph lines. He thought that with "little contrivance" a spoken message could be coded as keystrokes in one location which, through electromagnetic means, would set into action another of the machines to "speak" the message to an audience at a distant location. Another 30 years would pass before Alexander Graham Bell demonstrated his invention of the telephone, yet Henry had already conceived of the notion while witnessing Faber's machine talk. Further, unlike Bell's telephone, which transmitted an electrical analog of the speech pressure wave, Henry's description alluded to representing speech in *compressed* form based on slowly varying movements of the operator's hands, fingers, and feet as they formed the keystroke sequences required to produce an utterance, a signal processing technique that would not be implemented into telephone transmission systems for nearly another century.

It is remarkable that, at this moment in history, a talking machine had been constructed that was capable of transforming a type of phonetic representation into a simulation of speech production, resulting in an acoustic output heard clearly as intelligible speech – and this same talking machine had inspired the idea of electrical transmission of low-bandwidth speech. The moment is also ironic, however, considering that no one seized either as an opportunity for scientific or technological advancement. Henry understandably continued on with his own scientific pursuits, leaving his idea to one short paragraph in an obscure letter to a colleague. In need of funds, Faber signed on with the entertainment entrepreneur P.T. Barnum in 1846 to exhibit his talking machine for a several months run at the Egyptian Hall in London. In his autobiography, Barnum (1886) noted that a repeat visitor to the exhibition was the Duke of Wellington, who Faber eventually taught to "speak" both English and German phrases with the machine (Barnum, 1886, p. 134). In the exhibitor's autograph book, the Duke wrote that Faber's "Automaton Speaker" was an "extraordinary production of mechanical genius." Other observers also noted the ingenuity in the design of the talking machine (e.g., "The Speaking Automaton," 1846; Athenaeum, 1846), but to Barnum's puzzlement it was not successful in drawing public interest or revenue. Faber and his machine were eventually relegated to a traveling exhibit that toured the villages and towns of the English countryside; it was supposedly here that Faber ended his life by suicide, although there is no definitive account of the circumstances of his death (Altick, 1978). In any case, Faber disappeared from the public record, although his talking machine continued to make sideshow-like appearances in Europe and North America over the next 30 years; it seems a relative (perhaps a niece or nephew) may have inherited the machine and performed with it to generate income ("Talking Machine," 1880; Altick, 1978).

Although the talking machine caught the serious attention of those who understood the significance of such a device, the overall muted interest may have been related to Faber's lack of showmanship, the German accent that was present in the machine's speech regardless of the language spoken, and perhaps the fact that Faber never published any written account of how the machine was designed or built – or maybe a mechanical talking machine, however ingenious its construction, was, by 1846, simply considered passé. Decades earlier, others had already developed talking machines that had impressed both scientists and the public.

Most notable were Christian Gottlieb Kratzenstein and Wolfgang von Kempelen, both of whom had independently developed mechanical speaking devices in the late 18th century.

Inspired by a competition sponsored by the Imperial Academy of Sciences at St. Petersburg in 1780, Kratzenstein submitted a report that detailed the design of five organ pipe-like resonators that, when excited with the vibration of a reed, produced the vowels /a, e, i, o, u/ (Kratzenstein, 1781). Although their shape bore little resemblance to human vocal tract configurations, and they could produce only sustained sounds, the construction of these resonators won the prize and marked a shift toward scientific investigation of human sound production. Kratzenstein, who at the time was a Professor of Physics at the University of Copenhagen, had shared a long-term interest in studying the physical nature of speaking with a former colleague at St. Petersburg, Leonhard Euler, who likely proposed the competition. Well known for his contributions to mathematics, physics, and engineering, Euler wrote in 1761 that "all the skill of man has not hitherto been capable of producing a piece of mechanism that could imitate [speech]" (p. 78) and further noted that "The construction of a machine capable of expressing sounds, with all the articulations, would no doubt be a very important discovery" (Euler, 1761, p. 79). He envisioned such a device to be used in assistance of those "whose voice is either too weak or disagreeable" (Euler, 1761, p. 79).

During the same time period, von Kempelen – a Hungarian engineer, industrialist, and government official – used his spare time and mechanical skills to build a talking machine far more advanced than the five vowel resonators demonstrated by Kratzenstein. The final version of his machine was to some degree a mechanical simulation of human speech production. It included a bellows as a "respiratory" source of air pressure and air flow, a wooden "wind" box that emulated the trachea, a reed system to generate the voice source, and a rubber funnel that served as the vocal tract. There was an additional chamber used for nasal sounds, and other control levers that were needed for particular consonants. Although it was housed in a large box, the machine itself was small enough that it could have been easily held in the hands. Speech was produced by depressing the bellows, which caused the "voice" reed to vibrate. The operator then manipulated the rubber vocal tract into time-varying configurations that, along with controlling other ports and levers, produced speech at the word level, but could not generate full sentences due to the limitations of air supply and perhaps the complexity of controlling the various parts of the machine with only two hands. The sound quality was child-like, presumably due to the high fundamental frequency of the reed and the relatively short rubber funnel serving as the vocal tract. In an historical analysis of von Kempelen's talking machine, Dudley and Tarnoczy (1950) note that this quality was probably deliberate because a child's voice was less likely to be criticized when demonstrating the function of the machine. Kempelen may have been particularly sensitive to criticism considering that he had earlier constructed and publicly demonstrated a chess-playing automaton that was in fact a hoax (cf., Carroll, 1975). Many observers initially assumed that his talking machine was merely a fake as well.

Kempelen's lasting contribution to phonetics is his prodigious written account of not only the design of his talking machine, but also the nature of speech and language in general (von Kempelen, 1791). In "On the Mechanism of Human Speech" [English translation], he describes the experiments that consumed more than 20 years and clearly showed the significance of using models of speech production and sound generation to study and analyze human speech. This work motivated much subsequent research on speech production, and to this day still guides the construction of replicas of his talking machine for pedagogical purposes (cf., Trouvain and Brackhane, 2011).

One person particularly inspired by von Kempelen's work was, in fact, Joseph Faber. According to a biographical sketch (Wurzbach, 1856), while recovering from a serious illness in about 1815, Faber happened onto a copy of "On the Mechanism of Human Speech" and became consumed with the idea of building a talking machine. Of course, he built not a replica of von Kempelen's machine, but one with a significantly advanced system of controlling the mechanical simulation of speech production. As remarkable as Faber's machine seems to have been regarded by some observers, Faber was indeed late to the party, so to speak, for the science of voice and speech had by the early 1800s already shifted into the realm of physical acoustics. Robert Willis, a professor of mechanics at Cambridge University, was dismayed by both Kratzenstein's and von Kempelen's reliance on trial-and-error methods in building their talking machines, rather than acoustic theory. He took them to task, along with most others working in phonetics at the time, in his 1829 essay titled "On the Vowel Sounds, and on Reed Organ-Pipes." The essay begins:

> The generality of writers who have treated on the vowel sounds appear never to have looked beyond the vocal organs for their origin. Apparently assuming the actual forms of these organs to be essential to their production, they have contented themselves with describing with minute precision the relative positions of the tongue, palate and teeth peculiar to each vowel, or with giving accurate measurements of the corresponding separation of the lips, and of the tongue and uvula, considering vowels in fact more in the light of physiological functions of the human body than as a branch of acoustics.
> *(Willis, 1829, p. 231)*

Willis laid out a set of experiments in which he would investigate vowel production by deliberately neglecting the organs of speech. He built reed-driven organ pipes whose lengths could be increased or decreased with a telescopic mechanism, and then determined that an entire series of vowels could be generated with changes in tube length and reeds with different vibrational frequencies. Wheatstone (1837) later pointed out that Willis had essentially devised an acoustic system that, by altering tube length, and hence the frequencies of the tube resonances, allowed for selective enhancement of harmonic components of the vibrating reed. Wheatstone further noted that multiple resonances are exactly what is produced by the "cavity of the mouth," and so the same effect occurs during speech production but with a nonuniformly shaped tube.

Understanding speech as a pattern of spectral components became a major focus of acousticians studying speech communication for much of the 19th century and the very early part of the 20th century. As a result, developments of machines to produce speech sounds were also largely based on some form of spectral addition, with little or no reference to the human speech organs. For example, in 1859 the German scientist Hermann Helmholtz devised an electromagnetic system for maintaining the vibration of a set of eight or more tuning forks, each variably coupled to a resonating chamber to control amplitude (Helmholtz, 1859, 1875). With careful choice of frequencies and amplitude settings he demonstrated the artificial generation of five different vowels. Rudolph Koenig, a well-known acoustical instrument maker in 1800s, improved on Helmholtz's design and produced commercial versions that were sold to interested clients (Pantalony, 2004). Koenig was also a key figure in emerging technology that allowed for recording and visualization of sound waves. His invention of the phonoautograph with Edouard-Léon Scott in 1859 transformed sound via a receiving cone, diaphragm, and stylus into a pressure waveform etched on smoked paper rotating about a cylinder. A few years later he introduced an alternative instrument in which a flame would flicker in response to a sound, and the movements of flame were captured on a rotating mirror, again producing a visualization of the sound as a waveform (Koenig, 1873).

These approaches were precursors to a device called the "phonodeik" that would be later developed at the Case School of Applied Science by Dayton Miller (1909) who eventually used it to study waveforms of sounds produced by musical instruments and human vowels. In a publication documenting several lectures given at the Lowell Institute in 1914, Miller (1916) describes both the analysis of sound based on photographic representations of waveforms produced by the phonodeik, as well as intricate machines that could generate complex waveforms by adding together sinusoidal components and display the final product graphically so that it might be compared to those waveforms captured with the phonodeik. Miller referred to this latter process as harmonic synthesis, a term commonly used to refer to building complex waveforms from basic sinusoidal elements. It is, however, the first instance of the word "synthesis" in the present chapter. This was deliberate to remain true to the original references. Nowhere in the literature on Kratzenstein, von Kempelen, Wheatstone, Faber, Willis, or Helmholtz does "synthesis" or "speech synthesis" appear. Their devices were variously referred to as talking machines, automatons, or simply systems that generated artificial speech. Miller's use of *synthesis* in relation to human vowels seems to have had the effect of labeling any future system that produces artificial speech, regardless of the theory on which it is based, a *speech synthesizer*.

Interestingly, the waveform synthesis described by Miller was not actually synthesis of sound, but rather synthesis of graphical representations of waveforms. To produce synthetic sounds, Miller utilized a bank of organ pipes, each of which, by design, possessed a different set of resonant frequencies. By controlling the amplitude of the sound produced by each pipe, he could effectively produce a set of nearly pure tones that were summed together as they radiated into free space. The composite waveform could then be captured with the phonodeik device and compared to the graphical synthesis of the same vowel. These were primarily vowel synthesizers, where production of each vowel required a different collection of pipes. There was little ability to dynamically change any aspect of the system except for interrupting the excitation of the pipes themselves; Miller did suggest such an approach to forming some basic words.

At this point in time, about a decade and a half into the 20th century, the mechanical and electro-mechanical era of speech synthesis was coming to a close. The elaborate talking machines of von Kempelen and Faber that simulated human speech production were distant memories, having been more recently replaced by studies of vowels using electro-mechanical devices that produced the spectral components of speech waveforms. Although there was much debate and disagreement about many details on the production of speech, primarily vowels, the ideas generated in this era were fundamental to the development of phonetics. It had become firmly established by now (but not universally accepted) that the underlying acoustic principle of speech production was that resonances formed by a given configuration of an air cavity enhanced or accentuated the spectral components of a sound source (Rayleigh, 1878). The enhanced portions of the spectrum eventually came to be known as "formants," a term that seems to have been first used by Ludimar Hermann in his studies of vowel production using phonograph technology (Hermann, 1894, 1895). Thus, the stage had been set to usher in the next era of speech synthesis.

The electrical and electronic era

A shift from using mechanical and electro-mechanical devices to generate artificial speech to purely electrical systems had its beginnings in 1922. It was then that John Q. Stewart, a young physicist from Princeton published an article in the journal *Nature* titled "An Electrical Analogue of the Vocal Organs" (Stewart, 1922). After military service in World War I, during which he was the chief instructor of "sound ranging" at the Army Engineering School, Stewart had spent two years as research engineer in the laboratories of the American Telephone and Telegraph Company and the Western Electric Company (Princeton Library). His article was a report of research he had completed during that time. In it he presents a diagram of a simple electrical circuit containing an "interrupter" or buzzer and two resonant branches comprised of variable resistors, capacitors, and inductors. Noting past research of Helmholtz, Miller, and Scripture, Stewart commented that "it seems hitherto to have been overlooked that a functional copy of the vocal organs can be devised . . . [with] audio-frequency oscillations in electrical circuits" (1922, p. 311). He demonstrated that a wide range of artificial vowels could be generated by adjusting the circuit elements in the resonant branches. Because of the ease and speed with which these adjustments could be made (e.g., turning knobs, moving sliders, etc.), Stewart also reported success in generating diphthongs by rapidly shifting the resonance frequencies from one vowel to another. Although the title of the article suggests otherwise, the circuit was not really an electrical analog of the vocal organs, but rather a means of emulating the acoustic resonances they produced. The design was essentially the first electrical formant synthesizer; interestingly, however, Stewart did not refer to his system as a *synthesizer*, but rather as an electrical analog of the vocal system.

Stewart moved on to a long productive career at Princeton as an astrophysicist and did not further develop his speech synthesizer. He did, however, leave an insightful statement at the end of his article that foreshadowed the bane of developing artificial speech systems for decades to come, and still holds today. He noted that:

> The really difficult problem involved in the artificial production of speech sounds is not the making of the device which shall produce sounds which, in their fundamental physical basis, resemble those of speech, but in the manipulation of the apparatus to imitate the manifold variations in tone which are so important in securing naturalness.
>
> *(Stewart, 1922, p. 312)*

Perhaps by "naturalness" it can be assumed he was referring to the goal of achieving natural human sound quality as well as intelligibility. In any case, he was clearly aware of the need to establish "rules" for constructing speech, and that simply building a device with the appropriate physical characteristics would not in itself advance artificial speech as a useful technology or tool for research.

A few years later, in 1928, a communications engineer named Homer Dudley – also working at the Western Electric Company (later to become Bell Telephone Laboratories) – envisioned a system that could be used to transmit speech across the transatlantic *telegraph* cable (Schroeder, 1981). Because it was designed for telegraph signals, however, the cable had a limited bandwidth of only 100 Hz. In contrast, transmission of the spectral content of speech requires a minimum bandwidth of about 3000 Hz, and so the telegraph cable was clearly insufficient for carrying an electrical analog of the speech waveform. The bandwidth limitation, however, motivated Dudley to view speech production and radio transmission analogously. Just as the information content carried by a radio signal is embedded in the relatively slow modulation of a carrier wave, phonetic information produced by movements of the lips, tongue, jaw, and velum could be considered to similarly modulate the sound wave produced by the voice source. That is, the speech articulators move at inaudible syllabic rates that are well below the 100 Hz bandwidth of the telegraph cable, whereas the voice source or carrier makes the signal audible but also creates the need for the much larger bandwidth. Understanding the difficulties of tracking actual articulatory movements, Dudley instead designed a circuit that could extract low frequency spectral information from an acoustic speech signal via a bank of filters, transmit that information along the low-bandwidth cable, and use it to modulate a locally supplied carrier signal on the receiving end to reconstruct the speech. This was the first *analysis-synthesis* system in which some set of parameters determined by analysis of the original signal could be sent to another location, or perhaps stored for later retrieval, and used to synthesize a new version of the original speech. Dudley had achieved almost exactly that which Joseph Henry had imagined in that letter he wrote long ago about linking together several of Faber's talking machines to communicate across a long distance.

Dudley's invention became known as the VOCODER, an acronym derived from the two words *VOice CODER* (to avoid the repetition of capital letters and to reflect its addition to our lexicon, "Vocoder" will be used in the remainder of the chapter). The Vocoder was demonstrated publicly for the first time on September 11, 1936 at the Harvard Tercentary Conference in Cambridge, Massachusetts (Dudley, 1936). During an address given by F.B. Jewitt, President of Bell Telephone Laboratories, Dudley was called on to demonstrate the Vocoder to the audience (Jewett, 1936) and showed its capabilities for analysis and subsequent synthesis of speech and singing. Dudley could also already see the potential of using the Vocoder for entertainment purposes (Dudley, 1939). He noted that once the low frequency spectral modulation envelopes had been obtained from speech or song, any signal with sufficiently wide bandwidth could be substituted as the carrier in the synthesis stage. For example, instrumental music or the sound of a train locomotive could be modulated with the spectral-phonetic information present in a sentence, producing a bizarre but entirely intelligible synthetic version of the original speech utterance (Dudley, 1940). Ironically, due to the international political and military events of the late 1930s and early 1940s, the first major application of the Vocoder was not to amuse audiences, but rather to provide secure, scrambled speech signals between government and military officials during World War II, particularly the conversations of Winston Churchill in London and Franklin D. Roosevelt in Washington, D.C.

One of the difficulties that prevented wide acceptance of Vocoder technology for general telephone transmission was the problem of accurately extracting pitch (fundamental frequency) from an incoming speech signal (Schroeder, 1993). Transmitting pitch variations along with the other modulation envelopes was essential for reconstructing natural sounding speech. It was not, however, necessary for transmitting *intelligible* speech, and hence could be acceptably used when the security of a conservation was more important than the naturalness of the sound quality. Even so, both Churchill and Roosevelt complained that the Vocoder made their speech sound silly (Tompkins, 2010), certainly an undesirable quality for world leaders. Eventually the pitch extraction problem was solved, other aspects were improved, and Vocoder technology became a viable means of processing and compressing speech for telephone transmission.

With the capability of isolating various aspects of speech, Dudley also envisioned the Vocoder as a tool for research in phonetics and speech science. In 1939, he and colleagues wrote,

> After one believes he has a good understanding of the physical nature of speech, there comes the acid test of whether he understands the construction of speech well enough to fashion it from suitably chosen elements.
>
> *(Dudley et al., 1939a, p. 740)*

Perhaps Dudley realized, much as Stewart (1922) had warned, that building a device to decompose a speech signal and reconstruct it synthetically was relatively "easy" in comparison to understanding how the fundamental elements of speech, whatever form they may take, can actually be generated sequentially by a physical representation of the speech production system, and result in natural, intelligible speech. With this goal in mind, he and colleagues modified the Vocoder such that the speech analysis stage was replaced with manual controls consisting of a keyboard, wrist bar, and foot pedal (Dudley, Riesz, and Watkins, 1939). The foot pedal controlled the pitch of a relaxation oscillator that provided a periodic voice source to be used for the voiced components of speech; a random noise source supplied the "electrical turbulence" needed for the unvoiced speech sounds. Each of the ten primary keys controlled the amplitude of the periodic or noise-like sources within a specific frequency band, which together spanned a range from 0 to 7500 Hz. By depressing combinations of keys and modulating the foot pedal, an operator of the device could learn to generate speech.

This new synthetic speaker was called the "VODER" (or "Voder") a new acronym that comprised the capitalized letters in "Voice Operation DEmonstratoR" (Dudley, Riesz, and Watkins, 1939). In a publication of the Bell Laboratories Record (1939), the machine's original moniker was "Pedro the Voder," where the first name was a nod to Dom Pedro II, a former Emperor of Brazil who famously exclaimed "My God, it talks!" after witnessing a demonstration of Bell's invention of the telephone in Philadelphia in 1876. The Bell publication ("Pedro the Voder," 1939) pointed out that the telephone did not actually talk, but rather transmitted talk over distance. In contrast, the Voder *did* talk and was demonstrated with some fanfare at the 1939 World's Fair in New York and at the Golden Gate Exposition in San Francisco the same year. It is interesting that this publication also states "It is the first machine in the world to do this [i.e., talk]" (Bell Labs Pubs, 1939, p. 170). If this was a reference to synthetic speech produced by an *electronic* artificial talker, it is likely correct. But clearly Joseph Faber had achieved the same goal by mechanical means almost a century earlier. In fact, the description of the Voder on the same page as a "little old-fashioned organ with a small keyboard and a pedal" could have easily been used to describe Faber's machine. In many ways, Dudley and colleagues at Bell Labs were cycling back through history with a new form of technology that would now allow for insights into the construction of speech that the machines of previous eras would not reveal to their makers.

One of the more interesting aspects of the Voder development, at least from the perspective of phonetics, was how people learned to speak with it. Stanley S.A. Watkins, the third author on the Dudley, Riesz, and Watkins (1939) article describing the Voder design, was charged with prescribing a training program for a group of people who would become "operators." He first studied the ways in which speech sounds were characterized across the ten filter bands (or channels) of Voder. Although this was found to be useful information regarding speech, it was simply too complex to be useful in deriving a technique for talking with the Voder. Various other methods of training were attempted, including templates to guide the fingers and various visual indicators, but eventually it was determined that the most productive method was for the operator to search for a desired speech sound by "playing" with the controls as guided by their ear. Twenty-four people, drawn from telephone operator pools, were trained to operate the Voder for the exhibitions at both sites of the 1939 World's Fair. Typically, about one year was required to develop the ability to produce intelligible speech with it. In fact, Dudley et al., wrote "the first half [of the year of training was] spent in acquiring the ability to form any and all sounds, the second half being devoted to improving naturalness and intelligibility" (Dudley, Riesz, and Watkins, 1939, p. 763). Once learned, the ability to "speak" with the Voder was apparently retained for years afterward, even without continued practice. On the occasion of Homer Dudley's retirement in 1961, one of the original trained operators was invited back to Bell Labs for an "encore performance" with a restored version of the talking machine. As recalled by James Flanagan, a Bell Labs engineer and speech scientist, "She sat down and gave a virtuoso performance on the Voder" (Pieraccini, 2012, p. 55).

In his article "The Carrier Nature of Speech," Dudley (1940) made a compelling analogy of the Voder structure to the human speech production system. But the Voder was really a spectrum shaping synthesizer: The cutoff frequencies and bandwidths of the ten filters associated with the keyboard were stationary, and so control was imposed by allowing the key presses to modulate the signal amplitude within each filter band. In effect, this provided the operator a means of continuously enhancing or suppressing the ten discrete divisions of the spectrum in some selective pattern such that an approximation of time-varying formants were generated. It can be noted that Faber's mechanical talking machine from a century earlier presented an operator with essentially the same type of interface as the Voder (i.e., keyboard, foot pedal), but it was the shape of cavities analogous to the human vocal tract that were controlled rather than the speech spectrum itself. In either case, and like a human acquiring the ability to speak, the operators of the devices learned and internalized a set of rules for generating speech by modulating a relatively high-frequency carrier signal (i.e., vocal fold vibration, turbulence) with slowly varying, and otherwise inaudible, "message waves" (Dudley, 1940). Although the ability of a human operator to acquire such rules is highly desirable for performance-driven artificial speech, it would eventually become a major goal for researchers in speech synthesis to explicate such rules in an attempt to understand phonology and motor planning in speech production, as well as to develop algorithms for transforming symbolic phonetic representations into speech via synthetic methods.

The research at Bell Labs that contributed to the Vocoder and Voder occurred in parallel with development of the "sound spectrograph" (Potter, 1945), a device that could graphically represent the *time-varying record of the spectrum* of a sound rather than the waveform. The output of the device, called a "spectrogram," was arranged such that time and frequency were on the x-axis and y-axis, respectively, and intensity was coded by varying shades of gray. It could be set to display either the *narrowband* harmonic structure of a sound, or the *wideband* formant patterns. Although development of the spectrograph had been initiated by Ralph Potter and colleagues just prior to the United States' involvement in World War II, it was given "official rating as a war project" (Potter, 1945, p. 463) because of its potential to facilitate military communications and message decoding. During the war, the spectrograph design was refined and used extensively to study the temporo-spectral patterns of speech based on the "spectrograms" that it generated. It wasn't until several months after the war ended, however, that the existence of the spectrograph was disclosed to the public. On November 9, 1945, Potter published an article in *Science* titled "Visible Patterns of Sound" in which he gave a brief description of the device and explained its potential application as a tool for studying phonetics, philology, and music. He also suggested its use as an aid for persons who are hearing impaired; the idea was that transforming speech from the auditory to the visual domain would allow a trained user to "read" speech. Other publications regarding the spectrograph soon followed with more detailed descriptions concerning its design (Koenig, Dunn, and Lacy, 1946; Koenig and Ruppel, 1948) and use (Kopp and Green, 1946; Steinberg and French, 1946; Potter and Peterson, 1948; Potter, 1949).

Just as instrumentation that allowed researchers to *see* acoustic speech waveforms had motivated earlier methods of synthesis (e.g., Miller, 1916), the spectrographic visualization of speech would rapidly inspire new ways of synthesizing speech, and new reasons for doing so. Following World War II, Frank Cooper and Alvin Liberman, researchers at Haskins Laboratories in New York City, had begun extensive analyses of speech using a spectrograph based on the Bell Labs design. Their goals, which were initially concerned with building a reading machine for the blind, had been diverted to investigations of the acoustic structure of speech, and how they were perceived and decoded by listeners. They realized quickly, however, that many of their questions could not be answered simply by inspection of spectrograms. What was needed was a means of modifying some aspect of the visual representation of speech provided by the spectrogram, and transforming it back into sound so that it could be presented to a listener as a stimulus. The responses to the stimuli would indicate whether or not the spectral modification was perceptually relevant.

In 1951, Cooper, Liberman, and Borst reported on the design of a device that would allow the user to literally draw a spectrographic representation of a speech utterance on a film transparency and transform it into a sound wave via a system including a light source, tone wheel, photocell, and amplifier. The tone wheel contained 50 circular sound tracks that, when turned by a motor at 1800 rpm, would modulate light to generate harmonic frequencies from 120–6000 Hz, roughly covering the speech spectrum. The photocell would receive only the portions of spectrum corresponding to the pattern that had been drawn on the film, and convert them to an electrical signal which could be amplified and played through a loudspeaker. The "drawn" spectrographic pattern could be either a copy or modification of an actual spectrogram, and hence the device came to be known as the "Pattern Playback." It was used to generate stimuli for numerous experiments on speech perception and contributed greatly to knowledge and theoretical views on how speech is decoded (cf., Liberman, Delattre, and Cooper, 1952, 1954, 1957; Liberman et al., 1957; Harris et al., 1958; Liberman, Delattre, and Cooper, 1967). The Pattern Playback was the first speech synthesizer used for large-scale systematic experimentation concerning the structure of speech, and proved to be most useful for investigations concerning isolated acoustic cues such as formant transitions at the onset and offset of consonants (Delattre et al., 1952; Borst, 1956).

The usefulness of speech synthesizers as research tools was summarized in a review article by Cooper (1961) in which he wrote:

> The essential point here, as in all of science, is that we must simplify Nature if we are to understand her. More than that: we must somehow choose a particular set of simplifying assumptions from the many sets that are possible. The great virtue of speech synthesizers is that they can help us make this choice.
>
> *(Cooper, 1961, p. 4)*

The Pattern Playback served the purpose of "simplifying Nature" by making the spectrotemporal characteristics of speech accessible and manipulable to the researcher. When used in this manner, a speech synthesizer becomes an experimenter's "versatile informant" that allows for testing hypotheses about the significance of various spectral features (Cooper, 1961, pp. 4–5). One of advantages of the Pattern Playback was that virtually anything could be drawn (or painted) on the film transparency regardless of the complexity or simplicity, *and* it could be heard. For example, all of the detail observed for a speech utterance in a spectrogram could be reconstructed, or something as simple as a sinusoid could be drawn as a straight line over time. The disadvantage was that the only means of generating an utterance, regardless of the accuracy of the prescribed rules, was for someone to actually draw it by hand.

The users of the Pattern Playback became quite good at drawing spectrographic patterns that generated intelligible speech, even when they had not previously seen an actual spectrogram of the utterance to be synthesized (Delattre et al., 1952; Liberman et al., 1959). Much like the operators of the speaking machines that preceded them, they had, through practice, acquired or internalized a set of rules for generating speech. Delattre et al. (1952) did attempt to characterize some speech sounds with regard to how they might be drawn spectrographically, but it was Frances Ingemann who formalized rules for generating utterances with the Pattern Playback (Ingemann, 1957; Liberman et al., 1959). The rules were laid out according to place, manner, and voicing, and could be presumably used by a novice to draw and generate a given utterance. Although the process would have been extremely time consuming and tedious, Mattingly (1974) notes that this was the *first* time that explicit rules for generating speech with a synthesizer had been formally documented.

Other types of synthesizers were also developed during this period that facilitated production of artificial speech based on acoustic characteristics observed in a spectrogram, but were based on different principles than the Pattern Playback. In 1953, Walter Lawrence, a researcher for the Signals Research and Development Establishment in Christchurch, England, introduced a speech synthesizer whose design consisted of an electrical circuit with a source function generator and three parallel resonant branches. The frequency of each resonance could be controlled by the user, as could the frequency and amplitude of the source function. Together, the source and resonant branches produced a waveform with a time-varying spectrum that could be compared to a spectrogram, or modified for purposes of determining the perceptual relevance of an acoustic cue. Because the parameters of the circuit (i.e., resonance frequencies, source fundamental frequency, etc.) were under direct control, Lawrence's synthesizer became known as the "Parametric Artificial Talker" or "PAT" for short. PAT was used by Peter Ladefoged and David Broadbent to provide acoustic stimuli for their well-known study of the effects of acoustic context on vowel perception (Ladefoged and Broadbent, 1957).

At about the same time, Gunnar Fant was also experimenting with resonant circuits for speech synthesis at the Royal Institute of Technology (KTH) in Stockholm. Instead of placing electrical resonators in parallel as Lawrence did in building PAT, Fant configured them in a series or "cascade" arrangement. Fant's first cascade synthesizer, called "OVE I," an acronym based on the words "Orator Verbis Electris," was primarily a vowel synthesizer that had the unique feature of a mechanical stylus that could be moved in a two-dimensional plane for control of the lowest two resonance frequencies. A user could then generate speech (vowels and vowel transitions) by moving the stylus in the vowel space defined by the first two-formant frequencies, a system that may have had great value for teaching and learning the phonetics of vowels. It may have had some entertainment value as well. Fant (2005) reminisced that one of the three "opponents" at his doctoral dissertation defense in 1958 was, in fact, Walter Lawrence who had brought his PAT synthesizer with him to Stockholm. At one point during the defense proceedings Fant and Lawrence demonstrated a synthesizer dialogue between PAT and OVE I. Eventually, Fant developed a second version of the cascade-type synthesizer called "OVE II" (Fant and Martony, 1962). The main enhancements were additional subsystems to allow for production of nasals, stops, and fricatives, as well as a conductive ink device for providing time-varying parameter values to the synthesizer.

The development of PAT and OVE set the stage for a category of artificial speech that would eventually be referred to as *formant* synthesis, because they provided for essentially direct control of the formants observed in a spectrogram. In a strict sense, however, they are *resonance* synthesizers because the parameters control, among other things, the frequencies of the electrical (or later, digital) resonators themselves. In most cases, though, these frequencies are aligned with the center frequency of a formant, and hence resonance frequency and formant frequency become synonymous. Although it may seem like a minor technological detail, the question of whether such synthesizers should be designed with parallel or cascaded resonators would be debated for years to come. A parallel system offers the user the largest amount control over the spectrum because both the resonator frequencies and amplitudes are set with parameters. In contrast, in a cascade system the resonance frequencies are set by a user, while their amplitudes are an effect of the superposition of multiple resonances, much as is the case for the human vocal tract (Flanagan, 1957). Thus, the cascade approach could potentially produce more natural sounding speech, but with somewhat of a sacrifice in control. Eventually, Lawrence reconfigured PAT with a cascade arrangement of resonators, but after many years of experimentation with both parallel and cascade systems, John Holmes of the Joint Speech Research Unit in the U.K. later made a strong case for a parallel arrangement (Holmes, 1983). He noted that replication of natural speech is considerably more accurate with user control of both formant frequencies and their amplitudes.

Simultaneous with the development of formant synthesizers in the 1950s, was another type of synthesis approach, also based on electrical circuits, but intended to serve as a model of the shape of the vocal tract so that the relation of articulatory configuration to sound production could be more effectively studied. The first of this type was described in 1950 by H.K. Dunn, another Bell Labs engineer. Instead of building resonant circuits to replicate formants, Dunn (1950) designed an electrical transmission line in which consecutive (and coupled) "T-sections," made up of capacitors, inductors, and resistors, were used as analogs of the pharyngeal and oral air cavities within the vocal tract. The values of the circuit elements within each T-section were directly related to the cross-sectional area and length of the various cavities, and thus the user now had parametric control of the vocal tract shape. Although this was an advance, the vocal tract configurations that could be effectively simulated with Dunn's circuit were fairly crude representations of the human system.

Stevens, Kasowski, and Fant (1953), in their article "An Electrical Analog of the Vocal Tract," describe a variation on Dunn's design using a similar transmission line approach; however, they were able to represent the vocal tract shape as a concatenation of 35 cylindrical sections, where each section was 0.5 cm in length. The purpose in pursuing a more detailed representation of the vocal tract shape was to be able to "study in detail the mechanism of speech production and to investigate correlations between the acoustic and articulatory aspects of speech" and noted that "a speech synthesizer would be required to simulate more closely the actual dimensions of the vocal tract" (p. 735). Fant also began work on his own version of a Line Electrical Analog (LEA) that he used for studies of speech sounds. Both Stevens and House (1955) and Fant (1960) used these very similar synthesizers to better understand vowel articulation by first developing a three parameter model of the vocal tract shape in which the location and radius of the primary vowel constriction were specified, along with the ratio of lip termination area to lip tube length. Their synthesizers allowed for a systematic exploration of the parametric space and resulted in nomographic displays that demonstrated the importance of the location (place) and cross-sectional area of the primary vocal tract constriction in vowels. Collectively, this work significantly altered the view of vowel production.

A limitation of both the Stevens, Kasowski, and Fant (1953) and Fant (1960) line analog synthesizers was that they could not generate time-varying speech sounds because they accommodated only static vocal tract configurations; i.e., they couldn't actually talk. Using a more complex line analog circuit system and a bank of switches, George Rosen, a doctoral student at the Massachusetts Institute of Technology, devised a means of transitioning from one vocal tract configuration to another (Rosen, 1958). This new system, known as "DAVO" for "**d**ynamic **a**nalog of the **vo**cal tract," could generate fairly clear diphthongs and consonant-vowel (CV) syllables, but was not capable of sentence-level speech.

It can be noted that the parametric models of the vocal tract shape developed by Stevens and House (1955) and Fant (1960) were independent of the transmission line analogs that were used to produce the actual synthetic speech. The limitation of only static vowels, or CVs in the case of DAVO, was entirely due to the need for a complicated electrical circuit to simulate the propagation of acoustic waves in the vocal tract. The vocal tract models themselves could have easily been used to generate time-dependent configurations over the time course of a phrase or sentence, but a system for producing the corresponding synthetic speech waveform with such temporal variation simply did not yet exist, nor did the knowledge of how to specify the time-dependence of the vocal tract parameters.

Yet another type of speech synthesizer was also under development during the 1950s. With significant improvements in the state of audio recording technology, particularly those related to storing speech waveforms on magnetic tape, it was now possible to consider synthesis – perhaps in the purest sense of the word – based on splicing together small segments of prerecorded natural speech. Harris (1953a) designed a system in which segments of tape were isolated that contained many instances (allophones) of each consonant and vowel. Then, with a recording drum, tape loop, and timing and selector circuits (Harris, 1953b), synthetic speech could be generated by piecing together a sequence of segments deemed to match well with regard to formant frequencies and harmonics. The speech produced was found to be fairly intelligible but quite unnatural, presumably because of the discontinuities created at the segment boundaries.

Rather than focusing on vowel and consonant segments, Peterson, Wang, and Sivertsen (1958) experimented with alternative segmentation techniques and determined that a more useful unit for synthesizing speech could be obtained from segments extending in time from the steady-state location of one phoneme to the next. Referring to this unit as a "dyad," they suggested that it preserved the acoustic dynamics of the transitions between phonemes, precisely the information lost when the segmentation unit is the phoneme itself. The potential of this method to generate intelligible speech was demonstrated by Wang and Peterson (1958) where they constructed a sentence from more than 40 dyad segments extracted from previously recorded utterances. Much care was required in selecting the segments, however, in order to maintain continuity of pitch, intensity, tempo, and vocal quality. The range of phonetic characteristics that can be generated in synthetic speech by concatenating segments is, of course, limited by the segment inventory that is available. Sivertsen (1961) conducted an extensive study of the size of inventory needed relative to the type of segmentation unit chosen. She considered various segments with a wide range of temporal extent that included phonemes, phoneme dyads, syllable nuclei, half syllables, syllables, syllable dyads, and words, and found that, in general, "the size of the inventory increases with the length of the segment" (Sivertsen, 1961, p. 57). That is, a few small units can be combined in many ways to generate hundreds or thousands of increasingly larger units, but if the starting point is a large temporal unit, an enormous number is needed because the possibilities for recombining them are severely limited.

This approach to synthesis clearly has played a major role in technological applications such as modern text-to-speech systems utilizing unit selection techniques (cf., Moulines and Charpentier, 1990; Sagisaka et al., 1992; Hunt and Black, 1996), but Sivertsen (1961) also made a strong case for the use of segment concatenation methods as a research tool. In particular, she noted that using stored segments of various lengths can be used for evaluating some theories of linguistic structure, as well as for investigating segmentation of speech signals in general. In fact, Sivertsen suggested that essentially all speech synthesis methods could be categorized relative to how the speech continuum is segmented. If the segmentation is conceived as "simultaneous components" then speech can be synthesized by controlling various parametric representations "independently and simultaneously." These may be physiological parameters such as vocal tract shape, location and degree of constriction, nasal coupling, and laryngeal activity, or acoustical parameters such as formant frequencies, formant bandwidths, fundamental frequency, voice spectrum, and amplitude. If, instead, the speech continuum is segmented in time, synthetic speech can be accomplished by sequencing successive "building blocks," which may be extracted from recorded natural speech or even generated electronically.

The advent of digital computing in the early 1960s would dramatically change the implementation of speech synthesizers, and the means by which they may be controlled. The underlying principles of the various synthesis methods, however, are often the same or least similar to those that motivated development of mechanical, electrical, or electronic talking devices. Thus, delineation of synthesizer type relative to the segmentation of the speech continuum is particularly useful for understanding the differences and potential uses of the wide range of synthetic speech systems that had so far been advanced at the time, and also for those yet to be developed.

The digital and computational era

As Stewart (1922) had suggested in the early days of electrical circuit-based synthesis, building a device capable of producing sounds that resemble speech is far less difficult than knowing how to impose the proper control on its parameters to make the device actually talk. Although much progress had been made in development of various types of systems, controlling electronic speech synthesizers by manipulating circuit parameters, whether they were vocal tract or terminal analog types, was cumbersome and tedious. This could now be mitigated to some degree, however, by engaging a digital computer to control speech synthesizers that were, themselves, still realized as electronic circuits. That is, commands typed on a keyboard could be transformed into control voltages that imposed parameter changes in the synthesis circuitry. In effect, this allowed the "computational load" for generating the speech waveform to remain in the analog circuit, while transferring the control of the system to a user via a computer interface. It would not be long, however, before the hardware synthesizers were replaced with software realizations of the same circuit elements, offering far greater flexibility and ease with which synthetic speech could be generated.

Digital control facilitated development of "speech synthesis by rule" in which an orthographic representation of an utterance could be transformed into artificial speech. Based on a set of "rules" embedded in a computer program, a series of symbols representing the phonetic elements of a word or phrase were converted to temporal variations of the parameters of a specific type of synthesizer. For example, Holmes, Mattingly, and Shearme (1964) described the rules and associated computer program that calculated the time course of the parameters of a parallel resonance (formant) synthesizer. These included, among other variables, frequencies and amplitudes of three resonances, and fundamental frequency. A word such as "you" (/ju/) might be produced with a simple interpolation of the second formant frequency, F_2, from a high value, say 2200 Hz, down to a much lower value, perhaps 400 Hz, while other parameters could be held constant. The interpolated F_2 would then be used to alter the settings of circuit elements over a particular period of time, resulting in a speech waveform resembling "you."

A similar goal of producing "synthetic speech from an input consisting only of the names of phonemes and a minimum of pitch and timing information" was pursued by Kelly and Lochbaum (1962, p. 1), but in their system a digital lattice filter, entirely realized as a computer algorithm, was used to calculate the effective propagation of acoustic waves in an analog of the vocal tract configuration. Control of the system required specification of 21 time-varying cross-sectional areas representing the vocal tract shape along the axis extending from the glottis to lips, as well as nasal coupling, fundamental frequency, aspiration, and affrication. Each phoneme was assigned a vocal tract shape (i.e., 21 cross-sectional areas) read from lookup table; change in tract shape was accomplished by linearly interpolating, over time, each cross-sectional area specified for one phoneme to those of the next phoneme. This design functioned essentially as a digital version of a synthesizer like George Rosen's DAVO; but because it was software rather than hardware, it allowed for more precise specification of the vocal tract shape and almost endless possibilities for experimentation with interpolation types and associated rules.

Kelly and Lochbaum expressed disappointment in the sound quality of the speech generated by their system, but attributed the problem to inadequate knowledge of the cross-sectional areas that were used as the vocal tract shapes corresponding to phoneme targets. Although based on Fant's (1960) well-known collection of vocal tract data obtained from X-ray images, it would not be until the 1990s when imaging methods would allow for three-dimensional reconstructions of vocal tract shapes produced by human talkers (cf., Baer et al., 1991; Story, Titze, and Hoffman, 1996, 1998), and hence, improve this aspect of analog vocal tract synthesis. The time-varying spatial characteristics of a linearly interpolated vocal tract shape were, however, also potential contributors to the undesirable quality of the synthesis. A more complex set of rules for control of a vocal tract analog was described a few years later by Nakata and Mitsuoka (1965), and resulted in intelligible speech with "fairly good naturalness." Nonetheless, they, along with others believed that significant improvements in vocal tract analog synthesis required more detailed knowledge of realistic articulatory movement from which better timing rules could be derived.

By the 1960s, X-ray cineradiography technology had developed to a point where the spatial and temporal resolution were suitable for studying the articulatory movements of speech in a sagittal projection image. Motion picture X-ray films collected for various speech utterances could be analyzed frame by frame to track the changing positions of articulators and the time-varying configuration of the vocal tract outline. Just as the instrumentation that allowed scientists to *see waveforms and spectrograms* had motivated earlier forms of synthetic speech, the ability to now *see the movement of the articulators* motivated development of a new type of synthesis paradigm called "articulatory synthesis."

In 1967, Cecil Coker of Bell Laboratories demonstrated a synthesis system based on a computational model of the speech articulators. Simplified positions of the tongue, jaw, lips, velum, and larynx were represented in the midsagittal plane, where each could be specified to move with a particular timing function. The result was a time-varying configuration of the midsagittal vocal tract outline. To produce the speech waveform, the distances across the vocal tract airspace from glottis to lips at each time sample first needed to be converted to cross-sectional areas to form the area function (cf., Heinz and Stevens, 1964). These were then used in a vocal tract analog model like that of Kelly and Lochbaum (1962) to calculate wave propagation through the system. The resonance frequencies could also be calculated directly from the time-varying area function and used to control a formant synthesizer

(Coker and Fujimura, 1966). Similar articulatory models were developed by Lindblom and Sundberg (1971) and Mermelstein (1973), but incorporated somewhat more complexity in the articulatory geometry. In any case, the temporal characteristics of the synthesized articulatory movement could be compared to, and refined with, data extracted from midsagittal cineradiography films (e.g., Truby, 1965). An articulatory synthesizer developed at Haskins Laboratories called "ASY" (Rubin, Baer, and Mermelstein, 1981), extended the Mermelstein model, incorporating several additional sub-models and an approach based on key frame animation for synthesizing utterances derived from control of the movement over time of the vocal tract. This was one of the earliest articulatory synthesis tools used for large-scale laboratory phonetic experiments (e.g., Abramson et al., 1981). It was later enhanced to provide more accurate representations of the underlying vocal tract parameters and flexibility in their control by a user (the Haskins Configurable Articulatory Synthesizer, or CASY; see Rubin et al., 1996).

Articulatory synthesis held much promise because it was assumed that the rules required to generate speech would be closer to those used by a human talker than rules developed for controlling acoustic parameters such as formant frequencies. While that may ultimately be the case, such rules have been difficult to define in such a way that natural sounding, intelligible speech is consistently generated (Klatt, 1987). Articulatory synthesizers have become important tools for research, however, because they can serve as a *model* of speech production in which the acoustic consequences of parametric variation of an articulator can be investigated. Using the ASY synthesizer (Rubin, Baer, and Mermelstein, 1981) to produce speech output, Browman et al. (1984), Browman and Goldstein (e.g., 1985, 1991), Saltzman (1986, 1991), and others at Haskins Laboratories embarked on research to understand articulatory control. Guiding this work was the hypothesis that phonetic structure could be characterized explicitly as articulatory movement patterns, or "gestures." Their system allowed for specification of an utterance as a temporal schedule of "tract variables," such as location and degree of a constriction formed by the tongue tip or tongue body, lip aperture, and protrusion, as well as states of the velum and glottis. These were then transformed into a task-dynamic system that accounted for the coordination and dynamic linkages among articulators required to carry out a specified gesture. Over the years, techniques for estimating the time course of gesture specification have continued to be enhanced. Recently, for example, Nam et al. (2012) reported a method for estimating gestural "scores" from the acoustic signal based on an iterative analysis-by-synthesis approach.

Some developers of articulatory synthesis systems focused their efforts on particular subsystems such as the voice source. For example, Flanagan and Landgraf (1968) proposed a simple mass-spring-damper model of the vocal folds that demonstrated, with a computational model, the self-oscillating nature of the human vocal folds. Shortly thereafter, a more complex two-mass version was described (Ishizaka and Flanagan, 1972; Ishizaka and Matsudaira, 1972) that clearly showed the importance of the vertical phase difference (mucosal wave) in facilitating vocal fold oscillation. Additional degrees of freedom were added to the anterior-posterior dimension of the vocal folds by Titze (1973, 1974) with a 16-mass model. Although the eventual goal of subsystem modeling would be integration into a full speech synthesis system (cf., Flanagan, Ishizaka, and Shipley, 1975; Sondhi and Schroeter, 1987), much of their value is as a tool for understanding the characteristics of the subsystem itself. Maeda (1988, 1990), Dang and Honda (2004), and Birkholz (2013) are all examples of more recent attempts to integrate models of subsystems into an articulatory speech synthesizer, whereas Guenther (cf., 1994) and Kröger et al. (2010) have augmented such synthesizers with auditory feedback and learning algorithms. The main use of these systems has been to study some aspect of speech production, but not necessarily the conversion of a symbolic representation of an utterance into speech. It can also be noted that a natural extension of articulatory synthesis is the inclusion of facial motion that coincides with speaking, and has led to development audiovisual synthetic speech systems that can be used explore multi-modal nature of both speech production and perception (cf., Yehia, Rubin, and Vatikiotis-Bateson, 1998; Massaro, 1998; Vatikiotis-Bateson et al., 2000). This area will be covered in the chapter entitled "New horizons in clinical phonetics."

Other researchers focused on enhancing models of the vocal tract analogs *without* adding the complexity of articulatory components. Strube (1982), Liljencrants (1985), and Story (1995) all refined the digital lattice filter approach of Kelly and Lochbaum (1962) to better account for the acoustic properties of time-varying vocal tract shapes and various types of energy losses. Based on the relation of small perturbations of a tubular configuration to changes in the acoustic resonance frequencies, Mrayati, Carré, and Guérin (1988) proposed that speech could be produced by controlling the time-varying cross-sectional area of eight distinct regions of the vocal tract. The idea was that expansion or constriction of these particular regions would maximize the change in resonance frequencies, thus providing an efficient means of controlling the vocal tract to generate a predictable acoustic output. Some years later a set of rules was developed by Hill, Manzara, and Schock (1995) that specified the transformation of text input into region parameters and were used to build a vocal tract-based text-to-speech synthesizer. In a similar vein, Story (2005, 2013) has described an "airway modulation model" of speech production (called "TubeTalker") in which an array of functions can be activated over time to deform the vocal tract, nasal tract, and glottal airspaces to produce speech. Although this model produces highly intelligible speech, its primary use is for studying the relation of structure and movement to the acoustic characteristics produced, and the perceptual response of listeners (cf., Story and Bunton, 2010).

In parallel with development of articulatory-type synthesizers was the enhancement of resonance or formant-based synthesis systems. Along with numerous colleagues, Dennis Klatt's research on digital resonators as well as his studies on the acoustic characteristics of nearly all aspects of speech, led to a comprehensive system of rule-based formant synthesis. With various names such as "Klattalk," "MITalk," "DecTalk," and later "KLSYN88," this type of text-to-speech system has become well known to the public, particularly because of its collection of standard voices (cf., Klatt, 1982, 1987; Klatt and Klatt, 1990). Perhaps best known today is "Perfect Paul," the voice that was synonymous with the late British physicist Stephen Hawking who used the synthesizer as an augmentative speaking device. Formant synthesis can also be combined with articulatory methods. "HLSyn," developed by Hanson and Stevens (2002), is a system designed to superimpose high level (HL) articulatory control on the Klatt formant synthesizer. This approach simplified the control scheme by mapping 13 physiologically based HL parameters to the 40–50 acoustic parameters that control the formant synthesis. The advantage is that the articulatory parameters constrain the output so that physiologically unrealistic combinations of the voice source and vocal tract filter cannot occur. This type of synthesizer can serve as another tool for studying speech production with regard to both research and educational purposes.

Throughout this chapter, it has been presumed that regardless of the reasons for developing a particular type of synthesizer, at some level, the goal was to generate high-quality, intelligible speech. Some synthesizers have been developed, however, for the explicit purpose of degrading or modifying natural, recorded speech. Such synthesizers are useful for investigating speech perception because they allow researchers to systematically remove many of the acoustic characteristics present in the signal while preserving only those portions hypothesized to be essential cues. Remez et al. (1981) described a synthesis technique in which the first three formant frequencies tracked over the duration of a sentence, were replaced by the summation of three tones whose frequencies were swept upward and downward to match the temporal variation of the formants. Although the quality of the synthesized sound was highly artificial (perhaps otherworldly), listeners were able to identify the sentences as long as the tones were played simultaneously, and not in isolation of one another, revealing the power of speech cues that are embedded in the dynamic spectral patterns of the vocal tract resonances. Shannon et al. (1995) showed that intelligible speech could alternatively be synthesized by preserving temporal cues, while virtually eliminating spectral information. Their approach was essentially the same as Dudley's Vocoder (1939) in which the speech signal was first filtered into a set of frequency bands, and time-varying amplitude envelopes were extracted from each band over the duration of the recorded speech. The difference was that the number of bands ranged from only one to four, and the amplitude envelopes were used modulate a noise signal rather than an estimation of the voice source. Shannon et al., showed that listeners were adept at decoding sentence-level speech with only three bands of modulated noise. Similarly designed synthesizers (e.g., Loizou, Dorman, and Tu, 1999) have been used simulate the signal processing algorithms in cochlear implant devices for purposes of investigating speech perception abilities of listeners under these conditions. Yet another variation on this type of synthesis was reported by Smith, Delgutte, and Oxenham (2002) who developed a technique to combine the spectral fine structure of one type of sound with the temporal variation of another to generate "auditory chimeras." These have been shown to be useful for investigating aspects of auditory perception.

Many other types of speech synthesis methods have been developed in the digital era whose primary purpose is to generate high quality speech for automated messaging or be embodied in a digital assistant that converses with a user. These systems typically make use of synthesis techniques that build speech signals from information available in a database containing many hours of recordings of one or more voice professionals who produced a wide range of spoken content and vocal qualities. The "unit selection" technique, also referred to as "concatenative synthesis," is essentially the digital realization of the tape splicing method of Harris (1953b) and Peterson, Wang, and Sivertsen (1958), but now involves a set of algorithms that efficiently search the database for small sound segments, typically at the level of diphones, that can be stacked serially in time to generate a spoken message. A different technique, called "parametric synthesis," relies on an extensive analysis of the spectral characteristics of speech recordings in a database to establish parametric representations that can later be used to reconstruct a segment of speech (Zen, Tokuda, and Black, 2009). Unit selection typically produces more natural sounding speech but is limited by the quality and size of the original database. Parametric synthesis allows for greater flexibility with regard to modification of voice characteristics, speaking style, and emotional content, but generally is of lower overall quality. Both techniques have been augmented with implementation of deep learning algorithms that improve the efficiency and accuracy of constructing a spoken utterance, as well as increasing the naturalness and intelligibility of the synthetic speech (Zen, Senior, and Schuster, 2013; Capes et al., 2017). More recently, a new approach called direct waveform modeling has been introduced that utilizes a deep neural network (DNN) to generate new speech signals based on learned features of recorded speech (cf., van den Oord et al., 2016; Arik et al., 2017). This method has the potential to significantly enhance the quality and naturalness of synthetic speech over current systems, even though it is currently computationally expensive. It can be noted, however, that because unit selection, parametric, and direct waveform synthesizers construct speech signals based on underlying principles that are not specifically related to the ways in which a human forms speech, they are perhaps less useful as a tool for testing hypotheses about speech production and perception than many of the other techniques discussed in this chapter.

Summary

For centuries, past to present, humans have been motivated to build machines that talk. Other than the novelty, what is the purpose of speech synthesis, and what can be done with it? Certainly, technological applications have resulted from development of these devices, many of them having a major impact on how humans communicate with each other. Mattingly (1974) seems to have hit it just about right when he suggested that the "traditional motivation for research in speech synthesis" has been simply the desire to explain the mystery of how we humans successfully use our vocal tracts to produce connected speech. In other words, the primary means of scientifically investigating speech production has been based on building artificial talking systems and collecting relevant data with which to refine them. Mattingly (1974) also points out that, regardless of the underlying principles of the synthetic speech system built, the scientific questions are almost always concerned with deriving the "rules" that govern production of intelligible speech. Such rules may be elaborate and explicitly stated algorithms for transforming a string of text into speech based on a particular type of synthesizer, or more subtly implied as general movements of structures or acoustic characteristics. In any case, achieving an understanding of the rules and all their variations, can be regarded as synonymous with understanding many aspects of speech production and perception.

As in any area of science, the goal in studying speech has been to first determine the important facts about the system. Artificial talkers and speech synthesizers embody these "facts," but they typically capture just the essential aspects of speech. As a result, synthesis often presents itself as an aural caricature that can be perceived as an unnatural, and sometimes amusing rendition of a desired utterance or speech sound. It is particularly unique to phonetics and speech science that the models used as tools to understand the scientific aspects of a complex system produce a signal intended to be heard as if it were a human. As such, the quality of speech synthesis can be rather harshly judged because the model on which it is based has not accounted for the myriad of subtle variations and details that combine in natural human speech. Thus, we should keep in mind that the degree to which we can produce convincing artificial speech is a measure of the degree to which we understand human speech production.

Acknowledgments

The research was supported in part by NIH R01 DC011275 and NSF BCS-1145011.

References

Abramson, A. S., Nye, P. W., Henderson, J. B., and Marshall, C. W., 1981. Vowel height and the perception of consonantal nasality, *The Journal of the Acoustical Society of America*, 70, pp. 329–339.

Altick, R. D., 1978. *The shows of London*, Cambridge, MA and London: Belknap Press of Harvard University Press, pp. 355–356.

Arik, S. O., Chrzanowski, M., Coates, A., Diamos, G., Gibiansky, A., Kang, Y., Li, X., Miller, J., Ng, A., Raiman, J., Sengupta, S., and Shoeybi, M., 2017. *Deep voice: Real-time neural text-to-speech*. arXiv:1702.07825 [Accessed 5 March 2018].

Athenaeum, 1846, Our weekly gossip, *British Periodicals*, July 25, 978, p. 765.

Baer, T., Gore, J. C., Gracco, L. C., and Nye, P. W., 1991. Analysis of vocal tract shape and dimensions using magnetic resonance imaging: Vowels, *The Journal of the Acoustical Society of America*, 90, pp. 799–828.

Baldwin Jewett, F., 1936. The social implications of scientific research in electrical communication, *The Scientific Monthly*, 43, pp. 466–476.

Barnum, P. T., 1886. *Life of P. T. Barnum written by himself*, Buffalo, NY: The Courier Company Printers, p. 134.

Birkholz, P., 2013. Modeling consonant-vowel coarticulation for articulatory speech synthesis, *PLoS One*, 84, e60603, pp. 1–17. https://doi.org/10.1371/journal.pone.0060603.

Borst, J. M., 1956. The use of spectrograms for speech analysis and synthesis, *Journal of the Audio Engineering Society*, 4, pp. 14–23.

Browman, C. P., and Goldstein, L. M., 1985. Dynamic modeling of phonetic structure, *Phonetic Linguistics*, pp. 35–53.

Browman, C. P., and Goldstein, L. M., 1991. Tiers in articulatory phonology, with some implications for casual speech, In J. Kingston and M. E. Beckman (Eds.), *Papers in laboratory phonology I, between the grammar and the physics of speech*, Cambridge, UK: Cambridge University Press, pp. 341–376.

Browman, C. P., Goldstein, L. M., Kelso, J. A. S., Rubin, P. E., and Saltzman, E., 1984. Articulatory synthesis from underlying dynamics, *The Journal of the Acoustical Society of America*, 75, p. S22.

Capes, T., Coles, P., Conkie, A., Golipour, L., Hadjitarkhani, A., Hu, Q., Huddleston, N., Hunt, M., Li, J., Neeracher, M., Prahallad, K, Raitio, T., Rasipuram, R., Townsend, G., Williamson, B., Winarsky, D., Wu, X., and Zhang, H., 2017. Siri On-device deep learning-guided unit selection text-to-speech system, *Proceedings of Interspeech 2017*, pp. 4011–4015.

Carroll, C. M., 1975. *The great chess automaton*, New York: Dover Publications.

Coker, C. H., 1967. Synthesis by rule from articulatory parameters, *Proceedings of the 1967 Conference on Speech Communication Processes*, Cambridge, MA: IEEE, A9, pp. 52–53.

Coker, C. H., and Fujimura, O., 1966. Model for specification of the vocal tract area function, *The Journal of the Acoustical Society of America*, 40(5), pp. 1271–1271.

Cooper, F. S., 1961. Speech synthesizers, *Proceedings of the 4th International Congress of Phonetic Sciences (ICPhS'61)*, pp. 3–13.

Cooper, F. S., Liberman, A. M., and Borst, J. M., 1951. The interconversion of audible and visible patterns as a basis for research in the perception of speech, *Proceedings of the National Academy of Sciences*, 37(5), pp. 318–325.

Dang, J., and Honda, K., 2004. Construction and control of a physiological articulatory model, *The Journal of the Acoustical Society of America*, 115, pp. 853–870.

Delattre, P., Cooper, F. S., Liberman, A. M., and Gerstman, L. J., 1952. Speech synthesis as a research technique, *Proceedings of the Vllth International Congress of Linguists*, London, pp. 543–561.

Dudley, H., 1936. Synthesizing speech, *Bell Laboratories Record*, 15, pp. 98–102.

Dudley, H., 1939. The vocoder, *Bell Laboratories Record*, 18(4), pp. 122–126.

Dudley, H., 1940. The carrier nature of speech, *Bell System Technical Journal*, 19(4), pp. 495–515.

Dudley, H., Riesz, R. R., and Watkins, S. S. A., 1939. A synthetic speaker, *Journal of the Franklin Institute*, 227(6), pp. 739–764.

Dudley, H., and Tarnoczy, T. H., 1950. The speaking machine of Wolfgang von Kempelen, *The Journal of the Acoustical Society of America*, 22(2), pp. 151–166.

Dunn, H. K., 1950. The calculation of vowel resonances and an electrical vocal tract, *The Journal of the Acoustical Society of America*, 22(6), pp. 740–753.

Euler, L., 1761. The wonders of the human voice, *Letters of Euler on different subjects in natural philosophy addressed to German Princess*, David Brewster, ed., New York: J.J. Harper (publisher in 1833), pp. 76–79.

Fant, G., 1960. *Acoustic theory of speech production*, The Hague: Mouton.

Fant, G., 2005. Historical notes, *Speech Transmission Laboratory Quarterly Progress and Status Report (KTH)*, 47(1), pp. 9–19.

Fant, G., and Martony, J., 1962. Speech synthesis instrumentation for parametric synthesis (OVE II), *Speech Transmission Laboratory Quarterly Progress and Status Report (KTH)*, 2, pp. 18–24.

Flanagan, J. L., 1957. Note on the design of "terminal-analog" speech synthesizers, *The Journal of the Acoustical Society of America*, 29(2), pp. 306–310.

Flanagan, J. L., Ishizaka, K., and Shipley, K. L., 1975. Synthesis of speech from a dynamic model of the vocal cords and vocal tract, *Bell System Technical Journal*, 54(3), 485–506.

Flanagan, J. L., and Landgraf, L., 1968. Self-oscillating source for vocal-tract synthesizers, *IEEE Transactions on Audio and Electroacoustics*, 16(1), pp. 57–64.

Guenther, F. H., 1994. A neural network model of speech acquisition and motor equivalent speech production, *Biological Cybernetics*, 72(1), 43–53.

Hanson, H. M., and Stevens, K. N., 2002. A quasiarticulatory approach to controlling acoustic source parameters in a Klatt-type formant synthesizer using HLsyn, *The Journal of the Acoustical Society of America*, 112(3), pp. 1158–1182.

Harris, C. M., 1953a. A study of the building blocks in speech, *The Journal of the Acoustical Society of America*, 25(5), pp. 962–969.

Harris, C. M., 1953b. A speech synthesizer, *The Journal of the Acoustical Society of America*, 25(5), pp. 970–975.

Harris, K. S., Hoffman, H. S., Liberman, A. M., Delattre, P. C., and Cooper, F. S., 1958. Effect of third formant transitions on the perception of the voiced stop consonants, *The Journal of the Acoustical Society of America*, 30(2), pp. 122–126.

Heinz, J. M., and Stevens, K. N., 1964. On the derivation of area functions and acoustic spectra from cineradiographic films of speech, *The Journal of the Acoustical Society of America*, 36(5), pp. 1037–1038.

Helmholtz, H., 1859. Ueber die Klangfarbe der Vocale [On the timbre of vowels], *Annalen der Physik*, 123, pp. 527–528.

Helmholtz, H., 1875. *On the sensations of tone as a physiological basis for the theory of music*, London: Longmans, Green, and Co.

Hermann, L., 1894. Nachtrag zur Untersuchung der Vocalcurven, *Pflügers Archiv European Journal of Physiology*, 58, pp. 264–279.

Hermann, L., 1895. Weitere Untersuchungen über das Wesen der Vocale, *Pflügers Archiv European Journal of Physiology*, 61(4), pp. 169–204.

Hill, D., Manzara, L., and Schock, C., 1995. Real-time articulatory speech-synthesis-by-rules, *Proceedings of AVIOS*, 95, pp. 27–44.

Holmes, J. N., 1983. Formant synthesizers: Cascade or parallel? *Speech Communication*, 2(4), pp. 251–273.

Holmes, J. N., Mattingly, I. G., and Shearme, J. N., 1964. Speech synthesis by rule, *Language and Speech*, 7(3), pp. 127–143.

Hunt, A. J., and Black, A. W., 1996. Unit selection in a concatenative speech synthesis system using a large speech database, *Acoustics, Speech, and Signal Processing, ICASSP-96, Conference Proceedings*, IEEE, 1, pp. 373–376.

Ingemann, F., 1957. Speech synthesis by rule, *The Journal of the Acoustical Society of America*, 29(11), pp. 1255–1255.

Ishizaka, K., and Flanagan, J. L., 1972. Synthesis of voiced sounds from a two? Mass model of the vocal cords, *Bell System Technical Journal*, 51(6), pp. 1233–1268.

Ishizaka, K., and Matsudaira, M., 1972. Fluid mechanical considerations of vocal cord vibration, *Speech Communications Research Laboratory Monograph.*

Kelly, J. L., and Lochbaum, C. C., 1962. Speech synthesis, *Proceedings of the Fourth International Congress of Acoustics*, G42, 1–4.

Kempelen, W. R. von, 1791. *Mechanismus der menschlichen Sprache nebst der Beschreibung seiner sprechenden Maschine*, Vienna: J. B. Degen.

Klatt, D. H., 1982. The Klattalk text-to-speech conversion system, *Acoustics, Speech, and Signal Processing, IEEE International Conference on ICASSP '82*, 7, IEEE, pp. 1589–1592.

Klatt, D. H., 1987. Review of text-to-speech conversion for English, *The Journal of the Acoustical Society of America*, 82(3), pp. 737–793.

Klatt, D. H., and Klatt, L. C., 1990. Analysis, synthesis, and perception of voice quality variations among female and male talkers, *The Journal of the Acoustical Society of America*, 87(2), pp. 820–857.

Koenig, R., 1873. I. On manometric flames, *The London, Edinburgh, and Dublin Philosophical Magazine and Journal of Science*, 45(297), pp. 1–18.

Koenig, W., Dunn, H. K., and Lacy, L. Y., 1946. The sound spectrograph, *The Journal of the Acoustical Society of America*, 18(1), pp. 19–49.

Koenig, W., and Ruppel, A. E., 1948. Quantitative amplitude representation in sound spectrograms, *The Journal of the Acoustical Society of America*, 20(6), pp. 787–795.

Kopp, G. A., and Green, H. C., 1946. Basic phonetic principles of visible speech, *The Journal of the Acoustical Society of America*, 18(1), pp. 244–245.

Kratzenstein, C. G., 1781. *Tentamen Resolvendi Problema ab Academia Scientiarum Imperiali Petroplitana ad annum 1780 Publice Problema*, Petropoli: Typis Academiae Scientiarium.

Kröger, B. J., Birkholz, P., Lowit, A., and Neuschaefer-Rube, C., 2010. Phonemic, sensory, and motor representations in an action-based neurocomputational model of speech production, *Speech motor control: New developments in basic and applied research*, Maassen, B. and Van Lieshout, P. eds., New York: Oxford University Press, pp. 23–36.

Ladefoged, P., and Broadbent, D. E., 1957. Information conveyed by vowels, *The Journal of the Acoustical Society of America*, 29(1), pp. 98–104.

Lawrence, W., 1953. The synthesis of speech from signals which have a low information rate, *Communication Theory*, pp. 460–469.

Liberman, A. M., 1957. Some results of research on speech perception, *The Journal of the Acoustical Society of America*, 29, 117–123. http://dx.doi.org/10.1121/1.1908635

Liberman, A. M., Cooper, F. S., Shankweiler, D. P., and Studdert-Kennedy, M., 1967. Perception of the speech code, *Psychological Review*, 74, pp. 431–461. http://dx.doi.org/10.1037/h0020279

Liberman, A. M., Delattre, P., and Cooper, F. S., 1952. The role of selected stimulus-variables in the perception of the unvoiced stop consonants, *The American Journal of Psychology*, 65, pp. 497–516. http://dx.doi.org/10.2307/1418032

Liberman, A. M., Delattre, P., Cooper, F. S., and Gerstman, L., 1954. The role of consonant-vowel transitions in the perception of the stop and nasal consonants, *Psychological Monographs: General and Applied*, 68, pp. 1–13. http:/dx.doi.org/10.1037/h0093673

Liberman, A. M., Harris, K. S., Hoffman, H. S., and Griffith, B. C., 1957. The discrimination of speech sounds within and across phoneme boundaries, *Journal of Experimental Psychology*, 54, pp. 358–368. http://dx.doi.org/10.1037/h0044417

Liberman, A. M., Ingemann, F., Lisker, L., Delattre, P., and Cooper, F. S., 1959. Minimal rules for synthesizing speech, *The Journal of the Acoustical Society of America*, 31(11), pp. 1490–1499.

Liljencrants, J., 1985. *Speech synthesis with a reflection-type line analog*. DS Dissertation, Dept. of Speech Comm. and Music Acous., Royal Inst. of Tech., Stockholm, Sweden.

Lindblom, B. E., and Sundberg, J. E., 1971. Acoustical consequences of lip, tongue, jaw, and larynx movement, *The Journal of the Acoustical Society of America*, 50(4B), 1166–1179.

Loizou, P. C., Dorman, M., and Tu, Z., 1999. On the number of channels needed to understand speech, *The Journal of the Acoustical Society of America*, 106(4), pp. 2097–2103.

Maeda, S., 1988. Improved articulatory model, *The Journal of the Acoustical Society of America*, 84, Sup. 1, S146.

Maeda, S., 1990. Compensatory articulation during speech: Evidence from the analysis and synthesis of vocal tract shapes using an articulatory model, *Speech production and speech modeling*, W.L. Hardcastle, W.L. and Marcha, A., eds. Dordrecht: Kluwer Academic Publishers, pp. 131–149.

Massaro, D. W., 1998. *Perceiving talking faces: From speech perception to a behavioral principle*, Cambridge, MA: MIT Press.
Mattingly, I. G., 1974. Speech synthesis for phonetic and phonological models, *Current trends in linguistics*, Sebeok, T.A., ed., The Hague: Mouton, pp. 2451–2487.
Mermelstein, P., 1973. Articulatory model for the study of speech production, *The Journal of the Acoustical Society of America*, 53(4), pp. 1070–1082.
Miller, D. C., 1909. The phonodeik, *Physical Review*, 28, p. 151.
Miller, D. C., 1916. *The Lowell lectures: The science of musical sounds*, New York: MacMillan and Co., pp. 215–262.
Moulines, E., and Charpentier, F., 1990. Pitch-synchronous waveform processing techniques for text-to-speech synthesis using diphones, *Speech Communication*, 9, pp. 453–467.
Mrayati, M., Carré, R., and Guérin, B., 1988. Distinctive regions and modes: A new theory of speech production, *Speech Communication*, 7, pp. 257–286.
Nakata, K., and Mitsuoka, T., 1965. Phonemic transformation and control aspects of synthesis of connected speech, *Journal of the Radio Research Laboratory*, 12, pp. 171–186.
Nam, H., Mitra, V., Tiede, M., Hasegawa-Johnson, M., Espy-Wilson, C., Saltzman, E., and Goldstein, L., 2012. A procedure for estimating gestural scores from speech acoustics, *The Journal of the Acoustical Society of America*, 132(6), pp. 3980–3989.
Pantalony, D., 2004. Seeing a voice: Rudolph Koenig's instruments for studying vowel sounds, *American Journal of Psychology*, pp. 425–442.
Patterson, R., 1845. Stated Meeting, December 19, *Proceedings of the American Philosophical Society*, 4(34), p. 222.
Pedro the voder: A machine that talks, 1939, *Bell Laboratories Record*, 17(6), pp. 170–171. (no author listed).
Peterson, G. E., Wang, W. S. Y., and Sivertsen, E., 1958. Segmentation techniques in speech synthesis, *The Journal of the Acoustical Society of America*, 30(8), pp. 739–742.
Pieraccini, R., 2012. *The voice in the machine*, Cambridge, MA: MIT Press.
Potter, R. K., 1945. Visible patterns of sound, *Science*, 102(2654), pp. 463–470.
Potter, R. K., 1949. Objectives for sound portrayal, *The Journal of the Acoustical Society of America*, 21(1), pp. 1–5.
Potter, R. K., and Peterson, G. E., 1948. The representation of vowels and their movements, *The Journal of the Acoustical Society of America*, 20(4), pp. 528–535.
Rayleigh, J. W. S., 1878. *The theory of sound, vol. II*, New York: MacMillan and Co., pp. 469–478.
Remez, R. E., 2005. Perceptual organization of speech, *The Handbook of speech perception*, Pisoni, D. B. and Remez, R. E., eds., Oxford: Blackwell, pp. 28–50.
Remez, R. E., Rubin, P. E., Pisoni, D. B., and Carrell, T. D., 1981. Speech perception without traditional speech cues, *Science*, 212, pp. 947–950.
Rosen, G., 1958. Dynamic analog speech synthesizer, *The Journal of the Acoustical Society of America*, 30(3), pp. 201–209.
Rothenberg, M., Dorman, K. W., Rumm, J. C., and Theerman, P. H., 1992. 1846 letter from Joseph Henry to Henry M. Alexander, *The papers of Joseph Henry: Volume 6*, Washington, DC: Smithsonian Institution Press, pp. 359–364.
Rubin, P., Baer, T., and Mermelstein, P., 1981. An articulatory synthesizer for perceptual research, *The Journal of the Acoustical Society of America*, 70, pp. 321–328.
Rubin, P., Saltzman, E., Goldstein, L., McGowan, R., Tiede, M., and Browman, C., 1996. CASY and extensions to the task-dynamic model, *Proceedings of the 4th Speech Production Seminar*, Grenoble, France, pp. 125–128.
Sagisaka, Y., Kaiki, N., Iwahashi, N., and Mimura, K., 1992. ATR m-TALK speech synthesis system, *Proceedings of the International Conference on Spoken Language Processing*, ISCA Archive, http://www.isca-speech.org/archive, pp. 483–486.

Saltzman, E., 1986. Task dynamic coordination of the speech articulators: A preliminary model, *Experimental Brain Research Series*, 15, pp. 129–144.

Saltzman, E., 1991. The task dynamic model in speech production, *Speech motor control and stuttering*, Peters, H. F. M., Hulstijn, W., and Starkweather, W., eds., *Excerpta Medica*, Speech Motor Control and Stuttering. Elsevier Science Publishers. Amsterdam, pp. 37–52.

Schroeder, M. R., 1981. Homer W. Dudley: A tribute, *The Journal of the Acoustical Society of America*, 69(4), p. 1222.

Schroeder, M. R., 1993. A brief history of synthetic speech, *Speech Communication*, 13(1–2), pp. 231–237.

Scott, E-L., 1859. The phonoautograph, *Cosmos*, 14, p. 314.

Shannon, R. V., Zeng, F-G., Kamath, V., Wygonski, J., and Ekelid, M., 1995. Speech recognition with primarily temporal cues, *Science*, 270, pp. 303–304.

Sivertsen, E., 1961. Segment inventories for speech synthesis, *Language and Speech*, 4(1), pp. 27–90.

Smith, Z. M., Delgutte, B., and Oxenham, A. J., 2002. Chimaeric sounds reveal dichotomies in auditory perception, *Nature*, 416, pp. 87–90.

Sondhi, M., and Schroeter, J., 1987. A hybrid time-frequency domain articulatory speech synthesizer, *IEEE Transactions on Acoustics, Speech, and Signal Processing*, 35(7), pp. 955–967.

The Speaking Automaton, 1846. *London Times*, August 12. p. 3. www.phonozoic.net/library.html

Steinberg, J. C., and French, N. R., 1946. The portrayal of visible speech, *The Journal of the Acoustical Society of America*, 18(1), pp. 4–18.

Stevens, K. N., and House, A. S., 1955. Development of a quantitative description of vowel articulation, *The Journal of the Acoustical Society of America*, 27(3), pp. 484–493.

Stevens, K. N., Kasowski, S., and Fant, C. G. M., 1953. An electrical analog of the vocal tract, *The Journal of the Acoustical Society of America*, 25(4), pp. 734–742.

Stewart, J. Q., 1922. An electrical analogue of the vocal organs, *Nature*, 110(2757), pp. 311–312.

Story, B. H., 1995. *Physiologically-based speech simulation using an enhanced wave-reflection model of the vocal tract*. Ph.D. Dissertation, University of Iowa, Ann Arbor, MI: University Microfilms International.

Story, B. H., 2005. A parametric model of the vocal tract area function for vowel and consonant simulation, *The Journal of the Acoustical Society of America*, 117(5), pp. 3231–3254.

Story, B. H., 2013. Phrase-level speech simulation with an airway modulation model of speech production, *Computer Speech and Language*, 27(4), pp. 989–1010.

Story, B. H., and Bunton, K., 2010. Relation of vocal tract shape, formant transitions, and stop consonant identification, *Journal of Speech, Language, and Hearing Research*, 53, pp. 1514–1528.

Story, B. H., Titze, I. R., and Hoffman, E. A., 1996. Vocal tract area functions from magnetic resonance imaging, *The Journal of the Acoustical Society of America*, 100(1), pp. 537–554.

Story, B. H., Titze, I. R., and Hoffman, E. A., 1998. Vocal tract area functions for an adult female speaker based on volumetric imaging, *The Journal of the Acoustical Society of America*, 104(1), 471–487.

Strube, H., 1982. Time-varying wave digital filters and vocal-tract models, *Acoustics, Speech, and Signal Processing, IEEE International Conference on ICASSP '82*, 7, IEEE, pp. 923–926.

Talking Machine, 1880. *London Times*, February 12. www.phonozoic.net/library.html

Titze, I. R., 1973. The human vocal cords: A mathematical model, *Phonetica*, 28(3–4), pp. 129–170.

Titze, I. R., 1974. The human vocal cords: A mathematical model, *Phonetica*, 29(1–2), pp. 1–21.

Tompkins, D., 2010. How to wreck a nice beach, *The Vocoder from World War II to Hip-Hop, the machine speaks*, Brooklyn, NY: Melville House.

Trouvain, J., and Brackhane, F., 2011. Wolfgang von Kempelen's speaking machine as an instrument for demonstration and research, *Proceedings of the 17th International Conference of Phonetic Sciences*, International Phonetic Association, https://www.internationalphoneticassociation.org/icphs-proceedings/ICPhS2011/index.htm, pp. 164–167.

Truby, H. M., 1965. Matching speech cineradiography with pseudospeech, *The Journal of the Acoustical Society of America*, 37(6), p. 1187.

Van den Oord, A., Dieleman, S., Zen, H., Simonyan, K., Vinyals, O., Graves, A., Kalchbrenner, N., Senior, A., and Kavukcuoglu, K., 2016. *Wavenet: A generative model for raw audio*. arXiv preprint arXiv:1609.03499. [Accessed 5 March 2018].

Vatikiotis-Bateson, E., Kuratate, T., Munhall, K. G., and Yehia, H. C., 2000. The production and perception of a realistic talking face, *Proceedings of LP'98: Item order in language and speech*, Fujimura, O., Joseph, B. D., and Palek, B., eds., Prague: Karolinum Press (Charles University, 2, pp. 439–460).

Wang, W. S. Y., and Peterson, G. E., 1958. Segment inventory for speech synthesis, *Journal of the Acoustical Society of America*, 30(8), pp. 743–746.

Wheatstone, C., 1837. Reed organ-pipes, speaking machines, etc., *The scientific papers of Sir Charles Wheatstone* (1879), London: Taylor and Francis, pp. 348–367. Originally published in the London and Westminster Review, No. xi and liv., October 1837.

Willis, R., 1829. On the vowel sounds, and on reed organ pipes, *Transactions of the Cambridge philosophical society*, 3, pp. 231–268.

Wurzbach, C., *Biographies of the Empire Austria: Containing life sketches of memorable people, who lived from 1750 to 1850 in the imperial state and in its crown lands*, 60, pp. 1856–1891, Vienna: Austrian Academy of Sciences Press.

Yehia, H., Rubin, P., and Vatikiotis-Bateson, E., 1998. Quantitative association of vocal-tract and facial behavior, *Speech Communication*, 26(1–2), pp. 23–43.

Zen, H., Senior, A., and Schuster, M., 2013. Statistical parametric speech synthesis using deep neural networks, *Acoustics, Speech and Signal Processing (ICASSP)*, IEEE, pp. 7962–7966.

Zen, H., Tokuda, K., and Black, A. W., 2009. Statistical parametric speech synthesis, *Speech Communication*, 51(11), pp. 1039–1064.

2

Advances in vocal tract imaging and analysis

Asterios Toutios, Dani Byrd, Louis Goldstein, and Shrikanth Narayanan

Introduction

Several techniques are available for the acquisition of data on the kinematics of speech production. Electromagnetic articulography (EMA) (Schönle et al., 1987) uses electromagnetic fields to track the positions of small coil sensors adhering to the articulators in two or three dimensions with sampling rates up to 500 Hz. Electropalatography (EPG) (Hardcastle et al., 1989) uses an artificial palate with embedded electrodes to record linguapalatal contact, typically at 100–200 Hz. Ultrasound can be used to image the tongue (Stone, 2006; Whalen et al., 2005) or larynx (Celata et al., 2017; Moisik, Lin and Esling, 2014) at 30–100 Hz. Despite their availability, these techniques are limited in their coverage of the vocal tract. EMA provides rich data about the movement of sensors on lingual and labial fleshpoints, but such sensors/markers cannot be easily placed at posterior locations on the tongue, on the velum, in the pharynx, or at the larynx; hence these technologies are limited in the spatial coverage of the complex vocal tract geometry. Additionally, EMA does not provide information as to the passive vocal tract structures such as the palate (both hard and soft) and pharyngeal wall that are important landmarks for constriction location and airway shaping. EPG is restricted to contact measurements of the tongue at the hard palate and typically does not exceed a 100 Hz sampling rate. Further, EPG does not record kinematic information of the tongue but rather the consequence of this movement for (obstruent) constriction formation. Ultrasound cannot consistently or reliably image the tongue tip, or opposing vocal tract surfaces such as the hard and soft palate and hence the airway shaping.

X-ray radiation has been used to image the sagittal projection of the entire vocal tract at rates typically between 10 and 50 frames per second (Badin et al., 1995; Delattre, 1971; Munhall, Vatikiotis-Bateson and Tohkura, 1995; Wood, 1982), providing rich dynamic data with superior coverage of the entire vocal-tract configuration. However, its use for speech research has today been abandoned for health and ethical reasons, since X-ray energy exposes subjects to unacceptable levels of radiation. Magnetic resonance imaging (MRI) has been used to capture images of static configurations of the vocal tract, also with very good coverage of its global configuration, but it does this while subjects sustain (and sometimes phonate) continuant speech sounds over unnaturally long periods of time, thus producing static airway shaping information rather than dynamic speech production information (Clément et al., 2007; Narayanan, Alwan and Haker, 1995; Story, Titze, and Hoffman, 1996). While MRI has for some time been considered to be a slow imaging modality, modern techniques that were largely developed to capture the motion of the heart can now yield temporal resolutions exceeding those available with X-ray or ultrasound. In tagged or triggered MRI acquisition methods, notably repetitive cine-MRI (Stone et al., 2001; Takemoto et al., 2006), articulatory dynamics of running speech can be reconstructed from large numbers of repetitions (which should ideally be identical) of short utterances.

Real-time magnetic resonance imaging

Currently, significant advances in MR acquisition software, reconstruction strategies, and customized receiver coil hardware development have allowed real-time MRI (rtMRI) to emerge as an important and powerful modality for speech production research (Bresch et al., 2008; Narayanan et al., 2004; Niebergall et al., 2013; Scott et al., 2014; Sutton et al., 2009). RtMRI provides dynamic information from the entire midsagittal (or other) plane of a speaker's upper airway during arbitrary, continuous spoken utterances with no need for repetitions. Sampling rates can now be achieved that are acceptable for running speech, and noise cancellation can yield an acceptable synchronized speech audio signal. RtMRI can capture not only lingual, labial and jaw motion, but also articulatory motion of the velopharyngeal mechanism and of the laryngeal articulatory mechanism, including shaping of the epilaryngeal tube and the glottis. Additionally, and in contrast to many other imaging or movement tracking modalities, rtMRI can acquire upper and rear airway structures such as the hard and soft palate, pharyngeal wall, and details of the structures of the laryngeal mechanism. Though EMA still has superior temporal resolution and audio quality (as well as price and accessibility), it cannot parallel rtMRI as a source of dynamic information about overall vocal tract movement and airway shaping.

An MRI scanner consists of electromagnets that surround the human body and create magnetic fields. MR images are formed through the interaction between externally applied magnetic fields and nuclear magnetic spins in hydrogen atoms present in the water molecules of the human body. A static magnetic field (typically 1.5, 3, or 7 Tesla) serves to polarize the hydrogen atoms. Atoms are then excited using a radiofrequency magnetic field and a set of linear magnetic field gradients that are dynamically changing over very short periods of time according to pre-designed *pulse sequences*. After excitation, as the hydrogen atoms return to equilibrium, they emit signals that represent samples in the spatial Fourier transform domain (which is referred to as *k-space*) of the excited area. Given enough samples, an inverse Fourier transform can reconstruct a map of the density of hydrogen atoms in the excited area. Typically, atoms in a single thin plane are excited, and the k-space and Fourier transforms are two-dimensional. The orientation of the slice is determined by the gradient fields.

In typical MRI applications, the k-space may be sampled for several seconds, or even minutes, in order to generate a single high-quality image. However, in order to capture the dynamics of speech production in fine temporal resolution, especially with no need of repetitions, the sampling needs to happen in amounts of time much shorter than a second (Lingala, Sutton, et al., 2016). For such *real-time* MRI, the k-space is sampled only partially (but in a highly principled manner) in order to generate images of sufficient quality for further analysis. Thus, real-time MRI is subject to a compromise between temporal resolution and image quality. Image quality mainly comprises two factors – spatial resolution and signal-to-noise ratio – that can to some extent be independently controlled.

An efficient way to sample the k-space is along spirals, as shown in Figure 2.1, which is achieved by appropriate pulse-sequence design (Narayanan et al., 2004). Samples covering such a spiral can be acquired in little more than 6 ms. Successive spirals are rotated by certain angles with respect to each other, and by combining samples from a few spirals, an image can be formed. In the visualization of Figure 2.1, an image is formed by combining k-space information from five successive spirals.

In a typical implementation of vocal-tract rtMRI that has been extensively used (Narayanan et al., 2014; Toutios and Narayanan, 2016), 13 spirals were combined to form an image, thus leading to a temporal resolution of 78 ms per image. Each image is comprised of 68 by 68 pixels, with a spatial resolution of 3 by3 mm per pixel. Videos of vocal production were generated by combining successive images, or frames.[1] New frames were generated by overlapping information from six spirals, which yielded videos with a frame rate of 23 frames per second.

The more recent and currently used rtMRI acquisition protocol applies a constrained reconstruction scheme (Lingala et al., 2017). This method exploits redundancy across

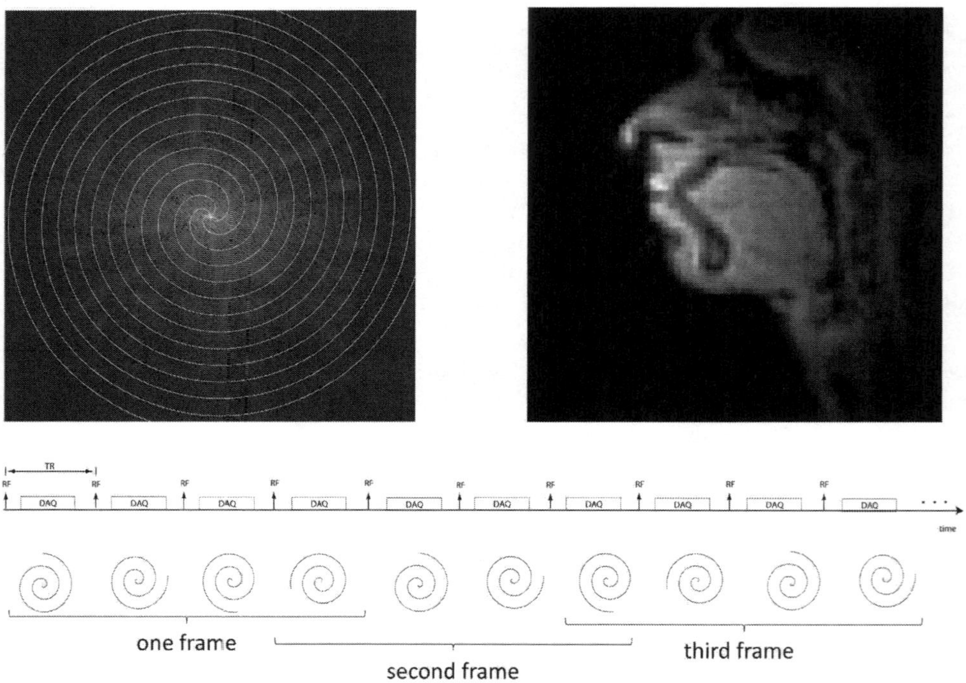

Figure 2.1 Left image shows the k-space transformation of the vocal-tract image shown on the right, with four spirals superposed on it. The k-space is sampled along such spirals. The bottom of the figure illustrates the principle by which samples from successive spirals, which are rotated with respect to each other, combine to form a video image frame. TR (repetition time) is the time between the application of two radiofrequency (RF) waves that excite hydrogen atoms after which data acquisition (DAQ) takes place. In this illustration, information from four spirals is combined to form an image frame, and one spiral is overlapped between successive frames. In the first of the reconstruction protocols discussed in the text, 13 spirals are combined to form a frame with an overlap of 7 frames. The more recent constrained reconstruction protocol effectively forms a video image frame from two spirals, without spiral overlap.

frames based on the fact that the critical dynamic information for speech production is concentrated at the edges between air and tissue, enabling a reconstruction with a temporal resolution of 12 ms, that is, a frame rate of 83 frames per second, with 84 by 84 pixels per image and 2.4 by 2.4 mm per pixel. A short example is shown in Figure 2.2. Crucial to the success of this method is the use of a custom array of coils surrounding the vocal tract that receive the signals emitted by the excited hydrogen atoms. These custom coils have superior sensitivity in regions corresponding to the pertinent vocal-tract structures (lips, tongue, velum, epiglottis, glottis) compared to receiver coils typically used in clinical MRI.

In most cases, rtMRI images a thin slice (~5 mm thick) at the mid-sagittal plane. However, it is possible to image any other plane, such as parasagittal, coronal, axial, or an arbitrary oblique plane. These views can offer particular insight to speech production research questions involving the shaping of constrictions, laterality, and stretching, compression, concavities/grooving and posturing of the tongue. It is also possible to image concurrently two or three slices, with the frame rate divided by a factor of two or three respectively – essentially switching slices rapidly between spiral acquisitions, giving rise to *multi-slice* dynamic videos. Figure 2.3 shows an example of such imaging. This technique can offer particular insight to the creation of more complex articulatory shaping and its concurrent larynx movement.

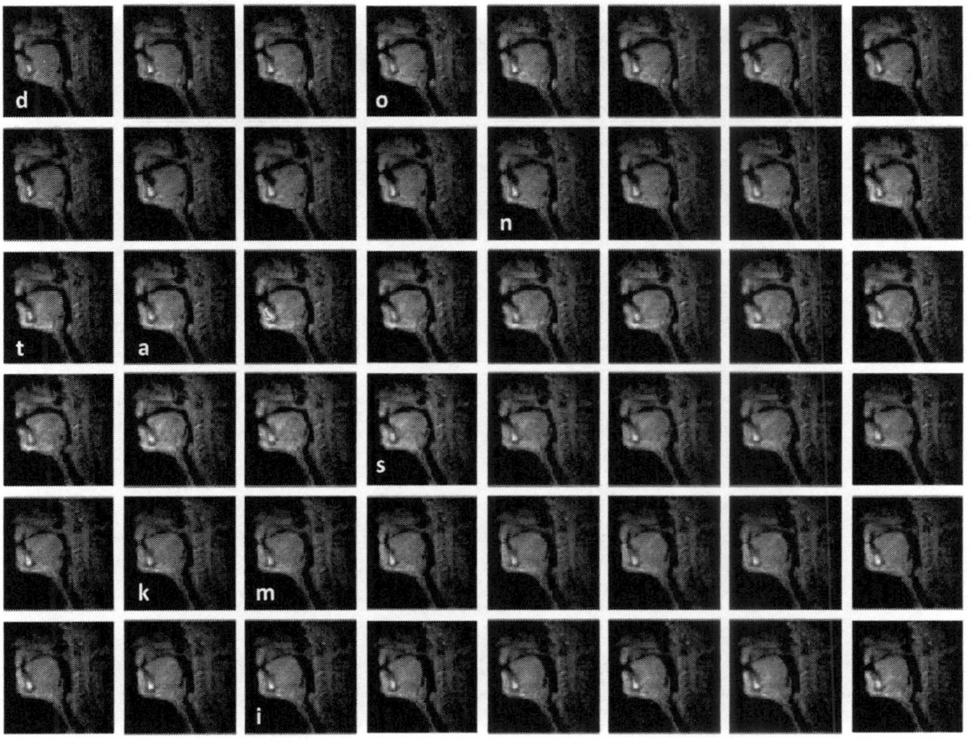

Figure 2.2 Successive midsagittal real-time MRI frames of a male speaker uttering "don't ask me." The 40 frames shown span about 480 ms (video reconstructed at 83 frames per second). The International Phonetic Alphabet (IPA) annotation serves as a rough guide for the segments being produced in the image sequence.

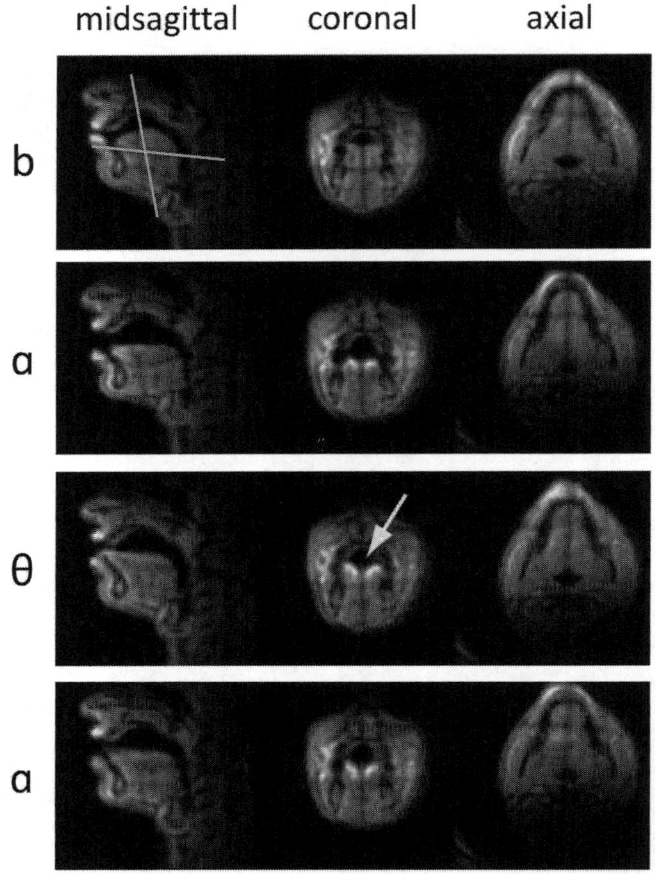

Figure 2.3 Concurrent multi-slice real-time MRI for the sequence /bɑθɑ/. The two lines on the top mid-sagittal image show the orientations of the axial and coronal slices. The arrow on the coronal image during /θ/ shows a tongue groove channel (which would be very difficult to observe with other imaging modalities).

Speech audio is typically recorded concurrently with rtMRI in articulatory research. Acquiring and synchronizing the audio with the imaging data presents several technical challenges. Audio can be recorded using a fiber-optic microphone (Garthe, 1991), but the overall recording setup typically needs to be customized (Bresch et al., 2006). Synchronization between audio and images can be achieved using a trigger signal from the MRI scanner. That said, a significant challenge in audio acquisition is the high level of noise generated by the operation of the MRI scanner. It is important that this noise be canceled satisfactorily in order to enable further analysis of the speech acoustic signal. Proposed audio de-noising algorithms specifically targeting the task can exploit the periodic structure of the MR noise generated by pulse sequences (Bresch et al., 2006), or not (Vaz, Ramanarayanan and Narayanan, 2013); the latter algorithms can be used even when the applied pulse sequence leads to non-periodic noise.

RtMRI image processing and analysis

Reconstructed rtMRI data have the form of high-frame rate videos depicting the hydrogen density of tissue in a thin vocal-tract slice, most usually the midsagittal. Some speech production phenomena may be studied simply by manually inspecting these videos and measuring the timing of articulatory events identified in the image sequences. To assist in this, our team at USC has developed and made freely available a graphical user interface (GUI) that allows users to browse the videos frame-by-frame, inspect synchronized audio and video segments in real time or at slower frame rates, and label speech segments of interest for further analysis with the supporting tool set.

Some speech production studies require more elaborate image processing and analysis of the rtMRI videos. Unsupervised segmentation of regions corresponding to the mandibular, maxillary and posterior areas of the upper airway has been achieved by exploiting spatial representations of these regions in the frequency domain, the native domain of MRI data (Bresch and Narayanan, 2009; Toutios and Narayanan, 2015). The segmentation algorithm uses an anatomically informed object model and returns a set of tissue boundaries for each frame of interest, allowing for quantification of articulator movement and vocal tract aperture in the midsagittal plane. The method makes use of alternate gradient vector flows, nonlinear least squares optimization, and hierarchically optimized gradient descent procedures to refine estimates of tissue locations in the vocal tract. Thus, the method is automatic and well-suited for processing long sequences of MR images. Obtaining such vocal-tract air-tissue boundaries enables the calculation of vocal-tract midsagittal cross-distances, which in turn can be used to estimate area functions via reference sagittal-to-area transformations (Maeda, 1990; McGowan, Jackson and Berger, 2012; Soquet et al., 2002). See Figure 2.4 for sample results deploying this processing method.

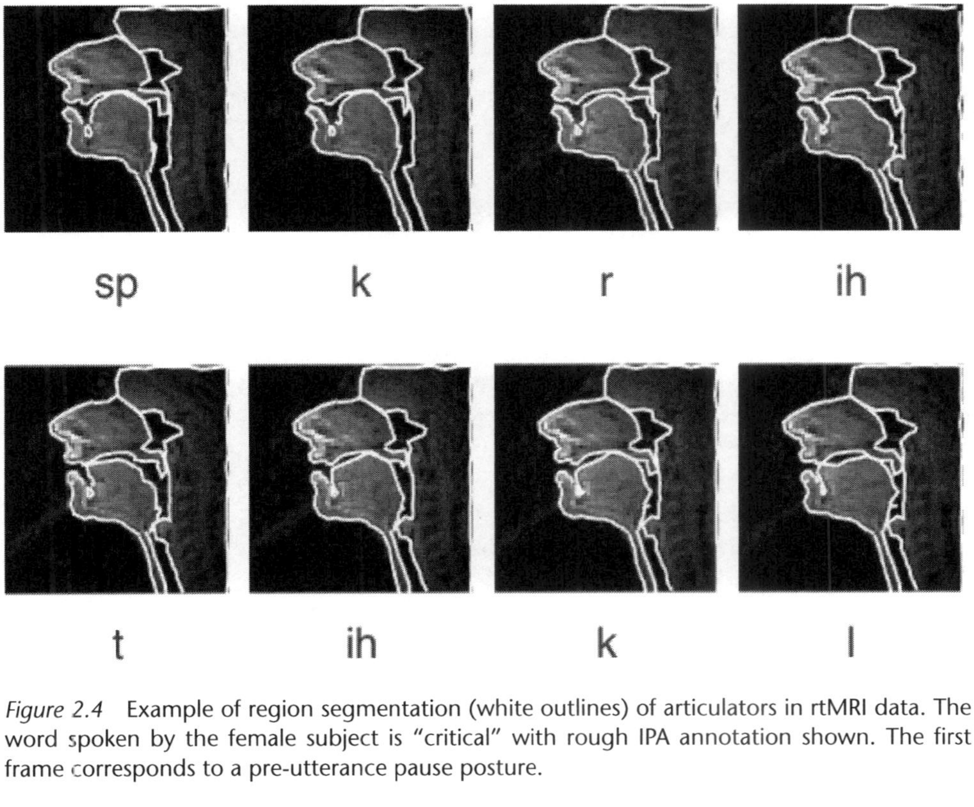

Figure 2.4 Example of region segmentation (white outlines) of articulators in rtMRI data. The word spoken by the female subject is "critical" with rough IPA annotation shown. The first frame corresponds to a pre-utterance pause posture.

A limitation of this unsupervised regional segmentation method is that it is slow, requiring significant computational resources. To address the issue of computational resources, our team has also started developing a convolutional deep neural network, trained on examples of video frames with corresponding air-tissue boundaries derived via the original segmentation method (Somandepalli, Toutios, and Narayanan, 2017). Once this neural network is in place and fully tested, deriving high-quality air-tissue boundaries from new rtMRI frames will be instantaneous.

While air-tissue boundary detection is important for capturing the posture of individual articulators over time, it is often enough to observe the dynamics of the formation and release of constrictions in a specific region of the vocal tract. As a faster (yet less accurate) alternative, a method of rapid semi-automatic segmentation of rtMRI data for parametric analysis has been developed that seeks pixel intensity thresholds distributed along tract-normal grid lines and defines airway contours constrained with respect to a tract-centerline constructed between the glottis and lips (Kim, Kumar et al., 2014; Proctor et al., 2010). A version of this rapid method has been integrated in the aforementioned GUI.

Pixel intensity in an MR image is indicative of the presence or absence of soft tissue; consequently, articulator movement into and out of a region of interest in the airway can be estimated by calculating the change in mean pixel intensity as the articulator of interest moves (increasingly) into and out of the region of interest. Using this concept, a direct image analysis method has been developed that bypasses the need to identify tissue boundaries in the upper airway (Lammert, Proctor, and Narayanan, 2010). In this approach to rtMRI speech dynamic image analysis, constriction location targets can be automatically estimated by identifying regions of maximally dynamic correlated pixel activity along the palate and at the lips, and constriction and release gestures (goal-directed vocal tract actions) can be identified in the velocity profiles derived from the smoothed pixel intensity functions in vocal tract regions of interest (Proctor et al., 2011). Such methods of pixel intensity-based direct image analysis have been used in numerous studies examining the compositionality of speech production, discussed in what follows.

Examining the compositionality of speech production

Speech is dynamic in nature: It is realized through time-varying changes in vocal tract shape that emerge systematically from the combined effects of multiple constriction events distributed over space (i.e., subparts of the vocal tract) and over time. Understanding the spatiotemporal dynamics of speech production is fundamental to linguistic studies.

Real-time MRI allows pursuing this goal through investigating the compositionality of speech into cognitively controlled goal-directed vocal tract action events, called gestures (Browman and Goldstein, 1992). Of specific interest are: (a) the compositionality in space, i.e., the deployment of gestures distributed spatially over distinct constriction effector systems of the vocal tract; (b) the compositionality in time, i.e., the deployment of gestures co-produced temporally; and (c) the characterization of articulatory setting, i.e., the postural configuration(s) that vocal tract articulators tend to be deployed from and return to in the process of producing fluent and natural speech. Each of these areas of study will exhibit differences among languages that reflect the range of biologically viable linguistic systems.

An example study on the compositionality of speech production in space examined retroflex stops and rhotics in Tamil (Smith et al., 2013). The study revealed that in some contexts these consonants may be achieved with little or no retroflexion of the tongue tip. Rather, maneuvering and shaping of the tongue so as to achieve post-alveolar contact varies across vowel contexts. Between back vowels /a/ and /u/, post-alveolar constriction involves the curling back of the tongue tip, but in the context of the high front vowel /i/, the same constriction is achieved by tongue bunching. Results supported the view that so-called retroflex consonants have a specified target constriction in the post-alveolar region but indicate that the specific articulatory maneuvers employed to achieve this constriction are not fixed. The superposition of the consonantal constriction task with the tasks controlling the shaping and position of the tongue body for the surrounding vowels (in keeping, for example, with Öhman, 1966) leads to retroflexion of the tongue in some cases and tongue bunching in others.

An example line of research on gestural compositionality in time examined the coordination of velic and oral gestures for nasal consonants. For English /n/ (Byrd et al., 2009), it was found that near-synchrony of velum lowering and tongue tip raising characterizes the timing for [n] in syllable onsets, while temporal lag between the gestures is characteristic for codas, supporting and extending previous findings for /m/ obtained with a mechanical velotrace (Krakow, 1993). In French – which, unlike English, contrasts nasal and oral vowels – the coordination of velic and oral gestures was found to be more tightly controlled, to allow for the distinction between nasal vowels and nasal consonants (Proctor, Goldstein, et al., 2013). But while the nature of the coordinative relation was different between French and English, the timing of the corresponding gestures as a function of prosodic context varied in the same way.

Regarding the characterization of articulatory setting, research using rtMRI of speech has supported the hypothesis that pauses at major syntactic boundaries (i.e., grammatical pauses) but not at ungrammatical pauses (e.g., word search) are planned by a high-level cognitive mechanism that also controls and modulates the rate of articulation around these prosodic junctures (Ramanarayanan et al., 2014). This work further hypothesizes that postures adopted during grammatical pauses in speech are more mechanically advantageous than postures assumed at absolute rest, i.e., that small changes in articulator positions during grammatical pauses would produce larger changes in speech task variables than small changes during absolute rest. This hypothesis was verified using locally weighted linear regression to estimate the forward map from low-level articulator variables to high-level task variables (Lammert et al., 2013). The analysis showed that articulatory postures assumed during grammatical pauses in speech, as well as speech-ready postures, are significantly more mechanically advantageous than postures assumed during absolute rest.

RtMRI data, complemented by speech audio, have afforded new insights into the nature and execution of speech production goals, the relationship between speech articulation and acoustics, and the nature of variability in speech motor control. Acquisition methodologies have now matured enough to enable speech production research across languages with a variety of articulatory shaping maneuvers and temporal patterning of articulation. Examples of studies enabled by rtMRI, from our team and other research groups, include, in addition to the aforementioned ones, work that has examined the production of nasals in English, French (Carignan et al., 2015; Proctor, Goldstein, et al., 2013), and Brazilian Portuguese (Barlaz et al., 2015; Meireles et al., 2015); liquids in English (Harper, Goldstein, and Narayanan, 2016; Proctor and Walker, 2012) and Korean (Lee, Goldstein, and Narayanan, 2015); English diphthongs (Hsieh and Goldstein, 2015), (Proctor et al., 2016); English and Spanish coronal stops (Parrell and Narayanan, 2014); Lebanese Arabic coronal "emphatic" (uvularized) consonants (Israel et al., 2012); Tamil retroflexes (Smith et al., 2013); Puerto Rican Spanish rhotics (Monteserín, Narayanan, and Goldstein, 2016); and Khoisan clicks (Proctor et al., 2016).

Finally, rtMRI can provide a unique view of speech compositionality in breakdown. Previous work has demonstrated the potential of rtMRI to study the characteristics of speech production of people suffering from verbal apraxia, i.e., the inability to execute a voluntary movement despite being able to demonstrate normal muscle function (Hagedorn et al., 2017), and people who have undergone surgical removal of part of their tongue (glossectomy) because of cancer (Hagedorn et al., 2014). Dynamical articulatory imaging can provide detailed and quantifiable characterizations of speech deficits in spatiotemporal coordination and/or execution of linguistic gestures and of compensatory maneuvers that are adopted by speakers in the face of such hurdles. This rtMRI data can have important potential benefits including for therapeutic and surgical interventions; additionally, an examination of the linguistic system in breakdown can contribute to a better understanding of the cognitive structure of healthy speech production.

A data-driven computational speech production framework

The collection of extensive amounts of rtMRI data enables computational modeling work that can advance the refinement of existing speech production models and the development of new ones. Of particular interest is modeling speech production across different individuals, in order to explore how individual vocal-tract morphological differences are reflected in the acoustic speech signal and what articulatory strategies are adopted in the presence of such morphological differences to achieve speech invariance, either perceptual or acoustic. One of the long-term objectives of this ongoing work is to improve scientific understanding of how vocal-tract morphology and speech articulation interact and to explain the variant and invariant aspects of speech properties within and across talkers. Initial work with rtMRI has focused on individual differences in the size, shape and relative proportions of the hard palate and posterior pharyngeal wall. Specific aims have been to characterize such differences (Lammert, Proctor, and Narayanan, 2013b), to examine how they relate to speaker-specific articulatory and acoustic patterns (Lammert, Proctor, and Narayanan, 2013a), and to explore the possibility of predicting them automatically from the acoustic signal (Li et al., 2013). Moreover, rtMRI may help characterize individual differences of other vocal-tract structures such as the epilaryngeal tube and the glottis (Moisik, Lin, and Esling, 2014)

In more recent work, a factor analysis was applied to air-tissue boundaries derived by the previously mentioned automatic segmentation algorithm (Bresch and Narayanan, 2009). The method, which was inspired by older articulatory models based on limited amounts of X-ray data (Harshman, Ladefoged, and Goldstein, 1977; Maeda, 1990), decomposes the vocal-tract dynamics into a set of articulatory parameter trajectories corresponding to relative contributions (degrees of freedom) of the jaw, tongue, lips, velum, and larynx, and operating on speaker-specific vocal-tract deformations (Toutios and Narayanan, 2015). Constrictions along the vocal tract were also measured from the segmentation results and a locally linear mapping from model parameters to constriction degrees was found using a hierarchical clustering process with a linearity test (Sorensen et al., 2016).

Having a locally linear mapping between linguistically critical constrictions along the vocal tract and the overall vocal-tract shaping, as represented compactly by the parameters of the articulatory model, enables the application of dynamical system modeling to animate the vocal tract towards the achievement of such constrictions. The assumption that deformations of the vocal-tract are governed by dynamical systems (more specifically, critically damped oscillators) that operate on the constrictions is a central concept in the theory of Articulatory Phonology (Browman and Goldstein, 1992) and Task Dynamics (Saltzman and

Munhall, 1989), its computational counterpart. The framework (factor analysis model; mapping between articulatory parameters and constrictions; animation with dynamical systems) was applied to a large number of English speakers to identify speaker-specific strategies that govern the tongue–jaw and lip–jaw coordinative synergies by which different individuals achieve vocal-tract constrictions (Sorensen et al., 2016).

Initial work has also been done toward using this framework for the synthesis of realistic vocal-tract dynamics from dynamical systems specifications. Critically damped oscillators involved in speech production (as proposed by Articulatory Phonology) are characterized by vectors of targets and stiffnesses, operating on *task variables* (constrictions along the vocal tract). The proposed framework enables casting the same dynamical systems to operate on the parameters of the articulatory model, which, in turn, can readily construct the midsagittal vocal tract shaping dynamics. The approach has been put forward for synthesizing vocal-tract dynamics for VCV sequences (where C was a voiced plosive), and these synthesized dynamics were used as inputs to an articulatory-to-acoustic simulator (Maeda, 1982), which generated satisfactory acoustic results (Alexander et al., 2017). Stiffness and target vectors in that work were set manually, but this is considered only as an essential first step toward fitting these parameters to the actual rtMRI data in an analysis-by-synthesis setup, which will be equivalent to uncovering the spatiotemporal structure of speech motor control commands, under the assumption of Task Dynamics (Saltzman and Munhall, 1989).

Extending the scope of Articulatory Phonology, one may forgo the assumption of critically damped oscillators and look instead to statistically decompose vocal-tract kinematics into a set of (free-form) spatiotemporal bases, or primitives, a small number of which are activated at any time in the course of a speech utterance. This has been achieved using a novel convolutive non-negative matrix factorization (NMF) algorithm (Vaz, Toutios, and Narayanan, 2016), in conjunction with the articulatory model and the parameter-to-constriction mapping. Vocal-tract dynamics were resynthesized efficiently from derived bases and activation patterns, however the association of these to phonological units remains challenging.

Strategies for modeling articulatory behavior can be beneficial towards goals beyond understanding linguistic control regimes and individual differences. These tools can help shed light to on paralinguistic aspects of articulatory behavior. One such case is the expression of emotion. The state-of-the-art in speech emotion research has predominantly focused on surface speech acoustic properties; there remain open questions as to how speech properties covary across emotional types, talkers, and linguistic conditions. Given the complex interplay between the linguistic and paralinguistic aspects of speech production, there are limitations to uncovering the underlying details just from the resultant acoustics. As will be discussed later in this chapter, a large rtMRI database of emotional speech has been collected, and analysis of this data using some of the tools described earlier is under way. Finally, rtMRI is being used to study different types of vocal performance, including Western Classical Soprano singing (Bresch and Narayanan, 2010) and Human Beatboxing performance (Proctor, Bresch, et al., 2013). This work investigates how human vocal organs are utilized in different performance styles, how performers adopt articulatory strategies to achieve specific acoustic goals, how their articulation in performance resembles or differs from that of spoken speech, and how percussive and linguistic gestures are coordinated.

Databases

In order to facilitate speech production research using rtMRI across the speech community, a body of rtMRI data, with synchronized and de-noised audio, has been made publicly available.[2] The USC-TIMIT database (Narayanan et al., 2014) includes rtMRI data from ten speakers (five male, five female), each producing a set of 460 phonetically balanced sentences from the MOCHA-TIMIT set.

The USC-EMO-MRI database includes rtMRI data from ten actors (five male, five female), each enacting four different emotions in the MRI scanner (neutral, happy, angry, sad) while repeating a small set of sentences multiple times (Kim, Toutios et al., 2014).

The USC Speech and Vocal Tract Morphology MRI Database (Sorensen et al., 2017) includes data from 17 speakers (eight male, nine female). In addition to rtMRI, the dataset also includes three-dimensional volumetric MRI data of vocal tract shapes during sustained speech sounds. The rtMRI data include consonant-vowel-consonant sequences, vowel-consonant-vowel sequences, read passages, and spontaneous speech. One of the passages was produced in five different speaking styles: normal, fast, slow, whispered and shouting. Volumetric MRI was acquired using an accelerated protocol that used 7 seconds to scan the full volume of the vocal tract. This (relatively) short scan time enabled the acquisition of volumetric MRI of the full set of vowels and continuant consonants of American English.

While rtMRI data in the aforementioned databases were collected using earlier acquisition protocols at 23 frames per second, the latest technology with improved temporal resolution is now showcased in a collection, available online, in which four expert phoneticians produce sounds of the world's languages as denoted in the IPA, with some supplementary English words and phonetically balanced texts (Toutios et al., 2016).

Open challenges

Real-time MRI for speech production research still presents challenges. First, rtMRI is currently done in a supine position, not the common upright posture for speech. Much literature has been devoted to the assessment of differences in speech articulation between the two positions (Kitamura et al., 2005; Stone et al., 2007; Tiede, Masaki, and Vatikiotis-Bateson, 2000; Traser et al., 2014). It has been suggested that positional differences are quite limited and that compensatory mechanisms, at least in healthy subjects, are sufficiently effective to allow the acquisition of meaningful speech data in a supine position (Scott et al., 2014). The potential use of upright or open-type scanners would fully remove this consideration, and there have been a few studies that demonstrate the utility of such scanners for upper-airway structures (Honda and Hata, 2007; Perry, 2010).

The MRI scanner is a very noisy environment, and subjects need to wear earplugs during acquisition, thus infringing on natural auditory feedback. Though it may be speculated the subjects would speak much louder than normal or that their articulation would be significantly affected as a result, it has been observed that these statements held true only rarely (Toutios and Narayanan, 2016). It is possible that somatosensory feedback compensates for the shortfall in auditory feedback (Katseff, Houde, and Johnson, 2012; Lametti, Nasir, and Ostry, 2012) and/or that the impairment in feedback is not exceedingly severe or perturbing.

Because of the large magnetic fields involved, people need to be excluded from being subjects in MRI research if they have prosthetics such as pacemakers, defibrillators, or (most) cochlear implants; these subjects can be identified and excluded in a screening process (Murphy and Brunberg, 1997). Otherwise, subject comfort is usually not an issue for adult healthy subjects and for scan durations (overall time spent in the scanner) of up to 90 minutes (Lingala, Toutios, et al., 2016).

Dental work is not a safety concern but may pose imaging issues. However, the disruptions associated with most dental work do not consistently degrade image quality. In general, image quality is subject-dependent (and in some cases it can be difficult to even maintain constant quality throughout the speech sample) (Lingala, Sutton, et al., 2016). It has been observed that the impact of dental work appears to be more prominent when such work resides on the plane that is imaged and that the impact is often quite localized around the dental work (Toutios and Narayanan, 2016). For example, orthodontic permanent retainers at the upper incisors result in loss of midsagittal visual information from a small circle (typically with diameter up to 3 cm) around the upper incisors.

The teeth themselves are not visible in MRI due to their chemical composition. Various methods have been used to superimpose teeth onto MRI images, including using data from supplementary Computed Tomography (CT) imaging (Story, Titze, and Hoffman, 1996), dental casts (Alwan, Narayanan, and Haker, 1997; Narayanan, Alwan, and Haker, 1997), or MRI data acquired using a contrast agent in the oral cavity such as blueberry juice (Takemoto et al., 2004) or ferric ammonium citrate (Ng et al., 2011) that leaves the teeth as signal voids. Recently, a method was proposed that reconstructs the teeth from a single three-dimensional MRI scan, where the speaker sustains a specially designed posture: Lips closed and tongue tightly in contact with the teeth (Zhang, Honda, and Wei, 2018)

Finally, even though MRI scanners are today commonplace (albeit expensive), they are not portable. Thus, rtMRI is not amenable to fieldwork studies. However, by providing unparalleled dynamic images of the entire vocal tract, rtMRI can help develop models that predict global tongue shaping from partial information, such as that provided by a portable ultrasound or EPG.

Conclusion

Research in the area of speech production has long sought to obtain accurate information about the movement and shaping of the vocal tract from larynx to lips. Dynamic, real-time articulatory data are crucial for the study of phonemic inventories, cross-linguistic phonetic processes, articulatory variability, and phonological theory. Such data afford insights into the nature and execution of speech production, the cognitive mechanisms of motor control, the relationship between speech articulation and acoustics, and the coordination of goals postulated in models of speech production. This chapter has presented an overview of recent advances in vocal tract imaging focusing on real-time MRI, and has reviewed examples of applications.

Real-time MRI presents an unprecedented opportunity for advancing speech production research. Current state-of-the-art in MR acquisition software, reconstruction strategies, and receiver coil development have allowed real-time MRI (rtMRI) to provide clear benefits in terms of spatial vocal tract coverage with very good temporal resolution as compared to other techniques for articulatory data acquisition (e.g., Bresch et al., 2008; Narayanan et al., 2004). RtMRI provides dynamic information from the entire midsagittal (or other) plane of a speaker's upper airway during arbitrary, continuous spoken utterances with no need for repetitions, and noise-cancellation techniques yield an acceptable synchronized speech audio signal. Many important early findings in speech production research were based on the study of X-ray videos of the vocal tract that collected limited amounts of data per speaker from a limited number of speakers, before being abandoned because of serious health concerns. Real-time MRI does not have such safety constraints. Real-time MRI further enables dynamic imaging of any arbitrary slice of interest (sagittal, coronal, axial, or oblique) in the vocal tract from larynx to lips, thus offering a most comprehensive means of observing the dynamics of vocal tract shaping. Finally, image processing and data analysis techniques are rapidly advancing the quantification and interpretation of this valuable real-time articulatory data.

Acknowledgments

Work supported by NIH grant R01DC007124 and NSF grant 1514544. The authors wish to thank Professor John Esling for valuable feedback on an earlier version of this chapter.

Notes

1 Visit Narayanan S. et al., SPAN: Speech Production and Articulation Knowledge Group, http://sail.usc.edu/span for example videos.
2 Narayanan S. et al., SPAN: Resources, http://sail.usc.edu/span/resources.html

References

Alexander, R., Sorensen, T., Toutios, A., and Narayanan, S. (2017). VCV synthesis using Task Dynamics to animate a factor-based articulatory model. In *Conference of the International Speech Communication Association (Interspeech)*. Stockholm, Sweden.

Alwan, A., Narayanan, S. S., and Haker, K. (1997). Toward articulatory-acoustic models for liquid approximants based on MRI and EPG data. Part II: The rhotics. *The Journal of the Acoustical Society of America, 101*(2), 1078–1089.

Badin, P., Gabioud, B., Beautemps, D., Lallouache, T., Bailly, G., Maeda, S., Zerling, J. P., and Brock, G. (1995). Cineradiography of VCV sequences: Articulatory-acoustic data for a speech production model. In *International Congress on Acoustics*. Trondheim, Norway.

Barlaz, M., Fu, M., Dubin, J., Shosted, R. K., Liang, Z., and Sutton, B. (2015). Lingual differences in Brazilian Portuguese oral and nasal vowels: An MRI study. In *International Conference of Phonetic Sciences*. Glasgow, UK.

Bresch, E., Kim, Y-C., Nayak, K. S., Byrd, D., and Narayanan, S. S. (2008). Seeing speech: Capturing vocal tract shaping using real-time magnetic resonance imaging. *IEEE Signal Processing Magazine, 25*(3), 123–132.

Bresch, E., and Narayanan, S. S. (2009). Region segmentation in the frequency domain applied to upper airway real-time magnetic resonance images. *IEEE Transactions on Medical Imaging, 28*(3), 323–338.

Bresch, E., and Narayanan, S. S. (2010). Real-time MRI investigation of resonance tuning in soprano singing. *The Journal of the Acoustical Society of America Express Letters, 128*(5), EL335–EL341.

Bresch, E., Nielsen, J., Nayak, K. S., and Narayanan, S. S. (2006). Synchronized and noise-robust audio recordings during realtime magnetic resonance imaging scans. *The Journal of the Acoustical Society of America, 120*(4), 1791–1794.

Browman, C. P., and Goldstein, L. (1992). Articulatory phonology: An overview. *Phonetica, 49*(3–4), 155–180.

Byrd, D., Tobin, S., Bresch, E., and Narayanan, S. (2009). Timing effects of syllable structure and stress on nasals: A real-time MRI examination. *Journal of Phonetics, 37*(1), 97–110.

Carignan, C., Shosted, R. K., Fu, M., Liang, Z. P., and Sutton, B. P. (2015). A real-time MRI investigation of the role of lingual and pharyngeal articulation in the production of the nasal vowel system of French. *Journal of Phonetics, 50*, 34–51.

Celata, C., Meluzzi, C., Moisik, S., and Esling, J. (2017). A lingual-laryngeal ultrasound view of aryepiglottic trills. In *International Conference Ultrafest VII*. Potsdam, Germany.

Clément, P., Hans, S., Hartl, D., Maeda, S., Vaissière, J., and Brasnu, D. (2007). Vocal tract area function for vowels using three-dimensional magnetic resonance imaging. A preliminary study. *Journal of Voice*, 21(5), 522–530.

Delattre, P. (1971). Pharyngeal features in the consonants of Arabic, German, Spanish, French, and American English. *Phonetica*, *23*, 129–155.

Garthe, D. (1991). A fiber-optic microphone. *Sensors and Actuators A: Physical*, *26*(1), 341–345.

Hagedorn, C., Lammert, A., Bassily, M., Zu, Y., Sinha, U., Goldstein, L., and Narayanan, S. S. (2014). Characterizing post-glossectomy speech using real-time MRI. In *International Seminar on Speech Production (ISSP)*. Cologne, Germany.

Hagedorn, C., Proctor, M., Goldstein, L., Wilson, S. M., Miller, B., Gorno-Tempini, M. L., and Narayanan, S. S. (2017). Characterizing articulation in apraxic speech using real-time magnetic resonance imaging. *Journal of Speech, Language, and Hearing Research*, *60*(4), 877–891.

Hardcastle, W., Jones, W., Knight, C., Trudgeon, A., and Calder, G. (1989). New developments in electropalatography: A state-of-the-art report. *Clinical Linguistics and Phonetics*, *3*(1), 1–38.

Harper, S., Goldstein, L., and Narayanan, S. (2016). L2 acquisition and production of the English rhotic pharyngeal gesture. In *Conference of the International Speech Communication Association (Interspeech)*. San Francisco, CA.

Harshman, R., Ladefoged, P., and Goldstein, L. (1977). Factor analysis of tongue shapes. *The Journal of the Acoustical Society of America*, *62*(3), 693–707.

Honda, Y., and Hata, N. (2007). Dynamic imaging of swallowing in a seated position using open-configuration MRI. *Journal of Magnetic Resonance Imaging*, *26*(1), 172–176.

Hsieh, F-Y., and Goldstein, L. (2015). Temporal organization of off-glides in American English. In *International Congress of Phonetic Sciences (ICPhS 2015)*. Glasgow, UK.

Israel, A., Proctor, M. I., Goldstein, L., Iskarous, K., and Narayanan, S. S. (2012). Emphatic segments and emphasis spread in Lebanese Arabic: A real-time magnetic resonance imaging study. In *Conference of the International Speech Communication Association (Interspeech)*. Portland, OR.

Katseff, S., Houde, J., and Johnson, K. (2012). Partial compensation for altered auditory feedback: A tradeoff with somatosensory feedback? *Language and Speech*, *55*(2), 295–308.

Kim, J., Kumar, N., Lee, S., and Narayanan, S. S. (2014). Enhanced airway-tissue boundary segmentation for real-time magnetic resonance imaging data. In *International Seminar on Speech Production (ISSP)*. Cologne, Germany.

Kim, J., Toutios, A., Kim, Y-C., Zhu, Y., Lee, S., and Narayanan, S. S. (2014). USC-EMO-MRI corpus: An emotional speech production database recorded by real-time magnetic resonance imaging. In *International Seminar on Speech Production (ISSP)*. Cologne, Germany.

Kitamura, T., Takemoto, H., Honda, K., Shimada, Y., Fujimoto, I., Syakudo, Y., Masaki, S., Kuroda, K., Oku-uchi, N., and Senda, M. (2005). Difference in vocal tract shape between upright and supine postures: Observations by an open-type MRI scanner. *Acoustical Science and Technology*, *26*(5), 465–468.

Krakow, R. A. (1993). Nonsegmental influences on velum movement patterns: Syllables, sentences, stress, and speaking rate. *Nasals, Nasalization, and the Velum*, *5*, 87–118.

Lametti, D. R., Nasir, S. M., and Ostry, D. J. (2012). Sensory preference in speech production revealed by simultaneous alteration of auditory and somatosensory feedback. *The Journal of Neuroscience*, *32*(27), 9351–9358.

Lammert, A., Goldstein, L., Narayanan, S. S., and Iskarous, K. (2013). Statistical methods for estimation of direct and differential kinematics of the vocal tract. *Speech Communication*, *55*, 147–161.

Lammert, A., Proctor, M. I., and Narayanan, S. S. (2010). Data-driven analysis of realtime vocal tract MRI using correlated image regions. In *Conference of the International Speech Communication Association (Interspeech)*. Makuhari, Japan.

Lammert, A., Proctor, M. I., and Narayanan, S. S. (2013a). Interspeaker variability in hard palate morphology and vowel production. *Journal of Speech, Language, and Hearing Research*, *56*, S1924–S1933.

Lammert, A., Proctor, M. I., and Narayanan, S. S. (2013b). Morphological variation in the adult hard palate and posterior pharyngeal wall. *Journal of Speech, Language, and Hearing Research*, *56*, 521–530.

Lee, Y., Goldstein, L., and Narayanan, S. S. (2015). Systematic variation in the articulation of the Korean liquid across prosodic positions. In *International Congress of Phonetic Sciences (ICPhS 2015)*. Glasgow, UK.

Li, M., Lammert, A., Kim, J., Ghosh, P. K., and Narayanan, S. S. (2013). Automatic Classification of palatal and pharyngeal wall shape categories from speech acoustics and inverted articulatory signals. In *ISCA Workshop on Speech Production in Automatic Speech Recognition (SPASR)*. Lyon, France.

Lingala, S. G., Sutton, B. P., Miquel, M. E., and Nayak, K. S. (2016). Recommendations for real-time speech MRI. *Journal of Magnetic Resonance Imaging*, *43*(1), 28–44.

Lingala, S. G., Toutios, A., Toger, J., Lim, Y., Zhu, Y., Kim, Y-C., Vaz, C., Narayanan, S., and Nayak, K. S. (2016). State-of-the-art MRI protocol for comprehensive assessment of vocal tract structure and function. In *Conference of the International Speech Communication Association (Interspeech)*. San Francisco, CA.

Lingala, S. G., Zhu, Y., Kim, Y-C., Toutios, A., Narayanan, S., and Nayak, K. S. (2017). A fast and flexible MRI system for the study of dynamic vocal tract shaping. *Magnetic Resonance in Medicine*, *77*(1), 112–125.

Maeda, S. (1982). A digital simulation method of the vocal-tract system. *Speech Communication*, *1*(3–4), 199–229.

Maeda, S. (1990). Compensatory articulation during speech: Evidence from the analysis and synthesis of vocal-tract shapes using an articulatory model. In W. J. Hardcastle and A. Marchal (Eds.), *Speech Production and Speech Modelling* (pp. 131–149). Dordrecht: Kluwer Academic.

McGowan, R. S., Jackson, M. T-T., and Berger, M. A. (2012). Analyses of vocal tract cross-distance to area mapping: An investigation of a set of vowel images. *The Journal of the Acoustical Society of America*, *131*(1), 424–434.

Meireles, A., Goldstein, L., Blaylock, R., and Narayanan, S. S. (2015). Gestural coordination of Brazilian Portuguese nasal vowels in CV syllables: A real-time MRI study. In *International Congress of Phonetic Sciences (ICPhS 2015)*. Glasgow, UK.

Moisik, S. R., Lin, H., and Esling, J. H. (2014). A study of laryngeal gestures in Mandarin citation tones using Simultaneous Laryngoscopy and Laryngeal Ultrasound (SLLUS). *Journal of the International Phonetic Association*, *44*(1), 21–58.

Monteserín, M. Ll., Narayanan, S., and Goldstein, L. (2016). Perceptual lateralization of coda rhotic production in Puerto Rican Spanish. In *Conference of the International Speech Communication Association (Interspeech)*. San Francisco, CA.

Munhall, K. G., Vatikiotis-Bateson, E., and Tohkura, Y. (1995). X-ray film database for speech research. *The Journal of the Acoustical Society of America*, *98*(2), 1222–1224.

Murphy, K. J., and Brunberg, J. A. (1997). Adult claustrophobia, anxiety and sedation in MRI. *Magnetic Resonance Imaging*, *15*(1), 51–54.

Narayanan, S. S., Alwan, A. A., and Haker, K. (1995). An articulatory study of fricative consonants using magnetic resonance imaging. *The Journal of the Acoustical Society of America*, *98*(3), 1325–1347.

Narayanan, S. S., Alwan, A. A., and Haker, K. (1997). Toward articulatory-acoustic models for liquid approximants based on MRI and EPG data. Part I. The laterals. *The Journal of the Acoustical Society of America*, *101*(2), 1064–1077.

Narayanan, S. S., Nayak, K. S., Lee, S., Sethy, A., and Byrd, D. (2004). An approach to real-time magnetic resonance imaging for speech production. *The Journal of the Acoustical Society of America*, *115*(4), 1771–1776.

Narayanan, S., Toutios, A., Ramanarayanan, V., Lammert, A., Kim, J., Lee, S., Nayak, K., Kim, Y-C., Zhu, Y., Goldstein, L., Byrd, D., Bresch, E., Ghosh, P., Katsamanis, N., and Proctor, M. (2014). Real-time magnetic resonance imaging and electromagnetic articulography database for speech production research (TC). *The Journal of the Acoustical Society of America*, *136*(3), 1307–1311.

Ng, I. W., Ono, T., Inoue-Arai, M. S., Honda, E., Kurabayashi, T., and Moriyama, K. (2011). Application of MRI movie for observation of articulatory movement during a fricative /s/ and a plosive /t/. *The Angle Orthodontist*, *81*(2), 237–244.

Niebergall, A., Zhang, S., Kunay, E., Keydana, G., Job, M., Uecker, M., and Frahm, J. (2013). Real-time MRI of speaking at a resolution of 33 ms: Undersampled radial FLASH with nonlinear inverse reconstruction. *Magnetic Resonance in Medicine*, *69*(2), 477–485.

Öhman, S. E. G. (1966). Coarticulation in VCV utterances: Spectrographic measurements. *The Journal of the Acoustical Society of America*, *39*(1), 151–168.

Parrell, B., and Narayanan, S. S. (2014). Interaction between general prosodic factors and language-specific articulatory patterns underlies divergent outcomes of coronal stop reduction. In *International Seminar on Speech Production (ISSP)*. Cologne, Germany.

Perry, J. L. (2010). Variations in velopharyngeal structures between upright and Supine positions using upright magnetic resonance imaging. *The Cleft Palate-Craniofacial Journal*, *48*(2), 123–133.

Proctor, M. I., Bone, D., Katsamanis, A., and Narayanan, S. S. (2010). Rapid semi-automatic segmentation of real-time magnetic resonance images for parametric vocal tract analysis. In *Conference of the International Speech Communication Association (Interspeech)*. Makuhari, Japan.

Proctor, M. I., Bresch, E., Byrd, D., Nayak, K. S., and Narayanan, S. S. (2013). Paralinguistic mechanisms of production in human "Beatboxing": A real-time magnetic resonance imaging study. *The Journal of the Acoustical Society of America*, *133*(2), 1043–1054.

Proctor, M. I., Goldstein, L., Lammert, A., Byrd, D., Toutios, A., and Narayanan, S. S. (2013). Velic coordination in French Nasals: A realtime magnetic resonance imaging study. In *Conference of the International Speech Communication Association (Interspeech)*. Lyon, France.

Proctor, M. I., Lammert, A., Katsamanis, A., Goldstein, L., Hagedorn, C., and Narayanan, S. S. (2011). Direct estimation of articulatory kinematics from real-time magnetic resonance image sequences. In *Conference of the International Speech Communication Association (Interspeech)*. Florence, Italy.

Proctor, M. I., and Walker, R. (2012). Articulatory bases of English liquids. In S. Parker (Ed.), *The Sonority Controversy* (Vol. 18, pp. 285–312). Berlin: De Gruyter.

Proctor, M., Zhu, Y., Lammert, A., Toutios, A., Sands, B., Hummel, U., and Narayanan, S. (2016). Click consonant production in Khoekhoe: a real-time MRI study. In S. Shah and M. Brenzinger (Eds.), *Khoisan Languages and Linguistics. Proc. 5th Intl. Symposium, July 13–17, 2014, Riezlern/Kleinwalsertal* (pp. 337–366). Cologne: Rüdiger Köppe.

Ramanarayanan, V., Lammert, A., Goldstein, L., and Narayanan, S. S. (2014). Are articulatory settings mechanically advantageous for speech motor control? *PLoS One*, *9*(8), e104168.

Saltzman, E. L., and Munhall, K. G. (1989). A dynamical approach to gestural patterning in speech production. *Ecological Psychology*, *1*(4), 333–382.

Schönle, P. W., Gräbe, K., Wenig, P., Höhne, J., Schrader, J., and Conrad, B. (1987). Electromagnetic articulography: Use of alternating magnetic fields for tracking movements of multiple points inside and outside the vocal tract. *Brain and Language*, *31*(1), 26–35.

Scott, A. D., Wylezinska, M., Birch, M. J., and Miquel, M. E. (2014). Speech MRI: Morphology and function. *Physica Medica*, *30*(6), 604–618.

Smith, C., Proctor, M. I., Iskarous, K., Goldstein, L., and Narayanan, S. S. (2013). Stable articulatory tasks and their variable formation: Tamil retroflex consonants. In *Conference of the International Speech Communication Association (Interspeech)*. Lyon, France.

Somandepalli, K., Toutios, A., and Narayanan, S. (2017). Semantic edge detection for tracking vocal tract air-tissue boundaries in real-time magnetic resonance images. In *Conference of the International Speech Communication Association (Interspeech)*. Stockholm, Sweden.

Soquet, A., Lecuit, V., Metens, T., and Demolin, D. (2002). Mid-sagittal cut to area function transformations: Direct measurements of mid-sagittal distance and area with MRI. *Speech Communication*, *36*(3), 169–180.

Sorensen, T., Skordilis, Z., Toutios, A., Kim, Y-C., Zhu, Y., Kim, J., Lammert, A., Ramanarayanan, V., Goldstein, L., Byrd, D., Nayak, K., Narayanan, S. (2017). Database of volumetric and real-time vocal tract MRI for speech science. In *Conference of the International Speech Communication Association (Interspeech)*. Stockholm, Sweden.

Sorensen, T., Toutios, A., Goldstein, L., and Narayanan, S. (2016). Characterizing vocal tract dynamics across speakers using real-time MRI. In *Conference of the International Speech Communication Association (Interspeech)*. San Francisco, CA.

Stone, M. (2006). Imaging and measurement of the vocal tract. In K. Brown (Ed.), *Encyclopedia of Language and Linguistics* (pp. 526–539). Oxford: Elsevier.

Stone, M., Davis, E. P., Douglas, A. S., NessAiver, M., Gullapalli, R., Levine, W. S., and Lundberg, A. (2001). Modeling the motion of the internal tongue from tagged cine-MRI images. *The Journal of the Acoustical Society of America, 109*(6), 2974–2982.

Stone, M., Stock, G., Bunin, K., Kumar, K., Epstein, M., Kambhamettu, C., Li, M., Parthasarathy, V., and Prince, J. (2007). Comparison of speech production in upright and supine position. *The Journal of the Acoustical Society of America, 122*(1), 532–541.

Story, B. H., Titze, I. R., and Hoffman, E. A. (1996). Vocal tract area functions from magnetic resonance imaging. *The Journal of the Acoustical Society of America, 100*(1), 537–554.

Sutton, B. P., Conway, C., Bae, Y., Brinegar, C., Liang, Z-P., and Kuehn, D. P. (2009). Dynamic imaging of speech and swallowing with MRI. In *International Conference of the IEEE Engineering in Medicine and Biology Society*. Minneapolis, MN.

Takemoto, H., Honda, K., Masaki, S., Shimada, Y., and Fujimoto, I. (2006). Measurement of temporal changes in vocal tract area function from 3D cine-MRI data. *The Journal of the Acoustical Society of America, 119*(2), 1037–1049.

Takemoto, H., Kitamura, T., Nishimoto, H., and Honda, K. (2004). A method of tooth superimposition on MRI data for accurate measurement of vocal tract shape and dimensions. *Acoustical Science and Technology, 25*(6), 468–474.

Tiede, M. K., Masaki, S., and Vatikiotis-Bateson, E. (2000). Contrasts in speech articulation observed in sitting and supine conditions. In *International Seminar on Speech Production (ISSP)*, Kloster Seeon, Bavaria (pp. 25–28).

Toutios, A., Lingala, S. G., Vaz, C., Kim, J., Esling, J., Keating, P., Gordon, M., Byrd, D., Goldstein, L., Nayak, K., and Narayanan, S. (2016). Illustrating the production of the International Phonetic Alphabet sounds using fast real-time magnetic resonance imaging. In *Conference of the International Speech Communication Association (Interspeech)*. San Francisco, CA.

Toutios, A., and Narayanan, S. S. (2015). Factor analysis of vocal-tract outlines derived from real-time magnetic resonance imaging data. In *International Congress of Phonetic Sciences (ICPhS 2015)*. Glasgow, UK.

Toutios, A., and Narayanan, S. S. (2016). Advances in real-time magnetic resonance imaging of the vocal tract for speech science and technology research. *APSIPA Transactions on Signal and Information Processing, 5*, e6.

Traser, L., Burdumy, M., Richter, B., Vicari, M., and Echternach, M. (2014). Weight-bearing MR imaging as an option in the study of gravitational effects on the vocal tract of untrained subjects in singing phonation. *PLoS One, 9*(11), e112405.

Vaz, C., Ramanarayanan, V., and Narayanan, S. S. (2013). A two-step technique for MRI audio enhancement using dictionary learning and wavelet packet analysis. In *Conference of the International Speech Communication Association (Interspeech)*. Lyon, France.

Vaz, C., Toutios, A., and Narayanan, S. (2016). Convex hull convolutive non-negative matrix factorization for uncovering temporal patterns in multivariate time-series data. In *Interspeech*. San Francisco, CA.

Whalen, D. H., Iskarous, K., Tiede, M. K., Ostry, D. J., Lehnert-LeHouillier, H., Vatikiotis-Bateson, E., and Hailey, D. S. (2005). The Haskins Optically Corrected Ultrasound System (HOCUS). *Journal of Speech, Language, and Hearing Research, 48*(3), 543–553.

Wood, S. A. J. (1982). *X-ray and Model Studies of Vowel Articulation*. Working Papers 23: 1–49. Department of Linguistics. Lund University.

Zhang, J., Honda, K., and Wei, J. (2018). Tooth visualization in vowel production MR images for three-dimensional vocal tract modeling. *Speech Communication*, 96, 37–48.

3

Under-researched languages

Phonetic results from language archives

D.H. Whalen and Joyce McDonough

Introduction

The upsurge in documentation of languages, especially endangered ones, that has occurred in the past decades has produced a large amount of potential data for linguistic research, including phonetic research. The increasingly common inclusion of spoken material in archived audio and video recordings potentially provides the means to document the sound and gesture patterns and phonetic properties of spoken and signed language, aspects of language not recoverable from written text. The utility of these recordings depends on several factors. First of all, the data need to be archived and accessible to a broad group of researchers, beyond those who originally collected the material. Second, methodologies and research questions need to be continually developed to use data that have not been collected specifically for phonetic research. Third, the needs of the various stakeholders – academics, community members, archivists and others – must be kept in balance. In this chapter, we will address the use of existing language archives of under-resourced or small language communities (henceforth "small languages") and the implications of this data for phonetic research.

At present, hundreds of languages are falling silent (Hale et al., 1992); indeed, entire language families are at risk (Whalen and Simons, 2012). Some languages can be, and have been, revived from documentary descriptions (Littledoe, 1998; Leonard, 2007; Hinton, 2001; Amery, 1995), but from a phonetician's point of view, phonetic detail is likely lost in the process. With an acoustic archive, however, patterns of sounds that link contemporary speakers to past generations can be recovered in revitalization efforts, if methodological phonetic analyses are performed.

In typical experimental phonetics, laboratory sessions are organized to elicit specific types of data related to research topics in phonetic description and theory. Experimental phonetics emerged at the end of the 19th century (Rousselot, 1897–1908), but limitations of equipment kept the amount of data small. Nonetheless, researchers have taken experimental methods into the field to collect phonetic data (Whalen and McDonough, 2015). In recent decades, the Phonetics Laboratory at the University of California, Los Angeles (UCLA), under Ladefoged and Maddieson produced an important body of knowledge on the phonetics of speech sounds in the languages throughout the world, working with academic linguists and community members, and using carefully constructed word lists and other materials in their fieldwork, to exemplify particular sound contrasts under investigation (archived at the UCLA Phonetics Lab Archive). The researchers who have contributed to this archive also developed field methods for collecting speech production data and performing speech perception experiments. Knowledge about sound systems in human language, the structure of the vowel space and consonant contrast patterns in phonemic inventories, came out of this work (Maddieson, 1984; Ladefoged and Maddieson, 1996b; Becker-Kristal, 2010; Schwartz et al., 1997; Lindblom, 1990). However, despite this work, and perhaps for historical reasons, phonetic documentation has not been fully incorporated into language documentation practices. Often, phoneticians are not included as part of more broadly aimed language documentation projects. To some extent, this is due to the small size of most documentation teams. Nonetheless, phoneticians are becoming more involved as linguists become aware of the importance and function of fine-grained phonetic detail in linguistic structures and phoneticians become more adept at analyzing the spontaneous speech that constitutes a large proportion of current corpora.

All types of speech corpora require careful transcription, translation, and annotation. The trend in recent language documentation efforts has emphasized the collection of "natural language," that is, narrative and other types of non-elicited "natural" speech. While this task is a challenge for spoken word corpora from any language, it is especially problematic for small and under-resourced languages, which are generally the focus of language documentation efforts. These projects in particular may not have sufficient resources to implement the translations and annotations necessary to produce useful corpora. The task of annotation and transcription is well known as a time-intensive task, one that requires training. Collection of spoken language corpora continues in spite of these challenges. There are opportunities for using these resources to undertake phonetic analyses that will both increase our knowledge of possible sound patterns occurring in linguistic systems, and provide an important asset to documentation efforts in language communities.

Small language communities are less studied and present difficulties that are not encountered in research on larger and better documented language groups. First, small languages can be typologically distinct from each other and from better-studied groups, presenting challenges to underlying assumptions about the proposed linguistic structures drawn exclusively from more commonly studied groups. Second because these projects often involve comparatively well-funded researchers working in communities with fewer monetary resources, this work involves tackling persistent and recalcitrant political, social and ethical issues. Third, significant issues arise in the analysis of data from communities with small numbers of speakers. While working with a small number of speakers itself in not uncommon in phonetic research, it is generally done within the context of language associated with a broad knowledge base. However, work on small languages lacks this base, underlining the value and importance of both the work and the development of field methodologies, archives and annotation practices that allow access to that data. Because speakers of small languages represent a more significant portion of the community as a whole, their requirements for the design and use of the material need greater attention than those from large languages. Data that suffer from any of the many problems that elicitation entails – poor recording conditions, inadequate design, unexpected interpretations by the speakers (Niebuhr and Michaud, 2015) – can be remedied at a later date for large languages. This may not be possible for small ones.

Linguistic theories and generalizations are based on data from a relatively small number of the world's languages, often ones spoken by large populations. In general, the languages and dialects that are rapidly disappearing are those that we know little about, and they frequently belong to small or disenfranchised communities of speakers. They may also be undergoing rapid generational change. Furthermore, a large portion of available language data is in written form, which is understandably a poor basis for information about the sound patterns of a speech community. Without spoken data, our knowledge of the phonetic structures found in human languages – the phonetic patterns and the relationship between phonetic structure and other linguistic phenomena – is limited by our dependence on an incomplete and typologically narrow set of data. Finally, spoken language recordings are difficult to collect and to archive, and accessibility to this data is a challenging issue. Standards of accessibility, for instance, can vary greatly depending on several intransigent factors from academic and community restrictions to the availability of professional archiving facilities.

In this chapter, we will provide an overview of the issues for phonetic science that arise in the collection, annotation, availability, and analysis of archival data along with a survey of published papers reflecting such analysis. Our chapter focuses on what we call a secondary use of archival data, in which the analysis postdates the archiving. This excludes cases where the data collected is by a phonetician and subsequently archived (as is the case, for instance, with most of the studies of the UCLA archive). This decision focuses attention on the need to develop practices that use language archives for phonetic analyses, as well as other linguistic research. While such archiving is essential for the continued expansion of our phonetic knowledge, we will focus on the use of archives on small languages by phoneticians, the issues encountered, and the work that has been done using these databases.

Our recommendations and assessment of the survey will illustrate our belief that analysis of existing archives is urgently needed. (Throughout this chapter, we use the term "archives" to refer by extension to the contents of archives, since archives themselves may use various designations for their contents, such as "collection," "records," "material," and "documents.") This use of the term also allows distinguishing archived materials from unarchived ones. There are two reasons supporting the immediate use of existing archives versus leaving the task to future users. First, although it is true that archives are intended to last indefinitely (and many print archives have lasted decades if not centuries), digital archives are inherently fragile, requiring more maintenance than print ones and a larger investment of time and money on the part of digital than print archives. (This issue is by no means limited to language documentation; see, e.g., Cottingham, 2008). In times of budget constraints, such expenditures are subject to examination in relation to the use of the archival material. The Digital Preservation Coalition, for example, suggests that "for items selected for permanent preservation it is anticipated that review and de-accessioning will occur in rare and strictly controlled circumstances" (Digital Preservation Coalition, 2015, Retention-and-review). Language archives may or may not fall into this category, depending on the institution and initial agreements. The DPC goes on to say: "For other collection levels such as mirrored or licensed resources review criteria may include: A sustained fall of usage to below acceptable levels." It is easy to imagine language archives having low usage values. Further, if archives begin to address the current limited accessibility of some audio archives, the added costs could come into play (Clement, 2014). Digital archives are so new a phenomenon that the issues about their fragile stability across time are only beginning to be understood and addressed. Second, many aspects of the recording situation are known to the depositor(s) that do not enter into the metadata for the archive. Being able to ask questions of the depositors while they are still active is often crucial to correct interpretation of the phonetic data.

Phonetic work on archives can sometimes be done with written text, to the extent that some phonetic/phonological aspects (subphonemic alternations, stress patterns) may be reconstructed from certain types of orthography and texts (such as poetry) but most analyses of phonetic patterns depend on acoustic recordings and associated transcriptions and annotations. Even imperfect transcriptions should be archived; some transcription is better than none. As examples, determination of stress versus pitch accent and meter in Latin has been argued to be derivable from poetry (e.g., Pulgram, 1954) as has the "darkness" of Latin /l/ (Sen, 2015). When acoustic analysis is possible, such secondary evidence does not make a significant contribution to theoretical debates.

Many current linguistic documentation practices tend to focus on the collection of spoken narratives and conversations, rather than specific elicitation techniques, such as word list recitation to elicit data on phoneme contrasts, or the methodologies of higher-level prosodic elicitations, for instance. As Pike (1947) pointed out, all elicitation techniques bring in their own set of biases, arguably including carefully controlled experiments. One advantage in the collection of narrative is that permits more natural speech and discourse related events. Moreover narratives also allow for the likelihood of providing documentation of higher-level prosodic phenomena such as utterance level prominence and intonation patterns (Fletcher and Evans, 2002; Bowern et al., 2012), as well as the effects of position-in-utterance on the realization of phonemic contrasts. With this in mind, information on the phonetics of phoneme inventories, including subphonemic details and potential information for perception of a contrast, can be extracted from narratives (DiCanio et al., 2015), and including, by extension, archived materials. By contrast, work in many small under-resourced communities that may lack a baseline description of their sound patterns, narrowly focused research questions or, for instance, perception experiments to test hypotheses that are performed in a lab setting, will need to have methodologies adapted to the knowledge available on a language (Remijsen and Ayoker, 2014, Remijsen, 2013). But this lab-in-the-field type work has much to contribute to general feature theories (Whalen and McDonough, 2015, Clements and Ridouane, 2011). With careful attention to the limitations of the data, a description of the main characteristics of phonetic realization of phonemic structure and prosodic patterns is possible from current archives and narratives, with the discussion and development of methods to do this work (see also Winter, 2015).

Phonetic description is ideally based on the productions of fluent speakers. Ideally, documentation would include both men and women, and at least six of each (Ladefoged and Maddieson, 1996a). (Of course, this does not cover all aspects of language, and sacred speech, child language, etc. would all require different populations.) Recording a variety of speakers allows the possibility of studying the range of individual variation and provides more support for the commonalities across speaker. For small languages, having data from a large number of speakers is often not a feasible goal. In communities where only a few speakers remain, or in which the remaining speakers no longer use the language, or are very elderly, or associate it with reduced status, the question of how many speakers to record is different and more subject to local conditions. The languages nonetheless remain examples of human language that deserve careful documentation.

Some statistical methods used on large corpora are not suitable for this latter type of data, given that the number of tokens will not provide sufficient power. Instead, good descriptive statistics and a transparent presentation of methods and results can provide a solid basis for all types of further language work well into the future (McDonough, 2003, Hargus, 2007).

The problem then is shifted to one of comparing the results and analyses done on large versus small language corpora and datasets, but this is hardly an issue for linguistic analysis alone. Comparisons with standard experimental phonetic work are also valuable. Archiving experimental results can serve to expand the knowledge base on a language (Whalen and McDonough, 2015) and increase our understanding of phonetic phenomena.

Acoustic data, though powerful, are limited to what can be inferred about the speech production process. Articulatory data provide another source of evidence and thus can also play a role in language documentation and revitalization efforts, as well as adding to our knowledge of speech and sound patterns (e.g., Miller, 2016). Obtaining data from speech production is more challenging than collecting acoustic recordings, and it is less frequently performed, especially in the field. This scarcity of production evidence persists despite the fact that it was done very early on in the history of experimental phonetics. Pliny Earl Goddard (1907, 1905) was a pioneer in taking articulatory measurement devices into the field. He showed, for example, that Hupa uses a more anterior articulation for /d/ than English, exemplified by static palatography from a bilingual speaker (1905:614). Only sporadic studies were performed for the next several decades, with more consistent efforts being spearheaded by Peter Ladefoged and Ian Maddieson, mostly using static palatography and airflow. Currently, those techniques continue to be used (Anderson, 2008; Flemming et al., 2008), but they have been augmented with electroglottography (EGG) (McDonough and Tucker, 2012; DiCanio, 2012; DiCanio, 2009; Kuang, 2013), electromagnetic articulometry (Wieling et al., 2016), and ultrasound (Gick et al., 2005; Miller, 2007; Whalen et al., 2011). The Pangloss Collection hosts EGG together with audio (see http://lacito.vjf.cnrs.fr/pangloss/corpus/list_rsc_en.php?lg=Na&aff=Na) The 40 documents with EGG recordings in that language are marked with a special icon with "EGG" written on it: EGG. The Archive of the Indigenous Languages of Latin America has recently received some EGG data from DiCanio's work on Itunyoso Trique (ISO 639–633 trq) (DiCanio, 2012) (see, e.g., https://ailla.utexas.org/islandora/object/ailla%3A243997). The increased ease of use of these techniques makes it likely that ever-increasing amounts of articulatory data will become available. Current phonetic archives, however, are still primarily acoustic in nature, and so the remainder of this chapter will focus on studies that make use of this modality.

While phoneticians are increasingly using large language corpora as a source of data for research questions to examine contemporary issues (for instance the finding of the uniform variability across speakers in realization of a phonetic property shared by multiple speech contrasts) (Chodroff and Wilson, 2017), the number of studies that make use of archival material from small languages is still small. As we have noted, the issues that arise in using small data are not unique to phonetics or linguistic research, nor is it intractable. The greater risk is not using the archives at all (Schmidt et al., 2006). We have underlined the importance of this type archived data in research; the issues that researchers encounter in using these databases will be discussed in the next section.

Archives

Language archives have seen a surge in submissions in recent years as the practice of language documentation has evolved to include archiving collected materials, including digital materials, and their associated metadata. The U.S. National Science Foundation now requires an archiving plan in its grant proposal submissions, for example. Large language archives such as the Linguistic Data Consortium provide corpora and allow access to various types (primarily through a payment schedule), but in small language archives such as the Endangered Language Archive, the Alaska Native Language Archive, or the Archive of the Indigenous Languages of Latin America, the relationship between the data, the researchers, and the language communities is more personal with concomitant and mutual obligations. Different types of issues arise in both depositing these materials as well as in general access to these archives, which must be responsive to cultural restrictions and constraints. But archiving also implicates access privileges. Across digital archives, access to material is quite variable, but restrictions on access are an important aspect of small language corpora. Access has been handled by access protocols, such as the tiered protocol access instituted by AILLA at the University of Texas at Austin, and this continues to be an important aspect of archives.

Not everything defined as a corpus resides in a digital archive, and we discuss only archival results here. An important criterion for being classified as an archive is being in a "trusted digital repository" (Research Libraries Group, 2002) that crucially aims to provide long-term curation for digital materials. Individual corpora on computers in laboratories, then, are not archives by definition. Curation of digital material in general is one of the biggest issues research libraries are now facing, and a dialogue between professional librarians and linguists is likely to be mutually beneficial in the continuing development of and access to these archives. In language documentation and description practices, such efforts as the OLAC standards (Bird and Simons, 2001), the GOLD ontology (Farrar and Lewis, 2007; Farrar et al., 2002), and META-SHARE OWL (McCrae et al., 2015) also work to standardize formats and metadata, but with variable results. Given the highly individual nature of the experience of fieldwork, it is unlikely that all but the broadest and most generous standards will be successfully adopted, such as the definition of metadata and enabling (both with funding and training) fieldworkers to archive field materials in trusted repositories. Flexible standards, then, can still result in greater transparency than a complete lack of standards.

In this spirit, we list some of the current prominent archives. Most of these archives are members of the Digital Endangered Languages and Musics Archives Network (DELAMAN; www.delaman.org/members), an international network of archives of data on linguistic and cultural diversity, in particular on small languages and cultures under pressure:

- Alaskan Native Language Archive (ANLA; www.uaf.edu/anla), at the University of Alaska, Fairbanks, focusing on Alaska Native languages
- Archive of Indigenous Languages of Latin America (AILLA; www.ailla.utexas.org), at the University of Texas at Austin, covering Latin America
- American Philosophical Society (APS) Digital Library (https://diglib.amphilsoc.org/audio/access), primarily focused on Native American languages of North America
- Archives of Traditional Music (ATM; www.indiana.edu/~libarchm), University of Indiana, Bloomington, containing various language recordings
- California Language Archive (CLA; http://cla.berkeley.edu), at the University of California, Berkeley, with material primarily from California languages but with other collections as well
- Documentation of Endangered Languages at the Max Plank in Nijmegen (DoBeS; http://dobes.mpi.nl/), funded by Volkswagen Foundation; now part of The Language Archive
- Endangered Languages Archive (ELAR; https://elar.soas.ac.uk/), part of the library at the School of Oriental and African Studies (SOAS), University of London, primarily

archiving results of research funded by the Endangered Languages Documentation Programme (ELDP; www.eldp.net)

- Linguistic Data Consortium (LDC; www.ldc.upenn.edu), a repository and distribution point for universities, companies and government research laboratories which creates, collects and distributes speech and text databases, lexicons, and other language resources
- Pangloss (formerly Lacito Archive) (http://lacito.vjf.cnrs.fr/pangloss/), itself part of the broader repository Cocoon (https://cocoon.huma-num.fr/exist/crdo/) containing varying amounts of data for more than 130 languages
- Pacific and Regional Archives for Digital Sources in Endangered Languages (Paradisec; www.paradisec.org.au/), a consortium of the University of Sydney, University of Melbourne, and Australian National University
- The Language Archive (TLA; https://corpus1.mpi.nl), containing material from Max Planck Institute for Psycholinguistics in Nijmegen and other sources (including DoBeS)
- UCLA Phonetics Lab Archive (http://archive.phonetics.ucla.edu/), an archive of the recordings of languages from around the world primarily collected by the Ladefoged-Maddieson team and their students, maintained by the Department of Linguistics

It should be noted that the *Illustration of the IPA* series in the *Journal of the IPA* typically has recordings associated with it. Issues from 2001 to three years before the present are publicly available (www.cambridge.org/core/journals/journal-of-the-international-phonetic-association/illustrations-of-the-ipa-free-content). (Note that to access the audio files, you have to click on the title of the article and then click on the "Supplementary Material" tab near the top of the page.) Most if not all of the examples in the text have an accompanying sound file, and all Illustrations have a connected text. This is often the story "The North Wind and the Sun," but some use an alternate text, such as the frog story. These are valuable examples, but are too limited for full phonetic analysis.

Nearly all of these archives contain spoken language corpora, though the data formats, metadata and access limits vary. Since digital data, as opposed to print, is subject to obsolescence and thus quite fragile data migration and updating must be implemented as an ongoing enterprise (e.g., Beagrie, 2008). But beyond these issues common to all digital databases, there are specific issues that arise in language archives.

Annotation

One of the most challenging issues that arises in spoken language corpora is the technical one of annotating speech. There are currently no satisfactorily accurate automated transcription systems that work to the level required by phoneticians and other linguists. The ideal of automating a usable transcription has been promoted since the beginning of the computer age, but it is not yet a reality. Strides have been made for major languages, including usable first-pass text-to-speech alignment algorithms. Advances are likely to help with work on small languages, as exemplified by Adams et al. (2017). However, for the present, an accurate job of transcription and annotation requires trained human annotators, a time-consuming enterprise, and an expensive commodity.

An acoustic signal that has a corresponding transcription and annotation, therefore, is necessary for phonetic analysis, but the level at which the two are aligned determines the types of analyses that can be performed. If a corpus is large enough to allow for substantial phonetic analysis, it will be too large to analyze by hand. The acoustic signal needs to be aligned to phonetic elements, and thus the detail of the phonetic annotation needs to match the scale of the proposed analysis. Locating the segments is a minimum. Identification of phonetic components (such as dividing stops into a closure portion and aspiration after release) is useful. Allowing overlapping annotations, such as those needed for tones, can also be useful. Automatic procedures can help here, as already demonstrated (Kempton and Moore, 2014; DiCanio et al., 2013), and the continuing progress in the field indicates that the tools will continue to improve.

Archive access and interpretation of transcription

Several issues arise in using archives based on data from small language communities for phonetic research. Often the expertise needed and difficulty of addressing these issues in the development of database archives may be vastly underestimated and can thus reduce their usefulness as crucial resources. The two main issues at this writing are, first, protocol and access to the data; and second, the practices used in the translation, transcription, and annotation of the speech. First, the databases almost by necessity vary widely, primarily due to the differences in the types of documentation undertaken and data collection practices that accompany the documentation. Second, in the archives, the type of data collected, the practices used in transcription and annotation, the research goals of the project and funder requirements on archiving and access of the data all determine the shape of the resulting database.

The terms "transcription" and "translation" refer to the act of providing a representation of digital speech recordings in some orthographic system (including the International Phonetic Alphabet, or IPA), and the translation of the speech into a commonly shared language such as English, Russian or French. The transcription itself may or may not be in the IPA, and it is subject to the orthographic conventions of IPA or the language community, if they exist. In general, this aspect of the process must be done in close collaboration with a native fluent speaker of the language who can provide the translation and help to correct the produced transcriptions. The speech can sometimes differ quite radically from a native speaker's more proper understanding and transcription of the spoken word, especially in "natural language" contexts such as conversations, lectures, or storytelling, which can contain pauses, idiolectal pronunciations, and expressions that are glossed over by the transcriber. Developing viable working relationships with language consultants and collaborators from small language communities is an important skill for fieldworkers; the role of these community consultants and advocates in developing these resources cannot be overestimated (Dwyer, 2006). This collaborative aspect of small language archive development is critical to small language archives, and is not as significant an issue in larger language archives because of the greater resources available, though it may well arise in the transcription of nonstandard dialects.

The term "annotation" refers to the addition of further analysis levels. Of particular use for phonetics is the alignment of this orthographic transcription to the physical speech signal. In contemporary work, the annotation to be aligned generally uses the IPA for a reasonably accurate phonemic representation. Several types of software exist that serve as platforms for doing these annotations by hand; currently the best developed and most used are ELAN and Praat, the latter especially developed for phonetic research. In both these programs, the annotations are deliverable as text files with time codes easily imported into other programs. The annotation of the speech signal generally proceeds in two steps depending on the type of annotation being done; as previously mentioned, first is the transcription of the speech and its translation, this is followed by the alignment of the orthographic transcription to the speech signal. This alignment allows the annotation of phrases and words, and – especially integral to phonetic research – ultimately the annotation of segmental and suprasegmental elements. There are, of course, other important types of annotation of speech, such as the annotation of syntactic and semantic units, morphological and part-of-speech parsing, phrasal groups and sentence types. These latter types require less fine-grained attention to alignment than do phonetic investigations, but all require alignment of text to the speech signal, whether gross or fine.

The practice of aligning a symbol with its specific realization as a consonant or vowel sound in the acoustic signal involves some arbitrary decisions, as boundaries are made to be non-overlapping even though the segments themselves influence overlapping portions (e.g., Liberman et al., 1967). For example, aligning the text symbol associated with the phoneme /a/ to the beginning and end of the vocalic segment of the phone [a] is standard practice, but it ignores the shared influence of adjacent consonants during the formant transitions. Nonetheless, such an alignment allows a good estimate of the major influence on the signal and can further carry the alignment of a pitch peak and a tone. Some boundaries are more difficult than others, even acknowledging the partially arbitrary nature of the decision. In a series of sonorants, for instance, the boundaries between segments are not clear and an annotator's skills are required in the recognition, and reporting, of the patterns in the speech that aid useful segmentation; delimiting fundamental frequency (f_0) is an even more elusive task, f_0 being subject to multiple influences across large time spans.

Annotation, therefore, is an acquired skill informed by training and practice to recognize and understand the patterns in the acoustic speech signal. The annotation of speech careful enough for linguistic research requires training in phonetics because these patterns differ from language to language and among dialects and speakers; they are critical to natural language structures and are at the crux of the phonetics/phonology interface. The transcriptional elements chosen reify the phoneme/allophone patterns (Errington, 2007: 23), and they thus evidence little recognition of the ubiquitous speech variability that confounds speech recognition.

Conversely, annotation and segmentation by hand is famously labor-intensive and time-consuming. Automatic transcription and alignment algorithms exist and can reduce some of the work but even the best automatic aligners are not accurate enough for some kinds of phonetic research, and require annotation by trained human annotators (but cf. Adda et al., 2016;). Finally, even archives that are developed for other types of analyses not directly related to phonetic research (such as syntactic or morphological analysis) will need careful phonetic transcriptions. Speech is the primary vehicle of communication, and the intersection of prosody and syntax is an area much in need of research.

Another issue that arises in using these archives for phonetic research is the archive's approach to protocol and access. This is partly due to the wide range of services these databases provide, which relate to their original purposes, funder requirements, and their growth patterns. While there is an increasing trend toward allowing access, practice still varies widely. Restriction of access seems to derive from the practice of print archives, where a single copy of a text would exist at a specific location. Although electronic formats can be duplicated without loss, many archives restrict them as much as print archives. Those that do allow copying have imposed graded access for those objects that have restrictions (cf AILLA's statement: www.ailla.utexas.org/site/howto_use.html#access), but there are still restrictions on some collections without such restraints, primarily an agreement not to use the data for commercial purposes. A major funder, the U.S. National Science Foundation (NSF) specifically requires data management plans for grantees "to share with other researchers, at no more than incremental cost and within a reasonable time, the primary data created or gathered in the course of work under NSF grants" (National Science Foundation 2010: 1). Although this is quite explicit, it contradicts another aspect of NSF policy: In North America especially, this policy can be in direct conflict with tribal requests to control access to their language data, which the NSF recognizes as intellectual property. Some datasets, such those in LDC, are created as intellectual property, and some of those are only available for an access fee, while others require payment of a media fee. Currently, these conflicting imperatives are settled on a case-by-case basis, resulting in a continuing inconsistency in access even in new acquisitions and new archives.

ELDP at the SOAS University of London has a firmer policy of archiving and access, requiring annual archiving and open access for registered users of ELAR to the majority of data collected during the duration of the grant, and this basic principle must be agreed upon at the time of the funding. Any access restrictions must be justified in the metadata, and ELDP and ELAR support flexible solutions in case of later encountered access issues. Compliance failures with regard to depositing – namely not depositing the documentary materials collected with ELDP funding at all – might result in barring future funding to both the grantee and the grantee's host institution.

Funding for language documentation by the German Volkswagen Foundation DoBeS project, another important source of past funding for work on small language communities, required that the data collected during funding follow a set of standardized metadata categories and be digitally archived according to open standards. The DoBeS Archive, presently part of TLA at Max Planck Institute for Psycholinguistics in Nijmegen, continues to implement upgrades to metadata and data formats. Additionally, DoBeS has provided funding for research projects based on use of the data in the archive, though very little of it has been used in phonetic research.

Archives not directly tied to funding usually have explicit access policies as well. Housed at the University of Texas at Austin and supported by the University of Texas Libraries, AILLA focuses specifically on indigenous languages south of the Rio Grande and contains copies of digitalized indigenous language recordings, field notes, photographs, and other research materials. AILLA was developed to make language resources openly accessible with a focus on the speakers of the languages represented in the archive. AILLA has a four-level access protocol system that is designed to protect intellectual property and indigenous community rights.

The best known archive for phonetic research remains the UCLA Phonetics Lab Archive, the archive developed by Ladefoged and Maddieson. It contains much of their material, collected on field trips funded by the NSF, as well as many recordings made by UCLA students and other researchers. It is presently maintained by the UCLA Linguistics Department. Its stated aim is to provide source materials for phonetic and phonological research, to illustrate phonetic structures found among human languages. This material may include phonetic transcriptions, which is significant because they were done by phoneticians. The archive's contents are all open access, under a Creative Commons license, for non-commercial use. Much of the phonetic work in existence done on endangered languages and small language communities is based on data found in this database. Many of these papers appeared in the *UCLA Working Papers in Phonetics*, and summaries appear in Ladefoged and Maddieson's (1996b) *Sounds of the World's Languages*. For the present survey, we are summarizing only papers that were done subsequently to the depositing in the archive, while most of the articles just mentioned were done by those who collected, analyzed and then archived the data.

Most of the archives listed here were designed for general use, not for phonetics specifically, but they have proven to be quite useful in that regard. Acoustic recordings are the most common means of accessing the phonetics of languages, providing evidence for many features. Recordings of various languages began soon after Edison's cylinder recording became available. A.L. Kroeber and J.P. Harrington, for example, recorded dozens of Native American languages of California. Some of the language material was in songs, which are challenging for phonetic analysis, but stories and conversations, often spanning several cylinders, were also recorded. Recent advances in laser technology have allowed the recovery of previously unusable cylinders and many archives include recordings of both elicited and narrative speech. The following section will outline many of the studies that have been performed to date.

Many of the studies to be summarized here make use of both archival and newly obtained material. This is due both to the gaps that are bound to occur in the sampling of speech sounds in spontaneous speech and to the typical use of highly controlled contexts for phonetic analysis. Indeed, Ladefoged (2003) downplays the usefulness of recorded texts for phonetic documentation:

> From a phonetician's point of view there is no point in making lengthy recordings of folk tales, or songs that people want to sing. Such recordings can seldom be used for an analysis of the major phonetic characteristics of a language, except in a qualitative way. You need sounds that have all been produced in the same way so that their features can be compared.
>
> *(p. 9)*

However, recordings of texts are exactly what we have for many endangered languages. In an explicit comparison of elicited and narrative vowel spaces, DiCanio et al. (2015) (summarized more fully next) found that the formants of elicited speech were somewhat more extreme than those in texts, but that both showed good separation between the categories. But combining the two techniques is common.

Challenges in using acoustic archives

Progress has been made in the textual analysis of large corpora (e.g., Kübler and Zinsmeister, 2015), but progress in phonetics remains slow. Despite the existence of a very useful handbook on procedures for doing large-scale acoustic analysis (Harrington and Cassidy, 1999), implementation of the techniques relies on the usefulness of the transcriptional data. If a corpus is annotated in practical orthography (as mentioned before) at the word or sentence level, a great deal of parsing remains to be done before acoustic analysis can take place. A range of challenges thus face a researcher approaching such a corpus.

Orthographies vary widely in their phonological transparency – but, fortunately, most recently devised orthographies are relatively shallow, allowing for fairly consistent grapheme-to-phoneme translation. One large challenge for even the most consistent orthography is allophonic variation. Underlying forms are often transcribed even though highly elided forms are the ones present in the speech signal. In narrative speech in Mixtec, for instance, voiceless obstruents (/t, tʃ, k/) are often produced as voiced and lenited variants (DiCanio et al., 2017). The orthographic system utilizes only the former, underlying forms.

Transcription errors are bound to occur in any large corpus, and they can also lead to sizable misalignments. (Examining such misalignments can be of use as a check on the transcription itself, however.) How to treat such errors is a matter of researcher choice, and certainly the number of errors is an important factor: The smaller the percentage, the less likely errors will influence the results. Some issues that introduce misalignments are not technically errors in the transcription. Hesitation sounds are often left out of transcriptions, but generally are interpreted as speech by forced aligners. In elicitation tasks, the matrix language is often left untranscribed, which leads to unusable alignments if no corrections are made.

Results from acoustic archives

This section presents summaries of the articles that we were able to find that analyze archives phonetically. We did not include analyses of material collected by the authors and then archived at a later date. Although this is the ideal approach to maintaining and sharing data, it is not our focus here. The list also excludes work on majority languages, of which there is a substantial amount. There are several works that make some use of the UCLA archive (e.g., Bradfield, 2014; Hsieh, 2007; Simas Frazão, 2013) or Pangloss (Schiering et al., 2010), but not to a large enough extent to count as phonetic studies. No doubt we have missed others, and we hope that many more will be added.

UCLA: Blankenship (2002)

Languages that contrast voice quality in their vowel systems have been under-studied, in part because the acoustic measurement techniques are not terribly robust. Blankenship (2002) studied four languages from the UCLA Phonetics Lab Archive – Mazatec (ISO 639–3 code maj), Tagalog (ISO 639–3 code tgl), Chong (ISO 639–3 code cog), and Mpi (ISO 639–3 code mpi) – to evaluate not only the presence of laryngealization but also the time course over the duration of the vocalic segment. Shifting from [ʔ] to [h] to modal could take place within 25 ms, and the various acoustic signatures of breathiness could occur singly or in one of many different combinations.

ANLA: Tuttle (2003)

The existence and discovery of archival material for the Salcha dialect of Tanana (ISO 639–3 code taa) made possible a phonetic comparison with the Minto dialect even though Salcha is no longer spoken (Tuttle, 2003). (The materials were in the ANLC collection – not ANLA at that time – and in the Oral History collection in the Alaska and Polar Regions Archives at the Elmer E. Rasmuson Library at the University of Alaska, Fairbanks.) Acoustic analysis revealed that, on the one hand, Minto had a difference in fundamental frequency (f_0) between "marked" syllables (syllables that are reconstructed as having constricted vowels in Proto-Athabaskan) while Salcha had no difference. Stress, on the other hand, was marked by f_0 in Salcha but not in Minto. (Duration signaled stress in both dialects.) Stress and intonation interacted: The frequent placement of verbs in sentence final position coupled with f_0 marking of stress (which is prominent on verbs) led to a reduction (to a non-significant level) of the intonational drop in f_0 at the end of sentences for Salcha but not Minto. Given the state of these dialects, only archival data could have shown these patterns.

UCLA: Esposito (2010)

Material from the UCLA Phonetics Lab Archive was used to test perception of voice quality distinctions in non-native speakers (Esposito, 2010; see also Keating and Esposito, 2007).

A first experiment used ten languages while a second used Mazatec (ISO 639–3 code maj). Of their three listener groups, Spanish- and English-speaking listeners were rather inconsistent, while Gujarati-speaking listeners were consistent but used three categories rather than the two used in the languages. This was confirmed with the larger sample from Mazatec, and it was further found that the best acoustic predictor of the Mazatec distinction was not used by any of the three listening groups.

CLA: Yu (2008)

Phonetic analysis revealed that quantity alternation in Washo (ISO 639–3 code was) is much more pervasive in the language than it was first described in the 1960s (Yu, 2008). Surprisingly, the current generation of Washo speakers retains subtle phonetic alternations, despite the fact they mostly grew up bilingual, if not English dominant.

UCLA: Keating et al. (2010)

Contrastive phonation types of four languages, one from the UCLA Phonetics Lab Archive were examined (Keating et al., 2010); the other three were archived in "Production and Perception of Linguistic Voice Quality" (at www.phonetics.ucla.edu/voiceproject/voice.html). When phonation categories with the same label (e.g., "breathy") were compared across languages, each category was found to differ from language to language on multiple acoustic measures. For example, breathy in Hmong (ISO 639–3 code mww) is distinct from breathy in Gujarati (ISO 639–3 code guj). This unexpected result suggests that language/speaker differences in voice quality are larger than the phonation category differences themselves.

UCLA: de Carvalho (2010)

The vowel characteristics of Pirahã (ISO 639–3 myp) were examined in the recordings of the UCLA archive (de Carvalho, 2010). This language has a three-vowel system, which allows for a test of the vowel dispersion theory (Liljencrants and Lindblom, 1972). Surprisingly, the dispersion in this three-vowel system was as large as has been found for larger inventories, putting limits on the dispersion theory. Some puzzling data on intrinsic fundamental frequency (Whalen and Levitt, 1995) were also presented.

UCLA: de Boer (2011)

Thirty languages from the UCLA archive were examined to determine whether the first formant for /i/ and /u/ were the same or not (de Boer, 2011). Both are described as being equally high in the vowel space, leading to the expectation that they would have the same F_1 value. However, /u/ consistently had a higher F_1, indicating a lower tongue position. A possible explanation based on the capabilities of the vocal tract was proposed. There was a trend for a smaller difference in females than in males, possibly due to differences in the size of the epilaryngeal tube.

UCLA: Garellek and Keating (2011)

San Felipe Jalapa de Díaz (Jalapa) Mazatec (ISO 639–3 code maj) has an unusual three-way phonation contrast crossed with a three-way level tone contrast that is independent of phonation (Garellek and Keating, 2011). Acoustic analysis found that the tone categories differ in f_0 over the course of the vowel, but that for laryngealized phonation, the beginning of the vowel loses the f_0 aspect of the tone contrast. This study shows that the acoustics support the three-way phonation and tone contrasts, even though individual parameters may merge.

UCLA: Coombs (2013)

Downstep in Ibibio (ISO 639–3 code ibb) was explored using previously recorded material (Coombs, 2013). These recordings were first found to be alignable with a tool trained on English (DiCanio et al., 2013). Ibibio shows a complex interaction of prosodic downdrift, phonological downstep, and a possible raising of high tones for enhancing contrast with low tones.

UCLA: Gordon (2015)

Using data from four languages, three in the UCLA archive, Gordon (2015) found that the effect of laryngeal setting, posited to be a major source of tonogenesis (Hombert et al., 1979), does not have a consistent effect on f_0. The languages were Hupa (ISO 639–3 code hup), Western Apache (ISO 639–3 code apw), Pirahã (ISO 639–3 code myp), and Banawá (ISO 639–3 code bnh). Even with the limited sample of four languages, many interactions between laryngeal setting and segmental organization were found. Surprisingly, the effects that were found were not smaller in magnitude for languages that had distinctive tone already.

ATM: Lawyer (2015)

Patwin (ISO 639–3 code pwi), a member of the small and underdescribed Wintuan language family, had aspects of its phonetics outlined from archival sources (Lawyer, 2015). Measures voice onset time (VOT), vowel space and duration provide phonetic detail to the phonological description of the paper.

ELAR: DiCanio and Whalen (2015)

The vowel formants in an Arapaho (ISO 639–3 code arp) speech corpus were found to differ in an expected direction with distinctive vowel length, with short vowels being more centralized and long vowels more peripheral (DiCanio and Whalen, 2015). However, the effect of speech style (elicited vs. narrative) was asymmetrical, with long vowels undergoing greater durational compression in narrative speech than short vowels, but with short vowels showing greater changes in quality. This was an unusual finding of speaking style affecting articulation beyond the operation of durational undershoot.

AILLA: DiCanio, Nam, Amith, Whalen, and Castillo García (2015)

Measurements of vowels in Yoloxóchitl Mixtec (ISO 639–3 code xty) (DiCanio, n.d.) indicated that vowel spaces can be recovered from narratives as well as elicited speech, even though there are differences in overall acoustic space between the two (DiCanio et al., 2015). Indeed, further separating the elicited tokens (by a median split) into short and long, and a three-way split of spontaneous tokens by duration showed that there was a fairly continuous expansion of the vowel space as duration increased, even for the elicited tokens. These findings have implications for the interpretation of measurements in majority languages as well.

Discussion and recommendations

The 13 papers cited have given us solid and often unexpected results, but this level of productivity is less than one might expect, given the great emphasis now put on archiving of linguistic data. We have already discussed some of the challenges to making use of archives, but we will outline those and others here along with recommendations for means of improving the use of these valuable resources. The first three would require resources that are not currently available, but we propose that they are worth considering for future initiatives. In particular, changes that return something of value to depositors would be an added incentive for the depositing of existing material.

Lack of phonetic transcription

A major bottleneck in the processing of language recordings is the labor-intensive, time-consuming process of transcription and annotation. Without at least a translation into a matrix language, recordings are of very limited value (Woodbury, 2003). Depending on the number of annotation levels and the amount of detail and rechecking employed, this process can take between 20 and 100 times real time (e.g., Auer et al., 2010). In general, transcriptions will be done using a practical orthography. This is useful both because such orthographies (when adequately designed) represent most of the important phonological content and because they are of immediate use to the communities using the language. Even the shallowest orthography, however, obscures some phonetic detail, making it difficult to use this level of description as a basis for phonetic analysis. The ideal would be to have, a phonological and a phonetic annotation level; this is seldom achieved, so other options need to be made available.

Recommendation: All recordings should, ideally, be transcribed. Further, phonetic use of archives would be enhanced if automatic creation of phonemic and phonetic layers from an orthographic layer were performed.

Benefits: Depositors receive something of value from depositing, both in being able to use the phonemic description and in seeing error in the transcription and/or the orthographic rules. Phonetic analysis will be easier.

Drawbacks: Relatively few such systems exist, and their development and implementation would require a substantial investment.

Coarse alignment of transcription to audio

The granularity of the alignment between a transcription and its audio signal varies greatly across corpora. Perhaps the most common is alignment at the sentence level, although even larger units (e.g., paragraph or entire text) are not unheard of. Alignment at the word level is reasonably common and allows some automatic phonetic analysis. Aligning to the phone level or the acoustic segment is the most useful for automatic phonetic analysis but is also the least common. We emphasize that only automatic analysis enables the major benefit of corpora, the ability to analyze a substantial number of examples. Producing these annotation layers by hand is itself time-consuming, though it can be automated to some extent (e.g., DiCanio et al., 2013).

Recommendation: Archived material would be more useful to phonetic analysis if they had an automatically generated alignment between phonemes and/or phones and the acoustic signal created upon deposit.

Benefits: The alignment will make phonetic analysis feasible with relatively little involvement of the depositor. Errors in transcription often stand out when alignment fails, allowing correction and thus improvement of the dataset.

Drawbacks: Alignment depends on the previously recommended construction of a phonemic level. Aligners have been made to work for many languages, even those with small corpora, but currently, "dictionaries" (lists of forms that occur in the data) must be made. Universal aligners are being developed (e.g., Strunk et al., 2014, Adda et al., 2016), but refinements are desirable. Archives are not currently able to provide this service, and it would require additional work by archive staff, which is typically a substantial cost.

Limited archiving of physiological measurements

Despite the long tradition of taking physiological measurements of endangered languages, there is virtually no tradition of archiving such data. Even for major languages, there are fewer such archives than we might expect at this point. The most heavily used is the X-Ray Microbeam dataset (Westbury, 1994). X-ray data from English and French (Munhall et al., 1995) and various languages (Sock et al., 2011) are also available but less frequently analyzed. Electromagnetic articulometry and real-time magnetic resonance imaging data are becoming available for English (Narayanan et al., 2014).

Recommendation: Begin to provide the data structures that archives would need to store physiological data in a way that is useful for further analysis.

Benefits: Aspects of phonetics that cannot be addressed by acoustics alone could be examined in greater detail.

Drawbacks: The design of metadata and data standards is more complex than those for audio signals, thus the amount of work needed to make the data interoperable is substantial. Migration to future platforms may also present a challenge. Storage requirements for physiological data are typically larger than those for audio, potentially requiring an increase in funding.

Require depositors to collect material for phonetic analysis

Elicited material for phonetic analysis is useful even when other speech samples are extensive. Phonetic results can be obtained from narratives and other continuous speech samples, as has been shown in several of the results summarized here, but targeted, elicited material can often be more easily analyzed. The phonemes of a language are relatively few and can be sampled with a relatively small word list (Ladefoged and Maddieson, 1996a). Sequences of phonemes are more numerous and also of interest, and sampling them requires a longer list. Prosodic and other larger contexts are similarly more numerous and require an even larger set of stimuli. In recommending this policy, we are, of course, thinking in terms of new collections; legacy material should be accepted in whatever state it exists. When researchers are planning to deposit their material in a particular archive (and many funders now require designation of the archive to be used), then they will have to address the elicitation requirements before making their recordings.

Recommendation: Require depositors to obtain an elicited set of stimuli for phonetic analysis.
Benefits: Phonetic analysis would be enhanced. Aspects of the phonology come to light even in the process of making the stimulus list.
Drawbacks: Archives do not have any means of enforcing this policy. Some archives do not allow multiple, small files, which are ideal for phonetic examples.

Conclusion

Archives hold great promise for future phonetic research. Substantial challenges exist in using archives as they are currently configured. Changes in the way that annotation tiers are implemented in archives can improve the accessibility of the data for phonetic research. Creating archives of articulatory and other physiological data is a large task that would have further sizable benefits; the costs are larger as well. The slow start to using archival data can be expected to seem less severe as greater and greater use is made of the archives. The ongoing expenses for digital archives, being greater than those for print archives, make for urgency in using digital archives. Further improvements, while desirable, generally would require even more financial support. Nonetheless, phonetic results can be obtained from these materials. We hope that our survey of those results will be hopelessly out of date in the near future.

Acknowledgments

We thank Siri Tuttle, Patricia A. Keating, Mandana Seyfeddinipur, Alexis Michaud, Susan Kung, Grace Kim-Lambert, and Nick Thieberger for helpful comments; mistakes remain our own.

References

Adams, O., Cohn, T., Neubig, G. & Michaud, A. 2017. Phonemic transcription of low-resource tonal languages. *In:* Wong, S-M. J. & Haffari, G. (eds.) *Proceedings of the Australasian Language Technology Association Workshop 2017*. Brisbane, Australia: Queensland University of Technology.

Adda, G., Adda-Decker, M., Ambouroue, O., Besacier, L., Blachon, D., Ene Bonneau-Maynard, H., Gauthier, E., Godard, P., Hamlaoui, F., Idiatov, D., Kouarata, G-N., Lamel, L., Makasso, E-M., Rialland, A., Stuker, S., Van de Velde, M., Yvon, F. & Zerbian, S. Innovative technologies for under-resourced language documentation: The BULB Project. *Workshop CCURL 2016 – Collaboration and Computing for Under-Resourced Languages – LREC, 2016–2005 2016*. Portoroz, Slovenia.

Amery, R. 1995. It's ours to keep and call our own: Reclamation of the Nunga languages in the Adelaide region, South Australia. *International Journal of the Sociology of Language*, 113, 63–82.

Anderson, V. B. 2008. Static palatography for language fieldwork. *Language Documentation and Conservation*, 2, 1–27.

Auer, E., Russel, A., Sloetjes, H., Wittenburg, P., Schreer, O., Masnieri, S., Schneider, D. & Tschöpel, S. 2010. ELAN as flexible annotation framework for sound and image processing detectors. *In:* Calzolari, N., Choukri, K., Maegaard, B., Mariani, J., Odijk, J., Piperidis, S., Rosner, M. & Tapias,

D. (eds.) *Proceedings of the Seventh Conference on International Language Resources and Evaluation (LREC'10)*. Valletta, Malta: European Language Resources Association (ELRA).

Beagrie, N. 2008. Digital curation for science, digital libraries, and individuals. *International Journal of Digital Curation*, 1, 3–16.

Becker-Kristal, R. 2010. Acoustic Typology of Vowel Inventories and Dispersion Theory: Insights from a Large Cross-Linguistic Corpus. Ph.D. dissertation, University of California, Los Angeles.

Bird, S. & Simons, G. F. 2001. The OLAC metadata set and controlled vocabularies. *Proceedings of the ACL 2001 Workshop on Sharing Tools and Resources – Volume 15*. France: Association for Computational Linguistics.

Blankenship, B. 2002. The timing of nonmodal phonation in vowels. *Journal of Phonetics*, 30, 163–191.

Bowern, C., McDonough, J. & Kelliher, K. 2012. Bardi. *Journal of the International Phonetic Association*, 42, 333–351.

Bradfield, J. 2014. Clicks, concurrency and Khoisan. *Phonology*, 31, 1–49.

Chodroff, E. & Wilson, C. 2017. Structure in talker-specific phonetic realization: Covariation of stop consonant VOT in American English. *Journal of Phonetics*, 61, 30–47.

Clement, T. 2014. The ear and the shunting yard: Meaning making as resonance in early information theory. *Information and Culture*, 49, 401–426.

Clements, G. N. & Ridouane, R. (eds.) 2011. *Where Do Phonological Features Come from? Cognitive, Physical and Developmental Bases of Distinctive Speech Categories*. Amsterdam, Philadelphia: John Benjamins Publishing.

Coombs, A. L. 2013. High tone processes in Ibibio. *Proceedings of Meetings on Acoustics*, 19, 060232.

Cottingham, K. 2008. Turning data graveyards into gold mines. *Journal of Proteome Research*, 7, 22.

De Boer, B. 2011. First formant difference for /i/ and /u/: A cross-linguistic study and an explanation. *Journal of Phonetics*, 39, 110–114.

De Carvalho, F. O. 2010. Vowel acoustics in Pirahã. *Revista de Estudos da Linguagem*, 18, 11–33.

DiCanio, C. T. n.d. Itunyoso Triqui collection of Christian DiCanio. ailla:243683. *The Archive of the Indigenous Languages of Latin America*. Available from: www.ailla.utexas.org/islandora/object/ailla%3A243683 [Accessed 7/1/2018].

DiCanio, C. T. 2009. The phonetics of register in Takhian Thong Chong. *Journal of the International Phonetic Association*, 39, 162–188.

DiCanio, C. T. 2012. The phonetics of fortis and lenis consonants in Itunyoso Trique. *International Journal of American Linguistics*, 78, 239–272.

DiCanio, C. T., Chen, Wei-Rong, Benn, J., Amith, J. D., & Castillo García, R. 2017. Automatic detection of extreme stop allophony in Mixtec spontaneous speech. Paper presented at the Annual Meeting on Phonology, New York City.

DiCanio, C. T., Nam, H., Amith, J. D., Whalen, D. H. & Castillo García, R. 2015. Vowel variability in elicited versus running speech: Evidence from Mixtec. *Journal of Phonetics*, 48, 45–59.

DiCanio, C. T., Nam, H., Whalen, D. H., Bunnell, H. T., Amith, J. D. & Castillo García, R. 2013. Using automatic alignment to analyze endangered language data: Testing the viability of untrained alignment. *The Journal of the Acoustical Society of America*, 134, 2235–2246.

DiCanio, C. T. & Whalen, D. H. 2015. The interaction of vowel length and speech style in an Arapaho speech corpus. *In:* The Scottish Consortium for ICPhS 2015 (ed.) *Proceedings of the 18th International Congress of Phonetic Sciences*. Glasgow, UK: University of Glasgow.

Digital Preservation Coalition. 2015. *Digital Preservation Handbook*. dpconline.org. Digital Preservation Coalition.

Dwyer, A. M. 2006. Ethics and practicalities of cooperative fieldwork and analysis. *In:* Gippert, J., Mosel, U. & Himmelmann, N. P. (eds.) *Essentials of Language Documentation*. Berlin: Mouton de Gruyter.

Errington, J. 2007. *Linguistics in a Colonial World: A Story of Language, Meaning and Power*. New York: Blackwell Publishing.

Esposito, C. M. 2010. The effects of linguistic experience on the perception of phonation. *Journal of Phonetics*, 38, 306–316.

Farrar, S. & Lewis, W. D. 2007. The GOLD Community of Practice: An infrastructure for linguistic data on the Web. *Language Resources and Evaluation*, 41, 45–60.

Farrar, S., Lewis, W. D. & Langendoen, D. T. 2002. An ontology for linguistic annotation. In: Semantic Web Meets Language Resources: Papers from the AAAI Workshop, Technical Report WS-02–16. AAAI Press, Menlo Park, CA.

Flemming, E., Ladefoged, P. & Thomason, S. 2008. Phonetic structures of Montana Salish. *Journal of Phonetics*, 36, 465–491.

Fletcher, J. & Evans, N. 2002. An acoustic phonetic analysis of intonational prominence in two Australian languages. *Journal of the International Phonetic Association*, 32, 123–140.

Garellek, M. & Keating, P. A. 2011. The acoustic consequences of phonation and tone interactions in Jalapa Mazatec. *Journal of the International Phonetic Association*, 41, 185–205.

Gick, B., Bird, S. & Wilson, I. 2005. Techniques for field application of lingual ultrasound imaging. *Clinical Linguistics and Phonetics*, 19, 503–514.

Goddard, P. E. 1905. Mechanical aids to the study and recording of language. *American Anthropologist*, 7, 613–619.

Goddard, P. E. 1907. *The Phonology of the Hupa Language*. Berkeley: University of California Press.

Gordon, M. 2015. Consonant-tone interactions: A phonetic study of four indigenous languages of the Americas. *In:* Avelino, H., Coler, M. & Wetzels, L. (eds.) *The Phonetics and Phonology of Laryngeal Features in Native American Languages*. Leiden/Boston: Brill.

Hale, K., Krauss, M., Watahomigie, L. J., Yamamoto, A. Y., Craig, C., Masayesva Jeanne, L. & England, N. 1992. Endangered languages. *Language*, 68, 1–42.

Hargus, S. 2007. *Witsuwit'en Grammar: Phonetics, Phonology, Morphology*. Vancouver: University of British Columbia Press.

Harrington, J. & Cassidy, S. 1999. *Techniques in Speech Acoustics*. Dordrecht: Kluwer Academic Publishers.

Hinton, L. 2001. Sleeping languages: Can they be awakened? *In:* Hinton, L. & Hale, K. (eds.) *The Green Book of Language Revitalization in Practice*. London: Academic.

Hombert, J-M., Ohala, J. J. & Ewan, W. G. 1979. Phonetic explanations for the development of tones. *Language*, 55, 37–58.

Hsieh, F-F. 2007. *Relational Correspondence in Tone Sandhi*. Ph.D. dissertation, Massachusetts Institute of Technology, Boston.

Keating, P. A. & Esposito, C. M. 2007. Linguistic voice quality. *UCLA Working Papers in Phonetics*, 105, 85–91.

Keating, P. A., Esposito, C. M., Garellek, M., Khan, S. U. D. & Kuang, J. 2010. Phonation contrasts across languages. *UCLA Working Papers in Phonetics*, 108, 188–202.

Kempton, T. & Moore, R. K. 2014. Discovering the phoneme inventory of an unwritten language: A machine-assisted approach. *Speech Communication*, 56, 152–166.

Kuang, J. 2013. The tonal space of contrastive five level tones. *Phonetica*, 70, 1–23.

Kübler, S. & Zinsmeister, H. 2015. *Corpus Linguistics and Linguistically Annotated Corpora*. London: Bloomsbury Publishing.

Ladefoged, P. 2003. *Phonetic Data Analysis: An Introduction to Fieldwork and Instrumental Techniques*. Malden, MA: Blackwell.

Ladefoged, P. & Maddieson, I. 1996a. Recording the phonetic structures of endangered languages. *UCLA Working Papers in Phonetics*, 93, 1–7.

Ladefoged, P. & Maddieson, I. 1996b. *The Sounds of the World's Languages*. Oxford, UK/Cambridge, MA: Blackwell.

Lawyer, L. C. 2015. Patwin phonemics, phonetics, and phonotactics. *International Journal of American Linguistics*, 81, 221–260.

Leonard, W. Y. 2007. *Miami Language Reclamation in the Home: A Case Study*. 3367487. Ph.D. dissertation, University of California, Berkeley.

Liberman, A. M., Cooper, F. S., Shankweiler, D. P. & Studdert-Kennedy, M. 1967. Perception of the speech code. *Psychological Review*, 74, 431–461.

Liljencrants, J. & Lindblom, B. 1972. Numerical simulation of vowel quality systems: The role of perceptual contrast. *Language*, 48, 839–862.

Lindblom, B. E. 1990. Explaining phonetic variation: A sketch of the H&H theory. *In:* Hardcastle, W. J. & Marchal, A. (eds.) *Speech Production and Speech Modeling*. Dordrecht: Kluwer Academic Publishers.

Littledoe, J. 1998. Wampanoag language reclamation project: First steps to healing the circle. *Thirtieth Algonquian Conference*, Boston, MA.

Maddieson, I. 1984. *Patterns of Sounds*. New York: Cambridge University Press.

McCrae, J. P., Labropoulou, P., Gracia, J., Villegas, M., Rodríguez-Doncel, V. & Cimiano, P. 2015. One ontology to bind them all: The META-SHARE OWL ontology for the interoperability of linguistic datasets on the Web. *In:* Gandon, F., Guéret, C., Villata, S., Breslin, J., Faron-Zucker, C. & Zimmermann, A. (eds.) *The Semantic Web: ESWC 2015 Satellite Events: ESWC 2015 Satellite Events, Portorož, Slovenia, May 31 – June 4, 2015, Revised Selected Papers*. Cham: Springer International Publishing.

McDonough, J. M. 2003. *The Navajo Sound System*. Dordrecht: Kluwer.

McDonough, J. M. & Tucker, B. V. 2012. Replicating Goddard: A contemporary airflow and EGG study of Dene SųŁiné *University of Rochester Working Papers in the Language Sciences*, 7, 1–17.

Miller, A. L. 2007. Guttural vowels and guttural co-articulation in Ju|'hoansi. *Journal of Phonetics*, 35, 56–84.

Miller, A. L. 2016. Posterior lingual gestures and tongue shape in Mangetti Dune !Xung clicks. *Journal of Phonetics*, 55, 119–148.

Munhall, K. G., Vatikiotis-Bateson, E. S. & Tohkura, Y. I. 1995. X-ray film database for speech research. *The Journal of the Acoustical Society of America*, 98, 1222–1224.

Narayanan, S., Toutios, A., Ramanarayanan, V., Lammert, A., Kim, J., Lee, S., Nayak, K., Kim, Y-C., Zhu, Y., Goldstein, L. M., Byrd, D., Bresch, E., Ghosh, P., Katsamanis, A. & Proctor, M. 2014. Real-time magnetic resonance imaging and electromagnetic articulography database for speech production research (TC). *The Journal of the Acoustical Society of America*, 136, 1307–1311.

National Science Foundation 2010. Data management for NSF SBE Directorate proposals and awards. Retrieved from https://www.nsf.gov/sbe/SBE_DataMgmtPlanPolicy.pdf

Niebuhr, O. & Michaud, A. 2015. Speech data acquisition: the underestimated challenge. *KALIPHO – Kieler Arbeiten zur Linguistik und Phonetik*, 3, 1–42.

Pike, K. L. 1947. Grammatical prerequisites to phonemic analysis. *Word*, 3, 155–172.

Pulgram, E. 1954. Accent and ictus in spoken and written Latin. *Zeitschrift für vergleichende Sprachforschung auf dem Gebiete der Indogermanischen Sprachen*, 71, 218–237.

Remijsen, B. 2013. Tonal alignment is contrastive in falling contours in Dinka. *Language*, 89, 297–327.

Remijsen, B. & Ayoker, O. G. 2014. Contrastive tonal alignment in falling contours in Shilluk. *Phonology*, 31, 435–462.

Research Libraries Group. 2002. *Trusted Digital Repositories: Attributes and Responsibilities*. Mountain View, CA: RLG.

Rousselot, P-J. 1897–1908. *Principes de phonétique expérimentale*. Paris: H. Welter.

Schiering, R., Bickel, B. & Hildebrandt, K. A. 2010. The prosodic word is not universal, but emergent. *Journal of Linguistics*, 46, 657–709.

Schmidt, T., Chiarcos, C., Lehmberg, T., Rehm, G., Witt, A. & Hinrichs, E. Avoiding data graveyards: From heterogeneous data collected in multiple research projects to sustainable linguistic resources. *6th E-MELD Workshop*, Ypsilanti, 2006.

Schwartz, J-L., Boë, L-J., Vallée, N. & Abry, C. 1997. The dispersion-focalization theory of vowel systems. *Journal of Phonetics*, 25, 255–286.

Sen, R. 2015. *Syllable and Segment in Latin*. Oxford: Oxford University Press.

Simas Frazão, K. 2013. *A sílaba no Akwẽ-Xerente (Jê)*. M.A. thesis, Universidade de Brasília, Brasília.

Sock, R., Hirsch, F., Laprie, Y., Perrier, P., Vaxelaire, B., Brock, G., Bouarourou, F., Fauth, C., Ferbach-Hecker, V. & Ma, L. *An X-ray Database, Tools and Procedures for the Study of Speech Production*. 9th International Seminar on Speech Production (ISSP 2011), 2011, 41–48.

Strunk, J., Schiel, F. & Seifart, F. 2014. Untrained forced alignment of transcriptions and audio for language documentation corpora using WebMAUS. *In:* Calzolari, N., Choukri, K., Declerck, T., Loftsson, H., Maegaard, B., Mariani, J., Moreno, A., Odijk, J. & Piperidis, S. (eds.) *Proceedings of LREC*. Reykjavik, Iceland: European Language Resources Association.

Tuttle, S. G. 2003. Archival phonetics: Tone and stress in Tanana Athabaskan. *Anthropological Linguistics*, 45, 316–336.

Westbury, J. R. 1994. *X-ray Microbeam Speech Production Database User's Handbook*. Madison, WI: Waisman Center, University of Wisconsin.

Whalen, D. H., DiCanio, C. T. & Shaw, P. A. 2011. Phonetics of endangered languages. *Acoustics Today*, 7, 35–42.

Whalen, D. H. & Levitt, A. G. 1995. The universality of intrinsic F0 of vowels. *Journal of Phonetics*, 23, 349–366.

Whalen, D. H. & McDonough, J. M. 2015. Taking the laboratory into the field. *Annual Review of Linguistics*, 1, 395–415.

Whalen, D. H. & Simons, G. F. 2012. Endangered language families. *Language*, 88, 155–173.

Wieling, M., Tomaschek, F., Arnold, D., Tiede, M. K., Bröker, F., Thiele, S., Wood, S. N. & Baayen, R. H. 2016. Investigating dialectal differences using articulography. *Journal of Phonetics*, 59, 122–143.

Winter, B. 2015. The other N: The role of repetitions and items in the design of phonetic experiments. *In:* The Scottish Consortium for ICPhS 2015 (ed.) *Proceedings of the 18th International Congress of Phonetic Sciences*. Glasgow, UK: University of Glasgow.

Woodbury, A. C. 2003. Defining documentary linguistics. *Language Documentation and Description*, 1, 35–51.

Yu, A. C. L. 2008. The phonetics of the quantity alternation in Washo. *Journal of Phonetics*, 36, 508–520.

Part II

Physiological basis of speech and hearing

4

The phonetics of voice[1]

Marc Garellek

Introduction

This chapter focuses on the phonetics of the voice. The term "voice" is used to mean many different things, with definitions varying both within and across researchers and disciplines. In terms of voice articulation, definitions can vary from the very narrow – how the vocal folds vibrate – to the very broad, where "voice" is essentially synonymous with "speech" – how the vocal folds and all other vocal tract articulators influence how we sound (Kreiman and Sidtis, 2011). In this chapter, I will use the term "voice" to refer to sound produced by the vocal folds, including but not limited to vocal fold vibration. I have chosen to focus only on a narrow conception of the voice in order to constrain the discussion; as we will see, the phonetics of voice – even when it concerns only vocal fold articulation – is remarkably complex and of great relevance to phonetic and linguistic research. In contrast, I will use the term "voice quality" to refer to the percept resulting from the voice: In other words, different vocal fold configurations have specific perceptual ramifications, which we will call changes in voice quality. The distinction between voice and voice quality adopted here is therefore analogous to that made between "fundamental frequency" (f_0) and "pitch."

Why should we be interested in the phonetics of the voice? Linguists are interested in how specific forms contribute to linguistic meaning; for spoken languages, phonetic and phonological research addresses this goal from the point of view of how sounds contribute to meaning. Because the vocal folds are part of the speech apparatus, a complete understanding of the sound-to-meaning relationship requires knowledge of how sounds produced by the vocal folds contribute to linguistic meaning.

There are two main contributions of the vocal folds: First, their movements can be used contrastively in languages. That is, in some languages changes in (a) the presence vs. absence of vocal fold vibration, (b) the rate of vibration, and (c) the quality of vibration can signal a change in lexical meaning: compare (a) English /ˈslɒpi/ "sloppy" vs. /ˈslɒbi/ "slobby"; (b) White Hmong /tɔ ˧/ "pierced" vs. /tɔ ˧/ "wait"; and (c) Jalapa Mazatec breathy-voiced [ⁿdæ̤ ˥] "horse," creaky-voiced [ⁿdæ̰ ˥] "buttock," and modal-voiced [ⁿdæ ˥] "seed" (Silverman et al., 1995; Garellek and Keating, 2011).[2]

Second, because of their position downstream from the trachea and upstream from the remainder of the vocal tract, all speech is first modulated by the vocal folds. This may seem counterintuitive at first, given that phoneticians tend to speak of two sources of sound excitation: voicing (produced by the vocal folds) and noise (produced in the vocal tract in all obstruents but [ʔ], [h], and [ɦ]). But even for sounds characterized by acoustic noise generated in the vocal tract (such as [t] and [s]), the vocal folds still assume a particular articulatory target; for example, voiceless obstruents (even when unaspirated) often show some degree vocal fold spreading (Munhall and Löfqvist, 1992), presumably to inhibit voicing and/or to facilitate the high airflow needed to generate turbulence for voiceless fricatives. The voice is thus part of the production of *all* speech sounds, regardless of whether it is used to make phonological contrasts. Aside from phonological meaning, the voice contributes to changes in prosody, syntax, discourse, as well as to speaker identity and emotional state (Choi et al., 2005; Zhuang and Hasegawa-Johnson, 2008; Gobl and Ní Chasaide, 2010; Esling and Edmondson, 2010; Kreiman and Sidtis, 2011; Yanushevskaya et al., 2011; Podesva and Callier, 2015; Park et al., 2016; Yanushevskaya et al., 2016). Changes in vocal fold vibration are also associated with differences in singing registers and with voice disorders (Sundberg, 1987; Titze, 1994; Kempster et al., 2011; Sapienza et al., 2011).

This chapter therefore takes as a starting point that the voice is ultimately used to convey information, which is transmitted between speakers and hearers in stages commonly known as the "speech chain" (Denes and Pinson, 1993). Although there have been many advancements over the years in understanding how the vocal folds are innervated, how they move and vibrate, and how different voice settings are manifested acoustically (for instance, see overviews in Titze, 1994; Baken and Orlikoff, 2000; Stevens, 2000; Gobl and Ní Chasaide, 2010; Hirose, 2010; Story, 2015), it is still unclear how these stages of the speech chain interact with one another to influence voice quality. Yet, ultimately one of the main goals of the study of the voice should be to answer two fundamental questions: (a) When we perceive a change in the voice, what caused that change? and (b) What are the acoustical and perceptual results of a change in voice production? In my research with colleagues (e.g., Kreiman et al., 2014), we address these questions by modeling how information about the voice is transmitted from speaker to hearer. Ideally, a unified theory of voice production, acoustics, and perception should be able to model any type of information that the voice can convey, including phonological, prosodic, discourse, sociolinguistic, and paralinguistic information, as well as talker identity. In this chapter, I focus largely on linguistic (especially phonological) meaning: how the voice is used to create sounds of the world's languages. Thus, the first goal of the phonetic study of the voice can be restated with respect to phonological meaning: when we perceive a *phonologically relevant* change in the voice (such as a switch between two sounds), what caused that change?

The past decade has seen a rapid increase in research on the role of the voice in sound systems, much of which will be reviewed in this chapter. This research will help outline the primary voice dimensions, defined here in articulatory terms, that are used in languages of the world to convey phonological meaning (see "Primary linguistic voice dimensions"). Readers will see that the study of the voice is essential for our understanding of phonetics and phonology, because *every* sound that we make involves an articulation of the vocal folds, which has specific acoustic attributes that listeners can hear and use in language.

What is covered in this chapter?

This chapter is largely theoretical in nature. The focus is on how we can model (within a unified framework) the three stages of the speech chain as it concerns the vocal folds and their use in sounds of the world's languages. Therefore, we will not review fine-grained details pertaining to voice anatomy and physiology (though see Titze, 1994; Stevens, 2000; Titze, 2006; Reetz and Jongman, 2008; Hirose, 2010; Kreiman and Sidtis, 2011; Gick et al., 2013; Story, 2015; Zhang, 2016b), as well as voice source modeling (Stevens, 2000; Gobl and Ní Chasaide, 2010; Story, 2012; Samlan et al., 2013; Kreiman et al., 2015; Moisik and Esling, 2014; Moisik et al., 2014; Story, 2015). Neither will we review instrumentation used to measure muscular and articulatory properties of the voice; I refer readers to Baken and Orlikoff (2000); Hirose (2010); Gick et al. (2013), among others. Given that this chapter focuses on linguistic meaning, readers who are especially interested in how the voice varies according to specific voice disorders, emotions, individuals, and singing styles should consult Laver (1980); Sundberg (1987); Titze (1994); Esling and Edmondson (2010); Gobl and Ní Chasaide (2010); Kreiman and Sidtis (2011); Sapienza et al. (2011), among others. However, this chapter should also be of use to these readers, in that we will review a theory of the voice that links vocal production, acoustics, and voice quality perception more generally. Moreover, we will discuss how the speech chain, as it concerns the vocal folds, relates to meaningful categories that must be accurately perceived in order for communication to be effective.

In the following section, I classify vocal fold articulations according to their primary phonological dimensions. I then review the psychoacoustic voice model by Kreiman et al. (2014) and how parameters of this model are perceived by listeners and relate to the phonological dimensions outlined in the previous section. In the next two sections, I discuss recent work showing how the parameters of Kreiman et al. (2014)'s voice model relate to voice source acoustics and vocal fold articulation as parameterized in a recent model by Zhang (2015, 2016a). I conclude with discussion of outstanding questions and areas for future research.

Primary linguistic voice dimensions

Vocal fold movements, despite being very complex, can be organized along two articulatory dimensions that are especially important in language (Table 4.1): How far apart the folds are from each other, and whether they are vibrating. (Further details on these articulations are

Table 4.1 Primary vocal fold movements and their use in sounds of the world's languages.

Dimension	*Articulatory description*	*Relevant sounds*
Approximation	How far apart the vocal folds are from each other	All voiced sounds All voiceless sounds, e.g., aspirated sounds, glottalized sounds, fricatives, trills, and ejectives
Voicing	Whether the vocal folds are vibrating	All voiced sounds, e.g., sonorant consonants (voiced) vowels
Rate	Rate of vibration	Tone Intonation Stress
Quality	Constriction of vibration Irregularity/noise	Register Contrastive voice quality ("phonation type")

presented in "Voice production.") In this chapter, I refer to this first dimension as *vocal fold approximation*, though it could likewise be called "abduction/adduction" and "spreading/constriction." The minimal vocal fold approximation in speech can be found during voiceless aspiration (e.g., for [h] and aspirated stops like [tʰ]), and the maximal vocal fold approximation, when the vocal folds are in full contact, can be found for a glottal stop [ʔ] as well as glottalized sounds and ejectives (e.g., [ʔ͡t, t']). Note that "minimal vocal fold approximation" is understood within the context of speech sounds; for example, during active breathing the vocal folds abduct even more than during aspirated speech sounds (Gick et al., 2013). Other voiceless sounds can be described as having incomplete vocal fold approximation that is nonetheless greater than that found for aspiration; this state of vocal fold approximation is sometimes called "prephonation" (Harris, 1999; Esling and Harris, 2003; Edmondson et al., 2011). Likewise, voiced sounds require some degree of vocal fold approximation, which can also vary in its degree. Thus, all sounds, regardless of whether they are "plain" voiceless sounds, aspirated, glottalized, or voiced, involve some degree of vocal fold approximation. A schematic of different states of vocal fold approximation for voiceless sounds is shown in Figure 4.1.

The second dimension, *vocal fold vibration,* is also often called "voicing." This dimension is dependent on vocal fold approximation: voicing can only be initiated with some amount of vocal fold approximation, and only certain degrees of vocal fold approximation can sustain voicing once it has begun (Titze, 1992; Kreiman and Sidtis, 2011). Consequently, all sounds with vocal fold vibration necessarily make use of both dimensions. Voicing is generally treated as being categorical: sounds produced with vocal fold vibration are "voiced," those without are "voiceless." (Voicing is sometimes also called "phonation," but this term is also used more generally to describe any sound generated in the larynx or the remaining components of the vocal tract.) Voicing is very important in languages' phonologies; voiced sounds, including vowels, sonorant consonants, and voiced obstruents, are found in every spoken language. About 80% of languages have voicing contrasts in obstruents (Maddieson et al., 2016).

Voicing can be further characterized along two dimensions that are very important for linguistic meaning. The first is *rate* (or "frequency") of vocal fold vibration, a continuous dimension that determines the fundamental frequency of the voice and is used to convey

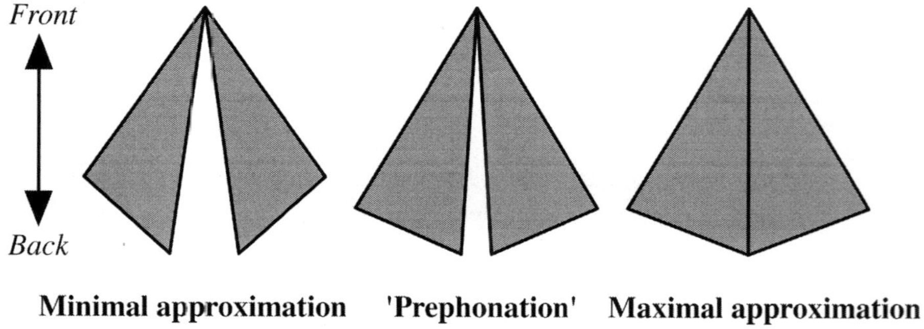

Figure 4.1 Schematized laryngoscopic (bird's-eye) view of the vocal folds showing different degrees of vocal fold approximation for voiceless sounds. In between minimal approximation (e.g., for a voiceless glottal fricative) and maximal approximation (e.g., for a glottal stop) is a state sometimes called "prephonation," which is found for voiceless unaspirated stops.

Source: Based on Harris, 1999; Esling and Harris, 2003; Edmondson et al., 2011.

lexical tone and intonation, and is one of the main correlates of lexical and phrasal stress (Gordon and Applebaum, 2010; Gordon, 2014; Garellek and White, 2015). The second dimension to voicing is the *quality* or "manner" of vocal fold vibration. Voice quality is also important for stress, tone, and intonation (Kreiman, 1982; Sluijter and van Heuven, 1996; Campbell and Beckman, 1997; Garellek and White, 2015; Mooshammer, 2010; Lancia et al., 2016); moreover, it is the primary dimension used for contrastive voice quality ("phonation type") and is important for voice registers, a multidimensional linguistic contrast involving a change in voice quality and other (laryngeal and supralaryngeal) changes (DiCanio, 2009; Brunelle, 2012; Abramson et al., 2015; Brunelle and Kirby, 2016; Tian and Kuang, 2016).

The most common voice qualities that are used in language are "modal," "breathy," and "creaky"; we will focus on these for the remainder of the chapter. They are defined relative to one another; thus, there is no "absolute" breathy voice, but certain voice qualities are "breathier" than others. It is partly due to their relative differences that many names for voice qualities exist: breathy voice qualities are sometimes called "lax," "slack," "murmured," "aspirated" while creaky qualities are "stiff," "tense," "laryngealized," "glottalized," "(vocal) fry," "pressed," to name but a few. Other terms, such as "rough," "strident," "sphincteric," "epiglottalized," or "harsh" voice, tend to be used for voice qualities that also necessarily involve supraglottal constriction (Laver, 1980; Traill, 1985; Gerratt and Kreiman, 2001; Edmondson and Esling, 2006; Miller, 2007; Moisik and Esling, 2011; Moisik, 2013) and thus fall outside the narrow definition of "voice" used here.

Although these different terms can sometimes refer to the same articulation, often researchers will use different terms to refer to distinct manners of vocal fold vibrations, acoustic characteristics, or perceptual voice qualities (Batliner et al., 1993; Gerratt and Kreiman, 2001; Redi and Shattuck-Hufnagel, 2001; Slifka, 2006; Kane et al., 2013; Kuang, 2013*b*; Keating et al., 2015). From an articulatory perspective, differences between breathy, modal, and creaky voice can minimally be described using a one-dimensional model of vocal fold approximation (Ladefoged, 1971; Gordon and Ladefoged, 2001): As we have already discussed, voiceless sounds can be made with minimal or maximal vocal fold approximation (as in [h] or [ʔ], respectively). In between these extremes, there is voicing. Voicing with less vocal fold approximation is "breathy," voicing with more approximation is "creaky," and voicing that is neither breathy nor creaky is "modal." ("Lax/slack" voice is sometimes considered intermediate to breathy and modal, and "tense/stiff" voice to creaky and modal; Keating et al., 2011; Kuang and Keating, 2014). This one-dimensional model of vocal fold approximation is schematized in Figure 4.2. It is conceptually simple and useful for describing the phonologically relevant relationship between voice qualities and categories of voiceless (consonantal) vocal fold approximation (Lombardi, 1991). However, it suffers from certain drawbacks. First, "modal" voice is defined in articulatory terms, relative to other states of vocal fold approximation; however, many researchers also use this term to refer to a speaker's default or "normal" voicing. Defined thus, if a speaker's normal voice quality is quite creaky, that speaker's "modal" voice would involve quite a bit of vocal

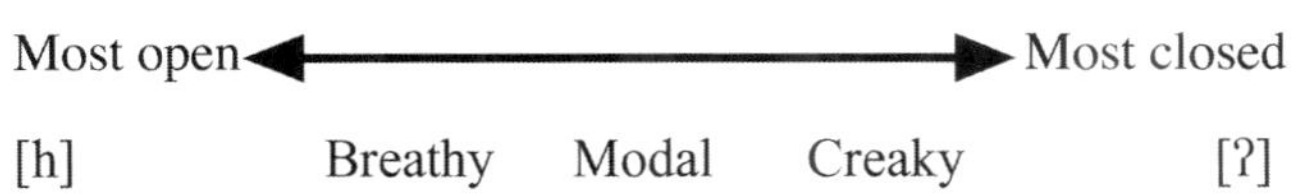

Figure 4.2 Simplified one-dimensional space for voice quality.

Source: Based on Ladefoged, 1971; Gordon and Ladefoged, 2001.

fold approximation, and thus should be captured under "creaky" in this model. The difference between these two definitions of "modal" (one articulatory and relative to non-modal voice, the other with reference to a speaker's normal quality) is generally thought to be of little practical importance, because we assume that speakers can always become creakier or breathier than their normal voice quality; for instance, a Jalapa Mazatec speaker whose normal voice quality is very creaky should be able to produce even creakier voice quality than her default in order to say a word with contrastive creaky voice in the language. But given that we still know very little about individual differences in voice quality – for example, if the degree of vocal fold approximation in a particular speaker's default voice quality has an effect on how that same speaker will produce non-modal voice – there may be an important distinction to be made between "modal" as defined articulatorily vs. speaker-dependently.

Second, although breathy and creaky voice are (generally) produced with different degrees of vocal fold approximation, creaky voice can involve additional supraglottal constriction (e.g., of the ventricular and aryepiglottic folds). The additional constrictions – and how these relate to linguistically relevant relationships between voice quality and supralaryngeal articulations (like tongue root advancement and vowel quality) – are captured more straightforwardly in a "valves" model of voice quality (see Table 4.2, after Esling and Harris, 2005; Edmondson and Esling, 2006). However, only Valve 1 from this model is involved in voice quality if the "voice" is narrowly defined as including only articulation of the vocal folds.

The third drawback to both continuum and valves models of the voice is that "creaky" voice – even if it is defined narrowly as a manner of vocal fold vibration with no additional supraglottal articulation – represents a cluster of voice qualities that share some perceptual attributes. In order to be perceived as creaky, the voice must be minimally low in pitch, irregular in pitch, or constricted-sounding (we will discuss what it means to be "constricted-sounding" in the following section), though not necessarily all three (Keating et al., 2015). For example, there are cases of creaky voice that are irregular and low in pitch, but also unconstricted (Slifka, 2000, 2006), which I call "unconstricted creaky voice." Further, there are two distinct types of creaky voice that are constricted in quality but can be regular in pitch: Vocal fry (which is low and regular in pitch) and tense (or "pressed") voice, which is constricted but with a high and (usually) regular pitch (Keating et al., 2015). Tense voice is often regular in pitch, but the increased constriction could result in sudden and irregular changes in voicing amplitude. Lastly, a very low-pitched voice (e.g., below 60 Hz) can also be perceived as creaky, despite not having any constriction or irregularity (Keating et al., 2015). Figure 4.3 illustrates the differences between prototypical creaky

Table 4.2 Valves of the throat and their functioning (from *Esling and Harris, 2005*; *Edmondson and Esling 2006*; see also *Figure 4.1* in *Edmondson and Esling 2006*). Valve 1 is similar to the continuum represented in *Figure 4.2*. The remaining valves pertain to structures above the vocal folds, and therefore would fall outside the narrow definition of "voice" used in this chapter.

Valve	*Description*
Valve 1	Vocal fold adduction and abduction
Valve 2	Ventricular fold adduction
Valve 3	Compression of the arytenoids and aryepiglottic folds epiglottal-pharyngeal
Valve 4	Constriction
Valve 5	Larynx raising
Valve 6	Pharyngeal narrowing

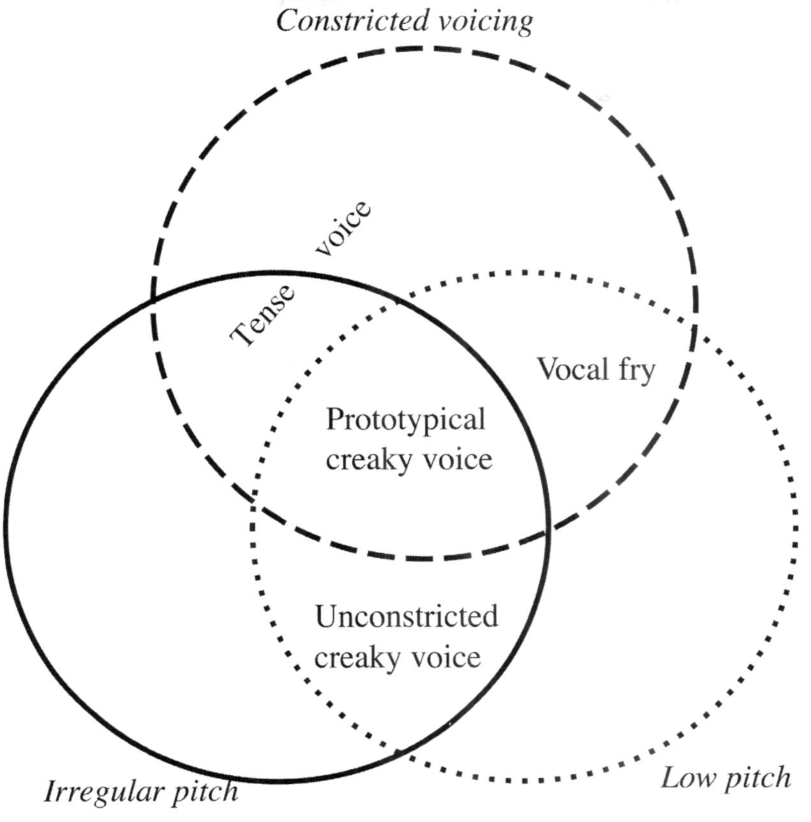

Figure 4.3 Three-dimensional space for creaky voice, with some subtypes shown.
Source: Based on Keating et al., 2015.

voice, unconstricted creaky voice, tense voice, and vocal fry according to pitch height, pitch regularity, and constricted quality.

Therefore, either a low pitch, an irregular pitch, or a constricted quality (regardless of pitch) is alone sufficient for listeners to perceive a voice as creaky, even if the articulatory origins and acoustic attributes underlying this percept can differ. However, much more work is needed to determine how perceptually distinct these subtypes can be (cf. Gerratt and Kreiman, 2001; Garellek, 2015), and how linguistically relevant they are. We have evidence that "prototypical" creaky voice (low-pitched, irregular in pitch, and constricted) is linguistically important, since it is commonly found for contrastive and allophonic creaky voice (Gordon and Ladefoged, 2001; Esposito, 2012; Garellek and Keating, 2011). Both of the other types of constricted voices listed in Figure 4.3 are of linguistic relevance: Vocal fry can be used to perceive a glottal stop [ʔ] (Hillenbrand and Houde, 1996; Gerfen and Baker, 2005), and tense voice can be used for the phonetic realization of contrastive creaky voice on a vowel with a high lexical tone, and is found more generally with higher-pitched lexical tones (Garellek and Keating, 2011; Kuang, 2013b, 2017a). Unconstricted creaky voice is found as a form of phrase-final creak (Kreiman, 1982; Redi and Shattuck-Hufnagel, 2001; Garellek, 2015) in utterance-final position when the subglottal pressure is low, at least for some speakers of American English (Slifka, 2000, 2006). If unconstricted creaky voice occurs due to low subglottal pressure, it should also occur in similar environments in other languages.

Given that creaky voice represents a cluster of vocal fold articulations and voice qualities, one might be inclined to ask whether phoneticians should retain the more general term "creaky" at all. I believe we should, because it is useful to have a word for the abstract phonological category, which may be realized (in different phonological environments and/or by different speakers) using different articulations. For instance, it is useful to have a "creaky" phonological category in Jalapa Mazatec, since this phonation type contrasts with more modal and breathy voice qualities. However, we know that the "creaky" voice type varies phonetically by lexical tone and preceding consonant in the language (Garellek and Keating, 2011; Kuang, 2013a), and likely also by prosodic position, talker, and other factors.

In sum, we can analyze languages' use of voice primarily in terms of vocal fold approximation and voicing, which in turn may differ by rate and quality. There are other dimensions of the voice, including whisper and vocal intensity, but these generally play smaller roles in phonologies of the world's languages (cf. Fulop and Golston, 2008 for the role of whispery voice in White Hmong). Vocal intensity, which is important for stress (Gordon and Applebaum, 2010), is controlled mostly by the subglottal pressure, but also by vocal fold and supralaryngeal adjustments (Sundberg, 1987; Zhang, 2016b). Having reviewed the primary dimensions of the voice used to make sounds of the world's languages, we will now turn to a model of how language users produce and perceive these dimensions.

A psychoacoustic model of the voice

One of the biggest challenges with modeling the voice is that voice articulation, acoustics, and perception are inherently multidimensional. The vocal folds have a complex structure and vibrate in a three-dimensional space. Acoustically, one can model the voice source in both temporal and spectral domains, and within each domain there are many different attributes to the voice that can be parameterized (Cumming and Clements, 1995; Gobl and Ní Chasaide, 2010; Kreiman et al., 2010; Kreiman et al., 2015). Voice perception is also extremely complex; there are dozens of ways of characterizing the voice (Kreiman and Sidtis, 2011), with terminologies and relevant taxonomies varying by discipline. For example, a whispery voice quality might not be a primary voice dimension in sounds of the world's languages, but it is common in speech and is associated with certain speech disorders (Laver, 1980; Sapienza et al., 2011; Gick et al., 2013). As discussed in the Introduction, models of voice articulation and acoustics may not be able to account for all perceptual changes in voice quality, or may have articulatory and acoustic parameters that are irrelevant for perception (Zhang et al., 2013; Kreiman et al., 2014; Garellek et al., 2016). Since our main goal in studying the voice is to link what speakers do with their voices with what listeners hear, models of the voice should link to voice perception; acoustic attributes are important only insofar as they are perceptible, and articulatory attributes only insofar as they result in perceptible acoustic changes.

For these reasons, Kreiman et al. (2014) propose a psychoacoustic model of the voice, shown in Table 4.3, which has the following parameters: Four pertaining to the harmonic structure of the voice source spectrum (the sound produced by the vocal folds, before being filtered by the vocal tract), another parameter for modeling the inharmonic component of the source spectrum (i.e., the noise), two temporal components of the voice source (f_0 and amplitude), and the vocal tract transfer function (which models the filtering from the vocal tract). Only the first three groups are relevant for the voice as it concerns the vocal folds;

Table 4.3 Components of the psychoacoustic model of voice quality and associated parameters (from Kreiman et al., 2014).

Model component	*Parameters*
Harmonic source	H1–H2 (see description in text)
spectral slope (Figure 4.4)	H2–H4
	H4–H2 kHz
	H2 kHz–H5 kHz
Inharmonic source noise	Harmonics-to-noise ratio (HNR)
Time-varying source characteristics	f_0 track
	Amplitude track
Vocal tract transfer function	Formant frequencies and bandwidths
	Spectral zeroes and bandwidths

though resonances and anti-resonances affect overall voice quality, they are here considered independent of the voice source parameters (cf. Cumming and Clements, 1995). This model makes several other important assumptions, notably that its parameters are both necessary and sufficient to model voice quality; thus, with one of these parameters missing, voice quality cannot be faithfully modeled, and no other measures are needed to model the voice.

The temporal parameters (the f_0 and amplitude tracks) relate to the presence of voicing, its rate of vibration, and its amplitude. The harmonic spectral slope parameters represent differences in harmonic amplitudes; thus, H1–H2 refers to the difference in amplitude between the first and second harmonic (Bickley, 1982), H2–H4 is the difference in amplitude between the second and fourth harmonics (Kreiman et al., 2007), H4–H2 kHz is the difference in amplitude between the fourth harmonic and the harmonic closest to 2000 Hz, and H2 kHz–H5 kHz is the difference in amplitude between the harmonic closest to 2000 Hz and the one closest to 5000 Hz (Kreiman et al., 2011). Together, they characterize the voice's "spectral tilt" in various harmonic and frequency bands.

The assumptions regarding the harmonic spectral slope model and its parameters warrant further discussion. The first main assumption is that the spectral tilt parameters can be articulatorily and perceptually independent of f_0, even though it is clear that f_0 changes are associated with changes in spectral tilt (Kuang, 2013a; Garellek et al., 2016; Kuang, 2017a). Thus, with a constant $f_0 = 100$ Hz, a measure like H2–H4 will have a frequency bandwidth of 200 Hz (between 200 Hz and 400 Hz), whereas with a constant f_0 of 200 Hz, the frequency bandwidth of H2–H4 will be 400 Hz (between 400 and 800 Hz). Frequency bandwidth can vary for H1–H2 and H2–H4, as well as well as H4–H2 kHz, though the latter parameter is bounded at the high end by a particular frequency of 2000 Hz. (The source spectrum model is therefore used only for f_0 values below 500 Hz; higher than that, and H4 will be equal to or surpass 2 kHz!) The final parameter H2 kHz–H5 kHz depends on frequency bandwidth alone, not harmonic bandwidth. Overall then, we assume in this model that voice quality is perceptually dependent on spectral tilt between fixed *harmonics* (regardless of their frequency) in the lower-frequency end of the spectrum, and that voice quality is perceptually dependent on spectral tilt between harmonics of fixed *frequencies* at the higher-frequency end of the spectrum. It should be noted here that spectral tilt measures over fixed frequency bands have also been shown to correlate with changes in quality (de Krom, 1995; Hartl et al., 2003; Samlan et al., 2013; Samlan and Kreiman, 2014).

The second main assumption is that we need four spectral tilt parameters. Kreiman et al. (2014) and Garellek et al. (2016) motivate a model of the harmonic source spectrum with four tilt parameters for several reasons. First, spectral tilt can vary independently according to frequency band; thus, spectral tilt can be negative in one portion of the spectrum, but positive in another (Kreiman et al., 2007; Garellek et al. 2016). Another reason for modeling spectral tilt in terms of multiple components is that distinct articulations might be responsible for different tilt components (Zhang et al. 2013). Moreover, source spectra share certain inflection points; for example, it is common for the harmonic slope to change abruptly around 2000 Hz. Finally, listeners are not equally sensitive to every component of spectral tilt (Garellek et al. 2016), and indeed sometimes the slope of one component can cancel out the perceptual effect of another (Garellek et al. 2013). We will also discuss the relevance of these parameters for linguistically relevant dimensions of the voice in the following section.

This model further assumes that it is the slope between harmonics, rather than amplitudes of individual harmonics, that is perceptually relevant for quality (Kreiman et al. 2014; Garellek et al. 2016). For instance, we assume that it is of no importance whether H3 is louder than either H2 or H4; the parameter H2–H4 depends only on the amplitudes of the harmonics adjacent to H3. In our use of this model, we therefore alter the amplitude of the intermediate harmonics to conform to the slope made between the two harmonic endpoints, as shown in Figure 4.4. Note also that the harmonic spectral slope model is based on our analysis of adult voices, and therefore it is unclear whether children's voices could and should be modeled similarly.

The final parameter of the model, the harmonics-to-noise ratio (HNR), refers to the difference in amplitude between the harmonic and inharmonic components of the source spectrum, as measured in the cepstral domain (de Krom, 1993). The choice of HNR as a means of measuring noise in this model assumes that spectral noise is psychoacoustically important (Kreiman and Gerratt, 2005; Shrivastav and Sapienza, 2006; Zhang et al. 2013; Garellek et al. 2016). Although there are many time-domain noise measures like jitter and shimmer, these are not included because they are not perceptually relevant independently of HNR (Kreiman and Gerratt, 2005). The current version of the model also assumes that

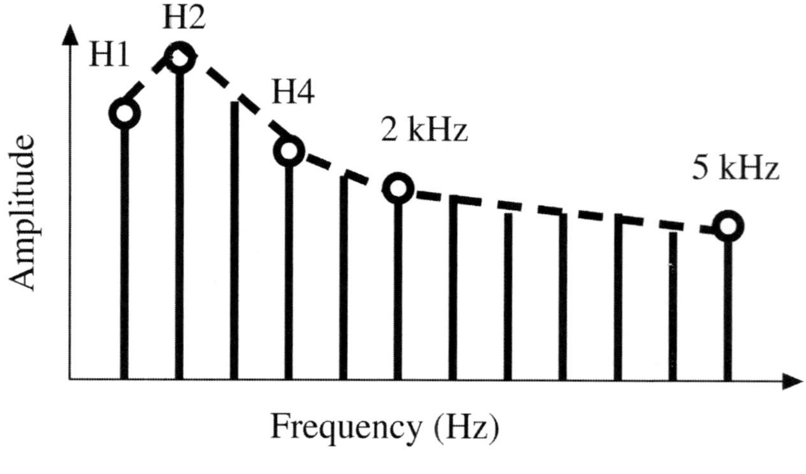

Figure 4.4 The four-parameter harmonic source spectrum model.

Source: Based on Kreiman et al., 2014.

HNR over the entire frequency range is sufficient to model the inharmonic component of the source spectrum. However, it is clear that noise interacts with harmonic components in different frequency bands in distinct ways (Kreiman and Gerratt, 2012; Garellek et al. 2016), and that changes in linguistic uses of voice quality are expressed with more narrowband noise measures (Garellek, 2012). Therefore, much more work is needed to determine how best to model noise and its role in causing changes in voice quality.[3]

A note on how to obtain measurements for these model parameters: Kreiman et al. (2014) and Garellek et al. (2016) calculate these model parameters using inverse filtering of audio recordings followed by analysis-by-synthesis. Although this allows for very accurate source and filter estimation, the main disadvantages of this process are that it is time-consuming and difficult to do on conversational speech (see Gobl and Ní Chasaide, 2010; Kreiman et al., 2010 for more discussion on the matter). However, these model parameters can be estimated from the audio signal if formant correction is used, e.g., with a program like VoiceSauce (Shue et al. 2011). This practice is often used in phonetic studies, but requires accurate formant measurements, which can be problematic with certain sounds. This is discussed in more detail in "Voice quality."

In the following sections, I will show how the primary linguistic dimensions of the voice can be expressed and measured using this psychoacoustic model, and how vocal fold articulation as it concerns these dimensions relates back to the model's parameters.

Acoustic properties of the primary phonological voice dimensions

The primary phonological voice dimensions (vocal fold approximation, voicing, rate of vibration, and quality of voicing) have clear acoustic ramifications that can be measured using the parameters of the psychoacoustic voice model outlined in "A psychoacoustic model of the voice."

Vocal fold approximation

Vocal fold approximation during voiceless sounds has both direct and indirect acoustic consequences. Direct consequences include the absence of periodic energy, and, for minimal vocal fold approximation (i.e., maximal abduction/spreading), the presence of aspiration noise, which in Kreiman et al. (2014)'s model can be measured using HNR (higher values of the measure indicate less noise). Aspiration noise can also be seen in spectra and spectrograms as broadband noise (though filtered by the shape of the vocal tract); in waveforms, aspiration noise is hard to distinguish from other sources of noise, such as frication from the vocal tract. Indirect consequences of vocal fold spreading can be seen on adjacent voiced sounds, which will be breathier, as discussed in "Voice quality."

Complete vocal fold approximation is hard to measure using parameters in Kreiman et al.'s (2014) model, and is hard to see directly in either temporal or spectral domains: If the vocal folds are constricted but not vibrating, then there is no acoustic energy that is produced during the constriction. However, as vocal folds transition from voicing to and from complete constriction, there are indirect consequences present in form of creaky voice on the adjacent sounds. In sum, vocal fold approximation can be measured indirectly through its effects on adjacent voicing, which we will discuss more next.

Voicing

Vocal fold vibration usually produces a complex (quasi-)periodic wave; that is, a wave with many frequency components (Stevens, 2000). The slowest component is the fundamental

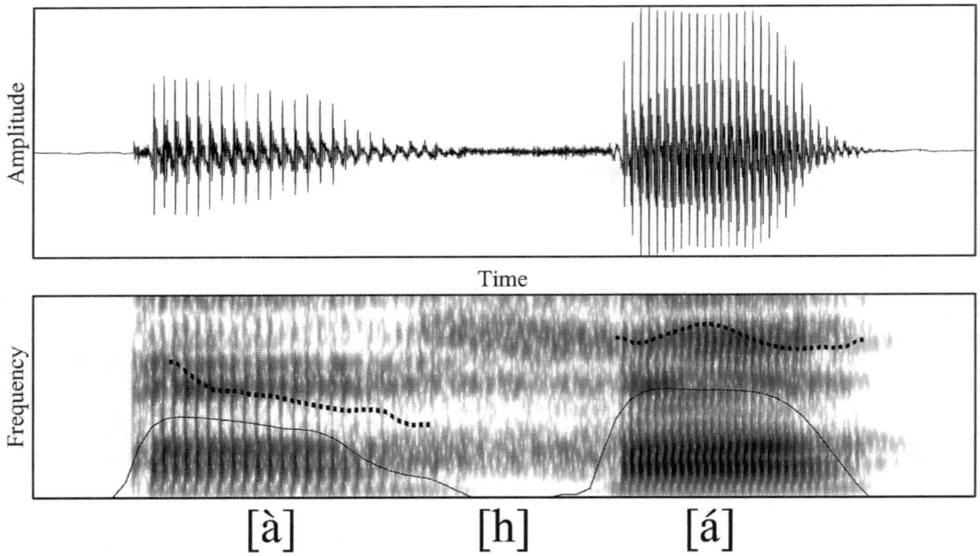

Figure 4.5 Waveform and spectrogram of the sequence [àhá]. The presence of voicing is indicated by the glottal pulses in both displays, as well as by the presence of an f_0 track (shown in the dashed line). The intensity track (the solid horizontal line in the display) provides information on the amplitude of the signal during voicing.

frequency (f_0), and the faster components are whole-integer multiples of the f_0 (see Figure 4.4). Thus, if voicing is present, there must be an f_0. Figure 4.5 illustrates how an f_0 track in the sequence [àhá] aligns with the presence of glottal pulses (the vertical striations) in the waveform and spectrogram. The intensity of voicing (roughly, "how loud" the voice is) can be measured by the psychoacoustic model using the amplitude track, also shown in Figure 4.5.

Rate of vibration

Differences in rate (or frequency) of vocal fold vibrations are reflected in the acoustic signal primarily through changes to the fundamental frequency and its change over time. In the temporal domain, this means that the periodic wave produced during voicing will recur more quickly or slowly, resulting in more closely or distantly spaced glottal pulses. This can be seen in Figure 4.5: Where the glottal pulses are closer together (i.e., in the second vowel), the f_0 track is higher. In the spectral domain, f_0 corresponds to the frequency of the first harmonic, though here temporal change in f_0 is not calculable. Using Kreiman et al. (2014)'s model, we can measure f_0 change using the f_0 track.

Voice quality

As discussed earlier, the three main voice qualities (breathy, modal, and creaky voice), as well as subtypes of creaky voice, can be described in terms of their degree of constriction (or spreading) and noise: Relative to modal voice, breathy voice is both more spread and noisier (because of the presence of aspiration noise), whereas prototypical creaky voice is more constricted and noisier because of irregular pitch.

These two basic dimensions to voice quality – spreading/constriction and noise – have specific acoustic attributes in the psychoacoustic model proposed by Kreiman et al. (2014). The most reliable correlate of increased spreading or constriction during voicing is through increased spectral tilt for spreading and decreased spectral tilt for constriction (Klatt and Klatt, 1990; Gordon and Ladefoged, 2001; Hanson et al., 2001; Kreiman et al., 2012; Chen et al., 2013; Samlan et al., 2013; Keating et al., 2015; Zhang, 2016a). For the four spectral tilt parameters discussed earlier (H1–H2, H2–H4, H4–H2 kHz, and H2 kHz–H5 kHz), greater spectral tilt due to breathy voice would be indicated by higher values of these measures. Of these four spectral slopes, it is clear on the one hand that at least H1–H2 and H2–H4 are relevant phonologically. For example, native speakers of White Hmong can use changes in either of these slopes to perceive their contrastive breathy-voiced tone (Garellek et al., 2013), and many other studies on a variety of languages have shown that breathy and creaky voice correlate with changes in H1–H2 (Bickley, 1982; Gordon and Ladefoged, 2001; Blankenship, 2002; Miller, 2007; DiCanio, 2009; Brunelle and Finkeldey, 2011; Garellek and Keating, 2011; Garellek, 2012; Esposito, 2012; Khan, 2012; Berkson, 2013; DiCanio, 2014; Yu and Lam, 2014; Abramson et al., 2015; Misnadin et al., 2015; Zhang and Yan, 2015; Tian and Kuang, 2016). Listeners of languages with contrastive or allophonic non-modal phonation show differing degrees of sensitivity to H1–H2 (Kreiman et al., 2010; Kreiman and Gerratt, 2010), and H2–H4 is also relevant for listeners' identification of speaker sex (Bishop and Keating, 2012). On the other hand, it is still unclear whether the higher-frequency slopes H4–H2 kHz and H2 kHz–H5 kHz contribute to linguistically relevant voice distinctions, though recent work suggests that they, along with H1–H2 and H2–H4, help differentiate creaky vowels from non-creaky ones in American English (Garellek and Seyfarth, 2016).

Other measures of spectral tilt over different frequency bands, such as H1–A1, H1–A2, and H1–A3 (differences in amplitude between the first harmonic and the harmonic closest to the first, second, and third formants) have proved useful for distinguishing voice qualities or registers in languages of the world (Ní Chasaide and Gobl, 1993; Hanson, 1997; Gordon and Ladefoged, 2001; Hanson et al., 2001; Wayland and Jongman, 2003; Gerfen and Baker, 2005; Andruski, 2006; Di-Canio, 2009; Esposito, 2010a, 2010b; Avelino, 2010; Garellek and Keating, 2011; Brunelle, 2012; Berkson, 2013; Kirby, 2014; Abramson et al., 2015; Tian and Kuang, 2016). There are several important remarks to make on the similarities and differences between these measures and the spectral tilt parameters proposed by Kreiman et al. (2014). First, both types of measures use harmonic-based bandwidths, rather than fixed frequency ranges (see discussion in "A psychoacoustic model of the voice"). Moreover, the harmonics closest to a formant (i.e., A1, A2, and A3) are not defined in a source model. One consequence of this is that measures like H1–A1, H1–A2, and H1–A3 are correlated and can even overlap with the source spectral tilt measures like H1–H2. For instance, the vowel [i] spoken by the average adult male speaker of American English has an F_1 at around 340 Hz (Hillenbrand et al., 1995). So if an adult male speaker of American English says [i] with an f_0 of 150 Hz, the harmonic closest to F_1 is H2. This means that, for this token, H1–H2 would be equal to H1–A1 (see the left panel of Figure 4.6). Thus, depending on context, it might not make sense to measure both H1–H2 and H1–A1 for the same token. However, this issue would not occur when using source spectral parameters like the kind found in Kreiman et al. (2014)'s model, because the model parameters can never overlap in frequency. Of more theoretical relevance is the fact that, for a measure like H1–A1, what counts as "A1" will vary by context. For instance, if the same adult male speaker from the previous example were to say the vowel [ɑ] with an $f_0 = 150$ Hz, then H1–A1 would be equal to the difference in amplitude between the first harmonic and the harmonic closest to roughly 770 Hz, which

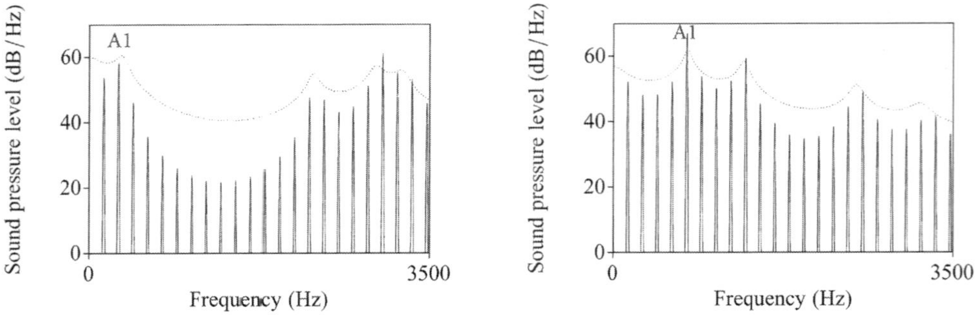

Figure 4.6 FFT and LPC spectra for synthetic [i] (left) and [ɑ] (right) with f_0 = 150 Hz and formants equal to that of an average adult male speaker of American English. For [i] (left), the second harmonic (H2) is also the harmonic closest to the first formant (A1), so H1–H2 equals H1–A1. For [ɑ] (right), H1–A1 equals H1–H5.

is H5 (at roughly 750 Hz, see the right panel of Figure 4.6). Measures like H1–A1, H1–A2, and H1–A3 vary in their harmonic bandwidth depending on the formant frequencies; however, *source* spectral tilt measures like H1–H2 and H2–H4 have fixed harmonic bandwidths and therefore do not depend on vowel quality. Thus, use of measures like H1–A1 assumes that the ways in which spectral tilt can determine voice quality necessarily depend on the vowel quality. For instance, if I compare Mazatec breathy vs. modal vowels of different qualities using H1–A1 (as in Garellek and Keating 2011), then I assume that a relevant way of distinguishing these voice qualities is by comparing the spectral tilt between H1 and the first formant, regardless of the harmonic that is most affected by that formant. But using measures such as H1–H2, H2–H4, H4–H2 kHz, and H2 kHz–H5 kHz implies that voice source characteristics are relevant independent of the filter; although Kreiman et al. (2014) assume that both the source and filter can influence voice quality, they further assume that measuring spectral tilt within fixed harmonic or frequency bands is a relevant way of distinguishing voice quality. It is still unclear which method of representing spectral tilt more closely reflects perception of voice quality: i.e., whether listeners perceive changes in quality more as a function of formant or harmonic-based differences in spectral tilt.

The second important dimension to voice quality is noise, which in the psychoacoustic voice model is calculated in the spectral domain as the HNR. Since breathy voice has aspiration noise (due to the increase in vocal fold spreading or lower vocal fold thickness, see "Voice production"), this will lower the HNR. Numerous studies have shown that HNR measures are useful for distinguishing breathy vs. non-breathy voice qualities used in language (Gordon and Ladefoged, 2001; Blankenship, 2002; Brunelle, 2012; Berkson, 2013; Esposito, 2012; Garellek, 2012; Khan, 2012; Kuang, 2012; Simpson, 2012; Tian and Kuang, 2016). Creaky voice also lowers HNR, but usually this is because of its irregular pitch: If the f_0 is not regular, the signal's noise will increase. Various studies also provide evidence for the use of HNR in distinguish creaky vs. non-creaky voice qualities in language (Blankenship, 2002; Esposito, 2012; Garellek, 2012, 2015; Keating et al., 2015; Garellek and Seyfarth, 2016). "Harsh" voice qualities – which are not reviewed in detail here because they necessarily involve supraglottal constriction (Edmondson et al., 2001; Edmondson and Esling, 2006) – can also have lower HNR (Miller, 2007), due at least in part to the supralaryngeal noise.

Phoneticians often use acoustic measures to categorize different voice qualities. For example, the lower values of H1–H2 in Category A compared with Category B might be used to justify an analysis in which Category A is creaky and Category B is modal. There are, however, two important things to keep in mind with regard to this practice. First, spectral tilt measures like H1–H2 vary continuously between more constricted creaky voice qualities (which have lower H1–H2) and less constricted or breathier voice qualities (which have higher H1–H2); modal voice's spectral tilt is somewhere in between that of constricted creaky and breathy voice. But raw values of spectral tilt measures do not index a precise voice quality; one person's creaky voice can have an average H1–H2 of −2 dB while another person's creaky voice averages 5 dB. Thus, if Category A has a higher H1–H2 than Category B, we cannot know whether the difference between A and B is one between more modal vs. creaky voice, between more breathy vs. modal voice, or between more breathy vs. more creaky voice. This is why spectral tilt measures are often interpreted with respect to noise measures like HNR (Blankenship, 2002; Garellek, 2012; Simpson, 2012; Garellek and White, 2015): if Category A has both a higher H1–H2 and a higher HNR than Category B, then we can assume A is more modal than B, because modal voice generally has higher H1–H2 and HNR values than creaky voice. But if Category A′ has a higher H1–H2 and a *lower* HNR than Category B, then we can assume A′ is breathier than B′, because breathy voice generally has higher H1–H2 and lower HNR values than modal voice (see Table 4.4). Figure 4.7 illustrates the relationship between breathy, modal, and (prototypical) creaky voice in a two-dimensional acoustic space consisting of spectral tilt and HNR.

The second caveat pertains to the fact that lower spectral tilt measures correlate with increased constriction. As we have discussed earlier, not all subtypes of creaky voice are more constricted or noisy than modal voice. For instance, tense voice is constricted, high in pitch, and usually regular in pitch, which means that we would not necessarily expect to find a decrease in HNR for tense voice relative to modal voice. The acoustic characteristics (in terms of both spectral tilt and noise) of various types of creaky voice are shown in Table 4.5.

Another difficulty with measuring voice quality is that when speech sounds travel through air, they bear evidence both of voice characteristics and of the supralaryngeal modulations of the vocal tract. It can sometimes be challenging to infer whether a particular acoustic property is due to voice or supralaryngeal vocal tract articulations: For instance, nasalized vowels (caused by velum lowering) and breathy vowels (caused by vocal fold spreading during voicing) both have higher spectral tilt (Klatt and Klatt, 1990; Simpson, 2012; Garellek et al., 2016). There are several options for researchers who wish to disentangle confounding effects of manner of voicing and supralaryngeal articulation. One can use "inverse filtering" to remove the acoustic effects of other articulators, and measure manner

Table 4.4 Sample H1–H2 and HNR values for two groups of Vowels A vs. B and A′ vs. B′. Even though Vowels A and A′ share the same H1–H2 value (as do B and B′), the HNR differences suggest that Vowel B is creakier than Vowel A, whereas Vowel A′ is breathier than Vowel B′.

	Vowel A	*Vowel B*	Vowel A′	*Vowel B′*
H1-H2	10	5	10	5
HNR	20	10	10	20
Interpretation	A has higher tilt, *less* noise than B. A = modal, B = creaky		A′ has higher tilt, *more* noise than B′. A′ = breathy, B′ = modal	

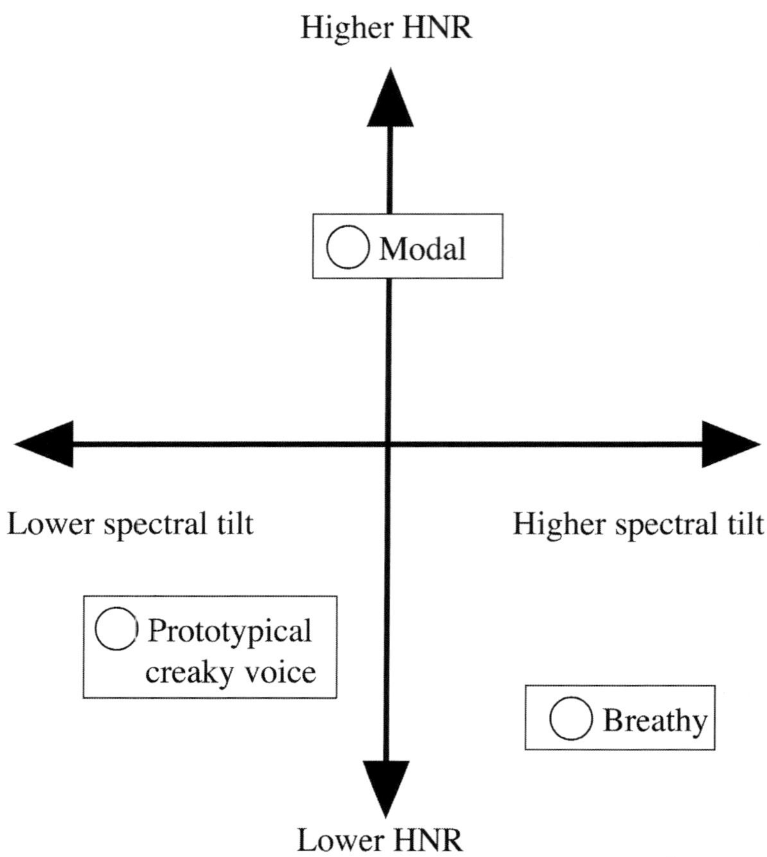

Figure 4.7 Relative acoustic differences between breathy, modal, and (prototypical) creaky voice, in terms of both spectral tilt and noise. The difference in position of breathy voice and prototypical creaky voice on the HNR scale is arbitrary (cf. Blankenship 2002 and Garellek 2012).

Table 4.5 Summary of psychoacoustic voice model's parameters according to primary phonological dimensions of voice.

Dimension	*Relevant model parameters*
Vocal fold approximation	Absence of f_0 track
	Aspiration noise (if vocal folds are spread)
	Voice quality changes on adjacent voiced sounds
Voicing	Presence of f_0 track
Rate of vibration	Frequency of f_0 track
Voice quality	**Breathy voice:**
(compared with modal)	Higher H1–H2, H2–H4, H4–H2 kHz, H2 kHz–H5 kHz
	Lower HNR
	Unconstricted creaky voice:
	Higher H1–H2 H2–H4, H4–H2 kHz, H2 kHz–H5 kHz
	Lower HNR Lower f_0
	Constricted creaky voice qualities
	(Prototypical creaky, tense voice, and vocal fry):
	Lower H1–H2 H2–H4, H4–H2 kHz, H2 kHz–H5 kHz
	Lower HNR (prototypical creaky voice)
	Lower f_0 (prototypical creaky voice and vocal fry)

of voicing from the source waveform (often with the additional step of modeling the waveform using a variety of voice source models; see Ní Chasaide and Gobl, 1993; Epstein, 2002; Gobl and Ní Chasaide, 2010; Kreiman et al., 2015). Another option is to measure spectral tilt and noise from the audio output spectrum, but to "correct for" or undo the effects of the supralaryngeal articulators (Hanson, 1995, 1997; Iseli et al., 2007). However, it should be noted that formant corrections are meant to undo the effects of vowel formants specifically; thus, they cannot remove the effects of nasalization or consonantal resonances (Simpson, 2012; Garellek et al., 2016). Of course, formant corrections will also fail whenever the formants are mistracked. This is especially common with high-pitched and breathy voices where the high frequency and energy of the first harmonic can be misidentified as a formant. It is thus recommended that researchers check the f_0 and formant frequencies to ensure that the spectral slope measures are not mistracked due to inaccurate tracking of f_0 or (for "corrected" measures) of the formants. Spectral slope measures whose harmonic amplitudes have been corrected for effects of formants and bandwidths are usually denoted with asterisks, e.g., H1*–H2*. Readers should therefore be aware that different researchers will use a label such as "H1–H2" to refer either to uncorrected spectral tilt derived from the output *audio* spectrum, or to the measure calculated directly from the *source* spectrum.

As mentioned at the start of this section, it is impossible to measure voice quality during a voiceless sound, which makes use of vocal fold approximation as its primary voice dimension. However, differences in vocal fold approximation can have ramifications for voice quality on an adjacent voiced sound. Numerous linguistic studies have shown that vowels adjacent to aspirated sounds are breathier than vowels adjacent to non-aspirated ones; conversely, vowels adjacent to glottalized sounds (including ejectives) tend to be creaky compared to vowels adjacent to nonglottalized ones (Löfqvist and McGowan, 1992; Ní Chasaide and Gobl, 1993; Blankenship, 2002; Vicenik, 2010; DiCanio, 2012; Esposito and Khan, 2012; Garellek, 2012; Gallagher, 2015; Misnadin et al., 2015; Garellek and Seyfarth, 2016). This relationship between voiceless consonants and voice quality during vowels is captured easily in Ladefoged's continuum model, because both voiceless vocal fold spreading/constriction and voice quality are modeled along a single dimension (analogous to our "vocal fold approximation" dimension, see Figure 4.2). For instance, in the sequence [ah], the vocal folds will have to transition from modal voicing to minimal vocal fold approximation, necessarily "passing through" breathy voice. This transition can be seen during the first vowel of [àhá] from Figure 4.5. Using VoiceSauce (Shue et al., 2011) to measure the four spectral tilt parameters from the audio spectra (but correcting for vowel formants), as well as HNR, it is clear that the vowel is breathier in the second half, nearest the [h] (see Figure 4.8): H1*–H2*, H2*–H4*, and H4*–H2 kHz* are higher, whereas HNR is lower (indicating greater noise). Instead, H2 kHz*–H5 kHz* is *lower* in the second half, which is likely due to interactions with high-frequency noise (Kreiman and Gerratt, 2012; Garellek et al., 2016).

Therefore, we can use various parameters of the psychoacoustic model described in "A psychoacoustic model of the voice" to measure acoustic changes in the voice associated with vocal fold approximation, voicing, and its rate and quality. The crucial parameters are f_0 (its presence vs. absence, and its value when present) as well as the source spectral tilt parameters and HNR. The formant parameters of Kreiman et al. (2014)'s model are also important for correcting for spectral tilt parameters like H1*–H2*, which are measured from the output audio spectrum, and when measuring a parameter like H1–A1, which makes reference to formants. In the next section, we show how a model of voice articulation can account for changes in these parameters.

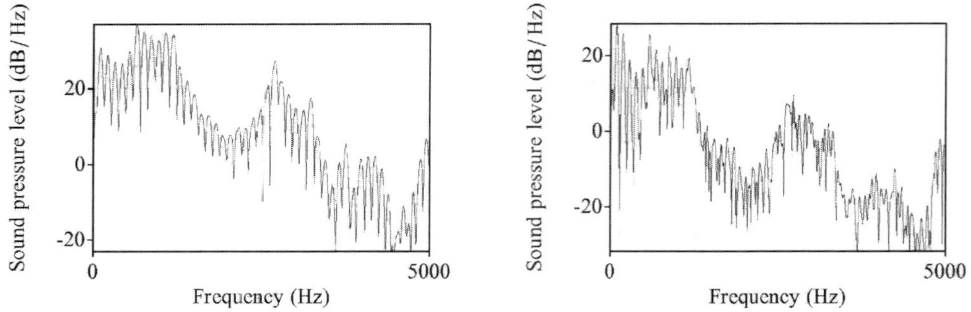

	First half	Second half
H1*–H2* (dB)	1.8	2.6
H2*–H4* (dB)	2.3	10.1
H4*–2 kHz*(dB)	19.1	27.4
2 kHz*–5 kHz* (dB)	0.9	–5.7
CPP (a measure of HNR, dB)	21.3	19.0

Figure 4.8 Top: audio spectra of the first vowel in the sequence [àhá]. The left panel is the spectrum taken over the first half of the vowel; the right panel over the second half. Bottom: spectral tilt parameters and CPP (Cepstral Peak Prominence, a measure of HNR). All acoustic measures but H2 kHz*–H5 kHz* indicate greater breathiness in the second half compared with the first.

Voice production

Voice production is remarkably complex and depends on lung pressure and several muscles that, working together, alter the shape and stiffness of the vocal folds, the distance between them and other laryngeal structures, and the position of the larynx as a whole. There currently exist numerous excellent sources on laryngeal anatomy and physiology as they pertain to speech (e.g., Titze, 1994; Stevens, 2000; Reetz and Jongman, 2008; Hirose, 2010; Kreiman and Sidtis, 2011; Gick et al., 2013), but in this section we will focus on the articulations of the vocal folds that are associated with the primary dimensions of the voice that are used in language (vocal fold approximation and voicing, the latter of which can be further characterized by its rate and manner), and how these relate back to the psychoacoustic voice model discussed in "A psychoacoustic model of the voice."

Measuring vocal fold articulation is fraught with challenges. The first main challenge is that the vocal fold dynamics are multidimensional, which makes it hard to determine what aspects of vocal fold articulation we should be measuring in the first place. For instance, many researchers have noted (via scoping) that individuals with voice disorders have asymmetric vocal fold vibration. Crucially though, asymmetric vibration is also very common in individuals with no voice disorders (Bonilha et al., 2012), and not all vocal fold asymmetries produce relevant changes in voice quality (Zhang et al., 2013; Samlan et al., 2014). The second main challenge is methodological: it is very hard to see and thus measure the vocal folds. Direct observation (e.g., via laryngoscopy) is invasive and limits the types of sounds speakers can make while being scoped and the types of sounds we can observe during imaging. While direct observation of the vocal folds provides extremely important information about vocal kinematics, it also only allows for a two-dimensional bird's-eye view of the superior part of the vocal folds.

Because of these challenges, there is a long-standing tradition (e.g., van den Berg and Tan, 1959) of using physical and, more recently, computational models of vocal fold articulation, which enable researchers to lower the degrees of freedom and determine how individual parameters affect vocal production, acoustics, and quality (Flanagan, 1972; for a recent overview, see Zhang, 2016b). In the remainder of this section, I will outline one such model, and show how its parameters can be used to understand how vocal articulation leads to linguistically relevant changes in voice quality.

Modeling voice articulation

Although the vocal folds are anatomically and physiologically complex, we can describe their linguistically relevant dimensions using a simplified model (Figure 4.9, after Zhang (2015, 2016a, 2017)). This three-dimensional model of the vocal folds has been used to simulate computationally the effects of various vocal fold parameters on voicing. Although there are many other models of vocal fold vibration (Isogai et al., 1988; Titze et al., 1995; Titze, 2006; Samlan and Story, 2011; Story, 2012; see also a recent overview in Zhang, 2016b), Zhang's model systematically relates model parameters to acoustic ones, some of which crucially appear in the psychoacoustic voice model described earlier. Therefore, it is particularly useful for assessing the cause-and-effect relationship between voice articulation, acoustics, and perception.

The relevant parameters are vocal fold stiffness in the front–back dimension (represented by the oblique arrow in Figure 4.9), medial surface thickness in the vertical direction, the angle between the vocal folds (the horizontal arrow), and subglottal pressure. This model makes several assumptions (which are described in detail in Zhang 2015, 2016a, 2017), and at present does not include interactions between the subglottal and supraglottal tracts. Though the vocal

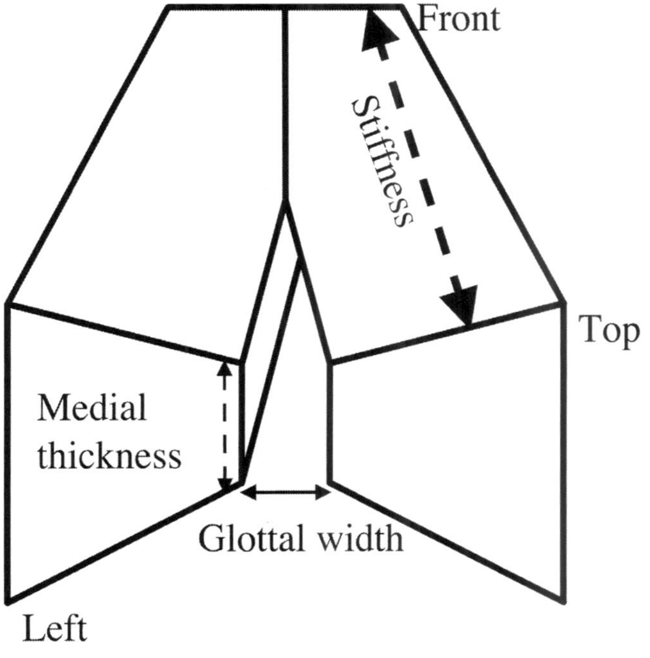

Figure 4.9 Simplified model of the vocal folds, after (Zhang, 2015, 2016a). The primary voice dimensions are influenced mainly by glottal width (the angle between the folds, thin unbroken arrow), their medial vertical thickness (thin dashed arrow), their stiffness from front to back (thick dashed arrow), and the interactions of these parameters with the subglottal pressure. Transverse stiffness is also included in later models (Zhang, 2017), but is less relevant for the primary voice dimensions in language (as discussed in text).

folds have multiple layers (Hirose, 1997; Kreiman and Sidtis, 2011; Gick et al., 2013; Zhang, 2016*b*) and are often simplified as a two-layered structure composed of a body and a cover (Hirano and Katika, 1985), Zhang (2016a) models the folds as a one-layer structure because the vocal fold body and cover rarely differ in stiffness (see also discussion for a two-layered version of the model in Zhang 2017). Moreover, Zhang (2016a) models only front–back stiffness because different degrees of muscular activation had strong effects on this dimension but much smaller effects on transverse stiffness (Yin and Zhang, 2013). Zhang (2017) also models transverse stiffness (set to identical values for body and cover layers), but its effects are mostly limited to phonation pressure threshold, where increasing transverse thickness results in an increase in the phonation pressure threshold, especially when the glottal width is large.

All of these parameters can vary in degree with changes in activation of laryngeal muscles as well as respiration. In the remainder of this section, I will review how these model parameters have been shown to, or might eventually be shown to, produce the primary linguistic dimensions of the voice that are used in sounds of the world's languages. A summary is shown in Table 4.6.

Table 4.6 Summary of Zhang (2015, 2016a, 2017)'s articulatory voice model's parameters according to primary phonological dimensions of voice. The initiation and sustaining of voicing depends on complex interactions between the four parameters (for more details, see Zhang 2016a). The precise model parameters required for some voice qualities are at present speculative (and are marked by an asterisk *), but are based on articulatory and acoustic characteristics described in previous studies, as described in "Primary linguistic voice dimensions."

Dimension	*Relevant model parameters*
Approximation	Glottal width
Voicing	Glottal width
	Medial vocal fold thickness
	Vocal fold stiffness
	Subglottal pressure
Rate of vibration	*To raise f_0:*
	Greater vocal fold stiffness
	Greater subglottal pressure
	Smaller glottal width
Voice quality	**Breathy voice:**
(compared with modal)	Less vocal fold thickness
	Larger glottal width
	***Unconstricted creaky voice**:
	Less vocal fold thickness
	Larger glottal width
	Less vocal fold stiffness
	Lower subglottal pressure
	Constricted creaky voice qualities
	(Prototypical creaky voice, tense voice, and vocal fry):
	More vocal fold thickness
	Smaller glottal width (Tense voice, vocal fry, and *prototypical creaky)
	Less vocal fold stiffness (Vocal fry and *prototypical creaky)
	Lower subglottal pressure (Vocal fry)

Vocal fold approximation

Zhang (2015, 2016*a*) models vocal fold articulation during voicing, and not voiceless vocal fold approximation used for aspirated and glottalized sounds. Nonetheless, we know that vocal fold approximation can be described by a continuum of glottal width, following the continuum and valves models described in "Primary linguistic voice dimensions." This dimension is indeed parameterized in Zhang (2015, 2016*a*)'s model as the angle between the two folds, or "glottal width" (the horizontal arrow in Figure 4.9). This should therefore be the primary parameter responsible for changes in vocal fold approximation that are used to make voiceless aspirated and glottalized consonants.

As we reviewed in "Primary linguistic voice dimensions," other voiceless sounds can be described as being in a "prephonation" state, during which the vocal folds are close together but not completely adducted, nor spread enough to produce much aspiration noise (Harris, 1999; Esling and Harris, 2003; Edmondson et al., 2011). This too can be modeled articulatorily using the glottal width parameter in Zhang (2015, 2016*a*)'s model. Yet we also know that voiceless unaspirated (and voiceless aspirated) stops are often followed by a rise in f_0 (Hombert et al., 1979). This may imply that the mechanisms involved in f_0 control (see "Rate of vibration") can also be involved in the production of voiceless stops. However, increased activation of the cricothyroid muscle (which results in increased vocal fold stiffness) is not clearly associated with production of voiceless stops (Hirose and Gay, 1972; Hombert et al., 1979); thus, Hombert et al. (1979) speculate that raising of the whole larynx, which indirectly affects vocal fold stiffness and thus f_0, can be responsible for this effect (see also Honda et al., 1999; Stevens, 2000; Brunelle, 2010).

Voicing

The mechanism of voicing is usually characterized by the myoelastic aerodynamic theory (van den Berg, 1958) and its more recent extensions (Titze, 2006). According to this theory, the combination of tissue elasticity (e.g., altering the stiffness of the intrinsic laryngeal muscles) and aerodynamic forces is responsible for initiating, sustaining, and ending the vibration of the folds. Vibration usually cannot start until after the vocal folds are brought together or nearly so, in order to build up the subglottal pressure (3–5 cm H_20 for modal voice, Titze, 1992). In his model simulations, Zhang (2016*a*) found that the most important parameter to voicing onset is the angle between the vocal folds: The greater the angle between the folds, the higher the pressure must be to initiate voicing (see also Titze, 1992). Vocal fold thickness also matters: The thinner the folds, the higher the pressure needed to initiate voicing, which Zhang (2016a) attributes to the difficulty of very thin vocal folds to maintain a degree of glottal opening that is conducive to voicing against the subglottal pressure. When the vocal folds are thin, their prephonatory glottal opening is much larger than the resting glottal opening, which makes it difficult to initiate voicing. But as vocal fold thickness increases, the resting glottal opening is easier to maintain. This enables voicing to begin at lower pressure, unless the vocal folds are so thick that additional pressure is needed to keep them from remaining closed.

The findings regarding voicing initiation pressure are also important for sounds of language, because at edges of utterances (when the subglottal pressure is low), voicing is accompanied by specific vocal fold changes. For instance, word-initial vowels in English and other languages are often glottalized (as in saying the word "after" with a glottal stop [ʔæftɚ]), especially phrase- and utterance-initially and when stressed (Nakatani and

Dukes, 1977; Umeda, 1978; Pierrehumbert and Talkin, 1992; Dilley et al., 1996; Davidson and Erker, 2014; Garellek, 2013, 2014). Since glottalization involves vocal fold approximation, it would be parameterized with a smaller angle between the vocal folds in this model. The smaller angle between the vocal folds is also associated with lower voicing initiation pressure, which would be beneficial for utterance-initial stressed vowels; these must be strongly voiced (to mark stress) despite the low subglottal pressure (Garellek, 2014).

Rate of vibration

Consistent with earlier work (e.g., Stevens, 2000), Zhang (2016a, 2017) found that rate of vibration depends on three parameters: f_0 increases with greater vocal fold stiffness, subglottal pressure, and vocal fold approximation. The role of increased vocal fold approximation in achieving higher f_0 is interesting for linguistic tonal patterns, because sounds with increased vocal fold adduction are often accompanied by higher f_0 (e.g., Korean fortis stops), and high tones are often accompanied by increased constriction (Kingston, 2005; Kuang, 2013b).

However, the articulatory parameters interact with one another in complicated ways that affect f_0 (and voice quality, which we discuss in the following section), because in human voices the vocal fold stiffness will covary with the other model parameters. For example, Zhang (2016a) finds that the f_0 can be raised by decreasing the glottal width (with or without an increase in the subglottal pressure), but that this is likely to come with greater vocal fold thickness and *low* front-to-back stiffness. The acoustic result is a higher f_0 with more constriction and decreased spectral tilt – essentially, the characteristics of tense voice. However, just raising the vocal fold stiffness parameter will likely be accompanied by decreased vocal fold thickness, which Zhang (2016a, p. 1506) says will be falsetto-like in quality. Falsetto voice is used as a singing register (Sundberg, 1987), but can also be used in language to index various emotions and types of sociolinguistic meaning (Callier, 2013; Stross, 2013; Zimman, 2013; Podesva and Callier, 2015; Starr, 2015). It may also be used for phonological purposes, e.g., as the phonetic implementation of very high-pitched tones such as the high-level tone in Black Miao and the falsetto tones of Hubei Chinese (Kuang, 2013b; Wang and Tang, 2012; Wang, 2015).

Voice quality

In Zhang (2016a)'s model, changes in voice quality are driven by vocal fold approximation, subglottal pressure, vocal fold thickness, and their interactions. Not surprisingly, lower vocal fold approximation (i.e., a greater angle of glottal width) is associated with higher noise (as measured by HNR); within limits, the more the vocal folds are spread, the more turbulent airflow is generated at the glottis. Lower subglottal pressure is also associated with higher noise, because voicing is weaker and less regular in this condition; not surprisingly, languages often have breathy and/or irregular creaky voicing at utterance edges, where the subglottal pressure is low (Rodgers, 1999; Ogden, 2001; Redi and Shattuck-Hufnagel, 2001; Slifka, 2003, 2006; Esling and Edmondson, 2010; Garellek, 2014, 2015; Di Napoli, 2015; Garellek and Seyfarth, 2016; Kuang, 2017b).

Interestingly, increasing vocal fold thickness has a strong influence on spectral tilt. Zhang (2016a) measures tilt using H1–H2, as well as larger frequency bands with reference to H1 (H1–H4, H1–H2 kHz, and H1–H5 kHz); aside from H1–H2, the other bands are not equivalent to the parameters from Kreiman et al. (2014)'s psychoacoustic model, though his results should be comparable to some extent. In his simulations, increasing vocal fold thickness results in lower spectral tilt in all frequency bands. Therefore, we would expect measures like H2–H4, H4–H2 kHz, and H2 kHz–H5 kHz to also be lower with increasing thickness. The combination of thick vocal folds with tight approximation, and very low stiffness and subglottal pressure, produces a voice quality that Zhang (2016a) describes as vocal fry-like, with a low f_0, spectral tilt, and noise.

Of the articulatory model's four parameters, only vocal fold thickness had a sizable effect on spectral tilt measures. This has implications for our understanding of linguistic voice quality, because breathy, modal, and creaky voices are usually analyzed and modeled in terms of glottal width (see the continuum and valves models in "Primary linguistic voice dimensions"). Instead, Zhang (2016a)'s results imply that vocal fold thickness should matter more than width in producing changes in voice quality associated with changes in spectral tilt. But because glottal width influences f_0, this parameter might be especially relevant for voice quality changes associated with specific lexical tones (Kingston, 2005; Kuang, 2013b) – and even though vocal fold thickness might contribute more to changes in spectral tilt in model simulations, in human voices this parameter is likely to covary with others in ways which we have yet to fully understand.

Summary of chapter and future work

This chapter provided an overview of the phonetics of voice, as defined narrowly by the activity of the vocal folds. I took as starting points an assumption and descriptive fact regarding the voice: First, I assumed that the study of voice should be driven by what humans can *hear* (rather than what we can *do*); and second, I assumed that the multidimensionality of voice production, acoustics, and perception necessitates a unified model of the voice that is driven by what we can hear.

In this chapter I narrowed considerably the discussion of "what we can hear" by focusing exclusively on linguistic properties of the voice, especially those that we know matter for languages' sound systems: Vocal fold approximation, voicing, rate of vibration, and quality of voicing. A combination of these four dimensions can be found in all sounds of language. Using the psychoacoustic model of the voice developed in Kreiman et al., 2014 and further (regarding the harmonic source spectrum) in Garellek et al., 2016, I showed how these linguistically relevant vocal dimensions can be modeled and measured. Recent articulatory modeling, such as that proposed by Zhang (2015, 2016a), also brings us closer to understanding the links between voice production, acoustics, and voice quality perception. By demonstrating how different aspects of vocal fold dynamics condition changes in the acoustic signal, articulatory and psychoacoustic models also enable us to better understand sound changes involving the different voice dimensions of language (Kirby, 2013, 2014; Kuang and Liberman, 2015; Ratliff, 2015; Brunelle and Kirby, 2016).

The articulatory and psychoacoustic models of the voice reviewed here are continuously being refined and improved; as I mentioned at various points in this chapter, many of their assumptions, and the predictions they make, have yet to be confirmed. Moreover, we are still far from knowing the relevant articulatory and psychoacoustic properties of all linguistically relevant aspects of the voice. For example, Keating et al. (2015) discuss other subtypes of creaky voice not reviewed here, and modeling the temporal characteristics of voice quality is still in its early stages, though temporal properties of the voice are extremely important in language (Nellis and Hollenbach, 1980; Silverman, 2003; DiCanio, 2009; Brunelle et al., 2010; Esposito and Khan, 2012; Garellek, 2012; Remijsen, 2013; Garellek and Seyfarth, 2016; Yu, 2017). Much further work is also needed to determine how to integrate other laryngeal and supralaryngeal structures with these models, since it is clear that the phonetics of the voice and its linguistic patterns cannot be separated completely from the rest of the vocal tract, or even the rest of the larynx (Edmondson and Esling, 2006; Moisik and Esling, 2011; Kuang, 2011; Brunelle, 2012; Story, 2012; Moisik and Esling, 2014; Samlan and Kreiman, 2014; Brunelle and Kirby, 2016; Garellek et al., 2016; Kuang and Cui, 2016; Carignan, 2017). For instance, recent modeling work by Story (2012) involves synthesis of voice (including aspiration) and supralaryngeal articulations, along with their time-varying characteristics. Moreover, the role of the voice in indexing non-phonological meaning (including differences based on age, sex, and gender) is also an important component to linguistic studies of the voice (Iseli et al., 2007; Zhuang and Hasegawa-Johnson, 2008; Esling and Edmondson, 2010; Kreiman and Sidtis, 2011; Mendoza-Denton, 2011; Callier, 2013; Zimman, 2013; Podesva and Callier, 2015; Starr, 2015; Park et al., 2016). Finally, through interdisciplinary research we stand to learn much more about how our voices convey different types of meaning.

Notes

1 I thank editors William Katz and Peter Assmann, an anonymous reviewer, Adam Chong, Pat Keating, Jody Kreiman, Yaqian Huang, and Robin Samlan for their thoughtful comments and suggestions on earlier versions of this chapter.
2 The transcriptions in Hmong and Mazatec include "Chao letters" (Chao, 1930) for differences in lexical tone: the vertical bar reflects the pitch range from lowest (Level 1) to highest (Level 5) in one's normal speaking range, and the horizontal lines perpendicular to the vertical bar represent pitch values along that range from the beginning to the end of the tone.
3 In fact, some current versions of this psychoacoustic voice model parameterize the spectral slope of the inharmonic noise in four frequency bands (Kreiman et al., 2016).

References

Abramson, A. S., Tiede, M. K. and Luangthongkum, T. (2015), 'Voice register in Mon: Acoustics and electroglottography', *Phonetica* **72**, 237–256.

Andruski, J. E. (2006), 'Tone clarity in mixed pitch/phonation-type tones', *Journal of Phonetics* **34**, 388–404.

Avelino, H. (2010), 'Acoustic and electroglottographic analyses of nonpathological, nonmodal phonation', *Journal of Voice* **24**, 270–280.

Baken, R. J. and Orlikoff, R. F. (2000), *Clinical Measurement of Speech and Voice*, Singular Publishing Group, San Diego.

Batliner, A., Burger, S., Johne, B. and Kießling, A. (1993), 'MÜSLI: A classifcation scheme for laryngealizations', *in Proceedings of ESCA Workshop on Prosody*, BMET, Lund, pp. 176–179.

Berkson, K. H. (2013), 'Phonation types in Marathi: An acoustic investigation', PhD thesis, University of Kansas.

Bickley, C. (1982), 'Acoustic analysis and perception of breathy vowels', *MIT Speech Communication Working Papers* **1**, 71–81.

Bishop, J. and Keating, P. (2012), 'Perception of pitch location within a speaker's range: Fundamental frequency, voice quality and speaker sex', *The Journal of the Acoustical Society of America* **132**, 1100–1112.

Blankenship, B. (2002), 'The timing of nonmodal phonation in vowels', *The Journal of Phonetics* **30**, 163–191.

Bonilha, H. S., Deliyski, D. D., Whiteside, J. P. and Gerlach, T. T. (2012), 'Vocal fold phase asymmetries in patients with voice disorders: A study across visualization techniques', *American Journal of Speech-Language Pathology* **21**, 3–15.

Brunelle, M. (2010), 'The role of larynx height in the Javanese tense ~ lax stop contrast', *in* R. Mercado, E. Potsdam and L. D. Travis, eds, *Austronesian and Theoretical Linguistics*, John Benjamins, Amsterdam, pp. 7–24.

Brunelle, M. (2012), 'Dialect experience and perceptual integrality in phonological registers: Fundamental frequency, voice quality and the first formant in Cham', *The Journal of the Acoustical Society of America* **131**, 3088–3102.

Brunelle, M. and Finkeldey, J. (2011), 'Tone perception in Sgaw Karen', *in Proceedings of the 17th International Congress of Phonetic Sciences*, Hong Kong, pp. 372–375. https://www.internationalphoneticassociation.org/icphs/icphs2011

Brunelle, M. and Kirby, J. (2016), 'Tone and phonation in Southeast Asian languages', *Language and Linguistics Compass* **10**, 191–207.

Brunelle, M., Nguyễn, D. D. and Nguyễn, K. H. (2010), 'A laryngographic and laryngoscopic study of Northern Vietnamese tones', *Phonetica* **67**, 147–169.

Callier, P. (2013), 'Linguistic context and the social meaning of voice quality variation', PhD thesis, Georgetown University.

Campbell, N. and Beckman, M. (1997), 'Stress, prominence, and spectral tilt', *in Intonation: Theory, Models, and Applications, International Speech Communication Association*, Athens, Greece, pp. 67–70.

Carignan, C. (2017), 'Covariation of nasalization, tongue height, and breathiness in the realization of F1 of Southern French nasal vowels', *Journal of Phonetics* **63**, 87–105.

Chao, Y. R. (1930), 'A system of "tone-letters" ', *Le Maître Phonétique* **45**, 24–27.

Chen, G., Kreiman, J., Gerratt, B. R., Neubauer, J., Shue, Y.-L. and Alwan, A. (2013), 'Development of a glottal area index that integrates glottal gap size and open quotient', *The Journal of the Acoustical Society of America* **133**, 1656–1666.

Choi, J-Y., Hasegawa-Johnson, M. and Cole, J. (2005), 'Finding intonational boundaries using acoustic cues related to the voice source', *The Journal of the Acoustical Society of America* **118**, 2579–2587.

Cumming, K. E. and Clements, M. A. (1995), 'Glottal models for digital speech processing: A historical survey and new results', *Digital Signal Processing* **5**, 21–42.

Davidson, L. and Erker, D. (2014), 'Hiatus resolution in American English: The case against glide insertion', *Language* **90**, 482–514.

de Krom, G. (1993), 'A cepstrum-based technique for determining harmonics-to-noise ratio in speech signals', *Journal of Speech and Hearing Research* **36**, 254–266.

de Krom, G. (1995), 'Some spectral correlates of pathological breathy and rough voice quality for different types of vowel fragments', *Journal of Speech and Hearing Research* **38**, 794–811.

Denes, P. B. and Pinson, E. N. (1993), *The Speech Chain: The Physics and Biology of Spoken Language*, 2nd edn, W. H. Freeman, New York.

Di Napoli, J. (2015), 'Glottalization at phrase boundaries in Tuscan and Roman Italian', *in* J. Romero and M. Riera, eds, *The Phonetics – Phonology Interface: Representations and Methodologies*, John Benjamins, Amsterdam.

DiCanio, C. T. (2009), 'The phonetics of register in Takhian Thong Chong', *Journal of the International Phonetic Association* **39**, 162–188.

DiCanio, C. T. (2012), 'Coarticulation between tone and glottal consonants in Itunyoso Trique', *Journal of Phonetics* **40**, 162–176.

DiCanio, C. T. (2014), 'Cue weight in the perception of Trique glottal consonants', *The Journal of the Acoustical Society of America* **119**, 3059–3071.

Dilley, L., Shattuck-Hufnagel, S. and Ostendorf, M. (1996), 'Glottalization of word-initial vowels as a function of prosodic structure', *Journal of Phonetics* **24**, 423–444.

Edmondson, J. A., Chang, Y., Hsieh, F. and Huang, H. J. (2011), 'Reinforcing voiceless finals in Taiwanese and Hakka: Laryngoscopic case studies', *in Proceedings of the 17th International Congress of Phonetic Sciences*, Hong Kong. https://www.internationalphoneticassociation.org/icphs/icphs2011

Edmondson, J. A. and Esling, J. H. (2006), 'The valves of the throat and their functioning in tone, vocal register and stress: Laryngoscopic case studies', *Phonology* **23**, 157–191.

Edmondson, J. A., Esling, J. H., Harris, J. G., Li, S. and Ziwo, L. (2001), 'The aryepiglottic folds and voice quality in the Yi and Bai languages: laryngoscopic case studies', *Mon-Khmer Studies*, 83–100.

Epstein, M. A. (2002), 'Voice quality and prosody in English', PhD thesis, UCLA.

Esling, J. H. and Edmondson, J. A. (2010), 'Acoustical analysis of voice quality for sociophonetic purposes', *in* M. D. Paolo and M. Yaeger-Dror, eds, *Sociophonetics: A student's guide*, Routledge, London, chapter 11.

Esling, J. H. and Harris, J. G. (2003), 'An expanded taxonomy of states of the glottis', *in Proceedings of the International Congress of Phonetic Science*, Barcelona, pp. 1049–1052. https://www.internationalphoneticassociation.org/icphs-proceedings/ICPhS2003/index.html

Esling, J. H. and Harris, J. G. (2005), 'States of the glottis: An articulatory phonetic model based on laryngoscopic observations', *in* W. J. Hardcastle and J. M. Beck, eds, *A Figure of Speech: A Festschrift for John Laver*, Lawerence Erlbaum Associates, Mahwah, NJ, pp. 347–383.

Esposito, C. M. (2010a), 'The effects of linguistic experience on the perception of phonation', *Journal of Phonetics* **38**, 306–316.

Esposito, C. M. (2010b), 'Variation in contrastive phonation in Santa Ana Del Valle Zapotec', *Journal of the International Phonetic Association* **40**, 181–198.

Esposito, C. M. (2012), 'An acoustic and electroglottographic study of White Hmong phonation', *Journal of Phonetics* **40**, 466–476.

Esposito, C. M. and Khan, S. (2012), 'Contrastive breathiness across consonants and vowels: A comparative study of Gujarati and White Hmong', *Journal of the International Phonetic Association* **42**, 123–143.

Flanagan, J. L. (1972), *Speech Analysis, Synthesis, and Perception*, Springer, Berlin.

Fulop, S. A. and Golston, C. (2008), 'Breathy and whispery voice in White Hmong', *Proceedings of Meetings on Acoustics* **4**, 060006.

Gallagher, G. (2015), 'Natural classes in cooccurrence constraints', *Lingua* **166**, 80–98.

Garellek, M. (2012), 'The timing and sequencing of coarticulated non-modal phonation in English and White Hmong', *Journal of Phonetics* **40**, 152–161.

Garellek, M. (2013), 'Production and perception of glottal stops', PhD thesis, UCLA.

Garellek, M. (2014), 'Voice quality strengthening and glottalization', *Journal of Phonetics* **45**, 106–113.

Garellek, M. (2015), 'Perception of glottalization and phrase-final creak', *The Journal of the Acoustical Society of America* **137**, 822–831.

Garellek, M. and Keating, P. (2011), 'The acoustic consequences of phonation and tone interactions in Jalapa Mazatec', *Journal of the International Phonetic Association* **41**, 185–205.

Garellek, M., Keating, P., Esposito, C. M. and Kreiman, J. (2013), 'Voice quality and tone identification in White Hmong', *The Journal of the Acoustical Society of America* **133**, 1078–1089.

Garellek, M., Ritchart, A. and Kuang, J. (2016), 'Breathy voice during nasality: A cross-linguistic study', *Journal of Phonetics* **59**, 110–121.

Garellek, M., Samlan, R., Gerratt, B. R. and Kreiman, J. (2016), 'Modeling the voice source in terms of spectral slopes', *The Journal of the Acoustical Society of America* **139**, 1404–1410.

Garellek, M. and Seyfarth, S. (2016), 'Acoustic differences between English /t/ glottalization and phrasal creak', *in Proceedings of Interspeech 2016*, ISCA, San Francisco, CA, pp. 1054–1058.

Garellek, M. and White, J. (2015), 'Phonetics of Tongan stress', *Journal of the International Phonetic Association* **45**, 13–34.

Gerfen, C. and Baker, K. (2005), 'The production and perception of laryngealized vowels in Coatzospan Mixtec', *Journal of Phonetics* **33**, 311–334.

Gerratt, B. R. and Kreiman, J. (2001), 'Toward a taxonomy of nonmodal phonation', *Journal of Phonetics* **29**, 365–381.

Gick, B., Wilson, I. and Derrick, D. (2013), *Articulatory Phonetics*, Blackwell, Oxford.

Gobl, C. and Ní Chasaide, A. (2010), 'Voice source variation and its communicative functions', *in* W. J. Hardcastle, J. Laver and F. E. Gibbon, eds, *The Handbook of Phonetic Sciences*, 2nd edn, Blackwell, Oxford, chapter 11, pp. 378–423.

Gordon, M. (2014), 'Disentangling stress and pitch accent: Toward a typology of prominence at different prosodic levels', *in* H. van der Hulst, ed, *Word Stress: Theoretical and Typological Issues*, Oxford University Press, Oxford, pp. 83–118.

Gordon, M. and Applebaum, A. (2010), 'Acoustic correlates of stress in Turkish Kabardian', *Journal of the International Phonetic Association* **40**, 35–58.

Gordon, M. and Ladefoged, P. (2001), 'Phonation types: a cross-linguistic overview', *Journal of Phonetics* **29**, 383–406.

Hanson, H. M. (1995), 'Glottal characteristics of female speakers', PhD thesis, Harvard University.

Hanson, H. M. (1997), 'Glottal characteristics of female speakers: Acoustic correlates', *The Journal of the Acoustical Society of America* **101**, 466–481.

Hanson, H. M., Stevens, K. N., Kuo, H-K. J., Chen, M. Y. and Slifka, J. (2001), 'Towards models of phonation', *Journal of Phonetics* **29**, 451–480.

Harris, J. G. (1999), 'States of the glottis for voiceless plosives', *in Proceedings of the International Congress of Phonetic Sciences*, San Francisco, CA, pp. 2041–2044. https://www.internationalphoneticassociation.org/icphs-proceedings/ICPhS1999/index.html

Hartl, D. M., Hans, S., Vessie're, J. and Brasnu, D. F. (2003), 'Objective acoustic and aerodynamic measures of breathiness in paralytic dysphonia', *European Archives of Oto-Rhino-Laryngology* **260**, 175–182.

Hillenbrand, J. M., Getty, L. A., Clark, M. J. and Wheeler, K. (1995), 'Acoustic characteristics of American English vowels', *The Journal of the Acoustical Society of America* **97**, 3099–3111.

Hillenbrand, J. M. and Houde, R. A. (1996), 'Role of F0 and amplitude in the perception of glottal stops', *Journal of Speech and Hearing Research* **39**, 1182–1190.

Hirano, M. and Katika, Y. (1985), 'Cover-body theory of vocal fold vibration', *in* R. G. Daniloff, ed, *Speech Science: Recent Advances*, College-Hill Press, San Diego, pp. 1–46.

Hirose, H. (1997), 'Investigating the physiology of laryngeal structures', *in* W. J. Hardcastle and J. Laver, eds, *The Handbook of Phonetic Sciences*, Blackwell, Oxford, pp. 116–136.

Hirose, H. (2010), 'Investigating the physiology of laryngeal structures', *in* W. J. Hardcastle, J. Laver and F. E. Gibbon, eds, *The Handbook of Phonetic Sciences*, 2nd edn, Blackwell, Oxford, pp. 130–152.

Hirose, H. and Gay, T. (1972), 'The activity of the intrinsic laryngeal muscles in voicing control', *Phonetica* **25**, 140–164.

Hombert, J-M., Ohala, J. J. and Ewan, W. G. (1979), 'Phonetic explanations for the development of tones', *Language* **55**, 37–58.

Honda, K., Hirai, H., Masaki, S. and Shimada, Y. (1999), 'Role of vertical larynx movement and cervical lordosis in F0 control', *Language and Speech* **42**, 401–411.

Iseli, M., Shue, Y-L. and Alwan, A. (2007), 'Age, sex, and vowel dependencies of acoustic measures related to the voice source', *The Journal of the Acoustical Society of America* **121**, 2283–2295.

Isogai, Y., Horiguchi, S., Honda, K., Aoki, Y., Hirose, H. and Saito, S. (1988), 'A dynamic simulation model of vocal fold vibration', *in* O. Fujimura, ed, *Vocal Physiology: Voice Production, Mechanisms and Functions*, Raven Press, New York, pp. 191–206.

Kane, J., Drugman, T. and Gobl, C. (2013), 'Improved automatic detection of creak', *Computer Speech and Language* **27**, 1028–1047.

Keating, P., Esposito, C., Garellek, M., Khan, S. and Kuang, J. (2011), 'Phonation contrasts across languages', *in Proceedings of the International Congress of Phonetic Sciences*, Hong Kong, pp. 1046–1049. https://www.internationalphoneticassociation.org/icphs/icphs2011

Keating, P., Garellek, M. and Kreiman, J. (2015), 'Acoustic properties of different kinds of creaky voice', in The Scottish Consortium for ICPhS 2015 (Ed.), *Proceedings of the 18th International Congress of Phonetic Sciences*, Glasgow, UK: The University of Glasgow. https://www.internationalphoneticassociation.org/icphs/icphs2011

Kempster, G. B., Gerratt, B. R., Abbott, K. V., Barkmeier-Kraemer, J. and Hillman, R. E. (2011), 'Consensus auditory-perceptual evaluation of voice: Development of a standardized clinical protocol', *American Journal of Speech-Language Pathology* **18**, 124–132.

Khan, S. (2012), 'The phonetics of contrastive phonation in Gujarati', *Journal of Phonetics* **40**, 780–795.

Kingston, J. (2005), *The Phonetics of Athabaskan Tonogenesis*, John Benjamins, Amsterdam, pp. 137–184.

Kirby, J. P. (2013), 'The role of probabilistic enhancement in phonologization', *in* A. C. L. Yu, ed, *Origins of Sound Change: Approaches to Phonologization*, Oxford University Press, Oxford, pp. 228–246.

Kirby, J. P. (2014), 'Incipient tonogenesis in Phnom Penh Khmer: Acoustic and perceptual studies', *Journal of Phonetics* **43**, 69–85.

Klatt, D. H. and Klatt, L. C. (1990), 'Analysis, synthesis, and perception of voice quality variations among female and male talkers', *The Journal of the Acoustical Society of America* **87**, 820–857.

Kreiman, J. (1982), 'Perception of sentence and paragraph boundaries in natural conversation', *Journal of Phonetics* **10**, 163–175.

Kreiman, J., Antoñanzas-Barroso, N. and Gerratt, B. R. (2010), 'Integrated software for analysis and synthesis of voice quality', *Behavior Research Methods* **42**, 1030–1041.

Kreiman, J., Antoñanzas-Barroso, N. and Gerratt, B. R. (2016), 'The UCLA voice synthesizer, version 2.0', *The Journal of the Acoustical Society of America* **140**, 2961.

Kreiman, J., Garellek, M., Chen, G., Alwan, A. and Gerratt, B. R. (2015), 'Perceptual evaluation of voice source models', *The Journal of the Acoustical Society of America* **138**, 1–10.

Kreiman, J., Garellek, M. and Esposito, C. (2011), 'Perceptual importance of the voice source spectrum from H2 to 2 kHz', *The Journal of the Acoustical Society of America* **130**, 2570.

Kreiman, J., Gerratt, B. and Antoñanzas-Barroso, N. (2007), 'Measures of the glottal source spectrum', *Journal of Speech, Language, and Hearing Research* **50**, 595–610.

Kreiman, J. and Gerratt, B. R. (2005), 'Perception of aperiodicity in pathological voice', *The Journal of the Acoustical Society of America* **117**, 2201–2211.

Kreiman, J. and Gerratt, B. R. (2010), 'Perceptual sensitivity to first harmonic amplitude in the voice source', *The Journal of the Acoustical Society of America* **128**, 2085–2089.

Kreiman, J. and Gerratt, B. R. (2012), 'Perceptual interaction of the harmonic source and noise in voice', *The Journal of the Acoustical Society of America* **131**, 492–500.

Kreiman, J., Gerratt, B. R., Garellek, M., Samlan, R. and Zhang, Z. (2014), 'Toward a unified theory of voice production and perception', *Loquens* **e009**.

Kreiman, J., Gerratt, B. R. and Khan, S. (2010), 'Effects of native language on perception of voice quality', *Journal of Phonetics* **38**(4), 588–593.

Kreiman, J., Shue, Y-L., Chen, G., Iseli, M., Gerratt, B. R., Neubauer, J. and Alwan, A. (2012), 'Variability in the relationships among voice quality, harmonic amplitudes, open quotient, and glottal area waveform shape in sustained phonation', *The Journal of the Acoustical Society of America* **132**, 2625–2632.

Kreiman, J. and Sidtis, D. (2011), *Foundations of Voice Studies*, Blackwell, Oxford.

Kuang, J. (2011), 'Production and perception of the phonation contrast in Yi', Master's thesis, UCLA.

Kuang, J. (2012), 'Registers in tonal contrasts', *UCLA Working Papers in Phonetics* **110**, 46–64.

Kuang, J. (2013a), 'Phonation in tonal contrasts', PhD thesis, UCLA.

Kuang, J. (2013b), 'The tonal space of contrastive five level tones', *Phonetica* **70**, 1–23.

Kuang, J. (2017a), 'Covariation between voice quality and pitch: Revisiting the case of Mandarin creaky voice', *The Journal of the Acoustical Society of America* **142**, 1693–1706.

Kuang, J. (2017b), 'Creaky voice as a function of tonal categories and prosodic boundaries', *in Proceedings of Interspeech 2017*, ISCA, Stockholm, pp. 3216–3220.

Kuang, J. and Cui, A. (2016), 'Relative cue weighting in perception and production of a sound change in progress', Talk presented at LabPhon 2016, Cornell, NY.

Kuang, J. and Keating, P. (2014), 'Vocal fold vibratory patterns in tense versus lax phonation contrasts', *The Journal of the Acoustical Society of America* **136**, 2784–2797.

Kuang, J. and Liberman, M. (2015), 'Influence of spectral cues on the perception of pitch height', in The Scottish Consortium for ICPhS 2015 (Ed.), *Proceedings of the 18th International Congress of Phonetic Sciences*, Glasgow, UK: The University of Glasgow. https://www.internationalphoneticassociation.org/icphs/icphs2011

Ladefoged, P. (1971), *Preliminaries to Linguistic Phonetics*, University of Chicago, Chicago.

Lancia, L., Voigt, D. and Krasovitskiy, G. (2016), 'Characterization of laryngealization as irregular vocal fold vibration and interaction with prosodic prominence', *Journal of Phonetics* **54**, 80–97.

Laver, J. (1980), *The Phonetic Description of Voice Quality*, Cambridge University Press, Cambridge.

Löfqvist, A. and McGowan, R. S. (1992), 'Influence of consonantal envelope on voice source aerodynamics', *Journal of Phonetics* **20**, 93–110.

Lombardi, L. (1991), 'Laryngeal features and laryngeal neutralization', PhD thesis, University of Massachusetts.

Maddieson, I., Flavier, S., Marsico, E. and Pellegrino, F. (2016), 'LAPSyD: Lyon-albuquerque phonological systems databases, version 1.0.', www.lapsyd.ddl.ish-lyon. cnrs.fr/lapsyd/. (Last checked on 2018–2006–2014).

Mendoza-Denton, N. (2011), 'The semiotic hitchhiker's guide to creaky voice: Circulation and gendered hardcore in a Chicana/o gang persona', *Journal of Linguistic Anthropology* **21**, 261–280.

Miller, A. L. (2007), 'Guttural vowels and guttural co-articulation in Ju|'hoansi', *Journal of Phonetics* **35**, 56–84.

Misnadin, Kirby, J. P. and Remijsen, B. (2015), 'Temporal and spectral properties of Madurese stops', in The Scottish Consortium for ICPhS 2015 (Ed.), *Proceedings of the 18th International Congress of Phonetic Sciences*, Glasgow, UK: The University of Glasgow. https://www.internationalphoneticassociation.org/icphs/icphs2011

Moisik, S. R. (2013), 'Harsh voice quality and its association with blackness in popular American media', *Phonetica* **69**, 193–215.

Moisik, S. R. and Esling, J. H. (2011), 'The "whole larynx" approach to laryngeal features', *in Proceedings of the 17th International Congress of Phonetic Sciences*, Hong Kong. https://www.internationalphoneticassociation.org/icphs/icphs2011

Moisik, S. R. and Esling, J. H. (2014), 'Modeling the biomechanical influence of epilaryngeal stricture on the vocal folds: A low-dimensional model of vocal-ventricular fold coupling', *Journal of Speech, Language, and Hearing Research* **57**, S687–S704.

Moisik, S. R., Lin, H. and Esling, J. H. (2014), 'A study of laryngeal gestures in Mandarin citation tones using simultaneous laryngoscopy and laryngeal ultrasound (SLLUS)', *Journal of the International Phonetic Association* **44**, 21–58.

Mooshammer, C. (2010), 'Acoustic and laryngographic measures of the laryngeal reflexes of linguistic prominence and vocal effort in German', *The Journal of the Acoustical Society of America* **127**, 1047–1058.

Munhall, K. and Löfqvist, A. (1992), 'Gestural aggregation in speech-laryngeal gestures', *Journal of Phonetics* **20**, 111–126.

Nakatani, L. H. and Dukes, K. D. (1977), 'Locus of segmental cues for word juncture', *The Journal of the Acoustical Society of America* **62**, 714–719.

Nellis, D. G. and Hollenbach, B. E. (1980), 'Fortis versus lenis in Cajonos Zapotec phonology', *International Journal of American Linguistics* **46**, 92–105.

Ní Chasaide, A. and Gobl, C. (1993), 'Contextual variations of the vowel voice source as a function of adjacent consonants', *Language and Speech* **36**, 303–330.

Ogden, R. (2001), 'Turn transition, creak and glottal stop in Finnish talk-in-interaction', *Journal of the International Phonetic Association* **31**, 139–152.

Park, S. J., Sigouin, C., Kreiman, J., Keating, P., Guo, J., Yeung, G., Kuo, F-Y. and Alwan, A. (2016), 'Speaker identity and voice quality: Modeling human responses and automatic speaker recognition', *in Proceedings of Interspeech 2016*, ISCA, San Francisco, CA, pp. 1044–1048.

Pierrehumbert, J. and Talkin, D. (1992), 'Lenition of /h/ and glottal stop', *in* G. J. Docherty and D. R. Ladd, eds, *Papers in Laboratory Phonology II*, Cambridge University Press, Cambridge, pp. 90–117.

Podesva, R. J. and Callier, P. (2015), 'Voice quality and identity', *Annual Review of Applied Linguistics* **35**, 173–194.

Ratliff, M. (2015), 'Tonoexodus, tonogenesis, and tone change', *in* P. Honeybone and J. Salmons, eds, *The Oxford Handbook of Historical Phonology*, Oxford University Press, Oxford, pp. 245–261.

Redi, L. and Shattuck-Hufnagel, S. (2001), 'Variation in the realization of glottalization in normal speakers', *Journal of Phonetics* **29**, 407–429.

Reetz, H. and Jongman, A. (2008), *Phonetics: Transcription, Production, Acoustics, and Perception*, Blackwell, Oxford.

Remijsen, B. (2013), 'Tonal alignment is contrastive in falling contours in Dinka', *Language* **89**, 297–327.

Rodgers, J. (1999), 'Three influences on glottalization in read and spontaneous German speech', *Arbeitsberichte des Instituts für Phonetik und digitale Sprachverarbeitung der Universität Kiel* **34**, 177–284.

Samlan, R. A. and Kreiman, J. (2014), 'Perceptual consequences of changes in epilaryngeal area and shape', *The Journal of the Acoustical Society of America* **136**, 2798–2806.

Samlan, R. A. and Story, B. H. (2011), 'Relation of structural and vibratory kinematics of the vocal folds to two acoustic measures of breathy voice based on computational modeling', *Journal of Speech, Language, and Hearing Research* **54**, 1267–1283.

Samlan, R. A., Story, B. H. and Bunton, K. (2013), 'Relation of perceived breathiness to laryngeal kinematics and acoustic measures based on computational modeling', *Journal of Speech, Language, and Hearing Research* **56**, 1209–1223.

Samlan, R. A., Story, B. H., Lotto, A. J. and Bunton, K. (2014), 'Acoustic and perceptual effects of left – right laryngeal asymmetries based on computational modeling', *Journal of Speech, Language, and Hearing Research* **57**, 1619–1637.

Sapienza, C., Hicks, D. M. and Ruddy, B. H. (2011), 'Voice disorders', *in* N. B. Anderson and G. H. Shames, eds, *Human Communication Disorders: An Introduction*, 8th edn, Pearson, Boston, pp. 202–237.

Shrivastav, R. and Sapienza, C. M. (2006), 'Some difference limens for the perception of breathiness', *The Journal of the Acoustical Society of America* **120**, 416–423.

Shue, Y-L., Keating, P. A., Vicenik, C. and Yu, K. (2011), 'VoiceSauce: A program for voice analysis', *in Proceedings of the International Congress of Phonetic Sciences*, Hong Kong, pp. 1846–1849. https://www.internationalphoneticassociation.org/icphs/icphs2011

Silverman, D. (2003), 'Pitch discrimination between breathy vs. modal phonation', *in* J. Local, R. Ogden and R. Temple, eds, *Phonetic Interpretation (Papers in Laboratory Phonology 6)*, Cambridge University Press, Cambridge, pp. 293–304.

Silverman, D., Blankenship, B., Kirk, P. and Ladefoged, P. (1995), 'Phonetic structures in Jalapa Mazatec', *Anthropological Linguistics* **37**, 70–88.

Simpson, A. (2012), 'The first and second harmonics should not be used to measure breathiness in male and female voices', *Journal of Phonetics* **40**, 477–490.

Slifka, J. (2000), 'Respiratory constraints on speech production at prosodic boundaries', PhD thesis, MIT Press.

Slifka, J. (2003), 'Respiratory constraints on speech production: Starting an utterance', *The Journal of the Acoustical Society of America* **114**, 3343–3353.

Slifka, J. (2006), 'Some physiological correlates to regular and irregular phonation at the end of an utterance', *Journal of Voice* **20**, 171–186.

Sluijter, A. M. C. and van Heuven, V. J. (1996), 'Spectral balance as an acoustic correlate of linguistic stress', *The Journal of the Acoustical Society of America* **100**, 2471–2485.

Starr, R. L. (2015), 'Sweet voice: The role of voice quality in a Japanese feminine style', *Language in Society* **44**, 1–34.

Stevens, K. N. (2000), *Acoustic Phonetics*, MIT Press, Cambridge.

Story, B. H. (2012), 'Phrase-level speech simulation with an airway modulation model of speech production', *Computer Speech and Language* **27**, 989–1010.

Story, B. H. (2015), 'Mechanisms of voice production', *in* M. A. Redford, ed., *Handbook of Speech Production*, Blackwell, Oxford, pp. 34–58.

Stross, B. (2013), 'Falsetto voice and observational logic: Motivational meanings', *Language in Society* **42**, 139–162.

Sundberg, J. (1987), *The Science of the Singing Voice*, Northern Illinois University Press, DeKalb, IL.

Tian, J. and Kuang, J. (2016), 'Revisiting the register contrast in Shanghai Chinese', *in Proceedings of Tonal Aspects of Languages 2016*, ISCA, Buffalo, NY, pp. 147–151.

Titze, I. R. (1992), 'Phonation threshold pressure: A missing link in glottal aerodynamics', *The Journal of the Acoustical Society of America* **91**, 2926–2935.

Titze, I. R. (1994), *Principles of Voice Production*, Prentice Hall Inc, Engelwood Cliffs, NJ.

Titze, I. R. (2006), *The Myoelastic Aerodynamic Theory of Phonation*, National Centre for Voice and Speech, Iowa City, IA.

Titze, I. R., Schmidt, S. S. and Titze, M. R. (1995), 'Phonation threshold pressure in a physical model of the vocal fold mucosa', *The Journal of the Acoustical Society of America* **97**, 3080–3084.

Traill, A. (1985), *Phonetic and Phonological Studies of the !Xóõ Bushmen*, Buske, Hamburg.

Umeda, N. (1978), 'Occurrence of glottal stops in fluent speech', *The Journal of the Acoustical Society of America* **64**, 88–94.

van den Berg, J. (1958), 'Myoelastic aerodynamic theory of voice production', *Journal of Speech and Hearing Research* **1**, 227–244.

van den Berg, J. and Tan, T. S. (1959), 'Results of experiments with human larynxes', *Practica Oto-Rhino-Laryngologica* **21**, 425–450.

Vicenik, C. (2010), 'An acoustic study of Georgian stop consonants', *Journal of the International Phonetic Association* **40**, 59–92.

Wang, C-Y. (2015), 'Multi-register tone systems and their evolution on the Jianghan plain', PhD thesis, Hong Kong University of Science and Technology.

Wang, C-Y. and Tang, C-J. (2012), 'The falsetto tones of the dialects in Hubei province', *in Proceedings of the 6th International Conference on Speech Prosody,* ISCA, Shanghai, China.

Wayland, R. and Jongman, A. (2003), 'Acoustic correlates of breathy and clear vowels: The case of Khmer', *Journal of Phonetics* **31**, 181–201.

Yanushevskaya, I., Murphy, A., Gobl, C. and Ní Chasaide, A. (2016), 'Perceptual salience of voice source parameters in signaling focal prominence', *in Proceedings of Interspeech 2016*, ISCA, San Francisco, CA, pp. 3161–3165.

Yanushevskaya, I., Ní Chasaide, A. and Gobl, C. (2011), 'Universal and language-specific perception of affect from voice', *in Proceedings of the 17th International Congress of Phonetic Sciences*, Hong Kong, pp. 2208–2211. https://www.internationalphoneticassociation.org/icphs/icphs2011

Yin, J. and Zhang, Z. (2013), 'The influence of thyroarytenoid and cricothyroid muscle activation on vocal fold stiffness and eigenfrequencies', *The Journal of the Acoustical Society of America* **133**, 2972–2983.

Yu, K. M. (2017), 'The role of time in phonetic spaces: temporal resolution in Cantonese tone perception', *Journal of Phonetics* **65**, 126–144.

Yu, K. M. and Lam, H. W. (2014), 'The role of creaky voice in Cantonese tonal perception', *The Journal of the Acoustical Society of America* **136**, 1320–1333.

Zhang, J. and Yan, H. (2015), 'Contextually dependent cue weighting for a laryngeal contrast in Shanghai Wu', *in* The Scottish Consortium for ICPhS 2015 (Ed.), *Proceedings of the 18th International Congress of Phonetic Sciences*, Glasgow, UK: The University of Glasgow, pp. 1–5. https://www.internationalphoneticassociation.org/icphs/icphs2011

Zhang, Z. (2015), 'Regulation of glottal closure and airflow in a three-dimensional phonation model: Implications for vocal intensity control', *The Journal of the Acoustical Society of America* **137**, 898–910.

Zhang, Z. (2016a), 'Cause-effect relationship between vocal fold physiology and voice production in a three-dimensional phonation model', *The Journal of the Acoustical Society of America* **139**, 1493–1507.

Zhang, Z. (2016b), 'Mechanics of human voice production and control', *The Journal of the Acoustical Society of America* **140**, 2614–2635.

Zhang, Z. (2017), 'Effect of vocal fold stiffness on voice production in a three-dimensional bodycover phonation model', *The Journal of the Acoustical Society of America* **142**, 2311–2321.

Zhang, Z., Kreiman, J., Gerratt, B. R. and Garellek, M. (2013), 'Acoustic and perceptual effects of changes in body layer stiffness in symmetric and asymmetric vocal fold models', *The Journal of the Acoustical Society of America* **133**, 453–462.

Zhuang, X. and Hasegawa-Johnson, M. (2008), 'Towards interpretation of creakiness in Switchboard', *in Proceedings of Speech Prosody*, ISCA, pp. 37–40.

Zimman, L. (2013), 'Hegemonic masculinity and the variability of gay-sounding speech: The perceived sexuality of transgender men', *Journal of Language & Sexuality* **2**, 1–39.

5
Articulatory phonetics

Bryan Gick, Murray Schellenberg, Ian Stavness, and Ryan C. Taylor

Articulatory phonetics is broadly concerned with understanding how humans use body structures to produce speech sounds. Articulatory phoneticians use a wide range of tools and techniques to study different aspects of these structures, from their physical form, function and control to their evolution, development and patterns of use. As such, the field of articulatory phonetics interacts with a wide range of other disciplines such as neuroscience, speech-language pathology, motor control, dentistry, cognitive science, biomedical engineering, developmental psychology, otolaryngology, and of course other subfields of phonetics and linguistics.

If articulatory phonetics as a field is indeed concerned with how speech is realized through physical actions, then it stands to reason that our models must include – or at least provide links to – parts of the body. Any attempt to study or describe a thing (such as a body part) is an attempt to reduce its complexity – and the speech apparatus is nothing if not complex. The human vocal tract is a continuous, high-dimensional space with practically unlimited degrees of freedom, and articulatory phoneticians have naturally come up with different ways of reducing the complexity of this space. Of course, when we reduce complexity we also remove or omit potentially important information, so it is important to consider carefully which parts our models and descriptions should include, and which they may leave out.

The present chapter explores some of the approaches traditionally used in the field of articulatory phonetics to describe the vocal tract, then goes on to consider the vocal tract from the lips to the larynx through the lens of a more embodied approach. We use the term "embodied" here in the sense of "situated in the body," where the body includes not just the "meat," but also all aspects of the nervous system including (but not limited to) both motor systems and internal and external sensory systems. Articulatory phonetics is in this sense inherently "embodied," as it attempts to make direct reference to body structures and their communicative functions. However, as articulatory phonetics is relatively young as a scientific (rather than descriptive) field, the broader implications of a more fully embodied approach to theories of speech sounds remain to be explored.

One of the predominant methods phoneticians have used to simplify the speech production system has been to reduce the vocal tract to a single central plane (the *midsagittal* plane). The midsagittal approach to reducing the dimensionality of the vocal tract has been reinforced over the past century by the development of tools such as X-ray that provide images of the midline of the vocal tract (Russell, 1933) and by the utility of the midsagittal approximation of vocal tract area for acoustic modeling (Serrurier et al., 2012; though this method of approximation is not without its challenges, e.g., Anderson et al., 2015). Figure 5.1 shows a two-dimensional outline of the vocal tract. The midsagittal outline, familiar to any student of phonetics, is fairly simple and appears to include all of the major "parts" commonly referred to by phoneticians (tongue, lips, velum, etc.). A serious limitation of the midsagittal reduction method is that it indiscriminately omits everything outside of that plane – indeed, being only an outline of the outer surfaces of the major structures along the midline, this representation omits reference even to any internal structure that may intersect this plane. The resulting outline contains no information about structures, for example, at the sides of the vocal tract, and no reference to any neurally accessible components of the system such as muscles and nerves. While the midsagittal section is certainly helpful for an initial descriptive presentation of the vocal apparatus, it is important to question whether it contains sufficient information to be useful as a scientific model of how the human body is used to articulate speech sounds.

Another way articulatory phoneticians have reduced the dimensionality of the vocal tract is by describing it in terms of a set of fixed, anatomically defined structures, often referred to using familiar body-part terms such as "lips" or "tongue tip." These terms are seldom given technical definitions, leaving it to the reader to interpret their precise meaning and

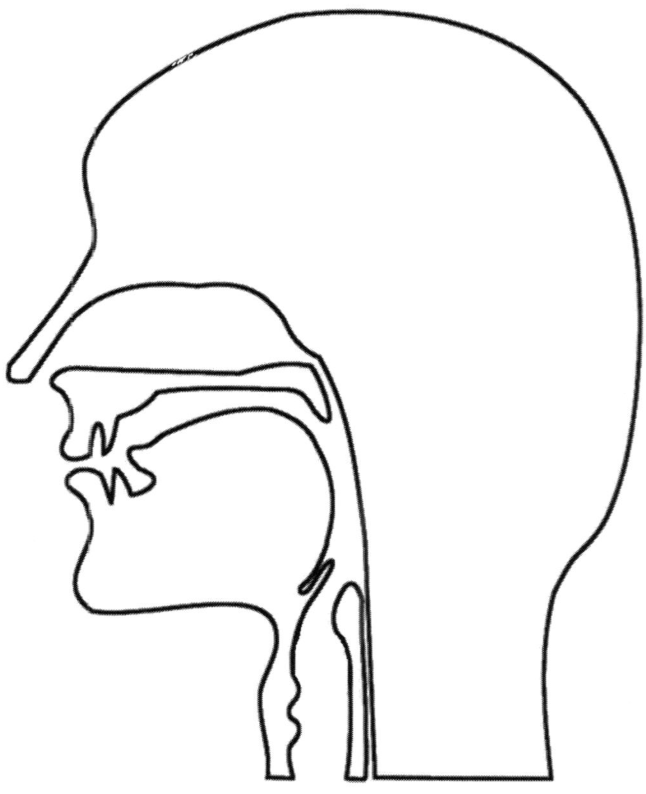

Figure 5.1 A two-dimensional outline of the vocal tract along the midsagittal plane.

scope. Not only does this leave our models open to significant cultural interpretation concerning the specific referents of body part terms (see, e.g., Enfield et al., 2006; Wierzbicka, 2007 for contrasting viewpoints on this subject), but dividing the vocal tract into anatomical articulators in this way raises the philosophical question of whether it is desirable or even possible to separate anatomical "body parts" from the muscular and neurological systems that control them. Wilson (1998) addresses this question in relation to the defining of hands:

> Should those parts of the brain that regulate hand function be considered part of the hand? . . . Although we understand what is meant conventionally by the simple anatomic term ['hand'], we can no longer say with certainty where the hand itself, or its control or influence, begins or ends in the body.
>
> *(Wilson, 1998: 9)*

This concept is by no means new to articulatory phonetics: In Cooper et al. (1958: 939) "action plans" were used as a way to link speech events to underlying muscular organization, with the goal "to describe speech events in terms of a rather limited number of muscle groups." Later, Liberman et al. (1967: 446) extended this concept to phonological features, arguing that "the distinctive features of a phoneme are closely linked to specific muscles and the neural commands that actuate them." Of course, while it is trivially true that any physical action can be realized only through neuromotor commands and concomitant muscle movements, the challenge is to explore which particular commands and movements are used, and more to the point, which (if any) are useful to us in understanding how speech works.

The following sections describe the "articulators" of speech in more embodied terms, allowing us to consider different regions of the vocal tract in turn, from the lips to the larynx. Each section develops concepts that emerge from a fuller description of the "parts" of speech as they help to deepen our understanding of the sound systems of human languages. It is important to note that, although the following sections have been given familiar anatomically based titles such as "Lips" and "Tongue," this usage should be taken as strictly descriptive.

Lips

The lips are the most visible part of the vocal tract, making them an easy place to start thinking about how the body makes speech sounds. Lips are associated with the production of bilabial speech sounds such as /b/, /m/ and /w/ and with labio-dental sounds such as /f/ and /v/. Despite the distinct structures and functions of the upper lip and the lower lip, the English language reserves a single term ("lip") for both structures, referring roughly to the fleshy parts immediately adjacent to the vermilion border (the often darker-hued bands immediately surrounding the mouth). In contrast, Jahai, a Mon-Khmer language spoken in Malaysia, uses a separate word for each lip, with *nus* "upper lip" including all the fleshy parts between the nose and mouth and *tnɨt* "lower lip" including all the fleshy parts of the lower lip and chin (Burenhult, 2006). Interestingly, defined in this way, the Jahai "articulators" could be said to reflect more accurately the underlying innervation, with the *nus* innervated by the buccal branches of the facial nerve and the *tnɨt* serviced by the marginal mandibular branches of the facial nerve. Anatomists have long since moved beyond trying to define the lips as a discrete and neatly contained anatomical structure (Lightoller, 1925). Rather, what we refer to as "lips" comprises a complex network of muscles and other tissues extending roughly from the chest to the cranium (see Figure 5.2), along with all of its associated skeletal, neural and metabolic structures, taking on different forms depending on its immediate function. So, where does one draw the line around "lips"?

The notion of "lips" becomes still more complicated as soon as we begin to use them to produce speech: Consider that the set of muscles recruited to produce the flat lip closure for /b/ (mainly marginal orbicularis oris [OOm], risorius [RIS] and mentalis [MEN]) is completely different from that recruited for the rounding of /w/ (mainly peripheral orbicularis oris [OOp]) (Gick et al., 2011), while /f/ and /v/ only use inferior OO (OOi) muscles to

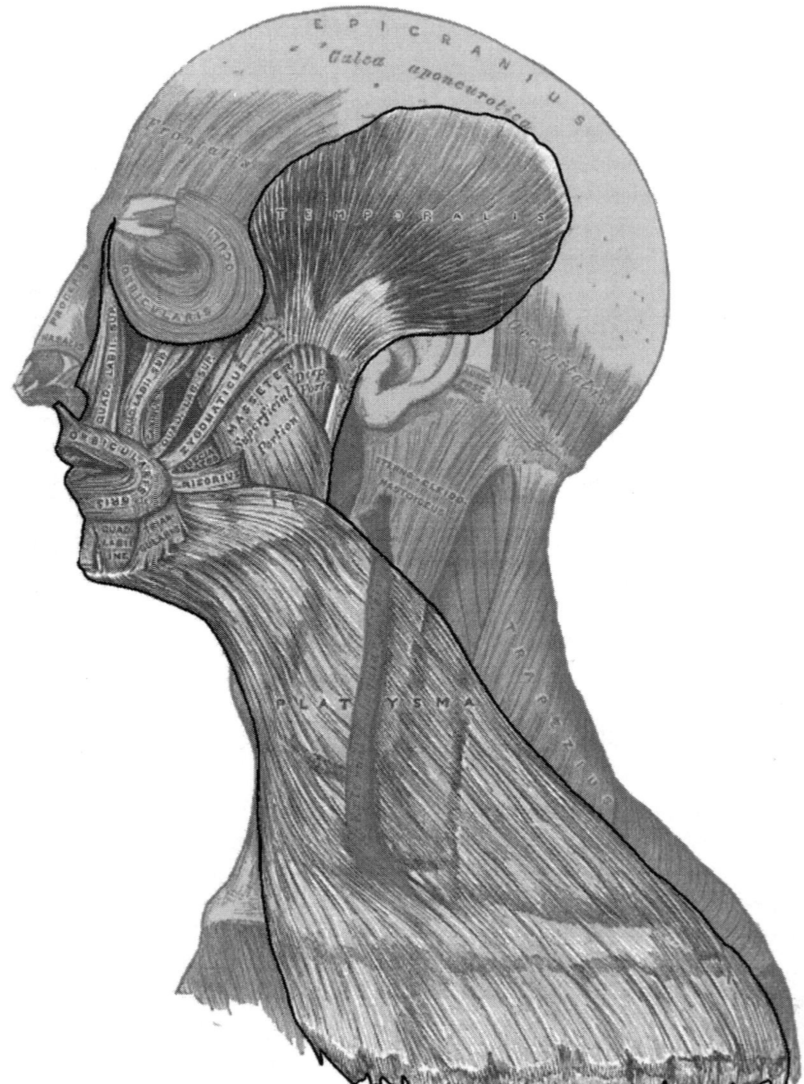

Figure 5.2 Muscles contributing to lip movement (outlined in black).[1]

Source: Adapted by B. Gick and R.C. Taylor, from Gray and Lewis (1918) Plate 378, [public domain]

close the bottom lip against the upper teeth (see Figure 5.3). That is to say, if articulators are defined so as to include the associated muscular and neural structures, then the "lips" we use to produce /b/ are quite literally a different body part from the "lips" we use to produce /w/ or the "lips" we use to produce /f/. At this point, the use of the term "lips" as a formal part of our phonetic description seems more of a liability than an aid. It would make more sense to define three separate structures that control these three separate sounds. Thus, if we really want to understand articulatory phonetics, we should ask not "what are lips?" or even "how do we control our lips?" but rather "how do the various systems of the body work together to produce the movements that result in the sound /w/?" This then raises other interesting questions, such as why do so many different languages realize /w/ (or /b/ or /f/) in similar ways?

When articulatory phonetics is viewed from an embodied point of view, we find that there are certain movements that our bodies can produce with particular efficiency and reliability – and that these robust movements appear in the phonetic inventories of language after language. These robust movements may be thought of as attractors or "sweet spots" in the action space that require less precise control while still producing consistent articulatory outputs. Examples of physical properties that permit consistent movement with imprecise control include situations of contact between body parts in which movement abruptly stops or changes, tissue stiffness that resists movement, and limits on muscle force-generating capacity. All of these are examples of the kind of "quantal" biomechanical-articulatory relations that have long been described for speech (e.g., Stevens, 1989; Fujimura, 1989; Schwartz et al., 1997) but seldom quantified; computer simulations representing the biomechanics of the body parts associated with speech articulation can be useful in elucidating these properties. Biomechanical simulations have shown quantal relations to correspond with the kinds of movements often used to make speech sounds (e.g., Buchaillard et al., 2009; Nazari et al., 2011; Gick et al., 2014, Moisik and Gick, 2017).

Three-dimensional biomechanical simulations of lip musculature and other structures can be useful in identifying the labial movements that show quantal properties, and the different groupings of muscles that drive these movements (e.g., Gick et al., 2011). The graph

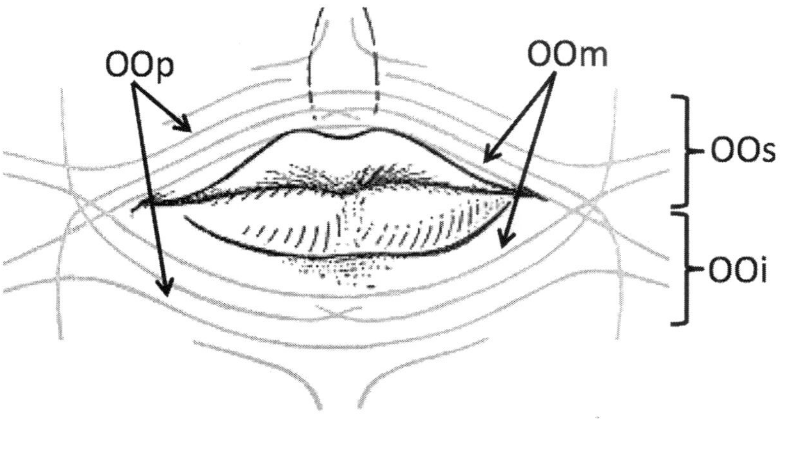

Figure 5.3 Schematic diagram illustrating the outer ring OOp (peripheral), inner ring OOm (marginal), upper half OOs (superior), and lower half OOi (inferior) of the orbicularis oris (OO) muscle.

Source: Adapted by B. Gick, from Gray and Lewis (1918), Plate 381 [public domain]

in Figure 5.4 illustrates how two different muscle groupings are used to produce reliable lip constrictions of different sizes (as for /b/ and /w/); in other words, each discrete lip movement (say, closure for /b/ or rounding for /w/) results from the action of a separate functional body structure, each having its own distinct musculature, innervation, and functional outcome. Semi-closed structures of this kind have sometimes been associated with the term "modules" or "muscle synergies" in the motor control literature (e.g., Safavynia and Ting, 2012), because they act as distinct and relatively autonomous functional units of action in the system. As these neuromuscular modules are built to take advantage of "biomechanical affordances" (Ting and Chiel, 2015), it is important to consider biomechanical properties of speech movements.

The term "modules" in this context refers to groupings of muscles and nerves whose activations result in robust, reliably produced movements (D'Avella and Bizzi, 2005). As Loeb et al. (2000:79) describe in their study of limb control:

> in the large space of simulated muscle combinations there exists a well-defined subset of synergies which will stabilize the limb despite activation noise, muscle fatigue, and other uncertainties – and these synergies stabilize the limb at predictable, restricted locations in the workspace.

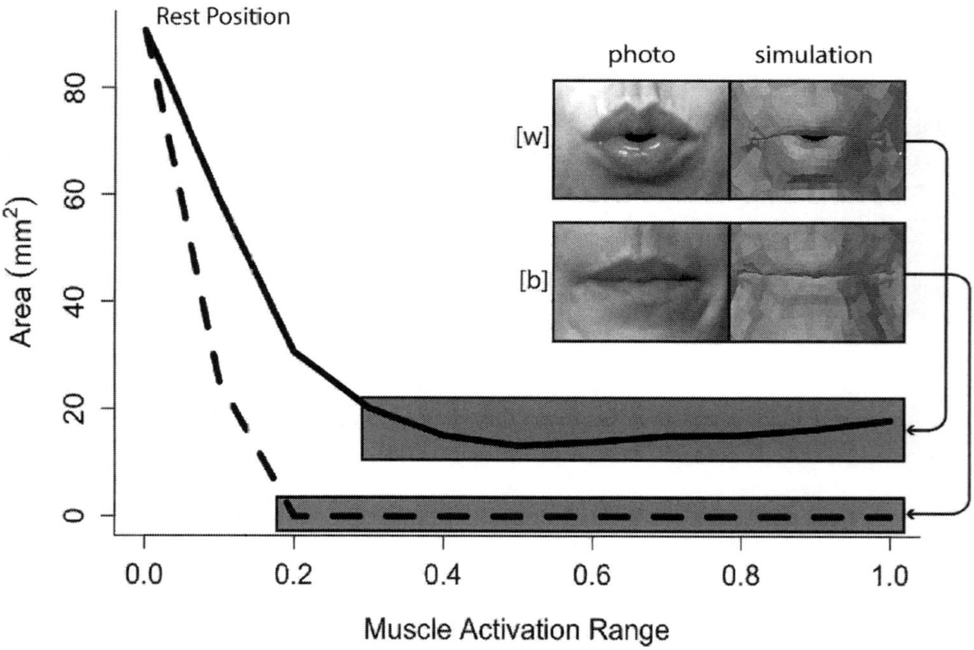

Figure 5.4 Area of lip opening as muscle activation increases; dashed line shows activation of a lip-closing module (OOM + RIS + MEN), solid line shows activation of a lip-rounding module (OOP). Note that each module stabilizes at its own natural size of opening after about 20–30% activation, with stable regions indicated in dotted boxes. Photos to the right show rounded and closed lip shapes for illustration.

Source: Graph adapted from (Gick et al., 2011) with permission. Images generated by C. Chiu using ArtiSynth; www.artisynth.org.

So, according to our model, these *robust* muscle synergies can be depended on to get the limb to the right place.

Groupings of this kind – of nerves and muscles and the structures they move, tuned by use and feedback, and organized to produce reliable speech movements – form the basis of actionable body parts of speech; these are the "articulators" of articulatory phonetics (see Gick and Stavness, 2013). A prediction of this approach is that there should be gaps in phonetic inventories corresponding to the absence of robust, reliable mechanisms at particular vocal tract locations. Insofar as our phonetic transcription systems, e.g., the International Phonetic Alphabet (IPA; see Figure 5.5), are representative of the phonetic variation observed in the languages of the world, these provide a good sense of what options are or are not available to speakers of a language. In fact, the IPA contains many gaps that are not judged physically impossible, but that are nevertheless unattested. For example, while it is entirely possible to produce a labio-dental stop by compressing the lower lip into the upper teeth with sufficient pressure, as evidenced by its occasional appearance as a blend of [p] and [f] in Belgian Dutch (Verhoeven, 2005) or in clinical speech (e.g., Hagedorn et al., 2014), this sound is not used contrastively in any language, presumably because the upper teeth simply provide a comparatively poor closure surface for the lower lip.

Note that as the structures we colloquially call "lips" may be involved in a variety of different speech sounds, their range of possible actions will potentially be governed by a large number of distinct neuromuscular modules specialized to produce different speech movements (as well as other modules for non-speech functions relating to ingestion, respiration, facial expression, and so on). Such modules make no formal reference to any predefined anatomical structure such as "lips," "upper lip," "lower lip," "jaw," etc. Importantly, what this means for articulatory phonetics is that each "articulator" identified in our model is an actionable unit with a built-in reliable function, enabling us to link every observable or measurable phonetic output with its concomitant embodied properties, including its kinematics, biomechanics, musculature, neural control, and the sensory structures through which it is trained and reinforced.

CONSONANTS (PULMONIC) © 2015 IPA

	Bilabial	Labiodental	Dental	Alveolar	Postalveolar	Retroflex	Palatal	Velar	Uvular	Pharyngeal	Glottal
Plosive	p b			t d		ʈ ɖ	c ɟ	k ɡ	q ɢ		ʔ
Nasal	m	ɱ		n		ɳ	ɲ	ŋ	ɴ		
Trill	ʙ			r					ʀ		
Tap or Flap		ⱱ		ɾ		ɽ					
Fricative	ɸ β	f v	θ ð	s z	ʃ ʒ	ʂ ʐ	ç ʝ	x ɣ	χ ʁ	ħ ʕ	h ɦ
Lateral fricative				ɬ ɮ							
Approximant		ʋ		ɹ		ɻ	j	ɰ			
Lateral approximant				l		ɭ	ʎ	ʟ			

Symbols to the right in a cell are voiced, to the left are voiceless. Shaded areas denote articulations judged impossible.

Figure 5.5 Excerpt from the IPA Chart, www.internationalphoneticassociation.org/content/ipa-chart, available under a Creative Commons Attribution-Sharealike 3.0 Unported License.

Source: Copyright 2015 International Phonetic Association

Tongue

The tongue is commonly thought of as the primary mover in speech articulation. It is perhaps the body's most flexible structure, interacting with other parts of the oral and pharyngeal tracts to produce a wide range of vowel and consonant sounds, including coronals (e.g., /t/, /n/, /l/), palatals (e.g., /i/, /j/, /c/), velars (e.g., /k/, /g/, /x/) and uvulars (e.g., /g/, /ɴ/, /ʀ/), to mention a few. Taken as a whole anatomical object, the tongue acts as a muscular hydrostat; that is, the volume of the tongue remains constant as it changes shape, so that when the tongue is squeezed in one area by the action of muscles we expect a corresponding passive expansion in another area to maintain the volume, as with a water balloon. Because of its hydrostatic properties, the human tongue has sometimes been compared with other muscular hydrostats in the animal kingdom, such as the octopus arm or squid tentacle (Kier and Smith, 2002). However, while tongues and tentacles may appear similar, and both do indeed have many degrees of freedom (DoF) – so many that it is hard to conceive how they can be controlled – the analogy largely ends here. Human tongues and octopus arms have very different internal structures and are controlled very differently. One way octopuses solve their DoF problem is by bending their arms only at specific locations (Sumbre et al., 2006), almost as if the arm contained bones and joints that help constrain its possible movements. This simplifies the control problem for the octopus's nervous system.

The tongue is also very flexible, but unlike an octopus arm, the tongue is surrounded by hard structures, and it interacts with these to produce its speech movements. Contrary to a "tentacle" analogy, which might lead us to imagine that the sides of the tongue move more-or-less in concert with the midline, the lateral edges of the tongue actually serve their own quite independent and important function – they are responsible for "bracing" the tongue against the upper molars and sides of the hard palate (Figure 5.6). This bracing greatly reduces the

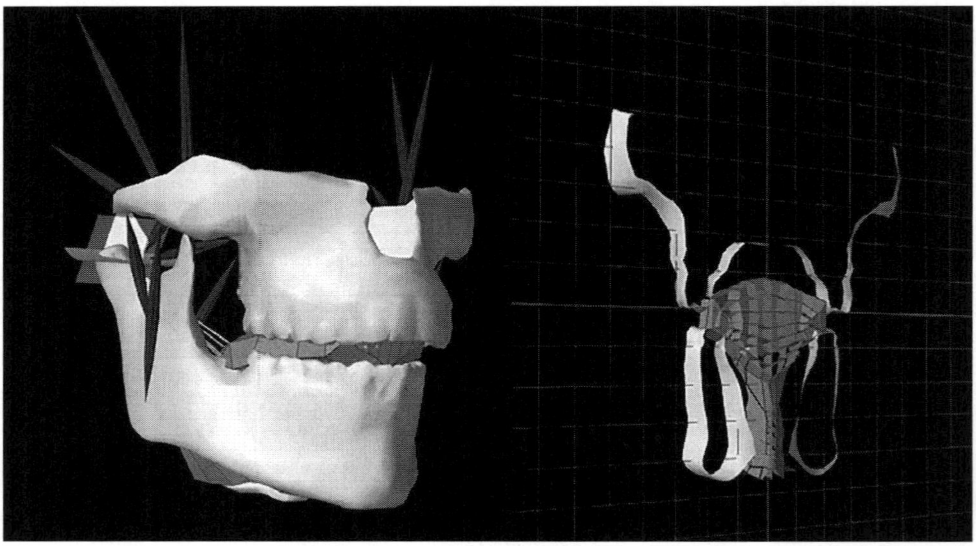

Figure 5.6 Computer simulation of oblique view of the tongue with surrounding skeletal structure (left) in the position to produce a coronal closure, with a coronal cross-section (right) showing the lateral tongue in contact with the molars.

Source: Images generated by I. Stavness using ArtiSynth; www.artisynth.org.

tongue's degrees of freedom and provides sensory feedback about the position of the tongue and, crucially, it forms the seal that keeps air from escaping into the cheeks, thus defining the aeroacoustic tube for speech. Because of its essential functions, with but few exceptions, bracing is maintained continuously throughout running speech (Gick et al., 2017).

Thus, for example, whenever the tongue tip moves upward to close for a /t/, the sides of the tongue are already braced against the teeth, holding in the air to allow pressure to build behind the tongue tip closure; likewise, in the case of a fricative like /s/, lateral bracing forms the central passageway through which air must travel, forcing the air forward through the narrow anterior passage to break against the teeth. This is not just true for coronal sounds, though, or for consonants: The tongue maintains this lateral bracing for vowels and consonants alike, suggesting a possible dedicated module for bracing that is kept constantly activated throughout speech, presumably as part of a language's pre-speech posture (Perkell, 1969) or articulatory setting (Gick et al., 2004). The notable exception to lateral bracing, of course, is the class of lateral sounds, such as English /l/, which are commonly associated with intentional lowering of the sides of the tongue. Acoustically, this lowering engages the side resonators of the buccal cavities, giving /l/ its characteristic sound. It is interesting to note that, when the tongue loses its lateral bracing during /l/, the anterior tongue normally makes contact with the alveolar ridge, providing anterior bracing for the tongue and ensuring that bracing at some location is maintained between the tongue and palate throughout running speech.

Bracing is an essential part of understanding tongue articulation, as it delineates the tongue's independently controllable functional regions (see Stone and Lundberg, 1996). For example, when the tongue is braced laterally, the tongue tip can function as a relatively simple valve. This simple valve is so efficient that the tongue tip is even capable of producing sequences of fast upward and downward motions in an oscillatory fashion, without active control; in speech, this dynamic can be seen in trilling of the tongue tip, as well as in sequential flaps in the word "Saturday" as produced by speakers of many dialects of English (Derrick et al., 2015). More posteriorly, as long as the lateral tongue remains braced, the mass of the tongue body cannot be raised and lowered as a single object by extrinsic muscles; rather, it must be raised and lowered through reshaping of the tongue, primarily through the action of muscles intrinsic to the tongue. Still farther back, the tongue dorsum interacts with the soft palate in complex ways to produce uvular sounds (such as the rhotic sounds in French or German); this complex interaction will be discussed in the following section on the soft palate. The tongue root likewise uses its own mechanisms to move anteroposteriorly (forwards and backwards) through combinations of intrinsic reshaping and as part of more general constriction maneuvers of the pharynx.

Considering the mechanics of the tongue in this light, its function looks less like that of a free-floating tentacle and more like a set of different – and tightly constrained – local mechanisms, some of which act like "valves" (Edmondson and Esling, 2006) or sphincters (Gick et al., 2013c). As with the lips, each such locality may be associated with a small number of dedicated neuromuscular modules, with the number depending on how many degrees of freedom (i.e., how many distinct configurations) need to be exploited at that location to realize a particular language's phonetic inventory.

Soft Palate

The soft palate (also referred to interchangeably as the velum) acts as the primary "gatekeeper" separating the oral, nasal, and pharyngeal cavities. Different parts of this highly flexible structure are responsible for controlling the velopharyngeal port (VPP; the passageway between the nasal and pharyngeal cavities) and the oropharyngeal isthmus (OPI; the passageway between the oral and pharyngeal cavities). This division of cavities by the soft palate is illustrated in Figure 5.7. In speech, the soft palate is sometimes characterized as functioning like a "trapdoor," which can adopt one of two positions: raised/open, to produce nasal sounds, or lowered/closed, to produce oral sounds; it is thus involved in creating both the oral/nasal distinction (as in /d/ vs. /n/ or /a/ vs. /ã/) and in interfacing with the tongue to form uvular constrictions for sounds such as /q/, /ɴ/ or /ʀ/ (Fujimura and Lindqvist, 1971).

The trapdoor model, however, does not account for the dual functions of the soft palate/velum as a simultaneously nasal and oral articulator. That is, if this structure can only be raised or lowered trapdoor-style, how can it participate in synchronous constrictions of the OPI and VPP? The answer lies in the complex structure and function of the soft palate (shown in Figure 5.7): These two distinct functions (closing the VPP to create oral sounds and interacting with the tongue dorsum to make various uvular constrictions for sounds such as the English /w/ or the French /ʁ/) are realized using independently controllable parts of the soft palate. Specifically, X-ray research has shown that, while the upper portion of the soft palate holds the VPP closed, the lower portion (the "veil" or "traverse" that hangs down in the back of the mouth, terminating with the uvula) functions independently from the rest of the soft palate, bending toward the tongue to form the uvular constriction for French /ʁ/

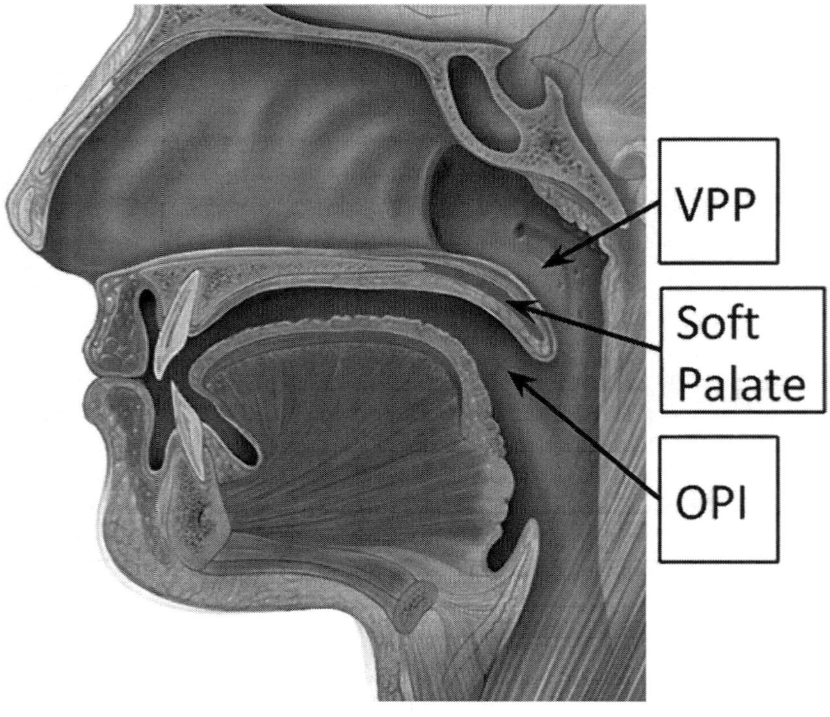

Figure 5.7 Midsagittal view of velopharyngeal port (VPP) and oropharyngeal isthmus (OPP) separated by the soft palate.

Source: Adapted from an image by Patrick J. Lynch, medical illustrator (CC BY 2.5 [http://creativecommons.org/licenses/by/2.5]), via Wikimedia Commons.

(Gick et al., 2014, 2013a). Considering its distinct structure and function – and the etymology of the term "velum" (Latin "veil") – it would make sense to reserve the term "velum" to refer exclusively to the veil-like structure that descends to interact with the tongue to form "velar" sounds.

An important lesson about articulatory phonetics that is perhaps most clearly demonstrated by the velum is that different speakers can use different – sometimes dramatically different – mechanisms for achieving similar outcomes. Well-known observations of this kind have been made about non-velar sounds, such as categorical variants of /r/ (e.g., Stavness et al., 2012) and /s/ (Dart, 1998). Similarly, the closure of the VPP has been shown to be achieved in one of four distinct ways (Biavati et al., 2009), as illustrated in Figure 5.8. Just over half of people are found to close the VPP with a relatively simple raising ("trapdoor") method where the velum raises mainly through constriction of the levator palati muscle, lifting the velum to the pharyngeal wall to close off the passageway; roughly 20% of people use not only the levator palati but also squeeze the VPP from the sides using the superior pharyngeal constrictor muscle; a further 15–20% of people add in constriction from the Passavant's Ridge in the pharyngeal wall to provide constriction from all four directions; finally, a small percentage of people close only laterally using the superior pharyngeal constrictor. Thus, distinct modules are not only important for describing different functions, but also for describing the various mechanisms individuals use to perform similar functions.

In the most widely attested VPP closure mechanism (Figure 5.8a), a distinctive "hump" is formed in the central posterior region of the velum, assisting in VPP closure. This hump is one example of how the soft palate functions more like a complex, tongue-like structure than like a simple trapdoor. Using computed tomography (CT) and magnetic resonance imaging (MRI) scans, Serrurier and Badin (2008) built a three-dimensional reconstruction of the soft palate that clearly shows the soft palate undergoing this intrinsic reshaping, apparently using intrinsic muscles to raise and retract the soft palate towards the rear pharyngeal wall. Subsequent simulation studies (Anderson et al., 2016) show that it is compression of the intrinsic portion of the levator veli palatini (LVP) muscle that hydrostatically produces this characteristic palatal hump (visible in Figure 5.9), similar to how the tongue raises to produce a palatal or dorsal constriction for sounds such as [j] or [k].

Our knowledge of the muscles involved in soft palate control has expanded considerably in recent years through the use of computer simulations. Simulations are an important tool for understanding a structure that is so difficult to observe in action using standard imaging techniques. Simulations such as the one shown in Figure 5.9 start with a detailed reconstruction of the three-dimensional geometry (shape) of bones, cartilage, ligaments,

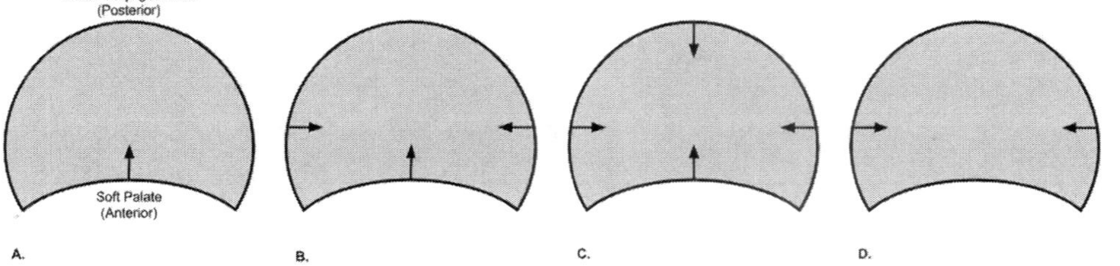

Figure 5.8 Variation in VPP closure: A. simple raising ("trapdoor") method; B. raising + lateral compression; C. raising + lateral compression + Passavant's Ridge; D. lateral compression only. Image by R. Taylor.

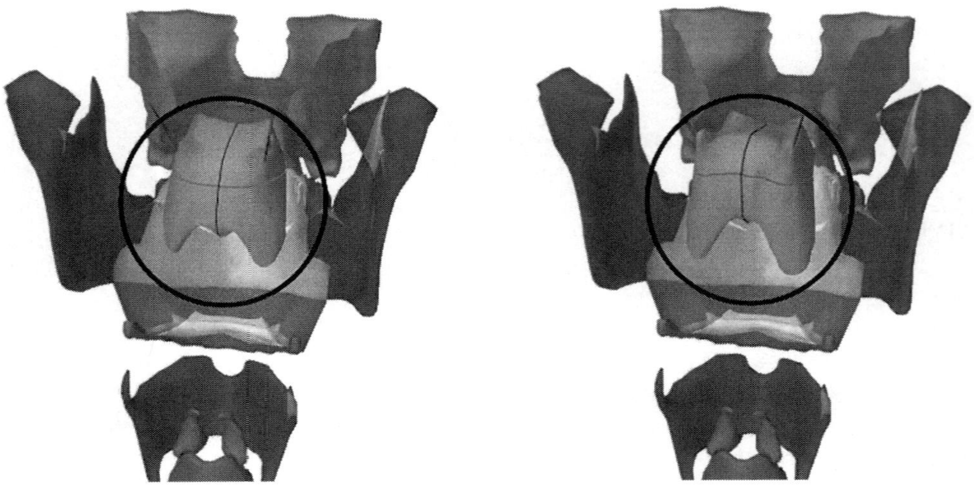

Figure 5.9 Computer simulation of posterior oblique views of soft palate, in relaxed (left) and raised/humped (right) position. The extrinsic portion of LVP muscles are shown as lines extending from the top corners of the soft palate. A horizontal gray intersect line roughly distinguishes the lower veil/velum portion from the rest of the soft palate, while a black line traces the midsagittal plane, highlighting the contour of the hump.

Source: Figure adapted by R.C. Taylor and Yadong Liu from images generated by P. Anderson using ArtiSynth (www.artisynth.org).

muscles, and other structures based on available medical image data from sources such as cryosection, CT and MRI; the resulting reconstructed structures are then broken into smaller elements that are assigned properties such as elasticity and stiffness based on known material properties. Simulations built from these structures can then be used to predict how, for example, contracting a particular muscle might modify the shape of that muscle and surrounding structures (see, e.g., Anderson et al., 2016; Gick et al., 2014). Computer simulations of the OPI have also shown that, as with the lips, different sizes and types of constrictions are produced using qualitatively different mechanisms, implying distinct neuromuscular modules. Gick et al.'s. (2014) simulation, for example, showed how the soft palate is an active contributor to making uvular sounds, with larger-area OPI constrictions (such as those for /u/ or /w/) produced using a mechanism depending mainly on the action of the palatoglossus muscle, while smaller-area constrictions (such as those for uvular fricatives) employ a strategy combining both palatoglossus and palatopharyngeus, which together form a "sling" effect that narrows the OPI as it pulls the velum toward the tongue.

Far from resembling a simple trapdoor, the soft palate/velum can be seen to exhibit the same qualitative properties as the tongue, with functionally independent substructures, essential speech and non-speech roles in multiple vocal tract cavities (oral, nasal, and pharyngeal), a high degree of speaker-specific variation, distinct functions for intrinsic and extrinsic musculature, hydrostatic control of shape, and modular neuromuscular organization. These properties enable the soft palate to participate in producing nearly every sound in the languages of the world.

Larynx

If there is any structure in the body that has a range and complexity of motion to rival the tongue, it is the larynx. While laryngeal phonetics has traditionally concentrated on the vocal folds, which act as the primary noise source for most speech vocalizations, a fuller picture of the larynx must include not just the vocal folds but also the epilarynx (which encompasses the epiglottis and the aryepiglottic folds; see Moisik, 2013). Different laryngeal states, or states of the glottis (Esling, 2006), have often been described as occurring on a continuum of glottal closure, from open to closed (Gordon and Ladefoged, 2001; Ladefoged, 1971):

(1) [open] voiceless – breathy – modal – creaky – glottal closure [closed]

The interpretation in (1) suggests that the larynx is controlled by a single "opening/closing" mechanism that produces different outputs by activating to different degrees. If this were correct, it would run counter to a modular approach. Note that, under this "single mechanism" view, the most widely attested type of phonation – modal voice – employs a potentially less stable intermediate state along a mechanical continuum of this kind (think of a light switch, with stable *up* and *down* "end state" positions at either end of its motion, but with any number of less stable positions in between).

Contrary to this view, laryngoscopic evidence (Esling, 1999) suggests that each state along the apparent continuum is produced by a quite distinct mechanism (Esling and Harris, 2005; Moisik and Esling, 2011), similar to those described earlier for the supralaryngeal articulators. These mechanisms may map to some degree onto the structures Edmondson and Esling (2006) term "valves." Moisik and Gick (2017) attribute these distinct laryngeal mechanisms to the actions of different muscle groupings, each of which is built to take advantage of a stable "sweet spot" in laryngeal biomechanics: By simulating the actions of a number of these structures, they find that each generates a different reliable outcome corresponding to a different speech sound, producing such varied output states as modal voice, creaky voice, glottal stop, and aryepiglotto-epiglottal fricative. Thus, each different degree of laryngeal aperture is the output of a distinct module rather than of gradual fine adjustments in aperture, so that every laryngeal state may be viewed (both in terms of description and potential stability) as an "end state" along its own continuum. In this way, "glottal" sounds are described here in the same terms as any other laryngeal and supralaryngeal sounds. To give an example, Moisik and Gick (2017) show that the ventricular folds are involved in producing a reinforced version of a glottal stop. Rather than relying simply on the true vocal folds for the closure, the ventricular folds act as a mass that supports the closure and dampens the vibration of the true folds (like a hand resting on a handbell to stop its ringing). This view of the larynx is analogous to our earlier description of the labial sounds, which result from discrete articulatory configurations as opposed to degrees along a continuum. The physical stability of each of these states is what allows speakers to accurately produce a specific articulatory configuration time and again in rapid speech.

The larynx is unlike the other structures we have observed in that it provides an exception to this "mechanical endpoint" control type when it is involved in one particular activity: inspiration. Moisik and Gick (2017) find that, unlike the vocal fold abduction that is used for speech sounds such as /h/ and plosive aspiration, the wider abduction used for inspiration operates in a variable, scalar way. That is, the more muscle activation that is used to open the vocal folds, the wider they open, in a more or less linear relationship. This flexibility in degree of glottal opening for inspiration allows the body to take in exactly as much oxygen as needed from one breath to another – an essential property for survival. The only specifically speech-related function that appears to possibly share this property of variable control is pitch (Moisik et al., 2017), though further research is needed to determine the mechanisms used by populations adept at producing a specific pitch target, such as professional singers and speakers of tone languages.

Putting articulations together

The previous sections have focused on identifying the basic structures and movements that make up speech. However, describing individual movements is of course insufficient for a model of how speech works, as even the simplest utterances combine strings of multiple overlapping actions. Coarticulation – how overlapping speech movements interact with one another – must thus be a central part of a complete model of speech.

Joos (1948) proposed an early embodied model of coarticulation in which he described local interactions between speech movements as the outputs of neurally mediated combinations of overlapping muscle activations. Joos argued that speech movements can be thought of as basically additive, but that the brain is needed to mediate such interactions to handle the complexity of coarticulation. The even-more-basic idea of unmediated additive muscle activations in motor control has since gained currency in the neurophysiology literature with Bizzi et al.'s. (1991) discovery of "superposition" of muscle activations in spinalized frogs. They show that overlapping movements can combine through simple addition of muscle activations, unmediated by higher structures in the nervous system. In this way, activations combine in different proportions to produce a large variety of movements. Subsequent work on humans has shown that, thus combined, only a half-dozen or so superposed modules are needed to describe a wide range of actions of the arm (D'Avella et al., 2006), the hand (Overduin, 2012), or even complex whole-body postures (Torres-Oviedo and Ting, 2007). This same mechanism has been proposed as a basis for combining speech movements in coarticulation (Gick and Stavness, 2013).

Some limited work has been done toward testing whether superposition is a plausible way to model coarticulation. Gick and colleagues (2013b) used biomechanical modeling to test superposition through simulations of coarticulatory interactions in VCV sequences. Comparing these simulation results with electromagnetic articulometry (EMA) results reported by Recasens and Espinosa (2009) resulted in characteristic patterns of coarticulation, obtained simply by temporally overlapping activations for canonical consonants and vowels. On the surface, these coarticulatory patterns can appear very complex: Not only do sounds coarticulate with one another differently under different conditions (at varying speech rates, for example), but each segment also seems to follow its own rules of coarticulation, with some segments described as more "resistant" to coarticulatory effects, or more "aggressive" in exerting their coarticulatory effects on nearby segments (e.g., Bladon and Al-Bamerni, 1976; Fowler and Brancazio, 2000).

It has often been observed that these two properties of coarticulation – resistance and aggressiveness – are positively correlated (e.g., Farnetani, 1990; Fowler and Saltzman, 1993; Recasens et al., 1997; Recasens and Espinosa, 2009). In biomechanical terms, this correlation is not surprising: Both "resistance" (i.e., the extent to which a movement may, or may not, be perturbed in response to another movement) and "aggressiveness" (i.e., the extent to which a movement perturbs other movements) are direct functions of the stiffness associated with each of the overlapping movements – and variable stiffness in the body is a function of muscle activation. Thus, a movement that employs more muscle activation – particularly intrinsic muscle activation – causes an increase in stiffness, which will effect an increase in both "resistance" and "aggressiveness" in coarticulation. Recasens and Espinosa (2009) observe that palatal segments exhibit both increased resistance and increased aggressiveness in their coarticulatory relations. Because of the absence of extrinsic muscles in the anterior mouth, palatal sounds have often been associated with comparatively high levels of intrinsic muscle activation (e.g., Stavness et al., 2012). While this intrinsic stiffness possibility remains to be more fully tested, an embodied approach offers a testable path forward towards a deeper understanding of how speech sounds work together.

An embodied approach to coarticulation treats instances of superposition the same, irrespective of the timescale of overlap. Thus, as muscle activations can be maintained over long periods of time (as in the tonic activations used in controlling body posture), we can construe any case of basic coarticulation as superposition, whether it appears to occur locally (as with immediately adjacent speech sounds), non-locally (as with the long-distance interactions observed in harmony systems), or globally (as with articulatory settings, where a setting may affect every sound in a language, see Gick et al., 2004). Of course, the extent to which any instance of coarticulation may be seen as "basic" is not known, but as technology has made these proposals testable, future work will enable researchers to uncover the extent to which additional factors come into play in determining the patterns of coarticulation in speech. It is likewise possible to construe other linguistic structures such as the syllable as being governed by the same basic principles of overlapping elements, as with other cases of coarticulation, provided these principles are accompanied by a theory specifying the relative timing of elements. Superposition with non-speech actions may also be captured using this approach (as with talking while chewing or smiling), providing a unified model for interactions both within and between speech and non-speech movements. This approach suggests that the built-in mechanics of the human body can go a long way towards handling local coarticulatory interactions in ways that may look quite complex on the surface, without reference to advance planning, contextual information or extrinsic models – indeed, with no specified model of coarticulation at all.

Conclusion

While there is a perennial appeal to looking for answers to questions about speech and language in the brain, every speech sound we produce is necessarily the result of the moving body. Humans are able to produce many of our most complex vocal tract behaviors (e.g., swallowing, vocalizing, suckling, breathing) at birth without experience beyond the womb, and indeed without a brain above the brainstem, as evidenced by studies of anencephalic newborns (Radford et al., 2019). Such observations reveal in vivid terms the degree to which the biomechanical and neural structures needed for complex vocal tract action appear to be built into the body, as is the case with other functions that are present from birth, such as locomotion (Dominici et al., 2011). It has long been argued that embodied structures of this kind are the basis not just of reflexive movement, but of all volitional movement – that is, that these are the only controllable discrete "body parts" our nervous systems can employ (e.g., Easton, 1972). Casting speech behavior in terms of these body-based structures offers researchers new ways of approaching some of the defining problems of articulatory phonetics (Gick, 2016; Gick and Stavness, 2013).

An apt model for speech sounds in such an embodied approach is not that we learn to control an inventory of sounds per se, but rather that we learn to build and control an inventory of highly specialized body parts, each of which is constructed and optimized to serve a specific phonetic function. Physical articulators thus cannot be divorced from the tasks they perform, combining both representation and action into primitives of the speech system. Identifying the movement primitives that make up this system has been a central enterprise in articulatory phonetics, where generations of phoneticians, phonologists, and speech researchers have described and cataloged in detail the minimal elements of the speech motor system; this tradition contrasts starkly with that of movement research in other areas, such as locomotion and posture, where primitives have been studied much less frequently, systematically, and comprehensively. This rich tradition in phonetics has grown out of the long-observed fact that humans have harnessed these physically stable movement primitives to form the basis of nature's most complex communication system. The field of articulatory phonetics thus deeply underlies theories of phonetics and phonology, speech evolution and acquisition, and sound change.

Acknowledgments

The authors wish to thank the many collaborators who have contributed to the studies and simulations that have fed into this paper. This work has been supported by NSERC Discovery grant RGPIN-2015-05099 to the first author, and by National Institutes of Health grant DC-002717 to Haskins Laboratories.

Note

1 Note that muscles that control the jaw (e.g., temporalis, masseter) are included here as these muscles are important in determining lip position. As the role of the jaw as a primary articulator in adult speech is controversial (see, e.g., Redford and van Donkelaar, 2008), the jaw will not be addressed independently in the present work.

References

Anderson, P., Fels, S., Stavness, I., Gick, B., 2016. Intrinsic and extrinsic portions of soft palate muscles in velopharyngeal and oropharyngeal constriction: A 3D modeling study. *Canadian Acoustics*. 44, 18–19.

Anderson, P., Harandi, N.M., Moisik, S.R., Stavness, I., Fels, S., 2015. A comprehensive 3D biomechanically-driven vocal tract model including inverse dynamics for speech research, in: *Proceedings of Interspeech 2015: 16th Annual Conference of the International Speech Communication Association*, Dresden, Germany, pp. 2395–2399.

Biavati, M.J., Sie, K., Wiet, G.J., Rocha-Worley, G., 2009. Velopharyngeal insufficiency. *Emedicine: Otolaryngology Facial Plastic Surgery*. pp. 1–21.

Bizzi, E., Mussa-Ivaldi, F.A., Giszter, S., 1991. Computations underlying the execution of movement: A biological perspective. *Science*. 253, 287–291.

Bladon, R.A.W., Al-Bamerni, A., 1976. Coarticulation resistance in English /l/. *Journal of Phonetics*. 4, 137–150.

Buchaillard, S., Perrier, P., Payan, Y. 2009. A biomechanical model of cardinal vowel production: Muscle activations and the impact of gravity on tongue positioning. *The Journal of the Acoustical Society of America*. 126, 2033–2051.

Burenhult, N., 2006. Body part terms in Jahai. *Language Science*. 28, 162–180.

Cooper, F.S., Liberman, A.M., Harris, K.S., Grubb, P.M., 1958. Some input-output relations observed in experiments on the perception of speech. *Proceedings of the 2nd International Congress on Cybernetics*. Namur, Belgium: International Association for Cybernetics. pp. 930–941.

Dart, S.N., 1998. Comparing French and English coronal consonant articulation. *Journal of Phonetics*. 26, 71–94.

D'Avella, A., Bizzi, E., 2005. Shared and specific muscle synergies in natural motor behaviors. *Proceedings of the National Academy of Science U. S. A*. 102, 3076–3081.

D'Avella, A., Portone, A., Fernandez, L., Lacquaniti, F., 2006. Control of fast-reaching movements by muscle synergy combinations. *Journal of Neuroscience*. 26, 7791–7810.

Derrick, D., Stavness, I., Gick, B., 2015. Three speech sounds, one motor action: Evidence for speech-motor disparity from English flap production. *The Journal of the Acoustical Society of America*. 137, 1493–1502. https://doi.org/10.1121/1.4906831

Dominici, N., Ivanenko, Y.P., Cappellini, R.E., G. d'Avella, A., Mondi, V., Cicchese, M., Fabiano, A., Silei, T., Di Paolo, A., Giannini, C., Poppele, R.E., Lacquaniti, F., 2011. Locomotor primitives in newborn babies and their development. *Science*. 334, 997–999.

Easton, T.A., 1972. On the normal use of reflexes. *American Scientist*. 60, 591–599.

Edmondson, J.A., Esling, J.H., 2006. The valves of the throat and their functioning in tone, vocal register and stress: Laryngoscopic case studies. *Phonology*. 23, 157–191.

Enfield, N.J., Majid, A., Van Staden, M., 2006. Cross-linguistic categorisation of the body: Introduction. *Language Sciences*. 28, 137–147.

Esling, J.H., 1999. The IPA categories,"Pharyngeal" and "Epiglottal" Laryngoscopic observations of Pharyngeal articulations and Larynx height. *Language and Speech*. 42, 349–372.

Esling, J.H., 2006. States of the glottis, in: Brown, K. (Ed.), *Encyclopedia of Language and Linguistics*. Oxford: Elsevier. pp. 129–132.

Esling, J.H., Harris, J.G., 2005. States of the glottis: An articulatory phonetic model based on laryngoscopic observations, in: Hardcastle, W.J., Beck, J. (Eds.), *A Figure of Speech: A Festschrift for John Laver*. Mahwah, NJ: Lawrence Erlbaum Associates, pp. 347–383.

Farnetani, E., 1990. VCV lingual coarticulation and its spatiotemporal domain, in: Netherlands, S. (Ed.), *Speech Production and Speech Modelling*, Dordrecht: Kluwer Academic Publishers, pp. 93–130.

Fowler, C.A., Brancazio, L., 2000. Coarticulation resistance of American English consonants and its effects on transconsonantal vowel-to-vowel coarticulation. *Language and Speech*. 43, 1–41.

Fowler, C.A., Saltzman, E., 1993. Coordination and coarticulation in speech production. *Language and Speech*. 36, 171–195.

Fujimura, O. 1989. Comments on "On the quantal nature of speech," by K. N. Stevens. *Journal of Phonetics*. 17, 87–90.

Fujimura, O., Lindqvist, J., 1971. Sweep-tone measurements of vocal-tract characteristics. *The Journal of the Acoustical Society of America*. 49, 541–558. https://doi.org/10.1121/1.1912385

Gick, B., 2016. Ecologizing dimensionality: Prospects for a modular theory of speech production. *Ecological Psychology*. 28, 176–181. https://doi.org/10.1080/10407413.2016.1195195

Gick, B., Allen, B., Roewer-Despres, F., Stavness, I., 2017. Speaking tongues are actively braced. *Journal of Speech, Language and Hearing Research*. 60, 494–506. https://doi.org/10.1044/2016_JSLHR-S-15-0141

Gick, B., Anderson, P., Chen, H., Chiu, C., Kwon, H.B., Stavness, I., Tsou, L., Fels, S., 2014. Speech function of the oropharyngeal isthmus: A modelling study. *Computer Methods in Biomechanics and Biomedical Engineering: Imaging & Visualization*. 2, 217–222.

Gick, B., Francis, N., Klenin, A., Mizrahi, E., Tom, D., 2013a. The velic traverse: An independent oral articulator? *The Journal of the Acoustical Society of America*. 133, EL208–EL213.

Gick, B., Stavness, I., 2013. Modularizing speech. *Frontiers in Psychology*. 4, 977.

Gick, B., Stavness, I., Chiu, C., 2013b. Coarticulation in a whole event model of speech production, in: *The Journal of the Acoustical Society of America – Proceedings of Meetings on Acoustics ICA2013*. ASA, 060207–060211.

Gick, B., Stavness, I., Chiu, C., Fels, S., 2011. Categorical variation in lip posture is determined by quantal biomechanical-articulatory relations, *Canadian Acoustics*. 39(3) pp. 178–179.

Gick, B., Wilson, I., Derrick, D., 2013c. *Articulatory Phonetics*. Oxford: John Wiley & Sons.

Gick, B., Wilson, I., Koch, K., Cook, C., 2004. Language-specific articulatory settings: Evidence from inter-utterance rest position. *Phonetica* 61, 220–233.

Gordon, M., Ladefoged, P., 2001. Phonation types: A cross-linguistic overview. *Journal of Phonetics*. 29, 383–406.

Gray, H., Lewis, W., 1918. *Anatomy of the Human Body*. New York, NY: Lea & Febiger.

Hagedorn, C., Lammert, A., Bassily, M., Zu, Y., Sinha, U., Goldstein, L., Narayanan, S.S., 2014. Characterizing post-glossectomy speech using real-time MRI, in: *Proceedings of the International Seminar on Speech Production*. Cologne.

Joos, M., 1948. Acoustic phonetics. *Language* 24, 5–136.

Kier, W.M., Smith, A.M., 2002. The structure and adhesive mechanism of octopus suckers. *Integrative and Comparative Biology*. 42, 1146–1153.

Ladefoged, P., 1971. *Preliminaries to Linguistic Phonetics*. Chicago: University of Chicago Press.

Liberman, A.M., Cooper, F.S., Shankweiler, D.P., Studdert-Kennedy, M., 1967. Perception of the speech code. *Psychological Review*. 74, 431–461.

Lightoller, G.H.S., 1925. Facial muscles: The Modiolus and Muscles surrounding the Rima Oris with some remarks about the Panniculus Adiposus. *Journal of Anatomy*. 60, 1–85.

Loeb, E.P., Giszter, S.F., Saltiel, P., Bizzi, E., Mussa-Ivaldi, F.A., 2000. Output units of motor behavior: An experimental and modeling study. *Journal of Cognitive Neuroscience*. 12, 78–97.

Moisik, S., 2013. *The Epilarynx in Speech*. Doctoral dissertation, University of Victoria.

Moisik, S.R., Esling, J.H., 2011. The "Whole Larynx" approach to laryngeal features, in: *Proceedings of the 17th International Congress of Phonetic Sciences*, pp. 1406–1409.

Moisik, S., Gick, B., 2017. The quantal larynx: The stable regions of laryngeal biomechanics and implications for speech production. *Journal of Speech, Language, and Hearing Research*, 60(3), 540–560. https://doi.org/10.1044/2016_JSLHR-S-16-0019

Moisik, S., Gick, B., Esling, J.H., 2017. The quantal larynx in action: Smooth and abrupt aspects of laryngeal motion observed in laryngoscopic videos, in: *Proceedings of the 11th International Seminar on Speech Production*. Tianjin, China, pp. 95–96.

Nazari, M.A., Perrier, P., Chabanas, M., Payan, Y., 2011. Shaping by stiffening: A modeling study for lips. *Motor Control* 15, 141–168.

Overduin, E., d'Avella, S.A., Carmena, A., Bizzi, J.M., 2012. Microstimulation activates a handful of muscle synergies. *Neuron* 76, 1071–1077.

Perkell, J.S., 1969. *Physiology of Speech Production: Results and Implications of a Quantitative Cineradiographic Study*. Cambridge, MA: MIT Press.

Radford, K., Taylor, R., Hall, J., Gick, B., 2019. Aerodigestive and communicative behaviours in anencephalic and hydranencephalic infants. *Birth Defects Research* 111(2). 41–52.

Recasens, D., Espinosa, A., 2009. Acoustics and perception of velar softening for unaspirated stops. *Journal of Phonetics*. 37, 189–211.

Recasens, D., Pallarès, M.D., Fontdevila, J., 1997. A model of lingual coarticulation based on articulatory constraints. *The Journal of the Acoustical Society of America*. 102, 544–561.

Redford, M.A., van Donkelaar, P., 2008. Jaw cycles and linguistic syllables in adult English, in: Davis, B.L., Zajdo, K. (Eds.), *The Syllable in Speech Production: Perspectives on the Frame/Content Theory*. London: Taylor & Francis, pp. 355–376.

Russell, G.O., 1933. First preliminary X-ray consonant study. *The Journal of the Acoustical Society of America*. 5, 247–251.

Safavynia, S.A., Ting, L.H., 2012. Task-level feedback can explain temporal recruitment of spatially fixed muscle synergies throughout postural perturbations. *Journal of Neurophysiology*. 107, 159–177.

Schwartz, J-L., Boë, L-J., Vallée, N., Abry, C. 1997. The dispersion-focalization theory of vowel systems. *Journal of Phonetics*. 25, 255–286.

Serrurier, A., Badin, P., 2008. A three-dimensional articulatory model of the velum and nasopharyngeal wall based on MRI and CT data. *The Journal of the Acoustical Society of America*. 123, 2335–2355.

Serrurier, A., Badin, P., Barney, A., Boë, L-J., Savariaux, C., 2012. The tongue in speech and feeding: Comparative articulatory modeling. *Journal of Phonetics*. 40, 745–763.
Stavness, I., Gick, B., Derrick, D., Fels, S., 2012. Biomechanical modeling of English /r/ variants. *The Journal of the Acoustical Society of America*. 131, EL355–EL360.
Stevens, K.N. 1989. On the quantal nature of speech. *Journal of Phonetics*. 17, 3–45.
Stone, M., Lundberg, A., 1996. Three-dimensional tongue surface shapes of English consonants and vowels. *The Journal of the Acoustical Society of America*. 99, 3728–3737.
Sumbre, G., Fiorito, G., Flash, T., Hochner, B., 2006. Octopuses use a human-like strategy to control precise point-to-point arm movements. *Current Biology*. 16, 767–772.
Ting, L.H., Chiel, H.J., 2015. Chapter 12: Muscle, biomechanics, and implications for neural control, in: Hooper, S.L., Büschges, A. (Eds.), *The Neurobiology of Motor Control: Fundamental Concepts and New Directions*. New York, NY: Wiley.
Torres-Oviedo, G., Ting, L.H., 2007. Muscle synergies characterizing human postural responses. *Journal of Neurophysiology* 98, 2144–2156. https://doi.org/10.1152/jn.01360.2006
Verhoeven, J., 2005. Belgian standard Dutch. *Journal of the International Phonetic Association*. 35, 243–247.
Wierzbicka, A., 2007. Bodies and their parts: An NSM approach to semantic typology. *Language Sciences*. 29, 14–65.
Wilson, F.R., 1998. *The Hand: How Its Use Shapes the Brain, Language, and Human Culture*. New York, NY: Pantheon Books.

6

Neural bases of speech production

Jason W. Bohland, Jason A. Tourville, and Frank H. Guenther

Introduction

Speech production is an effortless task for most people, but one that is orchestrated by the coordinated activity of a tremendous number of neurons across a large expanse of cortical and subcortical brain regions. Early evidence for the localization of functions related to speech motor output to the left inferior frontal cortex was famously provided by the French neurosurgeon Paul Broca (1861, 1865), and for many years associations between impaired behaviors and postmortem localization of damaged tissue offered our only window into the brain's speech systems. Starting in the 1930s, Wilder Penfield and his colleagues began to perfect and systematize electrical stimulation mapping in patients undergoing neurosurgery, providing a much finer picture of the localization of the upper motor neurons that drive the articulators and better defining the areas of the cerebral cortex that are important for speaking (Penfield and Roberts, 1959). The advent and availability of non-invasive brain imaging techniques, however, provided a critical turning point for research into the neural bases of speech, enabling the testing of hypotheses driven by conceptual and theoretical models in healthy and disordered populations.

Neuroimaging methods, which include positron emission tomography (PET), functional magnetic resonance imaging (fMRI), and electro- and magneto-encephalography (EEG/MEG), have provided substantial insight into the organization of neural systems important for speech and language processes (see reviews by Turkeltaub, 2002; Indefrey and Levelt, 2004; Demonet et al., 2005; Price, 2012). Research on speech production (distinct from language) focuses primarily on the motor control processes that enable rapid sequencing, selection, and articulation of phonemes, syllables, and words, as well as how the brain integrates incoming sensory information to guide motor output. We consider this domain to intersect the theoretical constructs of articulatory and auditory phonetics, encompassing how the brain enacts sound patterns and perceives and utilizes self-produced speech signals. Speech is also inherently coupled with phonology (the organization of speech sounds in the language) especially for planning multiple syllables and words. While this chapter touches on these aspects of language, the "extra-linguistic" aspects of speech production are its primary focus.

In this chapter we first present a brief overview of the mental processes proposed to underlie the brain's control of speech production, followed by a review of the neural systems that are consistently engaged during speech, with focus on results from fMRI. Finally, we review the DIVA (Directions Into Velocities of Articulators) model (Guenther, 1995, 2016; Guenther et al., 1998, 2006; Tourville and Guenther, 2011) and its extension as GODIVA (Gradient Order DIVA; Bohland et al., 2010), which provide frameworks for not only understanding and integrating the results of imaging studies, but also for formulating new hypotheses to test in follow-up experiments (Golfinopoulos et al., 2010).

Tapping into the mental processes underlying speech production

Influential conceptual models have delineated a series of stages involved in the process of speaking, from conceptualization to articulation (e.g., Garrett, 1975; Dell and O'Seaghdha, 1992; Levelt, 1999; Levelt et al., 1999). Such models propose a role for abstract phonological representations of the utterance to be produced, as well as somewhat lower-level auditory or motor phonetic and articulatory representations. These components are theoretically invoked after the specification of the phonological word form (i.e., a more abstract representation of the speech plan). The neural correlates of these different types of information may be, to a certain degree, anatomically separable, with distinct pools of neurons involved in representing speech in different reference frames or at different levels of abstraction. Additional groups of neurons and synaptic pathways may then serve to coordinate and transform between these different representations.

Different speech tasks naturally highlight different theoretical processes, and experiments investigating speech motor control vary accordingly in at least four key ways. First, in some studies, subjects are asked to produce speech overtly, involving articulation and the production of an audible speech signal, while in others speech is covert, involving only internal rehearsal without movement of the articulators; in each case, it is assumed that phonetic representations of speech are engaged during task performance. Covert speaking protocols have been used often to avoid contamination of images with movement-related artefacts, but a number of differences have been shown in comparing activation patterns in overt vs. covert speech in regions associated with motor control and auditory perception (Riecker, Ackermann, Wildgruber, Dogil, et al., 2000; Palmer et al., 2001; Shuster and Lemieux, 2005), including reduced activity in the motor cortex, auditory cortex, and superior cerebellar cortex for covert speech. Second, some studies use real words – entries in the speaker's mental lexicon[1] – while others use nonwords, typically comprising phonotactically legal phoneme sequences in the speaker's language (i.e., forming "pseudowords"). The latter are often used to control for effects related to lexical retrieval and/or semantic processes; such studies therefore may provide a purer probe for speech motor control processes. However, since pseudowords lack the *long-term* memory representations available for words, their production may also tax *short-term* phonological working memory more heavily than word production (Gathercole, 1995) and may thus increase task difficulty. These changes may result not only in a higher rate of speech errors during task performance but also in domain-general increases in cortical activity (e.g., Fedorenko, et al., 2013). Third, speech in the scanner may be guided by online reading processes, cued by orthographic display, repeated after auditory presentation of the target sounds, or triggered by other external cues such as pictures. Each of these cues leads to expected responses in different brain areas and pathways (such as those involved in reading or speech perception), and requires careful consideration of control conditions. Finally, the length of the speech stimulus can range from a single vowel or syllable to full sentences, with the latter engaging areas of the brain responsible for syntax and other higher-level language processes.

In most cases, the speech materials in speech production studies are parameterized according to phonological and/or phonetic variables of interest. For example, comparing the neural correlates associated with the production of sound sequences contrasted by their complexity (in terms of phonemic content or articulatory requirements) highlights the brain regions important for representing and executing complex speech patterns. Modern techniques such as repetition suppression fMRI (Grill-Spector et al., 2006) and multi-voxel pattern analysis (Norman et al., 2006) have recently been used to help determine the nature of speech-related neural representations in a given brain region, helping to tease apart domain-general activations from speech-specific neural codes.

An important additional focus involves the integration of sensory and motor processes, which is fundamental to acquiring and maintaining speech and to identifying and correcting errors online. The coupling of these neural components is described in more detail later in this chapter (see "Neurocomputational modeling of speech production"). Functional imaging studies have attempted to identify components underlying sensorimotor integration in speech by comparing activity while listening and producing or rehearsing speech (Buchsbaum et al., 2001; Hickok et al., 2003, 2009) and through the online use of altered auditory or somatosensory feedback (e.g., Hashimoto and Sakai, 2003; Tremblay et al., 2003; Heinks-Maldonado et al., 2006; Tourville et al., 2008; Golfinopoulos et al., 2011). Together, neuroimaging results have provided a detailed, though still incomplete, view of the neural bases of speech production.

Neural systems involved in speech production

Here we review current understanding of the neural bases of speech production in neurologically healthy speakers. Speaking engages a distributed set of brain regions across the cerebral cortex and subcortical nuclei in order to generate the signals transmitted along the cranial nerves that activate the muscles involved in articulation. In this section we first discuss key subcortical structures, followed by cortical regions that are activated during speech production tasks.

Subcortical structures

Subcortical brain regions reliably activated during speech production are illustrated in Figure 6.1, which shows regions of the basal ganglia and thalamus,[2] and Figure 6.2, which shows the cerebellum. Blood oxygenation level dependent (BOLD) fMRI responses in the brain regions shown in the dark gray continuum are significantly higher during speech production (reading aloud from an orthographic cue) than during a silent control task (viewing letter strings or non-letter characters approximately matched to the text viewed in the speech task). Statistical maps were derived from pooled analysis (Costafreda, 2009) of eight studies of speech production that includes data from 92 unique neurologically healthy speakers reading aloud one- or two-syllable words or nonwords. Not pictured are the cranial nerve nuclei that contain the motoneurons that activate the vocal tract musculature.

Cranial nerve nuclei

Neural signals are transmitted to the articulators along the cranial nerves, primarily involving 6 of the 12 cranial nerve bundles. These fibers originate in the cranial nerve nuclei

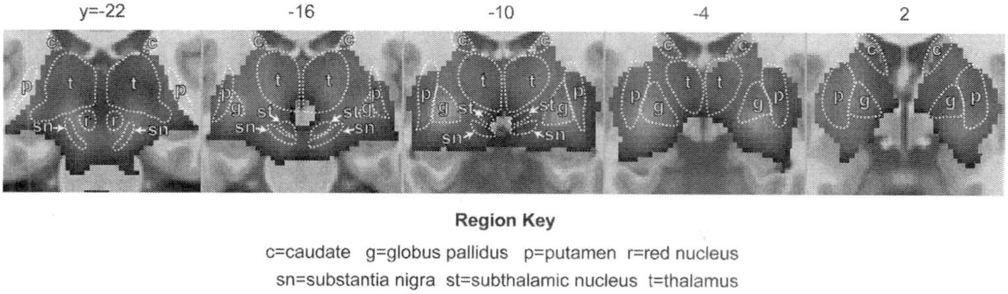

Figure 6.1 Regions of the basal ganglia and thalamus involved in speech production. Statistical parametric maps show subcortical regions (shaded in darker gray, with higher brightness indicating a larger overall effect) that are significantly more active during speech production than a silent baseline task (voxel-wise false discovery rate < .05). The statistical map is overlaid on a subset of coronal slices from the MNI152_2009a nonlinear symmetric template (Fonov et al., 2011). The MNI space *y*-coordinate for each image is listed; higher numbers correspond to more anterior slice positions. To aid in localizing functional-anatomical relationships, subcortical nuclei are outlined and labeled. Statistical maps were derived from a mixed-effects analysis of the *speech–baseline* contrast from 92 speakers that participated in one of 8 different speech production studies. Each participant produced single- or bi-syllabic words or pseudowords. Names for each outlined region are given by the Region Key.

Abbreviations: L = left hemisphere; R = right hemisphere.

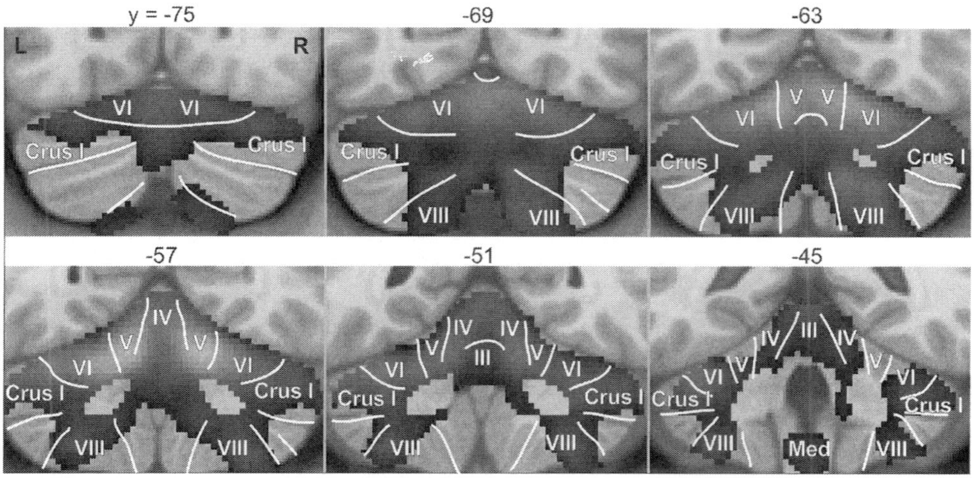

Figure 6.2 Cerebellar regions involved in speech production. Statistical parametric maps show cerebellar regions (shaded in darker gray, with higher brightness indicating a larger overall effect) that are significantly more active during speech production than a silent baseline task. Statistical maps were derived and plotted in the same manner as described in Figure 6.1. In each coronal image, the individual cerebellar lobules that contribute to speech production are labeled according to the protocol described by Schmahmann et al. (2000). White lines trace the cerebellar sulci that mark lobule boundaries.

Abbreviations: CrI = Crus I; Med = medulla.

within the brainstem. A primary anatomical subdivision can be made between control of vocal fold vibration, respiration, and articulation. The intrinsic laryngeal muscles are important during vocal fold opening, closure, and lengthening, and are innervated by motoneurons originating in the nucleus ambiguus, which form the external branch of the superior laryngeal nerve and the recurrent nerve. The extrinsic laryngeal muscles are primarily engaged in modulations of pitch, and receive projections from motoneurons located near the caudal hypoglossal nucleus (Jürgens 2002; Simonyan and Horwitz, 2011). Motoneuron signals project to the laryngeal muscles via the, Xth and XIth cranial nerves (Zemlin, 1998). Supralaryngeal articulatory information is carried via nerves originating in the trigeminal nucleus (forming the Vth nerve) and the facial motor nucleus (forming the VIIth nerve) in the pons, and from the hypoglossal nucleus in the medulla (forming the XIIth cranial nerve). These motor nuclei receive projections mainly from primary motor cortex, which provides the "instructions" for moving the articulators via a set of coordinated muscle activations. The VIIIth cranial nerve, which transmits auditory (as well as vestibular) information from the inner ear to the cochlear nucleus in the brainstem, is also relevant for speech production, forming the first neural component in the auditory feedback pathway involved in hearing one's own speech.

Brain imaging studies are limited by the available spatial resolution and rarely report activation of the small cranial nerve nuclei; furthermore, many studies do not even include these nuclei (or other motor nuclei located in the spinal cord important for respiratory control) within the imaging field of view. Activation of the pons (where many of the cranial nerve nuclei reside) is a relatively common finding in studies involving overt articulation (Paus et al., 1996; Riecker, Ackermann, Wildgruber, Dogil, et al., 2000; Bohland and Guenther, 2006; Christoffels et al., 2007), but these results typically lack the spatial resolution to resolve individual motor nuclei.

Basal ganglia and thalamus

The basal ganglia are a group of subcortical nuclei that heavily interconnect with the frontal cortex via a series of largely parallel cortico-basal ganglia-thalamo-cortical loops (Alexander et al., 1986; Alexander and Crutcher, 1990; Middleton and Strick, 2000). The striatum, comprising the caudate nucleus and putamen, receives input projections from a wide range of cortical areas. Prefrontal areas project mostly to the caudate, and sensorimotor areas to the putamen. A "motor loop" involving sensorimotor cortex and the SMA, passing largely through the putamen and ventrolateral thalamus (Alexander et al., 1986), is especially engaged in speech motor output processes. fMRI studies demonstrate that components of this loop are active even for production of individual monosyllables (Ghosh et al., 2008).

Figure 6.1 demonstrates that speech is accompanied by bilateral activity throughout much of the basal ganglia and thalamus, with a peak response in the globus pallidus, an output nucleus of the basal ganglia. Caudate activity is predominantly localized to the anterior, or head, region. Significant activation is shown throughout the thalamus bilaterally, with the strongest response in the ventrolateral nucleus (image at $y = -16$). An additional peak appears in the substantia nigra ($y = -22$), which forms an important part of the cortico-basal ganglia-thalamo-cortical loop, providing dopaminergic input to the striatum and GABAergic input to the thalamus.

The architecture of basal ganglia circuits is suitable for selecting one output from a set of competing alternatives (Mink and Thach, 1993; Mink, 1996; Kropotov and Etlinger, 1999), a property that is formalized in several computational models of basal ganglia function (e.g.,

Redgrave et al., 1999; Brown et al., 2004; Gurney et al., 2004). Due to the overall degree of convergence and fan-out of thalamo-cortical projections, basal ganglia circuits involved in speech are not likely to be involved in selecting the precise muscle patterns that drive articulation. Instead, as discussed later, the motor loop, which includes the SMA, is likely involved in the selection and initiation of speech motor programs represented elsewhere in the neocortex. A higher-level loop, traversing through the caudate nucleus and interconnecting with more anterior cortical areas, may also be involved in selection processes during speech planning and phonological encoding (as implemented in the GODIVA model described later in this chapter; Bohland et al., 2010).

While the precise functional contributions of the basal ganglia and thalamus in speech motor control are still debated, it is clear that damage and/or electrical stimulation to these regions is associated with speech disturbances. For example, Pickett et al. (1998) reported the case study of a woman with bilateral damage to the putamen and head of the caudate nucleus whose speech was marked by a general articulatory sequencing deficit, with a particular inability to rapidly switch from one articulatory target to the next. Electrical stimulation studies (for a review, see Johnson and Ojemann, 2000) have suggested involvement of the left ventrolateral thalamus (part of the motor loop described earlier) in the motor control of speech, including respiration. Schaltenbrand (1975) reported that stimulation of the anterior nuclei of the thalamus in some subjects gave rise to compulsory speech that they could not inhibit. Stimulation of the dominant head of the caudate has also been shown to evoke word production (Van Buren, 1963), and Crosson (1992) notes similarities between the results of stimulation in the caudate and the anterior thalamic nuclei, which are both components of a higher-level cortico-basal ganglia-thalamo-cortical loop with the prefrontal cortex. This suggests that these areas may serve similar functions, and that basal ganglia loops may be critical for the maintenance and release of a speech/language plan.

Functional imaging of the basal ganglia during speech has not always provided consistent results, but a few notable observations have been made. For example, striatal activity appears to decrease with increased speaking rate for both covert (Wildgruber et al., 2001) and overt speech (Riecker et al., 2006), which is in contrast to an approximately linear positive relationship between speech rate and BOLD response in cortical speech areas. Bohland and Guenther (2006) found an increased response in the putamen bilaterally when subjects produced three-syllable sequences overtly (compared to preparation alone). This coincided with additional motor cortical activation and is likely part of the motor loop described earlier. Furthermore, when stimuli were made more phonologically complex, activation increased in the anterior thalamus and caudate nucleus, as well as portions of prefrontal cortex. Similarly, Sörös et al. (2006) showed that caudate activity was increased for polysyllabic vs. monosyllabic utterances. Increased engagement of this loop circuit is likely due to the increased sequencing/planning load for these utterances. Basal ganglia circuits also appear to be critical for speech motor learning, as they are for non-speech motor skill learning (Doyon et al., 2009). For example, individuals with Parkinson's Disease exhibit deficits in learning novel speech utterances (Schulz et al., 2000; Whitfield and Goberman, 2017). Furthermore, in healthy adults learning to produce syllables containing phonotactically illegal consonant clusters (e.g., /gvazf/), activity in the left globus pallidus was greater when these syllables were novel than for syllables that had been previously practiced (Segawa et al., 2015).

While thalamic activation is often reported in neuroimaging studies of speech, localization of activity to specific nuclei within the thalamus is often imprecise due to their small size and close proximity. The spatial resolution of functional neuroimaging data is often insufficient to distinguish activity from neighboring nuclei. Additionally, the original data are often spatially smoothed, further limiting their effective resolution. Thus, the specific roles of individual nuclei within the larger speech production system remain somewhat poorly understood. Thalamic activations (primarily in the anterior and ventrolateral subregions) in neuroimaging studies have been associated with a number of processes relevant for speech including overt articulation (e.g., Riecker et al., 2005; Bohland and Guenther, 2006; Ghosh et al., 2008), volitional control of breathing (e.g., Ramsay et al., 1993; Murphy et al., 1997), swallowing (e.g., Malandraki et al., 2009; Toogood et al., 2017), and verbal working memory (Moore et al., 2013; e.g., Koelsch et al., 2009). While the thalamus is often viewed simply as a relay station for information transmitted to or from the cerebral cortex, analysis of the circuitry involved in nonhuman primates (Barbas et al., 2013) suggests this perspective is overly simplistic. Further work is needed to better delineate the contributions of the ventral lateral and ventral anterior portions of the thalamus to speech production.

Cerebellum

Cerebellar circuits have long been recognized to be important for motor learning and fine motor control, including control of articulation (Holmes, 1917). Cerebellar lesions can cause ataxic dysarthria, a disorder characterized by inaccurate articulation, prosodic excess, and phonatory-prosodic insufficiency (Darley et al., 1975). Damage to the cerebellum additionally results in increased durations of sentences, words, syllables, and phonemes (Ackermann and Hertrich, 1994; Kent et al., 1997). The classical view of the cerebellum's involvement in the control of speech is in regulating fine temporal organization of the motor commands necessary to produce smooth, coordinated productions over words and sentences (Ackermann, 2008), particularly during rapid speech. In addition to a general role in fine motor control, the cerebellum is implicated in the control of motor sequences (Inhoff et al., 1989), possibly in the translation of a programmed sequence into a fluent motor action (Braitenberg et al., 1997). Furthermore, it is considered to be an important locus of timing (Inhoff et al., 1989; Keele and Ivry, 1990; Ackermann and Hertrich, 1994; Ivry, 1997) and sensory prediction (Blakemore et al., 1998; Wolpert et al., 1998; Knolle et al., 2012). Like the basal ganglia, the cerebellum is heavily interconnected with the cerebral cortex via the thalamus, with particularly strong projections to the motor and premotor cortices.

Neuroimaging studies have helped provide a more refined picture of cerebellar processing in speech, with different loci of cerebellar activation associated with distinct functional roles. The most commonly activated portion of the cerebellum during speech is in the superior cerebellar cortex. This site may actually contain two or more distinct subregions, including an anterior vermal region in cerebellar lobules IV and V and a more lateral and posterior region spanning lobule VI and Crus I of lobule VII (Figure 6.2; Riecker, Ackermann, Wildgruber, Meyer, et al., 2000; Wildgruber et al., 2001; Riecker et al., 2002; Ghosh et al., 2008). Lesion studies implicate both the anterior vermal region (Urban et al., 2003) and the more lateral paravermal region (Ackermann et al., 1992) in ataxic dysarthria. Activation of the superior cerebellum appears to be particularly important for rapid temporal organization of speech, demonstrating a step-wise increase in response for syllable rates between 2.5 and 4 Hz (Riecker et al., 2005). These areas are also more active during overt compared to covert production and for complex syllables (i.e., those containing consonant clusters) compared to simple syllables (e.g., Bohland and Guenther, 2006).

The more lateral portions of the superior cerebellar cortex are likely involved in higher-order processes as compared to the phonetic-articulatory functions of the more medial regions (e.g., Leiner et al., 1993). This hypothesis is consistent with work by Durisko and Fiez (2010) suggesting that the superior medial cerebellum plays a role in general speech motor processing, with significantly greater activation during overt vs. covert speech, whereas no significant difference in activation was observed in the superior lateral cerebellum. Furthermore, the superior lateral region, as well as an inferior region (lobule VIIB/VIII, discussed further below), was more engaged by a verbal working memory task than the speaking tasks, suggesting their role in higher-level representations of the speech plan (Durisko and Fiez, 2010). The involvement of lateral regions of the cerebellar cortex in speech coding was also found in an experiment using fMRI repetition suppression[3] that showed adaptation to repeated phoneme-level units in the left superior lateral cerebellum, and to repeated supra-syllabic sequences in the right lateral cerebellum (Peeva et al., 2010).

Abundant evidence has shown that the cerebellum is engaged not just in motor learning and online motor control, but also for cognitive functions including working memory and language (Schmahmann and Pandya, 1997; Desmond and Fiez, 1998). Such a role is also supported by clinical cases in which cerebellar lesions give rise to deficits in speech planning and short-term verbal rehearsal (Silveri et al., 1998; Leggio et al., 2000; Chiricozzi et al., 2008). Ackermann and colleagues have suggested that the cerebellum serves two key roles in both overt and covert speech production: (a) temporal organization of the sound structure of speech sequences, and (b) generation of a pre-articulatory phonetic plan for inner speech (Ackermann, 2008). As noted throughout this chapter, each of these processes also likely engages a number of additional brain structures. Considerable evidence, however, points to the cerebellum being involved in pre-articulatory sequencing of speech, with the more lateral aspects engaged even during covert rehearsal (Riecker, Ackermann, Wildgruber, Dogil, et al., 2000; Callan et al., 2006).

A separate activation locus in the inferior cerebellar cortex (in or near lobule VIII, particularly in the right hemisphere) has been noted in some studies of speech and is evident in the pooled analysis results shown in Figure 6.2. Bohland and Guenther (2006) reported increased activity in this region for speech sequences composed of three distinct syllables, which subjects had to encode in short-term memory prior to production, compared to sequences composed of the same syllable repeated three times. In contrast with the superior cerebellar cortex, the inferior region did not show increased activity for more complex syllables (e.g., "stra" vs. "ta") compared to simple syllables, suggesting that it is involved in speech sequencing at the supra-syllabic level without regard for the complexity of the individual syllable "chunks." Further support for this view comes from the working memory studies of Desmond and colleagues. Desmond et al. (1997) reported both a superior portion (corresponding to lobule VI/Crus I) and an inferior portion (right-lateralized lobule VIIB) of the cerebellum that showed load-dependent activations in a verbal working memory task, but only the superior portions showed the load-dependent effects in a motoric rehearsal task (finger tapping) that lacked working memory storage requirements. Chen and Desmond (2005) extended these results to suggest that lobule VI/Crus I works in concert with frontal regions for mental rehearsal, while lobule VIIB works in concert with the parietal lobe (BA40) as a phonological memory store.

Increased activation of the right inferior posterior cerebellum (lobule VIII) was also noted in an experiment in which auditory feedback (presented over compatible headphones compatible with magnetic resonance imaging) was unexpectedly perturbed during speech (Tourville et al., 2008). A similar, bilateral, effect in lobule VIII was also observed during somatosensory perturbations using a pneumatic bite block (Golfinopoulos et al., 2011). While further study is required, these results suggest a role for lobule VIII in the monitoring and/or adjustment of articulator movements when sensory feedback is inconsistent with the speaker's expectations. However, it is not just inferior cerebellum that is sensitive to sensory feedback manipulations; using a multi-voxel pattern analysis approach, Zheng et al. (2013) demonstrated that bilateral superior cerebellum responds consistently across different types of distorted auditory feedback during overt articulation.

Cerebral cortex

The bulk of the neuroimaging literature on speech and language has focused on processing in the cerebral cortex. The cortical regions reliably active during our own speech production studies are demonstrated in Figure 6.3. The statistical maps were generated from the pooled individual *speech-baseline* contrast volumes described earlier. For the cerebral cortex, the *t*-test for significant differences was performed in a vertex-by-vertex fashion after mapping individual contrast data to a common cortical surface representation using FreeSurfer (Dale et al., 1999; Fischl et al., 1999).

Speech production recruits a large portion of the cortical surface, including lateral primary motor cortex (vMC, midMC, aCO in Figure 6.3; see Figure 6.3 caption and List of Abbreviations for the definitions of abbreviations), premotor cortex (midPMC, vPMC) somatosensory cortex (vSC, pCO), auditory cortex (Hg, PT, aSTg pSTg, pdSTs), medial prefrontal cortex (SMA, preSMA, dCMA, vCMA), and inferior frontal gyrus (dIFo, vIFo, aFO, pFO). This set of regions, referred to hereafter as the cortical "speech network," is consistently activated during speech production, even for simple, monosyllabic speech tasks (e.g., Sörös et al., 2006; Ghosh et al., 2008). The speech network is largely bilateral. In the detailed description that follows, however, evidence of lateralized contributions from some regions will be described. Bilateral activity in the middle cingulate gyrus (dCMA, vCMA) and the insula (aINS, pINS) is also apparent in Figure 6.3. While clear in this pooled analysis, significant speech-related activity in the cingulate and insula is noted less reliably in individual studies than the core regions listed earlier. After describing the most consistently activated cortical areas, we then discuss these and other regions that are less consistently active during speech and some of the factors that might contribute to this variability.

Additional prominent activations in Figure 6.3 appear in the bilateral medial occipital cortex (OC) extending into lingual gyrus (Lg), and the left superior parietal lobule (SPL). These activations likely reflect visual processes associated with reading stimuli and not speech production, and will not be addressed here.

Primary motor and somatosensory cortices (Rolandic cortex)

The strongest speech-related responses in Figure 6.3 (brightest values in the overlaid statistical map) are found along the central sulcus, the prominent anatomical landmark that divides the primary motor (BA 4) and primary somatosensory (BA 3, 1, and 2) cortices. This cluster of activity extends outward from the sulcus to include much of the lateral portion of the precentral and postcentral gyri, together referred to as Rolandic cortex, from deep within the opercular cortex dorso-medially to the omega-shaped bend in the central sulcus that marks the hand sensorimotor representation. Primary motor cortex lies anterior to the sulcus, sharing the precentral gyrus with premotor cortex (BA 6). Primary somatosensory cortex extends from the fundus of the central sulcus posteriorly along the postcentral gyrus. The representations of the speech articulators lie mostly in the ventral portion of the primary

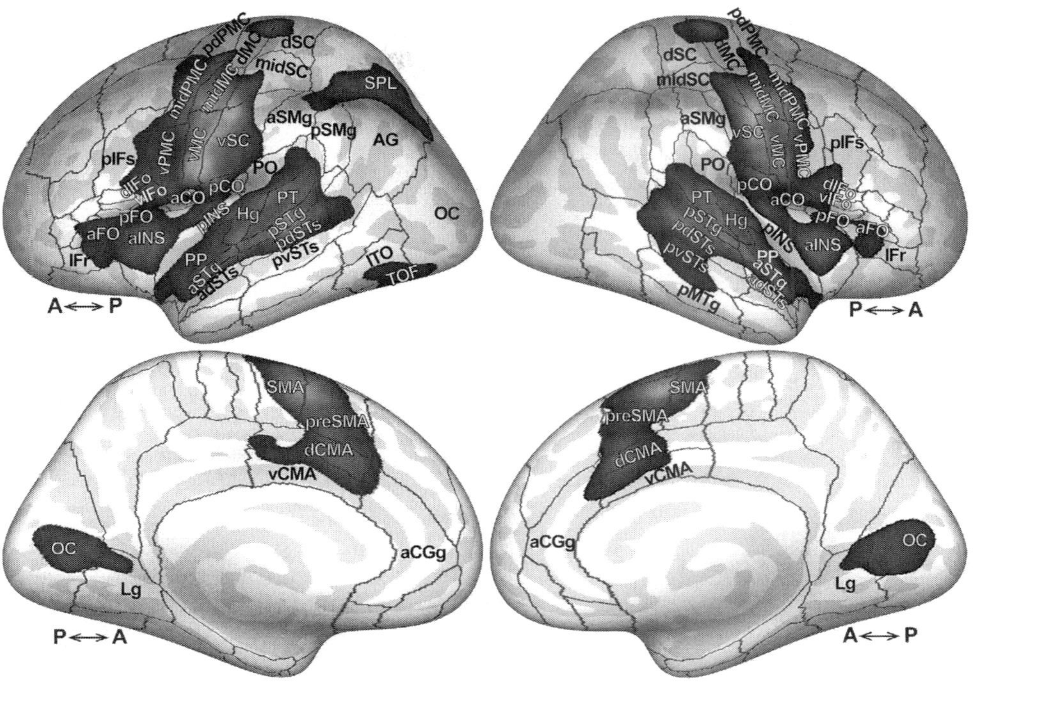

Figure 6.3 Cortical regions involved in speech production. Statistical parametric maps show cortical regions (shaded in darker gray, with higher brightness indicating a larger overall effect) that are significantly more active during speech production than during a silent baseline task (vertex-wise threshold: $p < .001$, cluster-wise threshold: $pFWE < .05$). Statistical maps are overlaid on the inflated "fsaverage" surface that is distributed with the FreeSurfer image processing software package (https://surfer.nmr.mgh.harvard.edu). Lateral (top) and medial (bottom) views of the left hemisphere are shown on the left, those of the right hemisphere are shown on the right. Anterior–posterior orientation is indicated below each surface by the A↔P icon. To localize functional activity to anatomical substrates, the SpeechLabel cortical regions of interest (Tourville and Guenther 2012) have also been overlaid on the cortical surface (black outlines).

Abbreviations: aCGg, anterior cingulate gyrus; aCO, anterior central operculum; adSTs, anterior dorsal superior temporal sulcus; aFO, anterior frontal operculum; Ag, angular gyrus; aINS, anterior insula; aSMg, anterior supramarginal gyrus; aSTg, anterior superior temporal gyrus; dCMA, dorsal cingulate motor area; dIFo, dorsal inferior frontal gyrus, *pars opercularis*; dMC, dorsal motor cortex; dSC, dorsal somatosensory cortex; Hg, Heschl's gyrus; Lg, lingual gyrus; midMC, middle motor cortex; midPMC, middle premotor cortex; midSC, middle somatosensory cortex; OC, occipital cortex; pCO, posterior central operculum; pdPMC, posterior dorsal premotor cortex; pdSTs, posterior dorsal superior temporal sulcus; pIFs, posterior inferior frontal sulcus; pINS, posterior insula; pMTg, posterior middle temporal gyrus; pFO, posterior frontal operculum; PO, parietal operculum; PP, planum polare; preSMA, pre-supplementary motor area; pSMg, posterior supramarginal gyrus; pSTg, posterior superior temporal gyrus; PT, planum temporale; pvSTs, posterior ventral superior temporal sulcus; SMA, supplementary motor area; SPL, superior parietal lobule; vCMA, ventral cingulate motor area; vIFo, ventral inferior frontal gyrus *pars opercularis*; vIFt, ventral inferior frontal gyrus, *pars triangularis*; vMC, ventral motor cortex; vPMC, ventral premotor cortex; vSC, ventral somatosensory cortex.

motor and somatosensory cortices, ranging approximately from the Sylvian fissure to the midpoint of the lateral surface of the cerebral cortex along the central sulcus.

Functional imaging studies involving overt articulation yield extremely reliable activation of the Rolandic cortex bilaterally. In our own fMRI studies, the ventral precentral gyrus is typically the most strongly activated region for any overt speaking task compared to a passive baseline task, a finding consistent with a meta-analysis of PET and fMRI studies involving overt single word reading, which found the greatest activation likelihood across studies along the precentral gyrus bilaterally (Turkeltaub, 2002). Like many areas involved in articulation, activations of the bilateral precentral gyri are strongly modulated by articulatory complexity (e.g., the addition of consonant clusters requiring rapid articulatory movements; Basilakos et al., 2017). These areas are also engaged, to a lesser extent, in covert speech or in tasks that involve preparation or covert rehearsal of speech items (e.g., Wildgruber et al., 1996; Riecker, Ackermann, Wildgruber, Meyer, et al., 2000; Bohland and Guenther, 2006).

The degree to which speech-related activation of the motor cortex is lateralized appears to be task-dependent. Wildgruber et al. (1996) identified strong left hemisphere lateralization during covert speech in the precentral gyrus. Riecker et al. (2000) confirmed this lateralization for covert speech, but found bilateral activation, with only a moderate leftward bias, for overt speech, and a right hemisphere bias for singing. Bohland and Guenther (2006) noted strong left lateralization of motor cortical activity during "no go" trials in which subjects prepared to speak a three-syllable pseudoword sequence but did not actually produce it, but on "go" trials, this lateralization was not statistically significant. This study also noted that the effect of increased complexity of a syllable sequence was significantly stronger in the left-hemisphere ventral motor cortex than in the right. These results offer the hypothesis that preparing speech (i.e., activating a phonetic/articulatory plan) involves motor cortical cells primarily in the left hemisphere, whereas overt articulation engages motor cortex bilaterally (Bohland et al., 2010).

Early electrical stimulation studies (Penfield and Rasmussen, 1950) suggested a motor homunculus represented along the Rolandic cortex and provided insight into the locations of speech-relevant representations. Functional imaging provides further evidence of these cortical maps. Figure 6.4 illustrates the results of recent meta-analyses of non-speech PET and fMRI tasks involving individual articulators (see also Takai et al., 2010; Guenther, 2016). Each panel shows peak (left-hemisphere) activation locations for individual articulators; the bottom right panel shows peak locations determined from two meta-analyses of speech production (Turkeltaub, 2002; Brown et al., 2005). The articulatory meta-analyses indicate a rough somatotopic organization consisting of (from dorsal to ventral) respiratory, laryngeal, lip, jaw, and tongue representations. Notably, however, representations for all of the articulators are clustered together in the ventral Rolandic cortex and overlap substantially; this overlap of articulatory representations in sensorimotor cortex likely contributes to the high degree of inter-articulator coordination present in fluent speech.

Supplementary and pre-supplementary motor areas

The supplementary motor area (SMA) is a portion of the premotor cortex located on the medial cortical surface anterior to the precentral sulcus (see Figure 6.3). It contains at least two subregions that can be distinguished on the basis of cytoarchitecture, connectivity, and function: The preSMA, which lies rostral to the vertical line passing through the anterior commissure, and the SMA proper (or simply SMA) located caudal to this line (Picard and

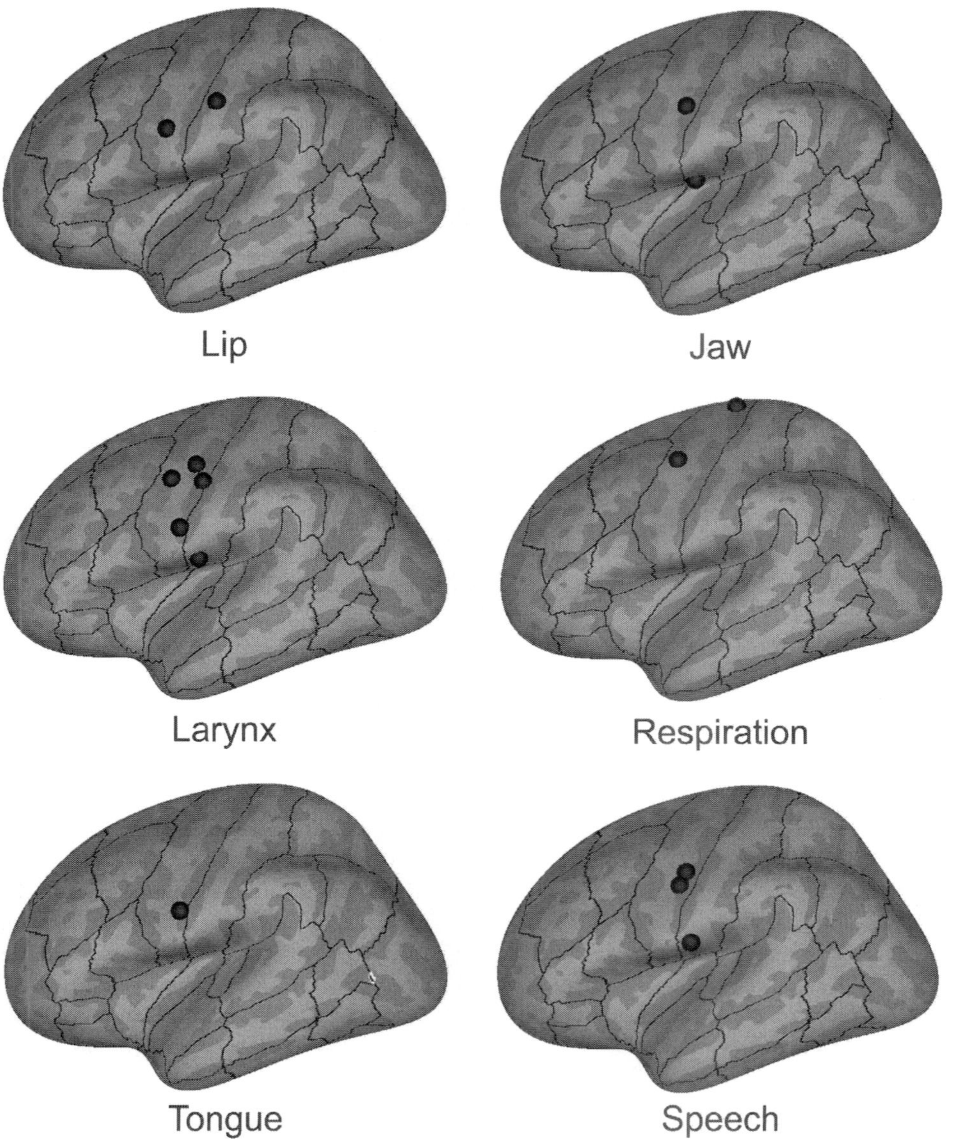

Figure 6.4 Speech articulator representations in left hemisphere Rolandic cortex. Locations shown in each of the first five panels were identified from an activation likelihood estimation meta-analysis of PET and fMRI studies of isolated articulator movements (Guenther, 2016, Appendix A). The sixth panel (bottom right) shows peaks from a meta-analysis of speech production (Turkeltaub, 2002; Brown et al., 2005).

Strick, 1996). Primate neurophysiological studies have suggested that the preSMA and SMA are differentially involved in the sequencing and initiation of movements, with preSMA acting at a more abstract level than the more motoric SMA (Matsuzaka et al., 1992; Tanji and Shima, 1994; Shima et al., 1996; Shima and Tanji, 1998a; Tanji, 2001). These areas also have distinct patterns of connectivity with cortical and subcortical areas in monkeys

(Jürgens, 1984; Luppino et al., 1993), a finding supported in humans using diffusion tensor imaging (Johansen-Berg et al., 2004; Lehéricy et al., 2004). Specifically, the preSMA is heavily connected with the prefrontal cortex and the caudate nucleus, whereas the SMA is more heavily connected with the motor cortex and the putamen, again suggesting a functional breakdown with preSMA involved in higher-level motor planning and SMA with motor execution.

Microstimulation of the SMA in humans (Penfield and Welch, 1951; Fried et al., 1991) often yields involuntary vocalization, repetitions of words or syllables, speech arrest, slowing of speech, or hesitancy, indicating its contribution to speech output. Speech-related symptoms from patients with SMA lesions have been described in the literature (e.g., Jonas, 1981, 1987; Ziegler et al., 1997; Pai, 1999). These often result in a transient period of total mutism, after which patients may suffer from reduced propositional (self-initiated) speech with non-propositional speech (automatic speech; e.g., counting, repeating words) nearly intact. Other problems include involuntary vocalizations, repetitions, paraphasias, echolalia, lack of prosodic variation, stuttering-like behavior, and variable speech rate, with only rare occurrences of distorted articulations. These outcomes are suggestive of a role in sequencing, initiating, suppressing, and/or timing speech output, but likely not providing detailed motor commands to the articulators. Based largely on the lesion literature, Jonas (1987) and Ziegler et al. (1997) arrived at similar conclusions regarding the role of the SMA in speech production, suggesting that it aids in sequencing and initiating speech sounds, but likely not in determining their phonemic content.

Recent neuroimaging studies have begun to reveal the distinct contributions made by the SMA and preSMA to speech production. For instance, Bohland and Guenther (2006) noted that activity in the preSMA increased for sequences composed of more phonologically complex syllables, whereas activity in the SMA showed no such effect for syllable complexity, but rather its response was preferentially increased when the sequence was overtly articulated. In a study of word production, Alario et al. (2006) provided further evidence for a preferential involvement of the SMA in motor output, and suggested a further functional subdivision within the preSMA. Specifically, these authors proposed that the anterior preSMA is more involved with lexical selection and the posterior portion with sequence encoding and execution. Tremblay and Gracco (2006) likewise observed SMA involvement across motor output tasks, but found that the preSMA response increased in a word generation task (involving lexical selection) as compared to a word reading task. Further evidence for a domain-general role of the left preSMA in motor response selection during word, sentence, and oral motor gesture production has been found using transcranial magnetic stimulation (Tremblay and Gracco, 2009) and fMRI (Tremblay and Small, 2011).

Collectively, these studies suggest that the SMA is more involved in the initiation and execution of speech output, whereas the preSMA contributes to higher-level processes including response selection and possibly the sequencing of syllables and phonemes. It has been proposed that the SMA serves as a "starting mechanism" for speech (Botez and Barbeau, 1971), but it remains unclear to what extent it is engaged throughout the duration of an utterance. Using an event-related design that segregated preparation and production phases of a paced syllable repetition task, Brendel et al. (2010) found that the medial wall areas (likely including both SMA and preSMA) became engaged when a preparatory cue was provided, and that the overall BOLD response was skewed toward the initial phase of extended syllable repetition periods; however, activity was not limited to the initial period but rather extended throughout the production period as well, suggesting some ongoing involvement throughout motor output. In a study probing the premotor speech areas using effective connectivity (which estimates the strength of influence between brain areas during a task), Hartwigsen et al. (2013) found that the optimal network arrangement (of 63 possible networks) placed the preSMA as the source of driving input (i.e., the starting mechanism) within the premotor network for pseudoword repetition. Bilateral preSMA was also more activated and provided significantly stronger faciliatory influence on dorsal premotor cortex during pseudoword repetition compared to word repetition, presumably due to an increased demand for sequencing speech sounds in unfamiliar pseudowords.

As more data accumulate, the overall view of the contribution of the medial premotor areas in speech motor control is becoming clearer, and is now being addressed in computational models. For example, the GODIVA model (Bohland et al., 2010) proposes that the preSMA codes for abstract (possibly syllable and/or word-level) sequences, while the SMA (in conjunction with the motor loop through the basal ganglia) is involved in initiation and timing of speech motor commands. This model is addressed in more detail in a later section ("The GODIVA model of speech sound sequencing").

Auditory cortex

Because speech production generates an acoustic signal that impinges on the speaker's own auditory system, speaking obligatorily activates the auditory cortex. As we describe in this section, this input is not simply an artifact of the speaking process, but instead it plays a critical role in speech motor control. The primary auditory cortex (BA 41), located along Heschl's gyrus on the supratemporal plane within the Sylvian fissure, receives (via the medial geniculate body of the thalamus) the bulk of auditory afferents, and projects to surrounding higher-order auditory cortical areas (BA 42, 22) of the superior temporal gyrus, including the planum temporale and planum polare within the supratemporal plane, and laterally to the superior temporal sulcus. These auditory areas are engaged during speech perception and speech production. It has been demonstrated with fMRI that covert speech, which does not generate an auditory signal, also activates auditory cortex (e.g., Hickok et al., 2000; Okada et al., 2003; Okada and Hickok, 2006). These results are consistent with an earlier MEG study demonstrating modulation of auditory cortical activation during covert as well as overt speech (Numminen and Curio 1999). It is notable that silent articulation (which differs from *covert speech* in that it includes overt tongue movemements) produces significantly increased auditory cortical activity bilaterally compared to purely imagined speech, despite no differences in auditory input (Okada et al., 2017).

Auditory and other sensory inputs provide important information to assist in the control problems involved in speech production. Specifically, hearing one's own speech allows the speaker to monitor productions and to make online error corrections as needed during vocalization. As described further in this chapter, modifications to auditory feedback during speech lead to increased activity in auditory cortical areas (e.g., Hashimoto and Sakai, 2003; Tourville et al., 2008; Niziolek and Guenther, 2013), and this has been hypothesized to correspond to an auditory error map that becomes active when a speaker's auditory feedback does not match his/her expectations (Guenther et al., 2006). The feedback-based control of speech is further described from a computational perspective in a later section ("The DIVA model of speech motor control").

A related phenomenon, referred to as "speech-induced suppression," is observed in studies using MEG or EEG. In this effect, activation in the auditory cortex (measured by the amplitude of a stereotyped potential ~100 ms after sound onset), is reduced for self-produced speech relative to hearing the speech of others or a recorded version of one's own voice when not speaking (Numminen et al., 1999; Curio et al., 2000; Houde et al., 2002). The magnitude of speech-induced suppression may be related to the degree of match of auditory expectations with incoming sensory feedback. This idea is further supported by studies that alter feedback (by adding noise or shifting the frequency spectrum) and report a reduced degree of suppression when feedback does not match the speaker's expectation (Houde et al., 2002; Heinks-Maldonado et al., 2006) and by a study demonstrating that less prototypical productions of a vowel are associated with reduced speech-induced suppression compared to prototypical productions (Niziolek et al., 2013). PET and fMRI studies have also demonstrated reduced response in superior temporal areas to self-initiated speech relative to hearing another voice, suggesting an active role in speech motor control (Hirano et al., 1996, 1997; Takaso et al., 2010; Zheng et al., 2010; Christoffels et al., 2011). Using multi-voxel pattern analysis, Markiewicz and Bohland (2016) found a region in the posterior superior temporal sulcus bilaterally whose response was predictive of the vowel that a subject heard and repeated aloud in an area consistent with the "phonological processing network" proposed by Hickok and Poeppel (2007). It is possible that this region encodes speech sounds at an abstract, phonological level, but this study could not specifically rule out a more continuous, auditory phonetic representation. For further discussion of the phonetics–phonology interface, see Chapter 13 of this volume.

An area deep within the posterior extent of the Sylvian fissure at the junction of parietal and temporal lobes (Area Spt) has been suggested to serve the role of sensorimotor integration in speech production (Buchsbaum et al., 2001; Hickok et al., 2003, 2009). This area, which straddles the boundary between the planum temporale and parietal operculum (PT and PO in Figure 6.3, respectively), is activated both during passive speech perception and during speech production (both overt and covert), suggesting its involvement in both motor and sensory processes. While not exclusive to speech acts, Area Spt appears to be preferentially activated for vocal tract movements as compared to manual movements (Pa and Hickok 2008). A recent state feedback control model of speech production proposes that this region implements a coordinate transform that allows mappings between articulatory and auditory phonetic representations of speech syllables (Hickok et al., 2011; Hickok, 2012). Such a role is largely consistent with proposals within the DIVA model (described in more detail in "The DIVA model of speech motor control"), although details differ in terms of the proposed mechanisms and localization.

Inferior frontal gyrus

The posterior portion of the inferior frontal gyrus (IFG) is classically subdivided into two regions: The *pars opercularis* (IFo; BA 44) and *pars triangularis* (IFt; BA 45). Left hemisphere IFo and IFt are often collectively referred to as "Broca's Area," based on the landmark study by Paul Broca that identified these areas as crucial for language production (Broca, 1861, see also Dronkers et al., 2007 for a more recent analysis of Broca's patients' lesions). Penfield and Roberts (1959) demonstrated that electrical stimulation of the IFG could give rise to speech arrest, offering direct evidence for its role in speech motor output. Later stimulation studies indicated the involvement of left inferior frontal areas in speech comprehension (Schäffler et al., 1993) in addition to speech production. The left IFG has also been implicated in reading (e.g., Pugh et al., 2001), grammatical aspects of language comprehension (e.g., Heim et al., 2003; Sahin et al., 2006), and a variety of tasks outside of the domain of speech and language production (see, for example, Fadiga et al., 2009).

Although likely also participating in higher-level aspects of language, the posterior portion of left IFG and the adjoining ventral premotor cortex (vPMC) are commonly activated in imaging studies of speech tasks as simple as monosyllabic pseudoword production (Guenther et al., 2006; Ghosh et al., 2008). The DIVA model (described in further detail in the next section) suggests that the left IFG and adjoining vPMC contain *speech sound map* cells that represent learned syllables and phonemes without regard for semantic content and that, when activated, generate the precise motor commands for the corresponding speech sounds. This view is consistent with the observation that activity in the left lateral premotor cortex decreases with learning of syllables containing phonotactically illegal consonant clusters, suggesting that practice with new sound sequences leads to the development of new, more efficient motor programs in this area (Segawa et al., 2015). This proposed role for left IFo/vPMC is similar, but not identical, to the view put forth by Indefrey and Levelt (2004), who suggested that this region serves as an interface between phonological and phonetic encoding, with the left posterior IFG responsible for syllabification (forming syllables from strings of planned phonological segments). This phonological role of the left IFG occurs in both the production and perception domains; for example, based on a large review of the PET and fMRI literature, Price (2012) suggested that both speech and non-speech sounds activate left IFG in tasks where they need to be segmented and held in working memory. Papoutsi et al. (2009) conducted an experiment using high and low frequency pseudoword production, aiming to clarify the role of the left IFG in either phonological or phonetic/articulatory processes in speech production. Their results revealed a differential response profile within the left IFG, suggesting that the posterior portion of BA 44 is functionally segregated along a dorsal–ventral gradient, with the dorsal portion involved in phonological encoding (consistent with Indefrey and Levelt, 2004), and the ventral portion in phonetic encoding (consistent with Hickok and Poeppel, 2004; Guenther et al., 2006). Further evidence that this region interfaces phonological representations with motoric representations comes from Hillis et al. (2004), who demonstrated that damage to the left (but not right) hemisphere posterior IFG is associated with apraxia of speech, a speech motor disorder that is often characterized as a failure or inefficiency in translating from well-formed phonological representations of words or syllables into previously learned motor information (McNeil et al., 2009).

While most evidence points to left-hemisphere dominance for IFo and IFt in speech and language function, a role for the right hemisphere homologues in speech motor control has also recently emerged. As previously noted, studies involving unexpected perturbations of either auditory (Toyomura et al., 2007; Tourville et al., 2008) or somatosensory (Golfinopoulos et al., 2011) feedback during speech (compared to typical feedback) give rise to differential sensory cortical activations, but also display prominent activations of right hemisphere ventral premotor cortex and posterior IFG. This activity is hypothesized to correspond to the compensatory motor actions invoked by subjects under such conditions, giving rise to a right-lateralized feedback control system (Tourville and Guenther, 2011), in contrast to a left-lateralized feedforward control system.

Thus far we have concentrated on cortical areas that are reliably active during speech tasks. Some regions of the cerebral cortex, however, appear to play a role in speech production but are not always significantly active compared to a baseline task in speech neuroimaging studies. These include the inferior frontal sulcus, inferior posterior parietal cortex, cingulate cortex, and the insular cortex. A number of factors may contribute to this, including variability in image acquisition, data analysis, statistical power, and precise speech and baseline tasks used. We next address several such areas.

Inferior frontal sulcus

The inferior frontal sulcus (IFS) separates the inferior frontal and middle frontal gyri in the lateral prefrontal cortex. In addition to a role in semantic processing (e.g., Crosson et al., 2001, 2003), the IFS and surrounding areas have been implicated in a large number of studies of language and working memory (Fiez et al., 1996; D'Esposito et al., 1998; Gabrieli et al., 1998; Kerns et al., 2004) and in serial order processing (Petrides, 1991; Averbeck et al., 2002, 2003). As previously noted, the dorsal IFG, which abuts the IFS,[4] appears to be more engaged by phonological than by motor processes; the IFS likewise appears to be sensitive to phonological parameters and specifically related to phonological working memory.

Bohland and Guenther (2006) showed that strongly left-lateralized activity within the IFS and surrounding areas was modulated by the phonological composition of multisyllabic pseudoword sequences. In this task, subjects were required to encode three-syllable sequences in memory prior to the arrival of a GO signal. IFS activity showed an interaction between the complexity of the syllables within the sequence (i.e., /stra/ vs. /ta/) and the complexity of the sequence (i.e., /ta ki ru/ vs. /ta ta/), which is consistent with this area serving as a phonological buffer (as hypothesized in the GODIVA model, described in more detail in the next section; Bohland et al., 2010). This area was previously shown to encode phonetic categories during speech perception (Myers et al., 2009), and recent work has shown that response patterns in the left IFS are predictive of individual phonemes (vowels) that a subject heard and must later produce in a delayed auditory repetition task (Markiewicz and Bohland 2016). These results argue that subjects activate prefrontal working memory representations as a consequence of speech perception processes (for maintenance or subvocal rehearsal of the incoming sounds), which may utilize an abstracted, phoneme-like representation in the left IFS.

Inferior posterior parietal cortex

The inferior posterior parietal cortex consists of the angular gyrus (BA 39) and supramarginal gyrus (BA 40). Although these areas were not found to be reliably active across word production studies in the meta-analysis of Indefrey and Levelt (2004),[5] they have been implicated in a number of speech studies. Speech production tasks with a working memory component can also activate the inferior parietal lobe and/or intraparietal sulcus (e.g., Bohland and Guenther, 2006). This observation fits in well with the view of inferior parietal cortex playing a role in verbal working memory (e.g., Paulesu et al., 1993; Jonides et al., 1998; Becker et al., 1999) and may also be related to the observation that damage to left supramarginal gyrus causes impairment on phonetic discrimination tasks that involve holding one speech sound in working memory while comparing it to a second incoming sound (Caplan et al., 1995). The left inferior parietal lobe has also been shown to be activated in syllable order judgments (compared to syllable identification), further suggesting its importance in encoding verbal working memory (Moser et al., 2009). Damage to the left supramarginal gyrus and/or temporal-parietal junction gives rise to difficulties in repetition tasks (Fridriksson et al., 2010), potentially compromising part of a "dorsal pathway" for acoustic-to-articulatory translation as suggested by Hickok and Poeppel (2007).

The anterior supramarginal gyrus has also been suggested to be involved in the somatosensory feedback-based control of speech (Guenther et al., 2006). This hypothesis was corroborated by results of an experiment showing increased activation in inferior parietal areas during speech when the jaw was unexpectedly perturbed compared to non-perturbed speech (Golfinopoulos et al., 2011). This topic will be discussed further in the next section (see "The DIVA model of speech motor control").

Cingulate cortex

Although not always identified in speech neuroimaging studies, activation of the middle cingulate gyrus is clearly illustrated in Figure 6.3 (dCMA, extending into vCMA). This activity peaks in the ventral bank of the cingulate sulcus, likely part of the cingulate motor area (cf. Paus et al., 1993). The cingulate motor area has been associated with providing the motivation or will to vocalize (e.g., Jürgens and von Cramon, 1982; Paus, 2001) and with processing reward-based motor selection (Shima and Tanji, 1998b). Bilateral damage to cingulate cortex can severely impact voluntary (but not innate) vocalizations in monkeys (Jürgens, 2009). In humans, bilateral damage to cingulate cortex can result in transcortical motor aphasia, marked by a dramatically reduced motivation to speak (including reduced ability to move or speak; Németh et al., 1988), but such damage does not impair grammar or articulation of any speech that is produced (Rubens, 1975; Jürgens and von Cramon, 1982).

Insular cortex

Buried deep within Sylvian fissure, the insula is a continuous sheet of cortex that borders the frontal, parietal, and temporal lobes. Because of its close proximity to several areas known to be involved in speech and language processes, it has long been considered a candidate for language function (Wernicke, 1874; Freud, 1891; Dejerine, 1914, see Ardila, 1999 for a review). In the anterior superior direction, the insula borders speech motor areas in the frontal opercular region of the IFG (BA 44) and the inferior-most portion of the precentral gyrus (BA 4, 6), which contains the motor representation of the speech articulators. In the posterior superior direction, the insula borders the somatosensory representations of the speech articulators in the postcentral gyrus (BA 1, 2, 3), as well as the parietal operculum (BA 40). Inferiorly, the insula borders the auditory cortical areas of the superior temporal plane (BA 41, 42, 22). Figure 6.3 shows bilateral insula activity that extends to each of these speech-related areas. Activity is stronger and more widespread in the anterior portion (aINS) than the posterior portion (pINS), particularly in the left hemisphere.

Unlike the neocortical areas described thus far, the insular cortex is a phylogenetically older form of cortex known as "mesocortex" (along with the cingulate gyrus) and is considered a paralimbic structure. In addition to speech, a wide range of functions including memory, drive, affect, gustation, and olfaction have been attributed to the insula in various studies (Türe et al., 1999). Consistent with the placement of the insula in the paralimbic system, Benson (1979) and Ardila (1999) have argued that the insula is likely involved in motivational and affective aspects of speech and language. Damage to the insula has been shown previously to lead to deficits in speech initiation (Shuren, 1993) and motivation to speak (Habib et al., 1995).

As noted in the review by Price (2012), the opinion of the research community on the role of the insular cortex in speech has evolved several times. This area has received significant recent attention in both the neuroimaging and neurology literatures (Ardila, 1999; Türe et al., 1999; Ackermann and Riecker, 2004), largely following the lesion mapping study of Dronkers (1996). This study found that the precentral gyrus of the left insula was the only common site of overlap in a group of patients diagnosed with apraxia of speech, but was preserved in a second group with aphasia but not apraxia of speech. This region, therefore, was argued to be critical for motor programming, or translating a planned speech sound into articulatory action.[6] A number of neuroimaging studies have found activation of the insula in overt speaking tasks (Wise et al., 1999; Riecker, Ackermann, Wildgruber, Dogil et al., 2000; Sakurai et al., 2001; Bohland and Guenther, 2006), even for single syllables (Sörös et al., 2006; Ghosh et al., 2008). The relatively consistent finding of greater activation of the anterior insula (either bilateral or left-lateralized, which varies across studies) for overt vs. covert speech suggests its role may be in assisting articulatory control rather than in pre-articulatory planning processes (Ackermann and Riecker, 2004). There is evidence against a role for anterior insula in the detailed planning of articulator movements; for example, Bohland and Guenther (2006) noted that activity at the level of the precentral gyrus of the anterior insula was not modulated by phonological/phonetic complexity. A separate focus of activity at the junction of the anterior insula and adjoining frontal operculum, however, was strongly modulated by complexity, which is largely consistent with other reports (Riecker et al., 2008; Shuster, 2009). These results suggest that anterior insula may enable or modulate speech motor programs, rather than store them.

Although many speech neuroimaging studies have reported insula activation, others have not, at least for some speaking conditions (e.g., Lotze et al., 2000; Riecker, Ackermann, Wildgruber, Meyer et al., 2000; Sörös et al., 2006). Furthermore, other lesion-based studies have not replicated the results of Dronkers (Hillis et al., 2004). Sörös et al. (2006) have suggested that insula activation may depend on whether the speaking condition involves repeated production of the same sounds or production of different syllables/words on each trial. Relatedly, insula recruitment may hinge on the automaticity of the speaking task, with very simple or overlearned speech tasks not necessitating its involvement, whereas more complex sequential production tasks may recruit insular cortex during or prior to articulation (Ackermann and Riecker, 2004). This role is largely consistent with a recent study using voxel-based lesion symptom mapping in a group of 33 patients with left-hemisphere strokes that related lesion site to several measures of performance on speech production tasks (Baldo et al., 2011). This study found that the superior portion of the precentral gyrus of the insula was critical for complex articulations (e.g., consonant clusters, multisyllabic words) but not for simple syllable production. The importance of the insula for speech production, however, remains contentious, with a recent individual subject analysis demonstrating weak responses of the anterior insula to overt speech (in comparison, for example, to the posterior IFG), and enhanced responses to non-speech oral movements (Fedorenko et al., 2015). Additional efforts are necessary to carefully delineate and differentially test between the various proposals in the literature about the role of the insula in speech. Such efforts may also benefit from computational/simulation studies, which can help to formalize theoretical roles and generate specific hypotheses that can be tested using neuroimaging.

Neurocomputational modeling of speech production

The expansive library of results from neuroimaging studies provide important insight into the roles of many brain areas in speech motor control. In isolation, however, these results do not provide an integrated, mechanistic view of how the neural circuits engaged by speech tasks interact to produce fluent speech. To this end, computational models that both (a) suggest the neural computations performed within specific modules and across pathways that link modules, and (b) propose specific neural correlates for these computational elements, help to bridge this critical gap. These models further suggest specific hypotheses that may be tested in imaging and behavioral experiments, leading to a continuous cycle of model refinement that provides a unifying account of a substantial fraction of the relevant literature. Next we briefly describe the most influential and thoroughly tested neurocomputational account of speech motor control, the DIVA model, which has been developed, tested, and refined by Guenther and colleagues over the last two decades. We also provide an introduction to an extension of the DIVA model, termed "GODIVA," which begins to account for higher-level phonological processes involved in speech planning and their interface with speech motor control (see also Hickok, 2012; Roelofs, 2014).

The DIVA model of speech motor control

The *D*irections *I*nto *V*elocities of the *A*rticulators (DIVA) model (recent descriptions in Guenther et al., 2006; Golfinopoulos et al., 2010; Tourville and Guenther, 2011; Guenther, 2016) provides a computational account of the neural processes underlying speech production. The model, schematized in Figure 6.5, takes the form of an adaptive neural network whose components correspond to regions of the cerebral cortex and associated subcortical structures (some of which are not shown in the figure for clarity). Each box in Figure 6.5 corresponds to a set of neurons (or *map*) in the model, and arrows correspond to synaptic projections that transform one type of neural representation into another. The model is implemented in computer simulations that control an articulatory synthesizer (Maeda, 1990)

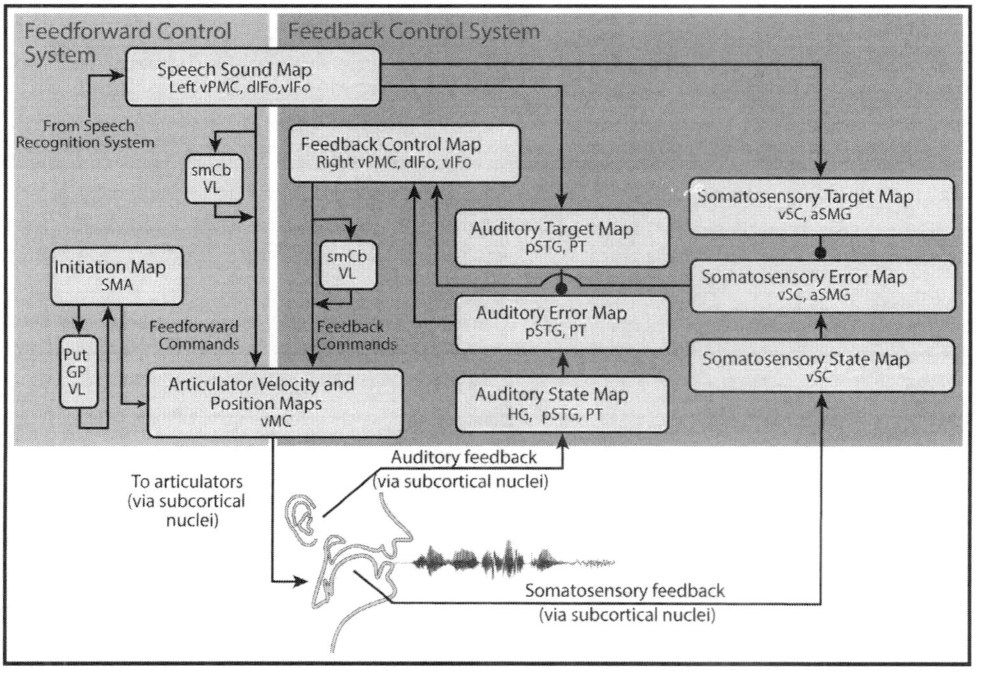

Figure 6.5 The *D*irections *I*nto *V*elocities of *A*rticulators (DIVA) neurocomputational model of speech motor control. Each component of the model (boxes) is associated with a specific brain region or set of regions, and all neural processing stages and their interactions via synaptic projections (arrows) are mathematically characterized. See text for details.

Abbreviations: GP, globus pallidus; Put, putamen; smCB, superior medial cerebellum; VL, ventrolateral thalamic nucleus. See Figure 6.3 caption for the definition of additional abbreviations.

in order to produce an acoustic signal. The articulator movements and acoustic signal produced by the model have been shown to account for a wide range of data concerning speech development and production (see Guenther et al., 1998, 2006 for reviews). The model's neurons (each meant to roughly correspond to a small population of neurons in the brain) are localized in a stereotactic coordinate frame to allow for direct comparisons between model simulations and functional neuroimaging experiments, and a number of model predictions about neural activity have been tested with fMRI (e.g., Ghosh et al., 2008; Tourville et al., 2008; Peeva et al., 2010; Golfinopoulos et al., 2011) and intracortical microelectrode recordings (Guenther et al., 2009). Although the model is computationally defined, the discussion here will focus on the hypothesized functions of the modeled brain regions without consideration of associated equations (see Guenther et al., 2006; Golfinopoulos et al., 2010 for mathematical details).

According to the DIVA model, production of speech starts with activation of neurons in a *speech sound map* in left ventral premotor cortex and an *initiation map* in SMA. How these neurons themselves may be activated by a representation of a multisyllabic speech plan is described further in "The GODIVA model of speech sound sequencing." The speech sound map includes a representation of each speech sound (phoneme or syllable) that the model has learned to produce, with the most commonly represented sound unit being the syllable (cf. the "mental syllabary" of Levelt and Wheeldon, 1994). Activation of speech sound map neurons leads to motor commands that arrive in motor cortex via two control subsystems: A *feedforward control subsystem* (left shaded box in Figure 6.5) and a *feedback control subsystem* (right shaded box). The feedback control subsystem can be further broken into two components: An auditory feedback control subsystem and a somatosensory feedback control subsystem.

The feedforward control system has two main components: One involving the ventral premotor and motor cortices along with a cerebellar loop, and one involving the SMA and associated basal ganglia motor loop. Roughly speaking, these two components can be thought of as a *motor program circuit* that generates the detailed muscle activations needed to produce phonemes, syllables, and words, and an *initiation circuit* that determines which motor programs to activate and when to activate them.

The first component of the feedforward control system involves projections from the left ventral premotor cortex to primary motor cortex, both directly and via a side loop involving the cerebellum[7] (feedforward commands in Figure 6.5). These projections encode stored motor commands (or motor programs) for producing the sounds of the speech sound map; these commands take the form of time-varying trajectories of the speech articulators, similar to the concept of a gestural score (see Browman and Goldstein, 1990). The primary motor and premotor cortices are well-known to be strongly interconnected (e.g., Passingham, 1993; Krakauer and Ghez, 1999). Furthermore, the cerebellum is known to receive input via the pontine nuclei from premotor cortical areas, as well as higher-order auditory and somatosensory areas that can provide state information important for choosing motor commands (e.g., Schmahmann and Pandya, 1997), and projects heavily to the primary motor cortex (e.g., Middleton and Strick, 1997). As previously noted (see "Neural systems involved in speech production"), damage to the superior paravermal region of the cerebellar cortex results in ataxic dysarthria, a motor speech disorder characterized by slurred, poorly coordinated speech (Ackermann et al., 1992), supporting the view that this region is involved in fine-tuning the feedforward speech motor commands, perhaps by information about the current sensorimotor state.

The second component of the feedforward system is responsible for the release of speech motor commands to the articulators. According to the model, the release of a motor program starts with activation of a corresponding cell in an initiation map that lies in the SMA. It is proposed that the timing of initiation cell activation, and therefore, motor commands, is governed by contextual inputs from the basal ganglia via the thalamus (see also "The GODIVA model of speech sound sequencing" for further details). The basal ganglia are well-suited for this role given their afferents from most cortical regions of the brain, including motor, prefrontal, associative, and limbic cortices. These nuclei are also strongly and reciprocally connected with the SMA (Romanelli et al., 2005).

The auditory feedback control subsystem involves axonal projections from speech sound map cells in the left ventral premotor cortex to the higher-order auditory cortical areas; these projections embody the auditory target region for the speech sound currently being produced. That is, they represent the auditory feedback that should arise when the speaker hears himself/herself producing the sound, including a learned measure of acceptable variability. This target is compared to incoming auditory information from the auditory periphery, and if the current auditory feedback is outside the target region, neurons in the model's *auditory error map*, which resides in the posterior superior temporal gyrus and planum temporale, become active. Auditory error cells project to a *feedback control map* in right ventral premotor cortex, which is responsible for transforming auditory errors into corrective movements of the speech articulators (feedback commands in Figure 6.5). Numerous studies suggest that sensory error representations in cerebellum influence corrective movements (e.g., Diedrichsen et al., 2005; Penhune and Doyon, 2005; Grafton et al., 2008), and the model accordingly posits that the cerebellum contributes to the feedback motor command.

The projections from the DIVA model's speech sound map to the auditory cortical areas inhibit auditory error map cells. If the incoming auditory signal is within the target region, this inhibition cancels the excitatory effects of the incoming auditory signal. If the incoming auditory signal is outside the target region, the inhibitory target region will not completely cancel the excitatory input from the auditory periphery, resulting in activation of auditory error cells. As discussed earlier, evidence of inhibition in auditory cortical areas in the superior temporal gyrus during one's own speech comes from several different sources, including recorded neural responses during open brain surgery (Creutzfeldt et al., 1989a, 1989b), MEG measurements (Numminen and Curio, 1999; Numminen et al., 1999; Houde et al., 2002), and PET measurements (Wise et al., 1999).

The DIVA model also posits a somatosensory feedback control subsystem operating alongside the auditory feedback subsystem. The model's *somatosensory state map* corresponds to the representation of tactile and proprioceptive information from the speech articulators in primary and higher-order somatosensory cortical areas in the postcentral gyrus and supramarginal gyrus of the inferior parietal lobe. The *somatosensory target map* represents the expected somatosensory consequences of producing the current sound; this target is encoded by projections from left ventral premotor cortex to the supramarginal gyrus. The model's *somatosensory error map* is hypothesized to reside primarily in the anterior supramarginal gyrus, a region that has been implicated in phonological processing for speech perception, and speech production (Geschwind, 1965; Damasio and Damasio, 1980). According to the model, cells in this map become active during speech if the speaker's tactile and proprioceptive feedback from the vocal tract deviates from the somatosensory target region for the sound being produced. The output of the somatosensory error map then propagates to motor cortex via the feedback control map in right ventral premotor cortex;

synaptic projections in this pathway encode the transformation from somatosensory errors into motor commands that correct those errors.

The DIVA model also provides a computational account of the acquisition of speech motor skills. Learning in the model occurs via adjustments to the synaptic projections between cortical maps (arrows in Figure 6.5). The first learning stage involves babbling movements of the speech articulators, which generate a combination of articulatory, auditory, and somatosensory information that is used to tune the feedback control system, specifically the synaptic projections that transform auditory and somatosensory error signals into corrective motor commands. The learning in this stage is not associated with specific speech sounds; instead these learned sensory-motor transformations will be used in the production of all speech sounds that are learned in the next stage.

The second learning stage is an imitation stage in which the model is presented with auditory sound samples of phonemes, syllables, or words to learn, much like an infant is exposed to the sounds and words of his/her native language. These sounds take the form of time-varying acoustic signals. Based on these samples, the model learns an auditory target for each sound, encoded in synaptic projections from left ventral premotor cortex to the auditory cortical areas in the posterior superior temporal gyrus (auditory target map in Figure 6.5). The targets consist of time-varying regions (or ranges) that encode the allowable variability of the acoustic signal throughout the syllable. The use of target *regions* rather than point targets is an important aspect of the DIVA model that provides a unified explanation for a wide range of speech production phenomena, including motor equivalence, contextual variability, anticipatory coarticulation, carryover coarticulation, and speaking rate effects (Guenther, 1995; Guenther et al., 1998). After the auditory target for a new sound is learned, the model then attempts to produce the sound. Initially the model does not possess an accurate set of feedforward commands for producing the sound, and sensory errors occur. The feedback control system translates these errors into corrective motor commands, and on each production attempt the commands generated by the feedback control system are incorporated into the feedforward command for the next attempt by adjusting the synaptic projections from the left ventral premotor cortex to the primary motor cortex (feedforward commands in Figure 6.5). This iterative learning process, which is hypothesized to heavily involve the cerebellum, results in a more accurate feedforward command for the next attempt. After a few production attempts, the feedforward command by itself is sufficient to produce the sound in normal circumstances. That is, the feedforward command is accurate enough that it generates very few auditory errors during production of the sound and thus does not invoke the auditory feedback control subsystem. As the model repeatedly produces a speech sound, it learns a somatosensory target region for the sound, analogous to the auditory target region mentioned earlier. This target represents the expected tactile and proprioceptive sensations associated with the sound and is used in the somatosensory feedback control subsystem to detect somatosensory errors.

As described earlier, cells in the speech sound map are activated both when perceiving a sound and when producing the same sound. This is consistent with studies that demonstrate recruitment of IFG and vPMC in speech perception (e.g., Wilson et al., 2004; D'Ausilio et al., 2009). In the model, these neurons are necessary for the acquisition of new speech sounds by infants. Here DIVA postulates that a population of speech sound map cells is activated when an infant hears a new sound, which enables the learning of an auditory target for that sound. Later, to produce that sound, the infant activates the same speech sound map cells to drive motor output. Individual neurons with such properties (i.e., that are active during both the performance and the comprehension of motor acts), have been found in the premotor Area F5 in monkeys (thought to be homologous with BA 44 in humans) and are commonly labeled "mirror neurons" (di Pellegrino et al., 1992; Gallese et al., 1996; Rizzolatti et al., 1996). See Rizzolatti and Arbib (1998) and Binkofski and Buccino (2004) for discussion of possible roles for mirror neurons in language beyond that proposed here.

The GODIVA model of speech sound sequencing

The DIVA model accounts for many aspects of the production of individual speech motor programs, with the most typical unit of motor programming being the syllable. Additional brain areas, particularly in the left prefrontal cortex, are involved in conversational speech, or for producing multisyllabic words or phrases. A large body of evidence, particularly from naturally occurring "slips of the tongue" (e.g., MacKay, 1970; Fromkin, 1971), indicates that speech involves substantial advanced planning of the sound sequences to be produced. The GODIVA model (Bohland et al., 2010) addresses how the brain may represent planned speech sequences, and how phonological representations of these sequences may interface with phonetic representations and the speech motor control circuits modeled by DIVA.

The model can be thought of, in some ways, as a neurobiologically grounded implementation of slots-and-fillers style psycholinguistic models (e.g., Shattuck-Hufnagel, 1979; Dell, 1986; Levelt et al., 1999). In these types of models, a phonological frame describes an arrangement of abstract, categorical "slots" that is represented independently of the segments that fill those slots. Thus, the word "cat," for example, could be jointly encoded by an abstract CVC (consonant-vowel-consonant) syllable frame and the string of phonemes /k/, /æ/, and /t/. During production, the slots in the phonological frame are "filled" by appropriate segments chosen from a buffer (i.e., phonological working memory). The segregation of frame and content is motivated in large part by naturally occurring speech errors, which are known to strongly preserve serial positions within syllables or words (i.e., the onset consonant from one forthcoming syllable may be substituted for the onset consonant from another, but very rarely for a vowel or coda consonant).

The GODIVA model specifically provides an account of how the preSMA, left posterior IFS, and basal ganglia implement these phonological representations and how they interact with the speech motor control networks described by DIVA. A simplified version of the GODIVA model is shown in Figure 6.6. According to the model, an upcoming multisyllabic utterance is represented simultaneously in two complementary modules within the prefrontal cortex. The sequential frame structure (syllable or word level) is hypothesized to be represented in the preSMA, without regard for the phonemes involved, whereas the phonological content of the utterance is represented in the left posterior inferior frontal sulcus (pIFS), organized by the location of the phonemes within the sequential frame. Each of these representations is modeled as a working memory, which can contain multiple co-active items (i.e., the model can simultaneously represent multiple forthcoming words or syllables). Each of these areas (preSMA and left pIFS) is modeled as containing both "plan cells" and "choice cells" arranged in a columnar architecture such that columns represent sequential frame structures (preSMA) or individual phonological units (left pIFS). The forthcoming order of the items in each buffer is represented using an activity gradient across multiple simultaneously active plan cells (Grossberg, 1978a, cf. 1978b; Hartley and Houghton, 1996; Bullock and Rhodes, 2003). During a selection process, winner-take-all dynamics allow a single choice cell to become active, effectively selecting the plan cell with the highest activity (i.e., the next item). The use of a gradient representation to maintain serial order gives rise to the model's name (Gradient Order DIVA). Such graded serial order

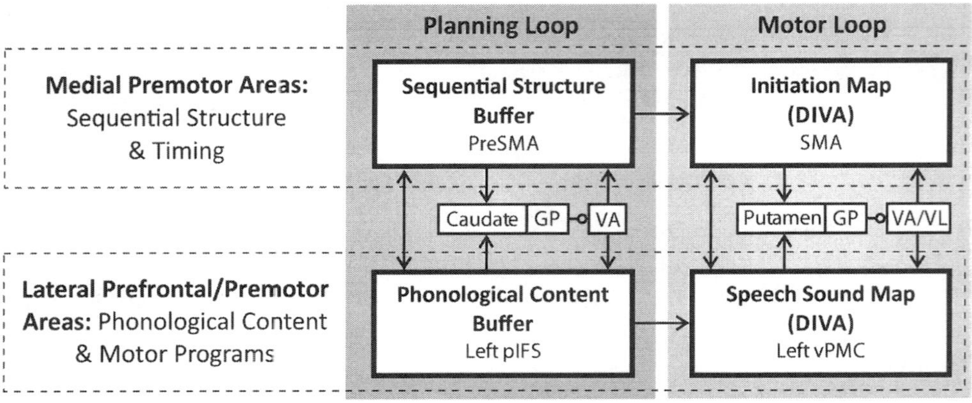

Figure 6.6 A simplified schematic of the GODIVA model of speech sound sequencing and its interface with the DIVA model of speech motor control. The GODIVA model implements components of the planning loop and their interactions with the motor loop, part of the DIVA model.

Abbreviations: GP, globus pallidus; pIFS, posterior inferior frontal sulcus; preSMA, pre-supplementary motor area; SMA, supplementary motor area; VA, ventral anterior nucleus of the thalamus; VL, ventrolateral thalamic nucleus; vPMC, ventral premotor cortex.

representations of complex movement sequences have been found in the lateral prefrontal cortex of nonhuman primates (Averbeck et al., 2002, 2003), and rank-order and sequence-selective cells have been identified in the preSMA (Clower and Alexander, 1998; Shima and Tanji, 2000). The primary subdivision within GODIVA – between pIFS and preSMA – can also be thought of as a computational implementation of the frame-content theory of speech production (MacNeilage, 1998).

The coordination of sequence structure and phonological content is proposed to involve a basal ganglia mediated "planning loop." The planning loop is hypothesized to involve the caudate nucleus and ventral anterior nucleus of the thalamus (whereas the "motor loop" involves the SMA, the putamen, and the ventral lateral nucleus of the thalamus). Production of an individual syllable (or word) begins by the selection of a winning sequential frame cell in the preSMA. Next, through interactions within the planning loop, phonemes are selected in the pIFS choice cells for each slot in the chosen sequential structure (see Bohland et al., 2010 for further details). The selection of phonetic/motor units to be produced (from those stored in DIVA's speech sound map, which are most typically syllable sized "chunks") is then made through projections from the left pIFS to left vPMC. These synaptic pathways specifically activate sensorimotor programs that match the sounds selected in the pIFS, with the best matching program (i.e., largest available matching unit) ultimately selected for execution. Production of that syllable (or word), however, will not commence until a second signal arrives at the ventral premotor cortex, arising from neurons in the SMA, which drive *initiation* (see initiation map in Figures 6.5 and 6.6). To coordinate timing, projections from preSMA to SMA activate, in the proper sequence, the appropriate neurons in the initiation map, which in turn leads to the readout of the feedforward commands for the next syllable via projections to the speech sound map. After a motor program has been initiated, its phonological representation in left pIFS is suppressed, and the circuit can, for example, begin selection of the next syllable in a multisyllabic utterance.

The GODIVA model provides a natural extension to DIVA, to account for multisyllabic planning, timing, and coordination, as well as their neural correlates as evidenced from clinical and neuroimaging studies. It also provides a means for addressing some aspects of speech disorders that may impact these levels of processing. For example, disruption of the pathway from left pIFS to left vPMC, responsible in the model for selecting syllable motor programs, would lead to many of the symptoms of apraxia of speech. Furthermore, the basic GODIVA framework has been extended to address the possible role of the basal ganglia in stuttering (Civier et al., 2013). In these computer simulations, which further elaborated the direct and indirect basal ganglia pathways within GODIVA, a hypothesized excess of the neurotransmitter dopamine (Wu et al., 1997) gives rise to reduced competition and delayed selection among competing speech motor programs, leading to dysfluencies similar to those observed in stuttering.

Conclusions and future directions

The history of scientific inquiry into the neural mechanisms underlying speech and language is a storied one, reaching back to the seminal lesion studies of Broca and his contemporaries in the mid-19th century. The advent of neuroimaging techniques such as PET and fMRI has greatly accelerated our knowledge of the neural bases of speech. Although the nature of the neural computations performed by different brain regions is still up for debate, there is general agreement regarding the involvement of a number of brain areas in speech articulation. In the cerebral cortex, these regions include the IFG, primary motor and somatosensory cortices, lateral premotor cortex, SMA, preSMA, and auditory cortex. Subcortical structures in the speech network include the cerebellum, basal ganglia, and thalamus. More complex speech and language tasks recruit additional areas, including a number of prefrontal and temporal association areas of the cerebral cortex. Cortical activities are modulated by two re-entrant loops with subcortical structures: A basal ganglia loop involved in action selection and initiation, and a cerebellar loop involved in generating the finely tuned motor commands that underlie fluent speech.

The formulation of neurocomputational models that provide both quantitative and neuroanatomical characterizations of the speech network is becoming increasingly important in order to make sense of an ever-increasing library of results based upon a broad and diverse set of methodologies. Although our focus herein was primarily on the DIVA model of speech motor control, a number of neurocomputational models have been formulated to address aspects of language production not specifically captured by DIVA. One of these (the GODIVA model of speech sound sequencing; Bohland et al., 2010) was described in some detail in this chapter. Other related models include, but are not limited to, the Weaver++ model of word form encoding (Roelofs, 1997; Roelofs and Hagoort, 2002), the ACT model of the motor "action repository" (Kröger et al., 2009), the state feedback control model (Houde and Nagarajan, 2011), and the hierarchical state feedback control model (Hickok, 2012). We expect efforts to build and test computational models of speech production to continue since these models provide coherence to a scientific literature that is prone to disconnection between sub-disciplines focusing on different experimental technologies.

Acknowledgments

Supported by the National Institute on Deafness and other Communication Disorders (R01 DC007683 and R01 DC002852) and the National Science Foundation (BCS 1655287).

Notes

1 The "mental lexicon" refers to a psycholinguistic construct that describes the store of information about the words in one's language. Many theoretical models (e.g., Levelt 1989) assume that phonological representations related to individual words are retrieved from this repository and used to drive typical language production.
2 Figure 6.1 also shows activity in the red nucleus, a midbrain structure whose role in speech is unclear as its primary influence is on limb-related motoneuron pools in the spinal cord (Duffy 1995).
3 The repetition suppression paradigm makes use of the idea that neural activity may be reduced when stimuli are repeated or, in particular, when repeated stimuli activate the same pools of neurons.
4 It is notable that activation results, particularly those analyzed volumetrically rather than in a surface-based framework, are often reported using brain atlases that do not distinguish gyri from their adjacent sulci. Thus, some activations that are focused within or extending into the IFS have likely been previously annotated as IFG.
5 This meta-analysis included single word production tasks based on four paradigms including picture naming, word generation, word reading, and pseudoword reading. While studies varied in terms of their lead-in processes, overt vs. covert production, and precise control tasks used, they generally did not place high demands on speech planning or working memory processes.
6 It should be noted that, although most agree it is a deficit with impact at the phonological–phonetic interface, the classification and theoretical explanations for apraxia of speech remain controversial (Ziegler et al., 2012). Dronkers (1996) required patients with apraxia of speech to have diagnoses from at least two clinicians according to a set of four criteria described by Wertz et al. (1991).
7 Though not shown in Figure 6.5 for clarity, this side loop passes through the pontine nuclei and thalamus on the way to and from the cerebellum, respectively.

References

Ackermann, H., 2008. Cerebellar contributions to speech production and speech perception: psycholinguistic and neurobiological perspectives. *Trends in Neurosciences*, 31 (6), 265–272.

Ackermann, H. and Hertrich, I., 1994. Speech rate and rhythm in cerebellar dysarthria: an acoustic analysis of syllabic timing. *Folia phoniatrica et logopaedica*, 46 (2), 70–78.

Ackermann, H. and Riecker, A., 2004. The contribution of the insula to motor aspects of speech production: a review and a hypothesis. *Brain and Language*, 89 (2), 320–328.

Ackermann, H., Vogel, M., Petersen, D., and Poremba, M., 1992. Speech deficits in ischaemic cerebellar lesions. *Journal of Neurology*, 239 (4), 223–227.

Alario, F-X., Chainay, H., Lehericy, S., and Cohen, L., 2006. The role of the Supplementary Motor Area (SMA) in word production. *Brain Research*, 1076 (1), 129–143.

Alexander, G.E. and Crutcher, M.D., 1990. Functional architecture of basal ganglia circuits: neural substrates of parallel processing. *Trends in Neurosciences*, 13 (7), 266–271.

Alexander, G.E., DeLong, M.R., and Strick, P.L., 1986. Parallel organization of functionally segregated circuits linking basal ganglia and cortex. *Annual Review of Neuroscience*, 9, 357–381.

Ardila, A., 1999. The role of insula in language: an unsettled question. *Aphasiology*, 13 (1), 79–87.

Averbeck, B.B., Chafee, M.V, Crowe, D.A., and Georgopoulos, A.P., 2002. Parallel processing of serial movements in prefrontal cortex. *Proceedings of the National Academy of Sciences of the United States of America*, 99 (20), 13172–13177.

Averbeck, B.B., Chafee, M.V, Crowe, D.A., and Georgopoulos, A.P., 2003. Neural activity in prefrontal cortex during copying geometrical shapes. I. Single cells encode shape, sequence, and metric parameters. *Experimental Brain Research*, 150 (2), 127–141.

Baldo, J.V, Wilkins, D.P., Ogar, J., Willock, S., and Dronkers, N.F., 2011. Role of the precentral gyrus of the insula in complex articulation. *Cortex*, 47 (7), 800–807.

Barbas, H., García-Cabezas, M.Á., and Zikopoulos, B., 2013. Frontal-thalamic circuits associated with language. *Brain and Language*, 126 (1), 49–61.

Basilakos, A., Smith, K.G., Fillmore, P., Fridriksson, J., and Fedorenko, E., 2017. Functional characterization of the human speech articulation network. *Cerebral Cortex*, 1–15.

Becker, J.T., MacAndrew, D.K., and Fiez, J.A., 1999. A comment on the functional localization of the phonological storage subsystem of working memory. *Brain and Cognition*, 41 (1), 27–38.

Benson, D., 1979. *Aphasia, Alexia, and Agraphia*. New York: Churchill Livingstone.

Binkofski, F. and Buccino, G., 2004. Motor functions of the Broca's region. *Brain and Language*, 89 (2), 362–369.

Blakemore, S.J., Wolpert, D.M., and Frith, C.D., 1998. Central cancellation of self-produced tickle sensation. *Nature Neuroscience*, 1 (7), 635–640.

Bohland, J.W., Bullock, D., and Guenther, F.H., 2010. Neural representations and mechanisms for the performance of simple speech sequences. *Journal of Cognitive Neuroscience*, 22 (7), 1504–1529.

Bohland, J.W. and Guenther, F.H., 2006. An fMRI investigation of syllable sequence production. *NeuroImage*, 32 (2), 821–841.

Botez, M.I. and Barbeau, A., 1971. Role of subcortical structures, and particularly of the thalamus, in the mechanisms of speech and language. A review. *International Journal of Neurology*, 8 (2), 300–320.

Braitenberg, V., Heck, D., and Sultan, F., 1997. The detection and generation of sequences as a key to cerebellar function: experiments and theory. *Behavioral and Brain Sciences*, 20 (2), 229–245–277.

Brendel, B., Hertrich, I., Erb, M., Lindner, A., Riecker, A., Grodd, W., and Ackermann, H., 2010. The contribution of mesiofrontal cortex to the preparation and execution of repetitive syllable productions: an fMRI study. *NeuroImage*, 50 (3), 1219–1230.

Broca, P.P., 1861. Perte de la parole, ramollissement chronique et destruction partielle du lobe antérieur gauche du cerveau. *Bulletin de la Société Anthropologique*, 2, 235–238.

Broca, P.P., 1865. Sur le siège de la faculté du langage articulé. *Bulletin de la Société Anthropologique*, 6, 337–393.

Browman, C. and Goldstein, L., 1990. Gestural specification using dynamically-defined articulatory structures. *Journal of Phonetics*, 18, 299–320.

Brown, J.W., Bullock, D., and Grossberg, S., 2004. How laminar frontal cortex and basal ganglia circuits interact to control planned and reactive saccades. *Neural Networks*, 17 (4), 471–510.

Brown, S., Ingham, R.J., Ingham, J.C., Laird, A.R., and Fox, P.T., 2005. Stuttered and fluent speech production: an ALE meta-analysis of functional neuroimaging studies. *Human Brain Mapping*, 25 (1), 105–117.

Buchsbaum, B.R., Hickok, G., and Humphries, C., 2001. Role of left posterior superior temporal gyrus in phonological processing for speech perception and production. *Cognitive Science*, 25 (5), 663–678.

Bullock, D. and Rhodes, B., 2003. Competitive queuing for serial planning and performance. *In*: M.A. Arbib, ed. *Handbook of Brain Theory and Neural Networks*. Cambridge, MA: MIT Press, 241–244.

Callan, D.E., Tsytsarev, V., Hanakawa, T., Callan, A.M., Katsuhara, M., Fukuyama, H., and Turner, R., 2006. Song and speech: brain regions involved with perception and covert production. *NeuroImage*, 31 (3), 1327–1342.

Caplan, D., Gow, D., and Makris, N., 1995. Analysis of lesions by MRI in stroke patients with acoustic-phonetic processing deficits. *Neurology*, 45 (2), 293–298.

Chen, S.H.A. and Desmond, J.E., 2005. Cerebrocerebellar networks during articulatory rehearsal and verbal working memory tasks. *NeuroImage*, 24 (2), 332–338.

Chiricozzi, F.R., Clausi, S., Molinari, M., and Leggio, M.G., 2008. Phonological short-term store impairment after cerebellar lesion: a single case study. *Neuropsychologia*, 46 (7), 1940–1953.

Christoffels, I.K., Formisano, E., and Schiller, N.O., 2007. Neural correlates of verbal feedback processing: an fMRI study employing overt speech. *Human Brain Mapping*, 28 (9), 868–879.

Christoffels, I.K., van de Ven, V., Waldorp, L.J., Formisano, E., and Schiller, N.O., 2011. The sensory consequences of speaking: parametric neural cancellation during speech in auditory cortex. *PLoS One*, 6 (5), e18307.

Civier, O., Bullock, D., Max, L., and Guenther, F.H., 2013. Computational modeling of stuttering caused by impairments in a basal ganglia thalamo-cortical circuit involved in syllable selection and initiation. *Brain and Language*, 126 (3), 263–278.

Clower, W.T. and Alexander, G.E., 1998. Movement sequence-related activity reflecting numerical order of components in supplementary and presupplementary motor areas. *Journal of Neurophysiology*, 80 (3), 1562–1566.

Costafreda, S.G., 2009. Pooling fMRI data: meta-analysis, mega-analysis and multi-center studies. *Frontiers in Neuroinformatics*, 3, 33.

Creutzfeldt, O., Ojemann, G., and Lettich, E., 1989a. Neuronal activity in the human lateral temporal lobe. II. Responses to the subjects own voice. *Experimental Brain Research*, 77 (3), 476–489.

Creutzfeldt, O., Ojemann, G., and Lettich, E., 1989b. Neuronal activity in the human lateral temporal lobe. I. Responses to speech. *Experimental Brain Research*, 77 (3), 451–475.

Crosson, B., 1992. *Subcortical Functions in Language and Memory*. New York: Guilford Press.

Crosson, B., Benefield, H., Cato, M.A., Sadek, J.R., Moore, A.B., Wierenga, C.E., Gopinath, K., Soltysik, D., Bauer, R.M., Auerbach, E.J., Gökçay, D., Leonard, C.M., and Briggs, R.W., 2003. Left and right basal ganglia and frontal activity during language generation: contributions to lexical, semantic, and phonological processes. *Journal of the International Neuropsychological Society*, 9 (7), 1061–1077.

Crosson, B., Sadek, J.R., Maron, L., Gökçay, D., Mohr, C.M., Auerbach, E.J., Freeman, A.J., Leonard, C.M., and Briggs, R.W., 2001. Relative shift in activity from medial to lateral frontal cortex during internally versus externally guided word generation. *Journal of Cognitive Neuroscience*, 13 (2), 272–283.

Curio, G., Neuloh, G., Numminen, J., Jousmäki, V., and Hari, R., 2000. Speaking modifies voice-evoked activity in the human auditory cortex. *Human Brain Mapping*, 9 (4), 183–191.

D'Ausilio, A., Pulvermüller, F., Salmas, P., Bufalari, I., Begliomini, C., and Fadiga, L., 2009. The motor somatotopy of speech perception. *Current Biology*, 19 (5), 381–385.

D'Esposito, M., Aguirre, G.K., Zarahn, E., Ballard, D., Shin, R.K., and Lease, J., 1998. Functional MRI studies of spatial and nonspatial working memory. *Cognitive Brain Research*, 7 (1), 1–13.

Dale, A.M., Fischl, B., and Sereno, M.I., 1999. Cortical surface-based analysis. I. Segmentation and surface reconstruction. *NeuroImage*, 9 (2), 179–194.

Damasio, H. and Damasio, A.R., 1980. The anatomical basis of conduction aphasia. *Brain*, 103 (2), 337–350.

Darley, F., Aronson, A., and Brown, J., 1975. *Motor Speech Disorders*. Philadelphia: W.B. Saunders.

Dejerine, J., 1914. *Sémiologie des affections du système nerveux*. Paris: *Masson*.

Dell, G.S., 1986. A spreading-activation theory of retrieval in sentence production. *Psychological Review*, 93 (3), 283–321.

Dell, G.S. and O'Seaghdha, P.G., 1992. Stages of lexical access in language production. *Cognition*, 42 (1–3), 287–314.

Demonet, J-F., Thierry, G., and Cardebat, D., 2005. Renewal of the neurophysiology of language : Functional neuroimaging. *Physiological Reviews*, 85, 49–95.

Desmond, J.E. and Fiez, J.A., 1998. Neuroimaging studies of the cerebellum: language, learning and memory. *Trends in Cognitive Sciences*, 2 (9), 355–362.

Desmond, J.E., Gabrieli, J.D., Wagner, A.D., Ginier, B.L., and Glover, G.H., 1997. Lobular patterns of cerebellar activation in verbal working-memory and finger-tapping tasks as revealed by functional MRI. *Journal of Neuroscience*, 17 (24), 9675–9685.

di Pellegrino, G., Fadiga, L., Fogassi, L., Gallese, V., and Rizzolatti, G., 1992. Understanding motor events: a neurophysiological study. *Experimental Brain Research*, 91 (1), 176–180.

Diedrichsen, J., Hashambhoy, Y., Rane, T., and Shadmehr, R., 2005. Neural correlates of reach errors. *Journal of Neuroscience*, 25 (43), 9919–9931.

Doyon, J., Bellec, P., Amsel, R., Penhune, V., Monchi, O., Carrier, J., Lehéricy, S., and Benali, H., 2009. Contributions of the basal ganglia and functionally related brain structures to motor learning. *Behavioural Brain Research*, 199 (1), 61–75.

Dronkers, N.F., 1996. A new brain region for coordinating speech articulation. *Nature*, 384 (6605), 159–161.

Dronkers, N.F., Plaisant, O., Iba-Zizen, M.T., and Cabanis, E.A., 2007. Paul Broca's historic cases: high resolution MR imaging of the brains of Leborgne and Lelong. *Brain*, 130 (Pt 5), 1432–1441.

Duffy, J., 1995. *Motor Speech Disorders: Substrates, Differential Diagnosis, and Management*. St. Louis: Mosby.

Durisko, C. and Fiez, J. A., 2010. Functional activation in the cerebellum during working memory and simple speech tasks. *Cortex; A Journal Devoted to the Study of the Nervous System and Behavior*, 46 (7), 896–906.

Fadiga, L., Craighero, L., and D'Ausilio, A., 2009. Broca's area in language, action, and music. *Annals of the New York Academy of Sciences*, 1169, 448–458.

Fedorenko, E., Duncan, J., and Kanwisher, N., 2013. Broad domain generality in focal regions of frontal and parietal cortex. *Proceedings of the National Academy of Sciences of the United States of America*, 110 (41), 16616–16621.

Fedorenko, E., Fillmore, P., Smith, K., Bonilha, L., and Fridriksson, J., 2015. The superior precentral gyrus of the insula does not appear to be functionally specialized for articulation. *Journal of Neurophysiology*, 113 (7), 2376–2382.

Fiez, J., Raife, E., and Balota, D., 1996. A positron emission tomography study of the short-term maintenance of verbal information. *Journal of Neuroscience*, 76 (2), 808–822.

Fischl, B., Sereno, M.I., and Dale, A.M., 1999. Cortical surface-based analysis. II: Inflation, flattening, and a surface-based coordinate system. *NeuroImage*, 9 (2), 195–207.

Fonov, V., Evans, A.C., Botteron, K., Almli, C.R., McKinstry, R.C., and Collins, D.L., 2011. Unbiased average age-appropriate atlases for pediatric studies. *NeuroImage*, 54 (1), 313–327.

Freud, S., 1891. *On Aphasia: A Critical Study (trans. 1953)*. Oxford: International Universities Press.

Fridriksson, J., Kjartansson, O., Morgan, P.S., Hjaltason, H., Magnusdottir, S., Bonilha, L., and Rorden, C., 2010. Impaired speech repetition and left parietal lobe damage. *Journal of Neuroscience*, 30 (33), 11057–11061.

Fried, I., Katz, A., McCarthy, G., Sass, K.J., Williamson, P., Spencer, S.S., and Spencer, D.D., 1991. Functional organization of human supplementary motor cortex studied by electrical stimulation. *Journal of Neuroscience*, 11 (11), 3656–3666.

Fromkin, V., 1971. The non-anomalous nature of anomalous utterances. *Language*, 47 (1), 27–52.

Gabrieli, J.D., Poldrack, R.A., and Desmond, J.E., 1998. The role of left prefrontal cortex in language and memory. *Proceedings of the National Academy of Sciences of the United States of America*, 95 (3), 906–913.

Gallese, V., Fadiga, L., Fogassi, L., and Rizzolatti, G., 1996. Action recognition in the premotor cortex. *Brain*, 119 (Pt 2), 593–609.

Garrett, M., 1975. The analysis of sentence production. *In*: G. Bower, ed. *Psychology of Learning and Motivation*, New York: Academic Press, 133–177.

Gathercole, S.E., 1995. Is nonword repetition a test of phonological memory or long-term knowledge? It all depends on the nonwords. *Memory & Cognition*, 23 (1), 83–94.

Geschwind, N., 1965. Disconnexion syndromes in animals and man. II. *Brain*, 88 (3), 585–644.

Ghosh, S.S., Tourville, J.A., and Guenther, F.H., 2008. A neuroimaging study of premotor lateralization and cerebellar involvement in the production of phonemes and syllables. *Journal of Speech, Language, and Hearing Research*, 51 (5), 1183–1202.

Golfinopoulos, E., Tourville, J.A., Bohland, J.W., Ghosh, S.S., Nieto-Castanon, A., and Guenther, F.H., 2011. fMRI investigation of unexpected somatosensory feedback perturbation during speech. *NeuroImage*, 55 (3), 1324–1338.

Golfinopoulos, E., Tourville, J.A., and Guenther, F.H., 2010. The integration of large-scale neural network modeling and functional brain imaging in speech motor control. *NeuroImage*, 52 (3), 862–874.

Grafton, S.T., Schmitt, P., Van Horn, J., and Diedrichsen, J., 2008. Neural substrates of visuomotor learning based on improved feedback control and prediction. *NeuroImage*, 39 (3), 1383–1395.

Grill-Spector, K., Henson, R., and Martin, A., 2006. Repetition and the brain: neural models of stimulus-specific effects. *Trends in Cognitive Sciences*, 10 (1), 14–23.

Grossberg, S., 1978a. Behavioral contrast in short term memory: serial binary memory models or parallel continuous memory models? *Journal of Mathematical Psychology*, 17 (3), 199–219.

Grossberg, S., 1978b. A theory of human memory: self-organization and performance of sensory-motor codes, maps, and plans. *Progress in Theoretical Biology*, 5, 233–374.

Guenther, F.H., 1995. Speech sound acquisition, coarticulation, and rate effects in a neural network model of speech production. *Psychological Review*, 102 (3), 594–621.

Guenther, F.H., 2016. *Neural Control of Speech*. Cambridge, MA: MIT Press.

Guenther, F.H., Brumberg, J.S., Wright, E.J., Nieto-Castanon, A., Tourville, J.A., Panko, M., Law, R., Siebert, S.A., Bartels, J.L., Andreasen, D.S., Ehirim, P., Mao, H., and Kennedy, P.R., 2009. A wireless brain–machine interface for real-time speech synthesis. *PLoS One*, 4 (12), e8218.

Guenther, F.H., Ghosh, S.S., and Tourville, J.A., 2006. Neural modeling and imaging of the cortical interactions underlying syllable production. *Brain and Language*, 96 (3), 280–301.

Guenther, F.H., Hampson, M., and Johnson, D., 1998. A theoretical investigation of reference frames for the planning of speech movements. *Psychological Review*, 105 (4), 611–633.

Gurney, K., Prescott, T.J., Wickens, J.R., and Redgrave, P., 2004. Computational models of the basal ganglia: from robots to membranes. *Trends in Neurosciences*, 27 (8), 453–459.

Habib, M., Daquin, G., Milandre, L., Royere, M.L., Rey, M., Lanteri, A., Salamon, G., and Khalil, R., 1995. Mutism and auditory agnosia due to bilateral insular damage – role of the insula in human communication. *Neuropsychologia*, 33 (3), 327–339.

Hartley, T. and Houghton, G., 1996. A linguistically constrained model of short-term memory for nonwords. *Journal of Memory and Language*, 35 (1), 1–31.

Hartwigsen, G., Saur, D., Price, C.J., Baumgaertner, A., Ulmer, S., and Siebner, H.R., 2013. Increased facilitatory connectivity from the pre-SMA to the left dorsal premotor cortex during pseudoword repetition. *Journal of Cognitive Neuroscience*, 25 (4), 580–594.

Hashimoto, Y. and Sakai, K.L., 2003. Brain activations during conscious self-monitoring of speech production with delayed auditory feedback: an fMRI study. *Human Brain Mapping*, 20 (1), 22–28.

Heim, S., Opitz, B., and Friederici, A.D., 2003. Distributed cortical networks for syntax processing: Broca's area as the common denominator. *Brain and Language*, 85 (3), 402–408.

Heinks-Maldonado, T.H., Nagarajan, S.S., and Houde, J.F., 2006. Magnetoencephalographic evidence for a precise forward model in speech production. *Neuroreport*, 17 (13), 1375–1379.

Hickok, G., 2012. Computational neuroanatomy of speech production. *Nature Reviews Neuroscience*, 13 (2), 135–145.

Hickok, G., Buchsbaum, B., Humphries, C., and Muftuler, T., 2003. Auditory-motor interaction revealed by fMRI: speech, music, and working memory in area Spt. *Journal of Cognitive Neuroscience*, 15 (5), 673–682.

Hickok, G., Erhard, P., Kassubek, J., Helms-Tillery, A.K., Naeve-Velguth, S., Strupp, J.P., Strick, P.L., and Ugurbil, K., 2000. A functional magnetic resonance imaging study of the role of left posterior superior temporal gyrus in speech production: implications for the explanation of conduction aphasia. *Neuroscience Letters*, 287 (2), 156–160.

Hickok, G., Houde, J., and Rong, F., 2011. Sensorimotor integration in speech processing: computational basis and neural organization. *Neuron*, 69 (3), 407–422.

Hickok, G., Okada, K., and Serences, J.T., 2009. Area Spt in the human planum temporale supports sensory-motor integration for speech processing. *Journal of Neurophysiology*, 101 (5), 2725–2732.

Hickok, G. and Poeppel, D., 2004. Dorsal and ventral streams: A framework for understanding aspects of the functional anatomy of language. *Cognition*, 92, 67–99.

Hickok, G. and Poeppel, D., 2007. The cortical organization of speech processing. *Nature Reviews Neuroscience*, 8 (5), 393–402.

Hillis, A.E., Work, M., Barker, P.B., Jacobs, M.A., Breese, E.L., and Maurer, K., 2004. Re-examining the brain regions crucial for orchestrating speech articulation. *Brain*, 127 (Pt 7), 1479–1487.

Hirano, S., Kojima, H., Naito, Y., Honjo, I., Kamoto, Y., Okazawa, H., Ishizu, K., Yonekura, Y., Nagahama, Y., Fukuyama, H., and Konishi, J., 1996. Cortical speech processing mechanisms while vocalizing visually presented languages. *Neuroreport*, 8 (1), 363–367.

Hirano, S., Kojima, H., Naito, Y., Honjo, I., Kamoto, Y., Okazawa, H., Ishizu, K., Yonekura, Y., Nagahama, Y., Fukuyama, H., and Konishi, J., 1997. Cortical processing mechanism for vocalization with auditory verbal feedback. *Neuroreport*, 8 (9–10), 2379–2382.

Holmes, G., 1917. The symptoms of acute cerebellar injuries due to gunshot injuries. *Brain*, 40 (4), 461–535.

Houde, J.F. and Nagarajan, S.S., 2011. Speech production as state feedback control. *Frontiers in Human Neuroscience*, 5, 82.

Houde, J.F., Nagarajan, S.S., Sekihara, K., and Merzenich, M.M., 2002. Modulation of the auditory cortex during speech: an MEG study. *Journal of Cognitive Neuroscience*, 14 (8), 1125–1138.

Indefrey, P. and Levelt, W.J.M., 2004. The spatial and temporal signatures of word production components. *Cognition*, 92 (1–2), 101–144.

Inhoff, A.W., Diener, H.C., Rafal, R.D., and Ivry, R., 1989. The role of cerebellar structures in the execution of serial movements. *Brain*, 112 (Pt 3), 565–581.

Ivry, R., 1997. Cerebellar timing systems. *International Review of Neurobiology*, 41, 555–573.

Johansen-Berg, H., Behrens, T.E.J., Robson, M.D., Drobnjak, I., Rushworth, M.F.S., Brady, J.M., Smith, S.M., Higham, D.J., and Matthews, P.M., 2004. Changes in connectivity profiles define functionally distinct regions in human medial frontal cortex. *Proceedings of the National Academy of Sciences of the United States of America*, 101 (36), 13335–13340.

Johnson, M.D. and Ojemann, G.A., 2000. The role of the human thalamus in language and memory: evidence from electrophysiological studies. *Brain and Cognition*, 42 (2), 218–230.

Jonas, S., 1981. The supplementary motor region and speech emission. *Journal of Communication Disorders*, 14 (5), 349–373.

Jonas, S., 1987. The supplementary motor region and speech. *In*: E. Perecman, ed. *The Frontal Lobes Revisited*. New York: IRBN Press, 241–250.

Jonides, J., Schumacher, E.H., Smith, E.E., Koeppe, R.A., Awh, E., and Reuter-lorenz, P.A., 1998. The role of parietal cortex in verbal working memory. *Journal of Neuroscience*, 18, 5026–5034.

Jürgens, U., 1984. The efferent and afferent connections of the supplementary motor area. *Brain Research*, 300 (1), 63–81.

Jürgens, U., 2002. Neural pathways underlying vocal control. *Neuroscience and Biobehavioral Reviews*, 26 (2), 235–258.

Jürgens, U., 2009. The neural control of vocalization in mammals: a review. *Journal of Voice*, 23 (1), 1–10.

Jürgens, U. and von Cramon, D., 1982. On the role of the anterior cingulate cortex in phonation: a case report. *Brain and Language*, 15 (2), 234–248.

Keele, S.W. and Ivry, R., 1990. Does the cerebellum provide a common computation for diverse tasks? A timing hypothesis. *Annals of the New York Academy of Sciences*, 608, 179–207–211.

Kent, R.D., Kent, J.F., Rosenbek, J.C., Vorperian, H.K., and Weismer, G., 1997. A speaking task analysis of the dysarthria in cerebellar disease. *Folia phoniatrica et logopaedica : Official Organ of the International Association of Logopedics and Phoniatrics (IALP)*, 49 (2), 63–82.

Kerns, J.G., Cohen, J.D., Stenger, V.A., and Carter, C.S., 2004. Prefrontal cortex guides context-appropriate responding during language production. *Neuron*, 43 (2), 283–291.

Knolle, F., Schröger, E., Baess, P., and Kotz, S.A., 2012. The cerebellum generates motor-to-auditory predictions: ERP lesion evidence. *Journal of Cognitive Neuroscience*, 24 (3), 698–706.

Koelsch, S., Schulze, K., Sammler, D., Fritz, T., Müller, K., and Gruber, O., 2009. Functional architecture of verbal and tonal working memory: An FMRI study. *Human Brain Mapping*, 30 (3), 859–873.

Krakauer, J. and Ghez, C., 1999. Voluntary movement. *In*: E.R. Kandel, J.H. Schwartz, and T.M. Jessel, eds. *Principles of Neural Science*. New York: McGraw Hill, 756–781.

Kröger, B.J., Kannampuzha, J., and Neuschaefer-Rube, C., 2009. Towards a neurocomputational model of speech production and perception. *Speech Communication*, 51 (9), 793–809.

Kropotov, J.D. and Etlinger, S.C., 1999. Selection of actions in the basal ganglia-thalamocortical circuits: review and model. *International Journal of Psychophysiology*, 31 (3), 197–217.

Leggio, M.G., Silveri, M.C., Petrosini, L., and Molinari, M., 2000. Phonological grouping is specifically affected in cerebellar patients: a verbal fluency study. *Journal of Neurology, Neurosurgery, and Psychiatry*, 69 (1), 102–106.

Lehéricy, S., Ducros, M., Krainik, A., Francois, C., Van de Moortele, P-F., Ugurbil, K., and Kim, D-S., 2004. 3-D diffusion tensor axonal tracking shows distinct SMA and pre-SMA projections to the human striatum. *Cerebral Cortex*, 14 (12), 1302–1309.

Leiner, H.C., Leiner, A.L., and Dow, R.S., 1993. Cognitive and language functions of the human cerebellum. *Trends in Neurosciences*, 16 (11), 444–447.

Levelt, W.J., 1989. *Speaking: From Intention to Articulation*. Cambridge, MA: MIT Press.

Levelt, W.J., 1999. Models of word production. *Trends in Cognitive Sciences*, 3 (6), 223–232.

Levelt, W.J., Roelofs, A., and Meyer, A.S., 1999. A theory of lexical access in speech production. *Behavioral and Brain Sciences*, 22 (1), 1–38–75.

Levelt, W.J. and Wheeldon, L., 1994. Do speakers have access to a mental syllabary? *Cognition*, 50 (1–3), 239–269.

Lotze, M., Seggewies, G., Erb, M., Grodd, W., and Birbaumer, N., 2000. The representation of articulation in the primary sensorimotor cortex. *Neuroreport*, 11 (13), 2985–2989.

Luppino, G., Matelli, M., and Camarda, R., 1993. Corticocortical connections of area F3 in the macaque Monkey. *Journal of Comparative Neurology*, 338 (1), 114–140.

MacKay, D.G., 1970. Spoonerisms: the structure of errors in the serial order of speech. *Neuropsychologia*, 8 (3), 323–350.

MacNeilage, P.F., 1998. The frame/content theory of evolution of speech production. *Behavioral and Brain Sciences*, 21 (4), 499–511–546.

Maeda, S., 1990. Compensatory articulation during speech: evidence from the analysis and synthesis of vocal-tract shapes using an articulatory model. *In*: W. Hadcastle and A. Marchal, eds. *Speech Production and Speech Modelling*. Boston: Kluwer Academic, 131–149.

Malandraki, G.A., Sutton, B.P., Perlman, A.L., Karampinos, D.C., and Conway, C., 2009. Neural activation of swallowing and swallowing-related tasks in healthy young adults: an attempt to separate the components of deglutition. *Human Brain Mapping*, 30 (10), 3209–3226.

Markiewicz, C.J. and Bohland, J.W., 2016. Mapping the cortical representation of speech sounds in a syllable repetition task. *NeuroImage*, 141, 174–190.

Matsuzaka, Y., Aizawa, H., and Tanji, J., 1992. A motor area rostral to the supplementary motor area (presupplementary motor area) in the monkey: neuronal activity during a learned motor task. *Journal of Neurophysiology*, 68 (3), 653–662.

McNeil, M., Robin, D., and Schmidt, R., 2009. Apraxia of speech: Definition, differentiation, and treatment. *In:* M.R. McNeil, ed. *Clinical Management of Sensorimotor Speech Disorders*. New York: Thieme, 249–268.

Middleton, F.A. and Strick, P.L., 1997. Cerebellar output channels. *International Review of Neurobiology*, 41, 61–82.

Middleton, F.A. and Strick, P.L., 2000. Basal ganglia and cerebellar loops: motor and cognitive circuits. *Brain Research Reviews*, 31 (2–3), 236–250.

Mink, J.W., 1996. The basal ganglia: focused selection and inhibition of competing motor programs. *Progress in Neurobiology*, 50 (4), 381–425.

Mink, J.W. and Thach, W.T., 1993. Basal ganglia intrinsic circuits and their role in behavior. *Current Opinion in Neurobiology*, 3 (6), 950–957.

Moore, A.B., Li, Z., Tyner, C.E., Hu, X., and Crosson, B.B., 2013. Bilateral basal ganglia activity in verbal working memory. *Brain and Language*, 125 (3), 316–323.

Moser, D., Baker, J.M., Sanchez, C.E., Rorden, C., and Fridriksson, J., 2009. Temporal order processing of syllables in the left parietal lobe. *Journal of Neuroscience*, 29 (40), 12568–12573.

Murphy, K., Corfield, D.R., Guz, A., Fink, G.R., Wise, R.J., Harrison, J., and Adams, L., 1997. Cerebral areas associated with motor control of speech in humans. *Journal of Applied Physiology*, 83 (5), 1438–1447.

Myers, E.B., Blumstein, S.E., Walsh, E., and Eliassen, J., 2009. Inferior frontal regions underlie the perception of phonetic category invariance. *Psychological Science*, 20 (7), 895–903.

Németh, G., Hegedüs, K., and Molnár, L., 1988. Akinetic mutism associated with bicingular lesions: clinicopathological and functional anatomical correlates. *European Archives of Psychiatry and Neurological Sciences*, 237 (4), 218–222.

Niziolek, C.A. and Guenther, F.H., 2013. Vowel category boundaries enhance cortical and behavioral responses to speech feedback alterations. *Journal of Neuroscience*, 33 (29), 12090–12098.

Niziolek, C.A., Nagarajan, S.S., and Houde, J.F., 2013. What does motor efference copy represent? Evidence from speech production. *Journal of Neuroscience*, 33 (41), 16110–16116.

Norman, K.A., Polyn, S.M., Detre, G.J., and Haxby, J.V, 2006. Beyond mind-reading: multi-voxel pattern analysis of fMRI data. *Trends in Cognitive Sciences*, 10 (9), 424–430.

Numminen, J. and Curio, G., 1999. Differential effects of overt, covert and replayed speech on vowel-evoked responses of the human auditory cortex. *Neuroscience Letters*, 272 (1), 29–32.

Numminen, J., Salmelin, R., and Hari, R., 1999. Subject's own speech reduces reactivity of the human auditory cortex. *Neuroscience Letters*, 265 (2), 119–122.

Okada, K. and Hickok, G., 2006. Left posterior auditory-related cortices participate both in speech perception and speech production: Neural overlap revealed by fMRI. *Brain and Language*, 98 (1), 112–117.

Okada, K., Matchin, W., and Hickok, G., 2017. Neural evidence for predictive coding in auditory cortex during speech production. *Psychonomic Bulletin & Review*. 25 (1), 423–430.

Okada, K., Smith, K.R., Humphries, C., and Hickok, G., 2003. Word length modulates neural activity in auditory cortex during covert object naming. *Neuroreport*, 14 (18), 2323–2326.

Pa, J. and Hickok, G., 2008. A parietal-temporal sensory-motor integration area for the human vocal tract: evidence from an fMRI study of skilled musicians. *Neuropsychologia*, 46 (1), 362–368.

Pai, M.C., 1999. Supplementary motor area aphasia: a case report. *Clinical Neurology and Neurosurgery*, 101 (1), 29–32.

Palmer, E.D., Rosen, H.J., Ojemann, J.G., Buckner, R.L., Kelley, W.M., and Petersen, S.E., 2001. An event-related fMRI study of overt and covert word stem completion. *NeuroImage*, 14 (Pt 1), 182–193.

Papoutsi, M., de Zwart, J.A., Jansma, J.M., Pickering, M.J., Bednar, J.A., and Horwitz, B., 2009. From phonemes to articulatory codes: an fMRI study of the role of Broca's area in speech production. *Cerebral Cortex*, 19 (9), 2156–2165.

Passingham, R., 1993. *The Frontal Lobes and Voluntary Action*. Oxford: Oxford University Press.

Paulesu, E., Frith, C.D., and Frackowiak, R.S., 1993. The neural correlates of the verbal component of working memory. *Nature*, 362 (6418), 342–345.

Paus, T., 2001. Primate anterior cingulate cortex: where motor control, drive and cognition interface. *Nature Reviews Neuroscience*, 2 (6), 417–424.

Paus, T., Perry, D.W., Zatorre, R.J., Worsley, K.J., and Evans, A.C., 1996. Modulation of cerebral blood flow in the human auditory cortex during speech: role of motor-to-sensory discharges. *The European Journal of Neuroscience*, 8 (11), 2236–2246.

Paus, T., Petrides, M., Evans, A.C., and Meyer, E., 1993. Role of the human anterior cingulate cortex in the control of oculomotor, manual, and speech responses: a positron emission tomography study. *Journal of Neurophysiology*, 70 (2), 453–469.

Peeva, M.G., Guenther, F.H., Tourville, J.A., Nieto-Castanon, A., Anton, J-L., Nazarian, B., and Alario, F-X., 2010. Distinct representations of phonemes, syllables, and supra-syllabic sequences in the speech production network. *NeuroImage*, 50 (2), 626–638.

Penfield, W. and Rasmussen, T., 1950. *The Cerebral Cortex of Man*. New York: Palgrave Macmillan.

Penfield, W. and Roberts, L., 1959. *Speech and Brain Mechanisms*. Princeton: Princeton University Press.

Penfield, W. and Welch, K., 1951. The supplementary motor area of the cerebral cortex: a clinical and experimental study. *Archives of Neurology and Psychiatry*, 66 (3), 289–317.

Penhune, V.B. and Doyon, J., 2005. Cerebellum and M1 interaction during early learning of timed motor sequences. *NeuroImage*, 26 (3), 801–812.

Petrides, M., 1991. Functional specialization within the dorsolateral frontal cortex for serial order memory. *Proceedings of the Royal Society B: Biological Sciences*, 246 (1317), 299–306.

Picard, N. and Strick, P.L., 1996. Motor areas of the medial wall: a review of their location and functional activation. *Cerebral Cortex*, 6 (3), 342–353.

Pickett, E., Kuniholm, E., Protopapas, A., Friedman, J., and Lieberman, P., 1998. Selective speech motor, syntax and cognitive deficits associated with bilateral damage to the putamen and the head of the caudate nucleus: a case study. *Neuropsychologia*, 36 (2), 173–188.

Price, C.J., 2012. A review and synthesis of the first 20 years of PET and fMRI studies of heard speech, spoken language and reading. *NeuroImage*, 62 (2), 816–847.

Pugh, K.R., Mencl, W.E., Jenner, A.R., Katz, L., Frost, S.J., Lee, J.R., Shaywitz, S.E., and Shaywitz, B.A., 2001. Neurobiological studies of reading and reading disability. *Journal of Communication Disorders*, 34 (6), 479–492.

Ramsay, S.C., Adams, L., Murphy, K., Corfield, D.R., Grootoonk, S., Bailey, D.L., Frackowiak, R.S., and Guz, A., 1993. Regional cerebral blood flow during volitional expiration in man: a comparison with volitional inspiration. *The Journal of Physiology*, 461 (1), 85–101.

Redgrave, P., Prescott, T.J., and Gurney, K., 1999. The basal ganglia: a vertebrate solution to the selection problem? *Neuroscience*, 89 (4), 1009–1023.

Riecker, A., Ackermann, H., Wildgruber, D., Dogil, G., and Grodd, W., 2000. Opposite hemispheric lateralization effects during speaking and singing at motor cortex, insula and cerebellum. *Neuroreport*, 11 (9), 1997–2000.

Riecker, A., Ackermann, H., Wildgruber, D., Meyer, J., Dogil, G., Haider, H., and Grodd, W., 2000. Articulatory/phonetic sequencing at the level of the anterior perisylvian cortex: a Functional Magnetic Resonance Imaging (fMRI) study. *Brain and Language*, 75 (2), 259–276.

Riecker, A., Brendel, B., Ziegler, W., Erb, M., and Ackermann, H., 2008. The influence of syllable onset complexity and syllable frequency on speech motor control. *Brain and Language*, 107 (2), 102–113.

Riecker, A., Kassubek, J., Gro, K., Grodd, W., Ackermann, H., and Gröschel, K., 2006. The cerebral control of speech tempo: opposite relationship between speaking rate and BOLD signal changes at striatal and cerebellar structures. *NeuroImage*, 29 (1), 46–53.

Riecker, A., Mathiak, K., Wildgruber, D., Erb, M., Hertrich, I., Grodd, W., and Ackermann, H., 2005. fMRI reveals two distinct cerebral networks subserving speech motor control. *Neurology*, 64 (4), 700–706.

Riecker, A., Wildgruber, D., Dogil, G., Grodd, W., and Ackermann, H., 2002. Hemispheric lateralization effects of rhythm implementation during syllable repetitions: an fMRI study. *NeuroImage*, 16 (1), 169–176.

Rizzolatti, G. and Arbib, M.A., 1998. Language within our grasp. *Trends in Neurosciences*, 21 (5), 188–194.

Rizzolatti, G., Fadiga, L., Gallese, V., and Fogassi, L., 1996. Premotor cortex and the recognition of motor actions. *Cognitive Brain Research*, 3 (2), 131–141.

Roelofs, A., 1997. The WEAVER model of word-form encoding in speech production. *Cognition*, 64 (3), 249–284.

Roelofs, A., 2014. Integrating psycholinguistic and motor control approaches to speech production: where do they meet? *Language, Cognition and Neuroscience*, 29 (1), 35–37.

Roelofs, A. and Hagoort, P., 2002. Control of language use: cognitive modeling of the hemodynamics of Stroop task performance. *Cognitive Brain Research*, 15 (1), 85–97.

Romanelli, P., Esposito, V., Schaal, D.W., and Heit, G., 2005. Somatotopy in the basal ganglia: experimental and clinical evidence for segregated sensorimotor channels. *Brain Research Reviews*, 48 (1), 112–128.

Rubens, A.B., 1975. Aphasia with infarction in the territory of the anterior cerebral artery. *Cortex*, 11 (3), 239–250.

Sahin, N.T., Pinker, S., and Halgren, E., 2006. Abstract grammatical processing of nouns and verbs in Broca's area: evidence from fMRI. *Cortex*, 42 (4), 540–562.

Sakurai, Y., Momose, T., Iwata, M., Sudo, Y., Ohtomo, K., and Kanazawa, I., 2001. Cortical activity associated with vocalization and reading proper. *Cognitive Brain Research*, 12 (1), 161–165.

Schäffler, L., Lüders, H.O., Dinner, D.S., Lesser, R.P., and Chelune, G.J., 1993. Comprehension deficits elicited by electrical stimulation of Broca's area. *Brain*, 116 (3), 695–715.

Schaltenbrand, G., 1975. The effects on speech and language of stereotactical stimulation in thalamus and corpus callosum. *Brain and Language*, 2 (1), 70–77.

Schmahmann, J.D., Doyon, J., Petrides, M., Evans, A.C., and Toga, A.W., 2000. *MRI Atlas of the Human Cerebellum*. San Diego: Academic Press.

Schmahmann, J.D. and Pandya, D.N., 1997. The cerebrocerebellar system. *International Review of Neurobiology*, 41, 31–60.

Schulz, G.M., Sulc, S., Leon, S., and Gilligan, G., 2000. Speech motor learning in Parkinson disease. *Journal of Medical Speech-Language Pathology*, 8 (4), 243–248.

Segawa, J.A., Tourville, J.A., Beal, D.S., and Guenther, F.H., 2015. The neural correlates of speech motor sequence learning. *Journal of Cognitive Neuroscience*, 27 (4), 819–831.

Shattuck-Hufnagel, S., 1979. Speech errors as evidence for a serial order mechanism in sentence production. *In*: W.E. Cooper and E.C.T. Walker, eds. *Sentence Processing: Pscyholinguistic Studies Presented to Merrill Garrett*. Hillsdale, NJ: Lawernce Erlbaum Associates.

Shima, K., Mushiake, H., Saito, N., and Tanji, J., 1996. Role for cells in the presupplementary motor area in updating motor plans. *Proceedings of the National Academy of Sciences of the United States of America*, 93 (16), 8694–8698.

Shima, K. and Tanji, J., 1998a. Both supplementary and presupplementary motor areas are crucial for the temporal organization of multiple movements. *Journal of Neurophysiology*, 80 (6), 3247–3260.

Shima, K. and Tanji, J., 1998b. Role for cingulate motor area cells in voluntary movement selection based on reward. *Science*, 282 (5392), 1335–1338.

Shima, K. and Tanji, J., 2000. Neuronal activity in the supplementary and presupplementary motor areas for temporal organization of multiple movements. *Journal of Neurophysiology*, 84 (4), 2148–2160.

Shuren, J., 1993. Insula and aphasia. *Journal of Neurology*, 240 (4), 216–218.

Shuster, L.I., 2009. The effect of sublexical and lexical frequency on speech production: an fMRI investigation. *Brain and Language*, 111 (1), 66–72.

Shuster, L.I. and Lemieux, S., 2005. An fMRI investigation of covertly and overtly produced mono- and multisyllabic words. *Brain and Language*, 93 (1), 20–31.

Silveri, M.C., Di Betta, A.M., Filippini, V., Leggio, M.G., and Molinari, M., 1998. Verbal short-term store-rehearsal system and the cerebellum: evidence from a patient with a right cerebellar lesion. *Brain*, 121, 2175–2187.

Simonyan, K. and Horwitz, B., 2011. Laryngeal motor cortex and control of speech in humans. *The Neuroscientist*, 17 (2), 197–208.

Sörös, P., Sokoloff, L.G.L., Bose, A., McIntosh, A.R.A., So, P., Graham, S.J., and Stuss, D.T., 2006. Clustered functional MRI of overt speech production. *NeuroImage*, 32 (1), 376–387.

Takai, O., Brown, S., and Liotti, M., 2010. Representation of the speech effectors in the human motor cortex: somatotopy or overlap? *Brain and Language*, 113 (1), 39–44.

Takaso, H., Eisner, F., Wise, R.J.S., and Scott, S.K., 2010. The effect of delayed auditory feedback on activity in the temporal lobe while speaking: a positron emission tomography study. *Journal of Speech, Language, and Hearing Research*, 53 (2), 226–236.

Tanji, J., 2001. Sequential organization of multiple movements: involvement of cortical motor areas. *Annual Review of Neuroscience*, 24, 631–651.

Tanji, J. and Shima, K., 1994. Role for supplementary motor area cells in planning several movements ahead. *Nature*, 371, 413–416.

Toogood, J.A., Smith, R.C., Stevens, T.K., Gati, J.S., Menon, R.S., Theurer, J., Weisz, S., Affoo, R.H., and Martin, R.E., 2017. Swallowing preparation and execution: Insights from a delayed-response Functional Magnetic Resonance Imaging (fMRI) study. *Dysphagia*, 32 (4), 526–541.

Tourville, J.A. and Guenther, F.H., 2011. The DIVA model: A neural theory of speech acquisition and production. *Language and Cognitive Processes*, 26 (7), 952–981.

Tourville, J.A. and Guenther, F.H., 2012. Automatic cortical labeling system for neuroimaging studies of normal and disordered speech. 2012 Society for Neuroscience Meeting Planner. New Orleans, LA.

Tourville, J.A., Reilly, K.J., and Guenther, F.H., 2008. Neural mechanisms underlying auditory feedback control of speech. *NeuroImage*, 39 (3), 1429–1443.

Toyomura, A., Koyama, S., Miyamaoto, T., Terao, A., Omori, T., Murohashi, H., and Kuriki, S., 2007. Neural correlates of auditory feedback control in human. *Neuroscience*, 146 (2), 499–503.

Tremblay, P. and Gracco, V.L., 2006. Contribution of the frontal lobe to externally and internally specified verbal responses: fMRI evidence. *NeuroImage*, 33 (3), 947–957.

Tremblay, P. and Gracco, V.L., 2009. Contribution of the pre-SMA to the production of words and non-speech oral motor gestures, as revealed by repetitive transcranial magnetic stimulation (rTMS). *Brain Research*, 1268, 112–124.

Tremblay, P. and Small, S.L., 2011. Motor response selection in Overt sentence production: a functional MRI study. *Frontiers in Psychology*, 2, 253.

Tremblay, S., Shiller, D.M., and Ostry, D.J., 2003. Somatosensory basis of speech production. *Nature*, 423 (6942), 866–869.

Türe, U., Yaşargil, D.C., Al-Mefty, O., Yaşargil, M.G., Üre, U.R.T., As, D.I.C.H.Y., Sciences, M., and Rock, L., 1999. Topographic anatomy of the insular region. *Journal of Neurosurgery*, 90 (4), 720–733.

Turkeltaub, P., 2002. Meta-analysis of the functional neuroanatomy of single-word reading: method and validation. *NeuroImage*, 16 (3), 765–780.

Urban, P.P., Marx, J., Hunsche, S., Gawehn, J., Vucurevic, G., Wicht, S., Massinger, C., Stoeter, P., and Hopf, H.C., 2003. Cerebellar speech representation: lesion topography in dysarthria as derived from cerebellar ischemia and functional magnetic resonance imaging. *Archives of Neurology*, 60 (7), 965–972.

Van Buren, J., 1963. Confusion and disturbance of speech from stimulation in vicinity of the head of the caudate nucleus. *Journal of Neurosurgery*, 20, 148–157.

Wernicke, C., 1874. *Der aphasische Symptomencomplex*. Breslau: Cohn and Weigert.

Wertz, R., Lapointe, L., and Rosenbek, J., 1991. *Apraxia of Speech in Adults: The Disorder and Its Management*. San Diego, CA: Singular Publishing Group.

Whitfield, J. and Goberman, A., 2017. Speech motor sequence learning: Effect of Parkinson disease and normal aging on dual-task performance. *Journal of Speech, Language, and Hearing*, 60 (6S), 1752–1765.

Wildgruber, D., Ackermann, H., and Grodd, W., 2001. Differential contributions of motor cortex, basal ganglia, and cerebellum to speech motor control: effects of syllable repetition rate evaluated by fMRI. *NeuroImage*, 13 (1), 101–109.

Wildgruber, D., Ackermann, H., Klose, U., Kardatzki, B., and Grodd, W., 1996. Functional lateralization of speech production at primary motor cortex: a fMRI study. *Neuroreport*, 7 (15–17), 2791–2795.

Wilson, S.M., Saygin, A.P., Sereno, M.I., and Iacoboni, M., 2004. Listening to speech activates motor areas involved in speech production. *Nature Neuroscience*, 7 (7), 701–702.

Wise, R.J.S., Greene, J., Büchel, C., and Scott, S.K., 1999. Brain regions involved in articulation. *Lancet*, 353 (9158), 1057–1061.

Wolpert, D.M., Miall, R.C., and Kawato, M., 1998. Internal models in the cerebellum. *Trends in Cognitive Sciences*, 2 (9), 338–347.

Wu, J.C., Maguire, G., Riley, G., Lee, A., Keator, D., Tang, C., Fallon, J., and Najafi, A., 1997. Increased dopamine activity associated with stuttering. *Neuroreport*, 8 (3), 767–770.

Zemlin, W., 1998. *Speech and Hearing Science, Anatomy and Physiology*. 4th Edition. Needham Heights, MA: Allyn & Bacon.

Zheng, Z.Z., Munhall, K.G., and Johnsrude, I.S., 2010. Functional overlap between regions involved in speech perception and in monitoring one's own voice during speech production. *Journal of Cognitive Neuroscience*, 22 (8), 1770–1781.

Zheng, Z.Z., Vicente-Grabovetsky, A., MacDonald, E.N., Munhall, K.G., Cusack, R., and Johnsrude, I.S., 2013. Multivoxel patterns reveal functionally differentiated networks underlying auditory feedback processing of speech. *Journal of Neuroscience*, 33 (10), 4339–4348.

Ziegler, W., Aichert, I., and Staiger, A., 2012. Apraxia of speech: Concepts and controversies. *Journal of Speech Language and Hearing Research*, 55 (5), S1485.

Ziegler, W., Kilian, B., and Deger, K., 1997. The role of the left mesial frontal cortex in fluent speech: evidence from a case of left supplementary motor area hemorrhage. *Neuropsychologia*, 35 (9), 1197–1208.

7

Phonetics and the auditory system

Matthew B. Winn and Christian E. Stilp

Introduction

Why combine these topics?

Rosen and Fourcin (1986) wrote, "trying to understand the auditory processes involved in the perception of speech is likely to lead not only to a better understanding of hearing, but also, of speech itself" (p. 373). In this chapter, we review some basic principles of the auditory system so that the perception and processing of speech can be understood within a biological framework. There are some ways that traditional acoustic descriptions of speech fail to capture how sounds are handled by the auditory system; this chapter contains some advice on how to approach experimental phonetics with the auditory system in mind. Rather than a comprehensive review of the auditory system or acoustic phonetics, this chapter focuses on a few basic principles that would be (a) essential bits of knowledge for anyone doing auditory-perceptual work, (b) useful for design and analysis of phonetics experiments, and (c) helpful for an auditory scientist interested in how basic auditory functions like spectral and temporal coding could play a role in the encoding of speech information. The scope will be limited to the factors that affect segmental/phonetic aspects of perception rather than prosody, voice quality, or tone.

Sound frequency, intensity, and timing are all processed nonlinearly, meaning that equivalent changes in the acoustic input do not map onto equivalent changes in the perceptual interpretation. Furthermore, perception of each of these acoustic properties is dependent on each of the others, and the encoding of a signal can unfold dramatically differently depending on what came before or after it. The spectral and temporal processing of the auditory system has meaningful implications for the processing of speech in particular, since it is replete with meaningful changes that span wide frequency ranges, occur on multiple timescales, and with great fluctuation in amplitude. In the next sections, we will review some of the most fundamental aspects of nonlinear auditory processing.

Nonlinear processing of frequency

Sound frequency is an organizing principle throughout the entire auditory system. The cochlea – the signature structure of the inner ear – acts as a mechanical spectrum analyzer, separating and ordering the frequency components in a way that is similar to a spectrum or a piano. However, unlike a conventional spectrum on a computer screen, the frequencies in the cochlea are arranged mostly logarithmically, meaning that equal spacing along the cochlea corresponds to equivalent *proportional* changes in frequency, rather than equivalent raw changes in frequency (Figure 7.1). For example, the space between cochlear locations for 500 Hz and 1000 Hz is much larger (100% change) than the space between areas for 4000 Hz and 4500 Hz (12.5% change), despite the equal linear change of 500 Hz. For this reason, many auditory researchers compare frequencies based on cochlear space using the function specified by Greenwood (1990), perceptual space using equivalent rectangular bandwidths (Glasberg and Moore, 1990), the mel scale (Stevens et al., 1937), or the Bark frequency scale (Zwicker, 1961; Traunmüller, 1990). These scales account for the expanded representation of low frequencies in the cochlea that gradually tapers off for higher frequencies.

Phoneticians can consider auditory frequency spacing in the design and analysis of speech stimuli in perceptual experiments. For example, a continuum of first formant (F_1) frequencies might be easily generated as 300, 400, 500, 600, 700 and 800 Hz, but these steps are not equally spaced in the human auditory system. A continuum with values of 300, 372, 456, 554, 668 and 800 Hz would occupy equidistant intervals along a typical adult human cochlea. These numbers were generated using the Greenwood (1990) formula using standard parameters for an adult 35 mm-long human cochlea. One could translate frequencies and cochlear positions using these functions (written for the R programming language), with sensible default values for the formula parameters declared in the opening lines:

```
freq_to_mm = function(frequency=1000, A=165.4, a=2.1, length=35, k=0.88){
  mm = log10((frequency/A)+k)*length/a
  return(mm)
}
mm_to_freq = function(position=10, A=165.4, a=2.1, length=35, k=0.88){
  frequency=A*((10^(a * position/length))-k)
  return(frequency)
}
```

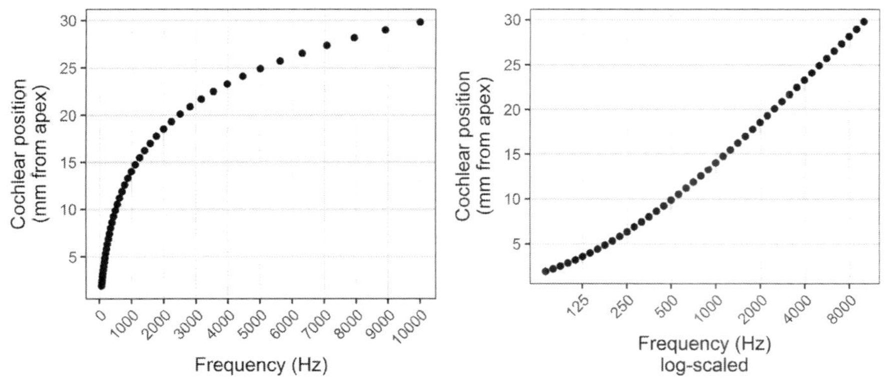

Figure 7.1 The place of cochlear excitation for various sound frequencies arranged on a linear scale (left panel) and a logarithmic scale (right panel), demonstrating that cochlear treatment of frequency is proportional rather than absolute.

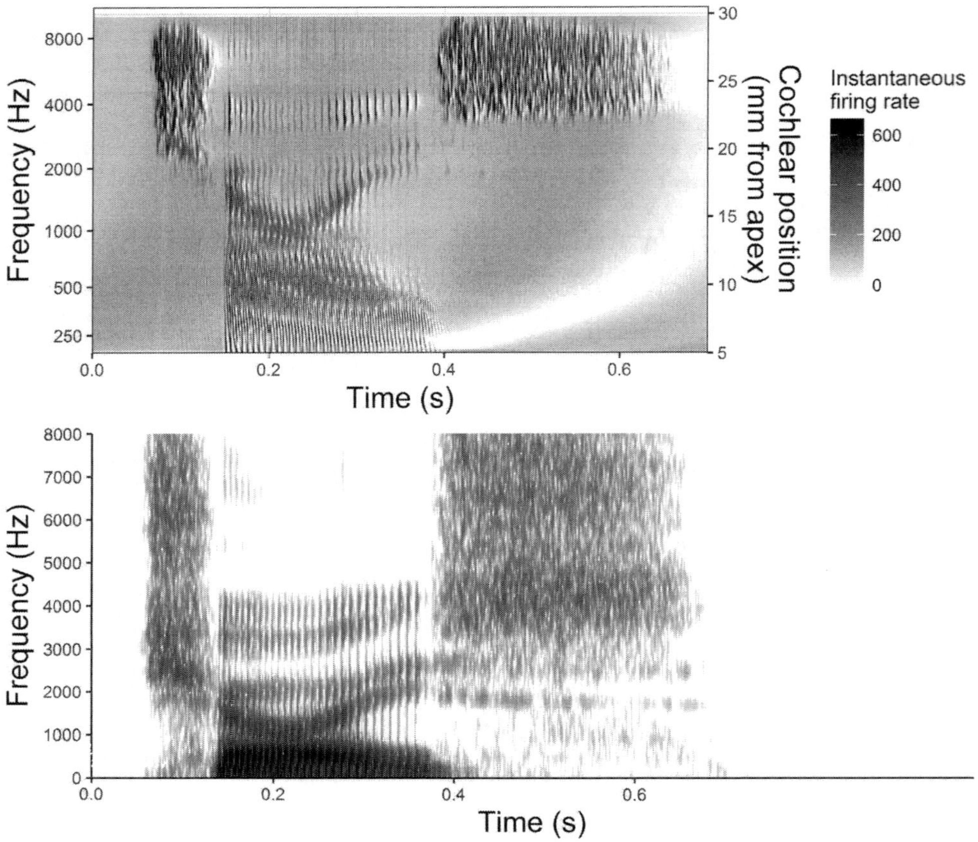

Figure 7.2 Neurogram (top) and spectrogram (bottom) of the word "choice."

The nonlinear arrangement of frequency and energy in the auditory system implies that the spectrogram – probably the most common way of viewing and analyzing speech signals – offers a distorted view of the signal in the ear. Scaling the spectrogram's frequency axis to correspond with cochlear spacing and expressing energy as neural activation rather than analytical signal energy produces a *neurogram*, which illustrates the signal from the perspective of the auditory system. Figure 7.2 shows a neurogram along with its corresponding spectrogram for the word "choice." The vowel dynamics, leading and trailing frication noise, and glottal pulses are visible in each image, but are spatially warped in the neurogram. Note also the "background" of resting state neural activity that allows the energy to both increase *and* decrease in order to signal change in the input.

Clearer understanding of frequency information is helpful not just for generating acoustic perceptual stimuli, but also for filtering or analyzing bands of frequency information (e.g., for contributions to intelligibility or other outcome measures). Suppose that the F_1 frequency varies between 300 and 1000 Hz, and the F_2 frequency varies between 1000 and 2500 Hz. The F_1 range seems smaller, but spans a distance of 6.84 mm in the standard adult cochlea, whereas the apparently larger 1000–2500 Hz spans just 6.06 mm. More cochlear space is dedicated to F_1 after all!

Pitch perception

Pitch is a complicated concept because it involves both spectral and temporal cues, and because related terms are sometimes used haphazardly. Individual components (e.g., sinusoids) of a complex sound have *frequency*, which is the measurable repetition rate. A complex sound with a large number of components at integer multiples of the fundamental frequency (like voiced speech) has a more complicated waveform pattern, but still a general rate of repetition, which is its *fundamental frequency* (f_0). f_0 can also be derived from the spacing between the harmonics, and usually from the frequency of the lowest harmonic component. *Pitch* has a more slippery definition; it is the *subjective* perceptual quality of a sound that scales closely with fundamental frequency, and which generally gives rise to melody.

Deriving pitch from the sound spectrum can be somewhat misleading. Even though the spectrum might cleanly distinguish all the harmonic components of a voice, the auditory system cannot encode every spectral component separately. Only the lowest seven or eight harmonics are proportionally far enough apart that they each activate a separate auditory filter (i.e., a separate place on the basilar membrane in the cochlea). The difference between the first and second harmonic is 100% (e.g., 100–200 Hz); the difference between the second and third is 50% (200–300 Hz), and the proportional change continues to decrease (33%, 25%, 20%, and so on). Around the eighth harmonic, the proportional difference is smaller than the proportional width of the resolving power of the cochlea (roughly 12–14%), so the higher harmonics are not represented distinctly in the auditory system, and are said to be *unresolved* (Moore et al., 1986). Interestingly, this upper limit holds true even for high-pitched voices, whose harmonics extend into higher-frequency regions of the cochlea, but are also spaced farther apart, therefore preserving resolution of only the first approximately seven harmonics.

f_0 is coded primarily by temporal cues. It is no coincidence that the upper limit of fundamental frequencies perceived to have tonal quality is around 5000 Hz, which is also the upper limit of the auditory system's ability to lock to the repetition rate of the sound waveform. For higher-order harmonics, the exact placement of excitation is not resolved, but the interaction of multiple components within one auditory filter creates amplitude fluctuations that repeat at the same rate as the fundamental (try adding sounds of 2000 and 2200 Hz; you will get a pattern that repeats 200 times per second). Therefore, one can derive the pitch by attending to temporal fluctuations in any part of the audible spectrum. However, pitch perception is markedly better when listeners have access to the lower-frequency resolved harmonics; the two cues appear to be complementary. Because cues for pitch are distributed across the whole spectrum, pitch information cannot be neutralized by simply removing or masking low-frequency components. Even without the first harmonic present, the fundamental (and therefore the pitch) remains the same, because the basic repetition rate of the complex wave remains the same. Consider how you can still identify different talkers and distinguish questions from statements when listening to an adult over the telephone, which filters out components below 300 Hz. Therefore, for an experimenter to control or neutralize the influence of pitch, it is not enough to filter out or mask out the fundamental and lowest harmonics (as done in numerous studies in the literature).

Listeners with typical ("normal") hearing can distinguish complex signals with just a 0.2% change in fundamental (Moore et al., 1984). Linguistically relevant acoustic contrasts generally do not require such fine-grained discrimination. Although listeners with typical hearing *can* perceive such miniscule changes in steady-state vowels (Klatt, 1973), this ability grows poorer – requiring about 6% change – when (synthetic) speech contains dynamic pitch movements ('t Hart, 1981). Rosen and Fourcin (1986) point out that there is also roughly 6% variance when talkers repeat the same speech segment, according to analysis of vowels from the classic study by Peterson and Barney (1952). Rosen and Fourcin's work demonstrates the power of perceptual analysis driven by analysis of the acoustic output itself. These studies collectively suggest that only frequency differences of 6% or more are likely to play a meaningful role in the transmission of speech information.

Pitch is an intensely studied aspect of audition partially because it serves as a mechanism to bind together multiple components of a complex sound so that they are perceived as a unified auditory stream (Culling and Darwin, 1993). When listening to two talkers simultaneously, intelligibility improves considerably when the two voices have greater separation of pitch (Brokx and Nooteboom, 1982), which partially explains why it is easier to hear one talker when a background talker is of a different gender (Brungart, 2001). Additionally, acoustic-phonetic cues that are carried by pitch are more robust to noise, even if they are ignored when the signal is in quiet (Wardrip-Fruin, 1985; Winn et al., 2013).

Perception of the spectrum becomes unclear when intensity is increased

At low sound intensities, active mechanisms of outer hair cells in the inner ear sharpen the peak of excitation in the cochlea, creating precise coding of frequency. Higher-intensity sounds activate a wider span of cochlear space, similar to the wide disturbance of a pond when a large stone is dropped in it. This means that frequency coding could be jeopardized when the sound is presented loudly. Figure 7.3 illustrates how auditory excitation in the cochlea grows to be not only wider (known as spread of excitation), but increasingly *asymmetrical* with greater intensity. Low-frequency sounds are relatively more disruptive than high-frequency sounds because the traveling wave of sound energy begins at the base of the cochlea (where high frequencies are encoded), and passes through lower-frequency regions on their way to their characteristic place of stimulation. This phenomenon is called "upward spread of masking." Illustration of excitation patterns in Figure 7.3 as well as other auditory responses elsewhere in this chapter were generated using the auditory periphery model of Zilany et al. (2014). The chaotic pattern at very high intensities is due to multiple modes of vibration in the basilar membrane response, in addition to the nonlinearities in inner hair cell discharge (modeled by Zilany and Bruce, 2007). These patterns are likely to contribute to the degradation in perception at very high intensities, known in audiology as the "roll-over" effect in speech when it is presented above normal conversational levels.

Upward spread of masking directly impacts perception of formants in speech. Like most other natural sounds, speech has greater energy in lower-frequency regions. The first formant can therefore spread excitation upward to mask the second and third formants. The amount of masking is extraordinary – about 40 dB – and was calculated originally by Rand (1974), who presented F_1 and the upper formants to opposite ears; in doing so, the 40 dB masking release was observed. A series of experiments using this principle eventually became part of the series of "duplex perception" studies, which played a role in the theoretical debate over the nature of phonetic representation and speech perception in general. But they began as a simple exploration of basic auditory principles.

Understanding the spread of cochlear excitation helps us to think of formants not as specific frequencies, but as regions that are less precise and more overlapping than a conventional spectrum would suggest. Zahorian and Jagharghi (1993) suggested a model of vowel recognition based on log-amplitude-scaled spectral shapes rather than formants.

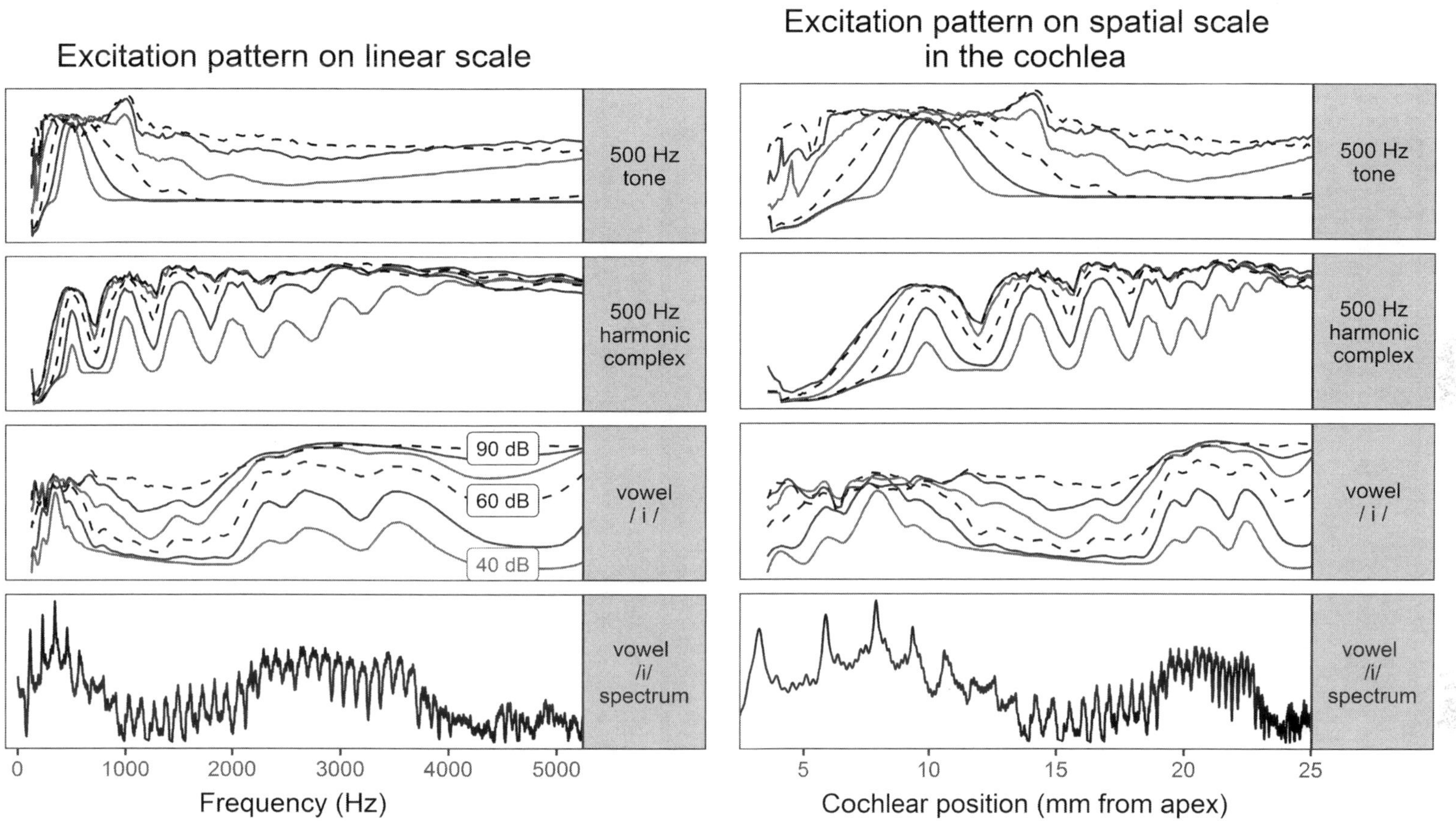

Figure 7.3 Auditory excitation patterns (inner hair cell discharge) for a simple 500 Hz pure tone, 500 Hz harmonic complex, and the vowel /i/ (with 115 Hz fundamental frequency), each labeled on the right band of each panel. The lowest panels show the analytical power spectrum of the /i/ vowel. Different lines represent different input intensity levels at 10-dB intervals. Larger intensities elicit smoother and less precise excitation patterns, including patterns with peaks unrelated to the original components.

The Bark frequency scale further aids the intuition for the frequency separation needed to perceive the vowel spectrum. Syrdal and Gopal (1986) suggested a framework whereby spectral peaks (formants) would be interpreted not as absolute values but in terms of relative distance to other peaks in auditory-perceptual space (or, arguably, physical space in the cochlea). A "critical distance" of 3–3.5 Bark was found to categorically distinguish vowel height (Bark f_0–F_1 distance) and advancement (Bark F_2–F_3 distance). Some papers provide very specific focus connecting the ideas of frequency integration and vowel perception (for reference, see Darwin and Gardner, 1986; Assmann and Nearey, 1987; Kiefte et al., 2010).

The biological framework of formants as broad areas of cochlear excitation can help to reconcile different proposed perceptual cues for phonemes. Consider the debate over acoustic cues for place of articulation in stops. Stevens and Blumstein described static cues according to gross spectral shape, which has good explanatory power in the acoustic (Stevens and Blumstein, 1978) and perceptual (Blumstein and Stevens, 1980) domains. Kewley-Port (1983) provided an account of this phonetic contrast by instead focusing on the dynamic transitions in formant frequencies. If upper formants are considered as areas of cochlear excitation, it is much easier to see the similarities between formants and the spectral shapes as described by Stevens and Blumstein: Regardless of the acoustic measurement, spectral components as high as F_2 or F_3 will necessarily be transformed by the cochlea into rather gross areas of excitation, or arguably "spectral shapes."

A more recent theory of vowel coding in the auditory system (Carney et al., 2015) shifts the focus away from formant *peaks* altogether. The high intensity of formant peaks would saturate inner hair cell discharge rates, and therefore not be coded robustly at higher levels in the auditory system (e.g., the inferior colliculus) that are selectively tuned to detect modulation rather than absolute energy. However, downward-sloping amplitude energy on the upper and lower edges of formants contain fluctuations in amplitude consistent with pitch periodicity, and would therefore project a fluctuating signal to which the auditory midbrain neurons would respond. The model and empirical data presented by Carney et al. (2015) suggest that the space *between* formants is the property most strongly represented at upper levels of the auditory system. This framework would be consistent with basic edge-detection principles that have prevailed in the visual sciences.

Not all frequencies are equally audible or equally loud

Different frequencies require different amounts of sound pressure level in order to be audible, or to be equal in loudness. Based on the current international standard (ISO 226) inspired by seminal work by Fletcher and Munson (1933) and Robinson and Dadson (1956), Figure 7.4 illustrates the dependence of loudness judgments on sound frequency. These *equal-loudness contours* have practical implications for normalizing sound levels and for delivering sound through specialized earphones. In situations where stimuli need to be shaped to match specific loudness perceptions, analysis of analytical sound pressure level is not sufficient; one must also consult the equal-loudness contours to ensure that the attenuation is reflective of the frequency of the signal being played. Equal loudness contours factor into frequency-specific energy weightings when estimating loudness of a broadband sound (using the dBA scale for low or moderate-intensity sounds and the dBC scale for loud sounds). The influence of frequency on loudness is less pronounced at higher levels; a high-intensity sound is loud, no matter what the frequency.

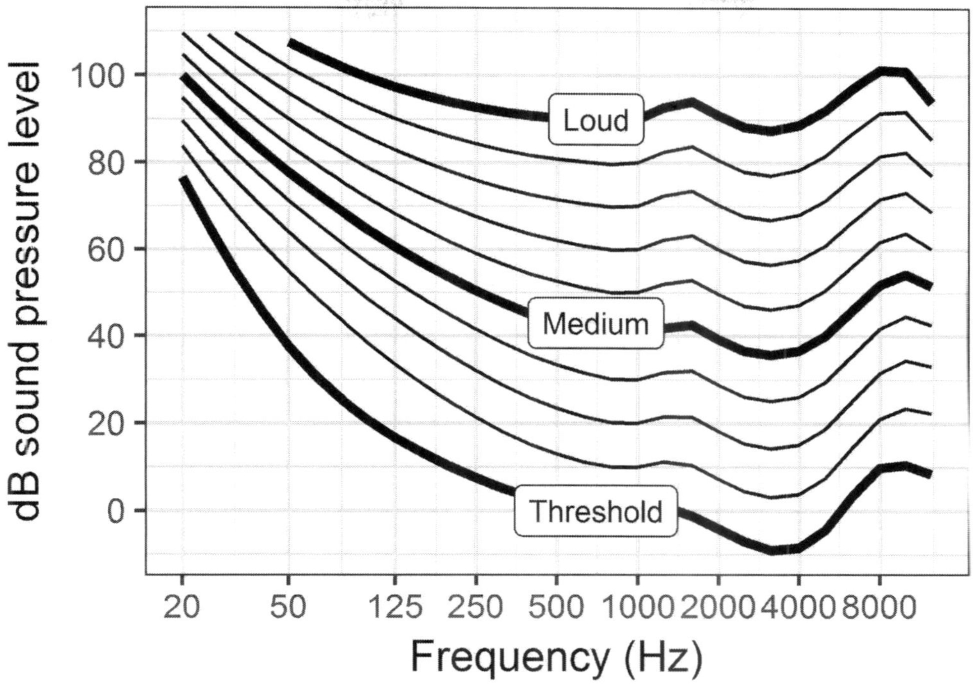

Figure 7.4 Equal loudness contours. Each line indicates the sound pressure intensities required at different frequencies to produce a fixed level of perceived loudness. The thickened lines correspond to uncomfortably loud sounds (top), medium-level sounds (middle), and the absolute thresholds for detection of different frequencies (bottom).

The interaction between spectrum and time

Perception of the sound spectrum becomes more accurate with increasing duration. Moore (2013) suggests that the gradual sharpening of spectral estimation unfolds over the course of a 30 ms time window, which happens to correspond to various meaningful time windows for phonetic perception. For example, it is the minimal stimulus duration required for accurate perception of sibilant fricatives (Jongman, 1989), formant trajectories in stop consonants (Blumstein and Stevens, 1979), vowel onglides and offglides (Assmann, 1996), and voicing distinctions in intervocalic or post-vocalic fricatives (Stevens et al., 1992). It was used by Dubno and Levitt (1981) in their detailed acoustic analysis of consonants in perceptual experiments. It is also close to the short "phonetic" auditory temporal window proposed by Poeppel and Hickok (2004) and the 20-ms boundary proposed to be a natural discontinuity in auditory temporal processing by Holt and colleagues (2004). Jongman (1989) points out that, at least among fricatives, place of articulation – traditionally thought to be cued spectrally – is much more affected by brevity of stimulus duration than other features such as voicing or manner. This observation is consistent with the cueing of velar consonants /g/ and /k/, which have a distinct relatively compact spectral peak in the mid-frequency range, which demands longer exposure to establish the precision of the spectrum. Fittingly, the duration of the burst and aspiration of these consonants is longer than their counterparts at other places of articulation (Blumstein and Stevens, 1980).

Temporal information

At its very core, speech is a temporal signal with multiple layers of amplitude modulations. Temporal cues are essential components of familiar phonetic contrasts such as voice onset time (VOT; duration of aspiration, temporal amplitude modulation between burst and vowel onset), word-medial contrasts in voiced and voiceless stops (duration of closure gap), fricative/affricate distinctions (presence or absence of silent closure gap, speed of frication rise time), word-final consonant voicing perception (duration of preceding vowel), and the speed of formant transitions (glide/stop contrasts), to name a few. Even cues that are seemingly spectral in nature – such as formants – can be described as temporally modulated energy in adjacent auditory filters.

Temporal cues can be classified into broad categories based on the speed of modulation. Rosen (1992) provided a thorough explanation of these categories and their translation to linguistic properties. Very slow (2–50 Hz) modulations comprise the signal *envelope*, which can convey information about syllable rate as well as manner of articulation and segment duration. Faster modulations, on the order of 50–500 Hz convey *periodicity*, and can transmit information about voice pitch. For this reason, a voiceless fricative /s/ that is artificially modulated at 100 Hz can sound like a voiced fricative /z/ even without the full complement of acoustic cues for glottal voicing. Waveform changes that happen faster than 500 Hz are generally described as *temporal fine structure*, and correspond to cues that are commonly thought to be "spectral" in nature, such as place of articulation. Different categories of waveform modulation are illustrated in Figure 7.5.

Although a storied history of speech perception research (namely, that which began at Haskins laboratories) focused on the spectral characteristics of speech, there are

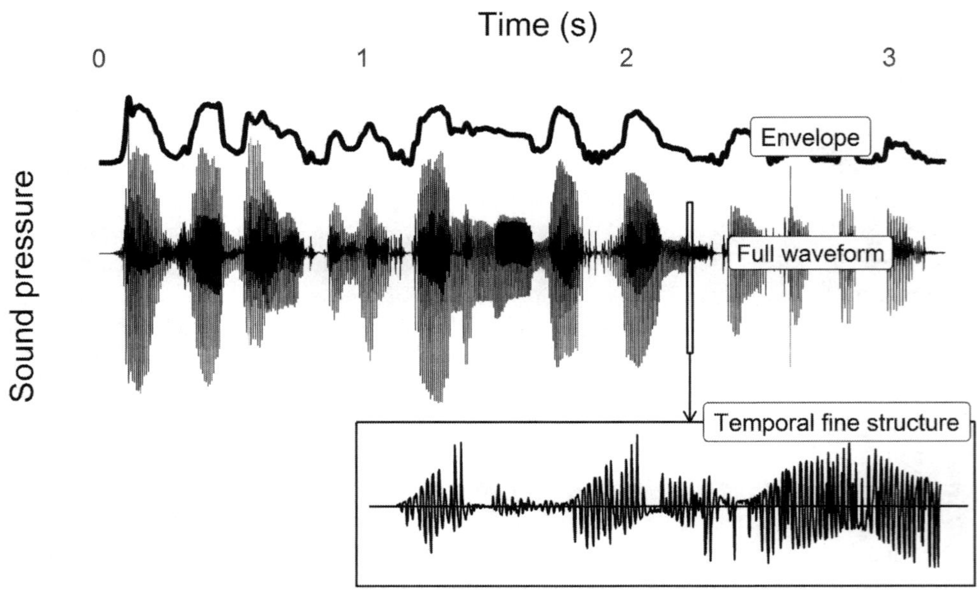

Figure 7.5 The sentence "A zebra is an animal that lives in Africa." The envelope is illustrated as a thick line above the full waveform, and the temporal fine structure for a 20-ms segment indicated by the narrow slice is illustrated in the zoomed-in inset box.

successful models of speech perception grounded in auditory principles that give special emphasis to temporal modulations (Dau et al., 1997). Furthermore, Giraud and Poeppel (2012) and Peelle and Davis (2012) describe how neural oscillations on different time-scales might facilitate speech perception (see also Chapter 8, this volume). They suggest that oscillations are entrained to fluctuations in the amplitude envelope of the speech signal at the levels of linguistic units like phonemes, syllables, etc. (but see Obleser et al., 2012 for a supportive but critical interpretation). These models suggest that when comparing sensitivity to different kinds of linguistic segments (e.g., syllables, fricative sounds, stop sounds), one must consider the general rate of change in the time domain. Apart from merely a descriptive tool, amplitude modulation spectra over very coarse frequency ranges have been used to efficiently model perception of consonants and vowels (Gallun and Souza, 2008).

The encoding of sound energy over time does not perfectly match the intensity of the sound waveform. First, the auditory system gives special emphasis to sound onsets and *changes* in amplitude, as will be further discussed later in the chapter. Also, the mechanical nature of the inner ear results in some sustained activation after a sound, called "ringing," that can interfere with perception of subsequent sounds presented in quick succession. This type of interference – called "forward masking" – can last upwards of 100 ms (Jesteadt et al., 1982), and can result in different detection thresholds for speech in isolation compared to speech in the context of other signals. Consonants – being relatively lower in intensity and shorter in duration – are more susceptible to forward masking than vowels (Fogerty et al., 2017). This might explain why consonants are relatively more difficult to perceive at syllable offset position compared to syllable onset position (Dubno et al., 1982).

Decomposing the temporal envelope

The complete waveform can be misleading. In the auditory system, it is decomposed by numerous auditory filters, and the output of each filter might look dramatically different from the full waveform you see on your computer screen. Figure 7.6 illustrates the word "sing," shown as a full waveform and after being sent through a small number of band-pass filters, each responsible for a narrow region of frequencies. With this in mind, it is useful to be skeptical of descriptions of complete waveforms, as they have no true corresponding biological representation beyond the middle ear.

Decomposing the signal into a small number of frequency bands with sparsely coded envelopes has been useful for the development of sound processing in cochlear implants (Loizou et al., 1998), whose processing strategies can be traced back directly to the development of the Vocoder (Dudley, 1939). It is a way of simplifying the signal since the fine structure is discarded in favor of a low-fidelity envelope that transmits only crude information about how the frequency bands change in amplitude over time. As long as there is no interfering noise, these simplified envelopes can support excellent speech recognition with as few as four to eight frequency bands (Shannon et al., 1995; Friesen et al., 2001).

Summary

With all of the transformations that occur in the auditory system, our knowledge of relevant acoustic cues for phonemes is seriously challenged by a need to translate acoustic measurements into properties that are actually encoded by the sensory system. The next section

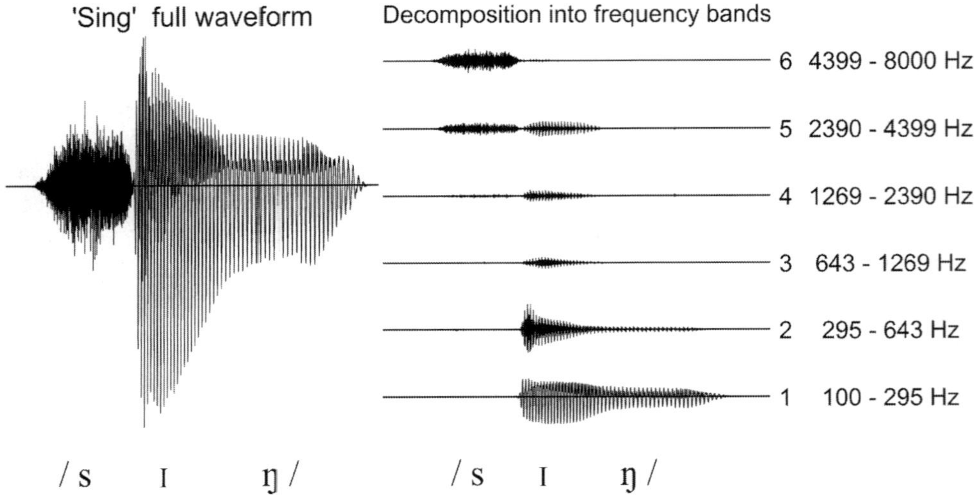

Figure 7.6 A complex sound decomposed into constituent frequency bands by the auditory system. Each band has its own envelope of energy over time, implying that the overall envelope on the composite waveform is typically not represented in the cochlea. The filter bands shown here are merely a six-channel view for simplicity, using frequency ranges of equal cochlear space. The typical auditory system would have many more frequency filters whose widths are narrower, but similarly proportional to their central frequencies.

walks us through how this can be accomplished, with the aid of decades of work in other sensory systems engaged in the same kind of computational problem.

Sensory systems as change detectors

Once the signal from the inner ear is transduced into action potentials at the auditory nerve, the auditory system gets quite complex. Information is relayed to the cochlear nucleus, superior olivary complex, inferior colliculus, and the medial geniculate body of the thalamus before reaching the brain. As further described in Chapter 8 of this volume, at every stage along the way, the neural code is repackaged so that more sophisticated aspects of the input can be represented. This is by far the most extensive subcortical processing in any sensory modality. Additionally, a dense network of feedforward, feedback, and lateral connections exists between auditory nuclei, so much so that nearly every figure depicting this network is noted as being highly simplified.

Given this complexity, how is one to understand how speech and other complex sounds are processed? This question has benefited from an unlikely source of inspiration: Claude Shannon's (1948) mathematical approach to information transmission in a communication system (i.e., "information theory"). In this approach, the amount of information transmitted is directly related to its predictability. If the transmitter's message is entirely predictable (e.g., "Thursday comes after Wednesday"), there is no new information for the receiver because it isn't anything she/he did not already know. However, if the transmitter's message is relatively unpredictable (e.g., "Audrey imagined a typhoon"), there is considerable potential information for the receiver.

These principal ideas in Shannon's information theory were originally conceived to describe communications systems, but they also do a very good job of describing sensation (Barlow, 1961) and perception (Attneave, 1954). When some stimulus in the environment is completely predictable or unchanging, it provides no new information for the perceiver. Conversely, when a stimulus is unpredictable or changing, it possesses potential information for the perceiver. Neurons exhibit efficient response strategies that optimize the amount of information they can transmit. Enhanced responses can indicate unexpected or changing inputs (high information content), whereas diminished responses can indicate expected or unchanging inputs (low information content). These notions form the foundation of the *efficient coding hypothesis* (Barlow, 1961, 2001; Simoncelli, 2003): Recoding the sensory input reduces its predictability and increases the informativeness of stimulus representations at later stages of sensory processing. By focusing on relative change, limited neural dynamic ranges adjust to maximize the amount of change detected in the environment (Kluender et al., 2003). The auditory system displays a variety of mechanisms for change detection, and these mechanisms can be highly informative for understanding how speech is processed and perceived.

Adaptation in the auditory nerve

In the presence of continued stimulation, neurons generally decrease their firing rate. This has been termed "firing rate adaptation," or "spike-frequency adaptation" (Figure 7.7). Adaptation is not mere neural fatigue, but instead an efficient way to code information about a stimulus that is not changing (Wark et al., 2007). Neurons are even observed to respond strongly to change *even when adapted* to previous stimuli (Smith, 1979; Smith and Zwislocki, 1975). There is a biological basis for viewing adaptation as an efficient response

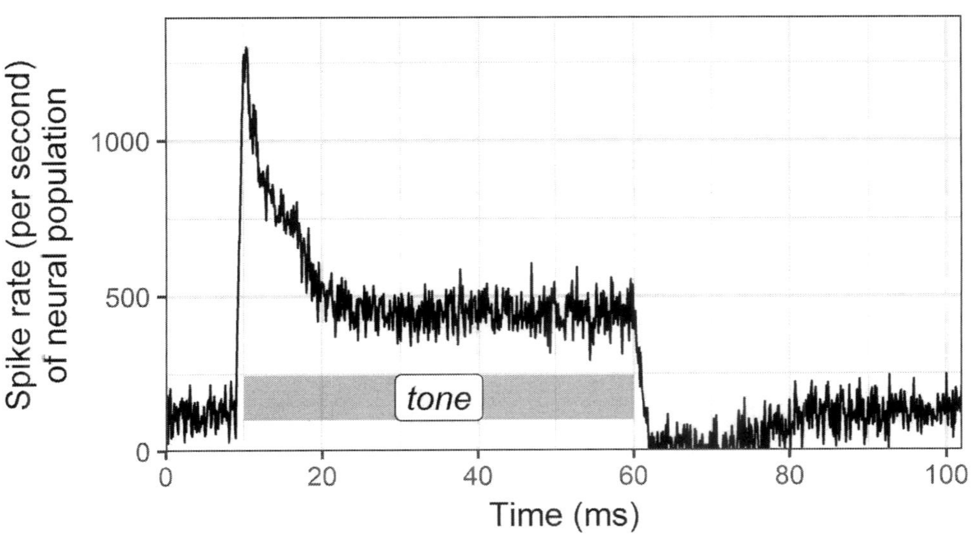

Figure 7.7 Firing activity of a population of auditory neurons in response to a 50-ms, constant-amplitude pure tone. The neural activity begins with a resting firing rate before any stimulus, represents the tone onset with disproportionately high firing that adapts within about 15 ms, and then remains steady through the end of the stimulus. At stimulus offset, activity decreases sharply before finally returning to its resting state.

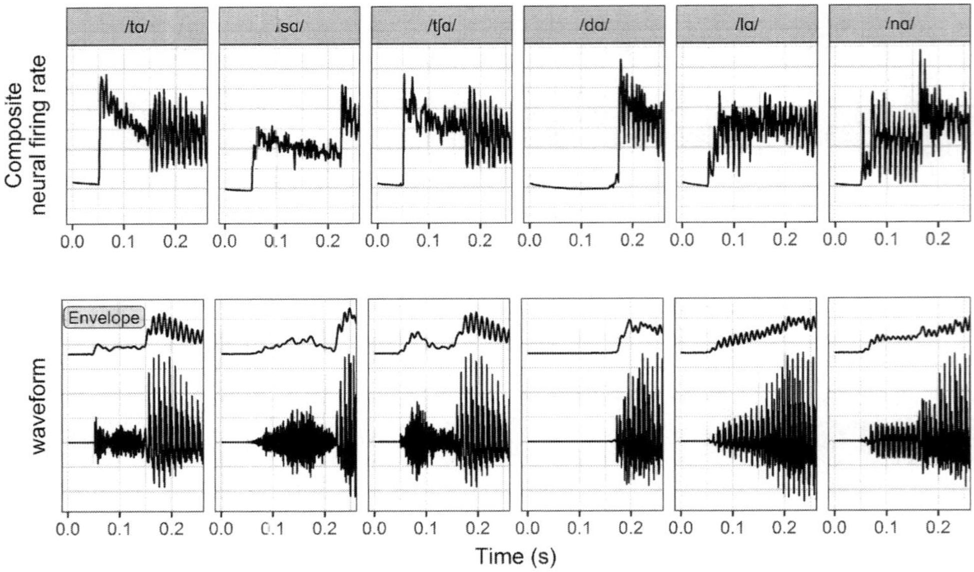

Figure 7.8 Overall neural firing response (akin to Figure 7.7) in response to phonemes with different manners of articulation.

strategy. Producing action potentials incurs a metabolic cost, and there are limitations on energy consumed by neural populations in the brain (Laughlin, 1981; Lennie, 2003). Thus, adaptation acts as a conservation of resources until they can be better deployed, such as when there is a change in the environment. Adaptation occurs throughout the auditory system to a wide range of stimulus properties, and it is reflected in other neural systems as well. Figure 7.7 illustrates the canonical neural activity over time in response to a simple pure tone, and Figure 7.8 expands this concept to phonemes with different manners of articulation, whose patterns of airflow are distinguished by their sound envelopes. Although the different manners are distinguished by their envelopes on the waveform (see Rosen, 1992), the neural representations of those envelopes are far less distinct, primarily because of the overrepresentation of onsets.

Neurons adapt if they are coding spectral energy that does not change substantially over time (such as formant frequencies in English vowels /i/ and /u/, and numerous other steady-state vowels in other languages). These adapted neurons remain sensitive to new information so that they can respond when these frequencies change, like during coarticulation into the next speech sound. In addition, adaptation is a strong candidate for producing spectral contrast effects (see section, "Speech perception as change detection").

Change detection in auditory cortex

Detection of sensory changes is also measured at the cortical level using mismatch negativity (MMN; Näätänen et al., 1978). MMN is an event-related potential elicited by neural populations in the brain. Studies of the MMN contrast the neural activity measured in response to a pattern of repetitive or predictable inputs (the "standard") against an unexpected stimulus that violates this pattern (the "deviant"). Mismatch responses occur automatically, even in the absence of attention, making them a popular tool for investigating central auditory function. They arise in response to changes in simple acoustic properties (e.g., frequency, duration, intensity, and spatial location; see Näätänen et al., 2007 for a thorough review), and they scale up to the level of phonetic contrasts as well (Aaltonen et al., 1987; Näätänen et al., 1997). MMNs have been reported for violations of cue covariance (Gomes et al., 1997; Takegata et al., 2005), which is highly relevant for phonetic categorization, given the abundance of covarying cues in phonemes (Repp, 1982). These cortical responses to stimulus changes are reliable predictors of speech intelligibility at segmental and sentence levels, and of language development (Koerner et al., 2016; Molfese and Molfese, 1997). Altogether, investigations of MMN paint a rich picture of how the auditory system is sensitive to changes, from simple (i.e., acoustic) to more complex (i.e., phonetic). This is consistent with the idea that deviance detection in audition is organized hierarchically (see Grimm et al., 2011; Escera and Malmierca, 2014 for reviews).

Speech perception as change detection

The acoustic complexity of speech is considerable, with important signal properties spanning narrow and broad frequency ranges as well as brief and long durations. It is both true and fortunate that the auditory system is constantly calibrating in order to be maximally sensitive to changes across variable frequency and temporal extents (Kluender et al., 2003). Considering the general principle of change detection that cuts across all sensory systems, it is unsurprising that it plays a significant role in speech perception. Some speech sounds can be defined by how they change over time. For example, the second formant (F_2) transition is a major cue for distinguishing voiced stop consonants (Delattre et al., 1955; Kewley-Port, 1983; Lahiri et al., 1984). Apart from this well-known case, there are other cases that deserve to be framed as change detection as well. Encoding spectral changes over time has proven to be fruitful in understanding speech perception by people with impaired auditory systems (Alexander and Kluender, 2009; Dorman and Loizou, 1996; Winn and Litovsky, 2015), and in highlighting the difference between automatic classification (Blumstein and Stevens, 1979) and human perception (Dorman and Loizou, 1996, Kewley-Port, 1983).

Vowel-Inherent Spectral Change

Although vowel recognition is typically described as depending primarily on the frequencies of the first two formants (and further formalized in the literature by mapping so-called steady-state formants onto a static two-dimensional space), there are extensive dynamics in play. Researchers often use tables of steady-state formant values from publications by Peterson and Barney (1952) and Hillenbrand et al. (1995) when preparing or analyzing their own speech stimuli. However, there is tremendous value in the authors' original commentaries surrounding these tables. For instance, Hillenbrand and colleagues suggested very strongly that English vowel categories should be defined not merely by a snapshot of steady-state values, but by the changes in those values over time. This point was earlier proposed and empirically verified in Canadian English by Nearey and Assmann (1986), with supporting evidence in American English contributed by Hillenbrand and Nearey (1999). In this latter report, automatic classification of F_1 and F_2 steady-state values was greatly enhanced by the addition of formant information from a second time point – much more so than the addition of duration, f_0, or F_3 information. Figure 7.9 depicts the movement of vowel formants in the production of English vowels by adult women recorded in the study by Hillenbrand

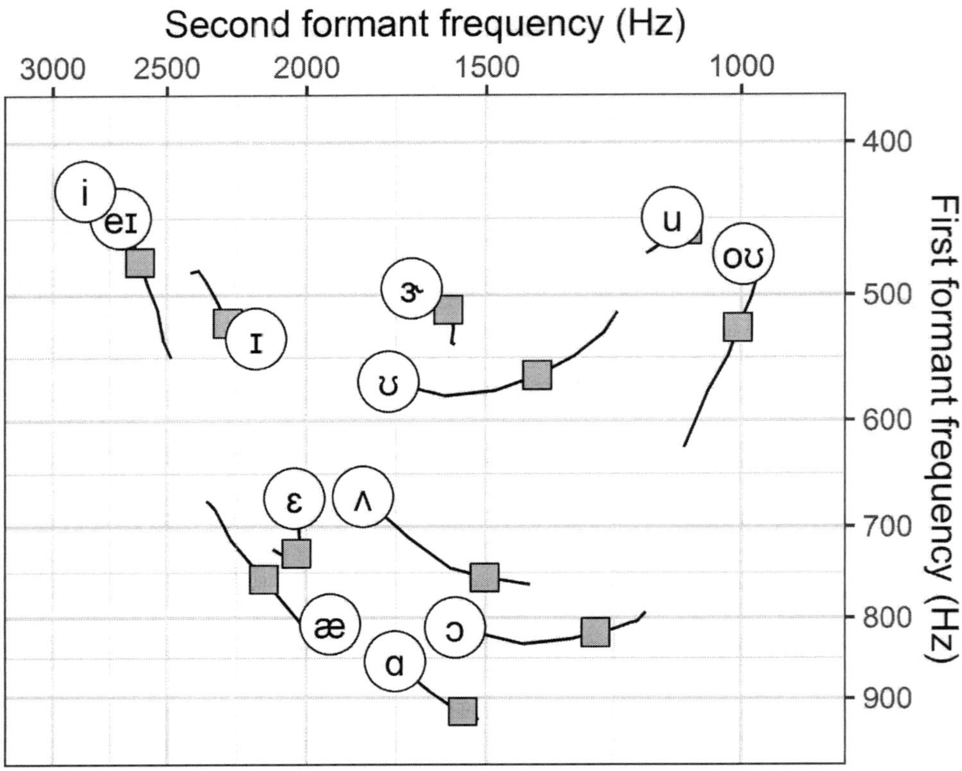

Figure 7.9 Formant dynamics in English vowels spoken by women recorded by Hillenbrand et al. (1995). Formant frequencies are measured at the 20% point (beginning of each line), 50% midpoint (gray boxes), and 80% point (circle with phonetic symbol) of vowel duration.

et al. (1995). This illustrates how much information is typically lost when only considering formants at vowel midpoints.

The concept of perceptually significant changes in formants across time has come to be known as vowel-inherent spectral change (VISC; Nearey and Assmann, 1986; Hillenbrand and Nearey, 1999; Morrison and Assmann, 2013). VISC plays an important role in vowel recognition, and not just for vowels traditionally labeled as being diphthongal. Accuracy of vowel perception drops considerably when formant trajectories are artificially flattened, for vowels spoken by adults (Hillenbrand and Nearey, 1999) and by children (ages 3, 5, and 7) (Assmann and Katz, 2000). It bears mention that while VISC is a perceptually salient cue that helps disambiguate vowels in American and Canadian English, this might be due to the crowded nature of these vowel spaces, contributing to the Adaptive Dispersion theory of vowel typology and the Dynamic Specification model of vowel perception (Jenkins and Strange, 2013). VISC has not been studied extensively in other languages, but languages with less-crowded vowel spaces might have less need for vowels to be disambiguated through VISC.

Recognition of other phonemes can be interpreted through the lens of change detection, but it is beyond the scope of this chapter to list them all. The earlier examples illustrate the importance of detecting changes in acoustic details within the phoneme (i.e., intrinsic cues to phoneme identity). However, surrounding sounds form an acoustic context whose properties can influence recognition of a given phoneme (i.e., extrinsic cues to phoneme identity). This distinction between intrinsic and extrinsic cues was originally raised for vowel perception (Ainsworth, 1975; Nearey, 1989), but it is appropriate for perception of any stimulus, speech or non-speech. Next, we briefly review how spectral and temporal context influences phoneme perception.

Short-term spectral contrast

Spectral properties of neighboring sounds can alter recognition of a phoneme, such that any differences in the spectra of two neighboring sounds will be perceptually magnified. If frequencies in the surrounding context are relatively lower, frequencies in a target sound may seem higher by comparison, and vice versa. The perceptual patterns that reveal the bias away from surrounding context are known as "spectral contrast effects." Such demonstrations date back at least to Lindblom and Studdert-Kennedy (1967), who studied identification of a target vowel as /ʊ/ or /ɪ/ in different consonantal contexts (/wVw/ or /jVj/). When F_2 transitions in the consonantal context started and ended at lower frequencies (/w/), the vowel was identified as the higher-F_2 /ɪ/ more often, and the opposite pattern emerged for the /jVj/ context. This pattern of results was later extended to stop consonant contexts (/bVb/, /dVd/) in perception of /o/–/ʌ/ and /ʌ/–/ɛ/ vowel continua (Nearey, 1989; Holt et al., 2000). Additionally, these results were replicated when consonantal contexts were replaced by pure tones and tone glides (Holt et al., 2000), suggesting that the contextual adjustment might be driven by general auditory contrast rather than phonemic or phonetic contrast.

Spectral context influences consonant recognition as well. Listeners are more likely to perceive /d/ (higher F_3 onset frequency) following /r/ (lower F_3 offset frequency), and more likely to perceive that same consonant as /g/ (lower F_3 onset frequency) following /l/ (higher F_3 offset frequency) (Mann, 1980, 1986; Fowler et al., 1990). Similar to the results of Holt and colleagues (2000), Lotto and Kluender (1998) replicated these effects by replacing the liquid consonant with pure tones and tone glides at the appropriate frequencies. The debate remains strong over whether these context effects can be described as general auditory phenomena or something more complicated (Lotto and Holt, 2006; Fowler, 2006; Viswanathan et al., 2009; Kingston et al., 2014).

Long-term spectral contrast

The influence of spectral context is not limited to the sound immediately adjacent to the target phoneme (Figure 7.10). Similar shifts in phoneme categorization occur when spectral properties are stable across a longer listening context like a sentence. Listeners are more likely to perceive a vowel with lower F_1 frequency (e.g., /ɪ/) when the preceding acoustic context features higher F_1 frequencies, and vice versa (Ladefoged and Broadbent, 1957). Such demonstrations are often referred to as "extrinsic normalization" or "vowel normalization" (e.g., Ainsworth, 1974; Nearey, 1989; Johnson, 1990), but similar effects have been reported in consonant recognition as well. Studies of speech and non-speech perception produced similar results using non-speech contexts (signal-correlated noise, Watkins, 1991; sine tones, Holt, 2005; string quintet, Stilp et al., 2010) and/or targets (brass instruments, Stilp et al., 2010), indicating that talker-specific information is not necessary in order to produce spectral contrast effects. This has led to suggestions that it is not talker information per se but the long-term average spectrum of preceding sounds that biased subsequent

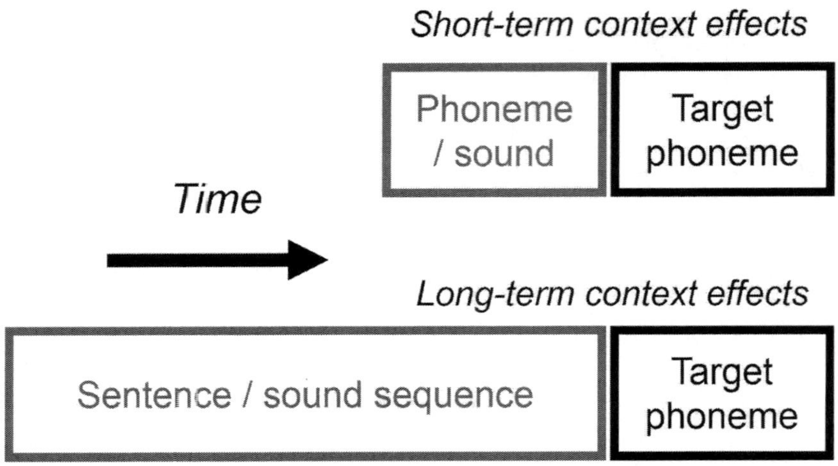

Figure 7.10 Different timescales of context (gray) influence phoneme categorization (black). The context can be the immediately preceding sound (top) or several seconds of sounds (bottom), whether they are speech or non-speech. This depicts "forwards" context effects (context precedes target phoneme), but "backwards" effects (phoneme precedes context) are also known to occur.

perception in these studies (Huang and Holt, 2012). However, it bears mention that similar effects have been reported without any influence from the long-term average spectrum of preceding sounds. Visual information about the talker's gender produced similar shifts in categorization boundaries (Glidden and Assmann, 2004), and expectations about talker gender can shift vowel categorization (Johnson et al., 1999).

Spectral contrast effects have been reported for recognition of phonemes cued by fundamental frequency, F_1, F_2, F_3, and overall spectral shape (see Stilp et al., 2015 for review). A series of experiments by Stilp and colleagues (2015) demonstrated the generality of long-term spectral contrast effects on categorization of /ɪ/ and /ɛ/. Perceptions were repeatedly influenced by spectral properties of the preceding sentence, whether those properties took the form of a narrow spectral peak (100 Hz bandwidth), a broader peak (300 Hz), or spanned the entire spectral envelope (after Watkins, 1991). Importantly, the size of the shift in phoneme categorization was correlated with the size of the spectral difference between the context sentence and subsequent target vowels (see also Stilp and Alexander, 2016). This relationship also exists in consonant categorization (Stilp and Assgari, 2017) and musical instrument categorization (Frazier et al., in press). Spectral contrast effects are a general principle of auditory perception, and the wide variety of examples in the literature suggest that they might play a widespread role in everyday speech perception as well.

Temporal contrast

Temporal properties of speech can also have contrastive effects on phoneme identification. Similar to the spectral contrast effects reported earlier, these effects occur on both shorter and longer timescales. Whether formant transitions are heard as fast (indicating a stop consonant) or slow (indicating a glide/semivowel) can be affected by temporal information from the surrounding speech context, such as speaking rate and the relative durations of consonant and adjacent vowel. Longer vowel duration makes the initial consonant sound shorter (i.e., more /b/ responses), and shorter vowel duration made the consonant sound longer (more /w/ responses; Miller and Liberman, 1979). Similar patterns emerge for other temporal contrasts, such as VOT for /b/ and /p/ (Green and Miller, 1985). Even a brief interval of silence can form a temporal context; an abrupt onset of the amplitude envelope is perceived to be shorter, leading to an increase in perception of affricates instead of fricatives (Dorman et al., 1979).

Temporal contrast effects can also occur across longer-duration listening contexts. Ainsworth (1973) reported that when preceding sounds had a slower tempo, a fixed-duration target consonant sounded faster; formant transitions normally slow enough to be perceived as /w/ were instead more likely to be heard as /b/. An analogous temporal contrast effect emerges for the perception of voicing in /ɡ/ and /k/ (Summerfield, 1981) and in the /ʃ/–/tʃ/ contrast (Haubert and Pichora-Fuller, 1999; Repp et al., 1978). The temporal category boundary between consonants essentially moves around to accommodate the momentary speaking rate and the exact syllable timing; listeners show sensitivity to changes in multiple timescales simultaneously. However, some controversy surrounds the consistency with which distal speech rate information affects speech perception (Heffner et al., 2017).

Together, these studies depict speech perception as being heavily influenced by detection of change relative to context. These changes can span narrow (a formant peak) to broad spectral bandwidths (spectral envelope) and narrow (tens of milliseconds) to broad temporal extents (several seconds). This acoustic diversity highlights the extent to which the auditory system is constantly adjusting its sensitivity to changes across frequency and across time in order to maximize the amount of information that can be transmitted to the perceiver. For a phonetician, this provides important perspective for evaluating phoneme perception. Not only do the (intrinsic) acoustic properties of a given phoneme affect its perception, but the (extrinsic) surrounding context plays a significant role as well.

Learning about the auditory system using speech sounds

Being conversant and knowledgeable about phonetics can be useful for auditory scientists. We highlight at least three benefits here: first, one can explore the performance of the auditory system using stimuli where signal properties translate into known meaningful differences in speech (as opposed to acoustic properties that are merely convenient and programmable). Second, we can explore cases where auditory cues permit categorization, rather than just discrimination. Finally, one can explore the effects of specific auditory deficits such as hearing loss on particular phonetic contrasts. In this section, we walk through some ways that acoustic phonetics can contribute to auditory science, and the challenges that remain.

Experimental control and external validity

There are some good reasons why psychoacousticians do not normally use speech stimuli. Speech acoustics are highly variable from one utterance to the next, so two experimenters might use different sounds even if they are nominally the same phoneme. Acoustic measurements of speech do not give an absolute template for speech perception in general. Even seminal papers on acoustic measurements such as Hillenbrand et al. (1995) warn readers against the tendency to use measurements as a framework for describing anything other than a snapshot in history in a particular region of a country (for further discussion, see Chapter 16 in this volume). There is no consensus on what constitutes an "ideal" speech stimulus,

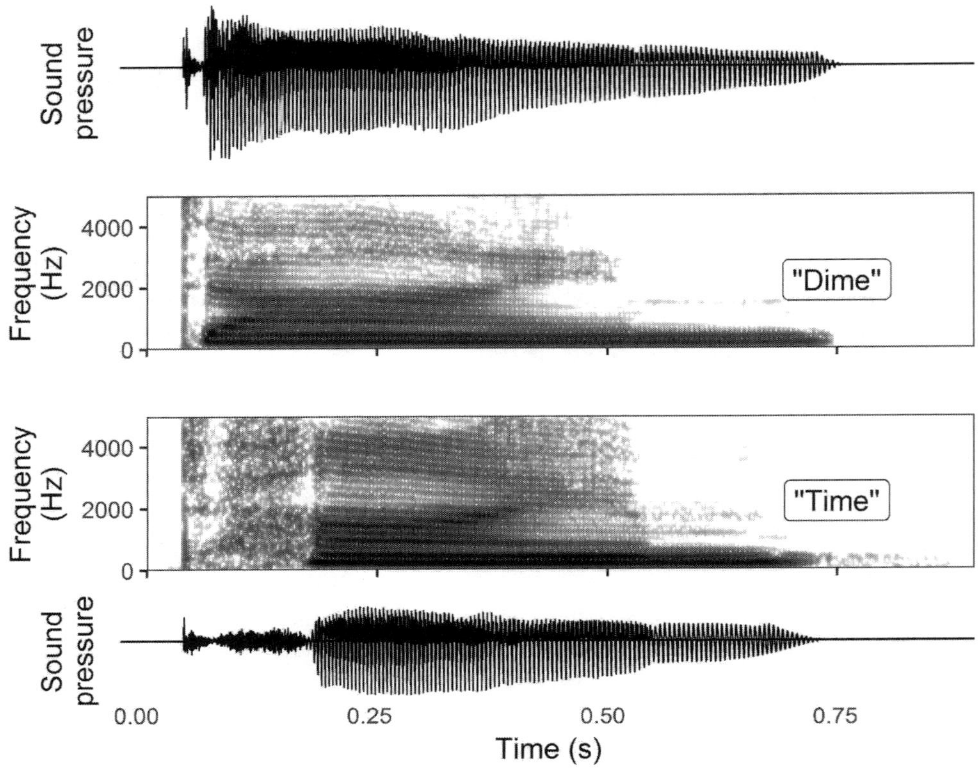

Figure 7.11 Waveforms and spectrograms for "dime" (top panels) and "time" (lower panels) showing that voicing contrast appears as differences in amplitude envelope/duration of consonant burst and aspiration, as well as formant frequencies at the onset of voicing.

or on how to properly control acoustic factors of interest (via synthesis, partial resynthesis, waveform editing, etc.). In the psychoacoustics world, everyone agrees on what constitutes a 1000 Hz tone of 300-ms duration and 70 dB SPL intensity. However, the pure tone might not represent any meaningful experience relating to communication. What we gain in stimulus acoustic control we also sacrifice in ecological validity, and vice versa.

Suppose one is interested in measuring auditory temporal processing because there are relevant phonetic cues that are temporal in nature. It can be tempting to use the classic "out-of-the box" psychoacoustic and phonetic tests such as gap detection and VOT categorization, respectively. However, there are at least two challenges worth noting. First (and most simply), the acoustic dimensions sometimes do not match up across different testing styles. For example, VOT is not a gap in the speech signal; it can arguably be described as an amplitude envelope modulation, or asynchrony in onset time of two crudely defined "high" and "low" frequency regions. Second, the prolonged aspiration of a voiceless English stop is not "added" onto the vowel but rather a progressive devoicing of the vowel; Figure 7.11 illustrates this principle by temporally aligning the contrastive pair "dime" and "time."

As stated earlier, it is reasonable to suspect that psychoacoustic tests probe abilities on a different scale than those needed for speech recognition. For example, while syllable-final stop sounds contain a gap whose duration is useful for voicing categorization (i.e., longer gaps typically correspond to voiceless stops), the duration of these gaps (30–150 ms) is an order of magnitude greater than just-noticeable gaps in psychoacoustic tests (2–5 ms).

Multidimensionality of phonetic contrasts

Phonetic contrasts cannot be completely described in only one acoustic domain at a time. The literature is replete with investigations of multiple acoustic parameters that covary with single linguistic features. Among them are Lisker's (1986) catalog of 16 cues for the /b/–/p/ contrast in word-medial position, and McMurray and Jongman's (2011) measures of 24 different cues for English fricative sounds. Although some of the cues are certainly more dominant than others in governing perception, we note these examples to highlight how synthetizing or manipulating speech must account for a high amount of complexity in order to retain natural acoustic quality.

Even when a temporal property is a salient cue for a phonetic contrast, its role can rarely be examined in isolation in the same way as in a classical psychoacoustic experiment. Consider the impact of vowel environment on VOT. Lower vowels (like /a/) are cued by higher F_1 values, and therefore contain a very salient up-sweeping F_1 transition. As stop consonant aspiration essentially devoices the transition into the following vowel, longer VOT results in a noticeably higher F_1 frequency at voicing onset. In experimental terms, this means the F_1 onset frequency (a spectral cue) can be strongly confounded with VOT (a nominally "temporal" cue), particularly in the context of low vowels like /a/. Incidentally, there are numerous examples of experiments that examined temporal perception using VOT stimuli in the /a/ context, with predictably mixed results. For example, Elangovan and Stuart (2005) found a relationship between gap detection and VOT boundary, but Mori et al. (2015) found no such pattern. It is likely that perception of temporal processing was diluted by a strong accompanying spectral cue in the /ba/–/pa/ series used in each study. Such mixed results are peppered throughout the literature on this topic, possibly because of an incomplete appreciation of the multiplicity of acoustic cues for the voicing feature. Barring a deep dive into the acoustics literature, a good practice for an auditory scientist interested in temporal processing would be to use a steady-state vowel context with low F_1, such as /i/, which affords ostensibly no extra spectral cues because there is no sweeping frequency transition.

Controlling acoustic-phonetic cues

Despite the inherent covariation among acoustic cues in speech, it is usually possible to manipulate speech sounds so that phonetic categorization mainly taps into a particular auditory domain. Detecting a stop following /s/, or detecting an affricate instead of a fricative at the end of a word is ostensibly the same as a psychoacoustic test of gap detection. Haubert and Pichora-Fuller (1999) examined the perception of word pairs that are differentiated by detecting the presence (the stop in "spoon" or the affricates in "catch" or "ditch") or absence of a short temporal gap (resulting in perception of "soon," "cash," or "dish"). For those interested in perception of frequency-specific peaks in the spectrum, there could be tests that rely on perception of low-frequency formants (as for vowel height distinction between "hoop" and "hope," or for F_1 transitions in "loss" and "laws"), mid-frequency formants (for vowel advancement distinctions like "shock" and "shack"), or high-frequency energy that distinguishes words like "key" and "tea." There are tests of amplitude modulation detection that have potential phonetic implications as well. Consider slow (2–10 Hz) rates of syllabicity and speech rate, or manner of articulation at slightly higher modulation rates (15–60 Hz).

Detection of faster (≈100–200 Hz) modulations in broadband noise is akin to detecting the presence (e.g., /z/) or absence (e.g., /s/) of voicing in fricatives. The list certainly does not end here; there are numerous other examples where simple or complex patterns in speech can be mapped to corresponding simple acoustic parameters in non-speech stimuli.

Discrimination and categorization

Even after identifying appropriate complementary psychoacoustic and phonetic tests, it is worthwhile to recall that the ability typically tested in non-linguistic psychoacoustic tests is *discrimination* while most phonetic perception tasks probe *categorization* (Holt and Lotto, 2010). A helpful guide to these abilities was written by Erber (1982) and to this day is still regarded as a useful framework for understanding development of audition in children. The paradigms used to test speech recognition demand processing that extends beyond the simple detection or discrimination of sounds. Speech sounds must be appropriately categorized, requiring listeners to derive meaning from superfluous variation, and to incorporate relevant contextual and linguistic knowledge. For people who use cochlear implants, word recognition is more strongly predicted by auditory categorization than by psychoacoustic discrimination (Winn et al., 2016).

Categorization depends on a host of methodological details that could have considerable implications for processing. For example, extremely fine discrimination of speech sounds (i.e., the "auditory" mode) emerges with short inter-stimulus comparison intervals, but more coarse category-level labeling, seemingly absent of fine discrimination at all (i.e., the "phonetic" mode) occurs at longer intervals (Pisoni, 1973). Early models of categorical perception (a well-known nonlinear mapping of acoustic cues into phonological categories) broadly equated discrimination and categorization: Sounds from two different categories were discriminable, and sounds from the same category were indiscriminable. However, subsequent work demonstrated that shared category membership does not render sounds indiscriminable (Pisoni and Lazarus, 1974; Massaro and Cohen, 1983), further highlighting important differences between these abilities.

Using speech stimuli to probe for auditory deficits

The utility of mapping simple acoustics parameters onto phonetic segments can be seen very clearly in experiments designed to test auditory *deficits* using speech sounds. Hearing loss in its most common form (high-frequency sensorineural hearing loss, resulting from damage to the cochlea) is not merely a reduction of loudness, but instead a distortion of the spectral representation of sound, as well as a drastic reduction of the wide dynamic range that is characteristic of typical hearing. These problems are exacerbated for those who wear cochlear implants, which are prosthetic devices that directly electrically stimulate the auditory nerve but fail to faithfully transmit all of the fine temporal or spectral details of real acoustic signals. Because of these less-intuitive aspects of hearing loss, the specific spectral and temporal structure of speech contrasts can lead to testable hypotheses about what kinds of perceptions (and misperceptions) will unfold from various deficits in the auditory system.

The temporal domain

Gordon-Salant et al. (2006) showed that older listeners generally have less efficient processing of temporal cues, even in the absence of any clinical hearing loss. Examples of this include poorer perception of affricate gaps, VOT, spectrotemporal transition speed (e.g., the /b/–/w/ contrast), and vowel duration (for the voicing contrast in syllable-final consonants). This study provides a very clean and thorough example of how speech contrasts can be used to target isolated auditory abilities normally constrained to psychoacoustic discrimination tests.

The spectral domain

Individuals who use cochlear implants frequently have their hearing tested for spectral resolution because of the sizable challenges that stand in the way of good spectral coding by their devices. Such testing can take many forms in both the psychoacoustic and phonetic realms. At a coarse level, vowels can be used to test perception of segments that are primarily defined in the spectral domain without many helpful cues in the temporal domain. Typically, such vowel testing is done with "hVd" words such as "heed," "hid," "head," etc., because the vowel is embedded in a consistent environment with virtually no confounding acoustic cues, each environment yields a valid word in English, and the acoustics of such vowels have been explored in numerous publications. Other studies examining dynamic cues in vowel perception generally found a lack of sensitivity to these crucial cues in cochlear implant users (see Iverson et al., 2006; Winn et al., 2012; Donaldson et al., 2013).

Vowels can be used to make specific predictions about how perception changes with local damage in the cochlea. DiNino et al. (2016) imposed frequency-specific degradation in a simulation of cochlear implants, where narrow regions of frequency information were either lost or redistributed, causing predictable warping of phonetic perceptual space. Vowel perceptions tended to gravitate away from the affected region. In cases where a mid-frequency region between 850 and 1850 Hz would carry F_2 information for back vowels spoken by a woman, perception of those vowels would be more "front" in nature (e.g., "hud" would be perceived as "head"). In this study and those mentioned in previous paragraphs, it is worth mentioning that the test stimuli were not chosen because words of hVd form are especially important in the lexicon, but because they provide a stable phonetic environment where some parameter of interest can be tested directly. Using this testing approach, one might be able to *diagnose* deficiencies or even localized sites of cochlear lesion by capitalizing on the acoustic structure of vowels and consonants (Winn and Litovsky, 2015).

Use of a cue vs. sensitivity to a cue

The perceptual weighting of an acoustic-phonetic cue (e.g., to distinguish between phonemes in a minimal pair) is not the same as psychoacoustic sensitivity. Work by Klatt (1982) and Rosen and Fourcin (1986) articulate the distinctions between these concepts in illuminating ways. Consider voice pitch, to which human listeners are exquisitely sensitive, but which is largely discarded when perceiving stop consonant voicing, despite being a natural cue (Abramson and Lisker, 1985). Exceptions occur only in circumstances of unnatural ambiguity (Haggard, 1978) and/or with harsh masking noise or band-limited conditions (Winn et al., 2013). The phonetic perception results do not necessarily imply that frequency discrimination is poor. Instead, they imply that the cue is not regarded as reliable enough to inform categorization of this contrast because some other cue takes priority. Following the framework established in vision science (Ernst and Banks, 2002; Jacobs, 2002), Toscano and McMurray (2010) modeled auditory cue weighting as a function of the *reliability* of the distribution of that cue as it appears in natural speech. For example, if VOT for two segments /b/ and /p/ is realized as two tightly constrained (low-variability) separate distributions, and some other cue (such as vowel duration) is realized as two wide (high-variability) and overlapping distributions, the secondary cue should be given much less perceptual weight on account of its lack of usefulness for the task at hand (regardless of whether it is perceptually discernible).

Conclusion

Basic properties of the auditory system play a vital role in the processing of speech sounds. Exploration of nonlinearities in frequency, intensity, and temporal processing offer insight into how speech is transformed from an acoustic signal to a neural signal. Consistent with other sensory systems, auditory processing shows special sensitivity to change over time, and handles information proportionally and with respect to context. Although speech sounds are multidimensional, phonetic contrasts can be found to rely relatively heavily on spectral or temporal cues, and can thus be used to probe the function of the auditory system in a fashion similar to classic psychoacoustics. Impairments of the auditory system lead to systematic deficits in phonetic perception, which can be revealed by experiments that treat the signal in an auditory framework. An examination of the auditory system and an equally rigorous examination of the acoustic structure of speech can contribute to refined methodology in phonetics, basic hearing sciences, and the study of speech perception by people with normal and impaired hearing.

References

Aaltonen, O., Niemi, P., Nyrke, T., & Tuhkanen, M. (1987). Event-related brain potentials and the perception of a phonetic continuum. *Biological Psychology*, 24(3), 197–207.

Abramson, A., & Lisker, L. (1985). Relative power of cues: F0 shift versus voice timing. In V. Fromkin (Ed.), *Linguistic phonetics* (pp. 25–33). New York: Academic Press.

Ainsworth, W. (1973). Durational cues in the perception of certain consonants. *Proceedings of the British Acoustical Society*, 2, 1–4.

Ainsworth, W. (1974). The influence of precursive sequences on the perception of synthesized vowels. *Language and Speech*, 17(2), 103–109.

Ainsworth, W. (1975). Intrinsic and extrinsic factors in vowel judgments. In G. Fant & M. Tatham (Eds.), *Auditory analysis and perception of speech* (pp. 10–113). London: Academic Press.

Alexander, J. M., & Kluender, K. R. (2009). Spectral tilt change in stop consonant perception by listeners with hearing impairment. *Journal of Speech, Language, and Hearing Research*, 52(3), 653–670.

Assmann, P. (1996). Modeling the perception of concurrent vowels: Role of formant transitions. *The Journal of the Acoustical Society of America*, 100(2 Pt 1), 1141–1152.

Assmann, P., & Katz, W. (2000). Time-varying spectral change in the vowels of children and adults. *The Journal of the Acoustical Society of America*, 108(4), 1856–1866.

Assmann, P., & Nearey, T. (1987). Perception of front vowels: The role of harmonics in the first formant region. *The Journal of the Acoustical Society of America*, 81(2), 520–534.

Attneave, F. (1954). Some informational aspects of visual perception. *Psychological Review*, 61(3), 183–193.

Barlow, H. (1961). Possible principles underlying the transformation of sensory messages. *Sensory Communication*, 217–234.

Barlow, H. (2001). The exploitation of regularities in the environment by the brain. *Behavioral and Brain Sciences*, 24(4), 602–671.

Blumstein, S., & Stevens, K. (1979). Acoustic invariance in speech production: Evidence from measurements of the spectral characteristics of stop consonants. *Journal of the Acoustical Society of America*, 66, 1001–1017.

Blumstein, S., & Stevens, K. (1980). Perceptual invariance and onset spectra for stop consonants in different vowel environments. *The Journal of the Acoustical Society of America*, 67(2), 648–662.

Brokx, J., & Nooteboom, S. (1982). Intonation and the perceptual separation of simultaneous voices. *Journal of Phonetics*, 10(1), 23–36.

Brungart, D. (2001). Informational and energetic masking effects in the perception of two simultaneous talkers. *The Journal of the Acoustical Society of America*, 109(3), 1101–1109.

Carney, L., Li, T., & McDonough, J. (2015). Speech coding in the brain: Representation of vowel formants by midbrain neurons tuned to sound fluctuations. *eNeuro*, 2(4), e0004–0015.2015 1–12.

Culling, J., & Darwin, C. (1993). Perceptual separation of simultaneous vowels: Within and across-formant grouping by F0. *The Journal of the Acoustical Society of America*, 93(6), 3454–3467.

Darwin, C., & Gardner, R. (1986). Mistuning a harmonic of a vowel: Grouping and phase effects on vowel quality. *The Journal of the Acoustical Society of America*, 79(3), 838–845.

Dau, T., Kollmeier, B., & Kohlrausch, A. (1997). Modeling auditory processing of amplitude modulation. II. Spectral and temporal integration. *The Journal of the Acoustical Society of America*, 102(5), 2906–2919.

Delattre, P., Liberman, A., & Cooper, F. (1955). Acoustic loci and transitional cues for consonants. *The Journal of the Acoustical Society of America*, 27(4), 769–773.

DiNino, M., Wright, R., Winn, M., & Bierer, J. (2016). Vowel and consonant confusions from spectrally-manipulated stimuli designed to simulate poor cochlear implant electrode-neuron interfaces. *The Journal of the Acoustical Society of America*, 140(6), 4404–4418.

Donaldson, G., Rogers, C., Cardenas, E., Russell, B., & Hanna, N. (2013). Vowel identification by cochlear implant users: Contributions of static and dynamic spectral cues. *The Journal of the Acoustical Society of America*, 134, 3021–3028.

Dorman, M. F., & Loizou, P. C. (1996). Relative spectral change and formant transitions as cues to labial and alveolar place of articulation. *The Journal of the Acoustical Society of America*, 100(6), 3825–3830.

Dorman, M., Raphael, L., & Liberman, A. (1979). Some experiments on the sound of silence in phonetic perception. *The Journal of the Acoustical Society of America*, 65(6), 1518–1532.

Dubno, J., Dirks, D., & Langhofer, L. (1982). Evaluation of hearing-impaired listeners test using a nonsense-syllable test II. Syllable recognition and consonant confusion patterns. *Journal of Speech and Hearing Research*, 25(March), 141–148.

Dubno, J., & Levitt, H. (1981) Predicting consonant confusions from acoustic analysis. *The Journal of the Acoustical Society of America*, 69, 249–261.

Dudley, H. (1939). Remaking speech. *The Journal of the Acoustical Society of America*, 11(2), 169–177.

Elangovan, S., & Stuart, A. (2005). Interactive effects of high-pass filtering and masking noise on word recognition. *Annals of Otology, Rhinology and Laryngology*, 114(11), 867–878.

Erber, N. (1982). *Auditory training*. Washington, DC: AG Bell Association for the Deaf.

Ernst, M., & Banks, M. (2002). Humans integrate visual and haptic information in a statistically optimal fashion. *Nature*, 415(6870), 429–433.

Escera, C., & Malmierca, M. (2014). The auditory novelty system: An attempt to integrate human and animal research. *Psychophysiology*, 111–123.

Fletcher, H., & Munson, W. (1933). Loudness, its definition, measurement and calculation. *Bell Labs Technical Journal*, 12(4), 377–430.

Fogerty, D., Bologna, W., Ahlstrom, J., & Dubno, J. (2017). Simultaneous and forward masking of vowels and stop consonants: Effects of age, hearing loss, and spectral shaping. *The Journal of the Acoustical Society of America*, 141(2), 1133–1143.

Fowler, C. A. (2006). Compensation for coarticulation reflects gesture perception, not spectral contrast. *Perception & Psychophysics*, 68(2), 161–177.

Fowler, C. A., Best, C., & McRoberts, G. (1990). Young infants' perception of liquid coarticulatory influences on following stop consonants. *Perception & Psychophysics*, 48(6), 559–570.

Frazier, J. M., Assgari, A. A., & Stilp, C. E. (in press). Musical instrument categorization is highly sensitive to spectral properties of earlier sounds. *Attention, Perception, & Psychophysics*.

Friesen, L., Shannon, R., Baskent, D., & Wang, X. (2001). Speech recognition in noise as a function of the number of spectral channels: Comparison of acoustic hearing and cochlear implants. *The Journal of the Acoustical Society of America*, 110(2), 1150–1163.

Gallun, F., & Souza, P. (2008). Exploring the role of the modulation spectrum in phoneme recognition. *Ear and Hearing*, 29(5), 800–813.

Giraud, A., & Poeppel, D. (2012). Cortical oscillations and speech processing: Emerging computational principles and operations. *Nature Neuroscience*, 15(4), 511–517.

Glasberg, B., & Moore, B. (1990). Derivation of auditory filter shapes from notched-noise data. *Hearing Research*, 47, 103–138.

Glidden, C. M., & Assmann, P. F. (2004). Effects of visual gender and frequency shifts on vowel category judgments. *Acoustics Research Letters Online* 5(4), 132–138.

Gomes, H., Bernstein, R., Ritter, W., Vaughan, H., & Miller, J. (1997). Storage of feature conjunctions in transient auditory memory. *Psychophysiology*, 34(6), 712–716.

Gordon-Salant, S., Yeni-Komshian, G., Fitzgibbons, P., & Barrett, J. (2006). Age related differences in identification and discrimination of temporal cues in speech segments. *The Journal of the Acoustical Society of America*, 119(4), 2455–2466.

Green, K., & Miller, J. (1985). On the role of visual rate information in phonetic perception. *Perception & Psychophysics*, 38(3), 269–276.

Greenwood, D. (1990). A cochlear frequency-position function for several species 29 years later. *The Journal of the Acoustical Society of America*, 87, 2592–2605.

Grimm, S., Escera, C., Slabu, L., & Costa-Faidella, J. (2011). Electrophysiological evidence for the hierarchical organization of auditory change detection in the human brain. *Psychophysiology*, 48(3), 377–384.

Haggard, M. (1978). The devoicing of voiced fricatives. *Journal of Phonetics*, 6(2), 95–102.

Haubert, N., & Pichora-Fuller, M. K. (1999). The perception of spoken language by elderly listeners: Contributions of auditory temporal processes. *Canadian Acoustics*, 27(3), 96–97.

Heffner, C., Newman, R., & Idsardi, W. (2017). Support for context effects on segmentation and segments depends on the context. *Attention, Perception, & Psychophysics*, 79(3), 964–988.

Hillenbrand, J., Getty, L., Clark, M., & Wheeler, K. (1995). Acoustic characteristics of American English vowels. *The Journal of the Acoustical Society of America*, 97(5), 3099–3111.

Hillenbrand, J., & Nearey, T. M. (1999). Identification of resynthesized vertical bar hVd vertical bar utterances: Effects of formant contour. *The Journal of the Acoustical Society of America*, 105(6), 3509–3523.

Holt, L. (2005). Temporally nonadjacent nonlinguistic sounds affect speech categorization. *Psychological Science*, 16(4), 305–312.

Holt, L., & Lotto, A. (2010). Speech perception as categorization. *Attention, Perception & Psychophysics*, 72(5), 1218–1227.

Holt, L., Lotto, A., & Diehl, R. (2004). Auditory discontinuities interact with categorization: Implications for speech perception. *The Journal of the Acoustical Society of America*, 116(3), 1763–1773.

Holt, L., Lotto, A., & Kluender, K. (2000). Neighboring spectral content influences vowel identification. *The Journal of the Acoustical Society of America*, 108(2), 710–722.

Huang, J., & Holt, L. (2012). Listening for the norm: Adaptive coding in speech categorization. *Frontiers in Psychology*, 3, 10.

Iverson, P., Smith, C., & Evans, B. (2006). Vowel recognition via cochlear implants and noise vocoders: effects of formant movement and duration. *The Journal of the Acoustical Society of America*, 120, 3998–4006.

Jacobs, R. (2002). What determines visual cue reliability. *Trends in Cognitive Science*, 6, 345–350.

Jenkins, W., & Strange, J. (2013) Dynamic specification of coarticulated vowels. In G. Morrison & P. Assmann (Eds.), *Vowel inherent spectral change* (pp. 87–116). Berlin: Springer.

Jesteadt, W., Bacon, S., & Lehman, J. (1982). Forward masking as a function of frequency, masker level, and signal delay. *The Journal of the Acoustical Society of America*, 71(4), 950–962.

Johnson, K. (1990). The role of perceived speaker identity in F0 normalization of vowels. *The Journal of the Acoustical Society of America*, 88(2), 642–654.

Johnson, K., Strand, E. A., & D'Imperio, M. (1999). Auditory – visual integration of talker gender in vowel perception. *Journal of Phonetics*, 27(4), 359–384.

Jongman, A. (1989). Duration of frication noise required for identification of English fricatives. *The Journal of the Acoustical Society of America*, 85(4), 1718–1725.

Kewley-Port, D. (1983). Time-varying features as correlates of place of articulation in stop consonants. *The Journal of the Acoustical Society of America*, 73(1), 322–335.

Kiefte, M., Enright, T., & Marshall, L. (2010). The role of formant amplitude in the perception of /i/ and /u/. *The Journal of the Acoustical Society of America*, 127(4), 2611–2621.

Kingston, J., Kawahara, S., Chambless, D., Key, M., Mash, D., & Watsky, S. (2014). Context effects as auditory contrast. *Attention, Perception, & Psychophysics*, 76, 1437–1464.

Klatt, D. H. (1973). Discrimination of fundamental frequency contours in synthetic speech: Implications for models of pitch perception. *The Journal of the Acoustical Society of America*, 53, 8–16.

Klatt, D. H. (1982). Prediction of perceived phonetic distance from critical-band spectra: A first step. *Proceedings – ICASSP, IEEE International Conference on Acoustics, Speech and Signal Processing*, 7(June), 1278–1281. doi:10.1109/ICASSP.1982.1171512

Kluender, K., Coady, J., & Kiefte, M. (2003). Sensitivity to change in perception of speech. *Speech Communication*, 41(1), 59–69.

Koerner, T., Zhang, Y., Nelson, P., Wang, B., & Zou, H. (2016). Neural indices of phonemic discrimination and sentence-level speech intelligibility in quiet and noise: A mismatch negativity study. *Hearing Research*, 339, 40–49.

Ladefoged, P., & Broadbent, D. (1957). Information conveyed by vowels. *The Journal of the Acoustical Society of America*, 29(1), 98–104.

Lahiri, A., Gewirth, L., & Blumstein, S. (1984). A reconsideration of acoustic invariance for place of articulation in diffuse stop consonants: Evidence from a cross-language study. *The Journal of the Acoustical Society of America*, 76(2), 391–404.

Laughlin, S. (1981). A simple coding procedure enhances a neuron's information capacity. *Zeitschrift Fur Naturforschung* C, 36(9–10), 910–912.

Lennie, P. (2003). The cost of cortical computation. *Current Biology*, 13(6), 493–497.

Lindblom, B., & Studdert-Kennedy, M. (1967). On the role of formant transitions in vowel recognition. *The Journal of the Acoustical Society of America*, 42(4), 830–843.

Lisker, L. (1986). 'Voicing' in English: A catalogue of acoustic features signaling /b/ versus /p/ in trochees. *Language and Speech*, 29, 3–11.

Loizou, P., Dorman, M., & Powell, V. (1998). The recognition of vowels produced by men, women, boys, and girls by cochlear implant patients using a six-channel processor. *The Journal of the Acoustical Society of America*, 103(2), 1141–1149.

Lotto, A., & Holt, L. (2006). Putting phonetic context effects into context: A commentary on Fowler. *Perception & Psychophysics*, 68(2), 178–183.

Lotto, A., & Kluender, K. (1998). General contrast effects in speech perception: Effect of preceding liquid on stop consonant identification. *Perception & Psychophysics*, 60(4), 602–619.

Mann, V. (1980). Influence of preceding liquid on stop-consonant perception. *Perception & Psychophysics*, 28(5), 407–412.

Mann, V. (1986). Distinguishing universal and language-dependent levels of speech perception: Evidence from Japanese listeners' perception of English "l" and "r." *Cognition*, 24(3), 169–196.

Massaro, D. W., & Cohen, M. M. (1983). Categorical or continuous speech perception: A new test. *Speech Communication*, 2(1), 15–35.

McMurray, B., & Jongman, A. (2011). What information is necessary for speech categorization? Harnessing variability in the speech signal by integrating cues computed relative to expectations. *Psychological Review*, 118, 219–246.

Miller, J., & Liberman, A. (1979). Some effects of later-occurring information on the perception of stop consonant and semivowel. *Perception & Psychophysics*, 25(6), 457–465.

Molfese, D., & Molfese, V. (1997). Discrimination of language skills at five years of age using event-related potentials recorded at birth. *Developmental Neuropsychology*, 13(2), 135–156.

Moore, B. (2013). *An introduction to the psychology of hearing* (6th ed.). Leiden: Brill.

Moore, B., Glasberg, B., & Peters, R. (1986). Thresholds for hearing mistuned partials as separate tones in harmonic complexes. *The Journal of the Acoustical Society of America*, 80(2), 479–483.

Moore, B., Glasberg, B., & Shailer, M. (1984). Frequency and intensity difference limens for harmonics within complex tones. *The Journal of the Acoustical Society of America*, 75(2), 550–561.

Mori, S., Oyama, K., Kikuchi, Y., Mitsudo, T., & Hirose, N. (2015). Between-frequency and between-ear gap detections and their relation to perception of stop consonants. *Ear and Hearing*, 36, 464–470.

Morrison, G., & Assmann, P. (Eds.). (2013). *Vowel inherent spectral change*. Berlin, Heidelberg: Springer-Verlag.

Näätanen, R., Gaillard, A., & Mäntysalo, S. (1978). Early selective-attention effect on evoked potential reinterpreted. *Acta Psychologica*, 42(4), 313–329.

Näätanen, R., Lehtokoski, A., Lennes, M., Cheour, M., Huotilainen, M., Iivonen, A., . . . Alho, K. (1997). Language-specific phoneme representations revealed by electric and magnetic brain responses. *Nature*, 385(6615), 432–434.

Näätanen, R., Paavilainen, P., Rinne, T., & Alho, K. (2007). The Mismatch Negativity (MMN) in basic research of central auditory processing: A review. *Clinical Neurophysiology*, 118(12), 2544–2590.

Nearey, T. (1989). Static, dynamic, and relational properties in vowel perception. *The Journal of the Acoustical Society of America*, 85(5), 2088–2113.

Nearey, T., & Assmann, P. (1986). Modeling the role of inherent spectral change in vowel identification. *The Journal of the Acoustical Society of America*, 80(5), 1297–1308.

Obleser, J., Herrmann, B., & Henry, M. (2012). Neural oscillations in speech: Don't be enslaved by the envelope. *Frontiers in Human Neuroscience*, 6, 250.

Peelle, J., & Davis, M. (2012). Neural oscillations carry speech rhythm through to comprehension. *Frontiers in Psychology*, 3, 320.

Peterson, G., & Barney, H. (1952). Control methods used in a study of the vowels. *The Journal of the Acoustical Society of America*, 24(2), 175–184.

Pisoni, D. (1973). Auditory and phonetic memory codes in the discrimination of consonants and vowels. *Perception & Psychophysics*, 13, 253–260.

Pisoni, D. B., & Lazarus, J. H. (1974). Categorical and noncategorical modes of speech perception along the voicing continuum. *The Journal of the Acoustical Society of America*, 55(2), 328–333.

Poeppel, D., & Hickok, G. (2004). Towards a new functional anatomy of language. *Cognition*, 92(1–2), 1–12.

Rand, T. (1974). Dichotic release from masking for speech. *The Journal of the Acoustical Society of America*, 55, 678–680.

Repp, B. (1982). Phonetic trading relations and context effects – new experimental evidence for a speech mode of perception. *Psychological Bulletin*, 92(1), 81–110.

Repp, B., Liberman, A., Eccardt, T., & Pesetsky, D. (1978). Perceptual integration of acoustic cues for stop, fricative, and affricate manner. *Journal of Experimental Psychology Human Perception and Performance*, 4(4), 621–637.

Robinson, D., & Dadson, R. (1956). A re-determination of the equal-loudness relations for pure tones. *British Journal of Applied Physics*, 7, 166–181.

Rosen, S. (1992). Temporal information in speech: Acoustic, auditory and linguistic aspects. Philosophical Transactions: *Biological Science*, 336, 367–373.

Rosen, S., & Fourcin, A. (1986). Frequency selectivity and the perception of speech. In B. Moore (Ed.), *Frequency selectivity in hearing* (pp. 373–488). London: Academic Press.

Shannon, C. (1948). A mathematical theory of communication. *The Bell System Technical Journal*, 27, 379–423.

Shannon, R., Zeng, F., Kamath, V., Wygonski, J., & Ekelid, M. (1995). Speech recognition with primarily temporal cues. *Science*, 270(5234), 303–304.

Simoncelli, E. (2003). Vision and the statistics of the visual environment. *Current Opinion in Neurobiology*, 13(2), 144–149.

Smith, R. (1979). Adaptation, saturation, and physiological masking in single auditory-nerve fibers. *The Journal of the Acoustical Society of America*, 65(1), 166–178.

Smith, R., & Zwislocki, J. (1975). Short-term adaptation and incremental responses of single auditory-nerve fibers. *Biological Cybernetics*, 17(3), 169–182.

Stevens, K., & Blumstein, S. (1978). Invariant cues for place of articulation in stop consonants. *The Journal of the Acoustical Society of America*, 64(5), 1358.

Stevens, K., Blumstein, S., Glicksman, L., Burton, M., & Kurowski, K. (1992). Acoustic and perceptual characteristics of voicing in fricatives and fricative clusters. *The Journal of the Acoustical Society of America*, 91(5), 2979–3000.

Stevens, S., Volkmann, J., & Newman, E. (1937). The mel scale equates the magnitude of perceived differences in pitch at different frequencies. *The Journal of the Acoustical Society of America*, 8(3), 185–190.

Stilp, C., & Alexander, J. (2016). Spectral contrast effects in vowel categorization by listeners with sensorineural hearing loss. *Proceedings of Meetings on Acoustics*, 26, 060003.

Stilp, C., Alexander, J., Kiefte, M., & Kluender, K. (2010). Auditory color constancy: Calibration to reliable spectral properties across speech and nonspeech contexts and targets. *Attention, Perception & Psychophysics*, 72(2), 470–480.

Stilp, C., Anderson, P., & Winn, M. (2015). Predicting contrast effects following reliable spectral properties in speech perception. *The Journal of the Acoustical Society of America*, 137(6), 3466–3476.

Stilp, C., & Assgari, A. (2017). Consonant categorization exhibits graded influence of surrounding spectral context. *The Journal of the Acoustical Society of America*, 141(2), EL153–EL158.

Summerfield, Q. (1981). Articulatory rate and perceptual constancy in phonetic perception. *Journal of Experimental Psychology: Human Perception and Performance*, 7(5), 1074–1095.

Syrdal, A., & Gopal, H. (1986). A perceptual model of vowel recognition based on the auditory representation of American English vowels. *The Journal of the Acoustical Society of America*, 79(4), 1086–1100.

't Hart, J. (1981). Differential sensitivity to pitch distance, particularly in speech. *The Journal of the Acoustical Society of America*, 69(3), 811–821.

Takegata, R., Brattico, E., Tervaniemi, M., Varyagina, O., Naatanen, R., & Winkler, I. (2005). Preattentive representation of feature conjunctions for concurrent spatially distributed auditory objects. *Cognitive Brain Research*, 25(1), 169–179.

Toscano, J., & McMurray, B. (2010). Cue integration with categories: Weighting acoustic cues in speech using unsupervised learning and distributional statistics. *Cognitive Science*, 34(3), 434–464.

Traunmüller, H. (1990). Analytical expressions for the tonotopic sensory scale. *The Journal of the Acoustical Society of America*, 88, 97.

Viswanathan, N., Fowler, C., & Magnuson, J. (2009). A critical examination of the spectral contrast account of compensation for coarticulation. *Psychonomic Bulletin & Review*, 16(1), 74–79.

Wardrip-Fruin, C. (1985). The effect of signal degradation on the status of cues to voicing in utterance-final stop consonants. *The Journal of the Acoustical Society of America*, 77(5), 1907–1912.

Wark, B., Lundstrom, B., & Fairhall, A. (2007). Sensory adaptation. *Current Opinion in Neurobiology*, 17(4), 423–429.

Watkins, A. (1991). Central, auditory mechanisms of perceptual compensation for spectral-envelope distortion. *The Journal of the Acoustical Society of America*, 90(6), 2942–2955.

Winn, M., Chatterjee, M., & Idsardi, W. (2012). The use of acoustic cues for phonetic identification: effects of spectral degradation and electric hearing. *The Journal of the Acoustical Society of America*, 131(2), 1465–1479.

Winn, M., Chatterjee, M., & Idsardi, W. (2013). Roles of voice onset time and F0 in stop consonant voicing perception: Effects of masking noise and low-pass filtering. *Journal of Speech, Language, and Hearing Research*, 56(4), 1097–1107.

Winn, M., & Litovsky, R. (2015). Using speech sounds to test functional spectral resolution in listeners with cochlear implants. *The Journal of the Acoustical Society of America*, 137, 1430–1442.

Winn, M., Won, J-H., & Moon, I-J. (2016). Assessment of spectral and temporal resolution in cochlear implant users using psychoacoustic discrimination and speech cue categorization. *Ear and Hearing*, 37, e377–e390.

Zahorian, S., & Jagharghi, A. (1993). Spectral-shape features versus formants as acoustic correlates for vowels. *The Journal of the Acoustical Society of America*, 94, 1966–1982.

Zilany, M., & Bruce, I. (2007). *Predictions of speech intelligibility with a model of the normal and impaired auditory periphery. Proceedings of the Third International IEEE/EMBS Conference on Neural Engineering*, 481–485.

Zilany, M., Bruce, I., & Carney, L. (2014). Updated parameters and expanded simulation options for a model of the auditory periphery. *The Journal of the Acoustical Society of America*, 135(1), 283–286.

Zwicker, E. (1961). Subdivision of the audible frequency range into critical bands. *The Journal of the Acoustical Society of America*, 33, 248.

8

The neural basis for auditory and audiovisual speech perception

Jonathan E. Peelle

Although much focus in phonetics is (understandably) on the acoustic speech signal, ultimately the sound waves produced by a speaker need to be interpreted by a listener's brain. This concept is beautifully illustrated in the classic "speech chain" (Denes and Pinson, 1993), a version of which is shown in Figure 8.1. As noted elsewhere in this volume, speech transmission is multisensory (see e.g., Chapter 19, "New horizons in clinical linguistics"). In this chapter, I review brain areas involved in the perception of various levels of spoken language, from isolated phonemes to narratives.

Basic principles

What do we mean by "speech"?

A fundamental challenge in discussing the neural basis for speech perception is defining what we mean by the term "speech": As illustrated in Figure 8.2, isolated phonemes, nonwords, words, and sentences are all associated with different (though frequently overlapping) patterns of language processing (Peelle, 2012). Thus, although it is common for researchers to talk about "speech perception" without specifying the category of speech they mean, in fact it is important to be specific regarding the types of acoustic and linguistic information listeners are processing. In the sections that follow I review these different levels of speech processing to make these distinctions clear. The full picture, of course, is slightly more complicated because of the overlapping levels of processing across different types of stimuli. Successfully isolating specific stages of sensory or linguistic processing requires careful attention to the experimental manipulations.

On a related point, when considering the results of neuroimaging studies, it is critical to consider the comparison or control condition to which speech is being compared. Processing acoustic stimuli that are not speech (such as pure tones, temporally modulated noise, or musical "rain") results in substantial activation in bilateral temporal cortex (Overath et al., 2010; Griffiths et al., 1998). This acoustic-related activity may occur in regions similar to those used for various levels of speech processing, and thus they make useful control conditions to better isolate activity that is preferential for auditory speech.

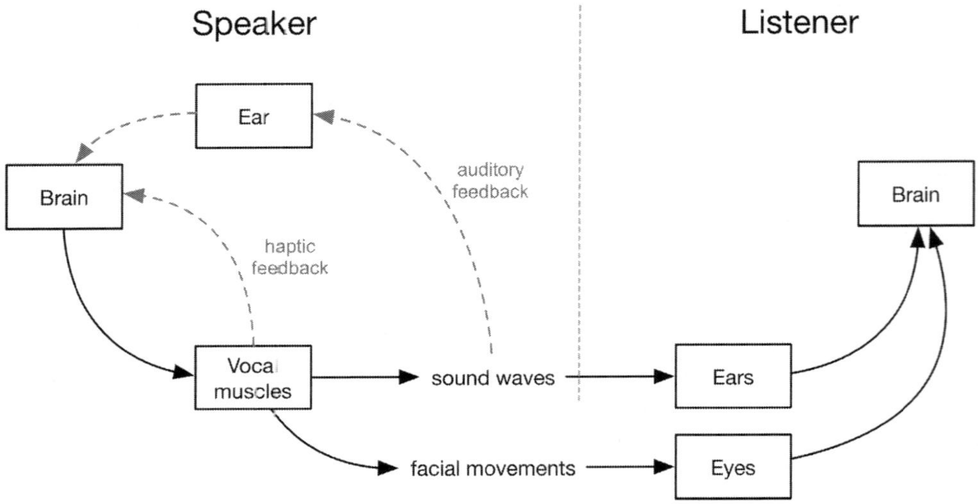

Figure 8.1 Re-creation of the classic speech chain of Denes and Pinson (1993). Speech functions to communicate a language message from the brain of the speaker to the brain of the listener, transmitted acoustically and visually, subject to a variety of constraints on its production, transmission, and reception.

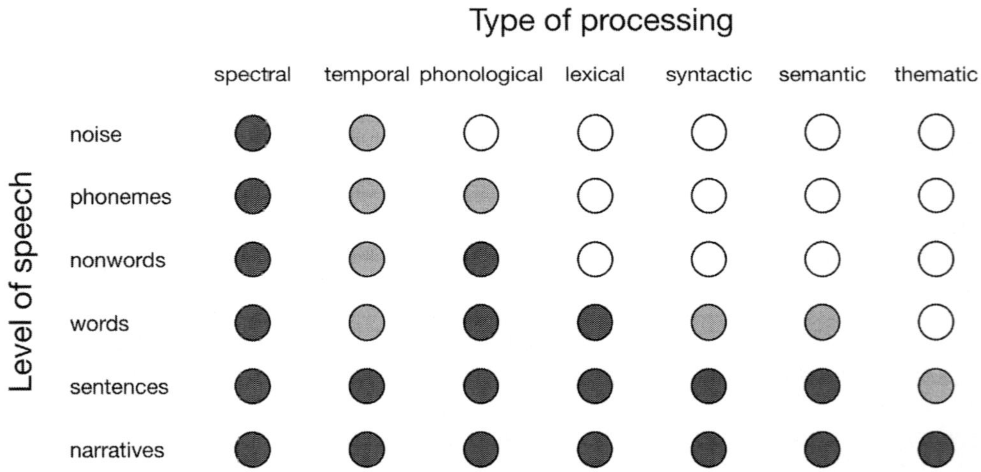

Figure 8.2 Illustration of some types of acoustic and linguistic processing (top) involved in various levels of speech perception (listed along the left). Darker circles indicate a stronger reliance on a particular type of processing. Although different types of speech stimuli have different processing requirements, there is also overlap in processing across different stages (for example, both single words and sentences require lexical and semantic processing, although the specific demands may differ). *Spectral* processing refers to information in multiple frequency ranges, and *temporal* processing refers to changing information over time. *Phonological* processing involves the arrangement or pattern of speech sounds. *Lexical* representations are learned word forms. *Syntactic* processing refers to understanding relationships between words; although typically thought of in the context of sentences, single words can also have syntactic information (for example, verbs that imply an actor and an object). *Semantic* processes are associated with concept representations of single words and are also important in interpreting connected speech. In this context, *thematic* processing refers to overarching organizing themes found in narratives that tie the story together across multiple sentences.

Anatomical connectivity

Before examining how the brain's activity changes when processing various types of speech, it is useful to consider the anatomical connectivity of speech-sensitive regions, starting with auditory cortex. These connections help outline a neural scaffolding that we might reasonably expect to be engaged in processing spoken language.

Data from nonhuman primates reveal a core auditory cortex that reflects tonotopic organization and responds to pure-tone stimuli (Kaas and Hackett, 2000). Outside the auditory core are belt and parabelt regions that show sensitivity to stimuli of increasing acoustic complexity, including broadband noise (Kaas et al., 1999).

Beyond auditory cortex, anatomical studies in primates have long emphasized the extensive and highly parallel anatomical coupling between auditory and frontal cortices (Petrides and Pandya, 2009; Hackett et al., 1999; Seltzer and Pandya, 1989). A summary figure of anatomical connectivity in monkey and cat is shown in Figure 8.3. Consistent with anatomical connectivity studies, electrophysiological findings in nonhuman primates show responses to auditory stimuli in frontal cortex, suggesting frontal involvement as a natural part of auditory processing (Romanski and Goldman-Rakic, 2002; Romanski et al., 1999).

These anatomical and functional connections have lent support to a dual-stream framework for speech processing (Hickok and Poeppel, 2007; Rauschecker and Scott, 2009; Hickok and Poeppel, 2000) consisting of a dorsal stream and a ventral stream. The dorsal

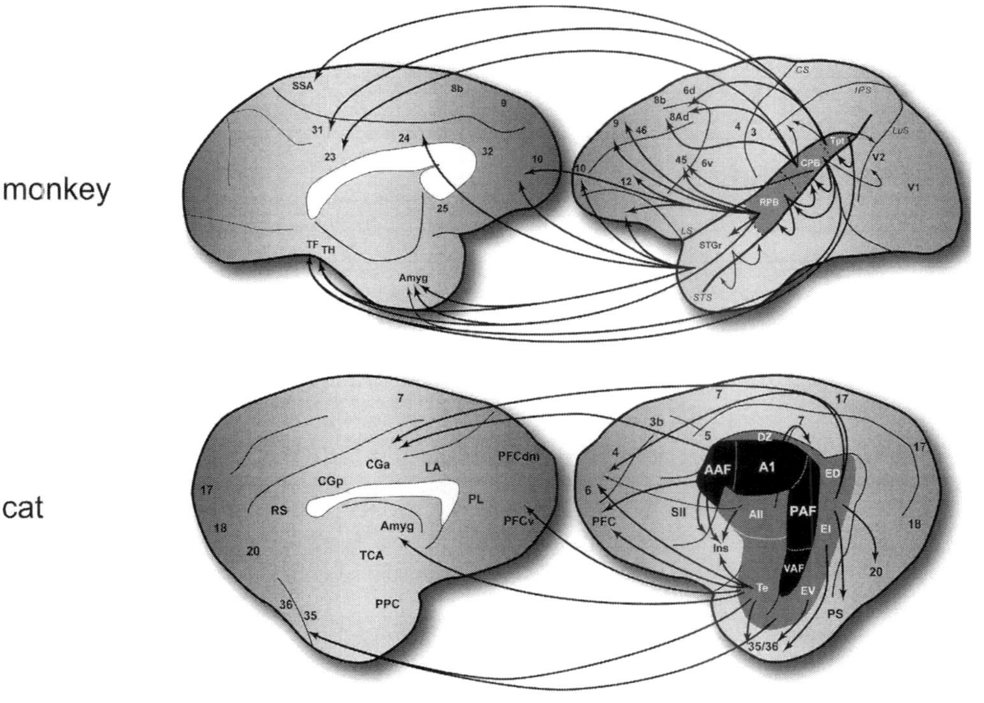

Figure 8.3 Summary figure of connectivity from auditory cortex in monkey (top) and cat (bottom). Numerous pathways exist to transmit information outside of auditory cortex in both the ipsilateral and contralateral hemispheres.

Source: Reproduced from Hackett (2011).

stream travels from auditory cortex along the arcuate fasciculus, through parietal lobe and into dorsal premotor cortex; the ventral stream proceeds from auditory cortex towards the anterior temporal lobe and through the uncinate fasciculus into ventral inferior frontal gyrus (IFG). Although animal data indicate more than these two pathways for information leaving auditory cortex (Hackett, 2011), the dual-stream model has proved to be a useful framework encompassing many of the main cortical areas involved in speech processing.

Neural systems supporting auditory speech perception

In the sections that follow, I review the brain regions involved in processing various levels of auditory speech, from isolated phonemes through narratives, following the distinctions outlined in Figure 8.2. A schematic of the main regions is shown in Figure 8.4.

Phoneme processing

Phonemes are implicitly involved in understanding words and sentences, but can also be studied in isolation. Phoneme perception requires processing an acoustically complex stimulus that can

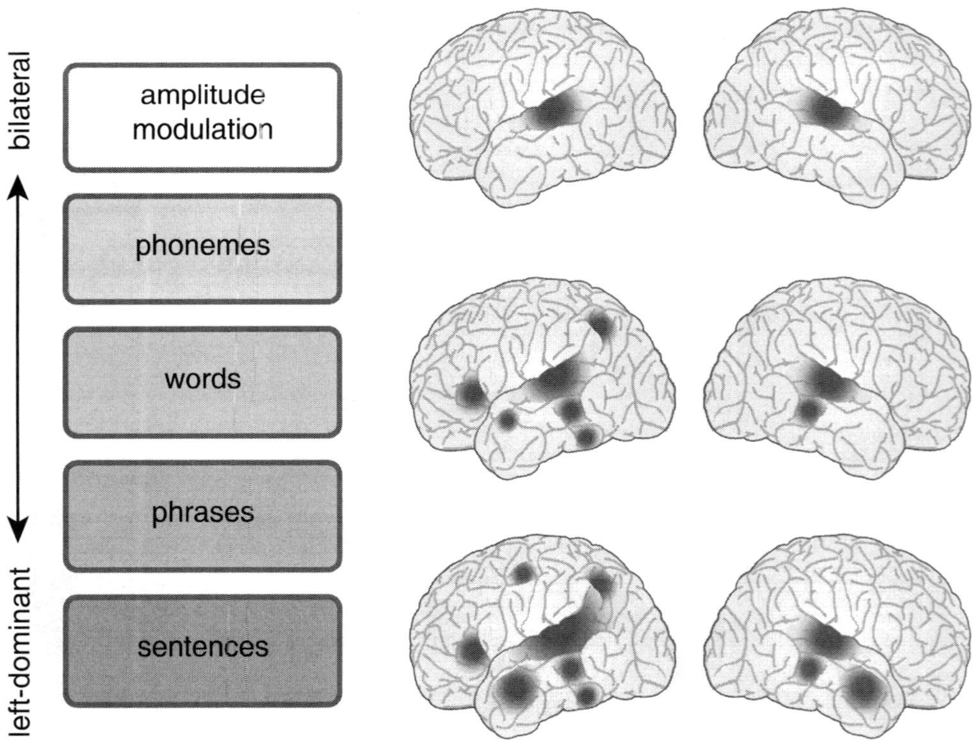

Figure 8.4 Schematic illustrating that the regions of the brain supporting speech perception depend on the type of acoustic and linguistic processing required, moving from primarily superior temporal regions for noise to an extended network of temporal, frontal, and parietal regions for more complex speech.

Source: From Peelle (2012).

be mapped to learned representations and thus reflects both auditory processing and memory, shaped by a listener's language experience.

A number of neuroimaging studies have investigated brain regions supporting phoneme processing. Rimol and colleagues (2005) used functional magnetic imaging (fMRI) to examine activity for consonant-vowel (CV) syllables and stop consonants, compared to a noise control condition. They found increased activation for both consonants and syllables relative to noise in posterior superior temporal sulcus (STS) and middle temporal gyrus (MTG) bilaterally, with some suggestion of greater activity in the left hemisphere (see also Obleser et al., 2007). In another fMRI study, Liebenthal and colleagues (2005) had listeners perform a two-alternative forced-choice discrimination task on either phonemes or carefully matched nonphoneme control sounds. The control sounds were created by spectrally inverting the first formant (F_1) of the phonemic stimuli, and were thus identical in duration and acoustic complexity, but did not involve phonemic representations. The authors found increased activity for the phonemes compared to nonphonemes in the left STS (see also Blumstein et al., 2005). It is important to emphasize that the activity seen for phonemes, in STS, is typically smaller in extent and more ventral than activity in auditory regions evoked by non-speech stimuli (Hall et al., 2002). This is consistent with a computational hierarchy for auditory processing in which learned representations (phonemes) are not stored in primary auditory cortex, but in later regions, presumably allowing for more flexibility in representing relationships between low-level features (Chang et al., 2010). Intercranial recordings from humans have shown that activity in posteriolateral temporal cortex can distinguish between different categories (Mesgarani et al., 2014; Nourski et al., 2014; Steinschneider et al., 2011).

Roles for both the left STS and left supramarginal gyrus in phoneme processing were also suggested by Jacquemot and colleagues (2003), who studied phonological processing in Japanese and French to dissociate acoustic properties (which were identical regardless of the native language of the listener) from phonological properties (which differed based on a listener's native language).They had listeners perform a discrimination task in which three pseudowords were presented: The first two identical, the third either matching or mismatching. The differences could be acoustic or phonological depending on the native language of the participant, allowing the authors to isolate activity due to phonological processing. Phonological change conditions were associated with regions of left superior temporal gyrus and left supramarginal gyrus.

Raizada and Poldrack (2007) used fMRI to study categorical processing, with a special focus on stimuli that bridged category boundaries. They found activity in several regions, most notably the left supramarginal gyrus, related to perceptual category boundaries. They interpret this finding as reflecting neural amplification of perceptually important stimulus changes. In a habituation paradigm, Joanisse and colleagues (2007) also found both superior temporal gyrus (STG) and inferior parietal cortex (near the supramarginal gyrus) responding to "deviant" phonemes, suggesting a role in novelty detection.

Finally, regions of left IFG have also been implicated in phoneme perception, including invariance to exemplars from the same phonetic category (Myers et al., 2009), multivariate responses that can predict categorical boundaries (Lee et al., 2012), and perceptual restoration of phonemes (Leonard et al., 2016). Rogers and Davis (2017) created continua of words (e.g., blade–glade), pseudowords (e.g., blem–glem), and word–pseudoword pairs (e.g., bone–ghone). They found increased responses in left IFG for real-word conditions with high phonetic ambiguity, suggesting the left IFG is important for phoneme discrimination, particularly when a decision is required about what has been heard.

Thus, phoneme processing relies on regions of the STS/STG, supramarginal gyrus, and IFG. The specific regions involved likely reflect not only the stimuli, but also the nature of the task (for example, passive listening vs. categorical judgments).

Single word processing

In addition to processing the formant transitions conveying phonemic information, processing single words involves both lexical and semantic representations.[1] At the lexical level, the appropriate word must be selected, taking into consideration the range of possible alternatives – i.e., all possible words – and acoustic and linguistic contextual cues that may make some words more likely than others.

Some of the earliest neuroimaging studies of speech processing showed bilateral temporal lobe activation when participants heard single words (Price et al., 1996; Price et al., 1992), a result that has been routinely replicated using a variety of different paradigms. In an fMRI study of word processing, Binder and colleagues (2000) compared activity for single words to a variety of control conditions including broadband noise, pure tones, nonwords, and reversed speech. They found that all stimuli elicited robust activation in bilateral superior temporal gyri. Smaller regions of bilateral superior temporal gyri showed a hierarchical progression, with responses to words being greater than to tones, which in turn were greater than to broadband noise. These findings support key roles for the STS and MTG in word processing, confirmed by many other studies using spoken words (Eckert et al., 2008; Bozic et al., 2010; Fonteneau et al., 2015; Sohoglu et al., 2012; Specht and Reul, 2003; Burton and Small, 2006).

One important point worth emphasizing is that although traditional neuroanatomical models of language focus on the left hemisphere, there is compelling converging evidence that both left and right temporal cortices support single-word processing. First, as already noted, neuroimaging studies routinely show activation in both left and right temporal cortex. Second, and perhaps more convincingly, patients undergoing a Wada procedure (anesthetizing one hemisphere for language lateralization) are able to perform single-word processing tasks with only their right hemisphere (McGlone, 1984). For example, Hickok and colleagues (2008) studied a group of patients who underwent the Wada procedure during presurgical evaluation for medically uncontrolled epilepsy. Participants were presented with auditory words, and were instructed to select which of four alternative pictures best matched the word. Foils could differ from the target word phonemically or semantically, allowing the authors to examine different types of errors. Although more errors were made during left-hemisphere anesthesia than for right-hemisphere anesthesia, most were semantic errors. Most importantly, even under conditions of left-hemisphere anesthesia, word perception performance was well above chance levels. This finding would not be expected if word processing were conducted exclusively by left-hemisphere regions. Of course, lateralization effects may well be a matter of degree. Additional research that quantitatively compares processing in left and right hemispheres of single words will be important in resolving this question.

Although the main brain regions involved in word level processing appear centered in bilateral superior temporal cortex, factors such as word frequency, the number of competitors, the conceptual meaning of a word, and other psycholinguistic considerations can all affect the brain networks involved, some of which I briefly touch on in the sections that follow.

Lexical competition

Most contemporary models of speech recognition operate in an activation-competition framework in which words whose stored representations are consistent with the incoming sensory input are considered possible candidates (Marslen-Wilson and Tyler, 1980; Norris and McQueen, 2008; Luce and Pisoni, 1998). Words that are acoustically similar to the target word make the task of selecting the correct word more difficult, particularly if the sensory input is degraded (for example, due to background noise). Thus, even words that are correctly perceived can differ in the amount of competition resolved during perception. Although behavioral effects of lexical competition have been demonstrated for some time, only recently have the neural networks required to deal with increased competition been investigated.

Zhuang and colleagues (2014) presented listeners with nonwords, constructed such that at the stimulus onset, an item could potentially be a word. The point at which the item became a nonword could occur early or late in the stimulus. The items also varied in their initial cohort size (related to lexical competition) and cohort dropout rate (related to lexical selection). They observed a cluster in left MTG and STG that showed increasing activity for items with late nonword points, consistent with the hypothesis that increasing matching results in greater processing demands in left hemisphere regions associated with lexical-semantic processing. Within the late nonword items, the authors looked for parametric effects of cohort competition and cohort selection. Competition effects were seen in bilateral ventral IFG (pars orbitalis), whereas selection effects were in more dorsal IFG (pars triangularis). These findings are supported by a magnetoencephalography (MEG) study from Kocagoncu and colleagues (2017) that showed effects of lexical competition occur relatively early after word onset in left STS/MTG followed by left IFG.

A particularly clever approach to lexical competition is to teach listeners new words that alter the competitors of existing items in the lexicon. For example, "cathedral" has few competitors; teaching participants that "cathedruke" is a word thus substantially increases the amount of competition. Interestingly, new words do not act as competitors until after sleeping (Dumay and Gaskell, 2007), presumably due to sleep-related consolidation processes (Davis and Gaskell, 2009). Increased competition effects related to word learning are seen in auditory cortex and hippocampus (Gagnepain et al., 2012; Davis et al., 2009), suggesting effects of consolidation on the representation of acoustic word forms.

Semantic representations

Although the nature of semantic representation is an area of active debate, many current approaches to semantic memory conform to a "hub and spoke" arrangement (Patterson et al., 2007; Reilly et al., 2016b). Evidence for modality-specific representations comes in part from a long history of category-specific semantic memory deficits that suggest representations for different categories (for example, animals vs. manufactured objects) are stored in anatomically separable locations in the brain (McCarthy and Warrington, 2016) (that is, if there were no anatomical distinctions between different categories, it would be impossible to impair knowledge about one category but not another following brain damage). In addition, studies suggest activity in modality-specific sensory and motor regions corresponding to specific types of information (for example, visual areas showing more activity for concepts relying on visual information) (Reilly et al., 2016a). Bonner and colleagues (2013) presented participants with written words in a lexical decision task. The words varied in their sensory-motor associations, being primarily visual (e.g., apple), primarily auditory (e.g., thunder), primarily motor (e.g., corkscrew), or abstract concepts (e.g., justice). The authors found increased activity (relative to nonwords) in the angular gyrus for all word categories. Provocatively, there were also suggestions of increases in modality-specific regions (for example, words with high auditory associations were associated with increased activity in auditory association cortex). These findings are in agreement with reports that patients with neurodegenerative disease who have gray matter atrophy in auditory association cortex perform more poorly on auditory concepts than other modalities (Bonner and Grossman, 2012). Thus, the nature of the concepts associated with individual words alters the brain regions involved in word comprehension.

Complementing evidence for distributed semantic representations is a rich history on amodal "hubs" that represent information from multiple modalities (or function to bind heteromodal information together). Traditionally, some of the strongest evidence comes from patients with semantic dementia (also referred to as the semantic variant of primary progressive aphasia, or svPPA). The most common areas of damage in svPPA are the left temporal pole and lateral anterior temporal lobe, extending back into the fusiform gyrus (Mummery et al., 2000; Gorno-Tempini et al., 2004). Patients with svPPA show impaired representation across semantic category, regardless of the modality of the input or output (Bozeat et al., 2000; Bozeat et al., 2003), suggesting these regions of left temporal cortex play a critical role in semantic memory. Complimentary evidence from fMRI implicates the angular gyrus as a second semantic hub: It is commonly activated in studies of semantic memory (Binder et al., 2009) and responds to combinations of word concepts (Price et al., 2015; Graves et al., 2010); gray matter volume in the angular gyrus relates to word learning (Lee et al., 2007).

Finally, it is worth noting the involvement of left IFG in semantic processing, particularly when decisions need to be made about a semantic property or category. For example, when selecting a target item from among a group of competing alternatives (Thompson-Schill et al., 1997) or making semantic judgments (Whitney et al., 2011), increased left IFG activity is seen. Thus, semantic representation relies on both modality-specific and amodal regions, with increased involvement of left IFG to resolve competition.

Sentence processing

In addition to the phonemic, lexical, and semantic processing required for understanding individual words, understanding sentences requires an appreciation for the conceptual and syntactic constraints that tie multiple words together. We have learned a great deal about the major brain networks involved in processing intelligible speech by observing the brain regions that are more active when listeners hear intelligible sentences compared to unintelligible control stimuli. One of the earliest and most influential demonstrations was conducted by Scott and colleagues (2000), who used positron emission tomography (PET) to measure neural responses to intelligible sentences compared to unintelligible spectrally rotated sentences. They found that regions of left temporal cortex (notably lateral anterior temporal lobe) showed a preferential response to intelligible speech. More recent investigations using similar stimuli have replicated (and extended) the main findings (Evans, 2017).

In a landmark study of auditory sentence processing, Davis and Johnsrude (2003) took a parametric approach to studying intelligibility. They used fMRI to monitor neural activity while participants listened to sentences that were presented at varying levels of intelligibility that had been arrived at through different forms of acoustic degradation (speech in noise, alternated speech, noise vocoded speech). This design thus helped identify regions that responded parametrically to speech intelligibility, and also the degree to which such regions were impacted by speech acoustics. They found that activity in bilateral superior temporal cortex and left ventral IFG correlated with speech intelligibility. In auditory cortex and nearby temporal lobe regions, these responses differed based on the type of acoustic manipulation performed, but in regions further removed – posterior and anterior to auditory cortex in the temporal lobe and IFG – responses were comparable regardless of the acoustic manipulation. These findings support a hierarchical organization to sentence processing in which information is transformed to more abstract representations as it travels away from auditory cortex along both the dorsal and ventral stream (Peelle et al., 2010a).

Given a general understanding of the main regions involved in understanding spoken sentences, we can again ask what functions may be supported by each of the areas, starting with primary auditory cortex. Although bilateral auditory cortex is naturally involved in low-level acoustic processing, recent studies have begun to identify features that have particular importance. One influential line of work focuses on how ongoing oscillatory activity in auditory cortex locks on to the acoustic envelope of connected speech (Giraud and Poeppel, 2012; Peelle and Davis, 2012). This research was inspired in part by studies using electrophysiology to examine auditory cortex responses to rhythmic stimuli in monkeys, as animal work shows phase locking to regular auditory stimuli (Lakatos et al., 2005). Human work using EEG and MEG is consistent with these observations: the phase of neural responses in auditory cortex discriminates between individual sentences (Luo and Poeppel, 2007). Oscillatory entrainment to the speech signal is enhanced for intelligible speech relative to less intelligible control stimuli (Peelle et al., 2013), suggesting that phase locking may play a role in language comprehension beyond acoustic processing (Ding et al., 2016).

Phase-locked responses reflect top-down attention (Lakatos et al., 2013; Lakatos et al., 2008), and during multi-talker listening more strongly reflect the target talker (Rimmele et al., 2015; Kerlin et al., 2010; Mesgarani and Chang, 2012; Zion Golumbic et al., 2013). Because phase-locked oscillations form a nested hierarchy (Gross et al., 2013), linking oscillations to the speech signal at one level (for example, 4–7 Hz) can potentially affect processing at many other timescales (Canolty and Knight, 2010; Jensen and Colgin, 2007), which may be important in breaking the continuous speech signal into manageable computational units (Ghitza, 2011). Thus, oscillatory activity in auditory cortex is well-suited to contribute to the comprehension of connected speech (Peelle and Davis, 2012).

Moving beyond the temporal lobe, left IFG is often active during sentence processing (Adank, 2012). Because left inferior frontal activity is not consistently observed for perception of single words or phonemes, a reasonable conclusion is that it reflects some aspect of sentence processing. One suggestion, which I cover in more detail later in the chapter, is that left IFG (sometimes including "Broca's Area") plays a specific role in syntactic processing (Grodzinsky and Santi, 2008). However, left IFG might support other processes during sentence comprehension that are not syntax-specific, including processes related to semantic integration (Hagoort, 2013), phrase building, or domain-general selection (Thompson-Schill et al., 1997). Thus, although there is widespread agreement that the left IFG is frequently active during sentence comprehension, the best way to characterize the processes engaged is still actively debated (Friederici and Gierhan, 2013; Fedorenko et al., 2012; Rogalsky and Hickok, 2011).

Although these studies help establish the *core* regions supporting intelligible speech processing, it is important to realize that everyday sentence comprehension requires solving a variety of linguistic challenges, and that doing so involves additional brain regions. Next I examine two illustrative examples: Syntactic complexity and semantic ambiguity.

Syntactic complexity

To correctly understand the meaning of a sentence, listeners must not only identify individual words but also determine the syntactic relationships between the words. For example, consider the following two sentences:

1 Kings that help queens are nice.
2 Kings that queens help are nice.

The words are identical, but changing their order alters the meaning of the sentence. In the first, kings are doing the helping, whereas in the second queens are doing the helping. There are many ways to change the syntactic processing demands of a sentence, which might rely on shared or separable neural systems. What regions are implicated in syntactic processing?

For several decades, the left IFG has been known to play an important role in syntactic processing. Although patients with Broca's aphasia have generally preserved language comprehension (i.e., production difficulties are a defining feature), they frequently have difficulty comprehending syntactically complex sentences (Love et al., 2008; Tyler et al., 2011; Papoutsi et al., 2011; Grodzinsky, 2000; Swinney and Zurif, 1995). This observation has been replicated in patients with nonfluent primary progressive aphasia (Peelle et al., 2008; Peelle et al., 2007), which is also associated with damage to the left inferior frontal cortex (Grossman, 2012).

In an fMRI study of spoken sentence processing in healthy adults (Peelle et al., 2010b), we examined activity for short sentences that contained center-embedded clauses that had a subject-relative ("Kings that help queens are nice") or object-relative ("Kings that queens help are nice") construction. Object-relative sentences have greater processing demands and are associated with poorer accuracy, longer response times (Wingfield et al., 2003), and/or increased brain activity (Lee et al., 2016; Peelle et al., 2004). We found syntax-related increases in many regions, most notably left IFG and dorsolateral prefrontal cortex, but also including middle temporal gyrus and inferior parietal cortex. These findings are in agreement with a number of studies of both auditory and visual sentence processing implicating left IFG in syntactic complexity (Hassanpour et al., 2015; Rodd et al., 2010; Tyler et al., 2010) and suggest left IFG plays a role in processing syntactically complex sentences.

Semantic ambiguity

Another frequently encountered challenge during sentence processing is that many words have multiple meanings, and the correct meaning must be inferred by the listener based on context. For example, the word "bark" can refer to the outer covering of a tree or the sound a dog makes, and in isolation its meaning is thus ambiguous. However, listeners have no difficulty understanding a sentence such as "Jamie was scared of the loud bark." Although we often subjectively experience this process of disambiguation as automatic, in fact it is not: When listeners hear sentences with ambiguous words, there are reliable increases in activity in left hemisphere regions associated with semantic processing, including fusiform gyrus, middle temporal gyrus, and IFG (Rodd et al., 2005; Rodd et al., 2012; Zempleni et al., 2007; Rodd et al., 2010).

Using multivariate techniques, Musz and Thompson-Schill (2017) investigated processing of homonyms that varied in the degree of meaning dominance in written language. For example, a word like "pen" has a highly dominant meaning (a writing implement), relative to other meanings (such as an enclosure for animals). A word like "pitcher," by contrast, has several meanings that are approximately equal in dominance (such as a container for liquid, or a position on a baseball team). These items were presented in sentences that biased interpretation towards a dominant or subordinate meaning, and subsequently read each word in isolation. The authors found that left IFG showed sensitivity to context (dominant vs. subordinate) and time disambiguating information was available (see also Rodd et al., 2012), and that left ventral anterior temporal lobe further varied in activity in relation to word-by-word variability in meaning dominance.

Finally, semantic disambiguation appears to depend on conscious attention, and neural responses associated with disambiguation disappear in mildly sedated listeners who still show robust cortical responses to acoustic stimulation (Davis et al., 2007), consistent with a reliance on active processing (for example, taking into account the surrounding context).

Spoken narrative comprehension

Understanding spoken language that spans multiple sentences is not uncommon and occurs during lectures and listening to stories. Neuroimaging studies of spoken narratives are particularly challenging because of the impact of scanner noise, which cannot be avoided using sparse imaging techniques as can be done for shorter stimuli (Edmister et al., 1999; Hall et al., 1999).

Data from narrative comprehension in quiet comes in part from PET studies. Crinion and colleagues (2003) played short children's stories for participants while measuring brain activity with PET. Compared to reversed speech, listening to the story resulted in stronger activity in bilateral temporal regions, most notably along the middle temporal gyrus, extending to the lateral anterior temporal lobe. It is somewhat surprising that no responses in frontal cortex were observed; this may have been due to either the modest number of participants, or the nature of the materials.

Additional data come from studies using continuous fMRI scanning, which are informative but must be interpreted in the context of the additional acoustic noise. To investigate temporal dependencies at different timescales, Lerner and colleagues (2011) played participants a 7-minute story in its original form, but temporally scrambled at the level of words, sentences, or paragraphs. They found that the reliability of inter-subject correlations varied, with regions near auditory cortex showing strong responses regardless of the temporal window (i.e., driven strongly by word-level processing). Regions further along in the hierarchy, in the frontal cortex, showed more reliable responses for longer temporal windows. These analyses suggest not only a role for the frontal cortex in narrative comprehension, but that frontal regions are required in particular for understanding the more complex structure (and longer temporal duration) of sentences and paragraphs.

Converging evidence in support of a role for frontal cortex in narrative processing comes from patients with frontotemporal dementia (FTD), a family of neurodegenerative diseases associated with progressive damage in circumscribed brain regions (Peelle and Grossman, 2008). Patients with behavioral variant FTD (bvFTD) are of particular interest because language impairment is not a primary symptom, and they have damage to large regions of bilateral frontal cortex. When trying to tell a short story, patients with bvFTD have difficulty organizing the story and are more likely to miss the main point of the story (Ash et al.,

2006). This behavior contrasts with FTD patients diagnosed with primary progressive aphasias, who have significant difficulties with language processing but not in these narrative-level operations. Similar narrative difficulties are seen in patients with amyotrophic lateral sclerosis (ALS) that are also related to damage in prefrontal cortex (Ash et al., 2014).

Thus, the brain networks involved in understanding a spoken narrative largely overlap the core sentence processing network. However, regions of frontal cortex may play an additional important role in maintaining thematic relationships over long timescales.

Neural systems supporting audiovisual speech perception

The focus so far has been on the brain systems involved in understanding auditory speech. However, in everyday conversation we can frequently see the speaker's face, providing an additional source of speech information. Speech perception, particularly in noise, is almost always more accurate when listeners can both hear and see a talker compared with listening alone (Erber, 1975; Sumby and Pollack, 1954). This clear behavioral finding raises challenges for neuroscience models of speech processing: How does information that necessarily enters the brain through different sensory receptors become integrated to form a single percept?

There are three anatomical regions that have been the focus of the neural basis for multisensory speech understanding, reflecting differing theoretical views of the underlying processes. The first is primary auditory cortex, which may represent temporal properties in connected speech (i.e., the amplitude envelope). The second is a heteromodal region of lateral posterior temporal cortex that is well-positioned to perform multisensory integration. The third is motor or premotor cortex as a way to retrieve articulatory representations. These mechanisms are not mutually exclusive, but have been suggested based on results from different experimental paradigms and theoretical motivations. I discuss each in turn.

Temporal predictions in auditory cortex

As noted previously, evidence from electrophysiology studies in nonhuman primates shows that oscillations in auditory cortex entrain to periodic stimuli, creating systematic fluctuations in population neural excitability (Lakatos et al., 2005). Importantly, the phase of neural oscillations in the ~3–7 Hz range have also been shown to entrain to human speech (Luo and Poeppel, 2007), with stronger entrainment for intelligible speech (Peelle et al., 2013). The entrainment of cortical oscillations to the acoustic speech envelope suggests a mechanistic role in auditory speech perception (Peelle and Davis, 2012) and a mechanism to affect hierarchical processing through nested oscillatory activity (Gross et al., 2013). Such a role is supported by the effects of attention on phase-locked oscillations in multi-talker situations (Zion Golumbic et al., 2013), understanding speech in background noise (Ding and Simon, 2013), and phoneme-level representations (Di Liberto et al., 2015).

More relevant for audiovisual speech processing are the multimodal effects observed in auditory cortex. Haptic stimulation can reset auditory oscillations, increasing sensitivity to motor inputs that follow (Lakatos et al., 2007). These findings lend support to the hypothesis that cortical oscillations can act as instruments of attentional selection, biasing perception to be more sensitive to behaviorally relevant inputs (Lakatos et al., 2013; Schroeder and Lakatos, 2009). Together, these observations suggest that oscillatory entrainment may play an important role in audiovisual speech perception (Schroeder et al., 2008).

Luo and colleagues (2010) played audiovisual movies to participants while recording brain activity with MEG. As might be expected, they found that oscillations in primary sensory cortices followed modality-specific information (i.e., oscillations in auditory cortex tracked acoustic information in the movies, and oscillations in visual cortex tracked visual information in the movies). Critically, however, they also found that visual information modulated acoustic entrainment in auditory cortex. A related finding was reported by Crosse and colleagues (2015), who found that visual information improved representation of the acoustic speech envelope in auditory cortex. This cross-modal modulation suggests that human speech perception conforms to principles of multisensory integration identified in animal studies.

What information might be provided by the visual stream, reflected in these oscillatory effects? One possibility is information regarding the acoustic envelope, which is typically strongly correlated with mouth opening (Chandrasekaran et al., 2009). Although envelope information may not be particularly informative regarding specific articulatory cues, it provides overall information about speech rhythm, and may therefore guide listeners towards extracting information from relatively more informative temporal windows.

It is worth noting that some, though not all, fMRI studies of visual or audiovisual speech perception have found changes in activity in auditory cortex associated with visual speech information (Calvert et al., 1997). Whether there is a link between altered oscillatory activity and fMRI activity in primary auditory cortex is unclear; however, both clearly implicate auditory cortex in audiovisual speech processing.

Although amplitude information may be useful in understanding connected speech, it likely plays less of a role in single words, as listeners have less opportunity to entrain to a talker's speech. And in all cases, the amplitude envelope does not provide a great deal of information to constrain phoneme perception, suggesting the need for complementary processes (Peelle and Sommers, 2015). Two primary candidates for these are posterior STS and premotor cortex, which I discuss next.

Posterior superior temporal sulcus as a site of multisensory integration

Posterior STS is a region of heteromodal association cortex with anatomical connections to both auditory and visual cortex (Seltzer et al., 1996). Although not consistently active in studies of auditory-only speech perception, posterior STS routinely appears in fMRI studies of audiovisual speech perception, particularly in studies using McGurk stimuli. The well-known McGurk effect (McGurk and MacDonald, 1976) provides a compelling demonstration of multisensory integration: When an auditory stimulus (e.g., /ba/) is presented with the face of a speaker articulating a different syllable (e.g., /ga/), listeners often perceive an illusory percept distinct from both sources (e.g., /da/). In many fMRI studies using McGurk stimuli, incongruent trials (i.e., trials eliciting a McGurk effect, and thus demonstrating multisensory integration) are compared to congruent trials. This comparison frequently reveals increased activity in left posterior STS (Jones and Callan, 2003; Sekiyama et al., 2003; Skipper et al., 2007; Matchin et al., 2014), suggesting this region plays a critical role for multisensory integration (Beauchamp, 2005; Desimone and Gross, 1979; Beauchamp et al., 2004).

In one particularly elegant study, Nath and Beauchamp (2011) presented listeners with McGurk stimuli that varied in the perceptual clarity of the auditory portion (by adding background noise) or the visual portion (by spatial blurring). The authors assessed functional connectivity between auditory and visual cortex and posterior STS, and found that functional connectivity increased as a function of the clearer input. That is, when the visual input was blurred, functional connectivity between posterior STS and auditory cortex increased, potentially reflecting a reweighting of multisensory input based on the reliability of the information provided (Ernst and Banks, 2002). Complementary evidence for this conclusion comes from a transcranial magnetic stimulation (TMS) study in which processing in posterior STS was disrupted, resulting in a disruption of the McGurk effect (Beauchamp et al., 2010).

Despite the intuitive appeal of McGurk-type stimuli for studying audiovisual speech perception, there are reasons to question whether the same processes operate during natural speech perception (Alsius et al., 2017). For example, McGurk stimuli require reconciling conflicting auditory and visual cues, which does not happen in natural speech, and in at least some studies individual differences in McGurk susceptibility do not relate to a listener's performance during audiovisual sentence perception (Van Engen et al., 2017).

Left frontal cortex as a pathway for motor representations to affect perception

Activity in the left premotor cortex is commonly observed during neuroimaging studies of speech perception (for example, listening to spoken words) (Binder et al., 2000), and stimulating motor cortex during perception has been suggested to influence speech perception (Schomers et al., 2015). Although the observation of premotor activity likely depends on factors such as the comparison condition or the acoustic environment (for example, quiet vs. background noise), this premotor activity has suggested to many researchers that premotor cortex may play a role in speech perception.[2] Here I will focus specifically on the potential role for motor representations in understanding audiovisual speech.

Fridriksson and colleagues (2008) used fMRI to investigate neural activation when participants performed a discrimination task on visual speech stimuli (without auditory information). They found increased activation in bilateral STG, left IFG, and left premotor cortex for visual speech compared to a visual non-speech control condition. Furthermore, activity in left IFG and premotor cortex increased when the visual speech was degraded (by decreasing the frame rate), an effect absent for the non-speech stimuli, suggesting a role for these regions of left frontal cortex in visual speech perception. Consistent with these results, Okada and Hickok (2009) presented participants with visual-only clips of single phonemes, and observed activation in bilateral STG, left IFG, and left premotor cortex.

Additional evidence supporting a role for motor representations in audiovisual speech processing comes from a role for visual speech in speech production. In one set of relevant studies, Fridriksson and colleagues (Fridriksson et al., 2012; Fridriksson et al., 2015) studied the degree to which viewing speech facilitated speech production in patients with nonfluent aphasia. Patients produced a greater variety of words when viewing audiovisual speech compared to auditory speech alone, and showed benefit to speech fluency with training.

In an fMRI study, Venezia and colleagues (2016) used a covert repetition paradigm with consonant-vowel (CV) syllables (e.g., /ba/) to test whether using visual-only or audiovisual stimuli to cue repetition recruited different networks compared to auditory-only input. Activity was observed both in posterior STS and premotor cortex. Importantly, speech motor regions were more active when the stimulus included visual speech, despite identical rehearsal requirements. These results suggest that processing visual speech entailed recruitment of a specific network of sensorimotor brain regions. If perceiving visual speech indeed involves motor regions, it would provide a straightforward mechanism to explain the speech entrainment results mentioned earlier.

Finally, there are results linking motor representations to speech-related cortical oscillations introduced previously. Park and colleagues (2016) used MEG to measure oscillatory activity while participants viewed audiovisual speech clips (narrative speech). They identified a significant coherence between oscillatory activity and visual cortex and a speaker's lip movements. More interestingly, they also observed significant coherence between a speaker's lip movements and oscillations in a listener's left motor cortex that was positively correlated with comprehension accuracy.

In summary, it is unlikely that motor speech representations are necessary for either auditory-only or audiovisual speech perception, as stroke patients with damage to these regions are able to perceive speech (Rogalsky et al., 2011). However, converging evidence points towards at least a supporting role for motor regions, which may contribute to the integration of multisensory information during audiovisual speech perception.

How acoustic challenge affects the brain networks supporting speech understanding

In everyday experience, we often listen to speech in less-than-ideal acoustic circumstances, including in the presence of background noise, competing talkers, foreign accents, or hearing loss (Mattys et al., 2012). There is now considerable evidence that acoustic challenges of this sort change the cognitive processes listeners engage during speech understanding (Peelle, 2018), further modulated by the motivation a listener has to understand what they are hearing (Pichora-Fuller et al., 2016).

Beyond the core speech regions already discussed, listening to acoustically degraded speech is routinely associated with increased brain activity, commonly in regions of frontal cortex. Davis and Johnsrude (2003) presented listeners with spoken sentences that were acoustically degraded in three ways: With background noise, through noise vocoding (Shannon et al., 1995), or as interrupted speech. They found areas of left prefrontal and premotor cortex that showed increased activity for degraded speech relative to clear speech, consistent with an increase in reliance on executive processes to successfully extract meaning from the acoustic signal. Increased frontal activity has also been seen to correlate with variability within the range of normal hearing in adults with clinically normal hearing (Lee et al., 2018).

A particularly relevant network for understanding degraded speech is the cingulo-opercular network, an executive attention network associated with task maintenance and error monitoring (Dosenbach et al., 2008; Neta et al., 2015; Power and Petersen, 2013). As with other tasks, during speech processing activity in the cingulo-opercular network is elevated following incorrect trials (i.e., incorrect perception of words in noise) (Wild et al., 2012; Erb et al., 2013; Eckert et al., 2009). Interestingly, trial-by-trial variations in activity in the cingulo-opercular network relate to memory for specific items (Vaden Jr. et al., 2017) and the intelligibility of the following word (Vaden Jr. et al., 2013), both suggesting a functional role for the cingulo-opercular network and speech intelligibility.

In addition to background noise, one common example of difficult speech processing comes from listening to speech in a non-native accent. Although there is ample behavioral evidence that this type of accented speech can be more difficult to process (Van Engen and Peelle, 2014), there is less evidence regarding the neural underpinnings of accented speech processing (Adank et al., 2015). In one study, Adank and colleagues (2012) examined neural processing for native speech and a novel accent. In contrast to speech in noise – which was associated with increased activity in the cingulo-opercular network – accented speech was associated with increased activity in the left anterior lateral temporal cortex. However, much remains unknown about the factors that affect perceptual and cognitive processing of accented speech.

It is clear that acoustic challenges of many sorts drastically change the cognitive resources listeners require to understand sentences. In this context, it is worth pointing out that fMRI scanning is associated with significant acoustic noise, in the range of 80–120 dBA or higher (Price et al., 2001; Ravicz et al., 2000; Foster et al., 2000). Although ear-plugs can help reduce the effects, hearing protection cannot fully block external sound, nor can it stop conduction through a listener's bones. Thus, when using fMRI to study speech processing, special sequences are often used to minimize scanner noise, and the acoustic scanning environment must always be considered when interpreting results (Peelle, 2014).

Summary

The brain networks required to understand human speech are widely distributed anatomically, and differ as a function of the specific acoustic and linguistic demands of a stimulus. Bilateral superior temporal cortex is engaged in phoneme and word processing, supplemented by left IFG during sentence comprehension. However, this core speech network is flexible, and during various types of linguistic or acoustic challenge, additional regions are frequently recruited, most notably executive attention networks. This neural flexibility highlights the importance of cognitive contributions to the sending and receiving ends of the speech chain.

Acknowledgments

This work was supported by NIH grants R01DC014281, R21DC015884, and the Dana Foundation. I am grateful to Aahana Bajracharya and Mike Jones for helpful comments on this chapter.

Notes

1 In some instances we may develop lexical representations without semantic representations. For example, I could instruct you that "negus" is a real word, without defining it. With training, these lexical representations show word-like effects (such as competing with similar sounding words) even though they lack a clear conceptual meaning (Davis et al., 2009). In everyday conversation these situations are rare, but still may occur (for example, someone might learn to recognize a new word they hear in conversation before learning its meaning).

2 It is worth noting some superficial similarities between these observations and the influential motor theory of speech perception (Liberman et al., 1967; Liberman and Mattingly, 1985), particularly in the context of mirror neurons. However, the modern cognitive neuroscience approach differs in important ways (Lotto et al., 2009; Rogalsky et al., 2011), and is my focus here.

References

Adank, P. 2012. Design choices in imaging speech comprehension: An activation likelihood estimation (ALE) meta-analysis. *NeuroImage*, 63, 1601–1613.

Adank, P., Davis, M. H. & Hagoort, P. 2012. Neural dissociation in processing noise and accent in spoken language comprehension. *Neuropsychologia*, 50, 77–84.

Adank, P., Nuttall, H. E., Banks, B. & Kennedy-Higgins, D. 2015. Neural bases of accented speech perception. *Frontiers in Human Neuroscience*, 9, 558.

Alsius, A., Paré, M. & Munhall, K. G. 2017. Forty years after hearing lips and seeing voices: The McGurk effect revisited. *Multisensory Research*, 31. https://brill.com/abstract/journals/msr/31/1-2/article-p111_7.xml

Ash, S., Menaged, A., Olm, C., McMillan, C. T., Boller, A., Irwin, D. J., McCluskey, L., Elman, L. & Grossman, M. 2014. Narrative discourse deficits in amyotrophic lateral sclerosis. *Neurology*, 83, 520–528.

Ash, S., Moore, P., Antani, S., McCawley, G., Work, M. & Grossman, M. 2006. Trying to tell a tale: Discourse impairments in progressive aphasia and frontotemporal dementia. *Neurology*, 66, 1405–1413.

Beauchamp, M. S. 2005. See me, hear me, touch me: Multisensory integration in lateral occipital-temporal cortex. *Current Opinion in Neurobiology*, 15, 145–153.

Beauchamp, M. S., Lee, K. E., Argall, B. D. & Martin, A. 2004. Integration of auditory and visual information about objects in superior temporal sulcus. *Neuron*, 41, 809–823.

Beauchamp, M. S., Nath, A. R. & Pasalar, S. 2010. fMRI-guided transcranial magnetic stimulation reveals that the superior temporal sulcus is a cortical locus of the McGurk effect. *Journal of Neuroscience*, 30, 2414–2417.

Binder, J. R., Desai, R. H., Graves, W. W. & Conant, L. L. 2009. Where is the semantic system? A critical review and meta-analysis of 120 functional neuroimaging studies. *Cerebral Cortex*, 19, 2767–2796.

Binder, J. R., Frost, J. A., Hammeke, T. A., Bellgowan, P. S., Springer, J. A., Kaufman, J. N. & Possing, E. T. 2000. Human temporal lobe activation by speech and nonspeech sounds. *Cerebral Cortex*, 10, 512–528.

Blumstein, S. E., Myers, E. B. & Rissman, J. 2005. The perception of voice onset time: An fMRI investigation of phonetic category structure. *Journal of Cognitive Neuroscience*, 17, 1353–1366.

Bonner, M. F. & Grossman, M. 2012. Gray matter density of auditory association cortex relates to knowledge of sound concepts in primary progressive aphasia. *Journal of Neuroscience*, 32, 7986–7991.

Bonner, M. F., Peelle, J. E., Cook, P. A. & Grossman, M. 2013. Heteromodal conceptual processing in the angular gyrus. *NeuroImage*, 71, 175–186.

Bozeat, S., Lambon Ralph, M. A., Graham, K. S., Patterson, K., Wilkin, H., Rowland, J., Rogers, T. T. & Hodges, J. R. 2003. A duck with four legs: Investigating the structure of conceptual knowledge using picture drawing in semantic dementia. *Cognitive Neuropsychology*, 20, 27–47.

Bozeat, S., Lambon Ralph, M. A., Patterson, K., Garrard, P. & Hodges, J. R. 2000. Non-verbal semantic impairment in semantic dementia. *Neuropsychologia*, 38, 1207–1215.

Bozic, M., Tyler, L. K., Ives, D. T., Randall, B. & Marslen-Wilson, W. D. 2010. Bihemispheric foundations for human speech comprehension. *Proceedings of the National Academy of Science*, 107, 17439–17444.

Burton, M. W. & Small, S. L. 2006. Functional neuroanatomy of segmenting speech and nonspeech. *Cortex*, 42, 644–651.

Calvert, G. A., Bullmore, E. T., Brammer, M. J., Campbell, R., Williams, S. C. R., McGuire, P. K., Woodruff, P. W. R., Iversen, S. D. & David, A. S. 1997. Activation of auditory cortex during silent lipreading. *Science*, 276, 593–596.

Canolty, R. T. & Knight, R. T. 2010. The functional role of cross-frequency coupling. *Trends in Cognitive Sciences*, 14, 506–515.

Chandrasekaran, C., Trubanova, A., Stillittano, S., Caplier, A. & Ghazanfar, A. A. 2009. The natural statistics of audiovisual speech. *PLoS Computational Biology*, 5, e1000436.

Chang, E. F., Rieger, J. W., Johnson, K., Berger, M. S., Barbaro, N. M. & Knight, R. T. 2010. Categorical speech representation in human superior temporal gyrus. *Nature Neuroscience*, 13, 1428–1432.

Crinion, J. T., Lambon Ralph, M. A., Warburton, E. A., Howard, D. & Wise, R. J. S. 2003. Temporal lobe regions engaged during normal speech comprehension. *Brain*, 126, 1193–1201.

Crosse, M. J., Butler, J. S. & Lalor, E. C. 2015. Congruent visual speech enhances cortical entrainment to continuous auditory speech in noise-free conditions. *Journal of Neuroscience*, 35, 14195–14204.

Davis, M. H., Coleman, M. R., Absalom, A. R., Rodd, J. M., Johnsrude, I. S., Matta, B. F., Owen, A. M. & Menon, D. K. 2007. Dissociating speech perception and comprehension at reduced levels of awareness. *Proceedings of the National Academy of Sciences*, 104, 16032–16037.

Davis, M. H., Di Betta, A. M., Macdonald, M. J. E. & Gaskell, M. G. 2009. Learning and consolidation of novel spoken words. *Journal of Cognitive Neuroscience*, 21, 803–820.

Davis, M. H. & Gaskell, M. G. 2009. A complementary systems account of word learning: Neural and behavioural evidence. *Philosophical Transactions of The Royal Society B*, 364, 3773–3800.

Davis, M. H. & Johnsrude, I. S. 2003. Hierarchical processing in spoken language comprehension. *Journal of Neuroscience*, 23, 3423–3431.

Denes, P. B. & Pinson, E. N. 1993. *The speech chain: The physics and biology of spoken language*. Long Grove, IL: Waveland Press, Inc.

Desimone, R. & Gross, C. G. 1979. Visual areas in the temporal cortex of the macaque. *Brain Res Cogn Brain Res*, 178, 363–380.

Di Liberto, G. M., O'Sullivan, J. A. & Lalor, E. C. 2015. Low-frequency cortical entrainment to speech reflects phoneme-level processing. *Current Biology*, 25, 2457–2465.

Ding, N., Melloni, L., Zhang, H., Tian, X. & Poeppel, D. 2016. Cortical tracking of hierarchical linguistic structures in connected speech. *Nature Neuroscience*, 19, 158–164.

Ding, N. & Simon, J. Z. 2013. Adaptive temporal encoding leads to a background-insensitive cortical reprsentation of speech. *Journal of Neuroscience*, 33, 5728–5735.

Dosenbach, N. U. F., Fair, D. A., Cohen, A. L., Schlaggar, B. L. & Petersen, S. E. 2008. A dual-networks architecture of top-down control. *Trends in Cognitive Sciences*, 12, 99–105.

Dumay, N. & Gaskell, M. G. 2007. Sleep-associated changes in the mental representation of spoken words. *Psychological Science*, 18, 35–39.

Eckert, M. A., Menon, V., Walczak, A., Ahlstrom, J., Denslow, S., Horwitz, A. & Dubno, J. R. 2009. At the heart of the ventral attention system: The right anterior insula. *Human Brain Mapping*, 30, 2530–2541.

Eckert, M. A., Walczak, A., Ahlstrom, J., Denslow, S., Horwitz, A. & Dubno, J. R. 2008. Age-related effects on word recognition: Reliance on cognitive control systems with structural declines in speech-responsive cortex. *Journal of the Association for Research in Otolaryngology*, 9, 252–259.

Edmister, W. B., Talavage, T. M., Ledden, P. J. & Weisskoff, R. M. 1999. Improved auditory cortex imaging using clustered volume acquisitions. *Human Brain Mapping*, 7, 89–97.

Erb, J., Henry, M. J., Eisner, F. & Obleser, J. 2013. The brain dynamics of rapid perceptual adaptation to adverse listening conditions. *Journal of Neuroscience*, 33, 10688–10697.

Erber, N. P. 1975. Auditory-visual perception of speech. *Journal of Speech and Hearing Disorders*, 40, 481–492.

Ernst, M. O. & Banks, M. S. 2002. Humans integrate visual and haptic information in a statistically optimal fashion. *Nature*, 415, 429–433.

Evans, S. 2017. What has replication ever done for us? Insights from neuroimaging of speech perception. *Frontiers in Human Neuroscience*, 11, 41.

Fedorenko, E., Duncan, J. & Kanwisher, N. G. 2012. Language-selective and domain-general regions lie side by side within Broca's area. *Current Biology*, 22, 2059–2062.

Fonteneau, E., Bozic, M. & Marslen-Wilson, W. D. 2015. Brain network connectivity during language comprehension: Interacting linguistic and perceptual subsystems. *Cerebral Cortex*, 25, 3962–3976.

Foster, J. R., Hall, D. A., Summerfield, A. Q., Palmer, A. R. & Bowtell, R. W. 2000. Sound-level measurements and calculations of safe noise dosage during EPI at 3 T. *Journal of Magnetic Resonance Imaging*, 12, 157–163.

Fridriksson, J., Basilakos, A., Hickok, G., Bonilha, L. & Rorden, C. 2015. Speech entrainment compensates for Broca's area damage. *Cortex*, 69, 68–75.

Fridriksson, J., Hubbard, H. I., Hudspeth, S. G., Holland, A. L., Bonilha, L., Fromm, D. & Rorden, C. 2012. Speech entrainment enables patients with Broca's aphasia to produce fluent speech. *Brain*, 135, 3815–3829.

Fridriksson, J., Moss, J., Davis, B., Baylis, G. C., Bonilha, L. & Rorden, C. 2008. Motor speech perception modulates the cortical language areas. *NeuroImage*, 41, 605–613.

Friederici, A. D. & Gierhan, S. M. E. 2013. The language network. *Current Opinion in Neurobiology*, 23, 250–254.

Gagnepain, P., Henson, R. N. & Davis, M. H. 2012. Temporal predictive codes for spoken words in auditory cortex. *Current Biology*, 22, 615–621.

Ghitza, O. 2011. Linking speech perception and neurophysiology: Speech decoding guided by cascaded oscillators locked to the input rhythm. *Frontiers in Psychology*, 2, 130.

Giraud, A-L. & Poeppel, D. 2012. Cortical oscillations and speech processing: Emerging computational principles and operations. *Nature Neuroscience*, 15, 511–517.

Gorno-Tempini, M. L., Dronkers, N. F., Rankin, K. P., Ogar, J. M., Phengrasamy, L., Rosen, H. J., Johnson, J. K., Weiner, M. W. & Miller, B. L. 2004. Cognition and anatomy in three variants of primary progressive aphasia. *Annals of Neurology*, 55, 335–346.

Graves, W. W., Binder, J. R., Desai, R. H., Conant, L. L. & Seidenberg, M. S. 2010. Neural correlates of implicit and explicit combinatorial semantic processing. *NeuroImage*, 53, 638–646.

Griffiths, T. D., Buchel, C., Frackowiak, R. S. & Patterson, R. D. 1998. Analysis of temporal structure in sound by the human brain. *Nature Neuroscience*, 1, 422–427.

Grodzinsky, Y. 2000. The neurology of syntax: Language use without Broca's area. *Behavioral and Brain Sciences*, 23, 1–21.

Grodzinsky, Y. & Santi, A. 2008. The battle for Broca's region. *Trends in Cognitive Sciences*, 12, 474–480.

Gross, J., Hoogenboom, N., Thut, G., Schyns, P., Panzeri, S., Belin, P. & Garrod, S. 2013. Speech rhythms and multiplexed oscillatory sensory coding in the human brain. *PLoS Biology*, 11, e1001752.

Grossman, M. 2012. The non-fluent/agrammatic variant of primary progressive aphasia. *Lancet Neurology*, 11, 545–555.

Hackett, T. A. 2011. Information flow in the auditory cortical network. *Hearing Research*, 271, 133–146.

Hackett, T. A., Stepniewska, I. & Kaas, J. H. 1999. Prefrontal connections of the parabelt auditory cortex in macaque monkeys. *Brain Research*, 817, 45–58.

Hagoort, P. 2013. MUC (Memory, Unification, Control) and beyond. *Frontiers in Psychology*, 12, 416.

Hall, D. A., Haggard, M. P., Akeroyd, M. A., Palmer, A. R., Summerfield, A. Q., Elliott, M. R., Gurney, E. M. & Bowtell, R. W. 1999. "Sparse" temporal sampling in auditory fMRI. *Human Brain Mapping*, 7, 213–223.

Hall, D. A., Johnsrude, I. S., Haggard, M. P., Palmer, A. R., Akeroyd, M. A. & Summerfield, A. Q. 2002. Spectral and temporal processing in human auditory cortex. *Cerebral Cortex*, 12, 140–149.

Hassanpour, M. S., Eggebrecht, A. T., Culver, J. P. & Peelle, J. E. 2015. Mapping cortical responses to speech using high-density diffuse optical tomography. *NeuroImage*, 117, 319–326.

Hickok, G., Okada, K., Barr, W., Pa, J., Rogalsky, C., Donnelly, K., Barde, L. & Grant, A. 2008. Bilateral capacity for speech sound processing in auditory comprehension: Evidence from Wada procedures. *Brain and Language*, 107, 179–184.

Hickok, G. & Poeppel, D. 2000. Towards a functional neuroanatomy of speech perception. *Trends in Cognitive Sciences*, 4, 131–138.

Hickok, G. & Poeppel, D. 2007. The cortical organization of speech processing. *Nature Reviews Neuroscience*, 8, 393–402.

Jacquemot, C., Pallier, C., LeBihan, D., Dehaene, S. & Dupoux, E. 2003. Phonological grammar shapes the auditory cortex: A functional magnetic resonance imaging study. *Journal of Neuroscience*, 23, 9541–9546.

Jensen, O. & Colgin, L. L. 2007. Cross-frequency coupling between neuronal oscillations. *Trends in Cognitive Sciences*, 11, 267–269.

Joanisse, M. F., Zevin, J. D. & McCandliss, B. D. 2007. Brain mechanisms implicated in the preattentive categorization of speech sounds revealed using FMRI and a short-interval habituation trial paradigm. *Cerebral Cortex*, 17, 2084–2093.

Jones, J. A. & Callan, D. E. 2003. Brain activity during audiovisual speech perception: An fMRI study of the McGurk effect. *Neuroreport*, 14, 1129–1133.

Kaas, J. H. & Hackett, T. A. 2000. Subdivisions of auditory cortex and processing streams in primates. *Proceedings of the National Academy of Sciences*, 97, 11793–11799.

Kaas, J. H., Hackett, T. A. & Tramo, M. J. 1999. Auditory processing in primate cerebral cortex. *Current Opinion in Neurobiology*, 9, 164–170.

Kerlin, J. R., Shahin, A. J. & Miller, L. M. 2010. Attentional gain control of ongoing cortical speech representations in a "cocktail party." *Journal of Neuroscience*, 30, 620–628.

Kocagoncu, E., Clarke, A., Devereux, B. J. & Tyler, L. K. 2017. Decoding the cortical dynamics of sound-meaning mapping. *Journal of Neuroscience*, 37, 1312–1319.

Lakatos, P., Chen, C-M., O'Connell, M. N., Mills, A. & Schroeder, C. E. 2007. Neuronal oscillations and multisensory interaction in primary auditory cortex. *Neuron*, 53, 279–292.

Lakatos, P., Karmos, G., Mehta, A. D., Ulbert, I. & Schroeder, C. E. 2008. Entrainment of neuronal oscillations as a mechanism of attentional selection. *Science*, 320, 110–113.

Lakatos, P., Musacchia, G., O'Connel, M. N., Falchier, A. Y., Javitt, D. C. & Schroeder, C. E. 2013. The specrotemporal filter mechanism of auditory selective attention. *Neuron*, 77, 750–761.

Lakatos, P., Shah, A. S., Knuth, K. H., Ulbert, I., Karmos, G. & Schroeder, C. E. 2005. An oscillatory hierarchy controlling neuronal excitability and stimulus processing in the auditory cortex. *Journal of Neurophysiology*, 94, 1904–1911.

Lee, H., Devlin, J. T., Shakeshaft, C., Stewart, L. H., Brennan, A., Glensman, J., Pitcher, K., Crinion, J., Mechelli, A., Frackowiak, R. S. J., Green, D. W. & Price, C. J. 2007. Anatomical traces of vocabulary acquisition in the adolescent brain. *Journal of Neuroscience*, 27, 1184–1189.

Lee, Y-S., Min, N. E., Wingfield, A., Grossman, M. & Peelle, J. E. 2016. Acoustic richness modulates the neural networks supporting intelligible speech processing. *Hearing Research*, 333, 108–117.

Lee, Y-S., Turkeltaub, P., Granger, R. & Raizada, R. D. S. 2012. Categorical speech processing in Broca's area: An fMRI study using multivariate pattern-based analysis. *The Journal of Neuroscience*, 32, 3942.

Lee, Y-S., Wingfield, A., Min, N. E., Kotloff, E., Grossman, M. & Peelle, J. E. 2018. Differences in hearing acuity among "normal-hearing" young adults modulate the neural basis for speech comprehension. *eNeuro*, ENEURO.0263–0217.2018.

Leonard, M. K., Baud, M. O., Sjerps, M. J. & Chang, E. F. 2016. Perceptual restoration of masked speech in human cortex. *Nature Communications*, 7, 13619.

Lerner, Y., Honey, C. J., Silbert, L. J. & Hasson, U. 2011. Topographic mapping of a hierarchy of temporal receptive windows using a narrated story. *Journal of Neuroscience*, 31, 2906–2915.

Liberman, A. M., Cooper, F. S., Shankweiler, D. P. & Studdert-Kennedy, M. 1967. Perception of the speech code. *Psychological Review*, 74, 431–461.

Liberman, A. M. & Mattingly, I. G. 1985. The motor theory of speech perception revised. *Cognition*, 21, 1–36.

Liebenthal, E., Binder, J. R., Spitzer, S. M., Possing, E. T. & Medler, D. A. 2005. Neural substrates of phonemic perception. *Cerebral Cortex*, 15, 1621–1631.

Lotto, A. J., Hickok, G. S. & Holt, L. L. 2009. Reflections on mirror neurons and speech perception. *Trends in Cognitive Sciences*, 13, 110–114.

Love, T., Swinney, D., Walenski, M. & Zurif, E. 2008. How left inferior frontal cortex participates in syntactic processing: Evidence from aphasia. *Brain and Language*, 107, 203–219.

Luce, P. A. & Pisoni, D. B. 1998. Recognizing spoken words: The neighborhood activation model. *Ear and Hearing*, 19, 1–36.

Luo, H., Liu, Z. & Poeppel, D. 2010. Auditory cortex tracks both auditory and visual stimulus dynamics using low-frequency neuronal phase modulation. *PLoS Biology*, 8, e1000445.

Luo, H. & Poeppel, D. 2007. Phase patterns of neuronal responses reliably discriminate speech in human auditory cortex. *Neuron*, 54, 1001–1010.

Marslen-Wilson, W. D. & Tyler, L. K. 1980. The temporal structure of spoken language processing. *Cognition*, 8, 1–71.

Matchin, W., Groulx, K. & Hickok, G. 2014. Audiovisual speech integration does not rely on the motor system: Evidence from articulatory suppression, the McGurk effect, and fMRI. *Journal of Cognitive Neuroscience*, 26, 606–620.

Mattys, S. L., Davis, M. H., Bradlow, A. R. & Scott, S. K. 2012. Speech recognition in adverse conditions: A review. *Language and Cognitive Processes*, 27, 953–978.

McCarthy, R. A. & Warrington, E. K. 2016. Past, present, and prospects: Reflections 40 years on from the selective impairment of semantic memory (Warrington, 1975). *Quarterly Journal of Experimental Psychology*, 69, 1941–1968.

McGlone, J. 1984. Speech comprehension after unilateral injection of sodium amytal. *Brain and Language*, 22, 150–157.

McGurk, H. & MacDonald, J. 1976. Hearing lips and seeing voices. *Nature*, 264, 746–748.

Mesgarani, N. & Chang, E. F. 2012. Selective cortical representation of attended speaker in multi-talker speech perception. *Nature*, 485, 233–237.

Mesgarani, N., Cheung, C., Johnson, K. & Chang, E. F. 2014. Phonetic feature encoding in human superior temporal gyrus. *Science*, 343, 1006–1010.

Mummery, C. J., Patterson, K., Price, C. J., Ashburner, J., Frackowiak, R. S. J. & Hodges, J. R. 2000. A voxel-based morphometry study of Semantic Dementia: Relationship between temporal lobe atrophy and semantic memory. *Annals of Neurology*, 47, 36–45.

Musz, E. & Thompson-Schill, S. L. 2017. Tracking competition and cognitive control during language comprehension with multi-voxel pattern analysis. *Brain and Language*, 165, 21–32.

Myers, E. B., Blumstein, S. E., Walsh, E. & Eliassen, J. 2009. Inferior frontal regions underlie the perception of phonetic category invariance. *Psychological Science*, 20, 895–903.

Nath, A. R. & Beauchamp, M. S. 2011. Dynamic changes in superior temporal sulcus connectivity during perception of noisy audiovisual speech. *Journal of Neuroscience*, 31, 1704–1714.

Neta, M., Miezin, F. M., Nelson, S. M., Dubis, J. W., Dosenbach, N. U. F., Schlaggar, B. L. & Petersen, S. E. 2015. Spatial and temporal characteristics of error-related activity in the human brain. *Journal of Neuroscience*, 35, 253–266.

Norris, D. & McQueen, J. M. 2008. Shortlist B: A Bayesian model of continuous speech recognition. *Psychological Review*, 115, 357–395.

Nourski, K. V., Steinschneider, M., Oya, H., Kawasaki, H., Jones, R. D. & Howard, M. A. 2014. Spectral organization of the human lateral superior temporal gyrus revealed by intracranial recordings. *Cerebral Cortex*, 24, 340–352.

Obleser, J., Zimmermann, J., Van Meter, J. & Rauschecker, J. P. 2007. Multiple stages of auditory speech perception reflected in event-related fMRI. *Cerebral Cortex*, 17, 2251–2257.

Okada, K. & Hickok, G. 2009. Two cortical mechanisms support the integration of visual and auditory speech: A hypothesis and preliminary data. *Neuroscience Letters*, 452, 219–223.

Overath, T., Kumar, S., Stewart, L., von Kriegstein, K., Cusack, R., Rees, A. & Griffiths, T. D. 2010. Cortical mechanisms for the segregation and representation of acoustic textures. *Journal of Neuroscience*, 30, 2070–2076.

Papoutsi, M., Stamatakis, E. A., Griffiths, J., Marslen-Wilson, W. D. & Tyler, L. K. 2011. Is left fronto-temporal connectivity essential for syntax? Effective connectivity, tractography and performance in left-hemisphere damaged patients. *NeuroImage*, 58, 656–664.

Park, H., Kayser, C., Thut, G. & Gross, J. 2016. Lip movements entrain the observers' low-frequency brain oscillations to facilitate speech intelligibility. *eLife*, 5, e14521.

Patterson, K., Nestor, P. J. & Rogers, T. T. 2007. Where do you know what you know? The representation of semantic knowledge in the human brain. *Nature Reviews Neuroscience*, 8, 976–987.

Peelle, J. E. 2012. The hemispheric lateralization of speech processing depends on what "speech" is: A hierarchical perspective. *Frontiers in Human Neuroscience*, 6, 309.

Peelle, J. E. 2014. Methodological challenges and solutions in auditory functional magnetic resonance imaging. *Frontiers in Neuroscience*, 8, 253.

Peelle, J. E. 2018. Listening effort: How the cognitive consequences of acoustic challenge are reflected in brain and behavior. *Ear and Hearing*, 39, 204–214.

Peelle, J. E., Cooke, A., Moore, P., Vesely, L. & Grossman, M. 2007. Syntactic and thematic components of sentence processing in progressive nonfluent aphasia and nonaphasic frontotemporal dementia. *Journal of Neurolinguistics*, 20, 482–494.

Peelle, J. E. & Davis, M. H. 2012. Neural oscillations carry speech rhythm through to comprehension. *Frontiers in Psychology*, 3, 320.

Peelle, J. E., Gross, J. & Davis, M. H. 2013. Phase-locked responses to speech in human auditory cortex are enhanced during comprehension. *Cerebral Cortex*, 23, 1378–1387.

Peelle, J. E. & Grossman, M. 2008. Language processing in frontotemporal dementia: A brief review. *Language and Linguistics Compass*, 2, 18–35.

Peelle, J. E., Johnsrude, I. S. & Davis, M. H. 2010a. Hierarchical processing for speech in human auditory cortex and beyond. *Frontiers in Human Neuroscience*, 4, 51.

Peelle, J. E., McMillan, C., Moore, P., Grossman, M. & Wingfield, A. 2004. Dissociable patterns of brain activity during comprehension of rapid and syntactically complex speech: Evidence from fMRI. *Brain and Language*, 91, 315–325.

Peelle, J. E. & Sommers, M. S. 2015. Prediction and constraint in audiovisual speech perception. *Cortex*, 68, 169–181.

Peelle, J. E., Troiani, V., Gee, J., Moore, P., McMillan, C., Vesely, L. & Grossman, M. 2008. Sentence comprehension and voxel-based morphometry in progressive nonfluent aphasia, semantic dementia, and nonaphasic frontotemporal dementia. *Journal of Neurolinguistics*, 21, 418–432.

Peelle, J. E., Troiani, V., Wingfield, A. & Grossman, M. 2010b. Neural processing during older adults' comprehension of spoken sentences: Age differences in resource allocation and connectivity. *Cerebral Cortex*, 20, 773–782.

Petrides, M. & Pandya, D. N. 2009. Distinct parietal and temporal pathways to the homologues of Broca's area in the monkey. *PLoS Biology*, 7, e1000170.

Pichora-Fuller, M. K., Kramer, S. E., Eckert, M. A., Edwards, B., Hornsby, B. W. Y., Humes, L. E., Lemke, U., Lunner, T., Matthen, M., Mackersie, C. L., Naylor, G., Phillips, N. A., Richter, M., Rudner, M., Sommers, M. S., Tremblay, K. L. & Wingfield, A. 2016. Hearing impairment and cognitive energy: The framework for understanding effortful listening (FUEL). *Ear and Hearing*, 37, 5S–27S.

Power, J. D. & Petersen, S. E. 2013. Control-related systems in the human brain. *Current Opinion in Neurobiology*, 23, 223–228.

Price, A. R., Bonner, M. F., Peelle, J. E. & Grossman, M. 2015. Converging evidence for the neuroanatomic basis of combinatorial semantics in the angular gyrus. *Journal of Neuroscience*, 35, 3276–3284.

Price, C. J., Wise, R. J. S., Ramsay, S., Friston, K., Howard, D., Patterson, K. & Frackowiak, R. 1992. Regional response differences within the human auditory cortex when listening to words. *Neuroscience Letters*, 146, 179–182.

Price, C. J., Wise, R. J. S., Warburton, E. A., Moore, C. J., Howard, D., Patterson, K., Frackowiak, R. S. J. & Friston, K. J. 1996. Hearing and saying: The functional neuro-anatomy of auditory word processing. *Brain*, 119, 919–931.

Price, D. L., De Wilde, J. P., Papadaki, A. M., Curran, J. S. & Kitney, R. I. 2001. Investigation of acoustic noise on 15 MRI scanners from 0.2 T to 3 T. *Journal of Magnetic Resonance Imaging*, 13, 288–293.

Raizada, R. D. S. & Poldrack, R. A. 2007. Selective amplification of stimulus differences during categorical processing of speech. *Neuron*, 56, 726–740.

Rauschecker, J. P. & Scott, S. K. 2009. Maps and streams in the auditory cortex: nonhuman primates illuminate human speech processing. *Nature Neuroscience*, 12, 718–724.

Ravicz, M. E., Melcher, J. R. & Kiang, N. Y.-S. 2000. Acoustic noise during functional magnetic resonance imaging. *The Journal of the Acoustical Society of America*, 108, 1683–1696.

Reilly, J., Garcia, A. & Binney, R. J. 2016a. Does the sound of a barking dog activate its corresponding visual form? An fMRI investigation of modality-specific semantic access. *Brain and Language*, 159, 45–59.

Reilly, J., Peelle, J. E., Garcia, A. & Crutch, S. J. 2016b. Linking somatic and symbolic representation in semantic memory: The dynamic multilevel reactivation framework. *Psychonomic Bulletin and Review*, 23, 1002–1014.

Rimmele, J. M., Zion Golumbic, E., Schröger, E. & Poeppel, D. 2015. The effects of selective attention and speech acoustics on neural speech-tracking in a multi-talker scene. *Cortex*, 68, 144–154.

Rimol, L. M., Specht, K., Weis, S., Savoy, R. & Hugdahl, K. 2005. Processing of sub-syllabic speech units in the posterior temporal lobe: an fMRI study. *NeuroImage*, 26, 1059–1067.

Rodd, J. M., Davis, M. H. & Johnsrude, I. S. 2005. The neural mechanisms of speech comprehension: fMRI studies of semantic ambiguity. *Cerebral Cortex*, 15, 1261–1269.

Rodd, J. M., Johnsrude, I. S. & Davis, M. H. 2012. Dissociating frontotemporal contributions to semantic ambiguity resolution in spoken sentences. *Cerebral Cortex*, 22, 1761–1773.

Rodd, J. M., Longe, O. A., Randall, B. & Tyler, L. K. 2010. The functional organisation of the fronto-temporal language system: Evidence from syntactic and semantic ambiguity. *Neuropsychologia*, 48, 1324–1335.

Rogalsky, C. & Hickok, G. 2011. The role of Broca's area in sentence comprehension. *Journal of Cognitive Neuroscience*, 23, 1664–1680.

Rogalsky, C., Love, T., Driscoll, D., Anderson, S. W. & Hickok, G. 2011. Are mirror neurons the basis of speech perception? Evidence from five cases with damage to the purported human mirror system. *Neurocase*, 17, 178–187.

Rogers, J. C. & Davis, M. H. 2017. Inferior frontal cortex contributions to the recognition of spoken words and their constituent speech sounds. *Journal of Cognitive Neuroscience*, 29, 919–936.

Romanski, L. M. & Goldman-Rakic, P. S. 2002. An auditory domain in primate prefrontal cortex. *Nature Neuroscience*, 5, 15–16.

Romanski, L. M., Tian, B., Fritz, J., Mishkin, M., Goldman-Rakic, P. S. & Rauschecker, J. P. 1999. Dual streams of auditory afferents target multiple domains in the primate prefrontal cortex. *Nature Neuroscience*, 2, 1131–1136.

Schomers, M. R., Kirilina, E., Weigand, A., Bajbouj, M. & Pulvermuller, F. 2015. Causal Influence of articulatory motor cortex on comprehending single spoken words: TMS evidence. *Cerebral Cortex*, 25, 3894–3902.

Schroeder, C. E. & Lakatos, P. 2009. Low-frequency neuronal oscillations as instruments of sensory selection. *Trends in Neurosciences*, 32, 9–18.

Schroeder, C. E., Lakatos, P., Kajikawa, Y., Partan, S. & Puce, A. 2008. Neuronal oscillations and visual amplification of speech. *Trends in Cognitive Sciences*, 12, 106–113.

Scott, S. K., Blank, C. C., Rosen, S. & Wise, R. J. S. 2000. Identification of a pathway for intelligible speech in the left temporal lobe. *Brain*, 123, 2400–2406.

Sekiyama, K., Kanno, I., Miura, S. & Sugita, Y. 2003. Auditory-visual speech perception examined by fMRI and PET. *Neuroscience Research*, 47, 277–287.

Seltzer, B., Cola, M. G., Gutierrez, C., Massee, M., Weldon, C. & Cusick, C. G. 1996. Overlapping and nonoverlapping cortical projections to cortex of the superior temporal sulcus in the rhesus monkey: double anterograde tracer studies. *Journal of Comparative Neurology*, 370, 173–190.

Seltzer, B. & Pandya, D. N. 1989. Frontal lobe connections of the superior temporal sulcus in the rhesus monkey. *Journal of Comparative Neurology*, 281, 97–113.

Shannon, R. V., Zeng, F-G., Kamath, V., Wygonski, J. & Ekelid, M. 1995. Speech recognition with primarily temporal cues. *Science*, 270, 303–304.

Skipper, J. I., van Wassenhove, V., Nusbaum, H. C. & Small, S. L. 2007. Hearing lips and seeing voices: How cortical areas supporting speech production mediate audiovisual speech perception. *Cerebral Cortex*, 17, 2387–2399.

Sohoglu, E., Peelle, J. E., Carlyon, R. P. & Davis, M. H. 2012. Predictive top-down integration of prior knowledge during speech perception. *Journal of Neuroscience*, 32, 8443–8453.

Specht, K. & Reul, J. 2003. Functional segregation of the temporal lobes into highly differentiated subsystems for auditory perception: an auditory rapid event-related fMRI-task. *NeuroImage*, 20, 1944–1954.

Steinschneider, M., Nourski, K. V., Kawasaki, H., Oya, H., Brugge, J. F. & Howard, M. A., 3rd 2011. Intracranial study of speech-elicited activity on the human posterolateral superior temporal gyrus. *Cerebral Cortex*, 21, 2332–2347.

Sumby, W. H. & Pollack, I. 1954. Visual contribution to speech intelligibility in noise. *The Journal of the Acoustical Society of America*, 26, 212–215.

Swinney, D. & Zurif, E. 1995. Syntactic processing in aphasia. *Brain and Language*, 50, 225–239.

Thompson-Schill, S. L., D'Esposito, M., Aguirre, G. K. & Farah, M. J. 1997. Role of left inferior prefrontal cortex in retrieval of semantic knowledge: A reevaluation. *Proceedings of the National Academy of Sciences*, 94, 14792–14797.

Tyler, L. K., Marslen-Wilson, W. D., Randall, B., Wright, P., Devereux, B. J., Zhuang, J., Papoutsi, M. & Stamatakis, E. A. 2011. Left inferior frontal cortex and syntax: function, structure and behaviour in patients with left hemisphere damage. *Brain*, 134, 415–431.

Tyler, L. K., Shafto, M. A., Randall, B., Wright, P., Marslen-Wilson, W. D. & Stamatakis, E. A. 2010. Preserving syntactic processing across the adult life span: The modulation of the frontotemporal language system in the context of age-related atrophy. *Cerebral Cortex*, 20, 352–364.

Vaden, K. I. Jr., Kuchinsky, S. E., Cute, S. L., Ahlstrom, J. B., Dubno, J. R. & Eckert, M. A. 2013. The cingulo-opercular network provides word-recognition benefit. *Journal of Neuroscience*, 33, 18979–18986.

Vaden, K. I. Jr., Teubner-Rhodes, S., Ahlstrom, J. B., Dubno, J. R. & Eckert, M. A. 2017. Cingulo-opercular activity affects incidental memory encoding for speech in noise. *NeuroImage*, 157, 381–387.

Van Engen, K. J. & Peelle, J. E. 2014. Listening effort and accented speech. *Frontiers in Human Neuroscience*, 8, 577.

Van Engen, K. J., Xie, Z. & Chandrasekaran, B. 2017. Audiovisual sentence recognition not predicted by susceptibility to the McGurk effect. *Attention, Perception, and Psychophysics*, 79, 396–403.

Venezia, J. H., Fillmore, P., Matchin, W., Isenberg, A. L., Hickok, G. & Fridriksson, J. 2016. Perception drives production across sensory modalities: A network for sensorimotor integration of visual speech. *NeuroImage*, 126, 196–207.

Whitney, C., Kirk, M., O'Sullivan, J., Lambon Ralph, M. A. & Jefferies, E. 2011. The neural organization of semantic control: TMS evidence for a distributed network in left inferior frontal and posterior middle temporal gyrus. *Cerebral Cortex*, 21, 1066–1075.

Wild, C. J., Yusuf, A., Wilson, D., Peelle, J. E., Davis, M. H. & Johnsrude, I. S. 2012. Effortful listening: The processing of degraded speech depends critically on attention. *Journal of Neuroscience*, 32, 14010–14021.

Wingfield, A., Peelle, J. E. & Grossman, M. 2003. Speech rate and syntactic complexity as multiplicative factors in speech comprehension by young and older adults. *Aging, Neuropsychology, and Cognition*, 10, 310–322.

Zempleni, M-Z., Renken, R., Hoeks, J. C. J., Hoogduin, J. M. & Stowe, L. A. 2007. Semantic ambiguity processing in sentence context: Evidence from event-related fMRI. *NeuroImage*, 34, 1270–1279.

Zhuang, J., Tyler, L. K., Randall, B., Stamatakis, E. A. & Marslen-Wilson, W. D. 2014. Optimially efficient neural systems for processing spoken language. *Cerebral Cortex*, 24, 908–918.

Zion Golumbic, E., Ding, N., Bickel, S., Lakatos, P., Schevon, C. A., McKhann, G. M., Goodman, R. R., Emerson, R., Mehta, A. D., Simon, J. Z., Poeppel, D. & Schroeder, C. E. 2013. Mechanisms underlying selective neuronal tracking of attended speech at a "cocktail party." *Neuron*, 77, 980–991.

Part III

Theories and models of speech perception and production

9

The acoustics and perception of North American English vowels

James M. Hillenbrand

Introduction

The purpose of this review is to summarize some of the literature on the acoustics and perception of vowels. In spite of the relative youth of this area of study, and of experimental phonetics more generally, the literature on the acoustics and perception of vowels is quite extensive. As a consequence, this review will be selective, and an attempt will be made to focus the discussion on those areas that seem to the author to be the most critical to understanding how vowels are spoken and recognized.

Source-filter theory and vowel production

Source-filter theory has served as the primary model that is used to understand the acoustics of speech production – both vowels and consonants – for a great many years. Figure 9.1 shows a simplified version of source-filter theory for the production of three monotone vowels with a static vocal tract posture. (Not shown in this simplified model is the radiation characteristic, a high-pass filter with a slope of about +6 dB per octave that accounts for the greater efficiency with which higher-frequency components are radiated from the enclosed vocal tract to the outside world.) In this figure, the same glottal source signal serves as the input to three different vocal tract filters whose shapes are controlled by the positions of the tongue, lips, and jaw. The peaks in the vocal tract frequency response curve (FRC) are responsible for the peaks that are seen in the envelope of the output spectrum.

What is a formant?

The term "formant" is the most widely used descriptive and explanatory term in acoustic and perceptual phonetics. Consequently, one would think that the term would have a clearly agreed upon meaning, and that any potential for misunderstanding the meaning of the term would be routinely addressed in introductory texts, but this is not the case. The central issue is that *formant* is sometimes used to refer to a peak in the envelope of an output spectrum, and the same term is sometimes used to refer to a peak in a vocal tract frequency response

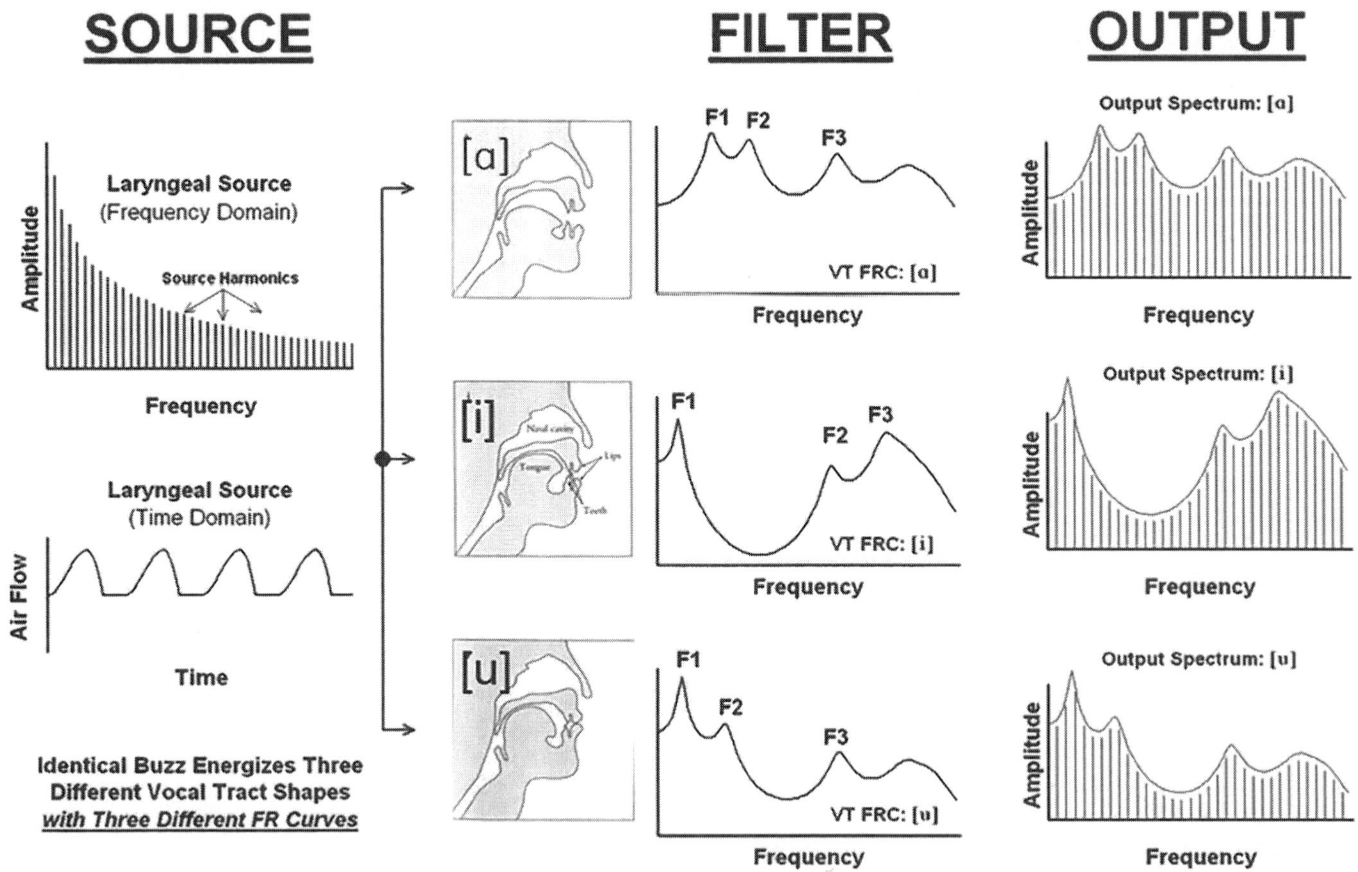

Figure 9.1 Slightly simplified version of source-filter theory for three static, phonated vowels. A single periodic glottal source signal serves as the input to three different vocal tract filters whose frequency response curves are controlled by the positions of the tongue, jaw, and lips. Amplitudes in the output spectrum are derived by multiplying the amplitudes at each frequency by the gain of the filter at those frequencies.

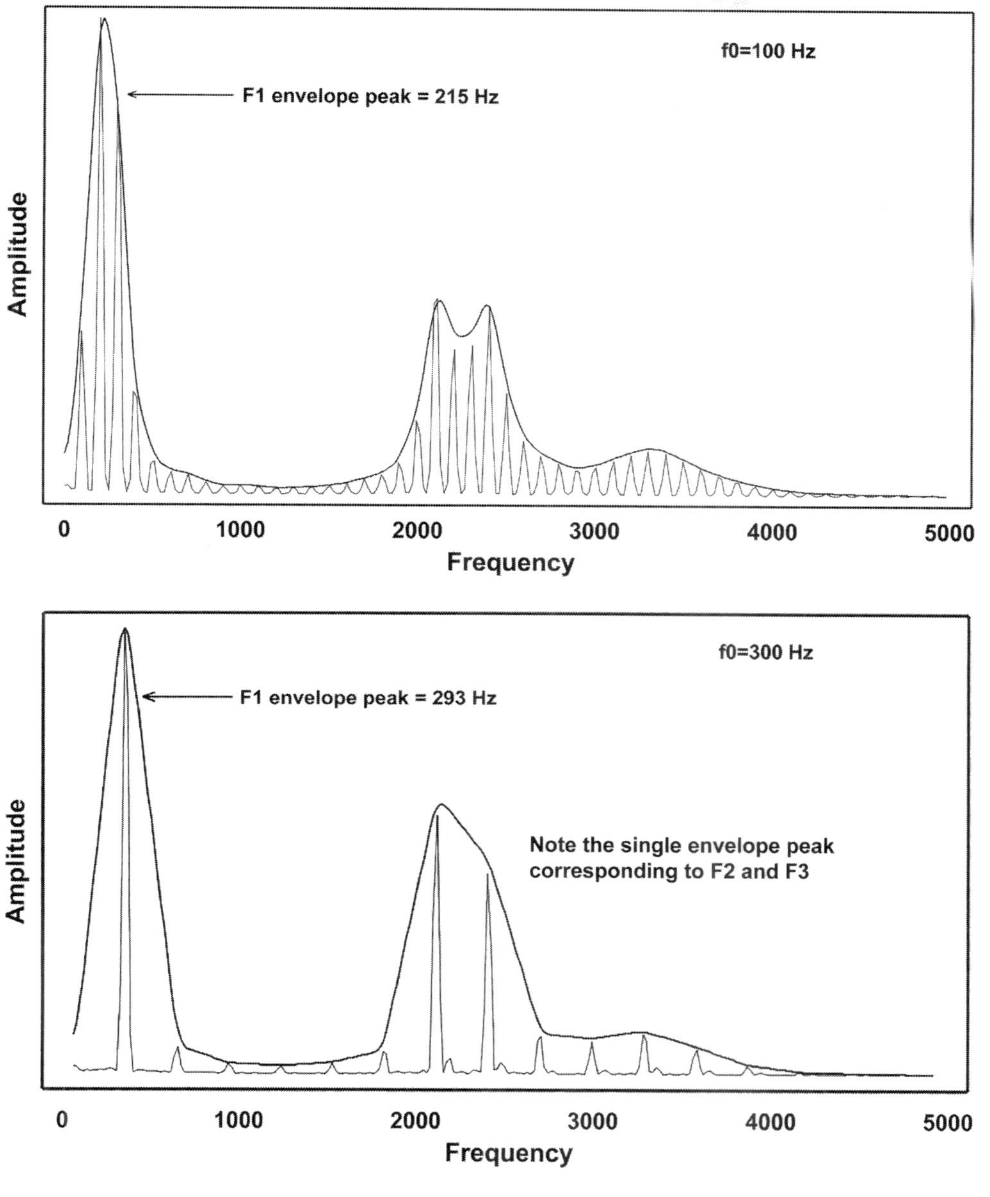

Figure 9.2 Formant-synthesized vowels with identical vocal tract resonances but different fundamental frequencies. The first three formant frequencies were set to 250, 2100, and 2400 Hz; resonator gains and bandwidths are identical for the two signals. The spectrum envelopes were computed by interpolating between adjacent harmonics (Paul, 1981), followed by smoothing with a 50 Hz Gaussian-weighted running average. Note that neither of the F_1 envelope peaks is especially close to the 250 Hz first resonance of the formant synthesizer. Further, the two envelope peaks differ from one another by 78 Hz, or a factor of 1.36. Also note the merger of F_2 and F_3 into a single envelope peak for the vowel with a 300 Hz f_0.

curve (quite often by the same writer). Fant (1960) explicitly defines formants as "the spectral peaks of the sound spectrum" (p. 20); however, later in the same book Fant appears to use the same term to refer to an FRC peak (e.g., p. 53). The view of a formant as a spectral peak is expressed in other widely read sources, such as Peterson and Barney (1952) and Flanagan (1972), who expresses the idea with exceptional clarity: "The *manifestations* of these normal modes as spectral peaks in the output sound are called formants" (p. 59) [emphasis added]. On the other hand, Stevens (2000) associates the term formant explicitly with the FRC rather than the output spectrum. Consistent with Stevens' view is the nearly universal use of the term "formant synthesis" to describe synthesis methods such as Klatt (1980; see also Klatt and Klatt, 1990). Implicit in *formant synthesis* is the view that a formant is a property of a filter since parameters such as F_1, F_2, etc., control the resonant frequencies of the filter. Also controlled are parameters such as A_1, A_2, etc. Although these parameters are referred to as formant *amplitudes* in Klatt and Klatt, the parameters that are being controlled in the synthesis settings are unambiguously *resonator gains*, not output amplitudes.

Peaks in FRCs and peaks in output spectra correspond closely in many cases, particularly for the three idealized vowels whose FRCs and output spectra are shown in Figure 9.1. Nevertheless, a peak in an FRC and a peak in the envelope of an output spectrum are not and cannot be the same thing. A simple example can be seen in Figure 9.2, which shows harmonic spectra and spectrum envelopes for two formant-synthesized vowels with identical settings of the formant-frequency control parameters (250, 2100, and 2400 Hz) but different fundamental frequencies (100 vs. 300 Hz). Envelopes of the output spectra were computed by interpolating between adjacent harmonics (Paul, 1981; Hillenbrand et al., 2006), followed by light smoothing. Note that the F_1 envelope peaks are not especially close to the 250 Hz setting of the first resonance of the synthesizer for either of the vowels. Further, the two envelope peaks corresponding to F_1 differ from one another by 78 Hz, or a factor of 1.36, despite identical resonator frequencies, gains, and bandwidths. Also note the merger of F_2 and F_3 into a single envelope peak for the vowel with a 300 Hz f_0. There is nothing special or contrived about the example in Figure 9.2; many others could be illustrated. The main point is that relationships between FRC peaks and peaks in the output spectrum are not always simple; as a consequence, the use of a single term to apply to two related but quite different concepts is far from ideal. Despite this, any change in the use or definition of the term "formant" at this late stage would appear to be out of the question. The term has been used to refer to two quite different phenomena for too long (but see Titze et al., 2015, for some history, discussion, and proposed solutions).

Some basic facts: Acoustic measurements and intelligibility

In what is almost certainly the most widely cited paper in the area, Peterson and Barney (1952; hereafter PB) measured the acoustic properties (f_0 and F_1-F_3) and the intelligibility of ten nominally monophthongal American English (AE) vowels (/i/,/ɪ/,/ɛ/,/æ/,/ɑ/,/ɔ/,/ʊ/, /u/,/ʌ/, and /ɚ/) spoken by a large group of talkers. While these kinds of measurements had been reported in previous studies, the scale of PB's work was unprecedented, and would remain so for several decades. Audio recordings were made of two repetitions each of the ten vowel types in /hVd/ words spoken by 76 talkers (33 men, 28 women, and 15 children). Relatively little is said about the dialect of the talkers, except that the women and children were raised primarily in the Mid-Atlantic area, while the dialect background of the men was more heterogeneous.

The 1,520 utterances (76 talkers × 10 vowels × 2 repetitions) were presented for identification in randomized order to 70 men and women, including 32 of the 76 talkers. The regional distribution of the listeners was said to be similar to that of the talkers. Identification results were relatively simple, at least in general terms. The average identification rate was 94.4%, with extremely low error rates for some vowels (e.g., /i/: 0.1%, /ɚ/: 0.3%, /u/: 0.8%). The only vowel type with a double-digit error rate was /ɑ/ (13%), confused mainly with /ɔ/. The primary finding, then, is that the utterances were overwhelmingly identified as the vowel that was intended by the talker, leaving open the obvious question of what information listeners are using to identify the vowels.

Formants and f_0 were measured at a single time slice that was judged by visual inspection of broadband spectrograms to be steady-state ("following the influence of the [h] and preceding the influence of the [d]," p. 177). The acoustic measurements were made from narrow band amplitude sections. Formant frequencies and amplitudes were estimated by calculating a weighted average using the frequencies and amplitudes of the harmonics comprising the formant peaks (Potter and Steinberg, 1950). A scatterplot of F_1 and F_2 is shown in Figure 9.3. It is clear from this familiar figure that there is a strong relationship between the F_1-F_2 values and the intended vowel category.

Figure 9.4 shows a scatterplot of F_1-F_2 values from a more recent study by Hillenbrand et al. (1995, hereafter H95). Recordings were made of 12 vowel types (/e/ and /o/ were added to the ten vowel types recorded by PB) in /hVd/ environment from 139 talkers (45 men, 48 women, and 46 10- to 12-year-old children). The general approach of the study was quite similar to PB, with the major departures consisting of: (a) The great majority of the talkers (87%) were from Southern Michigan, with most of the remaining talkers from other areas of the inland north that have been characterized by Labov et al. (1972) as part of the *Northern Cities*

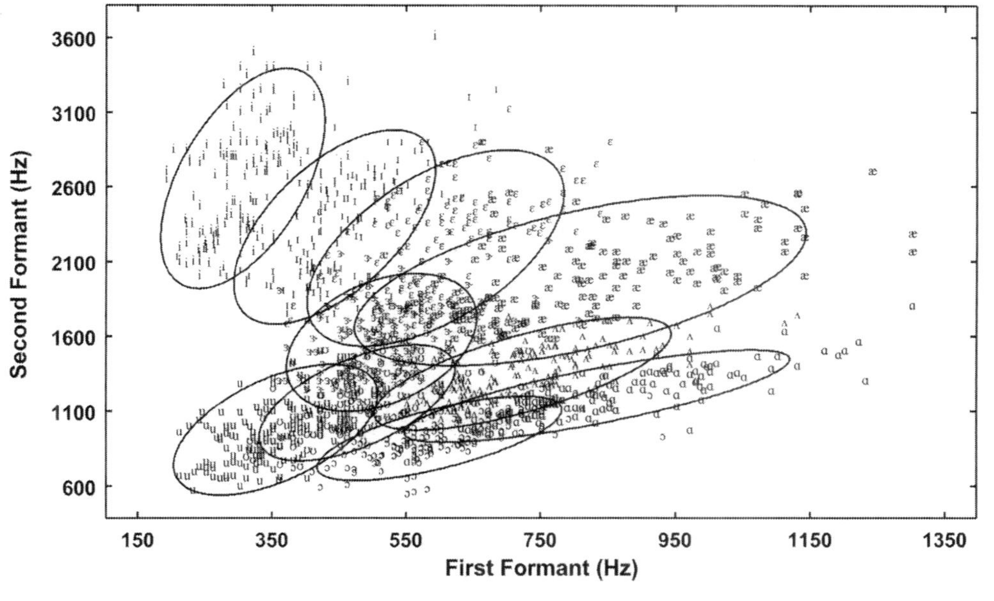

Figure 9.3 Formant frequency measurements at steady-state from Peterson and Barney (1952). The data have been thinned of redundant data points.

Source: Redrawn from Peterson and Barney (1952).

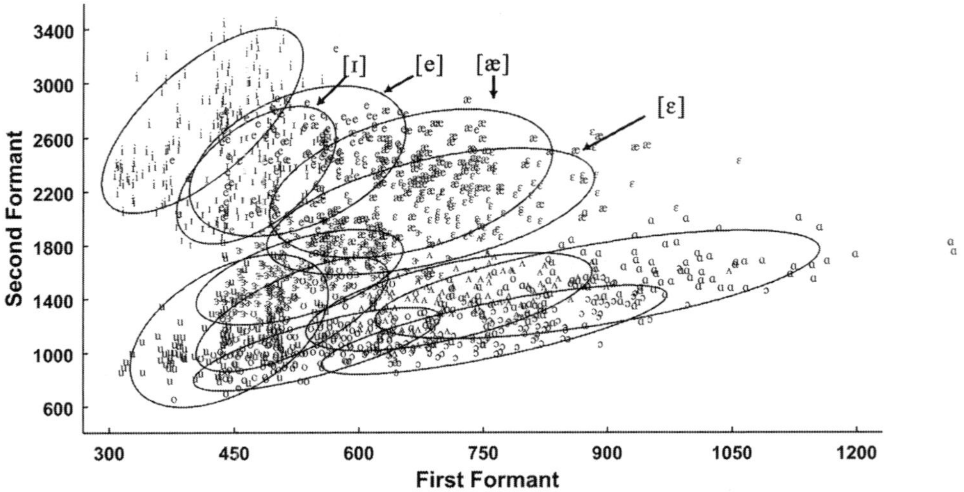

Figure 9.4 Formant frequency measurements at steady-state from Hillenbrand et al. (1995). The data have been thinned of redundant data points.

Source: Redrawn from Hillenbrand et al. (1995).

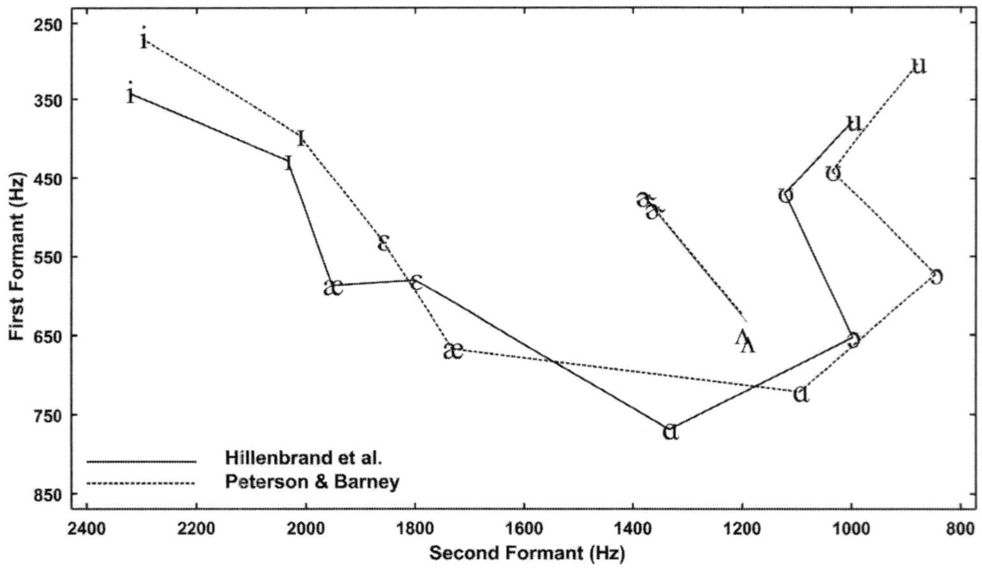

Figure 9.5 Acoustic vowel diagrams from Peterson and Barney (1952) and Hillenbrand et al. (1995). Note the raising of /æ/ and lowering/fronting of the back vowels (particularly /ɑ, ɔ/) in the Hillenbrand et al. Northern Cities vowels in relation to Peterson and Barney.

Source: Redrawn from Hillenbrand et al. (1995).

dialect group; and (b) measurements were made of the *contours* of f_0 and F_1, F_2 and F_3 (using linear predictive coding analysis) throughout the course of the vowel. To allow comparisons to PB, estimates of steady-state times were made by visual inspection of broadband spectrograms. While the formant values for some of the Michigan vowels differ from those of PB (Figure 9.5), mainly because of dialect differences, the two main features of the PB formant data are also observed in Figure 9.4: (a) There is a clear relationship between vowel category and the values of F_1 and F_2, but (b) there is a good deal of within-category variability and overlap among adjacent vowel types (see especially the overlap between /ɪ/–/e/ and /æ/–/ɛ/). In both PB and H95, some but by no means all of this variability is related to differences in vocal-tract length (Figure 9.6). Finally, as with PB, the utterances are overwhelmingly recognized as

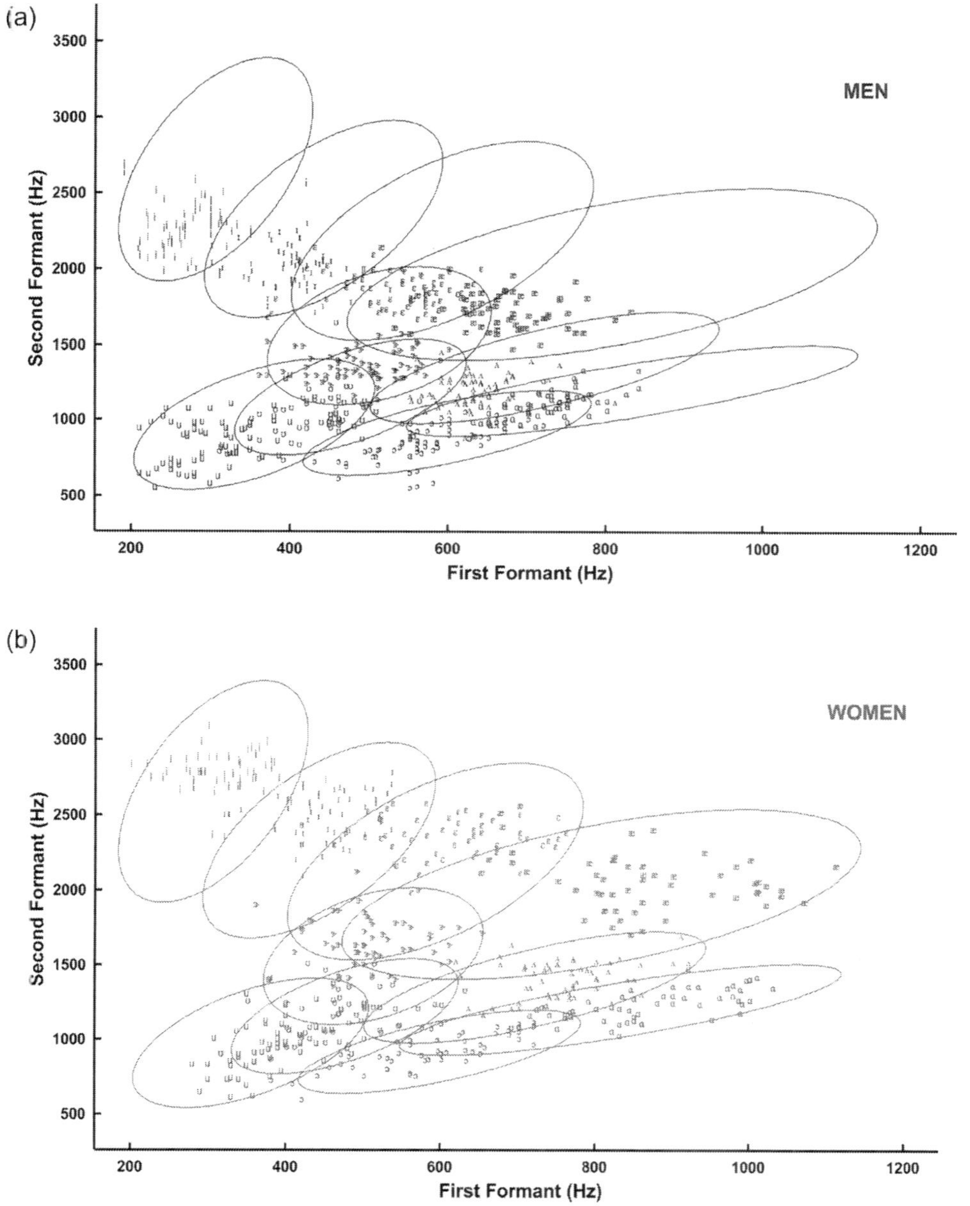

Figure 9.6 Formant frequency measurements for men, women, and children (Peterson and Barney, 1952). Note that, on average, formant frequencies increase from men to women to children. Some but not all of the within-vowel-category variability is clearly related to differences in vocal-tract length.

(c)

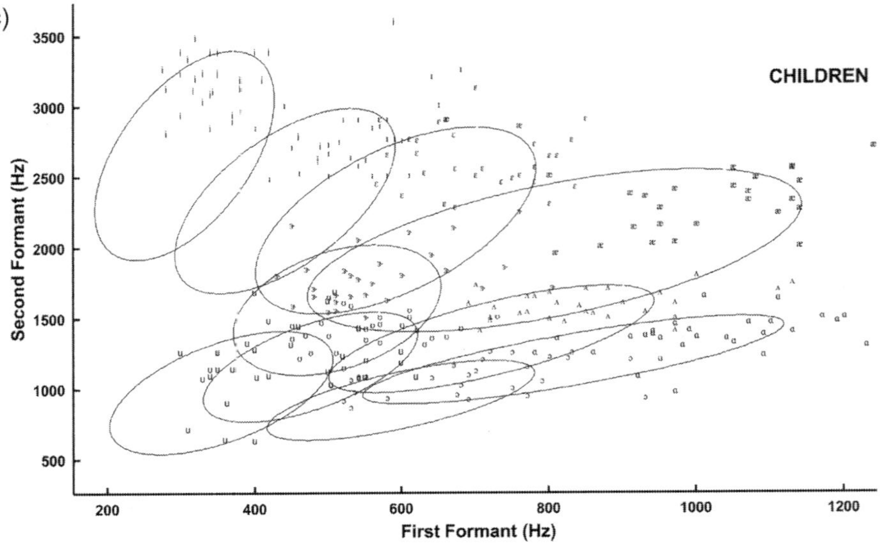

Figure 9.6 (Continued)

the vowel intended by the talker, with intelligibility that is very slightly higher (95.4%) than PB despite the addition of two vowel categories (/e/ and /o/).

In light of the excellent intelligibility of the vowels in both of these large-scale studies, it is clear that listeners must be identifying these speech sounds based on information in addition to (or perhaps in place of) F_1 and F_2. Some of these possibilities will be explored in later sections of the chapter.

Formants, spectral peaks, and spectral shape

An implicit assumption underlying experimental work such as PB is the idea that vowel identity is controlled not by the detailed shape of the spectrum but by the distribution of the two or three lowest formant frequencies. This assumption is so pervasive that it is only occasionally explicitly defended or even described. The alternative to formant theory – typically called a *whole spectrum* or *spectral shape* approach – presumes that vowel identity is determined by the gross shape of spectrum envelope. An important point that is sometimes made by advocates of whole spectrum models is that formants only seem to be important because spectral peaks have such a large effect on the overall shape of the spectrum envelope (e.g., Zahorian and Jagharghi, 1993; Rosner and Pickering, 1994).

A significant virtue of formant theory is that formant representations appear to account for a very large number of findings in the phonetic perception literature. A straightforward demonstration of this is the high intelligibility of speech that has been generated from the sparse set of control parameters that are needed to drive a formant synthesizer (e.g., Logan et al., 1989). Further, literature extending well into the 19th century (e.g., Mattingly, 1999) abounds with explanations of a wide variety of acoustic-phonetic phenomena that appeal to the concept of a formant. There are, however, several important problems with formant representations. Bladon (1982) referred to the most important of these as the *determinacy* problem: Quite simply, after many decades of concerted effort by many capable, imaginative investigators, no one has developed a fully reliable method to measure formant frequencies automatically from natural speech, even in the absence of challenging conditions such as noise or reverberation (see also Klatt, 1982). As is well known, the central problem is that formant tracking involves more than just extracting envelope peaks; it is necessary to assign each of the peaks to specific formant slots corresponding to F_1, F_2, F_3, etc., while rejecting envelope peaks that arise from sources other than vocal tract resonances.

A closely related problem is that the kinds of errors that are made by listeners do not appear to be consistent with the idea that the auditory system is tracking formants. As Klatt (1982) noted, even the best formant trackers are bound to make errors, and these errors are often large ones since they tend to involve either identifying spurious peaks as formants, or missing formants entirely (e.g., when closely spaced formants merge to form a single peak, as in F_1 and F_2 of /ɔ/, or F_2 and F_3 of /i/ or /ɚ/). Human listeners, on the other hand, nearly always hear a vowel that is very close in phonetic space to the vowel that was intended by the talker, as can be seen in virtually any vowel identification confusion matrix. This fact is more readily accommodated by whole spectrum models.

A sampling of findings that seem more consistent with a spectral shape model includes the following:

First, a statistical pattern classification study by Zahorian and Jagharghi (1993) showed that naturally spoken vowels in CVC syllables could be recognized with greater accuracy based on spectral shape than formants.

Second, a deceptively simple experiment by Lindqvist and Pauli (1968) showed that phonetic boundaries along a Swedish front-vowel continuum ([i]–[y]–[ʉ]) were unaffected by very large changes (as much as 25 dB at the extremes) in the level of F_1 in relation to F_2 and F_3 (see also Ainsworth and Millar, 1971).

Third, Ito and Yano (2001) created test signals in which either F_1 or F_2 was suppressed while maintaining spectral shape that was as close as possible to the original signals (see figure 1 from Ito and Yano). Listener responses to the formant-suppressed signals were largely similar to those of the original signals, suggesting that formant frequencies are not decisive in determining the vowel percept. (See Kiefte and Kluender, 2005, for related experimental work that led the authors to conclusions that are very different from Ito and Yano.)

Few whole-spectrum models have been specified as explicitly as Bladon and Lindblom (1981), who hypothesized that listener judgments of vowel quality are based on representations of loudness density versus pitch. Critical-band spectra derived from an auditory model (Schroeder et al., 1979) were used in combination with a metric of auditory-perceptual distance (Plomp, 1970) that could be used to predict the similarity of pairs of loudness-pitch spectra. To compare the model output to perceptual data, listeners heard pairs of signals consisting of four-formant /i/ or /y/ and one of seven versions of two-formant vowels with a fixed F_1 and with F_2 values ranging in third-octave steps between 1 and 4 kHz. Listeners were asked to judge the similarity in quality between different pairs of signals. The model output correlated well with the listener judgments (r = 0.89). However, in discussing their results, the authors noted that

> Our distance metric is overly sensitive to the ordinate dimension of the pseudo-auditory patterns [i.e., loudness]. . . . We evidently ought to look, at least in some cases, for a way of reinstating the spectral peak notion while not discarding the benefits that attach to our whole-spectrum measure.
>
> *(p. 1421)*

The issue of sensitivity to loudness differences was explored in an unusually insightful paper by Klatt (1982), which describes experimental work that was directed precisely at the formants/spectral-shape issue. Listeners were presented with pairs of synthetic signals consisting of a standard /æ/ and one of 13 comparison signals. The comparison signals were generated by manipulating one of two kinds of parameters: (a) those that affect overall spectral shape (e.g., high- or low-pass filtering, spectral tilt, changes in formant amplitudes or bandwidths, the introduction of spectral notches, etc.) – but without changing formant frequencies – or (b) formant frequencies, alone and in combination (e.g., F_1, F_2, F_1 and F_2, . . .). Listeners were asked to judge either (a) the overall psychophysical distance, or (b) the *phonetic* distance between the standard and comparison stimuli, "ignoring as much as they can any changes that are associated with a change in speaker or recording conditions" (Klatt, 1982, p. 1278). The results (Table 9.1) were quite clear in showing that formant frequencies were easily the most important parameters affecting phonetic quality. Other spectral differences – while readily audible to listeners – did not result in large changes in phonetic quality. The task was repeated with /ɑ/ and with whispered vowels, with very similar results. Klatt also showed that the metric used in Bladon and Lindblom correlated very poorly (r = 0.14, NS) with phonetic distance judgments made from the /ɑ/ test signals. Klatt summarized his findings in this way:

> Of the stimulus manipulations included in this study, only formant frequency changes induced large changes in phonetic distance. Even though filtering and spectral tilt conditions produce substantial changes in the spectrum [and in *psychophysical* distance judgements], these changes are apparently ignored when making phonetic judgements.
> *(p. 1278)*

Klatt did not see his findings as favoring formant theory, which he found implausible based on considerations such as those previously discussed. He argued that a spectral distance metric was needed that would be maximally sensitive to differences in spectral peaks

Table 9.1 Results from Klatt's (1982) experiment on perceived psychophysical (*Psy*) and phonetic (*Phon*) distances between pairs of vowels with a quality similar to /æ/.

	Psy	*Phon*
Spectral Shape Manipulations		
1. Random phase	20.0	2.9
2. High-pass filter	15.8	1.6
3. Low-pass filter	7.6	2.2
4. Spectral tilt	9.6	1.5
5. Overall amplitude	4.5	1.5
6. Formant bandwidth	3.4	2.4
7. Spectral notch	1.6	1.5
Formant Frequency Manipulations		
8. F_1 ±8%	6.5	6.2
9. F_2 ±8%	5.0	6.1
10. F_1, F_2 ±8%	8.2	8.6
11. F_1, F_2, F_3, F_4, F_5, ±8%	10.7	8.1

and minimally sensitive to spectral tilt, formant-level differences, and other spectral features that have little effect on phonetic distance judgments. Klatt proposed a measure in which, at each frequency, spectral slope rather than level differences are computed: "In this way, a formant peak with the same frequency location in each spectrum but a difference in peak height would have exactly the same (zero) slope at the peak and very similar slopes on the adjacent skirts" (Klatt, 1982, p. 1280). In addition, the slope-difference vector at each frame is multiplied by a weighting function such that greater weight is given to slope differences at envelope peaks, especially the peak with the highest amplitude. Klatt reported a correlation of 0.93 between the weighted slope measure and listener judgments of phonetic distance from the /ɑ/ experiment.

While Klatt did not believe that the proposed slope measure was the final word on the subject (see especially his Comment #5 under *Conclusions*), the weight of evidence suggests that neither formant representations nor a *psychophysically* motivated representation of envelope shape are capable of accounting for judgments of phonetic quality: "a metric is needed that attends to the locations of prominent energy concentrations, but does not attend greatly to their relative intensities, nor to the shape of the spectrum in the valleys between energy concentrations" (Klatt, 1982, p. 1281). Another peak-dominated spectral shape approach based on exactly this premise, but quite different in implementation, will be discussed in the next section.

Vowel recognition directly from harmonic spectra

Common to nearly all spectral shape models is the use of a smooth rather than a narrow band spectrum (i.e., a harmonic spectrum for the common case of phonated vowels) to represent the to-be-recognized input signal. In an insightful paper, de Cheveigné and Kawahara (1999) argue against smoothing. The centerpiece of their argument is illustrated in Figure 9.7. The dashed line in the top of panels *a–c* shows the idealized envelope shape for the vowel /ɑ/ at fundamental frequencies of 100, 200, and 300 Hz. The idealized envelopes are overlaid on harmonic spectra. As de Cheveigné and Kawahara note, the individual harmonics of the voice source effectively sample the idealized envelope shapes at discrete frequencies. At the bottom of each panel is the spectrum obtained through cepstral smoothing of the three harmonic spectra. It can be seen that the smoothed spectrum is a good fit to the idealized envelope at 100 Hz, only a reasonably good fit at 200 Hz, and a very poor fit at the moderately high f_0 of just 300 Hz. The authors point out that this occurs at the higher f_0s because the wide harmonic spacing undersamples the idealized envelope shape, resulting in alias-induced distortion in the same way that aliasing occurs in an undersampled audio signal.

In response to aliasing and other problems with smoothing, de Cheveigné and Kawahara proposed a *missing data model* of vowel identification in which narrow band rather than smoothed spectra serve as the input to the recognition algorithm. Harmonic input spectra are then directly compared to smooth templates for each vowel category, with spectral differences computed *only at harmonic frequencies* (i.e., there is no smoothing of input spectra and, consequently, no alias-induced distortion). Simulations were run using synthetic signals for five vowel types produced at f_0s between 20 and 300 Hz. Templates for each vowel were generated from known envelope shapes based on synthesis parameters. Findings showed good recognition rates for the missing data model across wide variation in f_0. On the other hand, an otherwise identical algorithm using smoothed spectra as inputs showed extreme sensitivity to f_0.

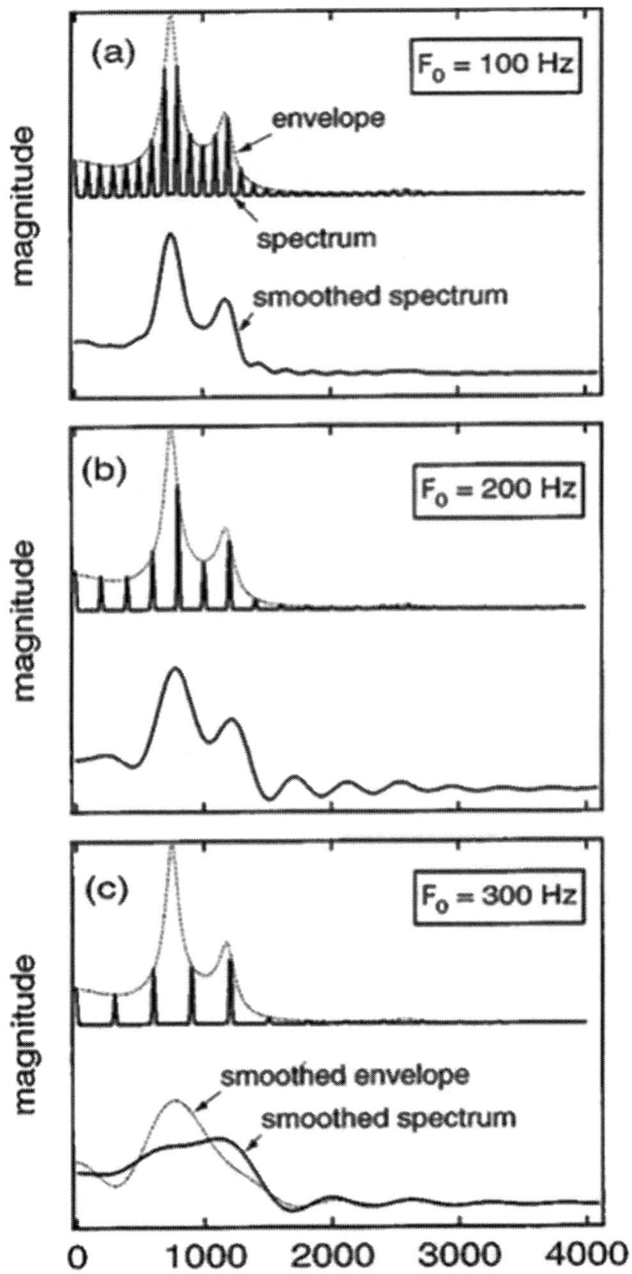

Figure 9.7 (a) Top: envelope (dotted line) and short-term magnitude spectrum of /ɑ/ at $f_0=100$ Hz (full line). Bottom: Smoothed short-term spectrum. Smoothing was performed by taking the Fourier transform of the magnitude spectrum, setting it to zero for lags larger than the Nyquist lag $T_0=1/2f_0$ (5 ms), and taking the inverse Fourier transform. The smoothed spectrum consists entirely of components below the Nyquist lag. (b) Same, at $f_0=200$ Hz. Note the ripples with a period corresponding to the inverse of the Nyquist lag (2.5 ms) that indicate that aliasing is taking place. (c) Same, at $f_0=300$ Hz, with the addition of the smoothed spectral envelope (dotted curve at bottom). The spectral envelope was smoothed by removal of lag components beyond the Nyquist lag. The difference between smoothed envelope and smoothed spectrum is the result of aliasing.

Source: Figure and caption reprinted from de Cheveigné and Kawahara (1999).

A *narrow band pattern-matching model* developed by Hillenbrand and Houde (2003) has features in common with Cheveigné and Kawahara, but the model was also strongly influenced by Klatt's (1982) findings on the disproportionate influence of spectral peaks in relation to other features of the spectrum in controlling phonetic quality. As with de Cheveigné and Kawahara, inputs to the recognition model consist of unsmoothed narrow band spectra that are compared to a set of smooth templates for each vowel category. Figure 9.8 shows the signal processing steps[1] that are used to prepare input spectra, beginning with a 64-ms Fourier spectrum using linear amplitudes. This is followed by spectrum level normalization (SLN): a gain function is computed as the *inverse* of a 1266 Hz Gaussian-weighted running average. The Fourier spectrum is then multiplied by this gain function, increasing the spectrum level in low energy regions and vice versa, thereby reducing (but not eliminating) variation in formant-level relationships and overall spectral tilt. Next, a masking threshold is calculated as a 328 Hz Gaussian-weighted running average. The masking threshold is then subtracted from the level-normalized spectrum, *with values below the masking threshold set to zero*. The purpose of the masking operation is to emphasize higher energy components (which lie above the masking threshold), to eliminate or reduce the level of spectral components in between harmonics and in the valleys between formant peaks, and to further reduce variation in spectral tilt. The final step involves scaling the peak amplitude in each spectrum to a constant.

The reference patterns that define each vowel category consist of a sequence of smooth spectra (Figure 9.9). A sequence of spectra is used rather than associating each vowel

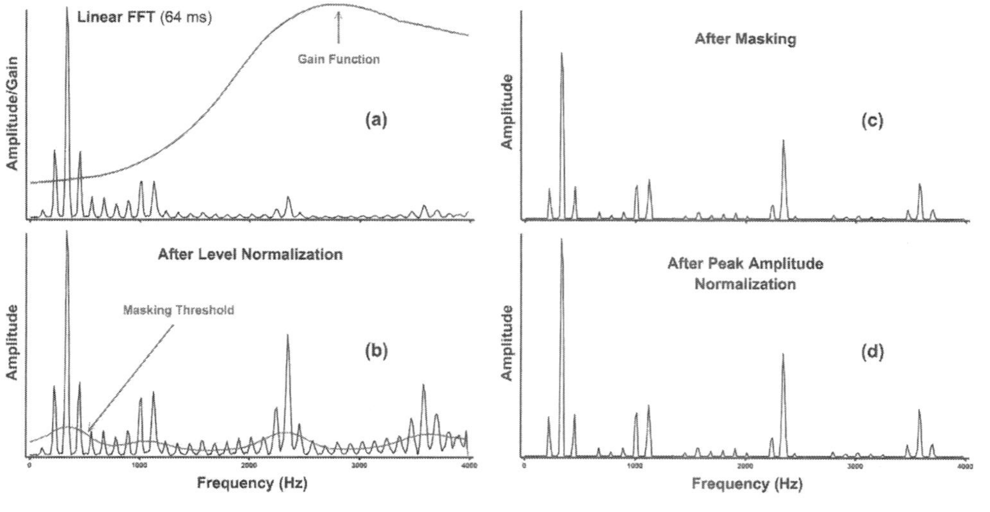

Figure 9.8 Signal processing steps used in the narrow band pattern matching model: (a) FFT computed over a 64-ms Hamming-windowed segment and broadband spectrum-level normalization (SLN) function computed as the inverse of a 1266-Hz Gaussian-weighted running average of spectral amplitudes; (b) spectrum after processing by the SLN operation and a masking (i.e., threshold) function computed as a 328-Hz Gaussian-weighted running average of spectral amplitudes; (c) spectrum after masking, i.e., after zeroing all spectral values that lie below the level of the masking function; and (d) amplitude normalization, implemented by scaling the largest peak in the spectrum to a constant.

Source: Redrawn from Hillenbrand and Houde (2003).

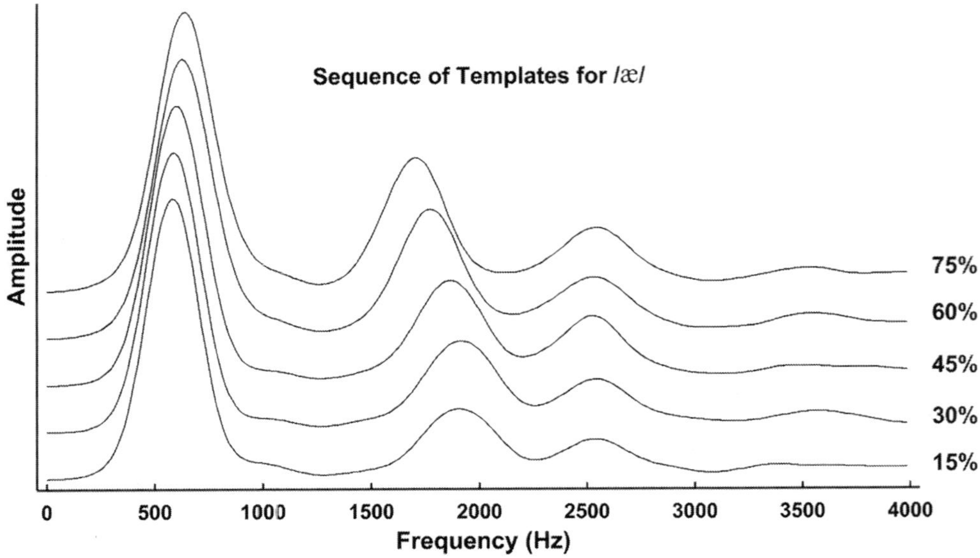

Figure 9.9 Sequence of five spectral shape templates for /æ/ computed at 15%, 30%, 45%, 60%, and 75% of vowel duration. The templates were derived by averaging the harmonic spectra of like vowels at similar times during the course of the vowel (e.g., 15%, 30%, . . .). Separate templates are computed for men, women, and children, based on an analysis of about 40 tokens per vowel category. The templates shown in this figure are from men. Note that successive templates have been offset on the amplitude scale so that the change in spectral shape over time can be seen more clearly.

Source: Reprinted from Hillenbrand and Houde (2003).

category with a single template because of the large body of evidence (discussed in the next section) implicating a significant role for spectral change in vowel perception. The templates are derived empirically simply by averaging the harmonic spectra of like vowels at similar times during the course of the vowel (e.g., 15%, 30%, . . .) – with each spectrum being processed using the steps that are illustrated in Figure 9.8 (i.e., SLN, masking, and peak amplitude normalization). Averaging is followed by light smoothing. Separate templates are computed for men, women, and children based on averaging about 40 tokens per vowel category.[2] Signals in the H95 database were used to create the templates, excluding the relatively small number of tokens with high identification error rates. Templates from the women's data for 6 of the 12 vowels sampled at 30% of vowel duration are shown in Figure 9.10. Note the merger of F_1 and F_2 in the /ɔ/ template and the merger of F_2 and F_3 in the /ɚ/ and /i/ templates. This means that the templates do not necessarily preserve formants in the traditional sense.

The recognition algorithm for a few vowel categories at a few time points is illustrated in Figure 9.11. The 256-point narrow band spectrum computed at 15% of vowel duration is subtracted point-for-point from each of the 12 vowel templates computed at that same time point (only four of which are shown here); the narrow band input spectrum at 30% of vowel duration (not shown) is then subtracted point-for-point from each the 12 vowel templates computed at 30% of vowel duration, and so on. It is important to note that spectral

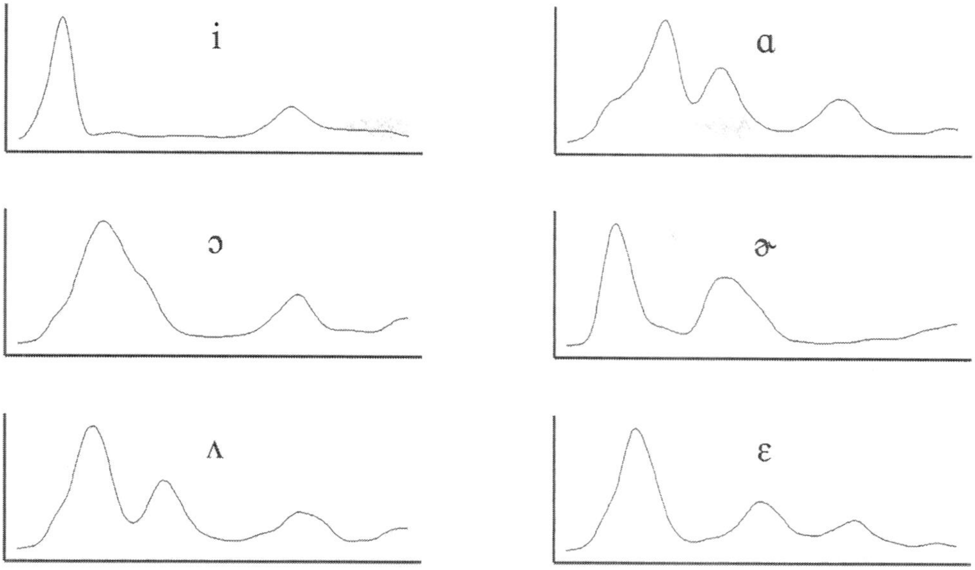

Figure 9.10 Vowel templates for women for 6 of the 12 vowels computed at 30% of vowel duration. The frequency scales are linear with a range of 0 to 4 kHz. Notice the merger of F_1 and F_2 for /ɔ/ and the merger of F_2 and F_3 for /ɚ/ and /i/.

differences are calculated at all 256 frequencies and not just at harmonic frequencies as in the de Cheveigné and Kawahara model. The vowel that is recognized is the template type (/i/, /ɪ/, . . .) that produces the smallest difference accumulated over the five time points (or two or three, or however many slices are used).

The recognition model was tested using the 139-talker, 1,668-token H95 database. The recognition rate averaged across all utterances was 91.4%, which compares with 95.6% intelligibility for the same signals.[3] Recognition rates were about two percentage points higher for the adults than the children, a pattern that was also shown by the listeners in H95. The confusion matrix resembled that of listeners (e.g., /ɑ/ was confused mainly with /ɔ/ and /ʌ/, /ɛ/ with /ɪ/ and /æ/, etc.), and individual tokens that were incorrectly recognized by the model tended to be the ones that were less intelligible to listeners.

The narrow band model was run (a) without SLN, (b) without masking, and (c) without either SLN or masking. Results were quite clear: Removal of SLN produced a modest drop of about two percentage points, while performance plunged from 91.4% to 59.9% with the removal of the masking operation. The dramatic drop in performance with the removal of masking reflects the importance of high-energy regions of the spectrum that are strongly emphasized through masking. Although the details of the recognition algorithm described here are quite different from Klatt's (1982) slope metric, both methods emphasize spectral peaks at the expense of other spectral details. It is not clear why the SLN produced such a modest improvement in performance, but the problem may well lie in the details of the implementation rather than the general concept.

In general, the narrow band model findings suggest the following: (a) Naturally spoken vowels can be recognized *directly* from narrow band spectra (i.e., without first recovering the envelope shape through smoothing); (b) vowels can be recognized accurately, and in

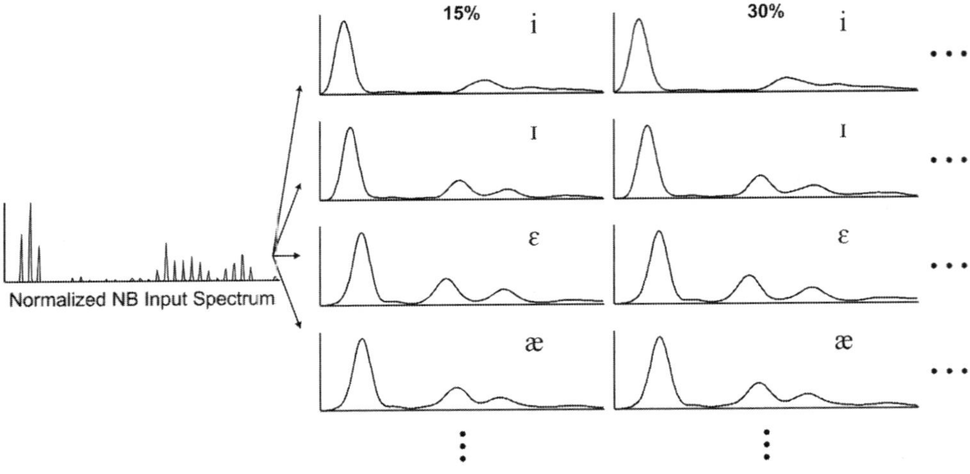

Figure 9.11 Illustration of the recognition algorithm used in the narrow band model. The narrow band spectrum computed at 15% of vowel duration is compared to the 12 vowel templates computed at the same time point (only four of which are shown here); the narrow band spectrum at 30% of vowel duration (not shown) is then compared to the 12 vowel templates computed at 30% of vowel duration, and so on.

Source: Redrawn from Hillenbrand and Houde (2003).

a way that generally resembles the behavior of listeners, without using formants; (c) accurate recognition is possible even when some of the templates do not preserve formants in the usual sense of the term; and (d) as in Klatt's (1982) study, recognition accuracy improves dramatically when steps are taken to emphasize the role of the spectral peaks that have been shown to have the greatest influence on judgments of phonetic quality. However, these peaks do not necessarily need to correspond to formants in the traditional sense.

The influence of spectral change on vowel perception

As discussed earlier, the acoustic measurements made by PB were sampled at a single time point at which the spectrum was judged by eye to be more-or-less stationary. It might be concluded from this measurement approach that investigators of that era made the tacit assumption that all of the information needed to identify a vowel was to be found in a single time slice. This view was summarized nicely by Tiffany (1953):

> It has been commonly assumed or implied that the essential physical specification of a vowel phoneme could be accomplished in terms of its acoustic spectrum as measured over a single fundamental period, or over a short interval including at most a few cycles of the fundamental frequency. That is to say, each vowel has been assumed to have a unique energy vs. frequency distribution, with the significant physical variables all accounted for by an essentially cross-sectional analysis of the vowel's harmonic composition.
>
> *(p. 290)*

Tiffany, however, questioned this assumption and suggested the possibility that changes in the spectrum throughout the course of a vowel may influence the percept. Similarly, in an early description of the PB vowels, Potter and Steinberg (1950) observed:

> It should be noted . . . that we are representing a vowel by a single spectrum taken during a particular small time interval in its duration. Actually, a vowel in the word situation . . . undergoes transitional movements from initial to final consonant. Not only does the spectrum of the vowel change with time, but the ear in identifying the word has the benefit of all of the changes.
>
> *(p. 815)*

Finally, the following statement is very nearly the last thing that PB say in their paper:

> It is present belief that the complex acoustical patterns represented by the words are not adequately represented by a single section, but require a more complex portrayal. The initial and final influences often shown in the bar movements of the spectrogram are of importance here. The evaluation of these changing bar patterns . . . is, of course, a problem of major importance in the study of the fundamental information bearing elements of speech.
>
> *(p. 184)*

In light of the early awareness of the potential importance of spectral change in characterizing vowels – clearly stated by several investigators in papers that received a good deal of attention – it is surprising that this issue did not receive much attention for many years. But despite the late start, there is now a significant body of evidence (mainly for the North American English vowels that have been most heavily studied) showing that spectral movement plays an important role in vowel perception. Evidence supporting this conclusion comes from several sources, including: (a) Measurement and pattern recognition studies showing that individual North American English (NAE) vowels have distinctive spectral change patterns, and that incorporation of this dynamic information in pattern recognition models significantly improves classification accuracy; (b) listening studies with excised signals showing that stationary targets are *not necessary* for vowels to be recognized accurately; and (c) listening studies with static vowels showing that stationary targets are *not sufficient* for accurate vowel recognition.

Spectral change 1: Measurement and pattern recognition

The top panel of Figure 9.12 shows average formant frequencies measured at the beginnings and ends of ten vowel types spoken in isolation by five men and five women from Western Canada (Nearey and Assmann, 1986). The bottom panel of this figure shows similar data from 12 vowel types in /hVd/ syllables spoken by 45 men from southern Michigan and other areas of the inland north (Hillenbrand et al., 1995; data from the H95 women and children show similar patterns). There are clearly some dialect-related differences between the two datasets, but also many similarities. There are a few vowels – mainly /i/ and /u/ – that show very little spectral movement, but most of the vowels show substantial diphthong-like changes over the course of the vowel, patterns that have been referred to as *vowel inherent spectral change* (VISC; Nearey and Assmann, 1986). The phonetic diphthongs /e/ and /o/ show precisely the kinds of spectral movements that are expected, but the degree

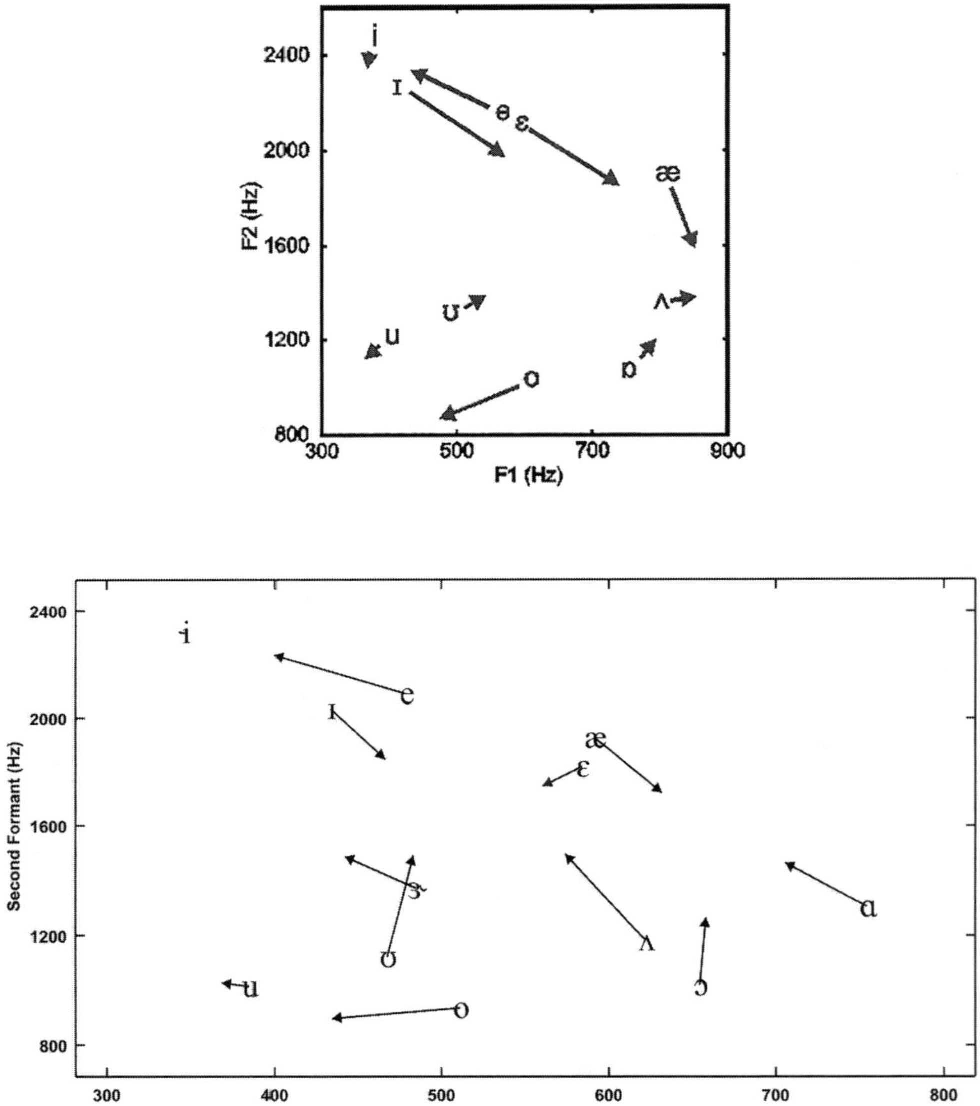

Figure 9.12 Top panel: Formant frequencies measured at the beginnings and ends of ten Western Canadian vowel types spoken in isolation by five men and five women (Nearey and Assmann, 1986). Arrow heads in both panels indicate vowel offsets. Bottom panel: Formant frequencies measured at the beginnings and ends of 12 American English vowel types in /hVd/ syllables (Hillenbrand et al., 1995). The utterances were spoken by 45 men.

Source: The top panel is reprinted from Nearey and Assmann (1986); the bottom panel is redrawn from Hillenbrand et al. (1995).

of spectral change shown for these two sounds is not unusual in relation to several of the nominally monophthongal vowels in both sets of data (see especially /ɪ/, /ɛ/, and /æ/ in the Western Canada data and all but a few of the vowel types in the Michigan data). The obvious possibility that is suggested by these measurements is that individual vowel types in the fairly crowded English vowel space are rendered more distinctive by differences in spectral change patterns. For example, in the Michigan data /æ/ is raised and fronted, creating a high degree of overlap between /æ/ and /ɛ/ when represented in static formant space (Figure 9.4). However, listeners in H95 showed an error rate of just 5% for these vowels, suggesting that the distinctive spectral change patterns (along with duration differences, which will be discussed later) enhance the intelligibility of these vowels. A similar role for spectral change is suggested for /ɪ/ and /e/, another pair of vowels that show a good deal of overlap in static formant space but show spectral change patterns that are quite different from one another (compare Figure 9.4 with the lower panel of Figure 9.12).

Evidence from pattern recognition studies shows conclusively that vowels can be classified with greater accuracy using features sets that incorporate spectral change as compared to otherwise comparable classification models that rely on measurements from a single time slice. For example, Zahorian and Jagharghi (1993) used a statistical pattern recognizer to classify nine vowel types in CVC syllables spoken by ten men, ten women, and ten children in the environment of nine initial consonants and eight final consonants (not fully crossed). The recognition algorithm was driven by features consisting of either formant frequencies or a discrete cosine transform representation of spectral shape. For both formant and spectral-shape features, the authors reported much better classification accuracy, and better agreement with listener data, when the classifier was driven by dynamic rather than static feature vectors. (They also reported better performance with spectral shape than formants.)

Similarly, using various combinations of f_0 and formants as features (e.g., F_1-F_2, F_1-F_2-F_3, f_0, F_1-F_2, etc.), H95 reported consistently better classification accuracy when the formant pattern was sampled twice (at 20% and 80% of vowel duration) than otherwise comparable models sampled once at steady-state (Table 9.2). Incorporating a third sample of the feature vectors at 50% of vowel duration produced little or no improvement in classification performance. A very similar finding using a different recognition model was reported by Hillenbrand and Houde (2003). These findings are consistent with the idea that listeners evaluate VISC based primarily on vowel onsets and offsets – the *dual-target model* proposed by Nearey and Assmann (1986).

A consistent advantage for dynamic rather than static features was also found in Hillenbrand et al. (2001) for formants measured from CVC syllables spoken by six men and six women using all combinations of seven initial consonants, eight vowel types, and six final consonants. As Stevens and House (1963) showed in a study using only symmetrical

Table 9.2 Accuracy in categorizing vowels using a quadratic discriminant classifier trained on one, two, or three samples of various combinations of f_0 and formant frequencies. From Hillenbrand et al. (1995).

Parameters	*1 sample*	*2 samples*	*3 samples*
F_1, F_2	76.1	90.3	90.4
F_1, F_2 and F_3	84.6	92.7	93.1
f_0, F_1, F_2	82.0	92.5	92.6
f_0, F_1, F_2 and F_3	87.8	94.1	94.8

consonant environments (/bVb/, /dVd/, /gVg/, etc.), there are many statistically reliable effects of consonant environment on vowel formants. In both studies, two of these effects were large (upward shifts in F_2 of ~500–700 Hz for /u/ and ~200–250 Hz for /ʊ/ in the environment of initial – but not final – alveolars), but most of the effects were not especially large in absolute terms. It is possible that complications due to these context effects would attenuate or even eliminate the performance advantage for dynamic feature sets. However, in Hillenbrand et al. (2001), pattern classification accuracy for features measured from these heterogeneous syllable types was consistently better with two rather than one sample of the formant pattern. The advantage in pattern classification accuracy, then, is not an artifact of simple, fixed consonant environments.

Spectral change 2: The non-essential nature of static targets

A series of experiments initially conducted at the University of Minnesota used a "silent center" technique to show conclusively that the static targets that might have been considered essential to the vowel percept were simply not needed. Shown in the top row of Figure 9.13, from Jenkins et al. (1983), are schematic representations of the original, naturally spoken /bVb/ syllables, with a shorter vowel on the left and a longer vowel on the right. In the middle row, the center 50% has been excised from the short vowel and the center 65% has been excised from the long vowel, leaving only the onsets and offsets. In the bottom row, the onsets and offsets have been edited out, leaving the center 50% (left) or 65% (right) of the syllable. Results of listening tests were unambiguous: the silent center signals were identified as well (92.4%) as the original utterances (93.1%); i.e., removal of the vowel centers had no measurable effect on vowel intelligibility. The variable centers were also well identified, with no statistically reliable differences among the identification rates for the three conditions.

A follow-up study by Nearey and Assmann (1986) excised 30-ms Hamming-windowed segments from isolated (but not static) vowels at 24% of vowel duration (nucleus) and at 64% of vowel duration (offglide). Listeners were asked to identify: (a) the unedited vowels, (b) the nucleus followed by the offglide, with 10 ms of silence separating the clips, (c) the nucleus segment repeated, and (d) the nucleus and offglide segments played in reverse order. Nearey and Assmann found that excised segments that were presented in natural order were as intelligible as the unedited vowels. However, error rates more than doubled for the repeated-nucleus and reverse-order conditions. The poor intelligibility of the reverse-order signals indicates that the key factor is not the presence vs. absence of spectral change, but rather a pattern of spectral change matching that which is typical of the vowel type that is being uttered. (For additional experimental work on excised vowels – all of it interesting – see Andruski and Nearey, 1992; Jenkins and Strange, 1999; Parker and Diehl, 1984; Strange, 1989; Strange et al., 1994).

Spectral change 3: The insufficiency of static targets

There is convincing evidence from several sources indicating that, for NAE vowels, very high identification rates of the kind reported by PB and H95 cannot be achieved using vowels with static spectral patterns. The most striking demonstration comes from a remarkable study by Fairbanks and Grubb (1961), who went to extraordinary lengths to record the highest quality and most representative examples of the nine static, sustained vowels that they studied (the vowel types studied by PB, excluding /ɚ/). A brief excerpt from a

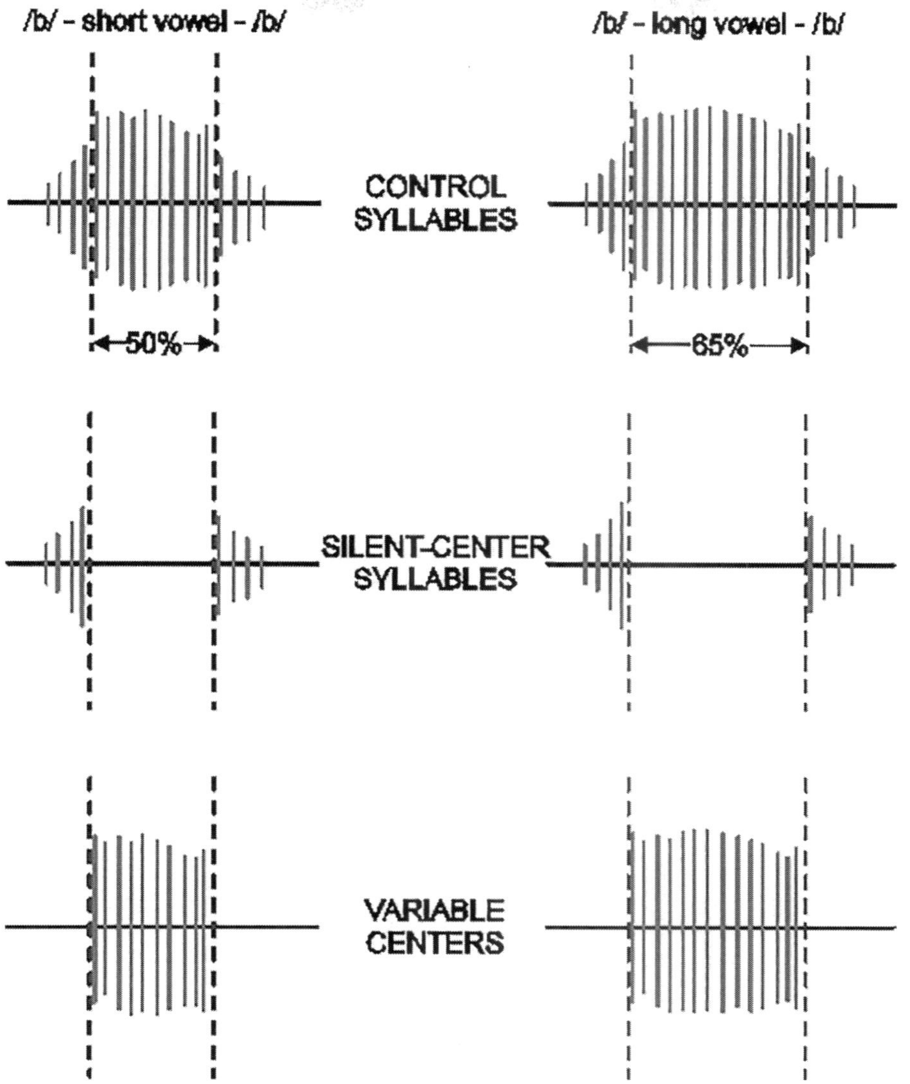

Figure 9.13 Control, silent-center, and variable-center conditions from Jenkins et al. (1983).

Source: Reprinted from Jenkins et al. (1983).

lengthy set of instructions that was given to their talkers will give the reader some idea of the extraordinary lengths to which the experimenters went to record prototypical instances of each vowel:

> Essentially what we are trying to do is to collect samples of each vowel that are as nearly typical or representative of that vowel as possible. More specifically, we are interested in samples that depict the central tendency of each vowel. . . . Another way of putting the problem is to say what we want you to do is to imagine the target on the basis of your experience in listening to speech, and then demonstrate what the target is

> by producing a vowel of your own that hits the target as you imagine it. You will understand from this that we are trying to get samples that are something more than merely acceptable and identifiable.
>
> *(p. 204)*

The seven talkers were all men, all phonetically trained, and all were faculty in the Speech and Hearing Department at the University of Illinois. Utterances were immediately auditioned by an experimenter, and talkers often recorded several tokens before an utterance was accepted. The full set of recordings was then auditioned a second time and talkers were asked to return to the lab to re-record any utterances that were judged by the experimenters to be unsatisfactory. The vowels were typically 1–2 s long and were intended to have stationary pitch and timbre; 300-ms segments were then excised from these recordings for presentation to listeners, who consisted of eight phonetically trained graduate students in the same department.

With that lengthy introduction to Fairbanks and Grubb, the results were quite simple: Despite the exacting procedures used by the experimenters to record the highest quality and most representative examples of each utterance, the average intelligibility was just 74.0% – more than 20 percentage points lower than the intelligibility of the /hVd/ utterances recorded by PB and H95, which were spoken by 76 untrained talkers (men, women, and children), and without the elaborate auditioning procedure used by Fairbanks and Grubb. Further, in PB the test signals were identified in a large auditorium by listeners with no phonetics training. Fairbanks and Grubb reported a good deal of variability in the intelligibility of individual vowel types, and these variations are revealing: the highest intelligibility (~91–92%) for these static vowels was seen for /i/ and /u/, vowels that tend to show the least spectral movement (see Figure 9.9). Much lower intelligibility (~53–66%) was reported for vowels that tend to show a good deal of spectral change for speakers in the Inland North (e.g., /ɪ/, /æ/, and /ʌ/). In addition to the static nature of the recordings, the absence of duration variability in the Fairbanks and Grubb vowels almost certainly contributed to the modest intelligibility of the utterances. Experimental work on the role of duration in vowel perception will be discussed in a separate section later in this chapter.

Evidence for the insufficiency of static targets also comes from Hillenbrand and Gayvert (1993), who used a formant synthesizer to generate 300-ms static versions of all 1,520 signals in the PB database using measured values of f_0 and F_1, F_2 and F_3. The average intelligibility of these static signals was 72.7%. Once again, this figure is more than 20 percentage points lower than the intelligibility of the original /hVd/ signals, and is quite similar to the value reported by Fairbanks and Grubb for their static vowels. Further, static vowels such as /i/ and /u/ tended to be identified much better (96.2% and 89.1%, respectively) than vowel types that typically show more spectral change. Findings leading to the same basic conclusion were reported by Hillenbrand and Nearey (1999), who asked listeners to identify three versions of 300 /hVd/ syllables drawn from the H95 recordings: (a) a naturally spoken signal (NAT), (b) an original-formant (OF) synthetic version of the same signal generated from the measured formant contours; and (c) a flat-formant (FF) version generated with formants fixed at the values measured at steady-state (Figure 9.14). Results for the critical OF–FF comparison were not subtle: The 88.5% average intelligibility for the OF signals dropped to 73.8% when the formants were flattened. It is striking how similar the intelligibility figures are for the static signals from Fairbanks and Grubb (74.0%), Hillenbrand and Gayvert (72.7%), and Hillenbrand and Nearey (73.8%). Further, as shown by both Fairbanks and Grubb and Hillenbrand and Gayvert, static vowels that typically show relatively

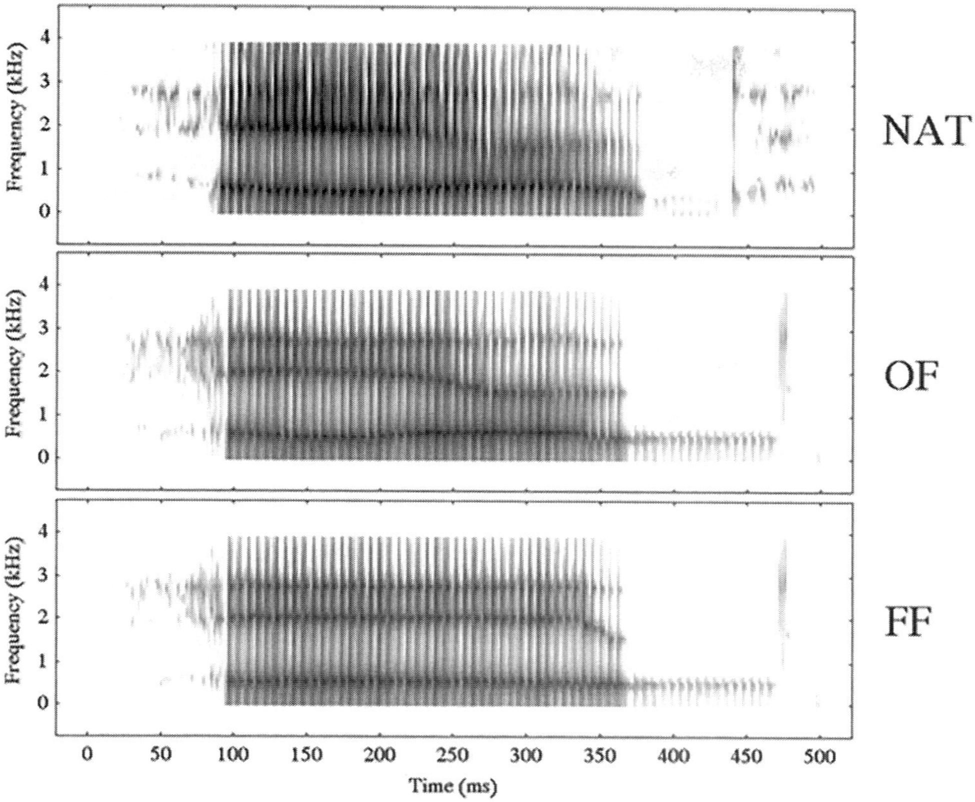

Figure 9.14 Three stimulus conditions from Hillenbrand and Nearey (1999). NAT: A naturally spoken /hVd/ syllable. OF: A formant-synthesized version of the same signal generated from the original measured formant contours. FF: A formant-synthesized version generated with formants fixed at the values measured at steady-state.

Source: Redrawn from Hillenbrand and Nearey (1999).

little spectral change are identified better than vowels that typically show more spectral change (Figure 9.15).

Although it is not relevant to the spectral change issue that is being discussed in this section, it is of some interest to note that the naturally spoken signals were significantly more intelligible (95.4%) than the OF formant-synthesized versions (88.5%). This difference of about seven percentage points, which is not trivial, is consistent with Bladon's (1982) *reductionism* argument against formant representations, the idea that formant representations discard information that may prove to be phonetically relevant.

In summary, a large body of evidence indicates that NAE vowels are better thought of as distinctive trajectories through acoustic-phonetic space rather than points in that space. In spite of this evidence, accumulated over several decades, the long-standing practice of characterizing vowels as points in acoustic-phonetic space rather than trajectories though that space remains exceedingly common. As we argue in Hillenbrand (2013), these static representations are not so much wrong as they are incomplete.

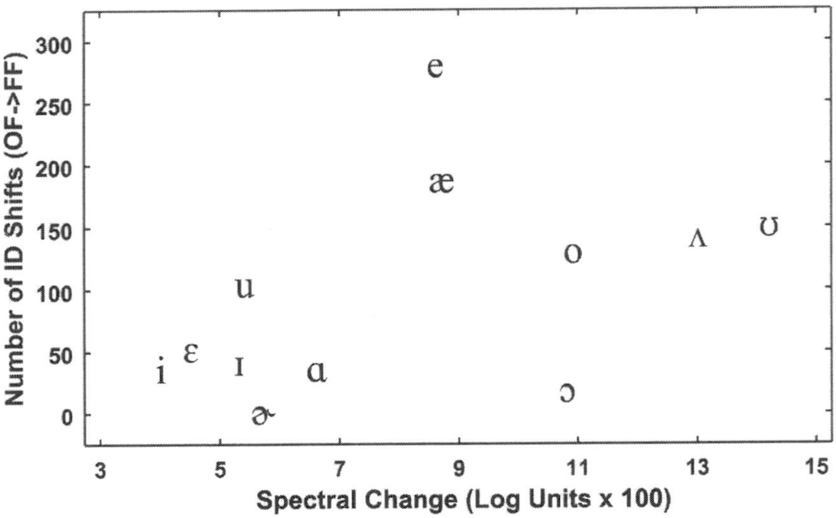

Figure 9.15 Total number of correct-to-incorrect changes in identification (OF to FF) as a function of the average magnitude of formant frequency change for each vowel. The magnitude of formant change for each vowel category was represented as the average length of a vector connecting formant measurements sampled at 20% and 80% of vowel duration. The vector was drawn in a three-dimensional space consisting of log-transformed values of F_1, F_2, and F_3.

Source: Redrawn from Hillenbrand and Nearey (1999).

The role of duration in vowel perception

There is good evidence that listeners make use of duration in identifying vowels, although there is less than perfect agreement on the details. The main source of the influence of duration on vowel identification can be seen in Table 9.3, which lists average durations and duration ratios for pairs of adjacent English vowels measured from connected speech by Crystal and House (1988). Generally similar findings have been reported for other kinds of speech material (e.g., Black 1949; van Santen, 1992; Hillenbrand et al., 1995). Most pattern recognition studies have shown better classification accuracy when duration is added to spectral parameter sets. Counterexamples include Zahorian and Jagharghi (1993), who reported non-significant improvements in classification accuracy of less than 1% when duration was added to spectral feature sets consisting of either formant frequencies or spectral shape. Watson and Harrington's (1999) study of Australian English vowels showed a small improvement in classification accuracy when duration was added to formant measurements, although the duration effect was seen mainly for diphthongs rather than monophthongs. In contrast, H95 reported consistent improvements in the accuracy of a quadratic discriminant classifier in recognizing vowels in /hVd/ syllables when duration measures were added to feature sets consisting of various combinations of f_0 and F_1, F_2 and F_3. Especially large improvements were seen for the /æ/–/ɛ/ pair. Similarly, Hillenbrand et al. (2000) reported modest but consistent improvements in classification accuracy with the addition of duration to parameter sets consisting of various combinations of f_0 and formant frequencies. The test signals consisted of CVC syllables formed by seven initial consonants, eight vowels, and six final consonants in all combinations spoken by six men and six women.

Table 9.3 Pairs of adjacent American English vowels that differ in inherent duration. Average duration ratios are shown in parentheses. Measurements were made from vowels in stressed syllables in connected speech (Crystal and House, 1988).

/e/	>	/ɪ/	(1.81)
/i/	>	/ɪ/	(1.59)
/æ/	>	/ɛ/	(1.50)
/u/	>	/ʊ/	(1.48)
/a/	>	/ʌ/	(1.36)
/e/	>	/ɛ/	(1.28)
/ɔ/	>	/ɑ/	(1.06)

Evidence that is more convincing than these pattern recognition studies comes from perceptual experiments in which listeners are asked to identify utterances in which vowel duration was directly manipulated. For example, Tiffany (1953) recorded 12 vowel types as long sustained vowels, which were later excised at four durations (80 ms, 200 ms, 500 ms, and 8 s). Several of Tiffany's findings were consistent with the idea that duration plays a role in vowel identification. For example, vowels with long inherent durations, such as /e/ and /ɑ/, were more likely to be correctly identified when presented at long durations, and vice versa for vowels such as /ɪ/ and /ʊ/ with short inherent durations. Stevens (1959) synthesized CVC syllables with the vowels /i/, /ɪ/, /ɛ/, /æ/, /u/, /ʊ/, /ʌ/, and /ɑ/ at durations between 25 ms and 400 ms. There were several effects that were consistent with Tiffany's findings and with the duration data in Table 9.3. For example, at short durations, vowels similar to /æ/ or /ɛ/ were heard more often as /ɛ/, and vowels similar to /ɑ/ or /ʌ/ tended to be heard as /ʌ/. However, the effect of duration on the identification of the /i/–/ɪ/ and /u/–/ʊ/ pairs was much weaker. (See also related work by Ainsworth, 1972, and the somewhat equivocal findings of Huang, 1986).

The experimental work discussed to this point used synthesized vowels that did not incorporate natural VISC patterns. It is now well established that the identity of NAE vowels is not conveyed well to listeners when spectral change patterns are not preserved, suggesting the possibility that the more ambiguous spectral properties of the static vowels that were used in early work may have invited greater reliance on duration, thereby overestimating its influence. Hillenbrand et al. (2000) synthesized 300 /hVd/ signals that were closely modeled on naturally spoken utterances drawn from H95. The synthesizer, which has features in common with McAuley and Quatieri (1986), is similar in general conception to inverse Fourier synthesis, with two major exceptions: (a) Phase relationships are not preserved and, more important, (b) sinusoidal components are synthesized only for (narrow band) spectral peaks, regardless of whether they are harmonic or inharmonic. The intelligibility of signals that are synthesized with this method is quite good, and duration can be artificially shortened or lengthened simply by analyzing the signal at one frame rate and synthesizing the signal at a different frame rate (e.g., duration can be increased by a factor of 1.5 by analyzing a signal with an 8-ms frame rate and synthesizing it at a 12-ms frame rate). When this method is used to alter the duration of a signal, the result is a pair of signals with the same sequence of spectra from one frame to the next, but the rate at which the spectra evolve over time is different from one duration condition to another. The vowels of 300 /hVd/ signals were synthesized: (a) at their original measured duration (OD), within the limits of the 8-ms frame rate that was used; (b) at a short duration (SD) of 144 ms (two standard deviations below the grand mean of all vowel durations); (c) at a long duration (LD) of 400 ms (two standard deviations above the grand mean); and (d) at a neutral duration (ND) of 272 ms, the grand mean of all vowel durations. Durations were modified during the vowel only and not during the /h/ and /d/ segments.

Table 9.4 shows the average intelligibility scores from 14 listeners. The 96.0% intelligibility for the OD signals is quite close to the 95.4% value reported by H95 for the full set of naturally spoken /hVd/ signals, indicating that the synthesis method preserves vowel identity. Artificially shortening or lengthening resulted in nearly symmetrical decreases in intelligibility of 4.6 and 5.1 percentage points, respectively. The ND condition, which did not prove to be very revealing, showed a modest drop of 1.9 percentage points.

The ~5% average drop in intelligibility resulting from either shortening or lengthening is not particularly revealing by itself since this figure is arrived at by averaging some cases in which pairs and clusters of vowels were strongly affected by duration with other cases in which duration effects that might have been expected almost never occurred. Confusion matrices were assembled that focused on instances in which the OD version of an utterance was identified correctly, but the SD or LD version was heard as some other vowel (e.g., the OD version might be correctly heard as /æ/ but the SD version as /ɛ/). Table 9.5 summarizes the most frequent labeling shifts resulting from shortening and lengthening. The most common identification shifts resulting from vowel shortening consisted of OD versions of /ɔ/ shifting to either /ɑ/ or /ʌ/, and /æ/ shifting to /ɛ/. As the table shows, the effects of vowel lengthening are nearly the mirror image of those for shortening. These findings, of course, are predictable based on the measurement data from studies such as Crystal and House (1988). However, conspicuously absent from this table are instances of shortened /i/ shifting to /ɪ/ (0.6%) or shortened /u/ shifting to /ʊ/ (0.0%) – in spite of large and reliable differences in typical duration for these pairs. The same was true for lengthened signals; e.g., lengthened /ɪ/ almost never shifted to /i/ (0.1%) and lengthened /ʊ/ rarely shifted to /u/ (1.3%). These findings indicate quite clearly that there is more going on with listeners' use (and non-use) of duration information than statistical learning based on the magnitude and reliability of measured duration differences in natural speech. As a simple illustration of this point, Crystal and House (1988) reported an inherent duration ratio of just 1.06 for /ɔ/:/ɑ/, but vowel shortening resulted in 41 /ɔ/→/ɑ/ shifts (14%). On the other hand, there were almost no shifts between /i/ and /ɪ/, despite an inherent duration ratio of 1.59, and *no* /u/–/ʊ/ shifts in spite of an inherent duration ratio of 1.48.

An account of these findings was offered suggesting that very little weight is given to duration for pairs such as /i/–/ɪ/ and /u/–/ʊ/ because these vowels can be identified with

Table 9.4 Average recognition rates for the four duration conditions (OD = original duration, ND = neutral duration, SD = short duration, LD = long duration). Standard deviations across listeners are shown in parentheses.

Duration	
Condition	*Intelligibility*
OD	96.0 (2.7)
SD	91.4 (5.2)
LD	90.9 (3.3)
ND	94.1 (2.9)

Table 9.5 The most frequent changes in vowel identity resulting from either vowel shortening or vowel lengthening. The percentages in the column to the right reflect the number of shifts in vowel identity (OD → SD or OD → LD) divided by the number of opportunities for such shifts to occur.

Effects of Vowel Shortening	
Vowel Shift	*Percentage*
/ɔ/ → /a/ or /ʌ/	43.0
/æ/→ /ɛ/	20.7
/a/→/ʌ /	9.4
Effects of Vowel lenghthening	
Vowel Shift	*Percentage*
/ʌ/ → /a/ or /ɔ/	36.0
/ɛ/ → /æ/	18.9

minimal ambiguity based on spectral information alone. On the other hand, /ɔ/ cannot be as reliably distinguished from /ɑ/ and /ʌ/, or /æ/ from /ɛ/, based solely on spectral information, increasing listeners' reliance on duration to identify these vowels. To test this idea, a statistical pattern classifier was trained on: (a) f_0, (b) two samples of F_1, F_2 and F_3 (at 20% and 80% of vowel duration), and (c) the original, measured duration values. The classifier was then tested using the same spectral measurements but durations that were either short or long by two standard deviations, as simulations of the SD and LD listening conditions. The pattern classifier produced vowel confusions that shared many features with the listener data in Table 9.5, such as large numbers of shifts in recognition involving /ɔ, ɑ, ʌ/ and /æ–ɛ/ but very few shifts involving /i/–/ɪ/ or /u/–/ʊ/.

In summary, duration plays a measurable role in vowel identification. The magnitude of the effect is a modest 5% averaged across all vowels, but the influence of this cue varies quite substantially across different pairs and clusters of vowels. Further, the weight that listeners give to duration appears to depend not only on the magnitude of measured differences in inherent duration for a given vowel pair but also on how accurately individual vowel types can be identified based on spectral information alone.

There is undoubtedly a good deal more to be learned about how listeners make use of duration in identifying vowels. The focus of this work has been on simple utterances such as isolated vowels or citation-form words. The role of duration in connected speech is less certain since it is well known that there is a large set of factors that influence segment duration in conversational speech. As discussed in Klatt's (1976) comprehensive review, the factors affecting segment duration run the gamut from global dimensions such as speaking rate to word- and phrase-final lengthening to lexical and sentential stress to phonetic details such as the influence of final-consonant voicing on the duration of the preceding vowel. Coming to some understanding of how listeners make use of duration in identifying vowels in the presence of this large and diverse set of competing factors that influence segment duration is a worthy topic for future work on this topic, though it is not likely to be an especially easy problem to address.

Talker normalization and frequency scaling

The acoustic characteristics of vowels (and other speech sounds) differ from one talker to the next, even when dialect is held constant, yet listeners typically have little difficulty recognizing speech across variation in talker characteristics. There is a long history of inquiry into the perceptual and cognitive mechanisms that might be involved in listeners' accommodation to variation in the characteristics of individual talkers. The literature in this area is vast, so it will be possible in this section to review just a sampling of the work on this problem. Ainsworth (1975) distinguishes intrinsic and extrinsic normalization processes. Intrinsic schemes derive normalizing information entirely from the to-be-recognized token.[4] With extrinsic normalization, calibrating information is derived from other speech sounds uttered by the same talker.

Intrinsic normalization

Many intrinsic normalization schemes have been proposed over the years. As Miller (1989) pointed out, many of these models are closely related to the *relative resonance* or *formant ratio* theory proposed by Lloyd in the late 19th century (e.g., Lloyd, 1890, 1892). Lloyd, who based his theory in large part on the central role that is played by frequency ratios in music, proposed that vowels with similar timbres have similar formant ratios. Lloyd's version of relative resonance theory is appealing in many respects, with the most significant virtue lying in the substantial reduction in variability that formant ratios produce when like vowels are spoken by talkers differing in sex or age (e.g., see Minifie, 1973, Figure 7.15). Formant ratio theory, however, is not without problems. The most important of these problems is the fact that there are pairs and clusters of vowels with distinct qualities but very similar formant ratios: e.g., /ɑ/-/ɔ/ and /u/-/ʊ/-/æ/.

A particularly influential model proposed by Miller (1984, 1989) uses three spectral distances: $\log F_3 - \log F_2$, $\log F_2 - \log F_1$, and $\log F_3 - \log SR$, where SR (sensory reference) is a transform of the fundamental frequency ($SR = 168/(f_0/168)^{1/3}$). The log formant differences, of course, are fully equivalent to Lloyd's formant ratios. The virtue of the third spectral difference is that vowel pairs with similar F_1–F_2 ratios (e.g., /ɑ/-/ɔ/ and /u/-/ʊ/) can be distinguished based on distinct distances between F_1 and f_0, addressing the most important problem with Lloyd's scheme. Miller tested his model using 435 utterances that were taken from several databases. Using hand-drawn "perceptual target zones" that were fit to the data by eye, Miller reported that vowel types could be recognized with 93% accuracy.

Many other versions of formant ratio theory have been proposed over the years, although as Miller (1989) points out, many of these authors do not appear to have been aware of Lloyd's early work. A model proposed by Syrdal (1985; Syrdal and Gopal, 1986) shares many features with Miller's model, except that spectral distances are calculated using the Bark scale rather than logs. The three parameters in this model are B_3–B_2 (B_3 = bark-transformed F_3, etc.), B_2–B_1, and B_1–B_0. Using measurements from PB and a linear discriminant classifier, Syrdal and Gopal reported a recognition rate of 85.7%. While this figure is substantially lower than the 94.5% intelligibility shown by PB's listeners, at least some of this difference is almost certainly related to the static nature of the PB measurements.

Disner (1980) argued that normalization methods should not only maximize differences between phonetically distinct vowel types, they should also minimize differences in the same vowel type spoken by different talkers. Syrdal (1985) evaluated this criterion by measuring the performance of a linear discriminant model in classifying the PB tokens by talker group (men vs. women vs. children), reasoning that an ideal normalization method would make it difficult to classify tokens of the same vowel type spoken by different talker groups. Syrdal found that the model was very good at classifying tokens by talker group when trained and tested on f_0 and F_1, F_2 and F_3 in Hz (89.9%), but classification accuracy for talker group fell to 41.7% when Bark spectral differences were used. The 41.7% correct identification figure for talker group is clearly above the ~33% that would be expected by chance, but Syrdal argued that at least some component of the above-chance performance might reflect dialect differences across the three talker groups (e.g., Byrd, 1992). However, the main point is that the Bark spectral difference representation was much better than absolute linear frequencies at minimizing differences across talker group. A large number of other intrinsic normalization schemes related to the formant-ratio concept have been proposed over the years. Of particular importance are thoughtful schemes described by Peterson (1961) and Nearey (1978, 1992; Nearey et al., 1979).

The work on intrinsic normalization discussed earlier consisted entirely of modeling studies. Modeling studies can be useful in suggesting logically possible perceptual mechanisms, but listening studies are needed to evaluate their validity. Of special interest is the question of whether listener judgments of vowel identity are, in fact, affected by f_0. There is no question that f_0 exerts a measurable effect on vowel identification, although the details are anything but simple. An early study of static, synthetic vowels by Miller (1953) reported an upward shift in F_1 of 80 Hz (16%) on an /ʊ/-/ʌ/ continuum as a result of doubling f_0 from 130 to 260 Hz. A much smaller shift of 30 Hz (6%) in the F_1 boundary was seen for the same one-octave f_0 change on an /ɪ/-/ɛ/ continuum. Among many other results of this kind, Fujisaki and Kawashima (1968) found a 14% F_1 shift for a one-octave change in f_0 for an /u/-/e/ continuum and a 21% shift for /o/-/ɑ/.

Using a different approach, Ryalls and Lieberman (1982) synthesized static versions of nine vowel types with formants set to the average values for PB's men and with f_0 set to (a) an average value (135 Hz), (b) a lower-than-average value (100 Hz, 5.2 semitones lower than the average value), or (c) a much higher than average value (250 Hz, 10.7 semitones higher than the average value). The authors reported no increase in the identification error rate when f_0 was decreased from 135 to 100 Hz, but an f_0 increase from 135 to 250 Hz produced significantly more identification errors. It is not entirely clear how this finding should be interpreted since, among other considerations, the increase in pitch from the average value to the high value was substantially greater than the decrease from the average value to the low value. A second experiment used average formant frequencies for PB's women. For reasons that are not entirely clear, the same three f_0 conditions (100, 135, and 250 Hz) were used for the women's signals as well. Results for these signals, which are not described in much detail, showed a higher error rate for the 250 Hz signals (inferential statistics are not reported for experiment 2). This finding is a bit surprising since the 250 Hz condition is only slightly higher than the 224 Hz average f_0 reported for PB's women. The main conclusion reached by the authors is that the error rate increased for the high f_0 condition because formants (or perhaps the envelope shape) are more poorly specified at higher f_0s due to the wider harmonic spacing. It is not entirely clear what the findings of this study might have to say about the role of f_0 in intrinsic normalization (and that does not appear to have been their purpose). However, for Experiment 1, the failure to find a difference in error rate between the average and low f_0 conditions would seem to be at odds with models such as Miller (1989) and Syrdal and Gopal (1986) that include some transform of the distance between F_1 and f_0 as a determinant of vowel identity.

An issue that goes unaddressed in a fair amount of the work in this area is the very basic question of why f_0 should play any role at all in vowel identification. In acoustic terms, distinctions between one vowel and another are determined largely by the filter, so it is not immediately obvious why f_0 should play any role in the perception of vowel identity. The most common (but not sole) explanation for the influence of f_0 on vowel identification suggests that it is a psychological effect in which decision criteria are adjusted based on learned associations between f_0 and formants; i.e., higher f_0s lead listeners to expect higher formant frequencies and vice versa (e.g., Assmann and Nearey, 2008; but see Irino and Patterson, 2002; Patterson et al., 2008, for a very different explanation).[5] Scale factors that relate different talker groups are substantially larger for f_0 than they are for formants. Using the PB data, average scale factors relating men and women are 1.16–11.19 for the first three formants, but nearly an octave (1.71) for f_0. Nevertheless, average f_0 values are strongly correlated with average values for F_1, F_2, and F_3 (r = 0.82–0.87).

There is a good deal of evidence showing that vowels are less intelligible when typical relationships between f_0 and formants are altered. For example, Slawson (1968) showed that changes in the quality of synthetic vowels occur when f_0 is shifted by an octave while leaving the formants unchanged. However, the number of shifts in vowel identity was significantly reduced when an increase in formant frequencies of just 10% accompanied the one-octave f_0 shift.

The most complete set of findings on this problem come from a series of studies by Assmann and colleagues (Assmann and Nearey, 2007, 2008; Glidden and Assmann, 2004). For example, Assmann and Nearey (2008) used a high-quality source-filter synthesizer (Kawahara, 1997; Kawahara et al., 1999) to resynthesize vowels excised from /hVd/ syllables spoken by men, women, and children. The spectral envelope and f_0 were then manipulated alone or in combination. Identification accuracy declined with increases in either envelope or f_0; however, identification rates remained high when both f_0 and envelope were increased in a manner that is consistent with the observed correlation between f_0 and formants. As Assmann and Nearey note, "performance is poorest in conditions where the formant pattern and f_0 violate expected patterns in natural speech" (p. 3205). A second experiment using utterances resynthesized from men, women, and children produced generally similar findings. While men's vowels were more vulnerable to downward frequency shifts and children's vowels were more vulnerable to upward shifts, the basic finding remained the same as the experiment using only adult male talkers: Labeling performance declined as the frequency-shifted utterances moved further away from a regression line relating f_0 and formant frequency.

The experiments by Assmann and colleagues, along with a series of related experiments by Smith, Patterson, and colleagues (e.g., Smith et al., 2005, 2005; Smith et al., 2007; Patterson et al., 2008), which are not discussed here, are consistent with the idea that f_0 plays a role in intrinsic normalization. However, there remain aspects of this idea that are not at all straightforward. As noted earlier, the most common explanation for the f_0 effect is based on learned associations across talkers between average f_0 and average formants (or some as-yet unspecified measure of "envelope height" based on the shape of the envelope). However, in recognizing speech in real-time based on intrinsic factors, listeners must make use of f_0 and formants over some short time interval rather than average values of these parameters. The consequences of this simple observation are not trivial. For example, even when restricting our attention to citation-form syllables, correlations between f_0 and formants are not very strong; e.g., using the PB data, correlations between f_0 and formants calculated across vowel type are just 0.22, 0.28, and 0.57 for F_1, F_2 and F_3, respectively. Further, ordinary conversational speech spoken by a single talker shows variation in f_0 extending over as much as an octave (Lieberman, 1967). Nearey (1989) asked whether it is possible that talkers adjust F_1 as f_0 varies in order to maintain a more nearly constant F_1–f_0 distance. The evidence for this is not particularly strong (Syrdal and Steele, 1985). (For an unusually thoughtful discussion of this and other issues related to the possible role of both f_0 and F_3 in vowel identification, see Nearey, 1989).

Extrinsic normalization

The basic idea underlying extrinsic normalization is that vowels are identified not simply by determining the position of that vowel in acoustic-phonetic space but rather by determining the relationship between a to-be-recognized vowel and a *frame of reference* that is established by listening to other vowels spoken by that talker. This idea was proposed by Joos (1948), who noted:

> On first meeting a person, the listener hears a few vowel phones, and on the basis of this small but apparently sufficient evidence he swiftly constructs a fairly complete vowel pattern to serve as a background (coordinate system) upon which he correctly locates new phones as fast as he hears them.
>
> *(Joos, 1948, p. 61)*

The idea is illustrated in Figure 9.16 (modeled after Barreda, 2013). The left panel shows formant frequencies for a typical adult male (based on PB averages) while the right panel shows the same kind of data for a typical child. The dot in each panel is an unknown vowel with F_1 = 580 Hz and F_2 = 1220 Hz. It can be seen that the unknown vowel is quite close to /ʌ/ in relation to the man's vowels but close to /ʊ/ for the child. Evidence that is relevant to extrinsic normalization comes from both modeling studies that test the feasibility of various algorithms for identifying vowels using extrinsic normalization and, more directly, from

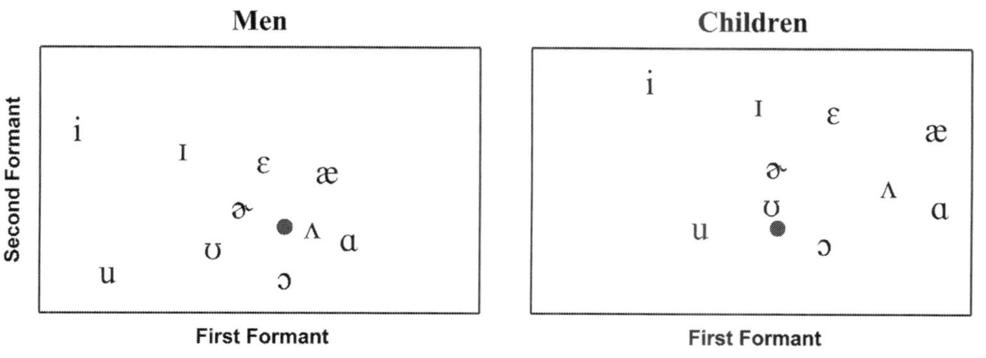

Figure 9.16 Average log-transformed formant frequency values for men (left) and children (right) based on the data from Peterson and Barney (1952). F_1 values vary between 270 and 1130 Hz and F_2 values vary between 845 and 3200 Hz. The dot in each figure represents a vowel of unknown identity with F_1 at 580 Hz and F_2 at 1220 Hz. If the vowel is recognized based on its relationship to each of the reference frames, it might be heard as /ʊ/ based on the reference frame on the left but /ʌ/ based on the reference frame on the right.

Source: The figure was modeled after Barreda (2013).

listening studies that seek to determine whether listeners appear to behave as though they are identifying vowels in relation to a frame of reference that is established by listening to other utterances spoken by a given talker.

A great deal of modeling work has been directed at developing extrinsic normalization methods. A small but reasonably representative sampling of this work will be described here. A widely cited method proposed by Gerstman (1968) for use in automatic speech recognition uses a simple linear rescaling of F_1 and F_2 values based on the minimum and maximum F_1 and F_2 values for each talker, independent of the vowel type that was spoken. Using the PB data – *from unanimously identified vowels only* – Gerstman reported that 97.5% of the vowels were classified correctly. This percent correct figure is slightly better than the 94.5% intelligibility shown by PB's listeners, although the algorithm was presented with measurements from unanimously identified words only, meaning that, by definition, the appropriate comparison figure for listener is 100%. Nevertheless, performance of the Gerstman algorithm was quite good.

A method developed by Lobanov (1971) is quite similar to Gerstman, except that formant frequencies are converted to *z* scores rather than proportions. The method was tested using Russian vowels spoken by three men in a wide variety of phonetic contexts. The method was successful in both minimizing within-vowel-category variability and maximizing the distances between vowel categories. Although the number of talkers used in the test was surprisingly small given that the main purpose was to address acoustic differences across talkers, the Lobanov procedure has been used successfully in a variety of areas of phonetics (e.g., Adank et al., 2004). A closely related method is the log-mean procedure described by Nearey (1978), which is also in common use.

Many other extrinsic models have been developed over the years, but as Nearey (1992) and others have noted, these data-analytic approaches to the problem can suggest logically possible perceptual strategies, but the findings can tell us little about whether listeners actually use strategies such as these. Further, some of these algorithms were explicitly developed to address problems in areas such as automatic speech recognition and were never intended to model human perception (e.g., Gerstman, 1968). In that context, listening studies have a more direct bearing on the role that might be played by extrinsic normalization. The best known study in this area is a demonstration by Ladefoged and Broadbent (1957) of what certainly appears to be extrinsic normalization of the kind that is illustrated in Figure 9.16. The authors synthesized four test words ("bit," "bat," "bet," "but") which were preceded by six versions of an introductory carrier phrase ("Please say what this word is . . ."). The six versions, which were intended to simulate different talkers, consisted of a standard phrase and five other versions with formant frequencies shifted in various ways (F_1 down, F_1 up, F_2 down, F_2 up, F_1 down and F_2 up). Listeners' identification of the test words was strongly affected by the acoustic characteristics of the carrier phrase, consistent with the view that, "the phonetic quality of a vowel depends on the relationship between the formant frequencies for that vowel and the formant frequencies of other vowels pronounced by that speaker" (Ladefoged and Broadbent, 1957, p. 99).[6] A brief demonstration of the Ladefoged and Broadbent experiment can be found at this link: https://engineering.purdue.edu/~malcolm/interval/1997-056/VowelQuality.html

There is a good deal of other experimental work that is consistent with the idea that listeners make use of information about a talker's speech in recognizing subsequent utterances spoken by that talker. For example, Creelman (1957) found that recognition accuracy for words presented in noise was significantly lower when the identity of the talker was unpredictable from one trial to the next. Similarly, a word recognition reaction time study by Summerfield and Haggard (1975) found longer latencies in word lists with mixed versus single talkers. The increased latencies are thought to reflect the processing overhead associated with talker normalization. In one of their conditions, Kato and Kakehi (1988) asked listeners to identify a series of Japanese monosyllables spoken by different talkers and presented in noise with an 8 dB signal-to-noise ratio. Recognition accuracy increased linearly from 70 to 76% from the first to the fifth syllable, with no further increases beyond that. The effect was not especially large in absolute terms, but it was statistically reliable. Finally, a series of experiments by Mullennix et al. (1989) showed that word recognition accuracy decreased and response latencies increased when talkers were mixed (seven men, eight women) versus segregated. Further, they reported significant effects for mixed vs. segregated talkers when the words were presented in noise (S/N = +10, 0, and −10 dB) and when they were presented in quiet.

An unusually interesting paper by Eklund and Traunmüller (1997) found that identification error rates for whispered Swedish vowels spoken by men and women were nearly five times higher on trials in which the sex of the speaker was misidentified than on the remaining trials. This would seem to be a clear indication that listeners were using a decision about the sex of the talker to identify the vowel. This finding is consistent with the idea that vowel identity is affected by listener judgments about the characteristics of the talker, a specific form of extrinsic normalization. However, Eklund and Traunmüller found that the reverse was also true: The error rate for identifying speaker sex was four times higher on trials in which the vowel was incorrectly identified. In phonated speech, the two most important cues in distinguishing the voices of men and women are f_0 and formants (e.g., Assmann et al., 2006; Hillenbrand and Clark, 2009), but in whispered vowels the only *major* cue to speaker sex is the spectrum envelope (or formants derived from it). The conclusion that appears inescapable is that vowel identification depends on a decision about speaker sex *and* that identification of the sex of the speaker depends on a decision about vowel identity. It is not obvious how this circular dependency might be implemented either by neurons or by a computer algorithm.

A frequently cited paper by Verbrugge et al. (1976) produced mixed results concerning extrinsic normalization. In one experiment, listeners identified /hVd/ syllables with 15 vowel types (the vowel types from H95 plus /aɪ/, /aʊ/, and /ɔɪ/) spoken by 30 talkers (men, women, and children). In one condition, the talkers were presented in random order with no precursor, while in a point-vowel precursor condition the test syllables were preceded by /kip/, /kɑp/, and /kup/ spoken by the same talker as the test syllable. (The idea that the point vowels may play a special role in talker normalization goes back at least as far as Joos, 1948.) The error rate for the no-precursor condition (12.9%) was not reliably different from that of the precursor condition (12.2%).[7] In a follow-up experiment, listeners were asked to identify /pVp/ syllables under four conditions: (a) Isolated syllables, mixed talkers; (b) isolated syllables, utterances grouped by talker; (c) test utterances from the mixed-talker set preceded by /hV/ syllables with the point vowels (/hi/, /hɑ/, /hu/)/ and (d) test utterances preceded by /hV/ syllables with non-point vowels (/hɪ/, /hæ/, /hʌ/). Results were mixed. The error rate was significantly higher for the mixed-talker condition (17.0%) than the segregated-talker condition (9.5%). However, exposure to a talker's speech did *not* result in a significant decrease in error rate for either point-vowel precursors (15.2%) or non-point-vowel precursors (14.9%). (See Morton et al., 2015, for different results on the effectiveness of precursors.) Further, there was no reliable difference between point-vowel and non–point-vowel precursors. In a third experiment, listeners were asked to identify /pVp/ syllables that had been excised from a rapidly spoken sentence. A relatively high error rate of 23.8% was reported, but the error rate for a separate group of listeners tested on syllables that were preceded by same-talker point-vowel precursors was significantly *higher* (28.6%). The authors suggested that the citation-form precursors led listeners to expect a more leisurely speaking rate which clashed with the briskly spoken /pVp/ syllables that had been excised from a sentence. The lowest error rate (17.3%) was observed in a third condition in which the test syllables were presented in the original sentence context. The authors concluded that the sentence frame, "aids vowel identification by allowing adjustment primarily to a talker's tempo, rather than to the talker's vocal tract" (Verbrugge et al., 1976, p. 198).

In a set of natural speech control conditions for an experiment on the perception of sinewave vowels, Hillenbrand et al. (2008) found no effect at all for an introductory carrier phrase (CP) on the identification of 16 monophthongs and diphthongs spoken by 20 talkers (10 men, 10 women). Listeners identified /hVd/ test syllables presented under three conditions: (a) isolated syllables, (b) a within-talker carrier phrase (CP) condition in which test syllables were preceded by a CP ("The next word on the list is . . .") spoken by the same talker who uttered the test syllable, and (c) a cross-talker condition in which the talkers who produced the CP and test syllables were paired randomly (with 20 talkers, this means that the CP and test-word talkers would differ on 95% of the trials). Identification rates for the three conditions were uniformly high and statistically indistinguishable from one another (isolated syllables: 95.5%, within-talker CP: 95.3%, across-talker CP: 96.4%).

A set of results that are only rarely cited within the context of extrinsic normalization is the commonplace finding that vowels spoken by a diverse group of talkers, and presented to listeners in random order, are highly identifiable. For example, consider the 94.5% identification rate for 10 vowel types spoken by 76 talkers in PB, the 95.4% identification rate for 12 vowel types spoken by 139 talkers in H95, and the ~96% identification rate reported by Abramson and Cooper (1959; cited in Verbrugge et al., 1976). Verbrugge et al., are among the few to comment on this point:

> there is reason to doubt whether a preliminary normalization step plays the major role in vowel perception that is commonly attributed to it. Remarkably low error rates have been found when human listeners identify single syllables produced by human talkers. Peterson and Barney (1952) and Abramson and Cooper (1959) found average error rates of 4% to 6% when listeners identified the vowels in h-vowel-d words spoken in random order by a group of talkers. The test words were spoken as isolated syllables and in most conditions the listeners had little or no prior experience with the talker's voice. On the face of it, these low observed error rates seem inconsistent with any theory that stresses the need for extended prior experience with a talker's vowel space.
>
> *(Verbrugge et al., 1976, p. 199)*

It is not a particularly simple matter to determine what the literature described in this section has to tell us about the status of extrinsic normalization. On the one hand, it appears undeniable that listeners are both more accurate and faster in recognizing speech when talkers are segregated rather than mixed. These effects tend not to be especially large, but they are real enough. On the other hand, it is not entirely clear what information listeners derive from the speech of these talkers, or how that information is put to use in recognizing subsequent speech. If utterances from a talker are used to derive a reference frame that is used in the manner described by Joos (1948), Ladefoged and Broadbent (1957), and others (and illustrated in Figure 9.16), then how could Verbrugge et al. (1976) – in two separate experiments – have failed to find that same-talker precursors improve vowel identification performance? Similarly, what explains why Hillenbrand et al. (2008) did not find even a hint of a difference in vowel recognition when comparing isolated syllables, syllables preceded by a within-talker carrier phrase, and syllables preceded by a cross-talker carrier phrase? Finally, as noted by Verbrugge et al., if the establishment of a reference frame is needed in order to recognize speech from a variety of talkers, what explains the very high vowel identification rates of ~94–96% when words spoken by large groups of men, women, and children are presented in random order, as in PB and H95?[8]

These negative findings with natural-speech carrier phrases or precursors might be seen as an indication that listeners rely on extrinsic normalization only when the speech has been degraded in some way, such as noise, reverberation, or filtering. However, Mullennix et al. (1989) reported clear evidence for increased accuracy and shorter latencies for segregated vs. mixed talkers when test words were presented in noise *and* when they were presented in quiet. More important, the central idea underlying extrinsic normalization of the kind proposed by Joos (1948) and Ladefoged and Broadbent (1957) is that a reference frame is needed to resolve the kind of ambiguity that is illustrated in Figure 9.16. Ambiguity problems such as these do not vanish under good listening conditions, so it is not easy to understand why listeners would fail to make use of an available reference frame when identifying clearly spoken utterances. There are, of course, the Ladefoged and Broadbent findings, which appear to show exactly these kinds of effects, but it is not at all obvious why these kinds of results should be seen only with synthetically generated speech and/or when talker variation is simulated by introducing somewhat arbitrary shifts in formant frequencies. A solution to these problems will not be offered here, but resolving these kinds of questions would appear to be a fit topic for further work on talker normalization.

Chapter summary

This chapter begins with an overview of source-filter theory as it applies to the production of phonated vowels. This is followed by a description of the spectral characteristics of NAE vowels, and the identification of these vowels by listeners. The most striking results, seen in studies such as PB and H95, are two findings that appear to be at odds with one another: (a) Acoustic measurements show a good deal of variability across talkers, and significant overlap among adjacent vowel categories; but (b) when presented to listeners for identification in random order, the utterances prove to be highly intelligible, with error rates of ~4.5–5.5%. These findings indicate that the most common method that is used to represent the acoustic properties of vowels – the two lowest formant frequencies – is either wrong or incomplete, and/or that there is more to the perceptual mechanisms underlying vowel identification than was initially imagined. The remainder of the chapter focuses on four research areas that have attracted a good deal of attention in the literature on vowel recognition: (a) Formants versus spectral shape, (b) the role of spectral change, (c) the role of duration, and (d) talker normalization.

Formants vs. spectral shape

Formant theory, which is more often implicitly assumed rather than explicitly stated, suggests that vowel identity is controlled by the frequencies of the two or three lowest formants rather than the detailed shape of the spectrum. *Spectral shape* or *whole spectrum* models, on the other hand, assume that vowel identity is controlled by the overall shape of the spectrum envelope. As one example of a spectral shape model, Bladon and Lindblom (1981) used an auditory model to derive critical band spectra for a set of synthetic vowels. An auditory distance metric was then used to predict perceptual distances between pairs of critical band spectra. The perceptual distances derived from the model correlated strongly with perceived distances between the same pairs of vowels. However, in what we believe is the most important experimental work on this question, Klatt (1982) showed conclusively, in three separate experiments, that the only way to induce a large change in the phonetic quality of synthetic vowels was to alter the formant-frequency pattern. Other changes in spectral shape, while quite audible to listeners, have very little effect on judgments of the phonetic distance between pairs of vowels. Klatt suggested that the evidence argued in favor of a spectral shape model that was dominated by high-energy regions of the spectrum, but without requiring formant tracking. Klatt proposed a phonetic distance metric that compared spectral slope rather than amplitude differences between input and reference spectra, with the goal of representing similarities and differences in peak frequencies rather than amplitude. Klatt reported a strong correlation ($r = 0.93$) between his weighted slope measure and listener judgments of phonetic distance from the first of his three listening experiments.

Consistent with Klatt's findings are vowel classification findings using a recognition algorithm that compared narrow band input spectra with a set of smoothed spectral shape templates that were empirically derived by averaging the narrow band spectra of like vowels spoken at similar time points throughout the course of the vowel (Hillenbrand and Houde, 2003). In preparing narrow band spectra for template generation, and to serve as input to the classifier, steps were taken to emphasize spectral peaks at the expense of spectral shape details such as formant amplitudes, overall spectral tilt, and spectral details in between harmonics. Using separate templates for men, women, and children, the algorithm classified 1,668 vowels from H95 with 91.4% accuracy. Significantly, the performance of the algorithm fell dramatically to just 59.9% when a simulation of masking was removed from the classifier. The masking simulation was designed to emphasize spectral peaks at the expense other aspects of spectral shape which contribute minimally to judgments of phonetic quality. Overall, findings in this area do not argue in favor of either formants or spectral shape, as the concept is typically conceived (e.g., Bladon and Lindblom, 1981). Although opinions on this issue vary, the argument made here is that the evidence is consistent with the idea that listeners base their judgments of vowel identity on a representation of spectral shape that is dominated by energy at or near spectral peaks, but without requiring the assignment of spectral peaks to specific formant slots (F_1, F_2, . . .) – i.e., without tracking formants.

The role of spectral change

Researchers were aware of the potential importance of spectral change in vowel identification as early as the 1950s (e.g., Potter and Steinberg, 1950; Peterson and Barney, 1952; Tiffany, 1953). For the NAE vowels that have received the most attention, this idea now has the status of established fact. Evidence comes from four overlapping sources. First, individual NAE vowel types have distinctive patterns of spectral change. A few vowel types, particularly /i/ and u/, show little spectral movement throughout the course of the vowel, but most others show diphthong-like movements called *vowel inherent spectral change*. Evidence from several statistical pattern classification studies shows that vowels can be classified with considerably greater accuracy when spectral change is included among the classification features (e.g., Zahorian and Jagharghi, 1993; Hillenbrand et al., 1995, 2001). Second, a series of experiments using silent-center vowels showed that vowel identification accuracy was unaffected when vowel centers were excised from CVC syllables (e.g., Jenkins et al., 1983; Parker and Diehl, 1984; Nearey and Assmann, 1986; Andruski and Nearey, 1992; Strange et al., 1994). These experiments indicate that the stationary targets that might have been thought of as essential to vowel identification are, in fact, not necessary. Third, several experiments indicate that static targets are not merely unnecessary, they are also insufficient for vowel identification. The most striking piece of evidence on this point comes from a remarkable study by Fairbanks and Grubb (1961), described at considerable length earlier. Briefly, the authors went to great lengths to record the highest quality examples of eight static vowel types spoken by just seven talkers, all men and all faculty members in Speech and Hearing Science. Elaborate procedures were in place to audition and re-record any utterances that were judged to be unsatisfactory. In spite of these and other steps that were taken to obtain the highest quality recordings, the average intelligibility was just 74%, much lower than the figures reported in PB and H95, who recorded more vowel types, with a much greater diversity of talkers, and without the elaborate auditioning procedures used by Fairbanks and Grubb. The main explanation for the high error rate in Fairbanks and Grubb is that the signals did not show the natural VISC patterns that are typical of NAE speech, although the use of fixed-duration vowels almost certainly played some role as well. Other evidence that static targets are not sufficient to explain the excellent intelligibility observed in studies such as PB includes Hillenbrand and Gayvert (1993), who used a formant synthesizer to generate 300-ms static versions of all 1,520 signals from PB based on their measurements of f_0 and F_1–F_3. The average intelligibility was 73.8%, similar to the figure reported by Fairbanks and Grubb. Similarly, Hillenbrand and Nearey (1999) asked listeners to identify three versions 300 /hVd/ drawn from the H95 signals: (a) Naturally spoken signals (NAT), (b) formant-synthesized versions generated from the original formant contours (OF), and (c) formant-synthesized versions generated from flattened formants (FF). The key OF–FF comparison showed a very large drop in intelligibility from 88.5% for the OF condition to 73.8% for the FF condition. In summary, the body of evidence in this area is quite clear in showing that NAE vowels are much better thought of as distinctive trajectories through acoustic-phonetic space rather than points in that space.

The role of duration in vowel identification

Although vowel duration is not phonemic in English, there is good evidence that listeners attend to duration in identifying vowels. Early studies using isolated, sustained vowels showed that listeners make use of vowel duration in a manner that is generally consistent with measured differences in inherent duration. For example, Tiffany (1953) showed that long vowels such as /ɑ/ and /e/ were more likely to be identified as the intended vowel when presented at longer durations, and vice versa for vowels with short inherent durations. Similar findings were reported by Stevens (1959), with the notable exception that the effect of duration on /i/–/ɪ/ and /u/–/ʊ/ was relatively weak, in spite of large and reliable inherent duration differences for these pairs. A more recent study (Hillenbrand et al., 2000) used /hVd/ syllables showing natural VISC patterns that were synthesized at original, shortened, and lengthened vowel durations. The original-duration signals were highly intelligible (96.0%); shortening or lengthening the vowels resulted in nearly symmetrical decreases in intelligibility of about five percentage points. However, this relatively modest drop in intelligibility was arrived at by averaging some cases in which vowels produced rather large effects (e.g., /æ/–/ɛ/ and /ɑ/–/ɔ/–/ʌ/) with other cases – notably /i/–/ɪ/ and /u/–/ʊ/ – in which duration produced almost no effect at all, in spite of large differences in inherent duration. Pattern recognition findings suggested that a likely explanation is that listeners give little weight to duration for vowels that can be identified well based on spectral features alone, and vice versa.

Talker normalization

The acoustic characteristics of a given vowel type vary across talkers, even when dialect is held constant. To many investigators, the fact that listeners have little difficulty recognizing the speech of many talkers suggests the operation of talker normalization mechanisms. Following Ainsworth, we distinguish between intrinsic normalization, in which all normalizing information is available directly in the to-be-recognized utterance, and extrinsic nomination, in which previous speech from a talker is used to establish a reference frame that is aids in the identification of later utterances.

Intrinsic normalization

As Miller (1989) noted, many intrinsic normalization schemes are variations of Lloyd's (1890, 1892) relative resonance theory, which suggests that vowels with similar qualities have similar formant ratios. Influential models developed by Miller (1984, 1989) and Syrdal (1985; Syrdal and Gopal, 1986) added a transform of the fundamental frequency to formant ratios to disambiguate vowel pairs with similar ratios. In addition to modeling work of this kind, there is clear evidence from listening experiments showing that judgments of vowel identity are affected by variations in f_0 when formants are held constant (e.g., Miller, 1953; Slawson, 1968; Fujisaki and Kawashima, 1968; Ryalls and Lieberman, 1982). There is disagreement about the critical issue of why f_0 should affect vowel recognition. A common (but note sole) suggestion is that f_0 plays an indirect role in vowel identification by affecting decision criteria based on learned associations between f_0 and formant frequencies (e.g., Assmann and Nearey, 2008; Barreda, 2013). These findings are consistent with the idea that f_0 plays an indirect role in vowel identification that is based on correlations between f_0 and formants in natural speech. However, as noted earlier, the idea is not with problems, including: (a) Even in citation-form speech, the relationship between f_0 and formants at the level of individual tokens (as opposed to averages across talkers) is not especially strong; and (b) instantaneous f_0 varies quite substantially in ordinary conversational speech.

Extrinsic normalization

One of the earliest pieces of experimental work in this area turns out to be one of the more interesting. Using a synthesizer that is far from the current state-of-the art, Ladefoged and

Broadbent (1957) created four test words that were preceded by either a standard introductory carrier phrase or one of five formant-shifted versions representing different talkers. Identification of the test words was affected by the acoustic properties of the carrier phrase in a manner that was generally consistent with the reference-frame hypothesis proposed by Joos (1948). Another major piece of evidence favoring a role for extrinsic normalization is the finding, replicated in many studies, that word recognition accuracy is higher, and/or latencies lower, when talkers are segregated versus mixed (e.g., Creelman, 1957; Summerfield and Haggard, 1975; Kato and Kakehi, 1988; Mullennix et al., 1989). Evidence from other studies has been either mixed or negative. For example, Verbrugge et al. (1976) replicated the common finding of higher recognition accuracy for segregated than mixed talkers, but found no evidence for higher recognition rates when test utterances were preceded by same-talker precursors consisting of either point- or non-point vowels. If the segregated-talker advantage is explained on the basis of extrinsic normalization, what accounts for the failure to find an improvement for same-talker precursors? In discussing these issues, Verbrugge et al., also asked the straightforward question of how extrinsic normalization could be essential to vowel recognition in light of the very high recognition rates of ~95% from studies such as PB in which utterances from a diverse group of talkers are presented for identification in random order. Finally, using naturally spoken utterances, Hillenbrand et al. (2008) found no difference in vowel recognition rates when carrier phrases were spoken by the same talker as the test syllable versus a different talker. Some of these findings would appear to be in conflict with others. Unfortunately, we are not in a position to offer a solution to these apparently conflicting findings.

Future directions

Vowel perception research has been dominated by studies using citation-form utterances such as isolated vowels or syllables/words with a simple and often fixed structure. Further, these utterances are typically longer and are almost certainly spoken with less pronounced coarticulatory patterns than are seen in ordinary conversational speech. There is an obvious reason for these constraints on speech material: These simpler utterances allow attention to be focused on a small and clearly specified set of underlying physical parameters. However, there are certain problems that cannot be understood with these kinds of utterances. One example, described earlier, concerns the influence of duration on vowel identity. The results of this work using isolated vowels and syllables seem clear enough, but in connected speech there is a large and complex set of factors that exert a systematic influence on segment duration (e.g., Klatt, 1976). It is not at all clear how listeners go about assigning duration variability to specific factors such as vowel identity, final-consonant voicing, speaking rate, word- and sentence-level stress, and the many other factors that influence vowel duration. A similar problem concerns how listeners go about assigning spectral change patterns to either vowel identity (i.e., treating the spectral changes as VISC patterns) or coarticulation. Research along these lines using connected speech would clearly require some ingenuity, but it would represent a useful avenue of research.

Notes

1 We are not suggesting that the signal processing steps described here literally take place when listeners recognize speech. These steps are intended as a proxy for psychological rather than physical processes that are involved in perception. For example, Klatt's (1982) findings clearly show that features such as spectral and formant amplitude relationships are quite audible to listeners, so it

cannot be that these features are literally removed from the input signal. However, these kinds of features play a limited role in judgments of phonetic quality.

2 We experimented with methods for normalizing input spectra and templates across talkers (Houde and Hillenbrand, 2007). These methods worked reasonably well, but we have not yet found anything that performs as well as separate templates for men, women, and children.

3 As will be discussed later, there is clear evidence that listeners make use of vowel duration in identifying vowels, indicating that at least some of the performance advantage for listeners is related to the fact that our algorithm does not incorporate duration information. We have not yet developed a method for combining the spectral information that is used in the current model with duration values.

4 Nearey (1989) makes the point that it is possible to argue that intrinsic schemes do not constitute normalization at all: "Although it is possible to formulate such approaches as normalization procedures the term is rarely used by this group. Instead, the invariance problem is deemed not to exist when the correct parametric representation of spectral properties of vowels is considered." (p. 2080).

5 Irino and Patterson (2002) have proposed that an obligatory transformation of input stimuli to a sensation of size takes place at an early stage of auditory analysis, and that this size sensation is not specific to speech or to human listeners. Further, Smith et al. (2005) have argued that the effects of frequency shifts on vowel identity cannot be explained on the basis of learned associations between f_0 and formants. See Assmann and Nearey (2008) for a discussion of this question.

6 The authors made what would seem to be surprising choices in the approach that was adopted for creating the five variations on the standard talker. In the formant data from both PB and H95, it can be seen that the main (though not sole) source of variation across individual talkers lies on a lower-left-to-upper-right diagonal, indicating the kinds of near-the-regression-line signals that produced the best intelligibility in the scaling studies by Assmann and colleagues. However, the manipulations that produced *all five* simulated talkers were in directions that moved the formants away this regression line. It is not at all clear what effect, if any, this approach to simulating talker differences may have had on their findings. But given the impact that this very interesting paper has had in this area, it might be worth finding out.

7 Statistics for a condition-by-vowel interaction were not reported, but even a casual inspection of their data (see their table I) indicates that results were quite different from one vowel type to the next. While these differences were discussed, a compelling explanation was not offered.

8 In one sense, even these very high identification rates underestimate how intelligible these utterances are. In the PB data, fully 55% of the errors come from just two vowels – /ɑ/ and /ɔ/ – which are confused mainly either with one another, or with /ʌ/. If data from these two vowels are removed, the identification rate rises to 96.9%. Data from H95 are similar.

References

Abramson, A. S., and Cooper, F. S. (1959). Perception of American English vowels in terms of a reference system. *Haskins Laboratories Quarterly Progress Report, QPR-32.*

Adank, P., Smits, R., and van Hout, R. (2004). A comparison of vowel normalization procedures for language variation research. *The Journal of the Acoustical Society of America, 116*, 3099–3107.

Ainsworth, W. A. (1972). Duration as a cue in the recognition of synthetic vowels. *The Journal of the Acoustical Society of America, 51*, 648–651.

Ainsworth, W. A. (1975). Intrinsic and extrinsic factors in vowel judgments. In G. Fant and M. Tatham (Eds.) *Auditory analysis and perception of speech*. London: Academic Press, 103–113.

Ainsworth, W. A., and Millar, J. (1971). The effect of relative formant amplitude on the perceived identity of synthetic vowels. *Language and Speech, 15*, 328–341.

Andruski, J. E., and Nearey, T. M. (1992). On the sufficiency of compound target specification of isolated vowels in /bVb/ syllables. *The Journal of the Acoustical Society of America, 91*, 390–410.

Assmann, P. F., and Nearey, T. M. (2007). Relationship between fundamental and formant frequencies in voice preference. *The Journal of the Acoustical Society of America, 122*, EL35–EL43.

Assmann, P. F., and Nearey, T. N. (2008). Identification of frequency-shifted vowels. *The Journal of the Acoustical Society of America, 124*, 3203–3212.

Assmann, P. F., Nearey, T. M., and Dembling, S. (2006). Effects of frequency shifts on perceived naturalness and gender information in speech. *Proceedings of the Ninth International Conference on Spoken Language Processing*, Pittsburgh, PA, 889–892.

Barreda, S. (2013). *Cognitively-active speaker normalization based on formant-frequency scaling estimation*. PhD dissertation, Department of Linguistics, University of Alberta, Edmonton, Alberta.

Bennett, D. C. (1968). Spectral form and duration as cues in the recognition of English and German vowels. *Language & Speech, 11*, 65–85.

Black, J. W. (1949). Natural frequency, duration, and intensity of vowels in reading. *Journal of Speech and Hearing Disorders, 14*, 216–221.

Bladon, A. (1982). Arguments against formants in the auditory representation of speech. In R. Carlson and B. Granstrom (Eds.) *The representation of speech in the peripheral auditory system*. Amsterdam: Elsevier Biomedical Press, 95–102.

Bladon, A., and Lindblom, B. (1981). Modeling the judgment of vowel quality differences. *The Journal of the Acoustical Society of America, 69*, 1414–1422.

Byrd, D. (1992). Sex, dialects, and reduction. In J. Ohala, T. M. Nearey, B. L. Derwing, M. M. Hodge, and G. E. Wiebe (Eds.) *Proceedings of the Second International Conference on Spoken Language Processing (ICSLP)*, Banff, Canada, 827–830.

Creelman, C. D. (1957). Case of the unknown talker. *The Journal of the Acoustical Society of America, 29*, 655.

Crystal, T. H., and House, A. S. (1988). The duration of American-English vowels: An overview. *Journal of Phonetics, 16*, 263–284.

de Cheveigné, A., and Kawahara, H. (1999). A missing data model of vowel identification. *The Journal of the Acoustical Society of America, 105*, 3497–3508.

Disner, S. F. (1980). Evaluation of vowel normalization procedures. *The Journal of the Acoustical Society of America, 76*, 253–261.

Eklund, I., and Traunmüller, H. (1997). Comparative study of male and female whispered and phonated versions of the long vowels of Swedish. *Phonetica*, 54, 1–21.

Fairbanks, G., and Grubb, P. (1961). A psychophysical investigation of vowel formants. *Journal of Speech and Hearing Research, 4*, 203–219.

Fant, G. (1960). *Acoustic theory of speech production*. The Hague: Mouton.

Flanagan, J. (1972). *Speech analysis, synthesis and perception*. New York: Springer-Verlag.

Fujisaki, H., and Kawashima, T. (1968). The roles of pitch and the higher formants in the perception of vowels. *IEEE Transactions on Audio and Electroacoustics, AU-16*, 73–77.

Gerstman, L. (1968). Classification of self-normalized vowels. *IEEE Transactions on Audio and Electroacoustics, AU-16*, 78–80.

Glidden, C. M., and Assmann, P. F. (2004). Effects of visual gender and frequency shifts on vowel category judgments. *Acoustics Research Letters Online, 5*, 132–138.

Hillenbrand, J. M. (2013). Static and dynamic approaches to vowel perception. In G. S. Morrison and P. F. Assmann (Eds.) *Vowel inherent spectral change*. Heidelberg: Springer-Verlag, 9–30.

Hillenbrand, J. M., and Clark, M. J. (2009). The role of f_0 and formant frequencies in distinguishing the voices of men and women. *Attention, Perception, & Psychophysics, 71*, 1150–1166.

Hillenbrand, J. M., Clark, M. J., and Houde, R. A. (2000). Some effects of duration on vowel recognition. *The Journal of the Acoustical Society of America, 108*, 3013–3022.

Hillenbrand, J. M., Clark, M. J., Houde, R. A., Hillenbrand, M. W., and Hillenbrand, K. S. (2008). Perceptual accommodation to sinewave speech. *The Journal of the Acoustical Society of America, 124*, 2435.

Hillenbrand, J. M., Clark, M. J., and Nearey, T. M. (2001). Effects of consonant environment on vowel formant patterns. *The Journal of the Acoustical Society of America, 109*, 748–763.

Hillenbrand, J. M., and Gayvert, R. T. (1993). Identification of steady-state vowels synthesized from the Peterson and Barney measurements. *The Journal of the Acoustical Society of America*, 94, 668–674.

Hillenbrand, J. M., Getty, L. A., Clark, M. J., and Wheeler, K. (1995). Acoustic characteristics of American English vowels. *The Journal of the Acoustical Society of America, 97*, 3099–3111.

Hillenbrand, J. M., and Houde, R. A. (2003). A narrow band pattern-matching model of vowel perception. *The Journal of the Acoustical Society of America, 113*, 1044–1055.

Hillenbrand, J. M., Houde, R. A., and Gayvert, R. A. (2006). Speech perception based on spectral peaks versus spectral shape. *The Journal of the Acoustical Society of America, 119*, 4041–4054.

Hillenbrand, J. M., and Nearey, T. N. (1999). Identification of resynthesized /hVd/ syllables: Effects of formant contour. *The Journal of the Acoustical Society of America, 105*, 3509–3523.

Houde, R. A., and Hillenbrand, J. M. (2007). Vocal tract normalization for vowel recognition. *The Journal of the Acoustical Society of America, 121*, 3189.

Huang, C. B. (1986). The effect of formant trajectory and spectral shape on the tense/lax distinction in American vowels. *IEEE ICASSP*, 893–896.

Irino, T., and Patterson, R. D. (2002). Segregating information about the size and shape of the vocal tract using a time-domain auditory model: The stabilised wavelet-Mellin transform. *Speech Communication, 36*, 181–203.

Ito, M., and Yano, J. (2001). On the effectiveness of whole spectral shape for vowel perception. *Journal of the Acoustical Society of America, 110*, 1141–1149.

Jenkins, J. J., and Strange, W. (1999). Perception of dynamic information for vowels in syllable onsets and offsets. *Perception and Psychophysics, 61*, 1200–1210.

Jenkins, J. J., Strange, W., and Edman, T. R. (1983). Identification of vowels in 'vowelless' syllables. *Perception and Psychophysics, 34*, 441–450.

Joos, M. A. (1948). Acoustic phonetics. *Language, 24*, Supplement 2, 1–136.

Kato, K., and Kakehi, K. (1988). Listener adaptability to individual speaker differences in monosyllabic speech perception. *The Journal of the Acoustical Society of Japan, 44*, 180–186.

Kawahara, H. (1997). Speech representation and transformation using adaptive interpolation of weighted spectrum: Vocoder revisited. *Proceedings of the ICASSP-1997*, 1303–1306.

Kawahara, H., Masuda-Katsuse, I., and de Cheveigné, A. (1999). Restructuring speech representations using a pitch-adaptive time-frequency smoothing and an instantaneous-frequency-based F0 extraction. *Speech Communication, 27*, 187–207.

Kiefte, M., and Kluender, K. (2005). The relative importance of spectral tilt in monophthongs and diphthongs. *The Journal of the Acoustical Society of America, 117*, 1395–1404.

Klatt, D. H. (1976). Linguistic uses of segmental duration in English: Acoustic and perceptual evidence. *The Journal of the Acoustical Society of America, 59*, 1208–1221.

Klatt, D. H. (1980). Software for a cascade/parallel formant synthesizer. *The Journal of the Acoustical Society of America, 67*, 971–995.

Klatt, D. H. (1982). Prediction of perceived phonetic distance from critical-band spectra: A first step. *IEEE ICASSP*, 1278–1281.

Klatt, D. H., and Klatt, L. C. (1990). Analysis, synthesis, and perception of voice quality variations among female and male talkers. *The Journal of the Acoustical Society of America, 87*, 820–857.

Ladefoged, P., and Broadbent, D. E. (1957). Information conveyed by vowels. *The Journal of the Acoustical Society of America, 29*, 98–104.

Labov, W., Yaeger, M., and Steiner, R. (1972). A quantitative study of sound change in progress. *Report to National Science Foundation Contract NSF-FS-3287*.

Lieberman, P. (1967). *Intonation perception and language*. Cambridge, MA: MIT Press.

Lindqvist, J., and Pauli, S. (1968). The role of relative spectrum levels in vowel perception. *STL-QPSR*, 2–3, 12–15.

Lloyd, R. J. (1890). *Some researches into the nature of vowel-sound*. Liverpool, England: Turner and Dunnett.

Lloyd, R. J. (1892). Speech sounds: Their nature and causation (V-VII). *Phonetische Studien*, *5*, 1–32, 129–141, 263–271.

Lobanov, B. M. (1971). Classification of Russian vowels spoken by different speakers. *The Journal of the Acoustical Society of America*, *49*, 606–608.

Logan, J., Greene, B., and Pisoni, D. (1989). Segmental intelligibility of synthetic speech produced by rule. *The Journal of the Acoustical Society of America*, *86*, 566–581.

Mattingly, I. G. (1999). A short history of acoustic phonetics in the U.S. *Proceedings of the XIVth International Congress of Phonetic Sciences*, 1–6.

McAuley, R. J., and Quatieri, T. F. (1986). Speech analysis/synthesis based on sinusoidal representation. *IEEE Transactions on Acoustics, Speech and Signal Processing, ASSP-22*, 330–338.

Miller, J. D. (1984). Auditory processing of the acoustic patterns of speech. *Archives of Otolaryngology*, *110*, 154–159.

Miller, J. D. (1989). Auditory-perceptual interpretation of the vowel. *The Journal of the Acoustical Society of America*, *85*, 2114–2134.

Miller, R. L. (1953). Auditory tests with synthetic vowels. *The Journal of the Acoustical Society of America*, *18*, 114–121.

Minifie, F. D. (1973). Speech acoustics. In F. D. Minifie, T. J. Hixon, and F. Williams (Eds.) *Normal aspects of speech hearing and language*. Englewood Cliffs, NJ: Prentice-Hall, 235–284.

Morton, J. R., Sommers, M. S., and Lulich, S. M. (2015). The effect of exposure to a single vowel on talker normalization for vowels. *The Journal of the Acoustical Society of America*, *137*, 1443–1451.

Mullennix, J. W., Pisoni, D. B., and Martin, C. S. (1989). The some effects of talker variability on spoken word recognition. *The Journal of the Acoustical Society of America*, *85*, 365–378.

Nearey, T. M. (1978). *Phonetic feature systems for vowels*. Bloomington, IN: Indiana University Linguistics Club.

Nearey, T. M. (1989). Static, dynamic, and relational properties in vowel perception. *The Journal of the Acoustical Society of America*, *85*, 2088–2113.

Nearey, T. M. (1992). Applications of generalized linear modeling to vowel data. In J. Ohala, T. M. Nearey, B. L. Derwing, M. M. Hodge, and G. E. Wiebe (Eds.) *Proceedings of the 1992 International Conference on Spoken Language Processing (ICSLP)*, Banff, Canada, 583–587.

Nearey, T. M., and Assmann, P. F. (1986). Modeling the role of vowel inherent spectral change in vowel identification. *The Journal of the Acoustical Society of America*, *80*, 1297–1308.

Nearey, T., Hogan, J., and Rozsypal, A. (1979). Speech signals, cues and features. In G. Prideaux (Ed.) *Perspectives in experimental linguistics*. Amsterdam, The Netherlands: John Benjamins.

Parker, E. M., and Diehl, R. L. (1984). Identifying vowels in CVC syllables: Effects of inserting silence and noise. *Perception and Psychophysics*, *36*, 369–380.

Patterson, R. D., Smith, D. R. R., van Dinther, R., and Walters, T. C. (2008). Size information in the production and perception of communication sounds. In W. A. Yost, R. R. Fay, and A. N. Popper (Eds.) *Auditory perception of sound sources*. New York: Springer.

Paul, D. B. (1981). The spectral envelope estimation vocoder. *IEEE Transactions on Acoustics, Speech and Signal Processing, ASSP-29*, 786–794.

Peterson, G. (1961). Parameters of vowel quality. *Journal of Speech and Hearing Research*, *4*, 10–29.

Peterson, G., and Barney, H. L. (1952). Control methods used in a study of the vowels. *The Journal of the Acoustical Society of America*, *24*, 175–184.

Plomp, R. (1970). Timbre as a multidimensional attribute of complex tones. In R. Plomp and G. Smoorenburg (Eds.) *Frequency analysis and periodicity detection in hearing*. Leiden: Sijthoff, 397–411.

Potter, R. K., and Steinberg, J. C. (1950). Toward the specification of speech. *The Journal of the Acoustical Society of America, 22*, 807–820.

Rosner, B. S., and Pickering, J. B. (1994). Vowel perception and production. In *Oxford Psychology Series, No. 23*. New York: Oxford University Press.

Ryalls, J., and Lieberman, P. (1982). Fundamental frequency and vowel perception. *The Journal of the Acoustical Society of America, 72*, 1631–1634.

Schroeder, M. R., Atal, B. S., and Hall, J. L. (1979). Objective measure of certain speech signal degradations based on masking properties of human auditory perception. In B. Lindblom and S. Ohman (Eds.) *Frontiers of speech communication research*. New York: Academic Press, 217–229.

Slawson, A. W. (1968). Vowel quality and musical timbre as functions of spectrum envelope and fundamental frequency. *The Journal of the Acoustical Society of America, 43*, 87–101.

Smith, D. R. R., Patterson, R. D., and Turner, R. (2005). The processing and perception of size information in speech sounds. *The Journal of the Acoustical Society of America, 117*, 305–318.

Smith, D. R. R., Patterson, R. D., Turner, R., Kawahara, H., and Irino, T. (2005). The processing and perception of size information in speech sounds. *The Journal of the Acoustical Society of America, 117*, 305–318.

Smith, D. R. R., Patterson, R. D., and Walters, R. C. (2007). Discrimination of speaker sex and size when glottal-pulse rate and vocal-tract length are controlled. *The Journal of the Acoustical Society of America, 122*, 3628.

Stevens, K. N. (1959). The role of duration in vowel identification. *Quarterly Progress Report, 52*, Research Laboratory of Electronics, MIT Press.

Stevens, K. N. (2000). *Acoustic phonetics*. Cambridge, MA: MIT Press.

Stevens, K. N., and House, A. S. (1963). Perturbation of vowel articulations by consonant context: An acoustical study. *Journal of Speech and Hearing Research, 6*, 111–128.

Strange, W. (1989). Dynamic specification of coarticulated vowels spoken in sentence context. *Journal of the Acoustical Society of America, 85*, 2135–2153.

Strange, W., Jenkins, J. J., and Miranda, S. (1994). Vowel identification in mixed-speaker silent-center syllables. *The Journal of the Acoustical Society of America, 95*, 1030–1043.

Summerfield, A. Q., and Haggard, M. P. (1975). Vocal tract normalisation as demonstrated by reaction times. In G. Fant (Ed.) *Auditory analysis and perception of speech*. New York: Elsevier, 115–141.

Syrdal, A. K. (1985). Aspects of a model of the auditory representation of American English vowels. *Speech Communication, 4*, 121–135.

Syrdal, A. K., and Gopal, H. S. (1986). A perceptual model of vowel recognition based on the auditory representation of American English vowels. *The Journal of the Acoustical Society of America, 79*, 1086–1100.

Syrdal, A. K., and Steele, S. (1985). Vowel F_1 as a function of speaker fundamental frequency. *The Journal of the Acoustical Society of America, 78*, Supplement 1, S56.

Tiffany, W. (1953). Vowel recognition as a function of duration, frequency modulation and phonetic context. *Journal of Speech and Hearing Disorders, 18*, 289–301.

Titze, I., Baken, R., Bozeman, K., Granqvist, S., Henrich, N., Herbst, C., Howard, D., Hunter, E., Kaelin, D., Kent, R., Kreiman, J., Kob, M., Lofqvist, A., McCoy, S., Miller, D., Noé, H., Scherer, R., Smith, B., Svec, Ternström, S., and Wolfe, J. (2015). Toward a consensus on symbolic notation of harmonics, resonances, and formants in vocalization. *The Journal of the Acoustical Society of America, 137*, 3005–3007.

van Santen, J. P. H. (1992). Contextual effects on vowel duration. *Speech Communication, 11*, 513–546.

Verbrugge, R. R., Strange, W., Shankweiler, D. P., and Edman, T. R. (1976). What information enables a listener to map a talker's vowel space? *The Journal of the Acoustical Society of America*, *60*, 198–212.

Watson, C. I., and Harrington, J. (1999). Acoustic evidence for dynamic formant trajectories in Australian English vowels. *The Journal of the Acoustical Society of America*, *106*, 458–468.

Zahorian, S., and Jagharghi, A. (1993). Spectral shape features versus formants as acoustic correlates for vowels. *The Journal of the Acoustical Society of America*, *94*, 1966–1982.

10

The phonetic properties of consonants

Marija Tabain

Whilst vowel quality can be described in terms of only two or three parameters – tongue height, front-back position, and rounding in articulatory terms, and F_1, F_2, and F_3 in acoustic terms – such is not the case for consonants. The International Phonetic Alphabet (IPA) suggests that consonants can be uniquely described using the properties of voicing, place, and manner, but as we shall see, these properties do not form a continuum in the same way that vowel height or vowel front–back specifications can be considered a continuum. Although it is true that consonants such as stops and nasals can have a particular place of articulation that can be accurately described in phonetic terms, how to categorize place for sounds such as fricatives or rhotics is much more problematic. Moreover, the role of overall tongue shape in determining the spectral output for sounds such as these is quite poorly understood, to the extent that it is not at all encoded in the IPA. In addition, the similarities in terms of dorsal constriction between rhotics and laterals are likewise not captured within the IPA.

In order to cover the wide variety of sounds that are considered consonants in the world's languages, this chapter will use the IPA as the organizing framework, working through the various (pulmonic) places and manners of articulation. It should be pointed out that, like consonant place, the category of consonant manner does not represent a continuum of sounds. Whilst it might be possible to say that a stop is lenited to a fricative-type sound at the same location, which in turn might be lenited to an approximant-type sound at this location, it is not necessarily the case, for example, that a particular fricative such as /s/ or /ʃ/ has a clear counterpart at the stop manner of articulation (as noted by Gordon 2016, the oral stops never lenite to /s/ or /ʃ/). Moreover, the articulatory and aerodynamic considerations involved in producing the different manners of articulation – nasal consonants, lateral consonants, stops, fricatives, approximants – result in acoustic outputs that require quite different measures and considerations for each of the different categories. The fact that these various manners of articulation can form coherent phonological categories is a challenge to phonetic research.

Stops

The IPA chart lists seven possible places of articulation for oral stop consonants (also known as "plosives"). A prototypical oral stop involves complete closure at some point along the oral cavity. In principle, such a closure involves a period of complete silence in a spectrogram display, although in practice a "voice bar" may be visible at the bottom of the spectrogram for at least part of the stop closure (voicing in stops will be discussed a little further later in this chapter). The exact duration of this closure depends on several factors, including prosodic factors (e.g., stops in stressed syllables have longer closures than stops in unstressed syllables), and on place of articulation and the active articulator involved. For instance, an alveolar stop (/t/, /d/) which is often produced with the rapidly moving tongue tip, often has a much shorter closure duration than a bilabial (p/, /b/) or a velar (/k/, /g/). In fact, it seems to be relatively difficult to achieve a complete closure in the velar region using the slower-moving tongue back/body, to the extent that phonemically velar stops are often realized with frication (see the section on Fricatives).

The three stop places of articulation just mentioned – bilabials (p/, /b/), alveolars (/t/, /d/), and velars (/k/, /g/) – are the most common stops across the world's languages, and are precisely the stops found in English and many other European languages. There is one respect, however, in which the bilabial stops differ from all other oral stop places of articulation, and this relates to the acoustic output. At the moment of release – i.e., at the moment that the closure is released – the portion of the oral cavity in front of the closure becomes acoustically "excited" by the acoustic energy built up behind the closure. This is because during the oral closure, as air continues to flow from the lungs into the oral cavity, pressure builds up behind the closure; and at the moment of release, air rushes into what was the front cavity, with the resulting burst of sound capturing the acoustic characteristics of this front cavity. For all oral stops except the bilabial, the cavity in front of the closure is within the oral cavity itself. However, for the bilabial stops, the "cavity" in front of the closure is the "outside world," and as such it is difficult for the relatively small amount of air flowing through the oral cavity to produce much acoustic energy in the large space beyond the lips. As a result, bilabials show much less acoustic energy at the moment of stop burst than do the other oral consonants, and this is particularly noticeable in the higher-frequency regions. For instance, in Figure 10.1, the stop burst for /p/, which is represented by the solid line, has a noticeable drop-off in energy across the frequency range, so that above 3 kHz it has very little energy overall. (The stop burst is the burst of energy that occurs in the first few milliseconds following the release of the stop closure.) The low-frequency energy that is seen for the bilabial comes from the cavity behind the constriction, and since in this case the entire oral and pharyngeal cavities are involved, the acoustic energy is at a very low frequency (the size of the cavity determines its resonance frequencies, with a larger cavity producing a lower-frequency resonance).

By contrast, the other stop places of articulation are very much shaped by the cavity in front of the constriction at the moment of release. Broadly speaking, this front cavity becomes smaller the more forward in the oral cavity the stop is articulated, and as a result, more high-frequency energy is typically present in the stop burst for stops that are articulated further forward in the oral cavity. Again looking at Figure 10.1, which shows the stop burst spectra for stops in four languages, it can be seen that the energy for /k/ is largely concentrated at lower frequencies than the energy for /t/. The energy for /k/ (shown as a dot-dash line) is noticeable at about 1500–2000 Hz, although for English the energy is spread across about 1000–3000 Hz. By contrast, the energy for /t/ (shown as a dotted line) is higher in the frequency range above 3 kHz, and this is particularly noticeable for Arrernte and Pitjantjatjara, where the alveolar /t/ and the "retroflex" /ʈ/ have a particularly broad spectral peak in the 2000–4000 Hz range.

Figure 10.1 also brings to light some other issues relating to "place" of articulation in consonants. As mentioned, this figure shows the alveolar and retroflex stops of the Australian

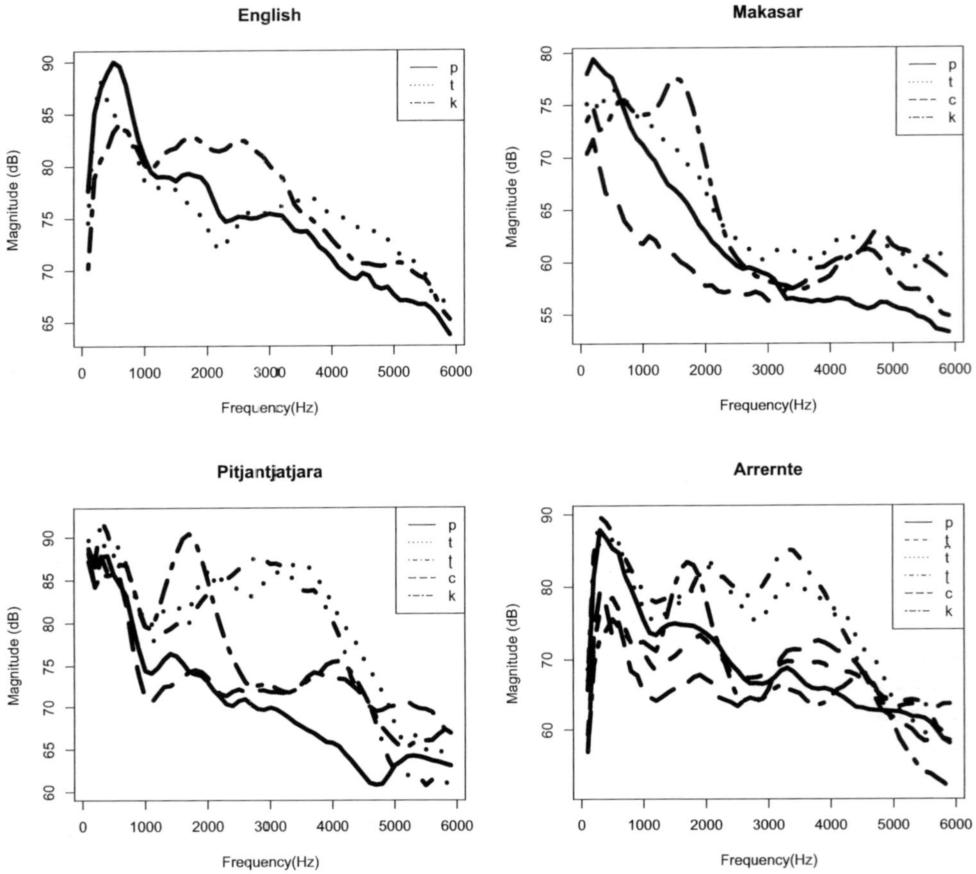

Figure 10.1 Stop burst spectra for four languages. English data are from five speakers (three female, two male), Makasar data are from seven speakers (three female, four male), Pitjantjatjara data are from three speakers (all female), and Arrernte data are from two speakers (both female). The data come from both stressed and unstressed syllables, but all are from a following /a/ vowel context. Each line represents an average spectrum for that particular speech sound. Total segment numbers in the plots are 630 for English, 1,506 for Makasar, 790 for Pitjantjatjara, and 622 for Arrernte. The English speakers are Australian; Arrernte and Pitjantjatjara are indigenous languages of Australia; and Makasar is an Indonesian language spoken in South Sulawesi.

languages Arrernte and Pitjantjatjara (the retroflex stops are shown as light blue lines). In Australian languages, both the alveolar and the retroflex are articulated with the tongue tip. In prototypical terms, the alveolar is produced as a "plateau" articulation – the tongue tip moves upwards to contact the alveolar ridge, and it releases at more or less the same point as initial contact. By contrast, the prototypical retroflex articulation involves a closure in the post-alveolar or pre-palatal region of the oral cavity, followed by a ballistic forward movement of the tongue that results in the closure being released towards the alveolar region. This highlights the fact that "retroflex" is not actually a *place* of articulation, but in a sense a *style* of articulation that relates to the direction of travel of the front part of the tongue. It is interesting that the IPA chart lists /t d/ as spanning the dental, alveolar and post-alveolar places of articulation, with various diacritics used to separate out these three places (a bridge for the dental /t̪/, and a minus sign below for the post-alveolar /t̠/, meaning retracted). There is in fact a tremendous amount of overlap between the alveolar and retroflex phonemic categories in Australian languages (Tabain, 2009), and discussion of this minimal phonemic contrast is beyond the scope of this chapter. However, it can be noted that some of the articulations might best be classed as the retracted /t̠/, since the point of contact is post-alveolar, but the ballistic forward movement of the tongue is not so apparent.

It may have been inferred from the preceding discussion that the prototypical alveolar and prototypical retroflex stops are very similar at the moment of stop burst release, since both are released at the alveolar region. However, there are some subtle differences between the two stop bursts, which suggest that the retroflex is not released quite as far forward as the alveolar. In general, the concentration of energy for the retroflex is at ever so slightly lower frequencies than for the alveolar, and this is most consistently reflected in differences at the right edge of the broad spectral peak – in Figure 10.1, it can be seen that for Pitjantjatjara, the /t/ has more energy than the /ʈ/ above about 3200 Hz, whereas for Arrernte this cross-over occurs at around 4000 Hz (for these particular speakers). The slightly greater higher-frequency energy for /t/ suggests that the cavity in front of the constriction release is slightly smaller for the alveolar than for the retroflex. It should, however, be noted that these apical consonants (i.e., made with the tongue tip) in the Australia languages have a lot more high-frequency energy than the English and Makasar alveolar stops. The exact reasons for these differences would require some careful articulatory-to-acoustic study, but the differences themselves are a reminder that each language must be treated in its own right when a particular symbol from the IPA is used to represent the sound in that language.

Figure 10.1 also shows the stop burst spectrum for the dental stop in Arrernte. Arrernte contrasts four coronal stops (coronal means sounds made with the tongue tip or blade), which can be divided into apicals (made with the tongue tip) and laminals (made with the tongue blade, which is just behind the tongue tip). The apicals are the alveolar and retroflex, just discussed, and the laminals are the palatal (discussed later in the chapter) and the dental. The Arrernte dental has very little contact between the tongue and the palate – the contact is primarily between the tongue and the upper front teeth. The tongue body is typically quite low, since contact at the teeth involves a relatively low point within the oral cavity. It can be seen that the stop burst spectrum for dental /t̪/ in Arrernte is really quite flat compared to the alveolar and retroflex spectra. Such a flat spectrum with a very broad spread of energy is typical of this sound. Part of the explanation for this broad spread of energy lies in the fact that there may not be a cavity as such in front of the constriction at the moment of release for the dental (perhaps comparable to the case of the bilabial). However, a more important consideration is the jaw movement related to these sounds. For the alveolar and for the retroflex, the jaw remains quite high at the moment of stop burst release, whereas for the dental this is not the case, with the jaw lowering before stop burst release in anticipation of the following vowel (Tabain, 2012). What is relevant here is that the lower teeth move together with the jaw, and the lower teeth can represent a significant obstacle to airflow at the moment of stop burst release. Such an obstacle serves to enhance the amplitude of any spectral peaks, and if this secondary obstacle is not present, the sound may not have as much energy. In fact, the presence of the teeth is what gives sibilant sounds such as /s/ and /ʃ/ (discussed later in the chapter) their characteristic noise. In the case of the stop bursts, if the lower teeth are in the path of the airstream at stop burst, the amplitude of spectral peaks is increased; this is the case for the alveolar and for the retroflex. However if the lower teeth are not in the path of the airstream, there is no overall increase in amplitude – this is the case with the dental, where the tongue tip is in contact with the upper teeth (it is presumably somewhat difficult to channel the air from this point at the upper teeth towards the lower teeth, at least for most speakers).

The other stop burst that can be seen in Figure 10.1 is for the palatal stop /c/ – or to be more precise, the alveo-palatal. The symbols that are used in the IPA – /c/ and /ɟ/ – are in fact ambiguous, and may represent a "proper" palatal sound that may be heard by native English speakers as /kj/ (that is, articulated just in front of the soft-palate/hard-palate juncture), and an alveo-palatal sound that can be heard by English speakers as /tj/. A typical characteristic of the alveo-palatal stop is that it is strongly affricated, and that is certainly the case for the languages shown in Figure 10.1. This is one reason why many researchers prefer to use the symbol /tɕ/ to denote the alveo-palatal stop. Indeed, English speakers may often hear this affricated /c/ as /tʃ/ (although there are important spectral differences as will be seen for /ʃ/). There is some variety in the /c/ spectra shown in Figure 10.1, but in all cases a spectral prominence can be seen at around 4000 Hz (about 4000–6000 Hz for Makasar, and about 3000–5000 Hz for Arrernte and Pitjantjatjara). Importantly, the balance of spectral energy is shifted upwards for the alveo-palatal – it will be seen that the stop burst for this sound has less energy in the spectral range below 3000 Hz than any of the other stops. It can be said that the palatal stop has a higher spectral "center of gravity" than the other stops, while the bilabial has a relatively low spectral center of gravity. It should be noted that the alveo-palatal stop, like the alveolar and retroflex, has a high jaw position at stop burst. This means that the high-frequency energy is enhanced by the teeth serving as an obstacle to the airflow. It is important to note that the concentration of energy is at higher frequencies for the alveo-palatal than it is for the alveolar, even though in principle one might expect that the smaller cavity in front of the alveolar closure would result in a higher-frequency spectral burst for the alveolar than for the alveo-palatal. A further discussion of this issue is beyond the scope of this chapter, but it suffices to say that the shape of the tongue at the moment of release, as well as shape characteristics of the cavity in front of the closure, and properties of the cavity behind the constriction, all contribute to the final spectral output. It would be fair to say that a better understanding of all of these contributing factors is much needed for the variety of sounds in the world's languages.

We now have only two stop "places" of articulation to consider on the IPA chart. The first is the uvular stops /q ɢ/, which are produced further back in the oral cavity than the velars. In languages that contrast velars and uvulars, it is typically the case that the uvulars induce a more back vowel quality on adjacent vowels; thus, a sequence /qa/ is more likely to sound like [qɑ]. The other stop – the glottal /ʔ/ – is not really oral, in the sense that it does not involve a closure in the oral cavity. This laryngeal consonant typically involves glottalization of adjacent vowels, and only prototypical glottal stop articulations involve a period of complete silence on a spectrogram.

Formant and other cues to place of articulation

Thus far, we have simply considered the stop burst as a cue to stop place of articulation, and in a sense, it is the presence of the burst that identifies the stop as being a stop. However, the actual place identity of the stop is cued by several aspects of the articulation, including the duration of the closure, the duration of the burst, and by formant transitions into and out of the stop itself.

The main formant to cue consonant place of articulation is F_2, although F_3 and perhaps even F_4 may play a role in certain instances (Ladefoged and Maddieson, 1996). F_1 is not usually considered a cue to stop place of articulation, although it is certainly a cue to stop manner (though see next paragraph regarding cues to post-velar places of articulation). F_1 is typically falling into a stop, and typically rising out of a stop (this includes nasal stops, as shown in Figure 10.2). This is because, theoretically, F_1 is at zero for a stop consonant, since the stop closure is an extreme case of a constriction in the oral cavity. In this case, the stop closure forms a constriction for a Helmholtz resonance – that is, the constriction can be considered the "neck" of a bottle-like resonator, and the cavity behind the constriction is the "bottle" itself. Since the cavity behind the constriction is quite large, it becomes the lowest resonance of the system, and hence is associated with F_1 in an adjacent vowel. In a Helmholtz resonance, the smaller the constriction, the lower the resonance frequency – at the point where there is no constriction, the resonance frequency is zero. This is why F_1 is typically falling into and rising out of a stop consonant.

However, other consonant effects on F_1 relating to coarticulation must not be discounted. For example, certain consonants result in modifications to F_1 at the midpoint of an adjacent vowel. For example, alveo-palatal stops require a relatively high jaw position due to the involvement of a large part of the tongue body in their articulation (the tongue body and the jaw are considered coupled articulators, cf. Keating et al., 1994). As a result, in a sequence such as /ca/, the tongue and jaw may not have time to reach the following low vowel target, and as a result, the sequence may (assuming no phonemic vowel constraints in the language) sound more like [ce] – that is, with a lower F_1 than might be expected for an /a/ vowel. This

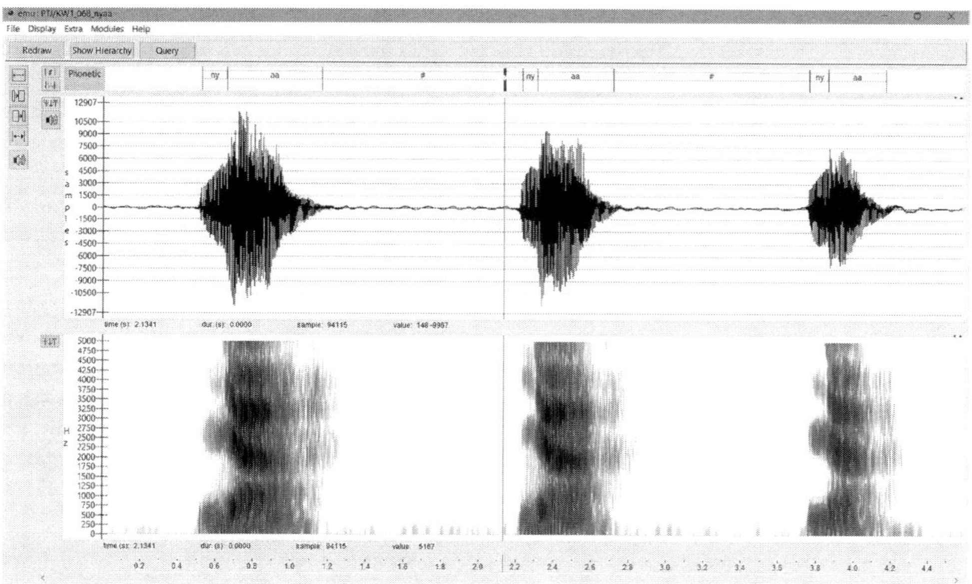

Figure 10.2 Waveform and spectrogram of Pitjantjatjara speaker Kathleen Windy (female) producing the word *nyaa* ("what?"). The segment "ny" denotes the palatal nasal /ɲ/. The frequency range of the spectrogram is 0–5 kHz, and the duration values along the y-axis are given in seconds.

is certainly the case following the alveo-palatal consonants in Arrernte. It was also mentioned that uvular consonants often result in a more back vowel articulation than would be expected for a given vowel phoneme – in this case, the effect of the consonant is on F_2 of the vowel (i.e., a lower F_2 adjacent to uvular consonants). However, post-velar consonants such as uvulars and pharyngeals also have a higher F_1 compared to more anterior consonants – if F_1 is treated as a Helmholtz resonance, then the shorter cavity behind the consonant constriction results in higher F_1 values, and thus a lower vowel. Notably, F_1 tends to be higher for pharyngeals than for uvulars (Alwan, 1989; Sylak-Glassman, 2014).

Nevertheless, as already mentioned, by far the most important cues to consonant place of articulation lie in the formant transitions into and out of the consonant itself. These transitions capture the changing shapes of the cavities in front of and behind the constriction as the articulators move from the consonant into the vowel (or the vowel into the consonant). It must be stressed that while the stop burst is defined primarily by the cavity in front of the constriction, the formant transitions are much more appropriately modeled as being vowel-like, and as such, both the cavity behind and the cavity in front of the constriction are relevant. As already noted that F_1 is associated with the constriction itself coupled with the back cavity. F_2 and F_3 are associated with the cavities behind and in front of the constriction. The cavity behind the constriction is modeled as a half-wavelength resonance – that is, the resonance is a function of twice the length of the cavity. A half-wavelength resonance is a resonance that is closed at both ends, and in this case, the resonance is deemed to be "closed" at both the glottis, and at the constriction. By contrast, the cavity in front of the constriction is modeled as a quarter-wavelength resonance – that is, the resonance is a function of four times the length of the cavity. A quarter-wavelength resonance is a resonance that is closed at one end, and open at the other. In this case, the resonance is deemed to be "closed" at the constriction, but open at the lips. F_2 is therefore assigned to whichever cavity has the lower resonance, and typically this is the back cavity; F_3 is then assigned to the cavity that has the higher resonance, which is typically the front cavity.

In the case of velar consonants, F_2 and F_3 are theoretically very close together. This is because the velar constriction often occurs at around two-thirds the length of the vocal tract length, as measured from the glottis to the lips. Since the cavity behind the velar constriction is in this case twice as long as the cavity in front of the constriction, the half-wavelength resonance behind the constriction is at theoretically the same frequency as the quarter-wavelength resonance in front of the constriction. In practice, however, the location of the velar constriction depends very much on the adjacent vowel context, with the constriction being further forward for front vowels and further back for back vowels. Nevertheless, a "velar pinch" is sometimes seen, where F_2 and F_3 come together leading into or out of a velar consonant (Johnson 2012). It should also be noted that F_2 and F_3 can be very close together for palatal consonants, as well.

When the consonant is further forward than this velar/palatal "two-thirds point," F_2 is affiliated with the back cavity, and F_3 with the front cavity (i.e.,. for the coronal consonants). When the consonant is further back than this velar "two-thirds point," F_2 is affiliated with the front cavity, and F_3 with the back cavity (i.e., for uvular consonants). For an alveolar, for example, F_2 is a back cavity resonance, even though the alveolar burst is associated with the front cavity. The alveolar "locus" for F_2 is typically around 2 kHz for adult female speakers (a bit lower for male speakers, and higher for children). However, it is important to note that the relative size of the front and back cavities for a given speaker depends not just on the location of the consonant constriction, but also on constriction length. For instance, alveolar and dental consonants have relatively similar constriction locations, but if one is an apical articulation (i.e., it uses only the smallest front portion of the tongue) and the other is a laminal articulation (i.e., it uses a larger portion of the front-most part of the tongue), the relative sizes of the front and back cavities may be affected. In Australian languages, alveolar and dental consonants tend to have similar F_2 values. However, dentals tend to have a higher F_3 value. Since dentals are laminal consonants, it is possible that the greater constriction length for the dental results in F_2 (the back cavity resonance) being similar to the alveolar consonants, but F_3 (the front cavity resonance) being higher than for the alveolar. F_1 for laminal articulations also tends to be lower than for apical articulations, and this is likely also related to the greater constriction length for laminals, since the F_1 Helmholtz resonance is lower when the constriction is longer. (I should stress at this point that for the sake of simplicity, I am using the tubes and resonators approach to modeling speech production, whereas in some instances an approach that uses perturbation theory [Chiba and Kajiyama, 1941] may be more appropriate. The reader is referred to Johnson (2012) for further discussion of perturbation theory.)

The question of laminal versus apical articulations raises another issue that concerns formant transitions, and that is transition duration. All else being equal, apical articulations reach their vowel target more quickly than do laminal articulations, so that transitions into and out of apical articulations tend to be quite short, while transitions into and out of laminal articulations (and also into and out of velars) tend to be a bit longer (cf. Dart, 1991). This is because the tongue tip on its own is quite a rapidly moving articulator; in addition, a laminal articulation typically recruits a large part of the tongue body, and the release of the longer (in length) constriction may take longer (in duration). This observation is particularly relevant for palatal consonants (which are never apical articulations!), where the transitions into and out of the vowel tend to be quite long. Palatals have a very high F_2 and also F_3 (which as already mentioned may be quite close together). This is because the cavity behind the constriction (F_2) is relatively short compared to the cavity behind the constriction for an alveolar. At the same time however, due to the large amount of tongue-palate contact for palatals, the front cavity (F_3) is also relatively small. Due to the involvement of large portions of the tongue, and also to the relatively high point of contact within the oral cavity, palatal transitions tend to be very long and very noticeable on a spectrogram, as they move from the high F_2 locus for the consonant (often above 2.5 kHz even for adult male speakers) to the F_2 for the vowel target (see the palatal nasal consonant in Figure 10.2 for an example).

As a point of contrast, we might consider the retroflex consonants. These are consonants that are articulated with the tongue tip, and so involve a relatively thin band of contact between the tongue and the palate. As discussed earlier, initial contact for the retroflex is further back than for the alveolar consonants. Since the cavity in front of the retroflex constriction is longer for the retroflex than for an alveolar articulated with the same active articulator, F_3 is lower for the retroflex than for the alveolar *at the onset of contact*. Indeed, a low F_3 is considered a defining characteristic of a retroflex articulation. The important point to note, however, is that F_3 is noticeably lower for the retroflex than for the alveolar only for the transition *into* the consonant. It is not always the case that F_3 is lower for the retroflex than for the alveolar for the transition *out of* the consonant, since as already mentioned, the ballistic forward movement of the tongue that is seen during the closure for a prototypical retroflex results in the retroflex consonant being released very close to the alveolar zone. Differences in F_2 between alveolars and retroflexes are often non-significant, and this may be due to a slightly different tongue configuration at the point of contact, resulting in the back cavity having relatively similar proportions for both of these consonant sounds.

Finally, we consider the bilabial consonant transitions (the glottal stop does not have a transition as such, since it does not involve a constriction at any point along the oral cavity). Bilabials are particular in that a lip constriction means that the tongue is free to articulate any adjacent vowels without being biomechanically constrained by the articulation for the consonant. This means that bilabial formant transitions do not tend to have very long durations. The theoretical F_2 and F_3 locus for bilabial consonants is quite low. This can be explained if one considers that at the moment of bilabial closure or release, the oral cavity forms one long tube, with the formants arising at multiples of the fundamental tube resonance. This tube can be modeled as a tube open at one end, and so as a quarter-wavelength resonance, although it is also possible that at the point of closure and release, the tube is more appropriately modeled as a tube closed at both ends, and so a half-wavelength resonance. The F_2 locus for a bilabial consonant is typically around 1 kHz for an adult male speaker.

Nasals

We turn now to the nasal consonants, or more properly, the nasal stop consonants. Nasal consonants are often conceived of as being the exact place-of-articulation counterparts of the oral stop consonants, and there are many phonetic and phonological reasons for this conception – for instance, in many languages, the only consonant clusters that are allowed are nasal + stop clusters with the same place of articulation (i.e., homorganic clusters), and indeed the presence of a nasal in the phoneme inventory implies a stop at the same place of articulation (Gordon, 2016). Nasal stops and oral stops both involve a complete closure within the oral cavity, but nasal stops differ from oral stops in that the primary airflow is in principle through the nasal cavity: The velum is lowered in order to allow for this airflow to happen. For this reason, there are no nasal consonants that are articulated further back than the uvular place of articulation. Indeed, the pharyngeal and glottal places of articulation are blocked out on the IPA chart, in order to indicate that if air is flowing through the nasal cavity, there cannot be a complete constriction at the pharyngeal or glottal places of articulation.

The manner class of nasals is primarily characterized by a noticeable reduction in spectral energy (Dang, Honda, and Suzuki, 1994; Dang and Honda, 1996). This loss in acoustic energy arises from two main sources: From losses within the nasal cavity itself, and from losses arising from the interaction between the oral and nasal cavities. We first consider the losses within the nasal cavity. Since in theory the primary airflow for nasal stops is through the nasal cavity, it is generally thought that energy is lost via the four pairs of para-nasal sinuses (maxillary, sphenoidal, frontal and ethomoidal). The para-nasal sinuses are very small side-branches from the main nasal cavity, with little openings (ostia) that result in the sinuses acting as Helmholtz (i.e., bottle-like) resonators that "trap" acoustic energy from the main nasal airflow. This means that the resonant frequencies at which the various para-nasal sinuses vibrate are removed from the spectral output – that is, the sinuses introduce anti-resonances (in signal processing terms these anti-resonances are often called "zeros") into the spectral output. The larger sinuses have Helmholtz resonances of around 500 Hz, while the smaller sinuses have Helmholtz resonances of 1500 Hz or more than 3000 Hz. The exact values of the sinus resonances vary dramatically from speaker to speaker, and are thought to contribute to individual speaker characteristics. Empirical studies also find zeros in the nasal spectrum well above 5 kHz, resulting in a heavily dampened spectrum above this frequency range. The important point to note from the phonetic point of view is that energy is lost across a wide range of frequency values, purely due to the presence of these sinuses. In addition, the presence of nasal hairs and mucus can also contribute to losses in the spectral output of nasal consonants (damping of acoustic energy), as can the presence of any asymmetries between the two nasal pathways as the airflow approaches the nares.

The second source of energy loss in nasals arises from acoustic energy being trapped within the oral cavity while the main airflow is (theoretically) through the nasal cavity. In this case, the exact frequency of the anti-resonance is dependent upon place of articulation and on the length of the constriction. Since the main path of the airflow is through the pharyngeal cavity and the nasal cavity, the pocket of air behind the constriction in the oral cavity forms a side-branch to the main airflow, just as the sinuses do within the nasal cavity. For a bilabial nasal, the side-branch is comparatively long, and estimates of the anti-resonance arising from the nasal cavity tend around 1000 Hz for an adult male (based on treating the side-branch as a quarter-wavelength resonator of about 8–9 cm, closed at the bilabial constriction). This anti-resonance becomes progressively higher in frequency as the constriction becomes further back (estimates of the anti-resonance frequency for velar /ŋ/ tend around 3500 Hz). At the point of a uvular constriction for the nasal /ɴ/, the side-branch theoretically disappears, as the air flows along the pharyngeal and nasal cavities only. However, it must be stressed that the size of the oral cavity side-branch depends not just on the passive place-of-articulation, but on the active articulator as well – for instance, in Australian languages, where the dental is a laminal articulation and the alveolar is an apical articulation, the anti-resonance for the dental may be higher than the anti-resonance for the alveolar, since the more extensive tongue–palate contact for the dental may result in a comparatively smaller back cavity. In addition, for some speakers, a retroflex nasal may have a higher anti-resonance than a palatal nasal, if for that speaker the tongue tip contacts the roof of the mouth at a point further back than the contact for the palatal.

The combined effect of all of these losses in acoustic energy is evident in Figure 10.2, which shows an example of a palatal nasal /ɲ/ followed by the low vowel /a:/ in the Pitjantjatjara word *nyaa* ("what?"). Since the nasal is word-initial, there seems to be much less energy for the first half of the consonant than for the second half, especially in the higher frequencies. Overall, it can be seen that there is much less energy for the nasal than there is for the following vowel, at all frequency ranges. Some energy is visible from 0 to 1 kHz, and from 2 to 3 kHz. However, there are large gaps in the spectrum between about 1 kHz and 2 kHz, and above 4 kHz, which represent the combined effects of the oral and sinus anti-resonances (note that the anti-resonance from the oral side-branch also has harmonics at odd multiples, so that for instance, an anti-resonance of 1000 Hz has another anti-resonance at 3000 Hz).

Two other points can be noted based on Figure 10.2. The first is that F_1 is clearly rising in the transition from nasal to vowel. This is because at the moment of nasal stop release, the tongue is still in the configuration for an oral stop consonant, and the normal F_1 transition that is seen for oral stops is also usually seen for nasal stops (assuming that the velopharyngeal port has been sufficiently closed to prevent nasal airflow, as appears to be the case in this spectrogram). At the same time in this spectrogram, F_2 is clearly falling, from about 2500 Hz at the nasal-vowel boundary, to about 1500 Hz for the vowel. F_3 falls from about 3500 Hz to about 3000 Hz. These are typical transitions for palatal consonants of all different manners of articulation.

As a side note, Australian languages such as Pitjantjatjara seem to show minimal nasalization of segments surrounding nasal consonants. This is thought to be so in order to maintain strong formant cues to consonant place of articulation, given that nasalization of vowels significantly alters vowel formant frequencies and bandwidths (nasalization of vowels is particularly common cross-linguistically when the nasal is in syllable coda position, making it very difficult to find boundaries between the vowel and the following nasal in the spectrogram). Altered formant cues may compromise access to place of articulation information in Australian languages, which have up to six places of articulation in oral stops, nasals and laterals. It is therefore important to note that despite the presence of the nasal "murmur," the main cues to place of articulation for nasals still lie in the formant transitions into and out of adjacent segments. To a certain extent, it could be argued that the presence of the nasal murmur simply serves to cue nasal manner itself, since it is very hard to distinguish nasal place of articulation based on the nasal murmur alone (Harrington, 1994; see also Malecot, 1956; Nakata, 1959; Fujimura, 1962; Recasens, 1983; Huffman and Krakow, 1993). Indeed, due to the low spectral energy of the nasal murmur, these sounds are all the more difficult to distinguish in noise, since any cues to place of articulation from the oral anti-resonance are compromised by the presence of background noise (because the anti-resonance cue to place of articulation is actually a spectral minimum, not a peak, and so is masked by background noise).

Thus far, we have focused on the anti-resonances that define the nasal consonants. This is because there is perhaps greater agreement among researchers as to exactly how these anti-resonances arise (see Fant, 1970, and Stevens, 1998). However, nasal consonants are also defined by their resonances, and exactly how these arise is not quite so clear – a lack of cross-language research on nasal consonants certainly doesn't help matters. In terms of spectral energy, nasal consonants often have a very low first formant, around 200–400 Hz for an adult male speaker and a little higher for an adult female speaker (such a low first nasal formant – usually labeled N1 – can be seen in Figure 10.2 for the female speaker). Theoretically, a second nasal formant may be seen at about 1000 Hz, with a third nasal formant at about 2000–2500 Hz. Nasal formants are characterized by very wide bandwidths. For the low first nasal formant, the bandwidth is about 100 Hz. For the higher formants, the bandwidth values tend around 300 Hz.

Some researchers consider that the first formant is a Helmholtz resonance formed by the pharyngeal cavity and by the constriction at the velopharyngeal port; the wide bandwidth is a result of the losses that arise within the nasal cavity. As a result of the low frequency of N1, it is often difficult to distinguish this first nasal formant from the fundamental frequency, with the two combining to form a significant spectral prominence in the low-frequency region. The second nasal formant (and its odd multiple, which may become the fourth formant) may arise as the natural resonance of the nasal cavity itself, while the third formant may arise as the natural resonance of the pharyngeal cavity (see Stevens, 1998; Fant, 1970; Tabain, Butcher, Breen, and Beare, 2016b). In contrast, other researchers consider that the entire nasal and pharyngeal tract forms one long resonating cavity, with no significant constriction at the velopharyngeal port. In this case, the nasal resonances are simply odd multiples of the quarter-wavelength resonance that extends from the glottis to the nares, albeit with the oral and sinus side-braches producing anti-resonances.

All of these modeling approaches to nasal consonants, however, fail to account for results from several empirical studies (on languages as diverse as the European languages Catalan, Polish, Czech, German, Hungarian, Russian and Swedish, and the Australian languages Yanyuwa, Yindjibarndi, Arrernte, Pitjantjatjara and Warlpiri) that find significant differences in the nasal formants based on place of articulation. The first nasal formant, N1, is found to be significantly lower for bilabials and significantly higher for velars, with the coronal consonants in between. Moreover, the bilabial nasal has the lowest N2, N3, and N4, and these higher nasal formants have similarly low values for the velar nasal. Given that acoustic models of nasals do not consider the possibility that place of articulation within the oral cavity has any influence on the spectral output other than via the introduction of anti-formants, these consistent empirical results are surprising, and suggest that oral resonances (and not just anti-resonances) play an important role in the output of nasal consonants. Interestingly, at least for the Australian languages, the palatal nasal /ɲ/ has a low N1 (like the bilabial /m/), but very high N2 and N3 (note that this low N1 does not seem to be replicated in European language data, where the palatal N1 instead patterns between the alveolar and the velar). As we saw earlier, a low F_1, and a high F_2 and F_3, are important cues to palatal place of articulation for the vowel formant transition, so the very high N2 and N3 in the nasal murmur suggest a significant contribution from the oral resonances to the nasal consonant output. There are also significant differences in bandwidth values between the various nasal places of articulation – for instance, the velar has by far the greatest bandwidth for N1, whereas the palatal has the greatest bandwidth for N2, N3, and N4.

So what might be some of the sources for these various differences in the places of articulation for nasals? It is certainly true that the presence of anti-resonances in the spectrum affects any nearby resonances, shifting them slightly in frequency, and broadening their bandwidths. However, this cannot account for all of the differences observed. One possibility for palatal nasals is that the proximity of the tongue body and the lowered uvula sets up a special coupling relationship between the oral and pharyngeal cavities. By contrast, for anterior coronal sounds such as the dental /n̪/, the alveolar /n/ and the retroflex /ɳ/, the back of the tongue may form a Helmholtz-like constriction with the lowered uvula, likewise leading to a greater contribution from the oral formants. The bilabial /m/, by contrast, should not involve any proximity between the tongue and the uvula (at least for most vowel contexts), and it is possible that the nasal formants for the bilabial nasal are simply harmonic multiples of the nasal cavity. Overall, the picture for where resonances arise for nasal consonants is a very murky one, and despite some good work on determining the resonance properties of the nasal and para-nasal cavities, the question of how/why the resonances in nasal consonants arise is one that requires much further articulatory-to-acoustic modeling.

Laterals

Lateral consonants are similar to nasal consonants in that they both involve a reduction of spectral energy due to the presence of anti-resonances in the spectrum. However, in the case of laterals, the importance of these anti-resonances is much diminished, since they only arise from within the oral cavity, and not from within the nasal and para-nasal cavities.

Laterals involve continuous airflow through the oral cavity, along the side(s) of the tongue. A constriction is formed at some point along the roof of the mouth, and the side(s) of the tongue are lowered in order to allow air to escape laterally. It is not clear whether the sides of the tongue are actively lowered, or whether the tongue is lengthened in order to shorten the width of the tongue (Ladefoged and Maddieson, 1996). Regardless of the exact mechanism, due to the volume-preserving nature of the tongue, when air is allowed to flow along the sides of the tongue, another part of the tongue must be displaced in order for this to happen. We will return to this issue later in the chapter, in relation to the class of liquids (i.e., laterals and rhotics).

According to the IPA chart, the central constriction for a lateral consonant may occur at any point from the dental place of articulation to the uvular place of articulation. However, the only official lateral (non-fricative) symbols are /l/, the retroflex /ɭ/, the palatal /ʎ/, and the velar /ʟ/. The dental or alveolar /l/ is by far the most common lateral in the world's languages, while the retroflex and palatal are not uncommon. The velar /ʟ/ is very rare; it occurs in some languages of Papua New Guinea, and it may occur allophonically in some dialects of English. It is not a sound that is well understood as yet, and to many English speakers it may simply sound like [gl̠]. It is possible that it is comparatively difficult to produce a full closure centrally in the velar or uvular region, while at the same time allowing air to flow along the sides of the tongue.

One important consequence of the central constriction for a lateral is that there is a pocket of air trapped behind the constriction. This pocket of air is considered to be the main source of any anti-resonances that occur in the lateral spectrum. The main airflow is along the side(s) of the tongue, and the pocket of air behind the constriction serves as a cavity to trap any acoustic energy at the resonant frequency of the cavity. The cavity is treated as a quarter-wavelength resonance (closed at the constriction), and as may be inferred from previous discussions, the exact length of this cavity will vary greatly depending on the place of articulation and on the active articulator (as an aside, it is not clear whether this cavity is of any appreciable size behind a velar constriction, as opposed to a more anterior constriction). The frequency of this anti-resonance may be less than 1000 Hz, or it may be as high as 4000 Hz – it is really not clear for the different lateral places of articulation. Additional anti-resonances may also arise when the left and right pathways for the lateral airflow are not symmetrical, and this may vary greatly from speaker to speaker.

Figure 10.3a shows a spectrogram of the Pitjantjatjara word *palyaṉi* /paʎaɳi/ ("to make/fix"). It can be seen that like the nasal, the lateral has somewhat less energy relative to the adjacent vowel, although it has more energy than the nasal in this same word. Some other similarities can be seen between the palatal lateral in this figure, and the palatal nasal in

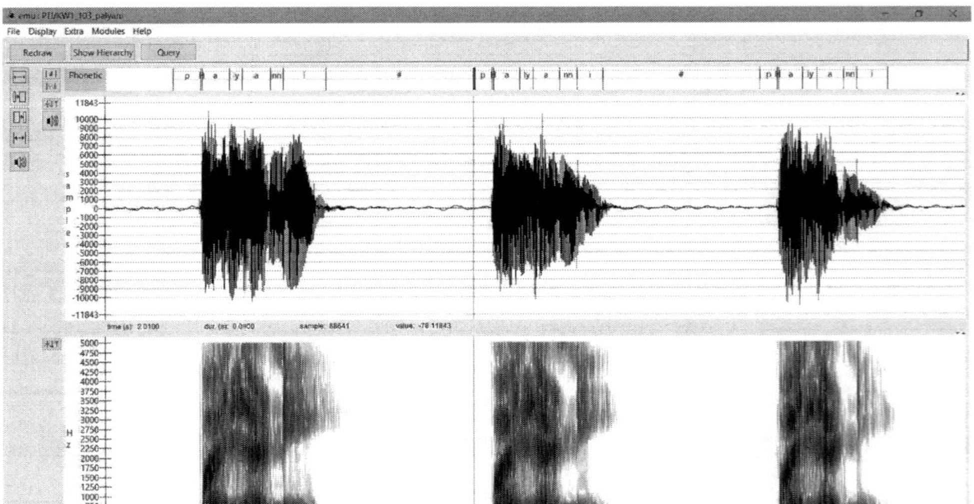

Figure 10.3a Waveform and spectrogram of Pitjantjatjara speaker Kathleen Windy (female) producing the word *palyaṉi* ("to make/fix"). The segment "ly" denotes the palatal lateral /ʎ/ and "nn" denotes a retroflex nasal. The frequency range of the spectrogram is 0–5 kHz, and the duration values along the y-axis are given in seconds.

Figure 10.2. In both figures, there is a large gap in spectral energy in the mid-frequencies; in the case of the lateral, this gap is between about 500 Hz and about 2000 Hz. However, the lateral has more energy than the nasal in the higher frequencies, above 4 kHz, and this is most likely due to the fact that there are no losses from the para-nasal sinuses. The lowest resonance for the lateral is at or below 500 Hz, and this is typical for all lateral sounds. It is thought that this lowest lateral resonance is due to a Helmholtz resonance formed between the lateral constriction along the side(s) of the tongue, and the large cavity behind the constriction. The lateral F_1 is lower for laminal articulations than for apical articulations. This is most likely due to a longer constriction or a smaller cross-sectional area for the constriction in the case of a laminal articulation (laminal articulations involve a higher tongue body position and a higher jaw position than do apical articulations).

As regards the higher frequency lateral resonances in Figure 10.3a, formants can be seen at about 2250 Hz, about 3250 Hz, and about 4200 Hz. These values are very typical for palatal laterals, the high second formant being a defining characteristic of all palatal consonants, as already seen. A high F_4 (above rather than below 4 kHz) seems to be a characteristic of laminal laterals. Since as already mentioned, laminals are characterized by a longer constriction than apicals, it is likely that F_4 arises from a back cavity resonance, which is presumably smaller for a laminal articulation than for an apical articulation.

Figure 10.3b shows spectrograms of an Arrernte speaker producing the minimal pair *alheme* /al̪əmə/ ("goes") followed by *aleme* /aləmə/ ("liver"), which shows the (laminal) dental versus (apical) alveolar contrast in this language. It can be seen that the lateral formants for these sounds are a little more evenly spaced than for the palatal. Some researchers

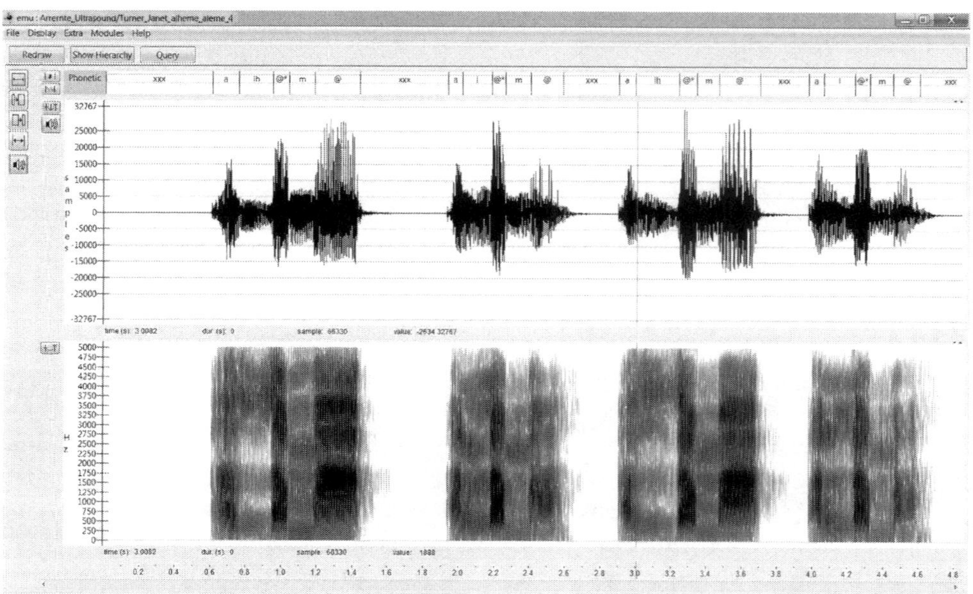

Figure 10.3b Waveform and spectrogram of Arrernte speaker Janet Turner (female) producing the minimal pair *alheme* ("goes") followed by *aleme* ("liver"). The segment "lh" denotes the dental lateral /l̪/ and "@" denotes the schwa vowel. The frequency range of the spectrogram is 0–5 kHz, and the duration values along the y-axis are given in seconds.

have suggested that the relatively even spacing of the upper formants, with a large gap between F_1 and F_2, is what gives laterals their “ringing” quality (Fant, 1970). In Figure 10.3b, the first lateral formant is once again below about 500 Hz, and it might be seen that this formant is a little higher for the laminal “lh” /l̪/ than for the apical /l/. For both of these sounds, the second formant sits at around 1700 Hz, and this is also typical for the retroflex /ɭ/, which is not shown here (recall that for the palatal, the second formant was above 2 kHz). A third formant is visible at about 3000 Hz in both cases, although there seems to be movement in the lateral F_2 and F_3 for the alveolar. This may relate to the marginal phonemic contrast between alveolars and retroflexes in this language, whereby the phonemic alveolar may show articulatory characteristics of a post-alveolar or retroflex consonant, as previously mentioned. F_3 in a retroflex lateral “ring” is a little lower than in the alveolar. It can also be seen in Figure 10.3b that F_4 in the lateral ring is higher in the laminal dental than in the alveolar, as mentioned earlier (although whether or not this is perceptible is a question for further research).

One final point worth commenting on in regards to the lateral figures is the sharp change in amplitude between the lateral and the vowel (Stevens, 1998). However, in many languages there is no such abrupt onset to the lateral when it is in coda position (Tabain, Butcher, Breen and Beare, 2016a). This is because lateral consonants are prone to vocalization (e.g., Hardcastle and Barry, 1989; Recasens, 1996). When the central constriction is released, the articulatory configuration very much resembles a vowel articulation. Indeed, many researchers have commented on the similarity between a lateral configuration and an /i/ vowel configuration. In both cases there is a Helmholtz resonance producing the first formant, with the second formant arising from the cavity behind the constriction (with the multiple of this resonance becoming the fourth formant), and the third formant arising from the cavity in front of the constriction. The main difference between the /i/ articulation and the lateral articulation is the presence of the anti-resonances, which may slightly shift the frequency of the formants and increase their bandwidths. It is perfectly possible to synthesize a lateral sound without any anti-resonances at all, simply by manipulating the resonance frequencies and bandwidths. We may note in passing that some researchers have suggested that the anti-resonance may cancel any resonances in front of the lateral constriction, but this result does not seem likely based on empirical data which shows a lower F_3 for retroflexes, for example.

Thus far, we have been considering a relatively “clear” lateral sound – namely with a relatively high F_2 in the lateral ring. However, in “dark” laterals, F_2 is considerably lower, and this is due to the presence of a second constriction within the oral cavity. In the case of Russian, which has a phonemic contrast between dark and light (i.e., velarized versus palatalized) consonants, it is possible to say that due to the small cross-sectional area of the velar constriction, a second Helmholtz resonance is formed between the back part of the tongue and the soft palate, thereby producing a much lower second formant.[1] In this case, it could be said that the “dark” lateral articulation somewhat resembles the articulation for an /u/ vowel, with a dorsal constriction, and an anterior constriction in the alveolar region rather than at the lips. Thus, if in coda position a dorsal constriction is formed for the lateral, but the anterior lateral constriction is not formed, or is formed a little later, the exact boundary between the vowel nucleus and the coda lateral can be a little difficult to determine visually on a spectrogram (this is often the case in many varieties of English, where the vocalized lateral usually sounds like the unrounded back vowel [ɯ]).

It should be noted that labial laterals are not considered possible in the IPA chart. It is certainly possible to allow air to flow only out of one corner of the mouth, so the reason for this theoretical restriction may be that it is not clear how a pocket of air could be trapped behind a central constriction involving the lips. Pharyngeal laterals are also considered impossible, since it is not clear that the root of the tongue could modify the airflow in the correct manner for a lateral. Finally, glottal laterals are not possible, since laterals necessarily involve a supralaryngeal modification of the airflow. In conclusion, it seems that a particular tongue configuration is needed for the class of lateral sounds.

Rhotics and other pulmonic consonants

Before we consider the class of fricative sounds, a few words are needed regarding the other pulmonic consonant sounds on the IPA chart. The IPA lists trill, tap/flap[2] lateral-fricative, and approximant manners of articulation (in addition to the oral stop, nasal, lateral, and fricative manners of articulation). Perhaps the most significant grouping of this rather miscellaneous collection of manners of articulation is the class of rhotics. Rhotics are /r/-like sounds, and it has been a point of some phonetic and phonological mystery as to why such a diverse range of sounds pattern together across the world's languages. Most researchers would agree that rhotic sounds are characterized by a comparatively low third formant, and that this low third formant is brought about by a constriction towards the uvular or pharyngeal region of the oropharyngeal space.

Figure 10.4 shows a spectrogram example for the two phonemic rhotic sounds of Arrernte in a minimal pair: *arreme* /arəmə/ ("louse") followed by *areme* /aɻəmə/ ("see"). The first rhotic is a trill, and phonologically it is considered to be alveolar. In this spectrogram, four periods of contact are visible (the last period of contact may not involve full closure). The

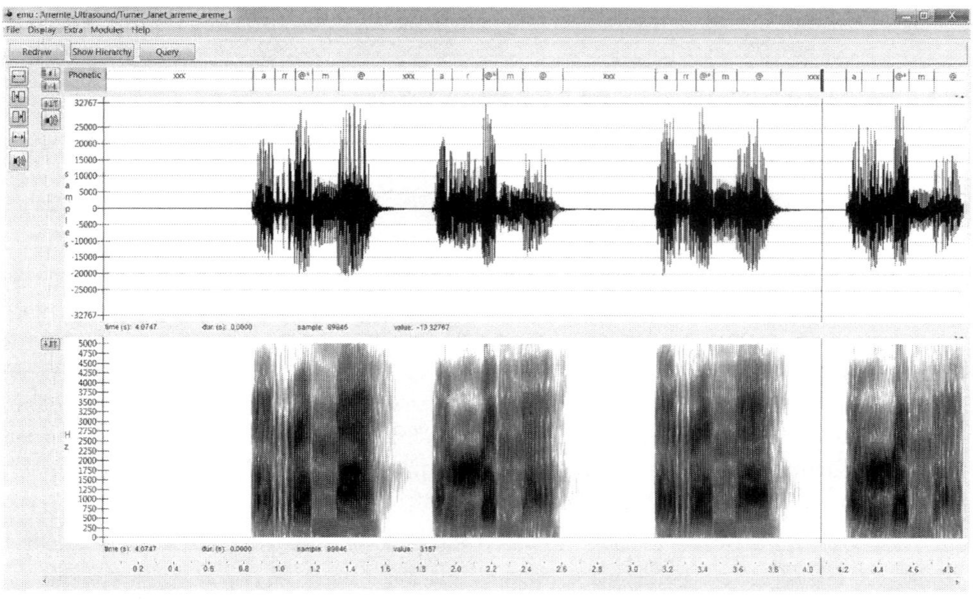

Figure 10.4 Waveform and spectrogram of Arrernte speaker Janet Turner (female) producing the minimal pair *arreme* ("louse") followed by *areme* ("see"). The segment "rr" denotes the alveolar /r/ and "r" denotes the retroflex glide /ɻ/. The frequency range of the spectrogram is 0–5 kHz, and the duration values along the y-axis are given in seconds.

second rhotic is an approximant or glide (the terms are often used interchangeably), and like the trill, it involves a sharp drop in energy from the adjacent vowels (note however that although this is typically the case in Arrernte, a rhotic glide does not always involve a clear drop in energy in all languages). The rhotic glide in this particular example has a very strong spectral prominence centered at about 1750 Hz. This is most likely the combined spectral prominence of F_2 and F_3 together. The other formants are comparatively much weaker for the glide in this particular spectrogram. Notably, however, both the trill and the glide induce a low F_3 in the adjacent vowels (perhaps a little less obvious in the case of the preceding vowel for the trill, but noticeable in all three other adjacent vowels).

In this particular example I have used the symbol for a retroflex glide /ɻ/, but some authors use the symbol for an alveolar glide /ɹ/ to denote the rhotic consonant in languages such as English. The exact articulatory differences between these two sounds are perhaps not terribly clear, but in general the retroflex symbol tends to be used for slightly "darker" sounds than the alveolar rhotic symbol ("dark" being a subjective measure dependent on the hearer's language background, but in general perhaps referring to just how low the F_2 + F_3 spectral prominence might be). In principle, the point of constriction for a "retroflex" rhotic glide should be a little further back than for an alveolar glide. In the case of the English rhotic, much research has shown that the low F_3 arises thanks to a combination of articulatory strategies: The dorsal constriction in the uvular or pharyngeal region, a coronal constriction in the alveolar or post-alveolar region, and a labial constriction as well. All of these constrictions target an anti-node in the standing wave of the third formant resonance of a schwa-like tube, each one of them serving to slightly lower the third formant, and together combining to significantly lower the third formant. (This approach to the English rhotic is based on perturbation theory, but other researchers have used tube models to account for the formant structure of this sound; see for example Zhou, 2009, and Zhou et al., 2008, for discussion of the retroflex versus bunched rhotic of English).

Perhaps somewhat surprisingly, the trill /r/ also involves a significant dorsal constriction in the pharyngeal region. It is thought that this constriction serves to brace the rear-most portion of the tongue, in order to facilitate trilling in the anterior portion of the tongue. The anterior portion for a trill is low in comparison to stop, nasal and lateral sounds at the same "place" of articulation. The other rhotic, the uvular /ʀ/ (sometimes realized in a fricated version as /ʁ/ or /χ/), by definition has a dorsal constriction in the uvular region.

As an aside, the dorsal constriction for the rhotics may be what brings these sounds together with the laterals in the natural class of liquids. It was mentioned earlier that the volume-preserving nature of the tongue leads to the rear-most portion of the tongue being more back for laterals than for stops or nasals with the same place of articulation. Whilst it is certainly not the case that all laterals are "dark" – that is, involving a significant dorsal constriction in the uvular or pharyngeal region – it may be the case that a sufficient number of laterals do involve some dorsal retraction, and that this is sufficient to systematically bring the class of laterals and the class of rhotics together into a natural class of liquid sounds. This is clearly an area for further cross-linguistic research.

Finally, it should be mentioned that the IPA chart recognizes other trill and approximant/glide sounds, such as the bilabial trill /ʙ/ and the glides /j/, /w/, /ɥ/ and /ɰ/. For a trill to be initiated, certain aerodynamic conditions must be met, which are not dissimilar to the conditions required for the initiation of voicing. The relevant trill articulator is set into vibration, and the volume of airflow that is required to maintain trilling leads to compromises between the duration of the trill and the continuation of voicing (see further below for discussion of voicing in fricatives and stops).

Glide articulations are the class of consonant articulations that are most similar to vowels. Air flows relatively unimpeded in the oral cavity, and indeed most glides are simply a relatively short version of a high vowel. The glide counterpart of the unrounded front (palatal) vowel /i/ is /j/; /w/ is the glide counterpart of the rounded back (velar) vowel /u/; /ɥ/ is the glide counterpart of the rounded front (palatal) vowel /y/; and /ɰ/ is the glide counterpart of the unrounded back (velar) vowel /ɯ/. In many languages, the unrounded glides serve as variants of stop or other manners of articulation at the same place of articulation. For instance, where there is not a complete closure for /g/, the sound may be lenited to [ɣ] or even to [ɰ]. In many languages, a palatal /ɲ/ or /ʎ/ may be realized over time as [j] – that is, the nasal or lateral components of the articulation are not realized.

Fricatives

Fricatives are characterized by a *critical* constriction in the oral cavity. By "critical" it is meant that the constriction creates turbulent airflow, and the resultant spectrum is characterized by noise (i.e., spectral energy is distributed randomly across the frequency range). The exact spectral properties of the fricative are dependent on both the location of the constriction and on the length of the constriction. The primary determiner of spectral characteristics of a fricative is the size of the cavity in front of the constriction. However, although constriction location and constriction length are relevant factors for the other consonant manners of articulation, as discussed earlier, they seem to be all the more critical for fricatives in ways that are not yet fully understood. Although by far the largest number of symbols in the IPA chart is for the class of fricatives, the precise articulatory and spectral differences between the various fricatives, in particular the typologically less common fricatives, is in need of further study. In this section I will consider some of the salient characteristics of fricatives, including those in some less well-studied languages.

Figure 10.5a shows an example of the glottal fricative /h/ in the word *hala* ("call to move buffalo") from the Indonesian language Makasar. It can be seen that the spectrum for the glottal is much noisier than the spectrum for the vowel, and the glottal has comparatively much less energy. The glottal fricative is not, strictly speaking, a fricative, since there is no constriction in the oral cavity that shapes the spectrum. Instead, the noise simply arises as a result of airflow through the glottis that has not been modified by voicing. (A breathy glottal "fricative" /ɦ/ is also possible, in which case vocal fold vibration is present, but closure at the vocal folds is not complete, resulting in a larger volume of air "leaking" through the glottis). It can be seen that the glottal fricative has a moderate amount of energy up to about 6 kHz in this spectrogram, and that the energy drops off greatly above this frequency range. Moreover, the peaks in the fricative noise correspond almost exactly to the formant peaks in the following vowel /a/. Indeed, this is the defining characteristic of a glottal fricative: It is effectively the voiceless version of an adjacent vowel.

Although not shown here, a labial fricative such as /f/ has a very similar spectrum to /h/ in the frequency range to about 5–6 kHz, but instead of dropping off above this range, the energy remains constant right up to the very highest frequencies (at least up to 20 kHz). This very constant, even spread of energy is a defining characteristic of the labial fricatives, and also of the dental fricative /θ/. Indeed, it is very difficult to distinguish the labio-dental fricative /f/ from the bilabial fricative /ɸ/, and /f/ from /θ/ in languages that have this contrast; studies have consistently shown that hearers rely on formant transition cues to distinguish place of articulation for these sounds, and also on visual cues. In the case of the labio-dental fricative, it is possible that a cavity exists between the upper teeth and the upper lip,

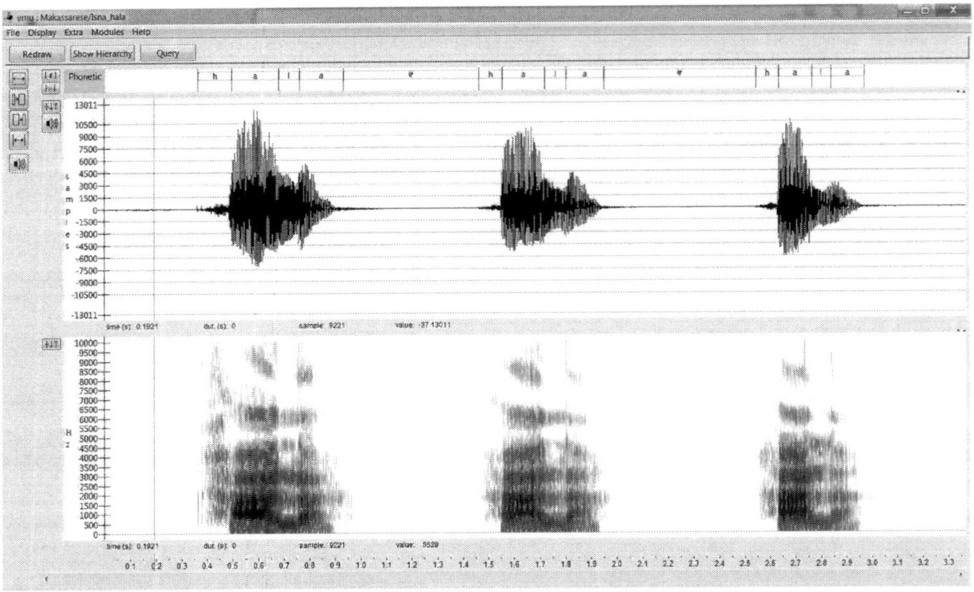

Figure 10.5a Waveform and spectrogram of Makasar speaker Isna Osman (female) producing the word *hala* ("call to move buffalo"). The frequency range of the spectrogram is 0–10 kHz, and the duration values along the y-axis are given in seconds.

particularly if the upper lip is slightly raised in production of this fricative. However, given that there are very few spectral differences between the anterior-most fricatives, it seems to be the case that any cavity in front of the constriction is negligible, and noise is simply generated at the constriction.

Figure 10.5b shows an example of the alveolar fricative /s/ in the word *sala* ("wrong/miss") by the same speaker of Makasar. It can immediately be seen that in comparison to /h/, there is very little energy below 4 kHz for /s/. By contrast, there is much energy above this frequency range, with a broad peak extending from about 5 kHz to 10 kHz. Although not shown here, the energy drops off above 10–11 kHz, where the energy levels for /s/ are comparable to the energy levels for the anterior fricatives /f/ and /θ/. (This particular instance of /s/ seems to have a little less energy around 7500 Hz, though this would not be typical of most instances of this sound). The strong spectral peak for the alveolar fricative /s/ is due to the presence of an obstacle downstream from the constriction. The main constriction for this sound is at the alveolar ridge, and involves a very narrow channel for airflow. Importantly, the airflow through the constriction is channeled towards the lower teeth (for this reason, sounds such as /s/, and /ʃ/ which is discussed next, have a very high jaw position), and these teeth act as an obstacle that increases the turbulence of the airflow, and thereby the amplitude of any spectral peaks. In the case of the alveolar, the cavity in front of the constriction is quite small, and as such the spectral peaks are at a very high frequency, as already seen. By far the most common fricative in the world's languages is /s/, and the salience of its noise is one reason why it is believed to be so common.

High-energy noise is the defining characteristic of fricative sounds that are termed "sibilants." The other fricative that can be termed sibilant is the sound that is spelled "sh" in

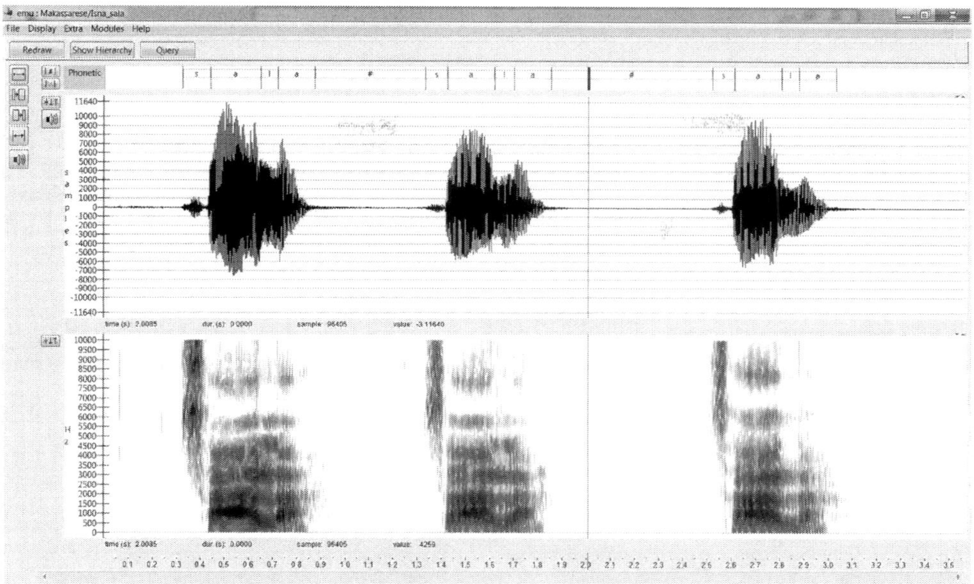

Figure 10.5b Waveform and spectrogram of Makasar speaker Isna Osman (female) producing the word *sala* ("wrong/miss"). The frequency range of the spectrogram is 0–10 kHz, and the duration values along the y-axis are given in seconds.

English, namely /ʃ/. On the IPA chart this sound is listed as post-alveolar, although some researchers use different terms for this sound, such as "palato-alveolar." As the name suggests, the place of constriction is slightly further back for the palato-alveolar/post-alveolar than it is for the alveolar, and the constriction is a little wider. However, as for the /s/, the lower teeth serve as an obstacle downstream of the constriction for /ʃ/, likewise amplifying any spectral peaks. Since the constriction for /ʃ/ is located further back in the oral cavity than the constriction for /s/, the spectral peaks for /ʃ/ are located at a correspondingly lower frequency. This can be seen in Figure 10.5c, which shows an utterance of the English word "shopping" /ʃɔpɪŋ/. It can be seen that there is very little energy below 2 kHz, and that there is a broad spectral peak between about 2.5 kHz and about 5.5 kHz, which is typical for this sound. Although there is less energy above 6 kHz, the amount of energy between 6 and 10 kHz is greater for /ʃ/ than for the non-sibilant sounds /f/ and /θ/. Above 10 kHz (not shown here), the energy in /ʃ/ continues to drop off, with the net result that /ʃ/ has less energy above 10 kHz than do the non-sibilant fricatives /f/ and /θ/. As an aside, the F_2 transition for /ʃ/ has a very high locus compared to the alveolar (or the dental), somewhat resembling a palatal (hence the term palato-alveolar used by some researchers).

Figure 10.5d shows an example of the retroflex fricative in the word /ʂʅ^{33}/ ("to die") from the Tibeto-Burman language Lisu. It can be seen that for this speaker, the retroflex fricative /ʂ/ has a strong spectral peak between about 2.5 and 3.5 kHz, with an extra, less intense peak between about 6 and 8 kHz (the energy gradually decreases above this range). The lower-frequency peak likely arises from the cavity in front of the constriction, and is lower than for the alveolar /s/, given that /ʂ/ likely has a longer front resonating cavity. The apparent extra, less-intense peak may arise from an additional cavity that is formed in a retroflex

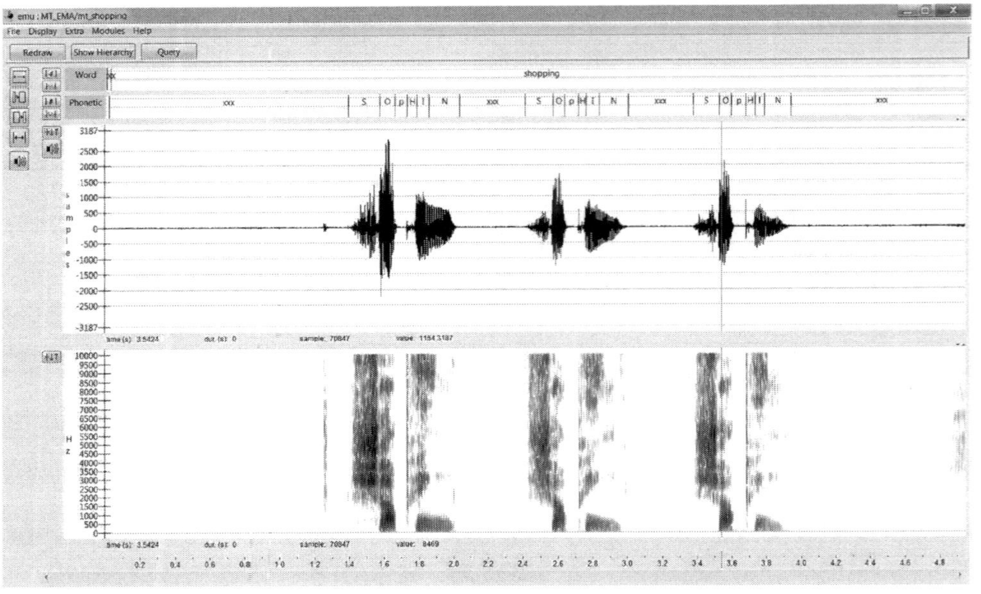

Figure 10.5c Waveform and spectrogram of Australian English speaker Marija Tabain (female) producing the word *shopping*. The segment "S" denotes the fricative /ʃ/ and "N" denotes the velar nasal /ŋ/. The frequency range of the spectrogram is 0–10 kHz, and the duration values along the y-axis are given in seconds.

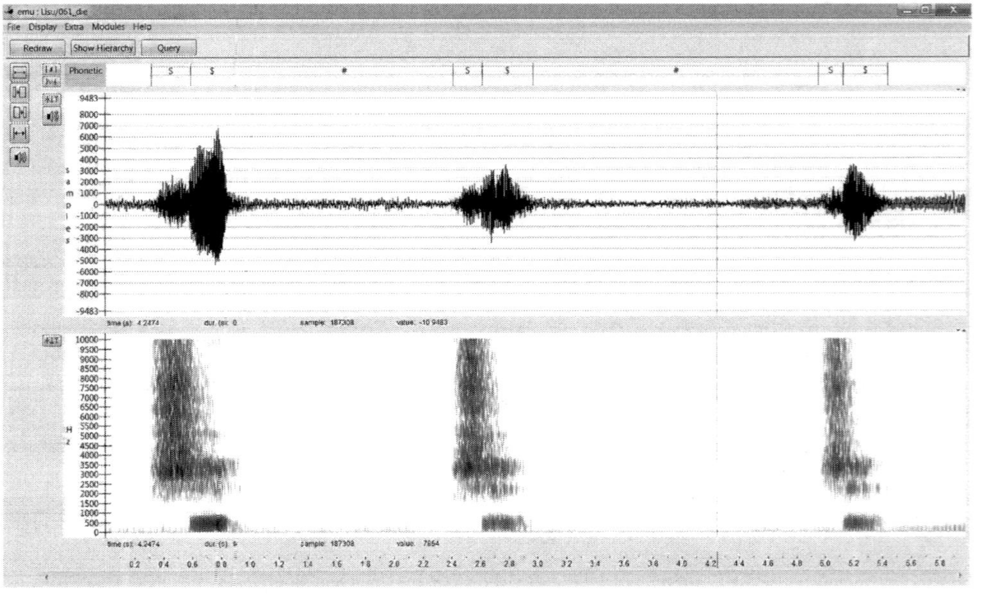

Figure 10.5d Waveform and spectrogram of Lisu speaker Defen Yu (female) producing the word /ʂʅ^{33}/ "(to die"). The segment "S" denotes the retroflex fricative /ʂ/ and "$" denotes the fricative vowel /ʅ/. The frequency range of the spectrogram is 0–10 kHz, and the duration values along the y-axis are given in seconds.

articulation, perhaps underneath the tongue. This is truly an area for extra articulatory-to-acoustic modeling.

Figure 10.5e shows an example of the alveo-palatal fricative in the word /ɕø^{21}/ ("walk"), also from Lisu. For this speaker it can be seen that there is a broad energy peak between about 6 and 10 kHz, and a narrower bandwidth peak at about 3 kHz. For this speaker the alveo-palatal /ɕ/ has less energy overall than the retroflex /ʂ/, although to what extent this is typical for Lisu or even cross-linguistically is not clear. Although the Lisu retroflex seems perceptually and acoustically similar to the same sound in Polish, the alveo-palatal seems to be different in the two languages. It is also not clear whether either the retroflex or the alveo-palatal sounds can be treated as a sibilant fricative. The amount of spectral energy for /ɕ/ suggests that it may be a sibilant, but further research is needed to determine exactly how the noise is channeled.

The back fricatives, such as the velar /x/, have much less energy overall than the coronal fricatives just described, although thanks to a large resonating cavity in front of the constriction, they do have a relatively larger amount of low frequency energy. As noted earlier, post-velar consonants tend to have a higher F_1 in adjacent vowels – with the pharyngeal consonants having an even higher F_1 than the uvular consonants – and often a lower F_2. It should be noted that the voiced pharyngeal fricative /ʕ/ is often realized without frication, as either an approximant or a stop; whereas the voiced uvular fricative /ʁ/ can be realized as either a fricative or as an approximant (Alwan, 1989).

Finally, it should be mentioned that lateral fricatives (voiceless /ɬ/ and voiced /ɮ/) are also possible if the air channel along the side(s) of the tongue forms a critical constriction

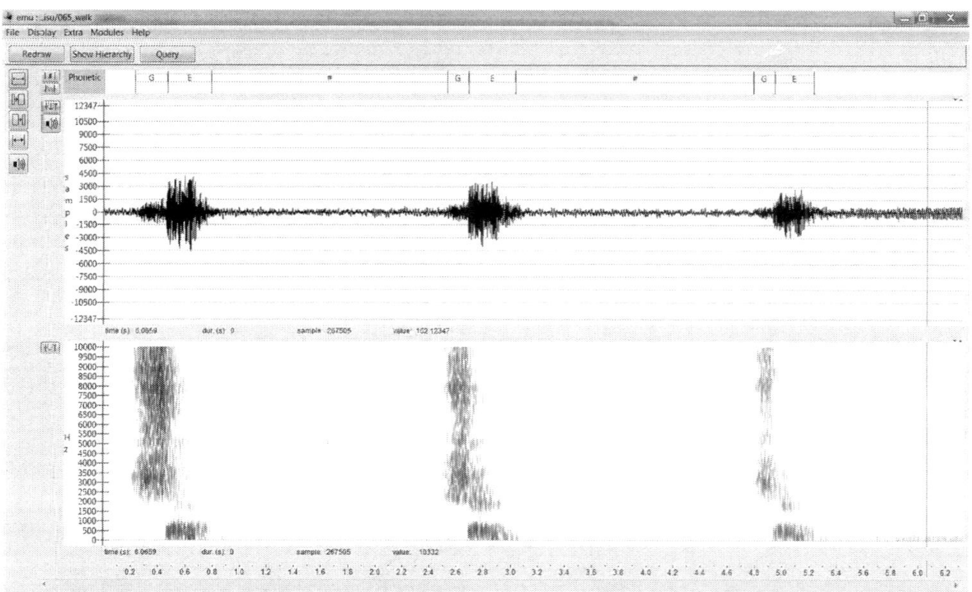

Figure 10.5e Waveform and spectrogram of Lisu speaker Defen Yu (female) producing the word /ɕø^{21}/ ("to walk"). "G" denotes the alveo-palatal fricative /ɕ/ and "E" denotes the front rounded vowel /ø/. The frequency range of the spectrogram is 0–10 kHz, and the duration values along the y-axis are given in seconds.

to generate turbulence. In addition, stops and fricatives may be combined to form affricates such as /ʦ/, /ʧ/ or /ʨ/, which are cross-linguistically relatively common. Articulatorily and spectrally affricates are very similar to stops + fricatives, but their timing characteristics are such that the overall duration is much shorter than for a stop and fricative produced separately.

A brief word on voicing in stops and fricatives

Before concluding this section on fricatives, it is worth emphasizing that the above discussion has focused on the voiceless stops and fricatives. This is because it is in the first instance simpler to consider the acoustic properties of these obstruent sounds without considering the consequences of voicing. In general, a certain amount of airflow is required to generate and maintain voicing, and a certain amount of airflow is required to generate noise within the oral cavity – this noise being necessary for accurate production of stop and fricative sounds, as seen earlier. At a certain point, these two requirements become incompatible. As a consequence, voicing rarely continues throughout the duration of a phonemically voiced stop or fricative consonant.

For voicing to continue, the air pressure below the glottis must be greater than the pressure above the glottis. When air flows freely through the oral or nasal cavity, as for a vowel, voicing may continue for quite some time, depending on the speaker's ability. However, when there is an obstruction in the oral cavity, the pressure above the glottis quickly becomes equal to the pressure below the glottis, and in this case voicing ceases. As a consequence, voicing ceases relatively quickly for a velar stop, since the cavity behind the velar constriction is relatively small. Voicing can continue for relatively longer in a bilabial stop, since the cavity behind the bilabial constriction is the entire oral cavity. In fact, speakers may recruit other articulatory strategies in order to enlarge the supralaryngeal cavities in order to maintain voicing, including expanding the cheeks, lowering the velum (to allow some nasal leakage), and lowering the larynx (to expand the pharyngeal cavity). Similarly for fricatives, voicing does not continue throughout the duration of phonemically voiced fricatives. In fact, since airflow is impeded by voicing, the pressure build-up required for the generation of turbulence at the fricative constriction, or for a high-energy stop burst, is not as great. As a result, the stop burst for voiced stops may be less intense than for voiceless stops, and spectral energy in voiced fricatives compared to voiceless fricatives may be reduced at higher frequencies. The presence of voicing in the spectrum therefore has important consequences for the spectral output of voiced stops and fricatives compared to voiceless stops and fricatives.

Summary

We have seen that there are many place of articulation contrasts that are encoded within the consonant portion itself – be it the stop burst, the nasal murmur, the lateral "ring," or the fricative noise. We have gained some insight into the various acoustic models that are used to understand these sounds, and yet the mystery remains that despite the very different acoustic results produced by the articulatory gestures, the cues to consonant place of articulation remain surprisingly constant across manner. There is no doubt that formant cues into and out of a consonant play a crucial role in identifying consonant place of articulation. However, even within a nasal murmur or a lateral "ring" (i.e., the lateral sound itself, akin to the nasal murmur), the palatal place of articulation is identified by a high second formant, and the retroflex "place" of articulation by a lowered third formant. Laminal articulations are routinely longer in duration and have a lower first formant value than apical articulations. Although we have not discussed more gross spectral measures such as spectral center of gravity or standard deviation of the spectrum in the present chapter, there are likewise remarkable similarities across manner classes for a given place of articulation. For instance, palatals have a higher spectral center of gravity, retroflexes have a lower spectral center of gravity compared to alveolars, and dentals have a much flatter spectrum than other places of articulation. Moreover, the study of dynamic cues to consonant production is only in its early stages (e.g., Reidy 2016, Holliday, Reidy, Beckman, and Edwards 2015, and Iskarous, Shadle, and Proctor 2011 on English fricatives for some examples), and this is another area for further research. Much acoustic modeling work has been based on major world languages such as English, and as empirical data keeps coming in from languages that have not yet enjoyed quite as much academic attention as the European languages, we may come to a better understanding of exactly why place of articulation is so robustly encoded across different manners of articulation.

Notes

1 Note that researchers working with English, however, prefer to view this dorsal constriction as a perturbation, and some even adopt a simple schwa-tube model for laterals, similar to the approach mentioned earlier for nasals.

2 A trill involves a vibration between two articulators, usually between an active and a passive articulator (as in the tongue tip and the alveolar ridge for an alveolar trill /r/, or the tongue dorsum and the uvula for the uvular trill /ʀ/), although bilabial trills are also possible. Taps and flaps involve only a single very brief closure – in the case of a flap the closure involves a ballistic forward movement of the tongue, whereas in the case of a tap the movement is more simply up and down.

References

Alwan, A. (1989). Perceptual cues for place of articulation for the voiced pharyngeal and uvular consonants. *The Journal of the Acoustical Society of America* **86** 549–556.

Chiba, T. & Kajiyama, M. (1941). *The Vowel: Its Nature and Structure*. (Kaiseikan, Tokyo).

Dang, J., Honda, K. & Suzuki, H. (1994). Morphological and acoustical analysis of the nasal and the paranasal cavities. *The Journal of the Acoustical Society of America* **96** 2088–2100.

Dang, J. & Honda, K. (1996). Acoustic characteristics of the human paranasal sinuses derived from transmission characteristic measurement and morphological observation. *The Journal of the Acoustical Society of America* **100** 3374–3383.

Dart, S. (1991). Articulatory and acoustic properties of apical and laminal articulations. *UCLA Working Papers in Phonetics*, 79.

Fant, G. (1970). *Acoustic Theory of Speech Production*, 2nd ed. (Mouton, The Hague).

Fujimura, O. (1962). "Analysis of nasal consonants." *The Journal of the Acoustical Society of America*, 34, 1865–1875.

Gordon, M. (2016). *Phonological Typology*. (Oxford University Press, Oxford).

Harrington, J. (1994). "The contribution of the murmur and vowel to the place of articulation distinction in nasal consonants." *The Journal of the Acoustical Society of America*, 96, 19–32.

Johnson, K. (2012). *Acoustic and Auditory Phonetics*, 3rd ed. (Wiley Blackwell, Maldon, Oxford, West Sussex).

Hardcastle, W. & Barry, W. (1989). "Articulatory and perceptual factors in /l/ vocalisations in English." *Journal of the International Phonetic Association*, 15, 3–17.

Holliday, J. J., Reidy, P. F., Beckman, M. E., & Edwards, J. (2015). "Quantifying the robustness of the English sibilant fricative contrast in children." *Journal of Speech, Hearing and Language Research*, 58, 622–637.

Huffman, M. & Krakow, R., eds. (1993). *Phonetics and Phonology: Nasals, Nasalization, and the Velum* (Academic Press, San Diego).

Iskarous, K., Shadle, C. H., & Proctor, M. I. (2011). "Articulatory acoustic kinematics: The production of American English /s/." *The Journal of the Acoustical Society of America* 129, 944–954.

Keating, P., Lindblom, B., Lubker, J. & Kreiman, J. (1994). "Variability in jaw height for segments in English and Swedish VCVs." *Journal of Phonetics*, 22, 407–422.

Ladefoged, P. & Maddieson, I. (1996). *The Sounds of the World's Languages*. (Wiley Blackwell, Oxford, UK, Cambridge, MA).

Malecot, A. (1956). "Acoustic cues for nasal consonants: An experimental study involving a tape-splicing technique." *Language*, 32, 274–284.

Nakata, K. (1959). "Synthesis and perception of nasal consonants." *The Journal of the Acoustical Society of America*, 31, 661–666.

Recasens, D. (1983). "Place cues for nasal consonants with special reference to Catalan." *The Journal of the Acoustical Society of America*, 73, 1346–1353.

Recasens, D. (1996). "An articulatory-perceptual account of vocalization and elision of dark /l/ in the Romance languages." *Language and Speech*, 39, 63–89

Reidy, P.F. (2016). Spectral dynamics of sibilant fricatives are contrastive and language specific. *The Journal of the Acoustical Society of America*, 140, 2518–2529.

Stevens, K. (1998). *Acoustic Phonetics* (Massachusetts Institute of Technology, Cambridge, MA).

Sylak-Glassman, J. (2014). Deriving Natural Classes: The Phonology and Typology of Post-velar Consonants. Ph.D., UC Berkeley.

Tabain, M. (2009). "An EPG study of the alveolar vs. retroflex apical contrast in Central Arrernte." *Journal of Phonetics*, 37, 486–501.

Tabain, M. (2012). "Jaw movement and coronal stop spectra in Central Arrernte." *Journal of Phonetics*, 40, 551–567

Tabain, M., Butcher, A., Breen, G. & Beare, R. (2016a). "An acoustic study of multiple lateral consonants in three Central Australian languages." *The Journal of the Acoustical Society of America*, 139, 361–372.

Tabain, M., Butcher, A., Breen, G. & Beare, R. (2016b). An acoustic study of nasal consonants in three Central Australian languages. *The Journal of the Acoustical Society of America* 139, 890–903.

Zhou, Xinhui, Carol Espy-Wilson, Suzanne Boyce, Mark Tiede, Christy Holland & Ann Choe (2008). A magnetic resonance imaging-based articulatory and acoustic study of "retroflex" and "bunched" American English /r/. *The Journal of the Acoustical Society of America* **123** 4466–4481.

Zhou, Xinhui. (2009). *An MRI-based articulatory and acoustic study of American English liquid sounds /r/ and /l/*. PhD thesis: University of Maryland.

11

Theories and models of speech perception

Michael Kiefte and Terrance M. Nearey

Introduction

Theories of speech perception attempt to explain how human listeners decode an acoustic waveform into those linguistic units they believe were intended by the speaker. Such theories attempt to answer two questions:

1 What are the units of speech being decoded?
2 What are the mechanisms by which listeners map the acoustic signal to these units?

Because spoken communication consists of at least two participants – a speaker and a listener[1] – there are two domains that have to be considered by any theory of speech perception: One is the *articulatory* or *gestural* domain which is tied directly to the physiology of the speech mechanism any speaker uses to produce speech sounds, including both the vocal tract and the neural structures that regulate it. The second is the *auditory* domain where the acoustic signal is transduced to an auditory representation that ultimately maps to the linguistic message that is ideally a close match to what the speaker intended. Although the term *speech perception* refers to a process that takes place in the listener, we cannot overlook the speaker's role: The speaker must first *encode* linguistic units to an acoustic waveform that a listener can *decode*.

Many theories of speech perception suggest that these two processes – encoding and decoding – are strongly related in some way; linguistic units have to be mapped both *to* and *from* an acoustic waveform. Some of these theories suggest that one of these pathways is much simpler and more direct than the other and that linguistic units are mapped to *either* auditory representations or articulatory gestures without any direct reference to the other.

The *spectrogram* in Figure 11.1 is a visual representation of the word "speech." A spectrogram is a spectrotemporal representation of a recorded sound that shows acoustic energy as a function of time along the x-axis, frequency along the y-axis, and amplitude as the grayscale intensity with darker patches representing relatively greater energy. The process by which a spectrogram is generated is not unlike how the auditory system delivers sound to the brain: Sound energy is analyzed by overlapping bandpass filters and the fluctuations in

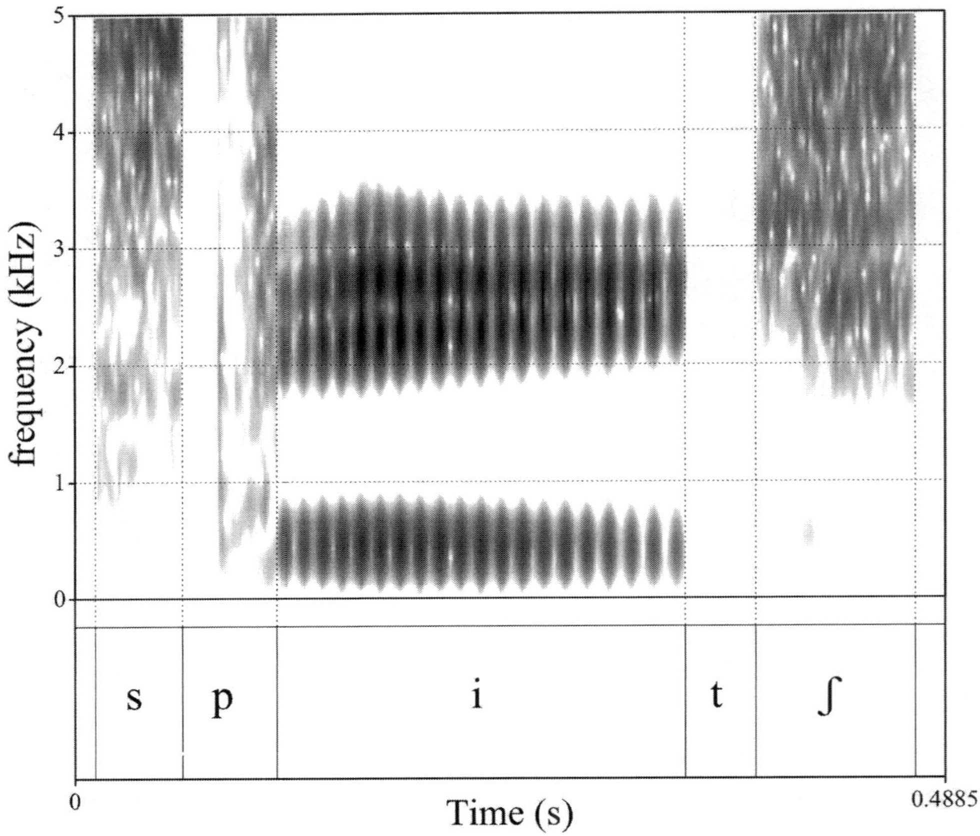

Figure 11.1 Spectrogram of the word "speech" with segmentation of phonemes /spitʃ/ generated by Praat (Boersma & Weenink, 2018).

energy within these bands are mapped to intensity levels as a function of both time and frequency. In the case of the auditory system, the bandpass-filter analysis is performed by the cochlea in which frequency-selective regions of the basilar membrane vibrate in response to incoming signals (Winn & Stilp, this volume). However, intensity level is mapped by the cochlea to neural impulses while, in the spectrogram, intensity is proportional to relative darkness of patches within the image.

Several pieces of information can be gleaned from the representation in Figure 11.1: The word-initial /s/ sound as well as the /ʃ/ at the end consist of largely high-frequency energy; the /p/ and /t/ sounds consist of a silent gap corresponding to closure at the lips or alveolar ridge, respectively. In the case of /p/, there is also a very brief noise burst and a period of noisy aspiration following closure. The vowel /i/ consists of mostly horizontal bands of relatively greater energy that correspond to formants or vocal-tract resonances – three such bands are visible: one below 500 Hz, and another two that appear almost merged above 2 kHz. The temporal extent of the speech sounds /s/, /p/, /i/, /t/, and /ʃ/ are not difficult to determine and their boundaries are also illustrated in the figure.

The prevailing view among many researchers is that the primary goal of speech perception is the correct identification of these individual speech sounds (although this view may, in itself, be too simplistic; Kluender & Kiefte, 2006; Kluender, Stilp & Kiefte, 2013). In addition, it is widely believed that the formants that extend throughout the duration of, e.g., /i/ in Figure 11.1 are also important in speech perception – not just for vowels but also for the adjacent consonants as well (see Kiefte, Nearey & Assmann, 2012, for a review). Throughout this chapter, we expand on these views.

How are these acoustic properties used by listeners to decode the acoustic waveform into something meaningful like the word "speech"? Can individual linguistic units be identified by matching the acoustic properties of the incoming sound directly to some internal representation? How does this internal representation relate to the physical properties of the speech sounds themselves? For example, is this internal representation defined by acoustics or the output of peripheral auditory structures? Or does the perceptual system first map the acoustic waveform systematically to articulatory patterns of a (real or virtual) vocal tract resembling those used by the speaker, which are, in turn, translated to an estimate of the intended speech sounds? Another possibility is that this internal representation is a compromise between auditory/acoustic and articulatory properties and that the direct relationships between these two domains can serve as important perceptual correlates. Since it is assumed that both speakers and listeners are in possession of a vocal tract capable of speech production through basic physiologic processes, it may seem reasonable that the first stage of speech perception is to map the acoustics onto the articulations that were used to generate them and then to identify individual speech sounds on the basis of those articulations. However, this *analysis by synthesis* is by no means straightforward. Conversely, if speech sounds are more directly represented by acoustics, then the speaker must determine the sequence of articulations that most closely produces the desired waveform which may also be a highly complex process.

Each of these positions suggests a tradeoff in the complexity of perception and production. If speech sounds are mapped directly to acoustic waveforms then it is the job of the speaker to navigate the complex relationship between articulation and acoustics. On the other hand, if speech perception is somehow mediated by articulation, then the listener must refer to a model of either the human vocal tract or neurological motor commands in order to map acoustics to the articulations intended by the speaker. The distinction between these two ideas lies primarily in how speech is represented in the mind of the listener. However, a third possibility is that the relationships or mappings between acoustics, perception *and* articulation are all relatively straightforward and that it is the job of speech researchers to discover these relationships. Intermediate positions also exist: It is also possible that all of these are true under certain circumstances and that listeners can make use of several types of information when decoding the speech signal.

An additional issue is whether there is perhaps a "special" phonetic mode of processing in either the articulatory or perceptual domain or whether the perceptual processes involved in human speech perception are based on fundamental psychoacoustic phenomena that are exploited in other domains. If it is the case that speech perception makes use of fundamental psychoacoustic processes that are well documented in other areas of perception, then there may be no need to suggest that there is something special or unique about speech perception that makes it fundamentally different from other types of auditory perception.

In this chapter, we give a broad overview of the theories that attempt to explain how the acoustic signal is converted into a linguistic message by the perceptual system of the listener. We will also provide a review of some of the perceptual phenomena that have influenced the development of these theories and which have been taken as key evidence for one or another.

In the following sections, we first describe evidence that the fundamental units of perception are basic speech sounds or phonemes which are a small finite set of building blocks from which all words or morphemes can be assembled. Then we explore some of the speech-related phenomena that theories of speech perception must address with respect to these building blocks – namely, context sensitivity, lack of invariance, and segmentability, which are all closely related. We will see that the acoustic and articulatory consequences of these basic linguistic units are widely overlapping in time: A given speech sound changes depending on the context in which it occurs, and acoustic correlates to individual speech categories can be shared between multiple speech sounds. Finally, we explore several theories of speech perception that attempt to explain how human listeners convert an acoustic signal into something potentially meaningful in spoken communication. Our discussion builds toward a discussion of both articulatory/gestural and acoustic/auditory perspectives and ends by advocating a "double-weak" approach wherein speech is viewed as being shaped by a kind of compromise between constraints on gestural and auditory complexity.

Units of speech perception

A common view among researchers is that the goal of human speech perception is to correctly identify some basic units of speech that are combined to make utterances. We referred to these units as "speech sounds," but what exactly are these basic units that are being transmitted from speaker to listener? Are they whole phrases, words, speech sounds or phonemes, or something even smaller, such as some fundamental acoustic or phonetic features?

In written language, a simplistic view is that the basic units or symbols of writing are letters or graphemes that can be assembled into arbitrarily long words or sentences. For example, in English, there are 26 small combinational units that can be rearranged to form novel, never-before-seen messages that can be reliably interpreted and repeated by a reader. In speech, we can understand novel phrases and sentences that violate basic grammatical rules such as *cat the dog bark jumped* which suggests that longer utterances can be composed from discrete words that can be rearranged at will and still be reliably repeated by a listener (even if they do not make sense). Likewise, we can hear and repeat well-formed nonsense words that have never been heard before, constructed by joining basic speech sounds or phonemes. We can invent novel words, such as *plim* /plɪm/, that listeners can reliably transcribe, either orthographically or phonetically. This can only be possible if we assume that basic speech sounds that correspond to, for example, /p/ or /l/, can be recombined to form words or syllables. However, due to coarticulation and lack of acoustic invariance as discussed in the following, the acoustic signal cannot be disassembled and rearranged as easily as can letters on a page (Harris, 1953; Cooper, Gaitenby, Mattingly & Umeda, 1969).

At a more fundamental level of linguistic description, listeners cannot, in general, understand new phonemes formed by altering or rearranging more basic acoustic properties. Studies have shown that adult listeners are not well suited for discriminating speech sounds that they have never heard before and which do not form part of their native phonology. For example, teaching new phonemic contrasts to second-language learners often poses challenges as the speech sounds of their native language interfere with both perception and production in the new language. Past the critical period of speech development, our perceptual systems are largely locked into a phonemic system specific to a native language (Flege, 1995; Best, 1995; Chang, this volume).

One theory of speech perception does, however, suggest that the fundamental units of speech are indeed very small and very general and that infants are tuned to these properties during the so-called critical period of language development (e.g., Stevens, 1989; Stevens & Keyser, 1989; Stevens & Blumstein, 1981). This small set of units, or distinctive features, are posited to be universal across all languages and are associated with well-defined psychoacoustic properties. On the opposite extreme of the theoretical spectrum, it has been suggested that speech perception is mediated by memory traces of previously heard utterances stored in an *episodic lexicon* which may consist of units as large as words or short phrases and that novel utterances are identified with reference to this broad store of acoustic experience (e.g., Goldinger, 1997; Johnson, 1997; Pisoni, 1997).

An intermediate view is that basic units of speech perception correspond to simple speech sounds such as /p/ or /u/. Although these symbolic units may have a fairly complex relationship to more fundamental acoustic elements, they are otherwise more general than the stored acoustic waves in an episodic lexicon (Nearey, 1990, 1992, 1997a, 1997b). Although speakers can rearrange these phonemes to form novel words or syllables, it is not the case that the acoustic waveforms corresponding to those phonemes can be arranged and rearranged by simply splicing them together.[2] It is well known that the acoustic properties associated with phonemes are widely overlapping in time (see the following). However, if we accept a theory of speech perception that posits phonemes as the fundamental symbolic units of speech, then we must also believe that there is a way for the auditory system to extract acoustic properties associated with different phonemes from widely overlapping acoustic segments.

There is good evidence that phonemes are the fundamental units of speech perception. It is known from early work in telecommunications that the correct identification of nonsense syllables over a noisy telephone channel can be predicted directly from the correct identification of the individual phonemes that make up the syllables themselves (see Allen, 1994; Fletcher, 1995). These syllables consisted of all possible combinations of consonant-vowel-consonant (CVC) sequences. It was found that the likelihood that a CVC syllable was correctly identified by a listener was the product of the likelihoods of the individual phonemes being correctly identified. This entails that the perception of individual phonemes is *statistically independent*, indicating that listeners identify syllables on the basis of their individual phonemes.

Although this observation holds true for nonsense syllables, it does not hold for real words and sentences. If listeners are presented with a mix of real and nonsense words in an open-set situation (e.g., "Write whatever you hear"), high-frequency real words are identified better than low-frequency ones, and those are better identified than nonsense words (Boothroyd & Nitrouer, 1988). However, the advantage of high-frequency real words can be eliminated altogether if listeners are presented with a *closed-set* choice, even with a very large number of possible items (Pollack, Rubenstein & Decker, 1959). A possible explanation for this range of behavior is that frequency effects and phonotactic patterns provide a kind of *a priori* bias toward certain words, even in the absence of any reliable sensory information. However, these biases are relatively labile and are not deeply wired into the representations themselves (for more discussion, see Bronkhorst, Bosman & Smoorenburg, 1993; Nearey, 2001; Luce & Pisoni, 1998; Broadbent, 1967).

Although Figure 11.1 seems to indicate that the temporal extent of individual phonemes is well defined, the waveforms associated with these speech sounds cannot be rearranged arbitrarily in a manner akin to an acoustic typewriter. For example, Mermelstein (1978) conducted an experiment with synthetic /bVC/ syllables, where the vowel ranged from /æ/ to /ɛ/ in the peak frequency of the first formant (F_1), while the consonant ranged from /t/ to /d/ in the duration of the vowel. Thus, the acoustic properties within the temporal extent of the vowel determined the identification of both the vowel itself as well as the following consonant. Indeed, when listeners identified these stimuli as one of *bad*, *bed*, *bat*, or *bet*, it was found that both F_1 and vowel duration influenced the identification of *both* the vowel and the consonant.

On the surface, the fact that the acoustic properties of the vowel determined the perception of both the vowel and the consonant appears to contradict the results of Fletcher (1995), who found that the perception of individual phonemes is statistically independent. Nonetheless, Nearey (1990, 1997b) found that stimulus properties produced *statistically independent* changes in the identification of consonants and vowels. Although there were response biases favoring *bat* and *bed*, these biases may be attributed to lexical or phonotactic frequency (*inter alia*, Nearey, 2004). When these bias effects are accounted for, listeners' identification of the vowel and consonant were still independent.

However, although the identification of individual phonemes is statistically independent, the acoustic information associated with each speech sound is still overlapping in time. Speech sounds are not "beads on a string" that can be rearranged in a manner similar to acoustic anagrams (e.g., Stetson, 1945). In the preceding example, exchanging vowels between words will also affect the perception of the final consonant. This overlap in acoustic information is seen as a problem of *segmentation* – i.e., speech sounds cannot be segmented from the waveform without potentially losing or distorting information.

Invariance, coarticulation, and trading relations

The fact that the acoustic counterparts of phonemes change depending on their context indicates that phonemes are not *invariant*. As one of the most influential publications in speech-perception research, a classic example of this was given by Liberman, Delattre and Cooper (1952) in their report on the identification of synthetic, voiceless stops in CV syllables. These syllables were generated by the Pattern Playback, which was capable of converting spectrograms – either photographic copies or hand-painted patterns – into sound (Cooper, 1950; Cooper, Delattre, Liberman, Borst & Gerstman, 1952). Liberman, Delattre & Cooper examined the perceptual effects of the initial stop bursts associated with the voiceless plosive consonants /p/, /t/, and /k/ by parametrically manipulating their spectral properties. A spectrogram of synthetic sounds similar to those used in the original study is given in Figure 11.2. When played, the stimuli approximate the sounds /pi ka pu/, despite the fact that the burst for all three syllables is completely identical. Specifically, the same burst is heard as /k/ before /a/, but as /p/ before /i/ and /u/.

In order to hear /k/ before either /i/ or /u/, instead of /p/, Liberman, Delattre and Cooper (1952) found that the center frequency of the burst had to be just higher than the frequency of F_2 of the following vowel, as illustrated in Figure 11.3.

This context dependence, or lack of *invariance* – i.e., the fact that the same acoustic waveform is identified as different speech sounds or that the same speech sound has very different acoustic properties depending on its surrounding context – has often been presented as a demonstration of the highly complex relationship between acoustics and perception of the speech signal: e.g., not only does place perception depend on the center frequency of the burst but also on the vowel context in which the burst occurs.

Two distinct acoustic properties in possibly non-overlapping time frames that correlate with the perception of the same phonetic contrast are said to share a *trading relation*. For example, the voicing distinction between, e.g., /b/ and /p/ correlates with voice onset time (VOT),[3] frequency of F_1 onset and frequency of voicing (f_0) for syllable-initial stops. For syllable-final stops, it also includes duration of the preceding vowel, while for intervocalic stops, it includes silence duration and the presence or absence of voicing during the closure

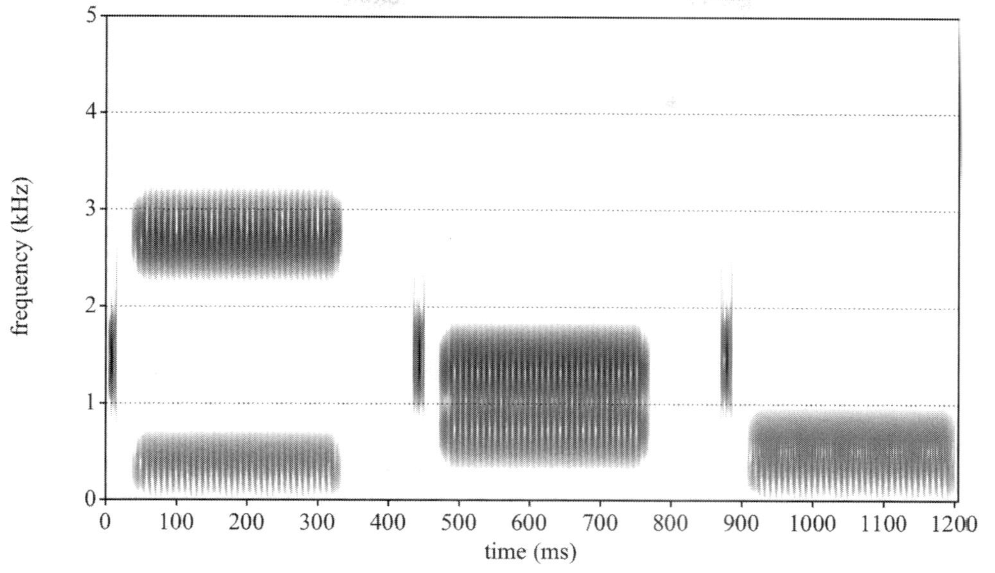

Figure 11.2 Spectrogram of stimuli similar to those used by Liberman, Delattre, and Cooper, (1952). Here the syllables /pi/, /ka/, and /pu/ are illustrated.

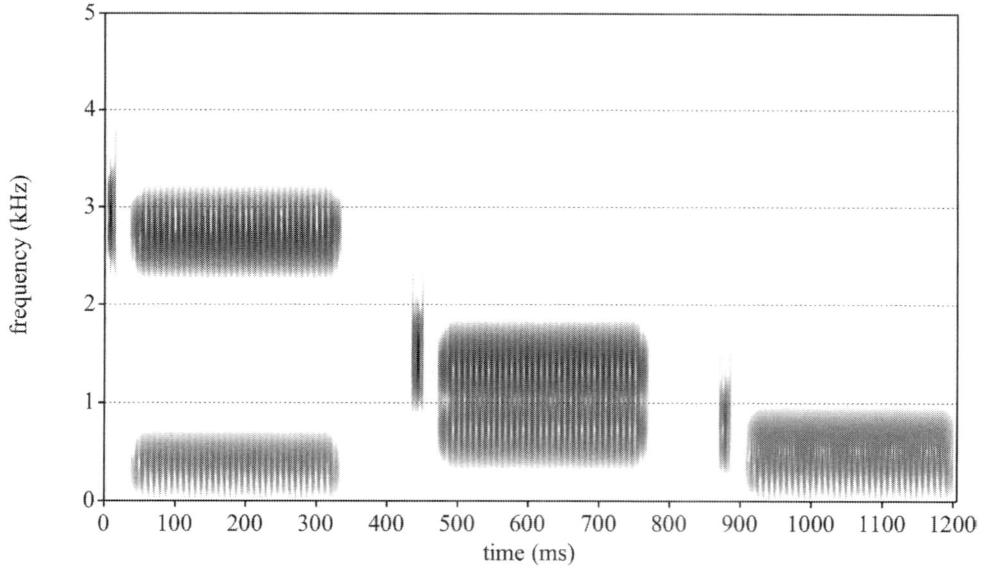

Figure 11.3 Spectrogram of stimuli similar to those used by Liberman, Delattre, and Cooper (1952). Here the syllables /ki/, /ka/, and /ku/ are illustrated.

interval (Repp, 1982). Changes in any one of these acoustic properties can result in a change in phonemic category. Additionally, changes in one of these properties can compensate for changes in another: For example, a longer closure duration is required to perceive a consonant as voiceless when voicing is present during closure than when it is not (Parker, Diehl & Kluender, 1986).

These complex patterns of context dependence encouraged models of speech perception that proposed "decoding" of the speech signal via speech production mechanisms (Liberman, Cooper, Shankweiler & Studdert-Kennedy, 1967). Other models of speech perception are able to capture some complex context dependency as well without reference to articulation (Nearey, 1990). While the data reported by Liberman, Delattre & Cooper might appear to be difficult to model using simple statistical methods, the original experiment (by Liberman, Delattre & Cooper, 1952) was replicated by Kiefte and Kluender (2005a) who found that, although there was clear context dependence for the perception of the initial consonant, it was not nearly as complex as originally found, and listeners' perception could be modeled adequately in terms of the acoustic properties alone.

Categorical perception

Problems of segmentability and lack of acoustic invariance are addressed to varying degrees by theories of speech perception. Another phenomenon that has been addressed by such theories is *categorical perception*, whereby listeners' ability to *discriminate* similar stimuli that differ in a single dimension along an acoustic continuum is determined largely by whether they label those stimuli as different categories. To demonstrate this phenomenon, two experiments are conducted: *identification* and *discrimination*. In the identification experiment, listeners are simply asked to identify each stimulus as one of a small number of categories: e.g., /ba/, /da/, or /ga/. In the discrimination experiment, listeners hear pairs of stimuli that are adjacent or nearly adjacent along the acoustic continuum and indicate whether they are same or different.[4]

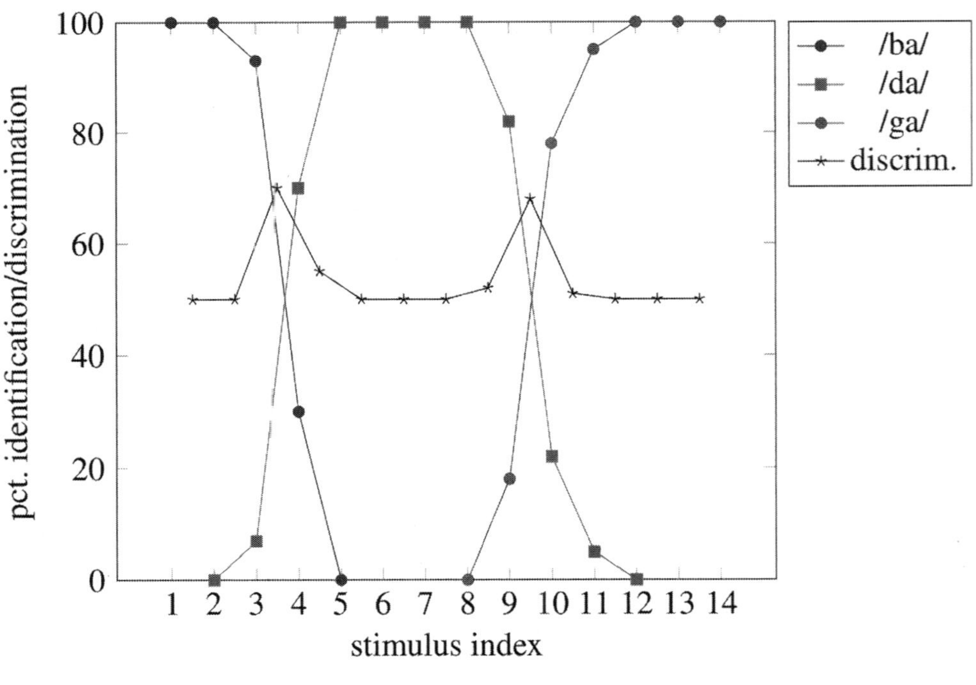

Figure 11.4 Hypothetical example illustrating the phenomenon of categorical perception. /ba/, /da/, and /ga/ show identification rates for the three categories as a function of stimulus index, while discrim. gives the predicted rate for adjacent stimuli (for details, see text).

Liberman, Harris, Hoffman and Griffith (1957) reported that when people listen to speech-like sounds that vary along a continuum of onset-F_2 transitions from /ba/ through /da/ to /ga/, they were much less able to hear differences between similar stimuli in those cases where they labeled both stimuli as belonging to the same category (e.g., both /ba/). However, if listeners tended to label them as different categories – e.g., one as /da/ and the other /ga/ – they could easily distinguish them. Another way to explain this phenomena is to imagine a boundary between each pair of adjacent categories /ba/–/da/ and /da/–/ga/: on one side of a boundary, listeners in the identification experiment are more likely to label the stimulus as, e.g., /ba/ and on the other side of the boundary, listeners identify the stimulus as /da/. If two stimuli fall on the same side of the boundary, however, listeners have greater difficulty distinguishing them *even if the absolute differences in the stimulus property between each pair are the same*. The consequences of this are that listeners' sensitivity to acoustic properties is nonlinear – i.e., equivalent changes in acoustic parameters are not heard as equivalent intervals by listeners.

Liberman et al. (1957) and Eimas (1963) found that listeners' ability to discriminate stimulus continua was just slightly better than could be predicted on the basis of identification responses alone – i.e., discrimination was much better *across* phoneme boundaries than within a single speech category. Eimas showed that this phenomenon was not found with non-speech stimuli and was therefore peculiar to speech perception. Similarly, McGovern and Strange (1977) found that a /ra/–/la/ continuum in which F_3 was varied was perceived categorically. However, if all but the third formant was removed from the stimuli, not only were the resulting sounds not heard as speech, but the stimuli were discriminated *continuously* instead of categorically. We return to these issues below.

In general, non-speech stimuli are perceived continuously in that listeners' sensitivity to small acoustic differences does not vary non-linearly across a continuum. Two conclusions were drawn from this (Liberman & Mattingly 1985). First, because this phenomenon only occurred with speech-like stimuli, it was thought that categorical perception could not be explained by general auditory processes. Second, it was thought that nonlinear discriminability in speech sounds reflected vocal-tract discontinuities between, e.g., different places of articulation, and it was therefore presumed that perception reflected these discontinuities. Because the presentation of speech stimuli resulted in discrimination behavior that was strikingly different from that found with non-speech tokens, many researchers were led to believe that a distinct neural structure existed for the sole purpose of decoding speech into phonetic units and that these structures were entirely separate from other forms of auditory perception. It was therefore suggested that categorical perception was unique to speech, and this fact was used as evidence in favor of *the Motor Theory of Speech Perception*, which posits that speech perception was somehow mediated by articulation.

According to the Motor Theory of Speech Perception, the reason listeners are more sensitive to differences between stimuli that represent different speech categories, such as /ba/ and /da/, or /da/ and /ga/, is that their perception of speech sounds is mediated directly by articulation. Although the stimuli may appear to vary continuously and linearly in the acoustic domain, the range of articulations required to produce those sounds is highly nonlinear. For example, the differences between /ba/ and /da/ are thought to be very large in terms of production, while differences between different articulations of /ba/ are relatively small.

Some researchers thought that categorical perception was a learned phenomenon – in the process of experimenting with their own vocal tracts through babbling, infants would learn the simple mapping between articulation and speech sounds. Although infants cannot label speech sounds directly, there are several techniques to determine if they can discriminate speech stimuli. For example, when a long series of stimuli are presented and which suddenly change by some small acoustic parameter, an infant who detects the difference might show an increase in sucking rate on an electronic pacifier – a technique known as the high-amplitude sucking (HAS) paradigm. Using this technique, Eimas, Siqueland, Jusczyk and Vigorito (1971) demonstrated that infants showed discrimination abilities that mirrored those of adults – i.e., they showed more sensitive discrimination for speech sounds that were in different categories. The fact that infants as young as one month exhibited this pattern of discrimination further suggested that, rather than being learned from experience with one's own vocal tract, speech perception resided in some special speech processing mechanism that was *innate* and special to humans (Liberman & Mattingly, 1985). This also resolved the problem of how nonverbal listeners could understand speech without the advantage of using their own speech in order to learn the mapping between articulation and speech sounds. However, we note in the following section that animals can also be trained to respond to speech stimuli in a manner similar to categorical perception, which suggests that this phenomenon does not, in fact, reflect any innate abilities in humans.

Gestural theories of speech perception

If, as suggested previously, the goal of speech perception is the correct identification of phonemes or simple speech sounds, then the next important question that must be answered by any theory of speech perception is how the acoustic signal relates to these fundamental symbolic units of speech (here, and in the next few sections, we adopt the overall taxonomy of Nearey, 1997b).

Three important observations led to what is now referred to as the *Motor Theory of Speech Perception* (Liberman, Cooper, Shankweiler & Studdert-Kennedy, 1967). First, the same sound can lead to the perception of different phonemes, depending on the context in which it occurs (e.g., Figure 11.2). Second, different sounds can lead to the perception of the same phoneme, again depending on the context in which it occurs (e.g., Figure 11.3). Finally, sensitivity to stimulus differences in speech sounds is highly nonlinear and is largely determined by listeners' ability to label phonemic categories that differ substantially in articulation.

Early attempts to find *invariant* acoustic counterparts to speech categories met with failure, and it was ultimately concluded that the relationship between perception and articulation may be simpler and more direct than that between perception and acoustics (e.g., Cooper, Delattre, Liberman, Borst & Gerstman, 1952). This was largely inspired by the complex mapping of relevant acoustic cues to particular phonetic distinctions that could only be understood with reference to their articulatory source (e.g., Liberman & Mattingly, 1985; Repp, 1982). The proposed simple relationship between perception and articulation was partly inspired by the context sensitivity of observed acoustic properties and the assumed context-invariance of articulation. It was therefore suggested that basic symbolic units or phonemes corresponded more closely to the articulatory or gestural domain.

Further examples of the segmentability problem and the lack of acoustic invariance are found in the voicing distinction in English CV syllables consisting of a plosive followed by a vowel: If the VOT is negative or zero, listeners generally perceive the plosive as voiced. However, listeners will also hear the plosive as voiced if the first formant or fundamental frequency has a low-frequency onset. Proponents of the Motor Theory have interpreted this relationship as the byproduct of relatively simple glottal gestures and, if the listener maps the acoustic signal to these relatively simple gestures, then the identification data can more easily be explained (see Kingston & Diehl, 1994, for a review).

As another example, the action of pressure release by the tongue dorsum at the velum or soft palate is generally heard as /g/ or /k/, regardless of the vowel that follows it. This simple relationship was clearly not evident between *acoustics* and perception (see Figures 11.2 and 11.3). Experiments showed that there was often a many-to-one or a one-to-many mapping between a perceived consonant and its associated acoustic stimulus parameters. For example, it was observed that the same burst centered at 1400 Hz was heard as /p/ before /i/ and /u/, but as /k/ before /a/ (Liberman, Delattre & Cooper, 1952; Schatz, 1954). Conversely, different bursts for /k/ were required before different vowels to generate a velar percept (Liberman, Delattre & Cooper, 1952). Although it has been suggested that the movement of the oral articulators can be perceived directly [e.g., Fowler's (1986) direct realist approach to speech perception], Liberman, Cooper, Shankweiler and Studdert-Kennedy (1967) instead claimed that the invariant component of speech was somehow *encoded* into the acoustic signal in a relatively complex manner.

Several observations were used to further illustrate the complexity of the acoustic signal relative to the articulations that produce it. First, a stream of "building blocks," in which discrete acoustic segments represented unique units of speech, would be very difficult to understand at the rates needed for the perception of continuous speech (*cf.* Liberman, 1984); communication by such means would be no more efficient than Morse code. In addition, basic acoustic properties typically associated with individual phonemes are in fact widely overlapping in natural speech. For example, we find acoustic properties relevant to the place of articulation of prevocalic stop consonants in the burst, formant transitions, and vowel formants, while vowel information can be found in the formant transitions and vowel formants. This lack of phoneme *segmentability* was seen as a consequence of the relative efficiency with which speech could be transmitted acoustically – i.e., several speech units could be conveyed simultaneously at any given moment.

The second observation that illustrated the complexity of the acoustic signal relative to its articulatory source and its perceptual representation was the nonlinear mapping between articulation and acoustics on the one hand, and the nonlinear mapping between acoustics and perception on the other. As has already been shown, very different stimuli are heard as the same speech unit. Although formant transitions for – e.g., /di/ and /du/ – are quite different (onset F_2 rising and falling respectively), they are nevertheless perceived as the same consonant.

Several other pieces of evidence were presented in support of the Motor Theory: Liberman, Isenberg and Rakerd (1981) demonstrated that when a speech stimulus was split into two parts and presented to different ears over headphones, the listeners hear one speech sound resulting from the integration across both ears as well as a non-speech sound. For example, if a single formant transition from a CV syllable is presented separately to one ear while the remaining stimulus, without that formant, is presented to the other, listeners hear both the original, integrated syllable and a chirp-like sound resulting from the isolated formant transition. Proponents of the Motor Theory took this as evidence that a special speech processor in the brain fuses speech-like stimuli, while a non-speech auditory module also processes the formant transition heard as a chirp.

Evidence for a special speech module in perception was also seen in what is now referred to as the *McGurk effect*: When the sound /ba/ is dubbed over a video of someone saying /ga/, the combined audiovisual stimulus produces the percept /da/. The fact that listeners perceive neither /ga/ nor /ba/ suggests that the audiovisual experience is processed in a special speech module and that listeners are attempting to determine speech gestures from the conflicting stimuli (McGurk & MacDonald, 1976). Thus, perception is neither completely auditory nor visual, but rather what is perceived is the (distorted) articulation itself.

However, the relationship between gestures and acoustics as suggested by the Motor Theory is not so straightforward; for example, the articulatory targets for the same vowel are quite varied across speakers (Ladefoged, DeClerk, Lindau & Papçun, 1972; Nearey, 1980; Johnson, Ladefoged & Lindau, 1993). Perkell, Matthies, Svirsky and Jordan (1993) have also shown that wide variation in tongue and lip position in the production of the vowel /u/ seems motivated by the production of a consistent *acoustic* output instead of a stable articulatory target. Some speakers appear to use varying articulatory means to achieve a relatively constant acoustic end in different phonetic contexts. Therefore, many have argued that, at least for some classes of sounds, the acoustic output produced by those gestures is much more invariant than the gestures themselves and that linguistically relevant properties are *acoustic* rather than gestural. If we assume that the auditory processing of acoustic events is relatively straightforward, then listeners may rely on the acoustic relationships to phonemes instead.

One of the early assumptions of the Motor Theory was that, even if acoustic properties are not invariant, articulations or gestures are. However, the lack of structural independence between articulators and coarticulation effects complicated the notion of articulatory invariance, which was only relatively obvious for bilabials such as /p/, /b/, and /m/. Liberman, Cooper, Shankweiler and Studdert-Kennedy (1967) therefore proposed that the *neuromotor rules* – or the neural signals that were used in production – held this simple one-to-one relationship with perception. This was viewed as advantageous since the listener could use the same neural mechanisms designed for speech production to decode the acoustic signal in perception, and it was suggested that perception was mediated in some way by these neuromotor correlates to articulatory gestures. The neural commands were assumed to be invariant across all contexts, despite the observed context dependencies found in acoustics and articulation. As more evidence was obtained regarding the exact nature of the neural mechanisms used in speech, the specification of invariance was weakened to merely the gestures *intended* by the speaker. For example, it was known that even a simple articulatory movement, such as the raising of the tongue dorsum to make contact with the velum, was the result of several complex neural commands. Such complexities were eventually accommodated by a form of Motor Theory that also strengthened the idea that speech processing was innate rather than learned and that speech perception was performed by a specialized speech module (Liberman & Mattingly, 1985). Motor Theory still maintained that perception and production are intimately linked.

In the last two decades, some results from neurophysiology have been interpreted by some as supporting a version of Motor Theory. It was discovered that neurons in the ventral premotor cortex of monkeys are active both when the monkey grasps an object as well as when it *observes* someone doing so (Rizzolatti & Arbib, 1998; Rizzolatti & Craighero, 2004). These neurons are referred to as *mirror neurons*; although they are primarily responsible for the regulation of motor commands, they also respond to the *perception* of those same actions and it was suggested that similar mirror neurons may play a role in speech perception, particularly within the framework of Motor Theory (Rizzolatti & Arbib, 1998; Lotto, Hickok & Holt, 2009). A similar result was later observed when the *sound* of an action resulted in an activation of the motor neurons associated with performing the action that produced the sound (Kohler, Keysers, Umilta, Fogassi, Gallese & Rizzolatti, 2002).

Therefore, these mirror neurons may represent the "missing link" between perception and production postulated earlier by Liberman and Mattingly (1985).

Although proponents of the Motor Theory maintained that the objects of perception were the intended gestures of the speaker, the issue of exactly *how* the perceptual system recovers these gestures from the waveforms has never been resolved (Kluender & Kiefte, 2006; Galantucci, Fowler & Turvey, 2006; Massaro & Chen, 2008). Therefore, much of the simplicity and elegance of the Motor Theory lies in the fact that the precise mechanism whereby listeners identify the symbolic units of speech is largely abstracted or completely ignored.[5]

Nearey (1992) refers to Motor Theory as a *strong gestural* position because of the strong links that are postulated between perception and articulation (see Figure 11.5). However, other theories regarding the relationship between articulation, auditory processing, and the symbolic units of language have been proposed as well. The next section presents *strong auditory* accounts which instead postulate a strong relationship between the auditory domain and perception.

Although Motor Theory claims that there is a direct relationship between speech sounds and the *intended* gestures of the speaker, Kingston and Diehl (1994, 1995) have argued that a number of properties claimed to be the natural fallout of the biophysical interaction of gestures instead result from *deliberate*, controlled actions (see also Diehl & Kluender, 1989). Specifically, they argue that many properties that may seem at first to simply covary automatically in production are, in fact, actively managed to produce an enhancement of the resultant auditory-perceptual properties. This perspective is described further in the following section.

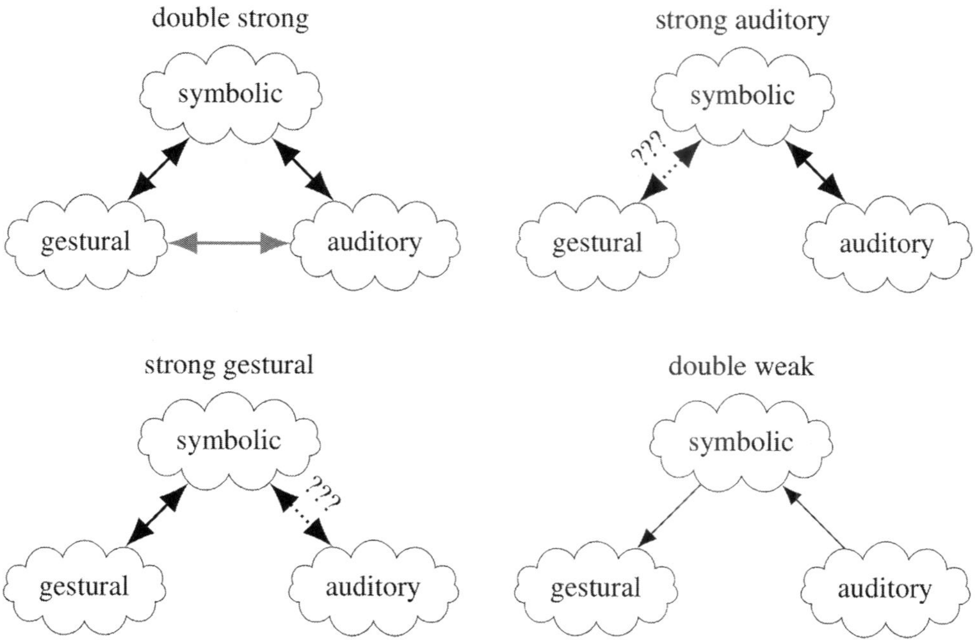

Figure 11.5 Schematic depiction of four patterns of strength of relationship among objects in the gestural, auditory, and symbolic domain.

Auditory/articulatory theories of speech perception

In auditory theories, it is assumed that there is a much stronger relationship between phonemes and basic auditory properties and that the identification of these linguistic units can be understood in terms of basic psychoacoustic processes that can be attested in other areas of auditory perception. Much of the evidence presented supporting Motor Theory was focused on the lack of acoustic invariance for coarticulated speech sounds such as CV syllables.

However, based on the Acoustic Theory of speech production, Fant (1970) suggested that a syllable-initial consonant could be identified from the release burst and the first few milliseconds thereafter, irrespective of coarticulatory effects. Several authors have taken this view and have subsequently proposed a set of cues based on grossly defined spectral properties. They also presuppose a direct and simple relationship between articulation and acoustics as well as between acoustics and perception. Expanding on these ideas, Stevens and Blumstein (1978) suggested that simple spectral properties drawn from brief frames of the waveform can contain context-invariant information regarding, e.g., stop-consonant-identity information (Stevens & Blumstein, 1978; Blumstein & Stevens, 1979). For example, they suggested that the stop burst and a very brief segment of vocalic formant transitions form a single integrated acoustic property that is essentially invariant within places of articulation: Bilabial releases were characterized by low-frequency formant energy resulting in a downward tilt in spectral shape; alveolar articulations were characterized by higher-frequency energy which resulted in a rising spectral tilt; and for velars, there should be a relatively pronounced peak of energy in the mid-frequency range, whereas bilabial and alveolar spectra were more diffuse. Hence it was thought that place of articulation could be discriminated entirely on the basis of very simple spectral parameters or *templates* without any need to refer directly to articulatory gestures. Blumstein and Stevens (1980) further suggested that even the deletion of release bursts which may occur for voiced stops or in rapid speech still does not substantially change these invariant global spectral properties.

Moreover, Stevens and Blumstein (1978) claimed that these templates reflected the articulatory configuration of the stop consonants at the moment of release. They proposed that not only do these acoustic properties have a direct one-to-one relationship with phonemes, but that they also have a simple one-to-one relationship with articulations. Nearey (1992) refers to this class of hypotheses as *double strong* theories because of the assumed direct links between all three domains: gestural, auditory, and phonemic (see Figure 11.5).

However, this model completely ignores contextual variability that is present in speech (e.g., Suomi, 1985). In particular, *formant transitions* between the release burst and the following vowel are determined by the identity of both the consonant and the vowel (e.g., see Sussman, Fruchter & Cable, 1995, for a review of *locus equations* which describe the correlation between formant frequencies at voicing onset and those of the following vowel). The position taken by Stevens and Blumstein (1978) was that these transitions serve no direct role in speech perception beyond what was abstracted into spectral templates and, similar to Cole and Scott (1974), they went on to suggest that the primary role of these formant transitions was to provide information regarding the *temporal order* of phonetic segments and to smooth out acoustic discontinuities between phonemes.

Similar to Stevens and Blumstein (1978) and Blumstein and Stevens (1979), Kewley-Port (1983) and Kewley-Port and Luce (1984) characterized stop consonants in terms of the global spectral tilt and compactness at stimulus onset. However, they also included time-varying relational acoustic features that spanned 20–40 ms beyond closure release which also included information regarding voicing as well as formant transitions. Based on the measurement of natural stimuli, as well as the results of synthesis experiments, Lahiri, Gewirth and Blumstein (1984) similarly concluded that it was not the absolute global spectral shape of the first few tens of milliseconds, but rather the *relative* change of this property over time that was best able to discriminate places of articulation. For example, it was hypothesized that there was a smaller change in high-frequency energy between the burst onset and the onset of voicing for alveolars than for bilabials.

Stevens (2002) proposed a model of speech perception in which words were specified by sequences of discrete symbols (phonemes) and that these speech categories were themselves described by relatively simple elements that were specified directly, both in terms of simple acoustic templates and gestures. Stevens (1989) had already suggested that vocal-tract gestures could be subdivided into discrete configurations and that small articulatory maneuvers can result in large changes in the acoustic output. He also added that there were broad regions of acoustic stability in vocal-tract configurations that speakers could exploit in speech production and that these regions corresponded to relatively invariant acoustic outputs. Further, because this acoustic model of speech perception relied on spectral templates that were so broadly defined that they could abstract away context sensitivity resulting in a highly schematized invariance, Stevens (2002) suggested that speech sounds could be aligned to acoustic landmarks such as abrupt onsets of energy or sudden changes in spectral composition.

This model was also heavily influenced by the notion of binary distinctive features in phonology (Halle & Stevens, 1991), which are a small set of universal properties that are sufficient to define all speech sounds of any human language. This notion of universal distinctive features suggests that phonemes are not arbitrarily different from one another, but vary along a small set of dimensions with the additional constraint that each of these dimensions can only have one of two values: present or absent. Although these features are often described in terms of articulation (e.g., *coronal*, *voiced*), it has been shown that perceptual errors most commonly occur along those dimensions as well (e.g., Miller & Nicely, 1955).

Auditory theories of speech perception

Although all of the observations described in the previous section showed some promise for invariant cues to speech categories in the acoustic waveform, none of the discussion so far has dealt with *how* these stimuli are processed by the auditory system. As mentioned previously, while the process of making a spectrogram is roughly similar to perceptual processing by the auditory periphery, its output is only a crude approximation of very first stages of neural encoding.

Several researchers have studied auditory-nerve responses to speech-like sounds (e.g., Young & Sachs, 1979; Sachs & Young, 1979; Recio, Rhode, Kiefte & Kluender, 2002). Much like the perception of speech by human listeners, Delgutte and Kiang (1984) found that these auditory-nerve responses are also context sensitive. For example, they found that the auditory-nerve responses to a recording of /da/ vary depending on the preceding context. The neurophysiological explanation for this phenomenon was *short-term peripheral adaptation* in which the response pattern of individual nerve fibers decays gradually over 100–150 ms – roughly the duration of a vowel. The effect of this adaptation is that spectral differences between adjacent segments of speech are enhanced by the auditory periphery. Delgutte, Hammond, Kalluri, Litvak and Cariani (1996) argued that these data demonstrate how adaptation serves to increase perceived spectral contrast between successive speech signals and that this effect enhances phonetically relevant spectral information.

Kluender, Coady and Kiefte (2003) and Kluender and Kiefte (2006) have suggested that the *only* information available to the auditory system is acoustic contrast. In support of this, they cite several studies demonstrating spectral-contrast effects between adjacent coarticulated consonants and vowels (e.g., Lotto & Kluender, 1998). For example, listeners are more likely to hear /dʌd/ than /dɛd/ when vowel-formant information (*here*, F_2) is ambiguous. However, when the consonants are replaced with /b/, listeners are more likely to hear /bɛb/ than /bʌb/, even for exactly the same vowel, demonstrating a lack of acoustic invariance for these vowels. When consonants are replaced by sine-wave analogs that are not heard as speech sounds but which contain similar spectral information, the same vowel-identification bias occurs. Lotto and Kluender argue that spectral contrast between successive acoustic segments largely determines perception, irrespective of whether elements of the acoustic context are heard as speech. For example, the differences between the second formant of the consonant and the F_2 of the vowel are perceptually exaggerated, resulting in more responses to /dʌd/ than /bɛb/, even when the second formant of the consonant is represented instead by a sinewave. Similarly, Stilp, Kiefte, Alexander, and Kluender (2010) demonstrated that a model of auditory contrast predicts changes in speech perception under several forms of acoustic distortion. Conversely, Darwin, McKeown and Kirby (1989), Watkins (1991), Watkins and Makin (1994), and Kiefte and Kluender (2008) demonstrated that listeners will *ignore* acoustic properties that do not change in a given acoustic context, even when those properties have been shown to be important for identification of speech sounds presented in isolation.

Kluender, Stilp, and Kiefte (2013) argue that examples that demonstrate a lack of acoustic invariance in speech result from the fact that the primary source of information in the speech signal is acoustic change and not absolute spectral properties. They further suggest that peripheral adaptation is one of the mechanisms by which the acoustic consequences of context sensitivity are decoded in auditory processing. For example, coarticulation increases acoustic similarity between neighboring speech sounds. However, peripheral adaptation emphasizes the remaining acoustic contrast such that perceived differences are magnified, thereby reversing the effects of coarticulation.

Kiefte and Kluender (2005b) further showed that listeners identify vowels primarily on the basis of *changing* acoustic properties and will ignore constant spectral characteristics (see Kiefte, Nearey & Assmann, 2012, for a review). This supports the view that changes in formant frequency are important in vowel perception. For example, Andruski and Nearey (1992), Nearey and Assmann (1986), and Hillenbrand, Getty, Clark and Wheeler (1995) showed that lax vowels, such as /ɪ/ and /ɛ/, may be characterized by the same magnitude of spectral change as observed for acknowledged diphthongs, such as /eɪ/. Later studies have shown that this vowel-inherent spectral change (VISC) is critical to vowel perception (e.g., Assmann & Katz, 2000).

If the lack of acoustic invariance for speech sounds is at least partly compensated for by relatively peripheral auditory structures, then these effects may not be specific to speech or even to human listeners. For example, Kuhl and Miller (1975) showed that when chinchillas[6] are trained to identify naturally produced tokens of /ta/ and /da/, they learn to categorize the voicing distinction between /t/ and /d/ in a manner very similar to that of human listeners. Further, Kuhl and Padden (1982) found that Japanese macaques, a small terrestrial monkey, showed a pattern of discrimination of VOT in prevocalic stops that was very similar to what is found in human listeners in experiments of categorical perception. In this case, the perceptual boundary for VOT between voiced and voiceless stops is different for each of the three places of articulation, /ba/–/pa/, /da/–/ta/, and /ga/–/ka/ (see Watson & Kewley-Port, 1988, for a discussion of the controversy over importance of "auditory proclivities" versus learned patterns in human VOT perception for stop consonants). Without any innate capacity for human speech, the macaques showed increased sensitivity to small changes in voice onset time at each of those boundaries observed in human listeners. Although we cannot call this "categorical perception" as the monkeys did not actually label any stimuli, the fact that they showed increased sensitivity at boundaries between human phonemes suggests a biological predisposition to distinguishing speech sounds at those locations in the stimulus continuum and that these differences across consonant contexts must be due to neural processing shared between primates. Similar results were also shown for distinctions between /b/, /d/, and /g/ by macaques along changes in onset frequency of F_2 (Kuhl & Padden, 1983). Although no one has proposed a specific auditory mechanism that explains these patterns of classification, the fact that they occur across species suggests that it is not specific to speech processing by human listeners.

Kluender, Diehl, and Killeen (1987) showed that Japanese quail learn context variability similar to that illustrated in Figures 11.2 and 11.3. The birds were first trained to discriminate /b/, /d/, and /g/ followed by one set of vowels and then tested on the same consonants when followed by a different set of vowels. Kluender, Diehl, and Killeen found that Japanese quail were able to generalize to the new vowel contexts despite context dependencies between consonants and vowels in CV syllables and even though the second set had never been heard before. In later experiments, Lotto, Kluender, and Holt (1997) found that quail compensated for coarticulation in /ar/ and /al/ before /ga/ and /da/ after being trained on /da/ and /ga/ in isolation. The authors concluded that there must be some very basic mechanism shared by the auditory systems of both birds and mammals that could account for this cross-contextual generalization.

So how are nonhuman animals able to unravel context sensitivity found in the speech signal? In direct opposition to the proposals laid out by proponents of the Motor Theory (Liberman & Mattingly 1985), Diehl and Kluender (1989) argue that the phonemic representation of the speech signal is primarily acoustic and that human listeners do not need to make reference to articulations or gestures to decode the speech signal.

Further, they claim that speakers, either directly or indirectly, *enhance* some of these auditory contrasts when speaking (Liljencrants & Lindblom, 1972). They note that in the vowel inventories of languages, vowels are maximally separated in formant frequencies to limit acoustic overlap. For example, in languages with only three vowels, vowel systems tend to consist of /i/, /a/, and /u/, which are the furthest apart that the human vocal tract will allow in terms of F_1 and F_2 frequency. For languages with five vowels, the additional vowels tend to be /e/ and /o/ which are acoustically intermediate. Further, the back vowels /u/ and /o/ are most frequently associated with lip rounding which lowers formant frequencies thereby increasing acoustic separation from the front vowels /i/, /e/, and /a/. In consonants, they also point out that differences in voice onset-time boundary between places of articulation serve only to maximize acoustic distinctiveness making it easier for both human – and nonhuman (e.g., Kuhl & Padden, 1982) – listeners to learn.

If the primary correlate to phoneme identity is auditory, it is then the task of the speaker to produce an appropriate acoustic signal that can be decoded by the auditory system of the listener. Diehl and Kluender (1989) point out that a number of examples of coarticulation are, in fact, *deliberately controlled* for the purpose of enhancing auditory contrast. In the last decade, researchers in neurophysiology have weighed in on the gestural versus auditory controversy from a new perspective (see Hickok, Houde & Rong, 2011, for discussion and extensive references to many aspects of the debate between proponents of these views of the primary "objects" of speech perception).

These auditory theories are contrasted with gestural theories in that they propose a strong relationship between the fundamental symbols of speech – i.e., phonemes – and basic acoustic properties whereas Motor Theory proposes a strong relationship between phonemes and the intended gestures of the speaker (see Figure 11.5).

Trading relations

All of these accounts, whether motivated by gestural or auditory processes, attempt to find invariant correlates to speech sounds in some domain of communication in the face of enormous context variability. In the case of Motor Theory, the invariants are to be found in the intended gestures of the speaker which must, somehow, be recovered by the listener. In auditory theories, the invariants are to be found in the outputs of fundamental auditory processes that are enhanced by this context variability, and it is the task of the speaker to produce these acoustic contrasts. Another position is that absolute invariants *do not exist* and that the *trading relations* or characteristic correlations between acoustic properties that are observed as part of these context effects are used directly in speech-sound identification (e.g., Lindblom, 1996).

In early experiments with the Pattern Playback, Cooper, Delattre, Liberman, Borst, and Gerstman (1952) and Liberman, Delattre, Cooper, and Gerstman (1954) found that listeners could identify /b/, /d/, and /g/ from second-formant transitions from the onset of the syllable to the vowel. However, they found that the direction and extent of these formant transitions also depended on the vowel context: while a rising F_2 was generally heard as /b/, a falling F_2 was identified as either alveolar or velar depending on the following vowel. To complicate matters further, Öhman (1966) found that formant transitions following *intervocalic* stops depended not only on the following vowel, but also on the preceding one. Because it was known that formant transitions reflected changes in the size and shape of the vocal tract and that these changes resulted primarily from the movement of the oral articulators, it was suggested at the time that these transitions merely gave the listener insight into the approximate configuration of the speaker's vocal tract (Delattre, Liberman & Cooper, 1955).

However, in apparent contradiction to his colleagues, Delattre (1969) suggested that these context-dependent but characteristic transitions for each place of articulation were defined in terms of *perception* and not production, in that phoneme identity was arrived at by perceptual means. Sussman, Fruchter, Hilbert, and Sirosh (1998) presented a summary of evidence that second formant transitions might serve as a *partly* invariant cue to the perception of stop consonants. It was originally found by Lindblom (1963) that the onset frequency of F_2 was strongly correlated with the F_2 of the following vowel and that the slope and y-intercept of the regression fit was specific to the consonant itself (see also Nearey & Shammass, 1987; Sussman, McCaffrey & Matthews, 1991; Sussman 1991). These correlations and their regression fits have been referred to as *locus equations*.

Not only did they suggest that perception of stop place was defined in purely acoustic terms, they even proposed a neurological mechanism whereby the human auditory system could take advantage of the observed correlations. They did so by drawing parallels between this language-specific ability and perceptual mechanisms that have been studied in specific mammalian and avian species. They also showed that this acoustic patterning was not merely a byproduct of human articulatory physiology, but that speakers actually exploited this acoustic correlation by specifically targeting the locus equation relations in articulation. It has also been shown that they provide good correlates to perception in synthetic speech (Fruchter & Sussman, 1997).

A double-weak framework for speech perception

While Stevens and Blumstein (1978) propose strong relationships between all three domains of speech – gestural, auditory, and symbolic – Nearey (1997b) proposes a significant compromise between these positions in which the relationship between phonemes and both acoustics and gestures is relatively weaker than that proposed elsewhere, but in which a relationship does indeed exist between all three of these domains, if only indirectly. It is clear that perception plays a role in speech production and that speakers monitor their own speech to correct for errors (Levelt, 1983). Similarly, if auditory feedback is distorted artificially in some manner, speakers will compensate articulatorily (e.g., Purcell & Munhall, 2006). Conversely, it has been suggested that mirror neurons in cortical regions of the brain associated with speech production have, at least, a limited role in speech perception (Hickok, Houde & Rong, 2011).

Nearey (1990, 1997b) proposes a *double-weak* approach to the study of speech perception. Nearey arrives at this position as by the force of the argument among opposing camps and he states: "I am genuinely impressed by the quality of the research by both the auditorists and the gesturalists that is critical of the other position. Each has convinced me that the others are wrong." In a talk to the Acoustical Society of America in 2016, he proposed the double-weak position as more of a framework than a true theory – one that postpones rumination on the deeper principles but rather adopts minimal assumptions about the relation among symbols, sounds and gestures. The framework might serve as a rationale for immediately pursuing empirical generalizations or primitive "laws." The hope is that some such generalizations will serve the role of Kepler's laws of planetary motion or eighteenth century "gas laws" which may also serve as grist for later, more deeply explanatory theories. A schematic depiction of the double-weak approach and its relation to other views is shown in Figure 11.5. In this figure, heavy, double-headed arrows indicate relatively strong and direct links. Thinner single-sided arrows indicate weaker (complex but otherwise *tractable*) links in the indicated direction. Dotted connections indicate a relationship the theory assumes but does not characterize, and which may be arbitrarily complex.

Advocates of the double-strong (both strong-auditory and strong-gestural) theory in the upper left claim that there are strong, direct ties between symbolic objects (e.g., distinctive features or phonemes) and auditory patterns on the one hand, but also a direct link from symbols to articulatory patterns (e.g., Stevens & Blumstein, 1978; Stevens & Blumstein, 1981). This seems to imply that there are also relatively strong, direct ties between auditory patterns and gestures, indicated by the gray double arrow. Strong gestural theory (e.g., that of Liberman & Mattingly, 1985), on the lower left, suggests that only the links between symbols and gestures are strong and relatively simple. Relations between symbols and acoustics in this theory are not direct, but must somehow infer gestual patterns from the auditory input and rely on the complex relationship between articulation and acoustics which are somehow mapped in the brain of the listener, at which point the symbols can be easily read off. However, Liberman and Mattingly make no attempt to characterize this latter relationship. Strong auditory theory (e.g., that of Kingston & Diehl, 1994), on the upper right, takes a diametrically opposed position and suggests that only the links between symbols and auditory patterns are strong and simple. Relations between symbols and articulation are not direct in this theory, but rather involve speakers finding ways to make sure that the gestures they choose will have the desired auditory effects and hence trigger the recognition of the correct symbols by the listener.

Double-weak theory gives up on the notion of any relation being strong or transparent. Rather, it contends the only things necessary for a successful speech communication system are:

1 For symbols to map into gestures that a speaker can manageably produce (i.e., the symbolic-to-gestural link)
2 For those same gestures to result in auditory patterns, that while not always transparently related to the symbols, can manageably be decoded into them (the auditory-to-symbolic link in Figure 11.5).

This implies (or at least readily allows) that gestural and auditory patterns are only indirectly linked by virtue of their relationship to acoustics. Neither requires a direct or fully transparent link to symbols: Rather,

> [The relations] . . . are assumed only to be tractably systematic, to lie within the range of the feasible for the (possibly speech-specialized) auditory and motor control systems. Longer-term and secular trends effectively impose a communicative natural selection, ensuring that the phonology of a language remains within easy reach of the vast majority of speakers and listeners.
>
> *(Nearey, 1997b, p. 3243)*

Although the double-weak approach is, in principle, about both production and perception, research in the framework has been limited to perception. Specifically, efforts have been directed at trying to explicitly characterize non-trivial, but relatively simple functions that can map cue patterns into listeners' choice behavior in categorization experiments (see Nearey, 1990, 1997b, for more details).

It is by no means clear to us what an analogously constrained double-weak approach to production would look like. However, we suspect it would involve organizing gestural patterns in some systematic way that produced appropriate acoustic reflexes, rather than patterns that were organized on the basis of motor or articulatory configurations and movements alone.

Notes

1 One of these can be replaced by a machine: either a speech synthesizer or an automatic speech-recognition system. However, these are merely simulations of processes that take place in humans.
2 However, careful selection of diphone (all combinations of two adjacent phonemes) or larger chunks of speech can serve as the basis of highly intelligible synthetic speech (Dutoit 1997).
3 The difference in time between the onset of laryngeal voicing and the release of the stop burst in plosives such as /p,t,k,b,d,g/
4 This is known as the AX design. Alternatively, in the ABX design, you can hear three sounds and say whether the third was identical to the first or second.
5 In the direct realist perspective of Fowler (1989), the inverse mapping from acoustics to gestures is not assumed to require any analysis-by-synthesis decoding, but is said to instead involve "direct perception" of gestures by listeners. While there is a very substantial difference in perspective compared to Motor Theory, we treat the empirical projections of the differences as quite subtle compared to differences with the non-gesturalist schools.
6 Chinchillas are an animal in the rodent order. Because their hearing has a frequency range similar to that of humans, they have been popularly used to test theories of auditory physiology.

References

Allen, J.B. (1994), 'How do humans process and recognize speech?', *IEEE Transactions on Speech and Audio Processing* **2**, 567–577.

Andruski, J.E. & Nearey, T.M. (1992), 'On the sufficiency of compound target specification of isolated vowels and vowels in /bVb/ syllables', *The Journal of the Acoustical Society of America* **91**, 390–410.

Assmann, P.F. & Katz, W.F. (2000), 'Time-varying spectral change in the vowels of children and adults', *The Journal of the Acoustical Society of America* **108**, 1856–1866.

Best, C.T. (1995), A direct realist view of cross-language speech perception, *in* W. Strange, ed., 'Speech Perception and Linguistic Experience: Issues in Cross-Language Research', York Press, Baltimore, MD, pp. 171–204.

Blumstein, S.E. & Stevens, K.N. (1979), 'Acoustic invariance in speech production: Evidence from measurements of the spectral characteristics of stop consonants', *The Journal of the Acoustical Society of America* **66**, 1001–1017.

Blumstein, S.E. & Stevens, K.N. (1980), 'Perceptual invariance and onset spectra for stop consonants in different vowel environments', *The Journal of the Acoustical Society of America* **67**, 648–662.

Boersma, P. & Weenink, D. (2018), 'Praat: Doing phonetics by computer', *Computer Program*. Version 6.0.37, Retrieved 3 February 2018 from www.praat.org

Boothroyd, A. & Nitrouer, S. (1988), 'Mathematical treatment of context effects in phoneme and word recognition', *The Journal of the Acoustical Society of America* **84**, 101–114.

Broadbent, D.E. (1967), 'Word-frequency effect and response bias', *Psychological Review* **74**, 1–15.

Bronkhorst, A.W., Bosman, A.J. & Smoorenburg, G.F. (1993), 'A model for context effects in speech recognition', *The Journal of the Acoustical Society of America* **93**, 499–509.

Cole, R.A. & Scott, B. (1974), 'The phantom in the phoneme: Invariant cues for stop consonants', *Perception & Psychophysics* **15**, 101–107.

Cooper, F.S. (1950), 'Spectrum analysis', *The Journal of the Acoustical Society of America* **22**, 761–762.

Cooper, F.S., Delattre, P.C., Liberman, A.M., Borst, J.M. & Gerstman, L.J. (1952), 'Some experiments on the perception of synthetic speech sounds', *The Journal of the Acoustical Society of America* **24**, 597–606.

Cooper, F.S., Gaitenby, J.H., Mattingly, I.G. & Umeda, N. (1969), 'Reading aids for the blind: A special case of machine-to-man communication', *IEEE Transactions on Audio and Electronics* **AU-17**, 266–270.

Darwin, C.J., McKeown, J.D. & Kirby, D. (1989), 'Perceptual compensation for transmission channel and speaker effects on vowel quality', *Speech Communication* **8**, 221–234.

Delattre, P. C. (1969), 'Coarticulation and the locus theory', *Studia Linguistica* **23**, 1–26.

Delattre, P.C., Liberman, A.M. & Cooper, F.S. (1955), 'Acoustic loci and transitional cues for consonants', *The Journal of the Acoustical Society of America* **27**, 769–773.

Delgutte, B., Hammond, B.M., Kalluri, S., Litvak, L.M. & Cariani, P.A. (1996), Neural encoding of temporal envelope and temporal interactions in speech, *in* W. Ainsworth & S. Greenberg, eds., 'Auditory Basis of Speech Perception', European Speech Communication Association, pp. 1–9.

Delgutte, B. & Kiang, N. Y.S. (1984), 'Speech coding in the auditory nerve: IV. Sounds with consonant-like dynamic characteristics', *The Journal of the Acoustical Society of America* **74**, 897–907.

Diehl, R.L. & Kluender, K.R. (1989), 'On the objects of speech perception', *Ecological Psychology* **1**, 121–144.

Dutoit, T. (1997), *An Introduction to Text-to-Speech Synthesis*, Kluwer, Dordrecht.

Eimas, P.D. (1963), 'The relation between identification and discrimination along speech and non-speech continua', *Language and Speech* **6**, 206–217.

Eimas, P.D., Siqueland, E.R., Jusczyk, P. & Vigorito, J. (1971), 'Speech perception by infants', *Science* **171**, 303–306.

Fant, G. (1970), *Acoustic Theory of Speech Production: With Calculations Based on X-Ray Studies of Russian Articulations*, second edn, Mouton, The Hague, the Netherlands.

Flege, J.E. (1995), Second language speech learning: Theory, findings, and problems, *in* W. Strange, ed., 'Speech Perception and Linguistic Experience: Issues in Cross-Language Research', York Press, Timonium, MD.

Fletcher, H. (1995), *Speech and Hearing in Communication*, American Institute of Physics, Woodbury, NY.

Fowler, C.A. (1986), 'An event approach to the study of speech perception from a direct-realist perspective', *Journal of Phonetics* **14**, 3–28.

Fowler, C.A. (1989), 'Real objects of speech perception: A commentary on Diehl and Kluender', *Ecological Psychology* **1**, 145–160.

Fruchter, D. & Sussman, H.M. (1997), 'The perceptual relevance of locus equations', *The Journal of the Acoustical Society of America* **102**, 2997–3008.

Galantucci, B., Fowler, C.A. & Turvey, M.T. (2006), 'The motor theory of speech perception reviewed', *Psychonomic Bulletin & Review* **13**, 361–377.

Goldinger, S.D. (1997), Words and voices: Perception and production in an episodic lexicon, *in* K. Johnson & J.W. Mullennix, eds., 'Talker Variability in Speech Processing', Morgan Kaufmann, San Francisco, CA, pp. 33–66.

Halle, M. & Stevens, K.N. (1991), Knowledge of language and the sounds of speech, *in* J. Sundberg, L. Nord & R. Carlson, eds., 'Music, Language, Speech and Brain', Springer, Berlin, pp. 1–19.

Harris, C.M. (1953), 'A study of the building blocks in speech', *The Journal of the Acoustical Society of America* **25**, 962–969.

Hickok, G., Houde, J. & Rong, F. (2011), 'Sensorimotor integration in speech processing: Computational basis and neural organization', *Neuron* **69**, 407–422.

Hillenbrand, J., Getty, L.A., Clark, M.J. & Wheeler, K. (1995), 'Acoustic characteristics of American English vowels', *The Journal of the Acoustical Society of America* **97**, 3099–3111.

Johnson, K. (1997), Speech perception without speaker normalization, *in* K. Johnson & J.W. Mullennix, eds., 'Talker Variability in Speech Processing', Morgan Kaufmann, San Francisco, CA, pp. 145–165.

Johnson, K., Ladefoged, P. & Lindau, M. (1993), 'Individual differences in vowel production', *The Journal of the Acoustical Society of America* **94**, 701–714.

Kewley-Port, D. (1983), 'Time-varying features as correlates of place of articulation in stop consonants', *The Journal of the Acoustical Society of America* **73**, 322–335.

Kewley-Port, D. & Luce, P.A. (1984), 'Time-varying features of initial stop consonants in auditory running spectra: A first report', *Perception & Psychophysics* **35**, 353–360.

Kiefte, M. & Kluender, K.R. (2005a), 'Pattern Playback revisited: Unvoiced stop consonant perception', *The Journal of the Acoustical Society of America* **118**, 2599–2606.

Kiefte, M. & Kluender, K.R. (2005b), 'The relative importance of spectral tilt in monophthongs and diphthongs', *The Journal of the Acoustical Society of America* **117**, 1395–1404.

Kiefte, M. & Kluender, K.R. (2008), 'Absorption of reliable spectral characteristics in auditory perception', *The Journal of the Acoustical Society of America* **123**, 366–376.

Kiefte, M., Nearey, T.M. & Assmann, P.F. (2012), Vowel perception in normal speakers, *in* M.J. Ball & F. Gibbon, eds., 'Handbook of Vowels and Vowel Disorders', Psychology Press, New York, pp. 160–185.

Kingston, J. & Diehl, R.L. (1994), 'Phonetic knowledge', *Language* **70**, 419–454.

Kingston, J. & Diehl, R.L. (1995), 'Intermediate properties in the perception of distinctive feature values', *Papers in Laboratory Phonology* **4**, 7–27.

Kluender, K.R., Coady, J.A. & Kiefte, M. (2003), 'Perceptual sensitivity to change in perception of speech', *Speech Communication* **41**, 59–69.

Kluender, K.R., Diehl, R.L. & Killeen, P.R. (1987), 'Japanese quail can learn phonetic categories', *Science* **237**, 1195–1197.

Kluender, K.R. & Kiefte, M. (2006), Speech perception within a biologically realistic information-theoretic framework, *in* M.A. Gernsbacher & M. Traxler, eds., 'Handbook of Psycholinguistics', second edn, Elsevier, London, pp. 153–199.

Kluender, K.R., Stilp, C.E. & Kiefte, M. (2013), Perception of vowel sounds within a biologically realistic model of efficient coding, *in* G. Morrison & P.F. Assmann, eds., 'Vowel Inherent Spectral Change', Springer, Berlin, pp. 117–151.

Kohler, E., Keysers, C., Umilta, M.A., Fogassi, L., Gallese, V. & Rizzolatti, G. (2002), 'Hearing sounds, understanding actions: Action representation in mirror neurons', *Science* **297**, 846–848.

Kuhl, P.K. & Miller, J.D. (1975), 'Speech perception by chinchilla: Voiced-voiceless distinction in alveolar plosive consonants', *Science* **190**, 69–72.

Kuhl, P.K. & Padden, D.M. (1982), 'Enhanced discriminability at the phonetic boundaries for the voicing feature in macaques', *Perception & Psychophysics* **32**, 542–550.

Kuhl, P.K. & Padden, D.M. (1983), 'Enhanced discriminability at the phonetic boundaries for the place feature in macaques', *The Journal of the Acoustical Society of America* **73**, 1003–1010.

Ladefoged, P., DeClerk, J., Lindau, M. & Papçun, G. (1972), 'An auditory-motor theory of speech production', *UCLA Working Papers in Phonetics* **22**, 48–76.

Lahiri, A., Gewirth, L. & Blumstein, S.E. (1984), 'A reconsideration of acoustic invariance for place of articulation in diffuse stop consonants: Evidence from a cross-language study', *The Journal of the Acoustical Society of America* **76**, 391–404.

Levelt, W.J. (1983), 'Monitoring and self-repair in speech', *Cognition* **14**, 41–104.

Liberman, A.M. (1984), On finding that speech is special, *in* 'Handbook of Cognitive Neuroscience', Springer, Boston, MA, pp. 169–197.

Liberman, A.M., Cooper, F.S., Shankweiler, D.P. & Studdert-Kennedy, M. (1967), 'Perception of the speech code', *Psychological Review* **74**, 431–461.

Liberman, A.M., Delattre, P. & Cooper, F.S. (1952), 'The rôle of selected stimulus-variables in the perception of the unvoiced stop consonants', *The American Journal of Psychology* **LXV**, 497–516.

Liberman, A.M., Delattre, P.C., Cooper, F.S. & Gerstman, L.J. (1954), 'The role of consonant-vowel transitions in the perception of the stop and nasal consonants', *Psychological Monographs: General and Applied* **68**(8), 1–13.

Liberman, A.M., Harris, K.S., Hoffman, H.S. & Griffith, B.C. (1957), 'The discrimination of speech sounds within and across phoneme boundaries', *Journal of Experimental Psychology* **54**, 358–368.

Liberman, A.M., Isenberg, D. & Rakerd, B. (1981), 'Duplex perception of cues for stop consonants: Evidence for a phonetic mode', *Perception & Psychophysics* **30**, 133–143.

Liberman, A.M. & Mattingly, I.G. (1985), 'The motor theory of speech perception revisited', *Cognition* **21**, 1–36.

Liljencrants, J. & Lindblom, B. (1972), 'Numerical simulation of vowel quality systems: The role of perceptual contrast', *Language* **48**, 839–862.

Lindblom, B. (1963), 'On vowel reduction', Technical Report 29, Speech Transmission Laboratory, Royal Institute of Technology, Stockholm, Sweden.

Lindblom, B. (1996), 'Role of articulation in speech perception: Clues from production', *The Journal of the Acoustical Society of America* **99**, 1683–1692.

Lotto, A.J., Hickok, G.S. & Holt, L.L. (2009), 'Reflections on mirror neurons and speech perception', *Trends in Cognitive Sciences* **13**, 110–114.

Lotto, A.J. & Kluender, K.R. (1998), 'General contrast effects in speech perception: Effect of preceding liquid on stop consonant identification', *Perception & Psychophysics* **60**, 602–619.

Lotto, A.J., Kluender, K.R. & Holt, L.L. (1997), 'Perceptual compensation for coarticulation by Japanese quail (*Coturnix coturnix japonica*)', *The Journal of the Acoustical Society of America* **102**, 1134–1140.

Luce, P.A. & Pisoni, D.B. (1998), 'Recognizing spoken words: The neighborhood activation model', *Ear and Hearing* **19**, 1–36.

Massaro, D.W. & Chen, T.H. (2008), 'The motor theory of speech perception revisited', *Psychonomic Bulletin & Review* **15**, 453–457.

McGovern, K. & Strange, W. (1977), 'The perception of /r/ and /l/ in syllable-initial and syllable-final position', *Perception & Psychophysics*, 162–170.

McGurk, H. & MacDonald, J. (1976), 'Hearing lips and seeing voices', *Nature* **264**, 746–748.

Mermelstein, P. (1978), 'On the relationship between vowel and consonant identification when cued by the same acoustic information', *Perception & Psychophysics* **23**, 331–336.

Miller, G.A. & Nicely, P.E. (1955), 'An analysis of perceptual confusions among some English consonants', *The Journal of the Acoustical Society of America* **27**, 338–352.

Nearey, T.M. (1980), 'On the physical interpretation of vowel quality: Cinefluorographic and acoustic evidence', *Journal of Phonetics* **8**, 213–241.

Nearey, T.M. (1990), 'The segment as a unit of speech perception', *Journal of Phonetics* **18**, 347–373.

Nearey, T.M. (1992), 'Context effects in a double-weak theory of speech perception', *Language and Speech* **35**, 153–171.

Nearey, T.M. (1997a), Modularity and tractability in speech perception, *in* K. Singer, R. Eggert & G. Anderson, eds., 'CLS 33: The Panels', Chicago Linguistic Society, Chicago, IL, pp. 399–413.

Nearey, T.M. (1997b), 'Speech perception as pattern recognition', *The Journal of the Acoustical Society of America* **101**, 3241–3254.

Nearey, T.M. (2001), 'Phoneme-like units and speech perception', *Language and Cognitive Processes* **16**, 673–681.

Nearey, T.M. (2004), 'On the factorability of phonological units in speech perception', *Laboratory Phonology* **6**, 197–221.

Nearey, T.M. & Assmann, P.F. (1986), 'Modeling the role of inherent spectral change in vowel identification', *The Journal of the Acoustical Society of America* **80**, 1297–1308.

Nearey, T. M. & Shammass, S. E. (1987), 'Formant transitions as partly distinctive invariant properties in the identification of voiced stops', *Canadian Acoustics* **15**, 17–24.

Öhman, S. E. G. (1966), 'Coarticulation in VCV utterances: Spectrographic measurements', *The Journal of the Acoustical Society of America* **39**, 151–168.

Parker, E.M., Diehl, R.L. & Kluender, K.R. (1986), 'Trading relations in speech and nonspeech', *Perception & Psychophysics* **39**, 129–142.

Perkell, J.S., Matthies, M.L., Svirsky, M.A. & Jordan, M.I. (1993), 'Trading relations between tongue-body raising and lip rounding in production of the vowel /u/: A pilot "motor equivalence" study', *The Journal of the Acoustical Society of America* **93**, 2948–2961.

Pisoni, D.B. (1997), Some thoughts on "normalization" in speech perception, *in* K. Johnson & J.W. Mullennix, eds., 'Talker Variability in Speech Processing', Morgan Kaufmann, San Francisco, CA, pp. 9–32.

Pollack, I., Rubenstein, H. & Decker, L. (1959), 'Intelligibility of known and unknown message sets', *The Journal of the Acoustical Society of America* **31**, 273–279.

Purcell, D.W. & Munhall, K.G. (2006), 'Compensation following real-time manipulation of formants in isolated vowels', *The Journal of the Acoustical Society of America* **119**, 2288–2297.

Recio, A., Rhode, W.S., Kiefte, M. & Kluender, K.R. (2002), 'Responses to cochlear normalized speech stimuli in the auditory nerve of cat', *The Journal of the Acoustical Society of America* **111**, 2213–2218.

Repp, B.H. (1982), 'Phonetic trading relations and context effects: New experimental evidence for a speech mode of perception', *Psychological Bulletin* **92**, 81–110.

Rizzolatti, G. & Arbib, M.A. (1998), 'Language within our grasp', *Trends in Neurosciences* **21**, 188–194.

Rizzolatti, G. & Craighero, L. (2004), 'The mirror-neuron system', *Annual Review of Neuroscience* **27**, 169–192.

Sachs, M.B. & Young, E.D. (1979), 'Encoding of steady-state vowels in the auditory nerve: Representation in terms of discharge rate', *The Journal of the Acoustical Society of America* **66**, 470–479.

Schatz, C.D. (1954), 'The role of context in the perception of stops', *Language* **30**, 47–56.

Stetson, R.H. (1945), *Bases of Phonology*, Oberlin College, Oberlin.

Stevens, K.N. (1989), 'On the quantal nature of speech', *Journal of Phonetics* **17**, 3–45.

Stevens, K.N. (2002), 'Toward a model for lexical access based on acoustic landmarks and distinctive features', *The Journal of the Acoustical Society of America* **111**, 1872–1891.

Stevens, K. N. & Blumstein, S. E. (1978), 'Invariant cues for place of articulation in stop consonants', *The Journal of the Acoustical Society of America* **64**, 1358–1368.

Stevens, K. N. & Blumstein, S. E. (1981), The search for invariant acoustic correlates of phonetic features, *in* P. D. Eimas & J. L. Miller, eds., 'Perspectives on the Study of Speech', Lawrence Erlbaum, Hillsdale, NJ, pp. 1–38.

Stevens, K. N. & Keyser, J. J. (1989), 'Primary features and their enhancement in consonants', *Language* **65**, 81–106.

Stilp, C. E., Kiefte, M., Alexander, J. M. & Kluender, K. R. (2010), 'Cochlea-scaled spectral entropy predicts rate-invariant intelligibility of temporally distorted sentences', *The Journal of the Acoustical Society of America* **128**, 2112–2126.

Suomi, K. (1985), 'The vowel-dependence of gross spectral cues to place of articulation of stop consonants in CV syllables', *Journal of Phonetics* **13**, 267–285.

Sussman, H. M. (1991), 'The representation of stop consonants in three-dimensional acoustic space', *Phonetica* **48**, 18–31.

Sussman, H. M., Fruchter, D. & Cable, A. (1995), 'Locus equations derived from compensatory articulation', *The Journal of the Acoustical Society of America* **97**, 3112–3124.

Sussman, H. M., Fruchter, D., Hilbert, J. & Sirosh, J. (1998), 'Linear correlates in the speech signal: The orderly output constraint', *Behavioral and Brain Sciences* **21**, 241–299.

Sussman, H. M., McCaffrey, H. A. & Matthews, S. A. (1991), 'An investigation of locus equations as a source of relational invariance for stop place categorization', *The Journal of the Acoustical Society of America* **90**, 1309–1325.

Watkins, A. J. (1991), 'Central, auditory mechanisms of perceptual compensation for spectral-envelope distortion', *The Journal of the Acoustical Society of America* **90**, 2942–2955.

Watkins, A. J. & Makin, S. J. (1994), 'Perceptual compensation for speaker differences and for spectral-envelope distortion', *The Journal of the Acoustical Society of America* **96**, 1263–1284.

Watson, C. & Kewley-Port, D. (1988), 'Some remarks on Pastore (1988)', *The Journal of the Acoustical Society of America* **84**, 2266–2270.

Young, E. D. & Sachs, M. B. (1979), 'Representation of steady-state vowels in the temporal aspects of the discharge patterns of populations of auditory-nerve fibers', *The Journal of the Acoustical Society of America* **66**, 1381–1403.

12

Prosody, tone, and intonation

Yi Xu

Introduction

Prosody refers to all suprasegmental aspects of speech, including pitch, duration, amplitude, and voice quality that are used to make lexical and post-lexical contrasts, and to convey paralinguistic meanings. Tone refers to pitch patterns that make lexical, grammatical, or morphological contrasts in many languages. Intonation refers to the melodic facet of prosody, although the two terms are sometimes interchangeable. Though often treated as separate research subjects, these three areas are heavily overlapped with each other not only in terms of the phenomena they cover, but also with regard to the underlying mechanisms they share. A common perspective that can link them all is the articulatory-functional principle, which views speech as a system for transmitting communicative meanings with the human articulators (Xu, 2005). From this perspective, lexical, post-lexical, affective, and social meanings are all conveyed in parallel, each encoded by its own unique imprints on the properties of various underlying articulatory targets. The articulation process turns these function-loaded targets into the acoustic patterns ultimately perceived by listeners, which consist of not only all the functional contributions, but also all the traces and artefacts of the articulation process itself.

This chapter first outlines the articulatory dynamics underlying the production of pitch, duration and voice quality, which serve as the basis for understanding how different functional components can be realized in parallel. Also introduced are various perturbations by a range of articulatory and aerodynamic effects that accompany the core articulatory process. The functional components are then introduced in terms of their respective contributions to the surface prosody as well as their communicative significance, ranging from making lexical contrasts through tone and stress, conveying post-lexical meanings such as focus, sentence modality and boundary marking, to expressing emotional and social meanings through paralinguistic prosody.

The heavy overlap of the communicative functions across the three areas makes it difficult to directly identify the unique contribution of each function to surface prosody. But the sharing of the common mechanisms makes it possible for findings in one area to be relevant to the others, provided that methods are used that can effectively separate the different sources of surface prosody. This chapter is therefore as much about methodology as about the state of the art in prosody research. Effective methodological techniques are illustrated throughout the discussion, and also highlighted at the end of the chapter. Also to be discussed is how the parallel encoding of the communicative functions is related to various prosodic phenomena, including, in particular, prosodic structures and rhythm. Throughout the chapter, various future research directions are suggested.

Articulatory mechanisms

Although multiple articulatory mechanisms are at play in the production of prosody, at the core is how the basic dynamics of articulation are used as a coding mechanism. Surrounding this core are sub-processes that affect various aspects of the overall coding dynamics. The effects of these processes are non-trivial, because they make up much of what we see as the prosodic patterns in the acoustic signal. Adequate knowledge about them is therefore crucial for our ability to separate the articulatory artefacts from the underlying targets that encode the communicative functions.

Basic articulatory dynamics

Speech conveys information by producing rapid alternation off acoustic patterns that represent meaning-carrying categories. In an ideal coding system, the shift between acoustic patterns would be instantaneous, so that surface patterns would directly reflect the underlying coding units without ambiguity. Take as an example fundamental frequency (f_0), the main acoustic correlate of tone and intonation, instantaneous pattern shifts would look like Figure 12.1a for a sequence of high and low tones. However, the human larynx is incapable of generating these kind of sudden shifts in f_0 because the larynx is a biomechanical system, subject to inertia. From Figure 12.1b, we can see that the articulated tones look like a series of transitions, each moving gradually toward the underlying register of the corresponding tone, without reaching a plateau.

These transitions seem to be rather slow relative to the normal speech rate of 5–7 syllables/s (Eriksson, 2012; Tiffany, 1980). The relatively slow movement is related to the maximum speed of pitch change (Xu & Sun, 2002). As shown in the formulae below (1–2), the time needed for pitch change of either direction increases quasi-linearly, and it takes about 100 ms to make even the smallest pitch change (i.e., when *d* approaches 0).

1 *Pitch rise:* $t_r = 89.6 + 8.7\,d$
2 *Pitch drop:* $t_f = 100.04 + 5.8\,d$

where t_r is minimum time needed for a full rise, t_f is the minimum time needed for a full fall, and *d* is the magnitude of the rise or fall in semitones.

From Figure 12.1b we can see that, for the most part, the transition toward each tonal target occurs *within* the temporal domain of the syllable that carries the tone rather than *between* the syllables. This becomes even clearer in Figure 12.2, where in each plot only the tones of the second syllable vary across four Mandarin tones: High (H), Rising (R), Low (L), and Falling (F). These tonal variations give the tones of the third syllable very different

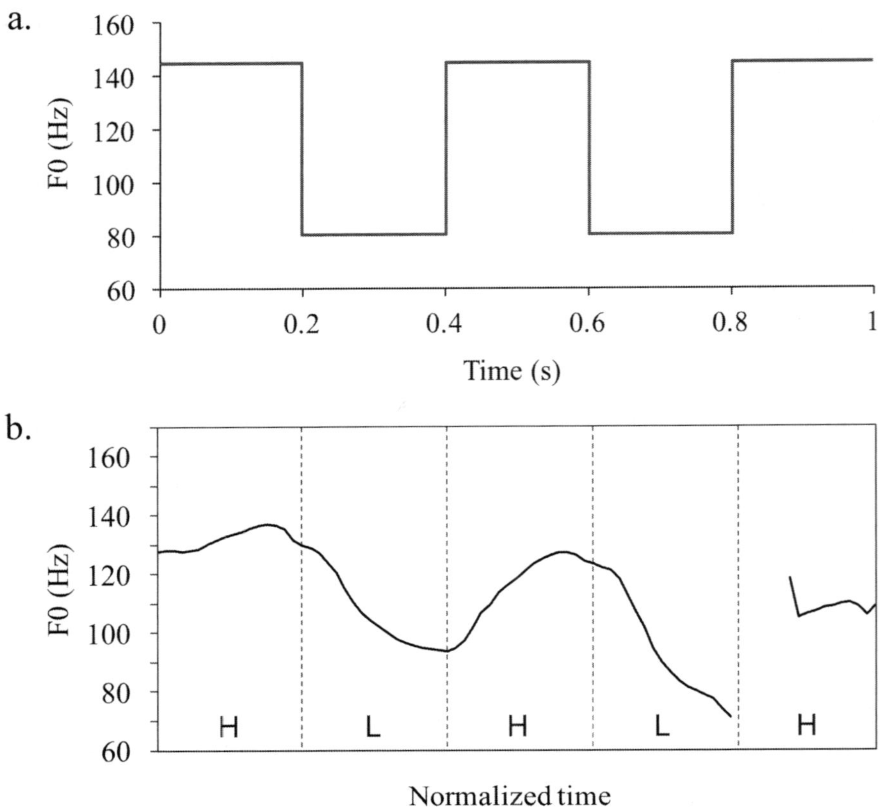

Figure 12.1 (a) A hypothetical f_0 contour of a sequence of high and low level tones with instantaneous transitions. (b) Mean f_0 contour of a sequence of high and low tones in Mandarin produced by four native male speakers.

Source: (data from Xu, 1999).

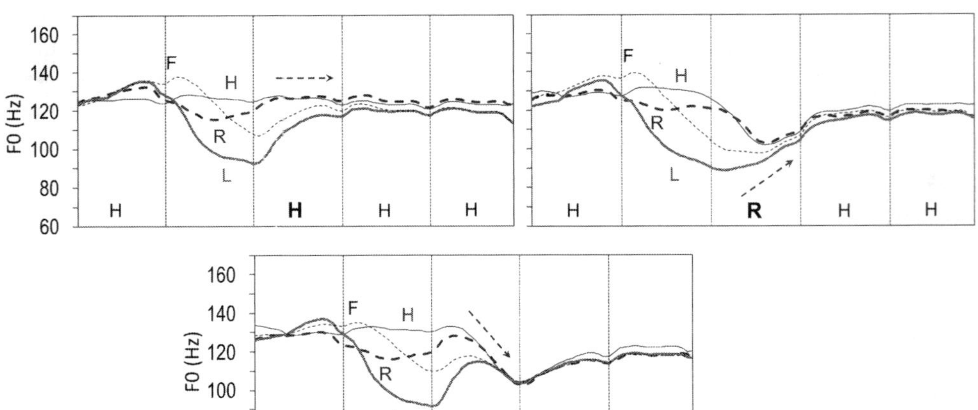

Figure 12.2 Mean f_0 contours of Mandarin tones in continuous speech, produced by four native male speakers. In each plot, only the tones of the second syllable vary across four tones. H = High, R = Rising, L = Low and F = Falling.

Source: Data from Xu (1999).

onsets in f_0. But the four contours in that syllable all converge to a linear shape that is consistent with the underlying form of these tones: high-level, rising and falling, as indicated by the arrows.

The convergence of the f_0 contours of the same tone after different preceding tones points to the basic dynamics of tone production: asymptotic approximation of an underlying pitch target during the host syllable, or *syllable-synchronized sequential target approximation* (Xu & Wang, 2001). That is, each tone has an underlying pitch target that can be as simple as a straight line with a specific height and slope. This pitch target is approached during articulation in synchrony with the syllable that carries the tone, and adjacent tones are produced by sequentially approaching their respective pitch targets.

f_0 perturbation by consonants

When a non-sonorant consonant occurs in a speech utterance, the vibration of the vocal folds is affected in two ways. First, voicing may be stopped, resulting in an interruption of otherwise continuous f_0 contours, or in other words, a *voice break*. Second, f_0 of the surrounding vowels is raised or lowered (Hombert et al., 1979), resulting in a *vertical perturbation*. The two effects are very different in nature, but they need to be considered together in order to identify their respective effects on f_0.

Figure 12.3 shows f_0 contours of (a) Mandarin (Xu & Xu, 2003) and (b) English phrases (Xu & Wallace, 2004) spoken in carrier sentences. For both languages, the contours of syllables with initial obstruents are displayed together with the contour in a syllable with an initial nasal. As can be seen, an obstruent introduces a gap at the beginning of the syllable. After the gap, f_0 first starts at a level well above that of the nasal, but then drops rapidly towards it. In the Mandarin case, there is almost full convergence with the nasal contour. In the English case the contours are higher than the nasal contours after a voiceless obstruent, but lower after a voiced obstruent. Thus there are at least two kinds of vertical perturbations,

(a)

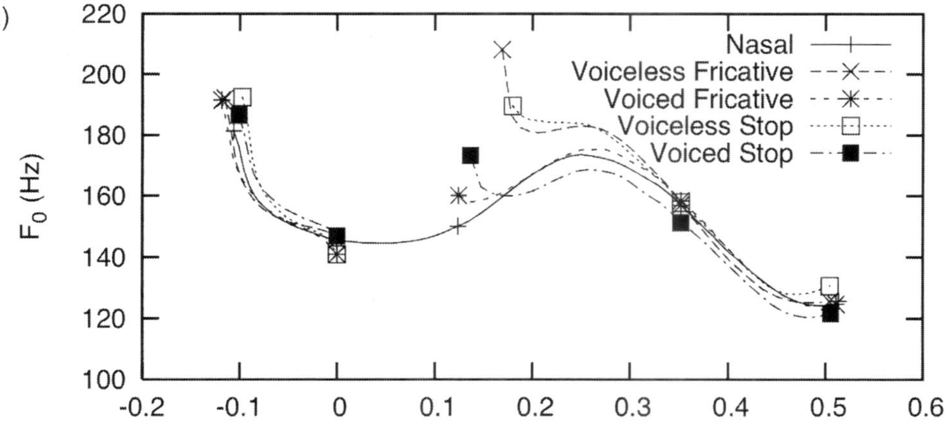

Figure 12.3 Mean f_0 contours of syllables with a nasal onset (continuous curves) and those with obstruent onsets in (a) Mandarin (Xu & Xu, 2003), where H = High tone, R = Rising tone, L = Low tone, and F = Falling tone, and (b) English (Xu & Wallace, 2004). All contours are time-normalized across the syllable.

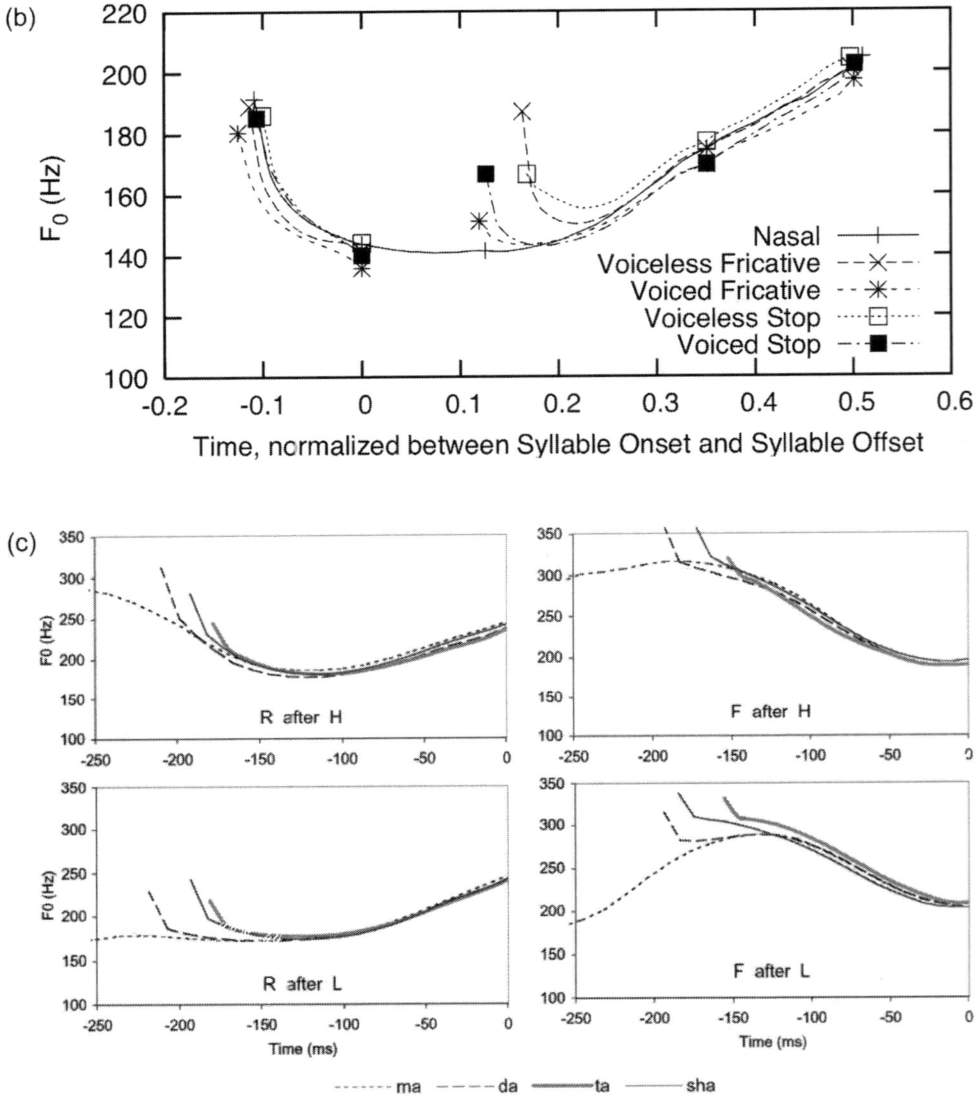

Figure 12.3 (Continued)

a *sharp upshift* after the voice break followed by a quick drop, and a *voicing effect* that can last till the end of the vowel.

As can be seen in Figure 12.3, the sharp upshift occurs at the release of any obstruent consonants. This means that the effect cannot be due to a high rate of airflow across the glottis at the release of a stop (Hombert et al., 1979). Rather, it is possible that the initial vibration at voice onset after an obstruent involves only the outer (mucosal) layer of the vocal folds, which has a higher natural frequency than the main body of the vocal folds, due to a smaller mass. Mucosal vibration (Giovanni et al., 1999) may also occur at voice offset, where f_0 is often seen to rise in breach of the main tonal or intonational contours, as shown in Figure 12.4. Here at the end of a declarative utterance, f_0 has dropped to a level of vocal fry. But the vibration suddenly shifts to a new mode at a frequency that is at odds with the general downtrend, and the overall intonation sounds perfectly complete without this final rise. The nature of this possible mucosal vibration (which occurs quite frequently, especially in female voice) and its potential link to the f_0 upshift by an obstruent are both in need of new research.

The longer-term perturbation effects, in contrast, seem to be more directly related to voicing. According to Halle and Stevens (1971), in the production of an obstruent consonant the tension of the vocal folds is adjusted to alter phonation threshold of the glottis (Titze, 1994). This helps to stop voicing in the case of voiceless consonants or to sustain voicing in the case of voiced consonants (Hanson & Stevens, 2002). These changes in vocal fold tension would affect f_0, raising it for the voiceless consonants, and lowering it for the voiced consonants.

Note that the three kinds of vertical effects are separable only when entire f_0 contours of syllables with obstruent consonants are directly compared to reference syllables with an onset nasal consonant. This comparison bears the assumption that, when an f_0 trajectory is interrupted by an obstruent, the adjustment of vocal fold tension for controlling f_0 does not stop. Continuous adjustment of f_0 without voicing is possible if f_0 and voicing are independently controlled. f_0 is mainly adjusted through vocal fold tension (Fujisaki, 1983), which is done by rotating the thyroid cartilage at its joints with the cricoid cartilage (Hollien, 1960). This involves the antagonistic contraction of the cricothyroid (CT) and the thyroarytenoid (TA) muscles, supplemented by adjustment of laryngeal height and subglottal pressure, with the contraction of the thyrohyoid, sternohyoid and omohyoid muscles (Atkinson, 1978; Erickson et al., 1995). Voicing control, on the other hand, is done by the abduction

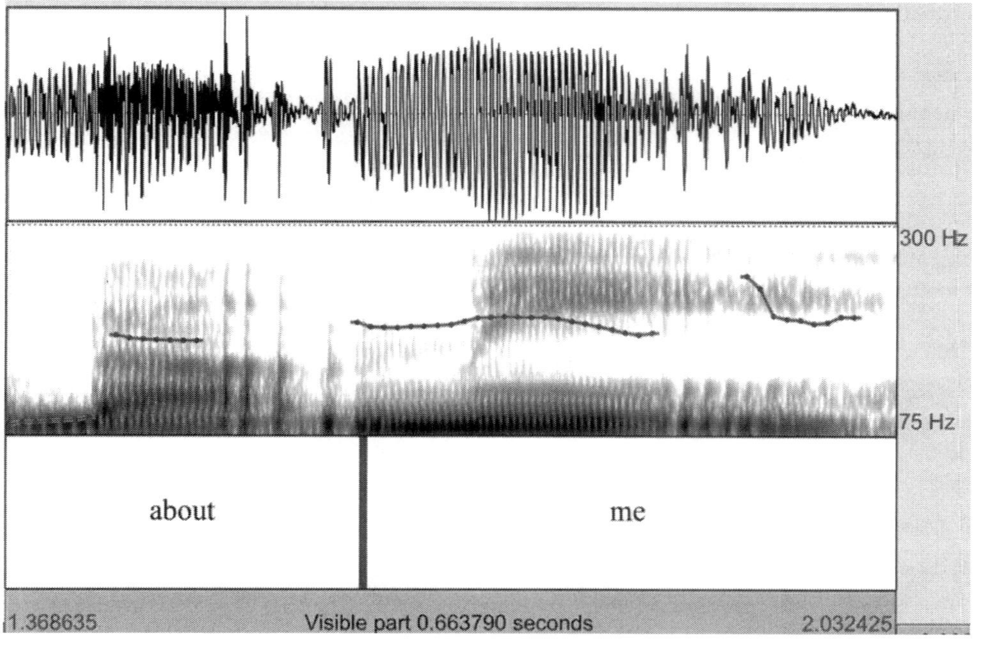

Figure 12.4 A case of likely mucosal vibration at voice offset. The words are ". . . about me" at the end of a declarative sentence in a falling intonation, spoken by a female speaker. Pitch track and spectrogram generated by Praat (Boersma, 2001).

Source: Data from Liu and Xu (2007).

and adduction of the vocal folds, which mainly involve the lateral cricothyroid (LCT) and the inter-cricoid muscles (Zemlin, 1998).

An additional minor effect is that of aspiration. In an aspirated obstruent, a high rate of airflow is needed to generate sufficient aspiration noise. As a result, part of the transglottal pressure is depleted by the time the glottis closes for the vowel. As a result, the amount of f_0 upshift at voice onset is smaller after aspirated consonants than after unaspirated consonants, as can be seen in Figure 12.3a for Mandarin (Xu & Xu, 2003). Note, however, this effect occurs very briefly and only at the voice onset. Thus, it is not the case that aspiration has a general f_0 lowering effect.

Pre-low raising

As shown in Figure 12.2, although the largest effects of the tonal alternation in the second syllable are on the following tone, some smaller effects can be also seen in the preceding syllable. The direction of these anticipatory effects, however, is mostly dissimilatory. That is, the f_0 of the first syllable is the highest when the tone of the second syllable is Low or Rising. This phenomenon, also known as anticipatory raising, anticipatory dissimilation, or H raising, has also been found for Yoruba (Connel & Ladd 1990; Laniran & Clements, 2003), Thai (Gandour et al., 1994), Igbo (Liberman et al., 1993), Fuzhou (Li, 2015), and many African languages (Schuh, 1978). There is even recent evidence that the height difference between accented and unaccented morae in Japanese could be due to anticipatory raising (Lee et al., 2017). The mechanism of this phenomenon is still unclear, but it is likely related to the production of low pitch, which involves a large downward movement of the larynx achieved by the contraction of the external laryngeal muscles, particularly the sternohyoids (Atkinson, 1978; Erickson et al., 1995; Honda et al., 1999). The laryngeal lowering shortens the vocal folds by pulling the larynx across a frontward spinal curvature at the neck, which tilts the cricoid cartilage forward, hence moving the arytenoids closer to the front tip of the thyroid cartilage. This shortening is partially passive, and so is in need of a counter contraction of an antagonist muscle. The only muscle that directly lengthens the vocal folds is the cricothyroids (CT) (Zemlin, 1998), whose preparatory contraction may thus raise pitch before it drops into the lower range. There are also other possible mechanisms that have been suggested (Gandour et al., 1994; Lee et al., 2017).

The perceptual effect of pre-low raising has not yet been extensively studied. However, there is evidence that speakers actually try to reduce its magnitude during normal production, because when under pressure of heavy cognitive load, the amount of pre-low raising is increased rather than decreased (Franich, 2015).

Post-low bouncing

Another mechanism closely related to the production of low pitch is *post-low bouncing* (Chen & Xu, 2006; Prom-on et al., 2012). This is the phenomenon that, after a tone with a very low pitch, f_0 sometimes *bounces back* before returning to a normal level. The bounce can take a few syllables to complete and is most likely to occur when the post-low syllable is weak, e.g., when it has the neutral tone (Chen & Xu, 2006), as shown in Figure 12.5. When the following syllable is not weak, the effect is observable only when the low-pitched syllable is under focus (Xu, 1999). Such a bouncing could be due to a temporary loss of antagonistic muscle balance when the cricoid cartilage returns up across the spinal curvature (Honda et al., 1999), resulting in an abrupt increase of vocal fold tension. This post-low

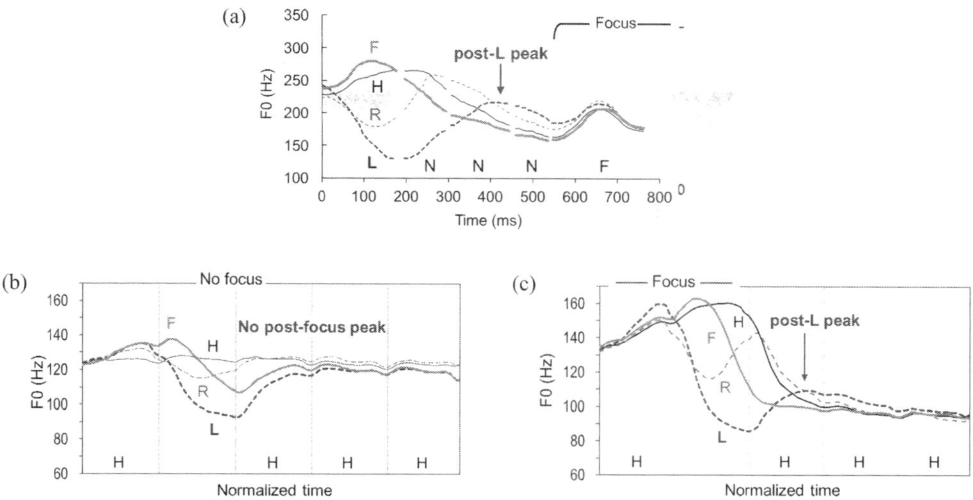

Figure 12.5 (a) Post-low bouncing in Mandarin neutral tone following the Low tone. (b) No post-low bouncing in Mandarin full tones. (c) Post-low bouncing in Mandarin full tones when the preceding Low tone is focused.

Source: Data from Chen and Xu (2006) and Xu (1999).

bouncing mechanism has been simulated by increasing the amount of pitch acceleration (second derivative of f_0) in the initial state of the tone that immediately follows the low tone (Prom-on et al., 2012).

Post-low bouncing may explain why the Mandarin neutral tone is high-pitched after the Low tone but relatively low-pitched after the other full tones (Chao, 1968). The bouncing mechanism could be behind some other tonal and intonational phenomena as well. For example, the distance between a very low-pitched tone in American English and the following f_0 peak remains largely constant (Pierrehumbert, 1980). This parallels the similar (though a bit longer) constant distance between the Low tone and the f_0 peak in the following neutral tone sequence (Chen & Xu, 2006). Further research in this direction should be able to assess the generality of this phenomenon.

Total pitch range

According to Zemlin (1998), a speaker's conversational pitch range spans about two octaves (24 semitones). Data from a more recent study show that the mean non-singing pitch range of American English speakers, even when not including the falsetto register (Svec et al., 1999), is about three octaves (35.4 semitones) (Honorof & Whalen, 2005).[1] In Mandarin, f_0 variations due to the four lexical tones span only about one octave at any particular sentence position (Xu, 1999). Also, the tonal pitch range is in the lower portion of the total pitch range. In Xu (1999), the highest mean pitch in sentences with no focus is about 140 Hz for males and 300 Hz for females. With focus it is about 164 and 342 Hz for males and females, respectively. These are still much lower than the highest mean f_0 in Honorof & Whalen (2005): 340 Hz for males and 500 Hz for females.

The lower pitch limit, in contrast, is frequently reached in normal speech, as is evident from the diverse strategies speakers employ at the low pitch extreme. For example, for the

Mandarin Low tone, as pitch continues to drop, some speakers engage a creaky voice, some use a voiceless whisper, and some even cease phonation altogether, replacing it with a glottal stop in the middle of the syllable (Zheng, 2006). The low-pitch-related non-modal phonations occur not only in the Low tone, but also in the lowest portion of the Rising tone, and they also become more frequent when the low portions of these tones become even lower under focus (Zheng, 2006). The creaky voice occurs in other languages as well when pitch becomes very low (Redi & Shattuck-Hufnagel, 2001). It thus seems that, in most of these cases, approaching the lower pitch limit leads to the changes in voice quality (Titze, 1994) rather than the latter being the primary property of the low lexical tone or boundary tone. In some languages, however, low-pitch related phonation could become the primary feature of some tones. Vietnamese tones, for example, have been argued to show more stable voice quality contrasts (modal, breathy, and creaky) than f_0 patterns (Pham, 2003).

The finding that there are about three octaves available to the speaker (Honorof & Whalen, 2005) may put to rest a dated, yet still somewhat influential belief that if a language is tonal, there is not much room left for intonation (Pike, 1948). But pitch range alone is not enough to explain the simultaneous encoding of so many suprasegmental functions. As will be discussed next, virtually all aspects of the dynamic coding mechanism are employed in one way or another by various functions, and even certain aspects of segmental articulation are involved.

Parallel encoding of multiple prosodic functions

While it is no secret that a rich set of meanings are conveyed suprasegmentally, it is often not fully obvious how many different functions are crowded into prosody, as they are typically investigated in separate studies. This section will provide an overview of the full scope of the multiplicity of the functions beyond consonants and vowels, and demonstrate how they are each effectively encoded via non-segmental means. The functions will be divided into three broad categories based on the kind of meanings they convey: *lexical contrast*, *post-lexical linguistic functions*, and *paralinguistic prosody*. As will be seen, most of the functions are multidimensional, but different functions may involve different combinations of the dimensions, and some may heavily rely on only one specific dimension.

Lexical contrast

This entry point into the prosodic domain of speech is actually overlapped with the segmental domain. Here the suprasegmental cues serve the same function as segments: to distinguish different words, or in some cases, different morphosyntactic categories. The best known of these cases are tone and pitch accent, which are used in roughly half of the world's languages (Yip, 2002). Much less emphasized is that word stress is also a lexical function that serves to make some lexical distinctions. What makes stress different from tone and pitch accent is that it is heavily multidimensional, involving vowel color, pitch, duration, and intensity all as important cues. The multiplicity of cues is best demonstrated by the classic study of Fry (1958), which examined the perception of near minimal noun-verb pairs in English that are distinguished mainly by stress, e.g., *subject*, *contract*. Interestingly, of the three suprasegmental cues examined – pitch, duration and intensity, pitch is by far the most robust. Only 5 Hz, which is about 0.87 semitones higher than the reference frequency of 97 Hz used in the study, is sufficient for listeners to *unambiguously* hear a word as either a noun (high-low pitch pattern) or a verb (low-high pitch pattern). Nevertheless, pitch is only one of the main cues for stress, beside duration and intensity as found by Fry (1958), and vowel color, as is well known, and the exact repertoire of cues is language dependent (de Jong & Zawaydeh, 2002; Ortega-Llebaria & Prieto, 2011; van Heuven & de Jonge, 2011).

The multiplicity of cues for lexical contrast will be further examined in the following subsections. In particular, given the basic articulatory mechanism of tone production outlined previously in this chapter, there are a number of degrees of freedom that are used by languages to make lexical contrasts. These include target strength, target shape, target timing, target shift, etc.

Target strength as lexical cue

In many cases, a phonological unit does not seem to have clearly specified phonetic properties, because its surface form depends heavily on the phonetic properties of adjacent units. A case in point is the neutral tone in Mandarin. As can be seen in Figure 12.6b, the f_0 of the neutral tone has very different contours when preceded by different tones. Traditionally, the neutral tone is therefore described as *toneless* (Chao, 1968) or tonally *unspecified* (Chen, 2000). But extensive f_0 variability is also seen at the beginning of the Falling tone in the second syllable after different tones in Figure 12.6a, which has been established earlier as due to inertia. By the end of the second syllable in Figure 12.6a (solid arrow), the diverse f_0 contours have all converged to a shape that resembles the phonological description of the Falling tone. A convergence trend can be also seen in the neutral tone on the second syllable in Figure 12.6b (dashed arrow), however. That is, well before the end of the syllable, all the f_0 contours have started to turn toward a common mid-level value, although full convergence is not achieved by the end of the second syllable. Figure 12.6c and 12.6d further show, however, that the convergence continues (dashed arrows) if the third and fourth syllables also have the neutral tone. The only exception is due to the post-low bouncing effect after the L tone as already discussed. But even in that case, when the effect is over, f_0 again turns toward the common mid-level height. By the end of the third neutral tone (rightmost arrow, Figure 12.6d), however, substantial differences related to the tone of the first syllable still remain. Thus, a key difference between the full tones and the neutral tone is that it takes much longer for the latter to reach a target.

These patterns suggest that the neutral tone also has a pitch target, which is at the mid-level of the tonal pitch range (Chen & Xu, 2006). This can be seen in Figures 6e and 6f, where the third neutral tone reaches a pitch level (indicated by the horizontal arrows) that is halfway between the highest point in the Falling tone and lowest point in the Low tone in the following syllable. However, the slow rate of approaching this target suggests that the tone is produced with a much weaker articulatory force than in the case of a full tone. Based on the estimate of a computational simulation, the strength of the neutral tone is less than half of the full tones (Xu & Prom-on, 2014). It has also been argued that the tone sandhi behavior of Shanghai Chinese involves a weak articulatory strength (Chen, 2008), because similar slow convergence as in Mandarin neutral tone is observed.

Weak articulatory strength may not be limited to lexical tones only. Evidence of weak articulatory strength is also found for unstressed syllables in English (Xu & Xu, 2005) in that although the f_0 of an unstressed syllable is extensively affected by the f_0 of the preceding syllable, the influence fades away over the course of the weak syllable. However, the rate of reduction of the carryover influence is much slower than in a stressed syllable. The same study also found evidence that the pitch target of an unstressed syllable is probably Mid, similar to the case of the Mandarin neutral tone. Weak articulatory strength may be

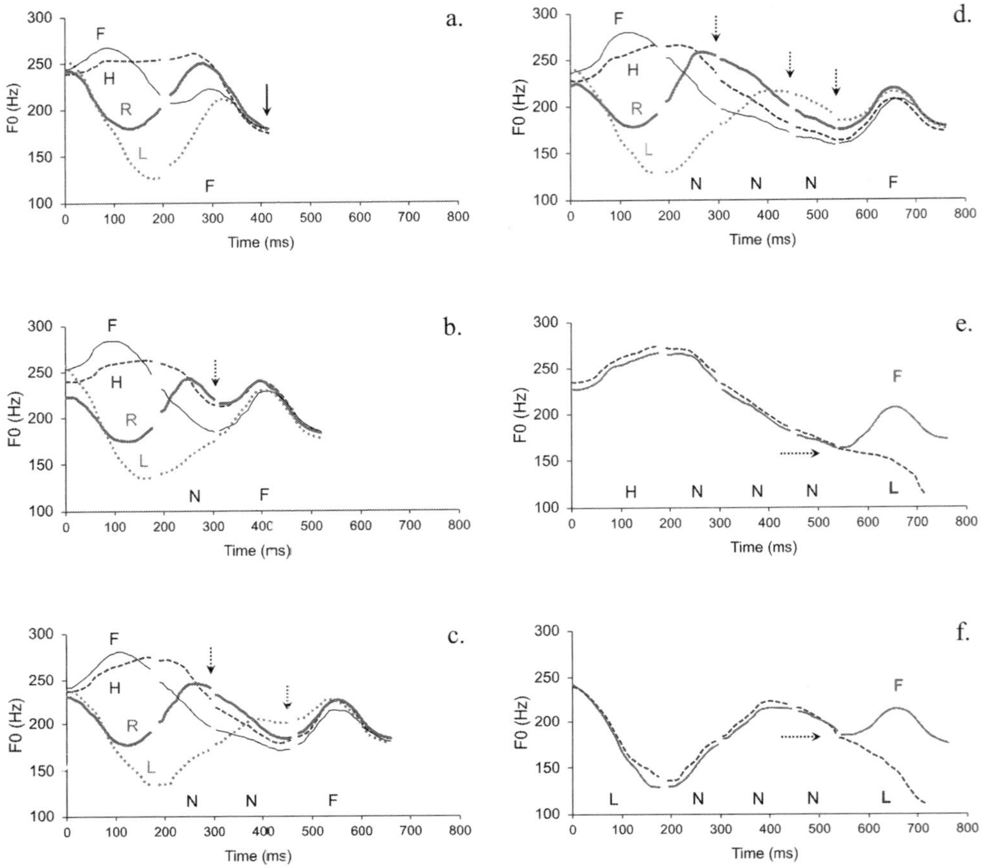

Figure 12.6 Mean f_0 contours of Mandarin sentences containing 0–3 neutral tone (N) syllables. In (a)–(d), the tone of the first syllable alternates across H, R, L and F. In (a) the tone of the second syllable is Falling. In (b)–(c), there are 1–3 neutral tone syllables after the first syllable. The vertical arrows point to the offsets of each neutral tone where variable degrees of convergence to the underlying level of the neutral tone can be seen. In (e) and (f) the tone sequences are the same except in the last syllable, which alternate between Falling and Low. The horizontal arrows point to a common height reached by the final neutral tone regardless of whether the following tone is Falling or Low. The gaps in the contours represent syllable boundaries.

Source: Data from Chen and Xu (2006).

used not only in of pitch production, but also in the articulation of segments. Target-like behavior is already demonstrated (Browman & Goldstein, 1992), but explorations as in Chen and Xu (2006) have never been done. This is partly due to an intrinsic difficulty in the segmental domain, because it is hard to have a sequence of unstressed vowels without intervening consonants. The frequent alternation of open and closed phases of the oral cavity would interrupt any continuous target approximation movement toward a neutral target. Thus, a clever design is needed to systematically study weak segmental targets.

Finally, despite the evidence for weak articulatory strength as a lexical cue as just discussed, it is not likely that greater than normal strength is used by any function as a major cue. This is because, as seen in the previous section on articulatory dynamics, maximum speed of pitch change is already often applied in the full tones, which means that maximum articulatory strength is already used. On the other hand, stressed syllables, as well as prosodic focus to be discussed in the next section, where a greater strength might reasonably be involved, are known to have increased duration. The duration increase would already provide sufficient time for the targets to be reached. If maximum articulatory strength is still applied, the target might be overshot, which would be undesirable. Given that so far there is no empirical evidence either way, however, further research is needed.

Target shape, contour tone, and alignment as cue

The basic dynamics of tone articulation outlined previously suggests that a target can be as simple as a linear function with an optional slope. This does not rule out the possibility that the target can be more complex. It is also possible that the target can simply be a turning point and its temporal alignment (Dilly & Brown, 2007; Remijsen & Ayoker, 2014). To determine whether a more complex or a simpler target is needed, however, the basic articulatory dynamics still needs to be taken into consideration. For example, due to inertia, the surface form of a unit cannot resemble its underlying form, because a significant portion of it, especially the early section, is likely to be still far away from the underlying form. This is particularly relevant for interpreting the presence and shape of a sizable movement in the early portion of a contour, and the presence and alignment of a turning point. In Figure 12.7, for example, the three Mandarin tones all show a sizable rising movement as well as a clear turning point when they are surrounded by two Low tones. However, a reexamination of Figure 12.2 tells us that the rising movement is optional for the High tone and the turning point is optional for both the High and Rising tones. Thus, it is unlikely that either the initial rise or the turning points are the main cue for differentiating these three tones.

It is possible, however, based on the observation of Figure 12.2, that the Rising and the Falling tones are each composed of two underlying pitch registers: LH and HL, respectively (Duanmu, 1994; Odden, 1995; Yip, 1989), instead of sloped linear functions as suggested by the arrows in the figure. In fact, composite representation of dynamic tones is a widely accepted norm in tonal phonology (Goldsmith, 1990; Hyman, 2007). Here again, the basic tonal dynamics could offer a way of testing the two accounts. Given that the production of a tone is to approximate its target(s) by overcoming inertia, if there are two consecutive targets, as the time available for a tone increases due to syllable lengthening, the separate approximations of the consecutive targets would become increasingly apparent, as illustrated by the dashed line in Figure 12.8a. If there is only a unitary sloping target, the slope itself will be increasingly better achieved. When speech rate is directly controlled, the latter is found to be the case for Mandarin Rising tone (Xu, 1998, 2001). That is, as the syllable became longer, it is the rising or falling slope of the dynamic tones that remains the most constant, and there is no sign of separate approximations of consecutive targets. Similar observations have been made for the dynamic tones in Cantonese (Wong, 2006b). Interestingly, in both cases, the dynamic portion of the tone is delayed to the end of the syllable, as illustrated by the solid line in Figure 12.8a.

The delayed realization of a sloping tone could be part of the basic dynamics of target approximation, because other alternatives may not really be viable, as illustrated in Figure 12.8b. There, the dashed line represents a simple slowing-down strategy, which would make the slope increasingly shallower as the syllable lengthens. The dotted line represents a strategy that faithfully realizes the target slope (represented by the arrow), but to do so as soon as it is articulatorily possible. This would result in an increasingly longer final plateau as the syllable continues to lengthen. Neither scenario has been observed so far. Instead,

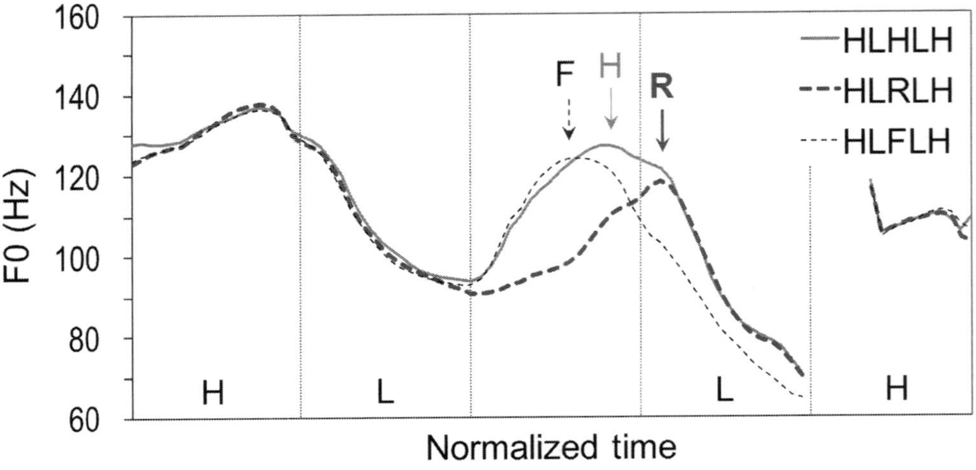

Figure 12.7 Time-normalized mean f_0 contours of five-tone sequences in Mandarin. The vertical arrows point to the f_0 peaks. All curves are averages of 24 repetitions by four male speakers.

Source: Data from Xu (1999).

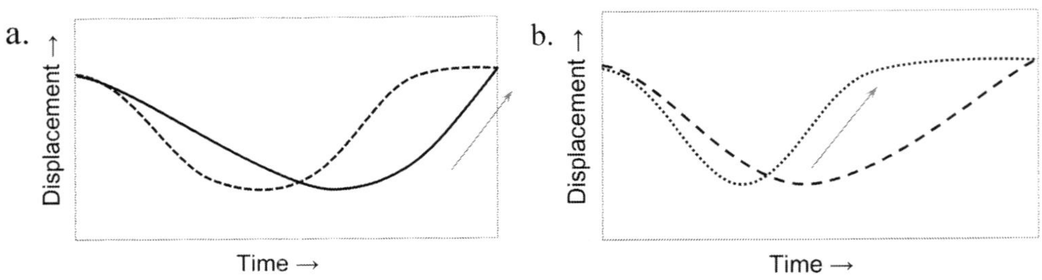

Figure 12.8 Hypothetical strategies for a contour tone. (a) The dashed line results from a sequential approximation of two successive targets; the solid line results from a delayed approximation of a sloping target. (b) The dashed line results from a simple slowing down of articulation rate; the dotted line results from a faithful realization of a sloping target at the earliest time allowed by the maximum speed of articulatory movement.

in Thai – a language with vowel length contrast, for example, the most characteristic portion of a tone is realized after a quasi-plateau when the vowel is long (Zsiga & Nitisaroj, 2007). This finding echoes what happens in Mandarin and Cantonese when a syllable with a dynamic tone is lengthened due to a change of speech rate (Xu, 1998; Wong, 2006b), as just mentioned. The delayed realization of a dynamic target may not be limited to tones. As found by Gay (1968), the final formant slope of a diphthong in English is also what remains the most constant as speech rate is reduced.

It is also possible that the delay of a dynamic target can itself be used as a distinctive cue. In Shilluk, for example, two falling tones differ from each other mainly in terms of the alignment of the sharpest fall in the syllable (Remijsen & Ayoker, 2014). This is consistent with the idea that speakers are able to delay the onset of a dynamic tone even if there is no alignment contrast (Figure 12.8a), which is a new direction that can be further explored.

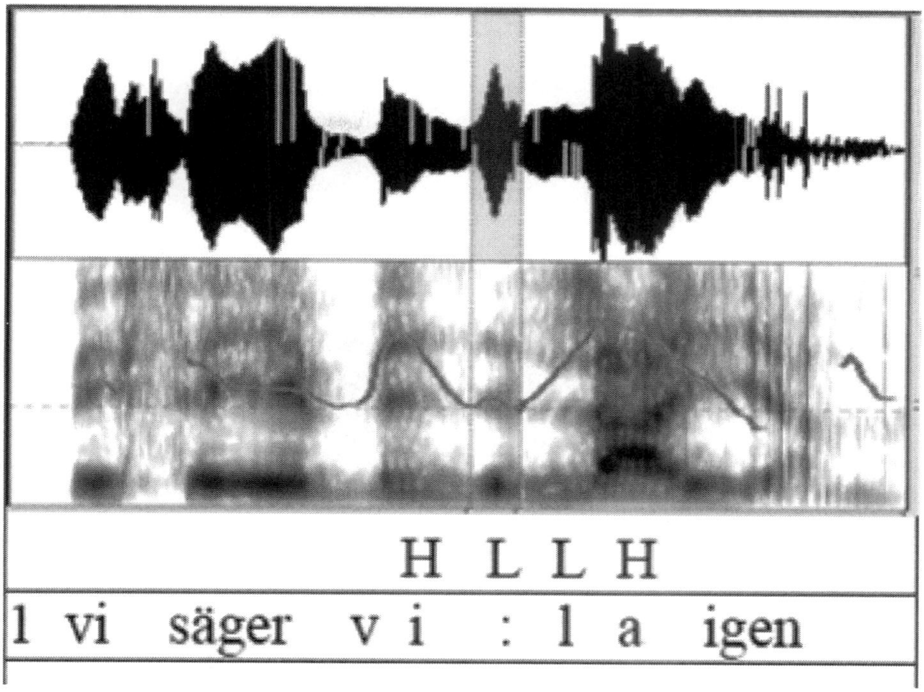

Figure 12.9 Swedish Accent II, where a Fall-Low sequence can occur within the same vowel [iː] in the word "vi:la." Curtesy of Antonis Botinis.

The basic articulatory dynamics of tone production also does not rule out the possibility that there may be cases of genuine consecutive targets within a syllable. An example is seen in Swedish (Figure 12.9), where the first part of accent II (HL) seems to show a fall followed by a low target (Botinis et al., 2014). The falling target is evident in that f_0 first goes up at the beginning of the syllable to reach a high peak, just like in a Falling tone (Figure 12.7), before dropping sharply. The subsequent low target is evident in that f_0 has dropped to the bottom of the pitch range and formed a low plateau, which is unlike the Falling tones in Mandarin and Thai that drop only to the middle of the pitch range and end with a high falling velocity at the syllable offset (Gandour et al., 1994; Xu, 1997), as can be seen in Figures 12.2 and 12.7. Again, this is yet another new direction for further research.

Target reassignment

The basic articulatory dynamics can also help to identify cases where tonal variations are *unlikely* to be due to inertia. A clear example is the Low-tone sandhi phenomenon in Mandarin (Chao, 1968), whereby the first Low in a Low-Low sequence is changed into a form that sounds indistinguishable from the Rising tone (Peng, 2000; Wang & Li, 1967). Despite many efforts, it has been difficult to identify a mechanism that can unequivocally derive this phenomenon. Detailed acoustic analyses show that the sandhied f_0 contour approaches a rising target even from the syllable onset, just as in an underlying Rising tone (Xu, 1997). Thus there seems to be a genuine *reassignment* of the underlying pitch target, although the exact reason for the reassignment is still unclear.[2]

The arbitrariness of the tone sandhi rules has been well recorded (Chen, 2000). Recent research is able to establish further that some of the arbitrary rules are still relatively transparent in that they are applied by speakers whenever the phonetic environment satisfies. In contrast, there are also sandhi rules that are *opaque*, as they are applied only to words that speakers are familiar with. The latter mechanism has been termed lexical or allomorph listing (Tsay & Myers, 1996; Zhang, 2014; Yip, 2004). It has been further demonstrated that different strategies may be involved in learning these types of tone sandhi rules. Currently this is a very active area of research (Zhang, 2014), which is likely to advance our knowledge significantly about the nature of tone sandhi.

What has been much less discussed is that tone-sandhi-like rules may apply in non-tone languages as well. In Figure 12.10a, for example, the monosyllabic word *job* shows a rise-fall contour. A similar rise-fall contour can be also seen in *Bloomingdales* in Figure 12.10b, but the shape is distributed across the whole word. This similarity may indicate a functional equivalence of the two contours (Arvaniti & Ladd, 2009; Ladd, 2008; Pierrehumbert, 1980). But the equivalence appears to be achieved by assigning a high-level or rising target to the stressed syllable, and a mid- or low-level target to the unstressed syllables. Thus, the fall in the monosyllabic word is split into a sequence of targets that are assigned to the individual syllables of a multi-syllabic word. Such target *reassignment* is therefore somewhat similar

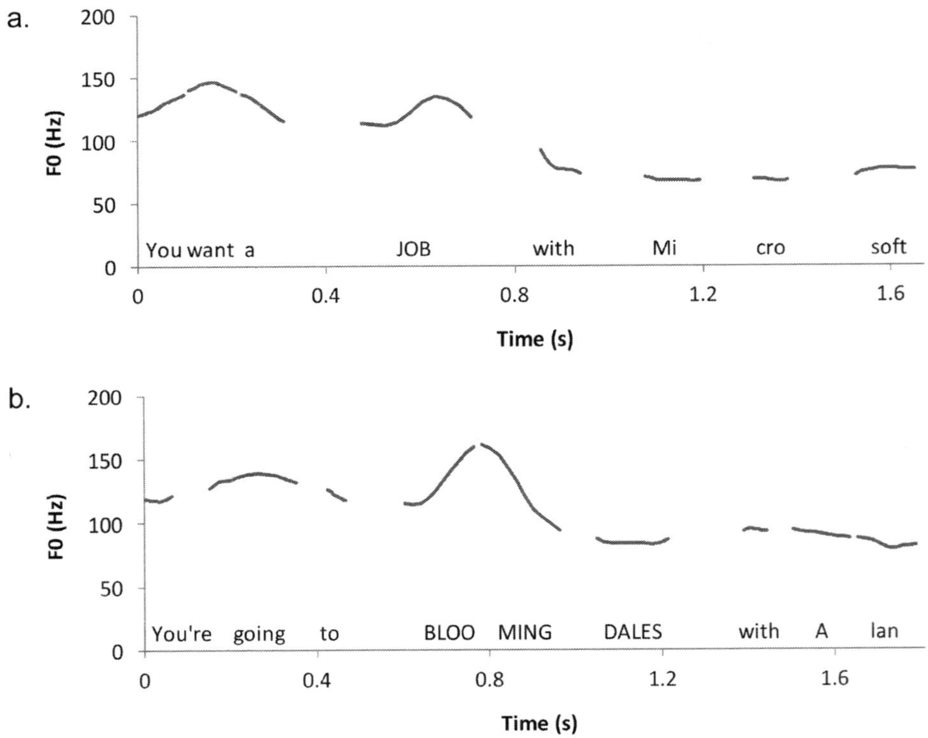

Figure 12.10 Mean f_0 contours of (a) "You want a JOB with Microsoft" and (b) "You're going to BLOOMINGDALES with Alan", averaged across eight repetitions by a male American English speaker. Capitalized words are in focus.

Source: Data from Liu et al. (2013).

to the target reassignment in tone sandhi. Evidence for similar target reassignment is found also for the interrogative intonation (Liu et al., 2013), as will be further discussed in connection with focus and sentence modality in later sections of this chapter.

The reassignment of the targets is likely necessitated by the nature of speech articulation. That is, it is impossible to separately articulate a sequence of pitchless syllables and a sequence of segmentless/syllableless f_0 contours and then somehow combine them later on, as assumed by some computational models of intonation (Fujisaki, 1983; van Santen et al., 2005). Instead, regardless of what a global contour may look like, each syllable in a multi-syllabic word or phrase has to have its own underlying pitch target while it is being articulated, just as it has to have its own consonantal and vocalic targets. Besides, the syllable-specific targets need to be specified in terms of stress-related articulatory strength, as discussed previously in the section on target strength, which cannot be part of the specifications of a functional equivalent global contour. Target reassignment is therefore probably much more widespread across languages than has been recognized. Further research may consider it as a possible factor when trying to account for various tonal and intonational phenomena.

Post-lexical linguistic functions

Prosody is also heavily involved in conveying meanings that are independent of lexical distinctions. As a result, the temporal domain of these functions is not limited to syllables or even words. Yet, for reasons just discussed in the previous section, even the prosody of larger temporal domains has to be ultimately realized via individual syllables. But here we are concerned mainly with the more global prosodic patterns, and the basic articulatory dynamics will be mentioned only in cases where it plays a critical role.

A main issue in regard to post-lexical prosody is that of function versus form. There is a strong form-oriented tradition which assumes that the understanding of prosody should start from a thorough description of the observable prosodic forms. The British school of intonation, for example, formulates a general scheme in which the intonation of any utterance consists of an obligatory nucleus and an optional head, prehead, and tail (O'Connor & Arnold, 1961; Palmer, 1922). Likewise, intonational phonology, also known as the Autosegmental-Metrical phonology theory of intonation (AM theory), formulates a scheme in which prosody is guided by a finite state grammar (Gussenhoven, 2004; Ladd, 1996; Pierrehumbert, 1980). In both cases, meanings are associated to the prosodic forms only *after the forms have been established* in terms of both their prosodic properties and rules that guide their alternation. As has become increasingly clear from the discussion so far, there seem to be many degrees of separation between the meaning-carrying functions and their associated prosodic form. First, due to inertia, an underlying target and its surface realization often only faintly resemble each other. Second, a function-specific form may often assign different underlying targets depending on various factors, as discussed in the previous section. Finally, there is also a third way of function-form separation, namely, the simultaneous encoding of multiple functions. Consequently, no temporal location of an utterance can be said to correspond to any single prosodic function. It is therefore ineffective to first categorize directly observable forms and then try to link each of them to a specific meaning-bearing function.

The discussion of post-lexical linguistic prosody in this section will follow, instead, a function-oriented approach. Each of the subsections will address whether and how a particular hypothetical function is encoded with specific prosodic cues. In addition, the evidence cited will be mainly from studies that have systematically controlled the prosodic functions being examined.

Focal contrast

Despite being one of the most widely discussed prosodic functions, focus still is in want of a precise definition. Earlier theories tend to associate focus with new information (Chaffe, 1976; Halliday, 1967), but exceptions such as the following make it untenable:

3 A: Did John or Mary have an operation? B: *Mary* had an operation.
4 A: Why did you miss the party? B: My *mother* got sick.

In (3) "Mary" is likely to be focused although it is already mentioned in the preceding question and thus is given. In (4) "got sick" is unlikely to be focused although it has not been mentioned before, as pointed out by Terken and Hirschberg (1994). Furthermore, new information is virtually everywhere if an utterance is to convey any meaning. A more sophisticated definition has been that focus is for indicating that there is an alternative relevant to the interpretation of a given linguistic expression (Krifka, 2008; Rooth, 1992). But an alternative-based definition would still over-predict focus because it is not the case that whenever there is an alternative interpretation in an utterance, focus has to occur. A more restricted definition would be based on the need to emphasize something. That is, when focus occurs, the speaker has felt a need to emphasize to the listener what is particularly important in the utterance, and is worthy of special attention. Evidence for this account is shown by recent studies using fMRI, ERP and eye-tracking technology (Chen et al., 2012; Chen et al., 2014; Kristensen et al., 2013). The findings of those studies suggest that focus is associated with attention allocation during discourse comprehension, while newness is associated only with memory retrieval.

For the purpose of empirical research, what is important is to have methods that can reliably elicit focus. Experimental studies have shown that mini dialogues are a highly reliable way of eliciting focus. In a mini dialogue, the leading sentence, or phrase, can be either a wh-question or a statement containing a piece of information to be negated in the target utterance. The former case is often referred to as information focus while the latter is contrastive focus.

One of the most fully controlled research studies in this area is that of Cooper, Eady and colleagues, which used the mini dialogue paradigm (Cooper et al., 1985; Eady & Cooper, 1986; Eady et al., 1986). These studies established that focus in American English is prosodically realized mainly by (a) consistently decreased peak f_0 of post-focus words, (b) consistently increased duration of the focused word, and (c) occasionally increased peak f_0 of the focused word. These are confirmed by later studies that examine continuous f_0 contours in greater detail (Xu & Xu, 2005; Liu et al., 2013). Some examples are shown in Figure 12.11a–b. Also using the mini dialogue paradigm, Jin (1996) and Xu (1999) found similar post-focus lowering of f_0 and on-focus increase of duration in Mandarin Chinese. But for the focused word in Mandarin, the effect is an *expansion* of the pitch range, consisting of increased f_0 maximum and decreased f_0 minimum, as can be seen in Figure 12.11c. Later studies further found intensity variations similar to those of f_0: on-focus increase and post-focus reduction (Chen et al., 2009; Lee et al., 2015). Thus, for both English and Mandarin, the most consistent correlates of focus are post-focus compression (PFC) of f_0, and on-focus increase of duration.

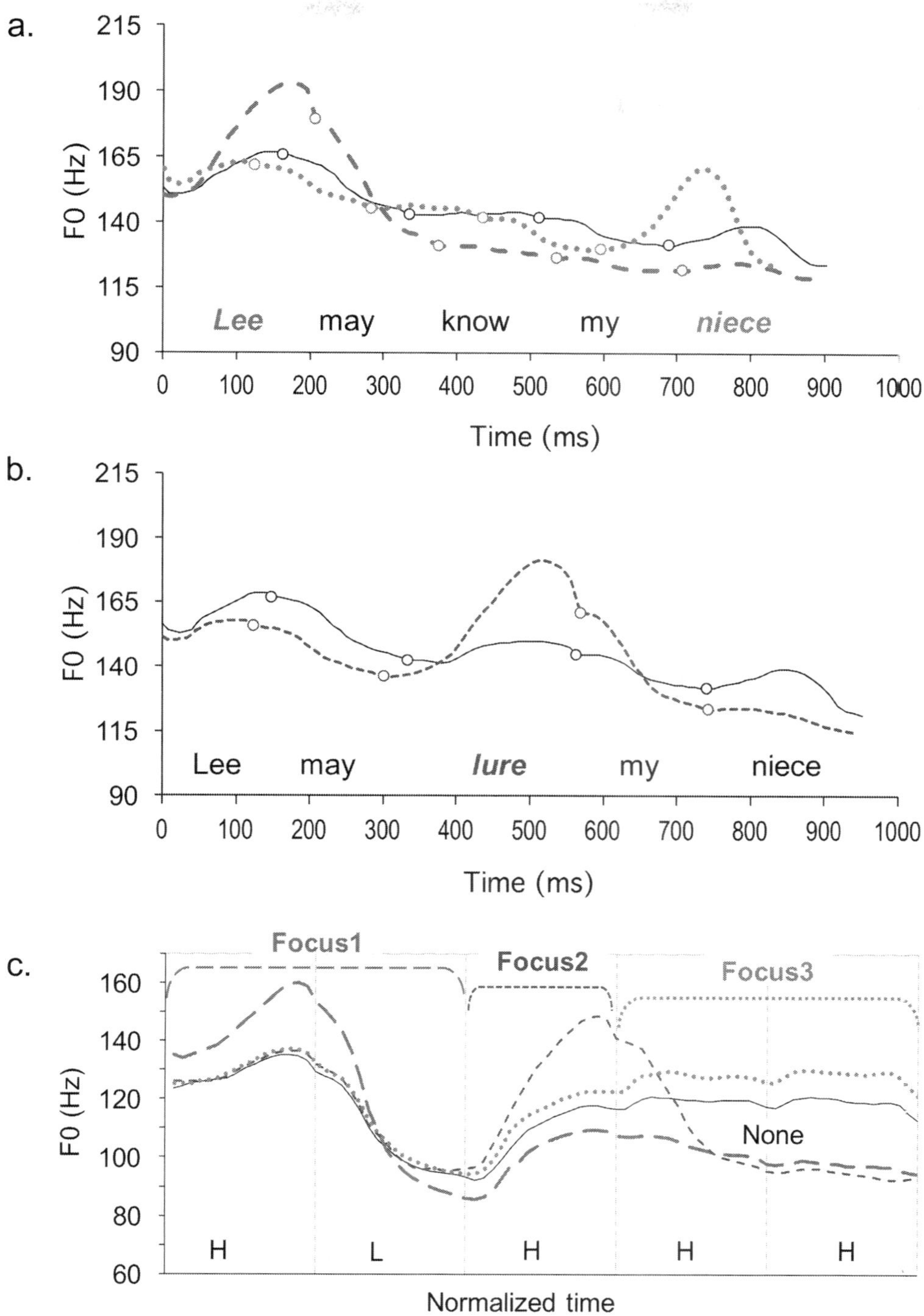

Figure 12.11 Focus prosody in English (a, b) and Mandarin (c).

Source: Data from Xu and Xu (2005) and Xu (1999).

Similar prosodic patterns, especially PFC of f_0, have been found in many other languages, including German (Féry & Kügler, 2008), Dutch (Rump & Collier, 1996), Swedish (Bruce, 1982), Japanese (Ishihara, 2002), Korean (Lee & Xu, 2010), Turkish (Ipek, 2011); Uygur (Wang et al., 2011), French (Dohen & Lœvenbruck, 2004), Arabic (Chahal, 2003), Hindi (Patil et al., 2008), Persian (Taheri-Ardali & Xu, 2012), and Finnish (Mixdorff, 2004). These languages all belong to major Euro-Asian language families: Indo-European, Uralic, Afro-Asiatic and Altaic. The only exceptions are Mandarin (Xu, 1999) and Tibetan (Wang et al., 2012), which belong to the Sino-Tibetan family. At least for some of these languages PFC is shown to be critical for focus perception: Finnish (Vainio et al., 2003), Dutch (Rump & Collier, 1996), English (Prom-on et al., 2009), Japanese (Ishihara, 2011; Sugahara, 2005), and Mandarin (Liu & Xu, 2005; Chen et al., 2009).

But PFC is absent in many other languages, including Southern Min (Chen et al., 2009), Cantonese (Wu & Xu 2010), Deang, Wa and Yi (Wang et al., 2011), Yucatec Maya (Kügler & Skopeteas, 2007), Chichewa, Chitumbuka, Durban Zulu, Hausa, Buli and Northern Sotho (Zerbian et al., 2010), and Wolof (Rialland & Robert, 2001). Some of these languages even show on-focus increase of pitch range, duration or intensity (Chen et al., 2009; Wu & Xu, 2010). Thus there seems to be a dichotomy in terms of whether a language uses PFC to mark focus, and the division seems to be partially related to language families: The non-PFC languages do not belong to any of the families of the known PFC languages: Indo-European, Uralic, and Altaic. The exceptions are the Sino-Tibetan and Afro-Asiatic families, which host both PFC (Mandarin, Arabic) and non-PFC languages (Cantonese, Taiwanese, Hausa). These distribution patterns have led to the hypothesis that languages with PFC are all related in that they are common descendants of a proto-language (Xu, 2011). Further motivating this *inheritance hypothesis* are two key findings. First, the distribution of PFC is not related to any language-specific features, such as tone or lexical stress (Chen et al., 2009). This means that PFC could not have emerged in a language due to these features. Second, PFC is hard to spread across languages, since (a) it is not transferred from a PFC language to a non-PFC language even when both languages are spoken natively by bilinguals (Wu & Chung, 2011), or near natively (Chen et al., 2014), b) it is hard to acquire by an L2 learner whose L1 has no PFC (Chen et al., 2014; Swerts & Zerbian, 2010), and (c) it is hard to acquire even by an L2 learner whose L1 already has PFC (Chen, 2015). This means that a language, e.g., Mandarin, could not have acquired PFC through contact with a neighboring PFC language, such as Mongolian or Manchurian (whose speakers ruled China for hundreds of years), but it itself has to be a descendent of a PFC language (Xu, 2011).

As for the identity of the common-protolanguage, the distribution of PFC across Indo-European, Uralic, Afro-Asiatic, and Altaic languages shows a resemblance to the hypothetical Nostratic macro family, according to which many of the Euro-Asian and Afro-Asiatic languages share a common proto-language that originated from the Fertile Crescent (Bomhard, 2008; Pedersen, 1931). The Nostratic macro family hypothesis is also largely consistent with the Farming/Language Dispersal Hypothesis (Diamond & Bellwood, 2003), according to which many of the major language families of the world dispersed along with the spread of agriculture, and the Fertile Crescent is the origin of the earliest agriculture, based mainly on wheat, barley, millet, and emmer (Diamond, 1998).

Probably the most radical aspect of the *inheritance hypothesis of PFC* is that it splits the Chinese languages into two groups, one consisting of many of the northern dialects with PFC, and the other consisting of many of the southern dialects/languages that lack PFC. Dialects in the northern group are likely descendants of Altaic languages, given the non-tranferability of PFC. Dialects/languages of the southern group, on the other hand, have two possible hereditary roots. Some could be descendants of a protolanguage (or protolanguages) originating from an area of rice-based agriculture (Diamond, 1998). Others may be close relatives of northern Chinese, but have lost PFC because of language shifts in southern populations that originally spoke various non-Chinese languages. Radical as it is, the inheritance hypothesis has generated some exciting new research that may shed light not only on speech prosody, but also on broader issues like language change, language typology, and language evolution.

There are three more issues about focus that are worth particular mentioning. First, despite the widely known division between various types of focus (Gussenhoven, 2007), especially between *information focus* – which is elicited by wh-question, and *contrastive focus* – which is used to correct a wrong piece of information, empirical research has not yet generated sufficient support for a clear distinction between them. Most studies have failed to find significant differences (Hanssen et al., 2008; Sityaev & House, 2003; Hwang, 2012; Katz & Selkirk, 2011; Kügler & Ganzel, 2014). But a few studies have found some small differences (Baumann et al., 2007; He et al., 2011; Sahkai et al., 2013). As will be discussed later, there is the possibility that even these small differences may not be due to focus type, but are attributable to paralinguistic functions that interact with focus.

Second, probably because of the critical role of PFC, final focus is often less effectively encoded than an earlier focus, as PFC is impossible to apply to the sentence-final location (Botinis et al., 1999; Liu & Xu, 2005; Rump & Collier, 1996). This finding is especially relevant for the controversial notion of *broad focus* that is used to refer to the prosody of sentences with no narrow focus, which are said to have a default sentence-final nuclear accent (Ladd, 1996, 2008). The weak prosodic cue for final focus may explain why utterances with no focus or neutral focus may have sounded as if there were a final accent, but it does not make them equivalent to final focus. The significant differences between broad and final focus has been clearly demonstrated (Katz & Selkirk, 2011; Xu, 1999; Xu & Xu, 2005). Besides, the idea that an entire sentence is focused when spoken as an answer to a question like *What happened?* seems to conflict with the idea of focus as selective highlighting, whether for the sake of pointing out the existence of alternatives (Krifka, 2008; Rooth, 1992) or directing listener's attention (Chen et al., 2014).

Finally, despite being an independent function in its own right, focus interacts with other functions in ways that may affect either the realization of focus itself or that of the other functions. For its own realization, focus is not effectively encoded in unaccented words in Japanese (Lee & Xu, 2012; Ishihara, 2011), and is less effectively realized on the Low tone in Mandarin than on the other tones (Lee et al., 2016). For the realization of other functions, in American English, a word-final stressed syllable (including that of a monosyllabic word) changes its target from a non-dynamic high to a dynamic fall when under focus (Xu & Xu, 2005; Liu et al., 2013). In Mandarin, in contrast, focus does not change the underlying targets of tone despite the changes in pitch range (Xu, 1999). As will be discussed in the next section, the interaction of focus with the modality function also involves changes in underlying pitch targets.

Modality

Modality, or sentence type, refers to whether an utterance is produced as a statement or a question. Much research has been done on the prosody of modality, but the general picture is not yet fully clear. On the one hand, there is a widely recognized cross-linguistic trend that a question often involves a rising intonation as opposed to a falling intonation in a statement (Bolinger, 1978; Greenberg, 1963; Ohala, 1983; Shattuck-Hufnagel & Turk, 1996). On the other hand, question-final pitch rise is often missing either in a language known to have rising question intonation, or absent in an entire language or dialect (Savino, 2012; Siemund 2001; Zerbian, 2010). Here again, systematic analysis of continuous pitch contours may help to identify phonetic details that can make the picture clearer. Figure 12.12 shows mean f_0 contours of Mandarin statements and questions consisting of words all with the same tones in each sentence (Liu & Xu, 2005). As can be seen, not all questions show sentence-final rises. Although f_0 rises sharply in both the Rising-tone and Low-tone questions, the Falling-tone question shows a sharp final fall just as in a statement, and the final rise in the High-tone question is not very sharp. What is common across all the tones, however, is the increasing pitch level throughout the sentence. As found in the study, the global difference between statements and questions can be fitted by a double exponential function, which can be considered as consisting of an *accelerating descent* in statements and an *accelerating ascent* in questions.

Therefore, for Mandarin the globally accelerating pitch level increase seems to be the *primary* cue for question prosody, which is "imposed" onto the tones of successive syllabic morphemes. Thus the local shape at the end of a sentence mainly reflects the lexical tones rather than being the question intonation proper. There is an exception to this simplistic account, however. That is, the L-tone sentence shows a simple drop of f_0 to the bottom at the end of a statement, but a low-rise contour at the end of a question. These two contour patterns are in fact two of the allophonic variances of the L tone (Chao, 1968). Thus, in addition to the accelerating pitch level, the interrogative function also interacts with the lexical tonal function to reassign the local tonal targets. Such interactions may be quite frequent across languages. In Cantonese, for example, all the tones change to a sharp rise in questions (Ma et al., 2006), which result in a reduction of tone identification (Fok-Chan, 1974; Ma et al.,

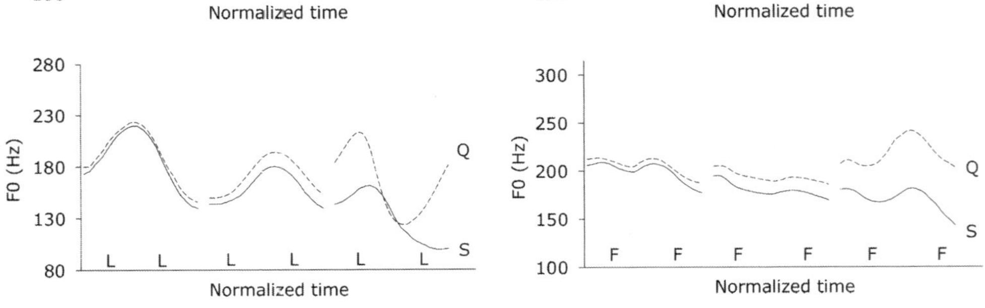

Figure 12.12 Mean f_0 contours averaged across eight speakers of Mandarin Chinese (five repetitions by each speaker).

Source: Data from Liu and Xu (2005).

2006). Languages, therefore, may differ in terms of whether modality or lexical contrast is given a greater weight in the control of sentence-final f_0 contours.

Even more dramatic interactions of the interrogative function with other functions can be seen in English (Liu et al., 2013). Figure 12.13a shows mean f_0 contours of two English sentences spoken as statements and questions, with focus in either medial or final positions. Here we can see three-way interactions between focus, modality, and lexical stress:

1. The pitch range of words are jointly determined by focus and modality. In a statement, pitch range is compressed and *lowered* after focus, but in a question, pitch range is compressed but *raised* after focus. Thus, post-focus compression applies to both modalities, but differs in terms of whether the compressed pitch range is raised or lowered.
2. The local contours of stressed syllables also vary depending on both focus and modality. Before and after focus, they are largely flat; under focus, they are either falling and rising depending on whether the sentence is a statement or a question, respectively.
3. There are also subtle changes in the local contour of stressed syllables that reflect a tendency for their underlying pitch targets to be slightly rising in questions but falling in statements even in pre-focal and post-focal words. This is revealed by both systematic acoustic analysis and modeling simulation in Liu et al. (2013).

These interaction patterns contrast with similar interactions in Mandarin as shown in Figure 12.13b in a number of ways. First, the post-focal pitch range is lowered in Mandarin even in questions. Second, as discussed earlier, the local tonal shapes in Mandarin do not vary in fundamental ways with changes in modality. But similar to Mandarin as mentioned earlier, the manifestation of modality in English is also global rather than limited only to the sentence final location. The early manifestation is perceptually relevant too. Both adults and 7–10-year-old children can identify sentence type correctly, often as early as from the first

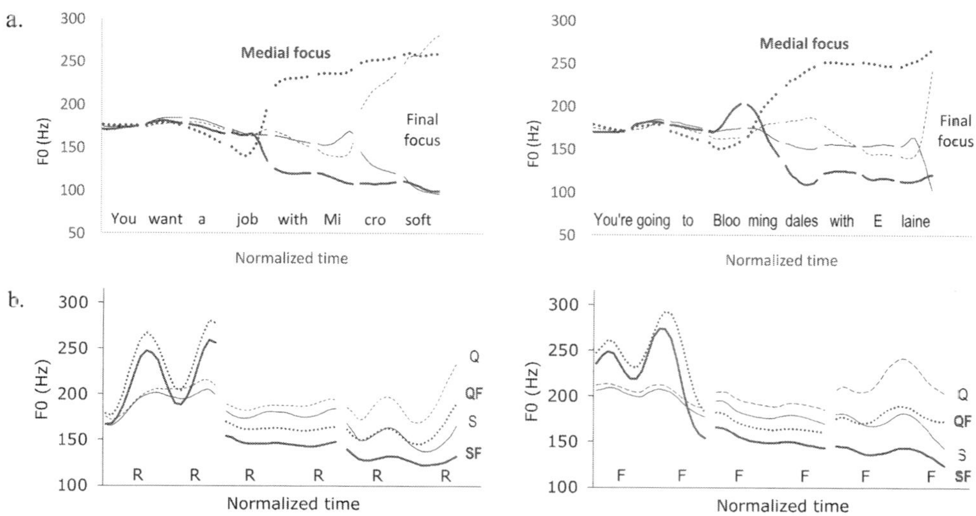

Figure 12.13 (a) Mean f_0 contours averaged across five speakers of American English (eight repetitions by each speaker). (b) Mean f_0 contours averaged across eight speakers of Mandarin (five repetitions by each speaker).

Source: Data from Liu et al. (2013).

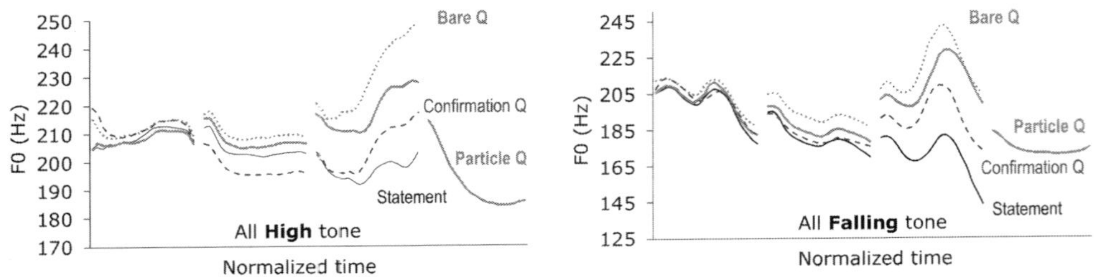

Figure 12.14 Mean f_0 contours averaged across eight speakers of Mandarin (five repetitions by each speaker).

Source: Data from Liu and Xu (2005).

word of a sentence (Saindon et al., 2017). Similar early identification of sentence type has been reported for other languages (Face, 2005; Thorsen, 1980; van Heuven & Haan, 2000).

Furthermore, the interaction of modality with pragmatic and paralinguistic functions introduces complications in the prosody of question intonation. In Figure 12.14, we can see that the pitch ranges of questions with various pragmatic connotations form a gradient, rather than clear-cut categories. Such a gradience cannot be fully accounted for in terms of linguistic prosody only. Also shown in Figure 12.14 is that sentences with a sentence-final particle have the second highest f_0 peak. This means that question particle and interrogative intonation are not in a trading relation (see also Abe (1998) for Japanese). Further discussion on this will be resumed later in this chapter in the section on paralinguistic prosody.

Finally, the accelerating global increase of pitch range in question intonation may be entirely absent in some languages. In three African language phyla: Niger-Congo, Nilo-Saharan, and Afro-Asiatic, questions are marked by *lax prosody* (Connell, 2017; Rialland, 2009; Salffner, 2010). Instead of sentence-final pitch increase, these languages use properties such as falling pitch contour, a sentence-final low vowel, vowel lengthening, and breathy utterance termination to mark questions. A remote yet intriguing possibility is that the accelerating pitch increase shared by so many of today's languages happened to be in the prosody of the language(s) spoken by people who came out of Africa tens of thousands of years ago, while the languages that remained in Africa always had a variety of question prosody. Thus, just like PFC, which may have split the modern languages from 13,000 years ago, lax prosody may have split languages even earlier, assuming that global prosody is among the most stable features of human speech.

Grouping/boundary marking by duration

The grouping function divides an utterance into chunks, presumably for the ease of production as well as perceptual processing (Cutler et al., 1997; Schafer et al., 2000). Although many prosodic cues have been reported, there is increasing evidence that it is the temporal domain of speech that provides the strongest and most reliable cues. Temporal cues consist of both the duration of articulated units (vowel, syllable, words, etc.) and the length of silent pauses. There is also evidence of cues in terms of pitch, in the form of pitch reset (Ladd, 1988; Swert, 1997). But they occur only in limited situations, and are often byproducts of communicative functions already discussed. There are also phenomena, such as rhythm metrics and hierarchical prosodic structures, that do not seem to serve any specific functions. But they are likely also byproducts of boundary marking as well as some other meaning-carrying functions (Arvaniti, 2012).

For temporal cues used as boundary marking, evidence comes from rather diverse sources, including domain-final lengthening, polysyllabic shortening and pausing. Domain-final lengthening, or final lengthening for short (also known as preboundary lengthening), refers to the fact that the duration of a syllable, syllable rhyme or the nuclear vowel increases at the end of increasingly larger syntactic/prosodic units (Klatt, 1976). Polysyllabic shortening refers to the finding that a stressed syllable tends to be increasingly shorter as the number of syllables in a word or phrase increases, e.g., in *sleep*, *sleepy*, *sleepily*, *sleepiness* (Lehiste, 1972; Klatt, 1976). Given that they seem to be complimentary to each other, the two phenomena could be reflections of the same trend of duration variation: the closer to the right edge of a unit, the longer the duration, and vice versa. This is partially evident in Figure 12.15a for American English (Nakatani et al., 1981). From right to left, syllable duration first decreases sharply, and then reaches a low plateau for within word positions. The same trend is also found in Mandarin (Xu & Wang, 2009), but even stronger, as can be seen in Figure 12.15b. Here, the increase in syllable duration occurs not only on the right edge between word/phrase-final syllable and non-final syllable, but also on the left edge, i.e., between word-initial and word-medial syllables.

There is a limit to how much a syllable can be lengthened to signal a boundary, however. The lengthening of a sentence-final syllable is found to be no greater than the lengthening of phrase-final syllables in American English (Klatt, 1975; Umeda, 1975; Wightman et al., 1992; Yang & Wang, 2002). This limit seems to be related to the second temporal cue for grouping, namely, silent pause. Silent pause refers to the full absence of phonation that lasts longer than the duration of any segment-intrinsic silence, e.g., a stop closure. There does not seem to be a limit on how long a silent pause can be. In fact, the length of a silent pause increases quasi-exponentially with the increase of perceived boundary strength, as can be seen in Figure 12.16 for Mandarin (Yang & Wang, 2002).

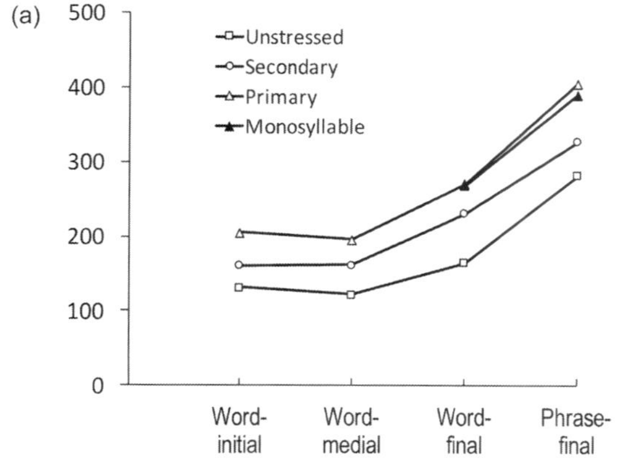

Figure 12.15 (a) Syllable duration as a function of position, stress level, and word length in English (redrawn based on data from Figure 12.4 of Nakatani et al., 1981). (b) Syllable duration as a function of position and word/phrase length in Mandarin. The numbers on the bars are in milliseconds.

Source: Adapted from Xu and Wang (2009).

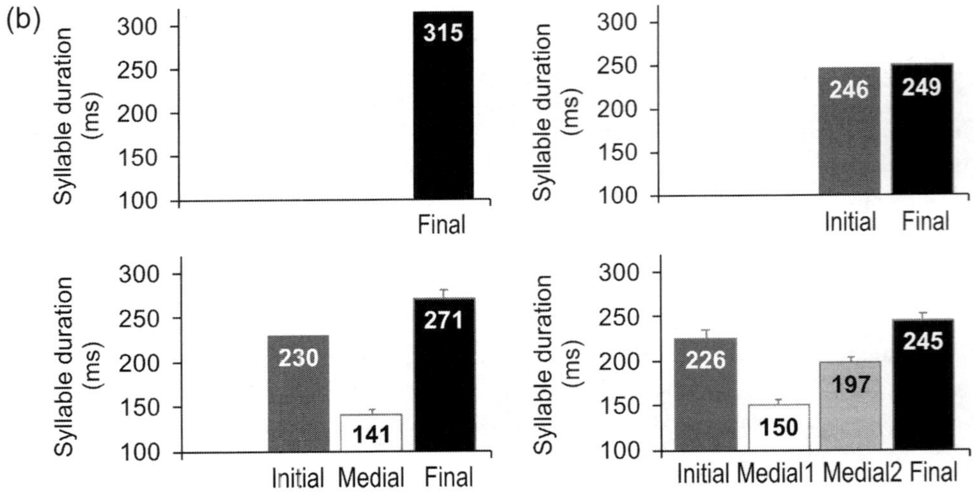

Figure 12.15 (Continued)

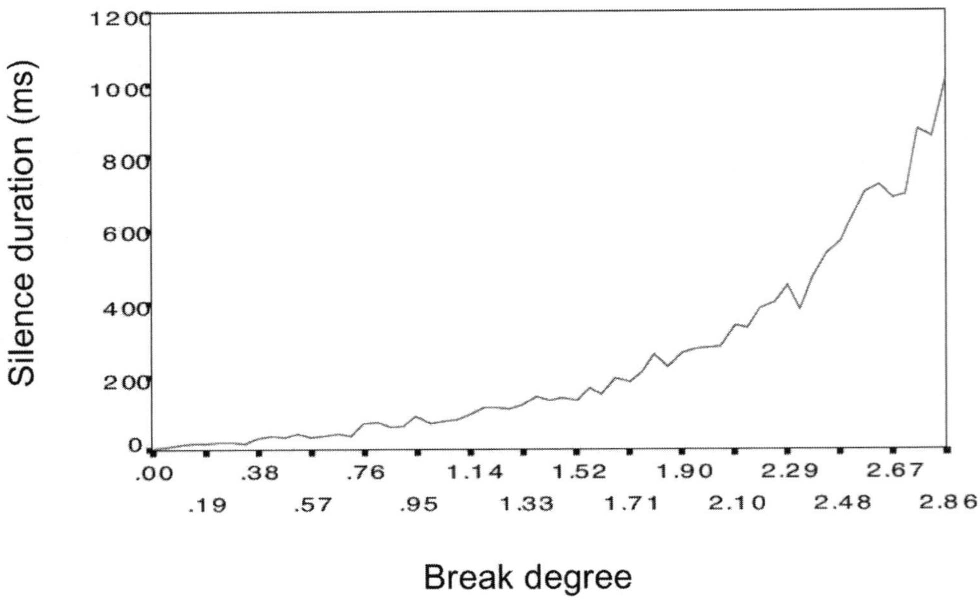

Figure 12.16 Duration of silence pause as a function of perceived prosodic boundary level (Yang & Wang, 2002).

Source: Courtesy of Bei Wang.

Thus, there seems to be a division of labor between final lengthening and silent pause in marking boundaries (Petrone et al., 2017). For weaker boundaries, only final lengthening is involved, while for stronger boundaries, e.g., groups larger than phrases, only silent pauses can indicate a further increase in boundary strength. At the phrase level, however, both cues are at work (Jeon & Nolan, 2013). It is therefore possible to combine final lengthening and pausing into a joint measurement of boundary strength, e.g., affinity index (Xu, 2009). Affinity refers to the fact that both domain-final syllable and silent pause increase the distance between the onset of final syllable and the onset of the upcoming syllable, and this distance seems to iconically encode the relational distance between the two adjacent domains: the closer the relation, the weaker the boundary between the two, and vice versa.

In addition, as it appears in Figure 12.16, and is argued by Wagner (2005) and Xu and Wang (2009), boundary strength is likely gradient rather than categorical. In Wagner (2005), listeners can identify up to seven levels of recursive syntactic relations, each with a boundary strength scaled by duration. In Xu and Wang (2009), even within a phrase, durational patterns reflected whether the phrase-internal grouping was 1+3 or 2+2. Similar sensitivity to boundary cues has also been shown by O'Malley et al. (1973) and Fant and Kruckenberg (1996).

The gradient nature of temporal marking of boundary strength discussed so far raises questions about the widespread notion of prosodic hierarchy (Beckman, 1996; Ladd, 2008; Selkirk, 1986). According to this notion, speech prosody is a hierarchical structure consisting of a limited number of levels: mora, prosodic word, foot, phrase, intonational phrase, and utterance. This structure not only governs its internal constituents, but also determines their relative prominence (Beckman, 1996; Liberman & Prince, 1977; Selkirk, 1980). The fine gradience of boundary strength makes it hard to find any fixed set of constituents to match a prosodic hierarchy. Furthermore, Figure 12.15a shows clearly that the effects of lexical stress in English are independent of durational variations due to boundary strength, without any cross interactions (Nakatani et al., 1981). Thus, grouping constituency is unlikely to govern word stress, which is lexically defined. Even further back, we have also seen that focus is functionally independent of lexical stress. It has also been shown that phrasal marking and focus are independently controlled in Japanese (Ishihara, 2011; Kubozono, 2007), and focus condition does not affect pauses in Swedish (Horne et al., 1995). Thus, there does not seem to be a functional need to use a hierarchical division of grouping to control either lexical stress or focus.

The temporal patterns related to boundary marking as well as lexical stress and focus also call into question the widely known rhythm class hypothesis (Abercrombie, 1967; Pike, 1945). The hypothesis divides languages into stress-timed (e.g., English, Arabic), syllable-timed (French, Italian, Yoruba) or mora-timed (Japanese), whereby the said timing unit is supposed to show a tendency of equal duration, i.e., equal temporal distance between stresses, syllables, and morae, respectively (Abercrombie, 1967; Port et al., 1987; Steever, 1987). Although such isochrony has been repeatedly demonstrated to be nonexistent (Dauer, 1983; Lehiste, 1977; Nakatani et al., 1981; Warner & Arai, 2001), the hypothesis is revived by the proposal of a number of rhythm metrics that can nevertheless divide or arrange languages along the dimensions defined by these metrics (Dellwo, 2006; Grabe & Low, 2002; Ramus et al., 1999). But the term stress-timing or syllable-timing should at least be indicative of a weak tendency toward isochronic recurrence of the said unit in the language. Yet even this tendency can be put into question. For example, based on the rhythm metrics, Grabe and Low (2002) and Lin and Wang (2007) have demonstrated that Mandarin firmly belongs to syllable-timed languages. Yet the data shown in Figure 12.15 indicate that Mandarin syllable duration varies more with position in phrase than English syllable duration, and Mandarin phrase-level units are more adjusted toward isochrony than English. The first trend is seen in the fact that phrase-medial syllables in Mandarin are shorter than the phrase-initial syllables, whereas in English, being word-medial does not further shorten the syllable at any specific stress level. The second trend is seen in the fact that, in Mandarin, a syllable in a monosyllabic word becomes much shorter when it is in a disyllabic word, even when it is still word final, whereas there is no significant shortening from monosyllabic word to multi-syllabic word in English. When the two trends are combined, Mandarin shows a greater tendency than English to equalize the total duration of a word or phrase, at the expense of syllable duration. This is exactly the opposite of what is predicted by a dichotomy of stress-timing versus syllable-timing.

The lack of compressibility of the syllable in some of the stress-timed languages is actually a consistent finding across studies. Crystal and House (1990) found that syllable duration has a quasilinear dependency on the number of phones in the syllable, and that the duration of stress groups has a quasilinear dependency on the number of syllables. Similar linearity patterns in English are found by van Santen and Shih (2000). For Swedish, Fant et al. (1989) found the correlation between stress interval and number of phones to be as high as 0.94. Interestingly, in van Santen and Shih (2000), which examined segmental duration in both English and Mandarin, there is already some evidence that segments and syllables are more compressible in Mandarin than in English, which is consistent with the finding of Xu and Wang (2009). Given that temporal patterns indeed provide critical cues for the grouping of segments and syllables into larger units, it is actually a good question for future research why some of the languages labeled as stress-timed actually show greater linearity of duration as a function of segments and syllables than some languages that are supposed to be syllable-timed, such as Mandarin.

Another often-reported boundary marking cue is pitch reset (Ladd, 1988; Swert, 1997). Pitch reset is defined as the difference in pitch across a boundary. But it is usually measured in terms of the amount of drop, or the lack thereof, of f_0 peaks or top lines across the adjacent units (Ladd, 1988; Swerts, 1997). Swerts (1997) found that pitch reset measured this way was related to the perceived boundary strength in Dutch, but the correlation was only 0.35. A major factor of uncertainty in this regard is that pitch is already used extensively for lexical contrast, focus and modality, as discussed in previous sections. Thus there is a question of how much pitch is also used as a boundary cue. Wang et al. (2018) examined the interaction between focus and boundary marking, and found that focus was signaled mainly by PFC, which can occur even across phrase breaks with silent pauses, whereas boundaries were mostly signaled by duration adjustments. The involvement of f_0 in boundary marking was only in terms of lowering of phrase-final f_0 minima and raising of phrase-initial f_0 minima at relatively strong boundaries, i.e., those with silent pauses.

The interaction of focus and boundary marking brings us to the relationship between syntactic/semantic and prosodic structure (Ladd, 2008). Much work has attempted to account for the mismatches between prosodic structure and syntactic/semantic constituency (Kratzer & Selkirk, 2007; Selkirk, 1980; Steedman, 2000). From a functional perspective, these mismatches are not really an issue, as what is important is how utterances are divided into smaller chunks for ease of comprehension. The chunking can be marked by syntax, prosody, or both. Evidence for this can been seen in a recent study that examined how listeners detect boundaries (Buxó-Lugo and Watson 2016). The findings are that (a) syntactic position predicted whether listeners reported hearing boundaries, (b) acoustic cues had a stronger effect for boundaries at syntactically unlicensed locations, and (c) listeners reported boundaries at licensed locations even when acoustic cues are weak. Thus both syntax and prosody provide useful cues for dividing utterances into smaller chunks, although there is also an incomplete division of labor. From this perspective, prosodic boundary marking is not for the sake of forming a prosodic structure for its own sake, but to either enhance a boundary already syntactically marked, or to provide boundary cues where syntax cues are ambiguous or absent (Allbritton et al., 1996; Lehiste, 1973; Price et al., 1991; Speer et al., 1996).

Paralinguistic prosody

Beyond post-lexical linguistic functions, there is a rich set of paralinguistic meanings conveyed by prosody that are related to emotion, attitude, and vocal traits. Emotion- and attitude-related prosody is known as *affective prosody*, *emotional prosody*, or *vocal expression of emotions and attitudes*. The latter (vocal-trait-related prosody) does not have a formal name, but covers things as variable as vocal attractiveness, charisma, dominance, sarcasm, irony, idiosyncratic prosody, etc. Though highly diverse, all these areas may be interconnected by a common mechanism first proposed for vocal calls in nonhuman animals by Morton (1977). This mechanism is extended to human speech through sound symbolism by Ohala (1983, 1984). Based on the analysis of calls by hundreds of bird and mammal species, Morton (1977) proposed that the calls are designed to mimic the acoustic properties of a large or small body size as a means to influence the behavior of the call receiver. When an animal is being aggressive, hostile, or is ready to attack, it would use calls with a low pitch and harsh quality to project a large body size in order to dominate the receiver. When being submissive, fearful, or friendly, it would use calls that are high-pitched and tone-like to project a small body size in order to appease the receiver. In the latter case, the acoustic properties may also mimic infant vocalization so as to elicit a parental instinct. Ohala (1984) extended Morton's theory to human vocalization, and also added a third acoustic dimension: vocal tract length. He further proposed that the smile is actually an expression derived from a strategy to shorten the vocal tract during vocalization by retracting the corners of the lips. In addition, he proposed that body size projection is also what drove the sexual dimorphism, whereby men's larynges are lower and vocal folds longer than women's for the sake of projecting a larger body size in competition with other males for attracting female mates.

The Morton-Ohala hypothesis of body size projection has been most successfully applied in research on sexually related vocal attractiveness. It has been shown that female listeners favor men's voice with lower pitch and more condensed formants (hence longer vocal tract) (Collins, 2000; Feinberg et al., 2005; Xu et al., 2013b), while male listeners prefer female voice with higher pitch and more dispersed formants (Collins & Missing, 2003; Feinberg et al., 2008; Xu et al., 2013b). Xu et al. (2013b) further found, however, that in terms of voice quality, both male and female listeners prefer the same from the opposite sex: *breathy* rather than *pressed* voice. The breathiness nudges the voice toward a pure tone, a quality associated with friendliness and non-aggression (Morton, 1977). Thus for an attractive male voice, intriguingly, the breathiness seems to soften the aggressiveness associated with low pitch and high formant density while preserving their association with masculinity (Xu et al., 2013b).

There is much less research applying the Morton-Ohala theory of body size projection to emotional prosody, however. A major difficulty seems to be that it is hard to find clear evidence from emotional speech through acoustic analysis (Scherer & Bänziger, 2004). This is presumably due to the heavy multidimensionality of emotional prosody in general, and the severe confound between pitch and loudness in particular, as will be discussed later. A method that is able to circumvent this difficulty is to use a perception paradigm in which the stimuli are generated either by direct speech synthesis or resynthesis of natural speech with manipulation of relevant acoustic dimensions, as suggested by Scherer and Bänziger

(2004). When carried out by a number of studies, the paradigm was shown to be highly effective. Chuenwattanapranithi et al. (2008) found, with articulatorily synthesized (Birkholz et al., 2006) isolated Thai vowels, anger and joy are associated with lowered or raised f_0 and lengthened or shortened vocal tract, respectively. Xu and Kelly (2010) replicated these findings with resynthesized British English numerals originally produced by a male speaker. The manipulation of formant dispersion (Fitch, 1994) was done by changing the spectral density with the PSOLA algorithm (Moulines & Charpentier, 1990). Similar findings were further made in Xu et al. (2013b), using a full sentence synthesized with an updated articulatory synthesizer capable of generating different voice qualities (Birkholz et al., 2011).

With the three specific acoustic parameters, namely, pitch, formant dispersion and voice quality, body size projection is a kind of dimensional approach to emotional prosody. But it is very different from the much better known dimensional theories of emotions (Russell, 1979, 2003; Schlosberg, 1954). Those theories are based on a depiction of how we *subjectively feel* when being emotional: do we feel pleasant or unpleasant? How emotionally aroused are we? Or do we feel that we are in control or want to approach or avoid the hearer? These are known as the *valence*, *arousal/activation* and *control/approach-avoidance* dimensions, respectively (Carver & Harmon-Jones, 2009; Davidson et al., 1990). Of these dimensions, however, only arousal/activation has been shown to have relatively consistent acoustic correlates (Bachorowski, 1999; Scherer et al., 1991). No consistent acoustic correlates have been identified for the other dimensions, as reviewed by Mauss and Robinson (2009). The lack of acoustic correlates with the emotional dimensions except arousal/activation therefore contrasts with clear correlations between body-size-related acoustic parameters and happiness and anger (Chuenwattanapranithi et al., 2008; Xu et al., 2013a).

However, the body size projection dimensions may not be adequate to separate emotions other than anger and happiness, such as sadness, fear, disgust, and surprise. Xu et al. (2013a) proposed that a wider range of vocal emotions can be encoded by a set of *bio-informational dimensions* (BIDs) that consist of the body size projection dimension and three additional dimensions: *dynamicity*, *loudness*, and *association* (Xu et al., 2013a). Like body size projection, the additional dimensions are also based on how they would influence the behavior of the receiver rather than how they are felt subjectively. *Dynamicity* is based on how vigorous the speaker wants to appear to the listener. *Audibility* controls the loudness of the vocalization, depending on whether it is beneficial for the vocalization to be heard only in close proximity. *Association* makes an associative use of sounds typically accompanying a non-emotional biological function in circumstances beyond the original ones, e.g., mirroring the sounds of vomiting to express disgust (Darwin, 1872). The BIDs would therefore allow an even richer multidimensional combination potentially used by many different emotions.

An initial test of BIDs was done by Xu et al. (2013a), using resynthesis of a full sentence in British English to generate a multidimensional matrix of combinations of parameters that are associated with body size projection and dynamicity. The former is done by varying formant shift ratio and pitch median, and the latter by varying pitch range and speech rate. Among the main findings are the following.

1. In addition to a wide formant dispersion (hence short vocal tract length) as mentioned previously, happiness also shows a large pitch range and fast speech rate, indicating high dynamicity.
2. Sadness show two highly distinct types: *depressed* and *grief-stricken*. While the depressed type shows similar characteristics as in most previous reports (Scherer, 2003; Williams & Stevens, 1972), with low values for virtually all parameters except for

neutral formant dispersion, the grief-stricken type shows high pitch median, narrow pitch range, slow speech rate, and, surprisingly, low formant dispersion. The lengthened vocal tract as indicated by the low formant dispersion suggests that the crying vocalization, which is best seen in children, is for making a harsh demand rather than a gentle plea, as many parents would attest.

3 The most prototypical fear vocalization showed, also surprisingly, a narrow formant dispersion. This was interpreted as evidence that fear is not equal to submission, contrary to Morton's original hypothesis. But his principle still applies. That is, with a low formant dispersion, fear vocalization probably expresses a threat to fight on, especially when faced by a predator, as total submission would mean being eaten.

4 Finally, the best anger vocalization was heard from stimuli with 50 Hz median pitch, which sounded as if they were uttered with a vocal fry. This suggests that rough voice quality, which was only accidentally generated in the study, may be critical for expressing anger.

The contribution of voice quality was explored in a number of perception studies, using two methods. One is to coach a speaker to say a sentence with breathy, modal, or tense voice. The other is to use VocalTractLab which by that time had incorporated a glottal modal for controlling voice quality (Birkholz et al., 2011). The first method is found to be effective only in limited ways, as it is sometimes difficult to coach speakers to produce desired voice qualities consistently (Noble & Xu, 2011). The second method was better in terms of consistency, but its effectiveness varied with specific paralinguistic functions. Nevertheless, Xu et al. (2013b) was able to find, as mentioned earlier, that voice quality was a major determinant of vocal attractiveness, not only for female voice but also for male voice.

Thus the bio-informational dimensions, due to their ability to link specific acoustic parameters to theory-motivated hypotheses, enable the construction of testable predictions about various paralinguistic functions, including emotions, attitudes, and vocal traits. They may also enable connection of previous findings that hitherto seem to be unrelated.

One major issue in need of investigation is the audibility dimension proposed in Xu et al. (2013a). Production studies have mostly found high pitch to be characteristic of angry voice (Mauss & Robinson, 2009; Scherer, 2003; Williams & Stevens, 1972). Perceptual studies, however, have consistently found angry voice to be associated with a lower pitch than happiness (Chuenwattanapranithi et al., 2008; Xu & Kelly, 2010; Xu et al., 2013a, 2013b). Likewise, charismatic speech (Niebuhr et al., 2016; Rosenberg & Hirschberg, 2009) and speech that is heard to signal a high social rank (Ko et al., 2014) are both found to have high f_0 even for male speakers, which again violates the prediction of body size projection. Here the potential confound is the natural correlation between f_0 and voice amplitude (Alku et al., 2002; Brumm & Zollinger, 2011): other things being equal, the higher the amplitude of the voice, the higher the f_0. This is true of not only human voice, but also bird songs, and is related to the well-known Lombard effect (Brumm & Zollinger, 2011; Nemeth et al., 2013). Thus it could be the case that the high f_0 of hot anger (Scherer, 2003) is closely related to a high loudness rather than for the sake of increasing pitch per se. The high loudness is already found in addition to high f_0 in the case of charismatic and high-rank speech (Ko et al., 2014; Niebuhr et al., 2016; Rosenberg & Hirschberg, 2009). But in general, the exact relationship between amplitude and f_0 in paralinguistic prosody is not yet clear, and so is in need of further research.

Finally, paralinguistic functions are likely to frequently interact with lexical and post-lexical linguistic functions, especially the latter. For example, the gradient pitch range variations related to the many modality types as shown in Figure 12.14 could well be partially due to the different paralinguistic connotations involved, e.g., uncertainty, surprise, incredulity, and assertiveness. In addition, the prosodic difference sometimes found between contrastive and informational focus (Baumann et al., 2007; He et al., 2011; Sahkai et al., 2013) could also be related to their paralinguistic connotations. The study of detailed interactions between linguistic and paralinguistic functions may therefore lead to exciting new findings in further research.

A methodological note

The multiple degrees of separation, mentioned previously, between prosodic functions and their underlying properties means that it is vital to apply methodological techniques that are effective in revealing potential causal relations. Some of these techniques have been illustrated throughout the chapter. This section will highlight two such techniques, with some elaboration.

Examining continuous prosody

As phoneticians often note, *the devil is in the fine phonetic details* (Hawkins, 2003; Nolan, 1999). For intonation, these details are frequently in continuous prosodic events such as f_0 contours. As shown in Figure 12.17a, if only a single f_0 measurement is taken from each syllable in an utterance (which is almost a common practice), the nature of the contextual tonal variation is not at all clear. Two to three measurements per syllable, as shown in Figure 12.17b and 12.17c, do improve the picture a bit further, but some important details are still missing. It is only when the contours appear fully continuous with eight points per syllable, as shown in Figure 12.17d, does the evidence of asymptotic target approximation become obvious.

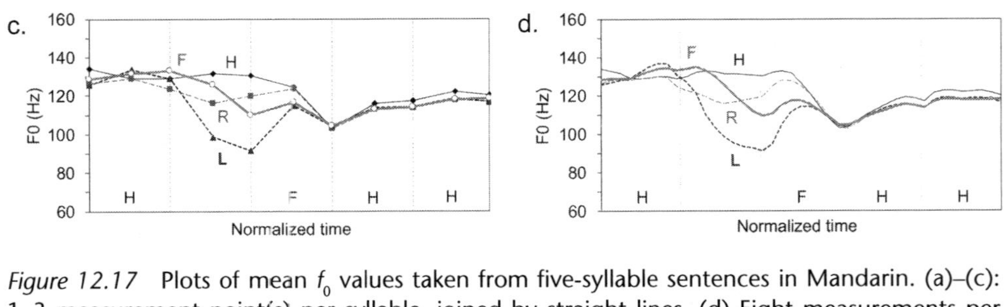

Figure 12.17 Plots of mean f_0 values taken from five-syllable sentences in Mandarin. (a)–(c): 1–3 measurement point(s) per syllable, joined by straight lines. (d) Eight measurements per syllable.

Source: Data from Xu (1999).

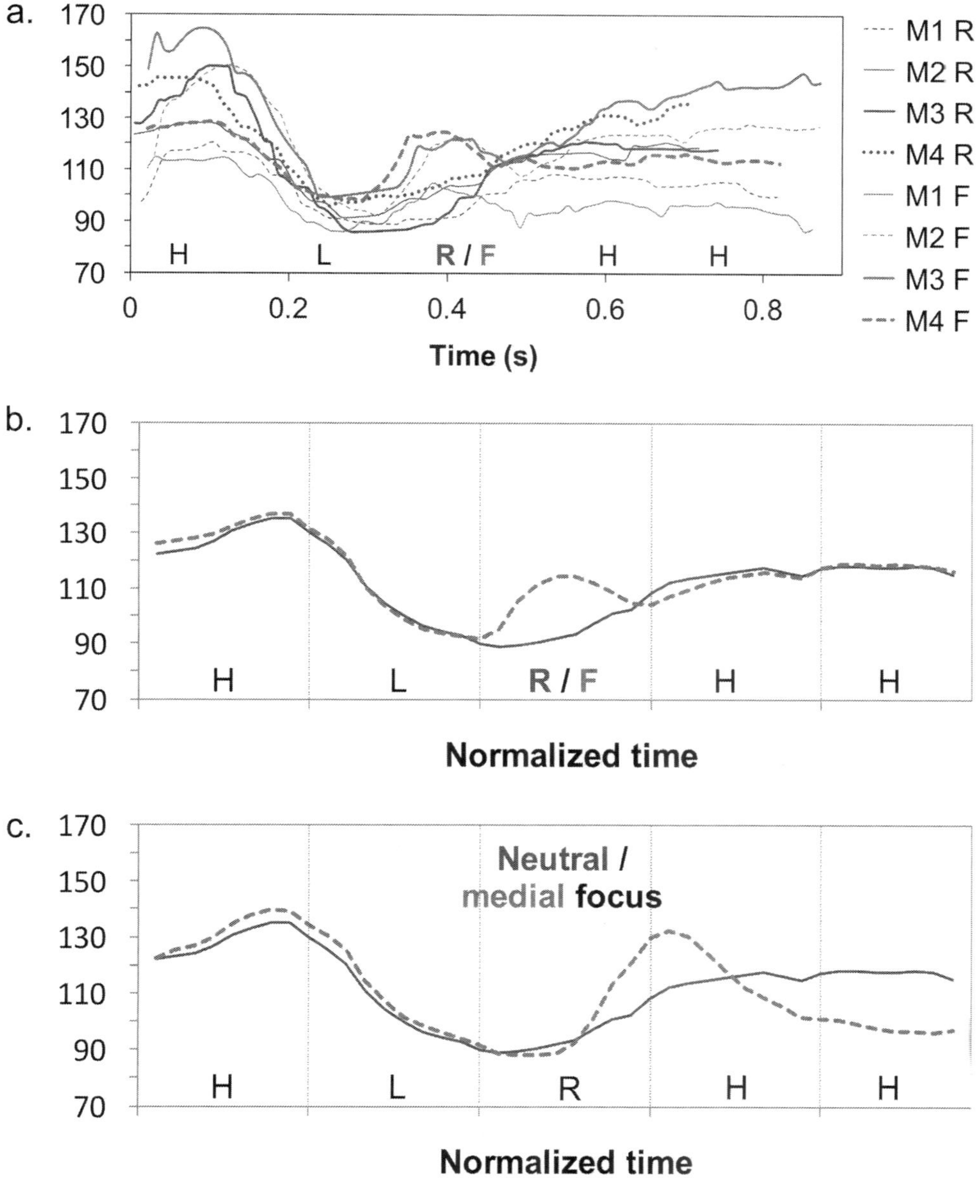

Figure 12.18 (a) f_0 contours of two Mandarin tone sequences differing in the tone of the third syllable, produced by four male speakers. (b) Mean f_0 contours time-normalized with respect to syllables, averaged across five repetitions each by four speakers. (c) Mean time-normalized f_0 contours averaged across five repetitions by four speakers each.

Source: Data from Xu (1999).

Making minimal pair comparisons

The example in Figure 12.17 not only shows the importance of observing continuous prosodic events, but also illustrates the need for minimal-pair comparisons at the level of continuous trajectories. The concept of minimal pair comparison is familiar to anyone who does statistical comparison in their research. But minimal pair comparisons at the level of fully continuous trajectories are still relatively rare in the segmental (Gelfer et al., 1989) as well as suprasegmental domains. A main reason is the difficulty in making the comparison. Figure 12.18a, for example, shows f_0 contours of two Mandarin five-tone sequences that differ only in the tone of the third syllable: Rising vs. Falling, produced by four male speakers. Because the utterances differ not only in f_0, but also in duration, it is hard to see the critical difference between the two sequences, although it is already a minimal pair design. In Figure 12.18b, the f_0 contours are time-normalized (i.e., with the same number of evenly spaced measurement points in each equivalent interval) with respect to the syllable and then averaged across five repetitions each by four speakers. The difference between the two sequences now becomes clear. In Figure 12.18c, the minimal-pair comparison is between neutral focus and medial focus. Again, the contrast is very clear thanks to the time normalization and averaging. It can also be seen clearly that due to the on-focus exaggeration of the Rising tone, the effect of the sharp rise does not fade away until halfway into the following syllable. This graphical information tells us that, if we were to capture the PFC effect, the measurement points have to be taken after the strong carryover effect of the Rising tone is largely over.

Concluding Remarks

This chapter has reviewed the literature on prosody, tone, and intonation with the aim of addressing the question: how is it possible that a vastly rich set of communicative meanings can be simultaneously conveyed through suprasegmental means? Past research has shown that articulatory mechanisms, lexical contrasts, post-lexical linguistic functions, and paralinguistic prosody all have their own unique domain-specific mechanisms. Recognizing the specific mechanisms turns out to be critical for understanding the highly diverse phenomena in all these areas. It is also shown that the individual processes can be all integrated into a framework that allows simultaneous transmission of multiple communicative meanings in parallel. Numerous questions, many of which were raised by the mechanistic-functional approach, still await answers, as mentioned throughout the chapter. Answering these questions in future research will no doubt significantly advance our understanding of the suprasegmental aspects of speech.

Notes

1 Courtesy of Douglas N. Honorof for the numerical data.
2 There is some evidence that this is a historical change that started centuries ago and slowly spread across many northern dialects (Mei, 1977). This makes the true mechanism of the change hard to unearth, as it is difficult to know the exact pitch value of the Low tone at that time.

References

Abe, I. (1998). Intonation in Japanese. In *Intonation systems – a survey of twenty languages*. D. Hirst and A. Di Cristo. Cambridge: Cambridge University Press, pp. 360–375.

Abercrombie, D. (1967). *Elements of general phonetics*. Edinburgh: Edinburgh University Press.

Alku, P., Vintturi, J. and Vilkman, E. (2002). Measuring the effect of fundamental frequency raising as a strategy for increasing vocal intensity in soft, normal and loud phonation. *Speech Communication* **38**: 321–334.

Allbritton, D. W., McKoon, G. and Ratcliff, R. (1996). Reliability of prosodic cues for resolving syntactic ambiguity. *Journal of Experimental Psychology: Learning, Memory, and Cognition* **22**(3): 714–735.

Arvaniti, A. (2012). The usefulness of metrics in the quantification of speech rhythm. *Journal of Phonetics* **40**(3): 351–373.

Arvaniti, A. and Ladd, D. R. (2009). Greek wh-questions and the phonology of intonation. *Phonology* **26**(01): 43–74.

Atkinson, J. E. (1978). Correlation analysis of the physiological factors controlling fundamental voice frequency. *The Journal of the Acoustical Society of America* **63**: 211–222.

Bachorowski, J. A. (1999). Vocal expression and perception of emotion. *Current Directions in Psychological Science* **8**(2): 53–57.

Baumann, S., Becker, J., Grice, M. and Mücke, D. (2007). Tonal and articulatory marking of focus in German. In *Proceedings of the 16th International Congress of Phonetic Sciences*, Saarbrucken, pp. 1029–1032.

Beckman, M. E. (1996). The parsing of prosody. *Language and Cognitive Processes* **11**: 17–67.

Birkholz, P., Jackèl, D. and Kröger, B. J. (2006). Construction and control of a three-dimensional vocal tract model. In *Proceedings of the 31st International Conference on Acoustics, Speech, and Signal Processing*, Toulouse, France, pp. 873–876.

Birkholz, P., Kröger, B. J. and Neuschaefer-Rube, C. (2011). Synthesis of breathy, normal, and pressed phonation using a two-mass model with a triangular glottis. In *Proceedings of Interspeech 2011*, Florence, Italy, pp. 2681–2684.

Boersma, P. (2001). Praat, a system for doing phonetics by computer. *Glot International* **5**(9/10): 341–345.

Bolinger, D. (1978). Intonation across languages. In *Universals of human language, Phonology V. 2*. J. H. Greenberg: Stanford University Press, pp. 471–523.

Bomhard, A. R. (2008). *Reconstructing proto-nostratic: Comparative phonology, morphology, and vocabulary*. Leiden: Brill.

Botinis, A., Ambrazaitis, G. and Frid, J. (2014). Syllable structure and tonal representation: Revisiting focal Accent II in Swedish. In *Proceedings from FONETIK 2014*, Stockholm, Sweden, pp. 65–70.

Botinis, A., Fourakis, M. and Gawronska, B. (1999). Focus identification in English, Greek and Swedish. In *Proceedings of the 14th International Congress of Phonetic Sciences*, San Francisco, pp. 1557–1560.

Browman, C. P. and Goldstein, L. (1992). Targetless schwa: An articulatory analysis. In *Papers in Laboratory Phonology II: Gesture, segment, prosody*. R. Ladd. Cambridge University Press, Cambridge, pp. 26–36.

Bruce, G. (1982). Developing the Swedish intonation model. *Lund University, Department of Linguistics Working Papers* **22**: 51–116.

Brumm, H. and Zollinger, S. A. (2011). The evolution of the Lombard effect: 100 years of psychoacoustic research. *Behaviour* **148**(11–13): 1173–1198.

Buxó-Lugo, A. and Watson, D. G. (2016). Evidence for the influence of syntax on prosodic parsing. *Journal of Memory and Language* **90**: 1–13.

Carver, C. S. and Harmon-Jones, E. (2009). Anger is an approach-related affect: Evidence and implications. *Psychological Bulletin* **135**(2): 183.

Chaffe, W. (1976). Givenness, contrastiveness, definiteness, subjects, topics and point of view. In *Subject and Topic*. C. Li. New York: Academic Press, pp. 25–55.

Chahal, D. (2003). Phonetic cues to prominence in Lebanese Arabic. In *Proceedings of the 15th International Congress of Phonetic Sciences*, Barcelona, pp. 2067–2070.

Chao, Y. R. (1968). *A grammar of spoken Chinese*. Berkeley, CA: University of California Press.

Chen, L., Li, X. and Yang, Y. (2012). Focus, newness and their combination: Processing of information structure in discourse. *PLoS One* **7**(8): e42533.

Chen, L., Wang, L. and Yang, Y. (2014). Distinguish between focus and newness: An ERP study. *Journal of Neurolinguistics* **31**: 28–41.

Chen, M. Y. (2000). *Tone sandhi: Patterns across Chinese dialects*. Cambridge: Cambridge University Press.

Chen, S. W., Wang, B. and Xu, Y. (2009). Closely related languages, different ways of realizing focus. In *Proceedings of Interspeech 2009*, Brighton, pp. 1007–1010.

Chen, Ying. (2015). Post-focus compression in English by Mandarin learners. In *Proceedings of the 18th International Congress of Phonetic Sciences*, Glasgow, UK.

Chen, Ying, Xu, Y. and Guion-Anderson, S. (2014). Prosodic realization of focus in bilingual production of Southern Min and Mandarin. *Phonetica* **71**: 249–270.

Chen, Yiya. (2008). Revisiting the phonetics and phonology of shanghai tone sandhi. In *Proceedings of Speech Prosody 2008*, Campinas, Brazil, pp. 253–256.

Chen, Yiya. and Xu, Y. (2006). Production of weak elements in speech – evidence from f0 patterns of neutral tone in standard Chinese. *Phonetica* **63**: 47–75.

Chuenwattanapranithi, S., Xu, Y., Thipakorn, B. and Maneewongvatana, S. (2008). Encoding emotions in speech with the size code – a perceptual investigation. *Phonetica* **65**: 210–230.

Collins, S. A. (2000). Men's voices and women's choices. *Animal Behaviour* **60**: 773–780.

Collins, S. A. and Missing, C. (2003). Vocal and visual attractiveness are related in women. *Animal Behaviour* **65**(5): 997–1004.

Connell, B. (2017). Tone and intonation in Mambila. *Intonation in African Tone Languages* **24**: 131.

Connell, B. and Ladd, D. R. (1990). Aspects of pitch realization in Yoruba. *Phonology* **7**: 1–29.

Cooper, W. E., Eady, S. J. and Mueller, P. R. (1985). Acoustical aspects of contrastive stress in question-answer contexts. *The Journal of the Acoustical Society of America* **77**: 2142–2156.

Crystal, T. H. and House, A. S. (1990). Articulation rate and the duration of syllables and stress groups in connected speech. *The Journal of the Acoustical Society of America* **88**: 101–112.

Cutler, A., Dahan, D. and van Donselaar, W. (1997). Prosody in the comprehension of spoken language: A literature review. *Language and Speech* **40**: 141–201.

Darwin, C. (1872). *The expression of the emotions in man and animals*. London: John Murray.

Davidson, R. J., Ekman, P., Saron, C., Senulis, J. and Friesen, W. (1990). Emotional expression and brain physiology I: Approach/withdrawal and cerebral asymmetry. *Journal of Personality and Social Psychology* **58**: 330–341.

Dauer, R. M. (1983). Stress-timing and syllable-timing reanalyzed. *Journal of Phonetics* **11**: 51–62.

de Jong, K. and Zawaydeh, B. (2002). Comparing stress, lexical focus, and segmental focus: Patterns of variation in Arabic vowel duration. *Journal of Phonetics* **30**: 53–75.

Dellwo, V. (2006). Rhythm and speech rate: A variation coefficient for ΔC. In *Language and language processing: Proceedings of the 38th Linguistic Colloquium. Piliscsaba 2003*. P. Karnowski and I. Szigeti. Frankfurt am Main: Peter Lang, pp. 231–241.

Diamond, J. M. (1998). *Guns, germs and steel: A short history of everybody for the last 13,000 years*. London: Vintage.

Diamond, J. M. and Bellwood, P. (2003). Farmers and their languages: The first expansions. *Science* **300**(5619): 597–603.

Dilley, L. C. and Brown, M. (2007). Effects of pitch range variation on f0 extrema in an imitation task. *Journal of Phonetics* **35**(4): 523–551.

Dohen, M. and Lœvenbruck, H. (2004). Pre-focal rephrasing, focal enhancement and post-focal deaccentuation in French. In *Proceedings of the 8th International Conference on Spoken Language Processing*, Jeju, Korea, pp. 1313–1316.

Duanmu, S. (1994). Against contour tone units. *Linguistic Inquiry* **25**: 555–608.

Eady, S. J. and Cooper, W. E. (1986). Speech intonation and focus location in matched statements and questions. *The Journal of the Acoustical Society of America* **80**: 402–416.

Eady, S. J., Cooper, W. E., Klouda, G. V., Mueller, P. R. and Lotts, D. W. (1986). Acoustic characteristics of sentential focus: Narrow vs. broad and single vs. dual focus environments. *Language and Speech* **29**: 233–251.

Erickson, D., Honda, K., Hirai, H. and Beckman, M. E. (1995). The production of low tones in English intonation. *Journal of Phonetics* **23**: 179–188.

Eriksson, A. (2012). Aural/acoustic vs. Automatic methods in forensic phonetic case work. In *Forensic Speaker Recognition*. New York: Springer, pp. 41–69.

Face, T. L. (2005). F0 peak height and the perception of sentence type in Castilian Spanish. *Revista internacional de Lingüística Iberoamericana* **3**: 49–65.

Fant, G. and Kruckenberg, A. (1996). On the quantal nature of speech timing. In *Proceedings, Fourth International Conference on Proceedings of Spoken Language, 1996. ICSLP 96*. IEEE, pp. 2044–2047.

Fant, G., Kruckenberg, A. and Nord, L. (1989). Stress patterns, pauses, and timing in prose reading. *STL-QPSR* **1**: 7–12.

Feinberg, D. R., DeBruine, L. M., Jones, B. C. and Perrett, D. I. (2008). The role of femininity and averageness of voice pitch in aesthetic judgments of women's voices. *Perception* **37**: 615–623.

Feinberg, D. R., Jones, B. C., Little, A. C., Burt, D. M. and Perrett, D. I. (2005). Manipulations of fundamental and formant frequencies influence the attractiveness of human male voices. *Animal Behavior* **69**: 561–568.

Féry, C. and Kügler, F. (2008). Pitch accent scaling on given, new and focused constituents in German. *Journal of Phonetics* **36**(4): 680–703.

Fitch, W. T. (1994). *Vocal tract length perception and the evolution of language*. Ph.D. Dissertation, Brown University.

Fok-Chan, Y. Y. (1974). *A perceptual study of tones in Cantonese*. Hong Kong: University of Hong Kong Press.

Franich, K. (2015). The effect of cognitive load on tonal coarticulation. In *Proceedings of the 18th International Congress of Phonetic Sciences*, Glasgow, UK.

Fry, D. B. (1958). Experiments in the perception of stress. *Language and Speech* **1**: 126–152.

Fujisaki, H. (1983). Dynamic characteristics of voice fundamental frequency in speech and singing. In *The production of speech*. P. F. MacNeilage. New York: Springer-Verlag, pp. 39–55.

Gandour, J., Potisuk, S. and Dechongkit, S. (1994). Tonal coarticulation in Thai. *Journal of Phonetics* **22**: 477–492.

Gay, T. J. (1968). Effect of speaking rate on diphthong formant movements. *The Journal of the Acoustical Society of America* **44**: 1570–1573.

Gelfer, C. E., Bell-Berti, F. and Harris, K. S. (1989). Determining the extent of coarticulation: Effects of experimental design. *The Journal of the Acoustical Society of America* **86**(6): 2443–2445.

Giovanni, A., Ouaknine, M., Guelfucci, B., Yu, P., Zanaret, M. and Triglia, J. M. (1999). Nonlinear behavior of vocal fold vibration: The role of coupling between the vocal folds. *Journal of Voice* **13**(4): 465–476.

Goldsmith, J. A. (1990). *Autosegmental and metrical phonology*. Oxford: Blackwell Publishers.

Grabe, E. and Low, E. L. (2002). Durational variability in speech and the rhythm class hypothesis. In *Papers in laboratory phonology 7*. C. Gussenhoven and N. Warner. The Hague: Mouton de Gruyter, pp. 515–546.

Greenberg, J. H. (1963). Some universals of grammar with particular reference to the order of meaningful elements. *Universals of Language* **2**: 73–113.

Gussenhoven, C. (2004). *The phonology of tone and intonation*: Cambridge: Cambridge University Press.

Gussenhoven, C. (2007). Types of focus in English. In *Topic and focus: Cross-linguistic perspectives on meaning and intonation*. C. Lee, M. Gordon and D. Büring. New York: Springer, pp. 83–100.

Halle, M. and Stevens, K. N. (1971). A note on laryngeal features. *Quarterly Progress Report, M.I.T. Research Laboratory of Electronics* **101**: 198–213.

Halliday, M. A. K. (1967). Notes on transitivity and theme in English: Part 1. *Journal of Linguistics* **3**(1): 37–81.

Hanson, H. M. and Stevens, K. N. (2002). A quasiarticulatory approach to controlling acoustic source parameters in a Klatt-type formant synthesizer using HLsyn. *The Journal of the Acoustical Society of America* **112**: 1158–1182.
Hanssen, J., Peters, J. and Gussenhoven, C. (2008). Prosodic effects of focus in Dutch declaratives. In *Proceedings of Speech Prosody 2008*, Campinas, Brazil, pp. 609–612.
Hawkins, S. (2003). Roles and representations of systematic fine phonetic detail in speech understanding. *Journal of Phonetics* **31**: 373–405.
He, X., Hanssen, J., van Heuven, V. J. and Gussenhoven, C. (2011). Phonetic implementation must be learnt: Native versus Chinese realization of focus accent in Dutch. In *Proceedings of the XVIIth International Congress of Phonetic Sciences*, Hong Kong, pp. 843–846.
Hollien, H. (1960). Vocal pitch variation related to changes in vocal fold length. *Journal of Speech and Hearing Research* **3**: 150–156.
Hombert, J. M., Ohala, J. and Ewan, W. (1979). Phonetic explanation for the development of tones. *Language* **55**: 37–58.
Honda, K., Hirai, H., Masaki, S. and Shimada, Y. (1999). Role of vertical larynx movement and cervical lordosis in F0 control. *Language and Speech* **42**: 401–411.
Honorof, D. N. and Whalen, D. H. (2005). Perception of pitch location within a speaker's F0 range. *The Journal of the Acoustical Society of America* **117**: 2193–2200.
Horne, M., Strangert, E. and Heldner, M. (1995). Prosodic boundary strength in Swedish: Final lengthening and silent interval duration. In *Proceedings of the XIIIth International Congress of Phonetic Sciences (ICPhS)*, Stockholm, pp. 170–173.
Hwang, H. K. (2012). Asymmetries between production, perception and comprehension of focus types in Japanese. In *Proceedings of Speech Prosody 2012*, Shanghai, pp. 326–329.
Hyman, L. M. (2007). Universals of tone rules: 30 years later. *Tones and Tunes* **1**: 1–34.
Ipek, C. (2011). Phonetic realization of focus with no on-focus pitch range expansion in Turkish. In *Proceedings of the 17th International Congress of Phonetic Sciences*, Hong Kong, pp. 140–143.
Ishihara, S. (2002). Syntax-phonology interface of wh-constructions in Japanese. In *Proceedings of Tokyo Conference on Psycholinguistics 2002 (TCP 2002)*, Tokyo, pp. 165–189.
Ishihara, S. (2011). Japanese focus prosody revisited: Freeing focus from prosodic phrasing. *Lingua* **121**: 1870–1889.
Jeon, H. S. and Nolan, F. (2013). The role of pitch and timing cues in the perception of phrasal grouping in Seoul Korean. *The Journal of the Acoustical Society of America* **133**(5): 3039–3049.
Jin, S. (1996). *An acoustic study of sentence stress in Mandarin Chinese*. Ph.D. Dissertation. The Ohio State University.
Katz, J. and Selkirk, E. (2011). Contrastive focus vs. discourse-new: Evidence from phonetic prominence in English. *Language* **87**(4): 771–816.
Klatt, D. H. (1975). Vowel lengthening is syntactically determined in a connected discourse. *Journal of Phonetics* **3**: 129–140.
Klatt, D. H. (1976). Linguistic uses of segmental duration in English: Acoustic and perceptual evidence. *The Journal of the Acoustical Society of America* **59**: 1208–1221.
Ko, S. J., Sadler, M. S. and Galinsky, A. D. (2014). The sound of power: Conveying and detecting hierarchical rank through voice. *Psychological Science* **26**(1): 3–14.
Kratzer, A. and Selkirk, E. (2007). Phase theory and prosodic spellout: The case of verbs. *The Linguistic Review* **24**(2–3): 93–135.
Krifka, M. (2008). Basic notions of information structure. *Acta Linguistica Hungarica* **55**(3): 243–276.
Kristensen, L. B., Wang, L., Petersson, K. M. and Hagoort, P. (2013). The interface between language and attention: Prosodic focus marking recruits a general attention network in spoken language comprehension. *Cerebral Cortex* **23**(8): 1836–1848.
Kubozono, H. (2007). Focus and intonation in Japanese: Does focus trigger pitch reset. In *Proceedings of the 2nd Workshop on Prosody, Syntax, and Information Structure (WPSI2)*, Potsdam: University of Potsdam, pp. 1–27.

Kügler, F. and Genzel, S. (2014). On the elicitation of focus – prosodic differences as a function of sentence mode of the context? In *Proceedings of TAL 2014*, Nijmegen, pp. 71–74.

Kügler, F. and Skopeteas, S. (2007). On the universality of prosodic reflexes of contrast: The case of Yucatec Maya. In *Proceedings of the 16th International Congress of Phonetic Sciences*, Saarbrücken, Germany.

Ladd, D. R. (1988). Declination "reset" and the hierarchical organization of utterances. *The Journal of the Acoustical Society of America* **84**: 530–544.

Ladd, D. R. (1996). *Intonational phonology*. Cambridge: Cambridge University Press.

Ladd, D. R. (2008). *Intonational phonology*. Cambridge: Cambridge University Press.

Laniran, Y. O. and Clements, G. N. (2003). Downstep and high raising: Interacting factors in Yoruba tone production. *Journal of Phonetics* **31**: 203–250.

Lee, A., Prom-on, S. and Xu, Y. (2017). Pre-low raising in Japanese pitch accent. *Phonetica* **74**(4): 231–246.

Lee, A. and Xu, Y. (2012). Revisiting focus prosody in Japanese. In *Proceedings of Speech Prosody 2012*, Shanghai, pp. 274–277.

Lee, Y. C., Wang, B., Chen, S., Adda-Decker, M., Amelot, A., Nambu, S. and Liberman, M. (2015). A crosslinguistic study of prosodic focus. In *2015 IEEE International Conference on Proceedings of Acoustics, Speech and Signal Processing (ICASSP)*. IEEE, pp. 4754–4758.

Lee, Y. C., Wang, T. and Liberman, M. (2016). Production and perception of tone 3 focus in Mandarin Chinese. *Frontiers in Psychology* **7**(1058).

Lee, Y. C. and Xu, Y. (2010). Phonetic realization of contrastive focus in Korean. In *Proceedings of Speech Prosody 2010*, Chicago, pp. 1–4.

Lehiste, I. (1972). The timing of utterances and linguistic boundaries. *The Journal of the Acoustical Society of America* **51**: 2018–2024.

Lehiste, I. (1973). Phonetic disambigation of syntactic ambiguity. *Glossa* **7**: 107–122.

Lehiste, I. (1977). Isochrony reconsidered. *Journal of Phonetics* **5**: 253–263.

Li, Y. (2015). Tone sandhi and tonal coarticulation in Fuzhou Min. In *Proceedings of the 18th International Congress of Phonetic Sciences*, Glasgow, UK.

Liberman, M. and Prince, A. (1977). On stress and linguistic rhythm. *Linguistic Inquiry* **8**: 249–336.

Liberman, M., Schultz, J. M., Hong, S. and Okeke, V. (1993). The phonetic interpretation of tone in Igbo. *Phonetica* **50**: 147–160.

Lin, H. and Wang, Q. (2007). Mandarin rhythm: An acoustic study. *Journal of Chinese Language and Computing* **17**: 127–140.

Liu, F. and Xu, Y. (2005). Parallel encoding of focus and interrogative meaning in Mandarin intonation. *Phonetica* **62**: 70–87.

Liu, F. and Xu, Y. (2007). Question intonation as affected by word stress and focus in English. In *Proceedings of the 16th International Congress of Phonetic Sciences*, Saarbrücken, pp. 1189–1192.

Liu, F., Xu, Y., Prom-on, S. and Yu, A. C. L. (2013). Morpheme-like prosodic functions: Evidence from acoustic analysis and computational modeling. *Journal of Speech Sciences* **3**(1): 85–140.

Ma, J. K., Ciocca, V. and Whitehill, T. L. (2006). Effect of intonation on Cantonese lexical tones. *The Journal of the Acoustical Society of America* **120**(6): 3978–3987.

Mauss, I. B. and Robinson, M. D. (2009). Measures of emotion: A review. *Cognition & Emotion* **23**(2): 209–237.

Mei, T. L. (1977). Tones and tone sandhi in 16th century Mandarin. *Journal of Chinese Linguistics* **5**: 237–260.

Mixdorff, H. (2004). Quantitative tone and intonation modeling across languages. In *Proceedings of International Symposium on Tonal Aspects of Languages: With Emphasis on Tone Languages*, Beijing, pp. 137–142.

Morton, E. S. (1977). On the occurrence and significance of motivation-structural rules in some bird and mammal sounds. *American Naturalist* **111**: 855–869.

Moulines, E. and Charpentier, F. (1990). Pitch-synchronous waveform processing techniques for text-to-speech synthesis using diphones. *Speech Communication* **9**(5–6): 453–467.

Nakatani, L. H., O'connor, K. D. and Aston, C. H. (1981). Prosodic aspects of American English speech rhythm. *Phonetica* **38**: 84–106.

Nemeth, E., Pieretti, N., Zollinger, S. A., Geberzahn, N., Partecke, J., Miranda, A. C. and Brumm, H. (2013). Bird song and anthropogenic noise: Vocal constraints may explain why birds sing higher-frequency songs in cities. In *Proceedings of the Royal Society B: Biological Sciences 280(1754): 20122798*.

Niebuhr, O., Voße, J. and Brem, A. (2016). What makes a charismatic speaker? A computer-based acoustic-prosodic analysis of Steve Jobs tone of voice. *Computers in Human Behavior* **64**: 366–382.

Noble, L. and Xu, Y. (2011). Friendly speech and happy speech – are they the same? In *Proceedings of the 17th International Congress of phonetic Sciences*, Hong Kong, pp. 1502–1505.

Nolan, F. (1999). The devil is in the detail. In *Proceedings of the 14th International Congress of Phonetic Sciences*, San Francisco, pp. 1–8.

O'Connor, J. D. and Arnold, G. F. (1961). *Intonation of colloquial English*. London: Longmans.

O'Malley, M. H., Kloker, D. R. and Dara-Abrams, B. (1973). Recovering parentheses from spoken algebraic expressions. *IEEE Transaction on Audio and Electroacoustics* **AU-21**: 217–220.

Odden, D. (1995). Tone: African languages. In *The handbook of phonological theory*. J. A. Goldsmith. Cambridge, MA: Blackwell, pp. 444–475.

Ohala, J. J. (1983). Cross-language uses of pitch: An ethological view. *Phonetica* **40**: 1–18.

Ohala, J. J. (1984). An ethological perspective on common cross-language utilization of F0 of voice. *Phonetica* **41**: 1–16.

Ortega-Llebaria, M. and Prieto, P. (2011). Acoustic correlates of stress in central Catalan and Castilian Spanish. *Language and Speech* **54**(00238309): 73–97.

Palmer, H. E. (1922). *English intonation, with systematic exercises*. Cambridge, MA: Heffer.

Patil, U., Kentner, G., Gollrad, A., Kügler, F., Féry, C. and Vasishth, S. (2008). Focus, word order and intonation in Hindi. *Journal of South Asian Linguistics* **1**: 55–72.

Pedersen, H. (1931). *The discovery of language: Linguistic science in the nineteenth century English,* translation by John Webster Spargo. Bloomington, IN: Indiana University Press.

Peng, S. H. (2000). Lexical versus 'phonological' representations of Mandarin Sandhi tones. In *Papers in laboratory phonology V: Acquisition and the lexicon*. M. B. Broe and J. B. Pierrehumbert. Cambridge: Cambridge University Press, pp. 152–167.

Petrone, C., Truckenbrodt, H., Wellmann, C., Holzgrefe-Lang, J., Wartenburger, I. and Höhle, B. (2017). Prosodic boundary cues in German: Evidence from the production and perception of bracketed lists. *Journal of Phonetics* **61**: 71–92.

Pham, A. H. (2003). The key phonetic properties of Vietnamese tone: A reassessment. In *Proceedings of the 15th International Congress of Phonetic Sciences*, Barcelona, pp. 1703–1706.

Pierrehumbert, J. (1980). *The phonology and phonetics of English intonation*. Ph.D. Dissertation, MIT Press, Cambridge, MA. [Published in 1987 by Indiana University Linguistics Club, Bloomington].

Pike, K. L. (1945). *The intonation of American English*. Ann Arbor, MI: University of Michigan Press.

Pike, K. L. (1948). *Tone Languages: A technique for determining the number and type of pitch contrasts in a language: With studies in tonemic substitution and fusion*. Ann Arbor, MI: University of Michigan Press.

Port, R. F., Dalby, J. and O'Dell, M. (1987). Evidence for mora timing in Japanese. *The Journal of the Acoustical Society of America* **81**: 1574–1585.

Price, P. I., Ostendorf, M., Shattuck-Hufnagel, S. and Fong, C. (1991). The use of prosody in syntactic disambiguation. *The Journal of the Acoustical Society of America* **90**: 2956–2970.

Prom-on, S., Liu, F. and Xu, Y. (2012). Post-low bouncing in Mandarin Chinese: Acoustic analysis and computational modeling. *The Journal of the Acoustical Society of America* **132**: 421–432.

Prom-on, S., Xu, Y. and Thipakorn, B. (2009). Modeling tone and intonation in Mandarin and English as a process of target approximation. *The Journal of the Acoustical Society of America* **125**(1): 405–424.

Ramus, F., Nesporb, M. and Mehlera, J. (1999). Correlates of linguistic rhythm in the speech signal. *Cognition* **73**: 265–292.

Redi, L. and Shattuck-Hufnagel, S. (2001). Variation in the realization of glottalization in normal speakers. *Journal of Phonetics* **29**: 407–429.
Remijsen, B. and Ayoker, O. G. (2014). Contrastive tonal alignment in falling contours in Shilluk. *Phonology* **31**(03): 435–462.
Rialland, A. (2009). African "lax" question prosody: Its realisations and its geographical distribution. *Lingua* **119**: 928–949.
Rialland, A. and Robert, S. (2001). The intonational system of Wolof. *Linguistics* **39**: 893–939.
Rooth, M. (1992). A theory of focus interpretation. *Natural Language Semantics* **1**(1): 75–116.
Rosenberg, A. and Hirschberg, J. (2009). Charisma perception from text and speech. *Speech Communication* **51**(7): 640–655.
Rump, H. H. and Collier, R. (1996). Focus conditions and the prominence of pitch-accented syllables. *Language and Speech* **39**: 1–17.
Russell, J. A. (1979). Affective space is bipolar. *Journal of Personality and Social Psychology* **37**(3): 345–356.
Russell, J. A. (2003). Core affect and the psychological construction of emotion. *Psychological Review* **110**: 145–172.
Sahkai, H., Kalvik, M. L. and Mihkla, M. (2013). Prosody of contrastive focus in Estonian. In *Proceedings of Interspeech 2013*, Lyon, France, pp. 315–319.
Saindon, M. R., Trehub, S. E., Schellenberg, E. G. and van Lieshout, P. H. (2017). When is a question a question for children and adults? *Language Learning and Development*, 1–12.
Salffner, S. (2010). *Tone in the phonology, lexicon and grammar of Ikaan*, Ph.D. Dissertation, SOAS, University of London.
Savino, M. (2012). The intonation of polar questions in Italian: Where is the rise? *Journal of the International Phonetic Association* **42**: 23–48.
Schafer, A. J., Speer, S. R., Warren, P. and White, D. (2000). Intonational disambiguation in sentence production and comprehension. *Journal of Psycholinguistic Research* **29**: 169–182.
Scherer, K. R. (2003). Vocal communication of emotion: A review of research paradigms. *Speech Communication* **40**: 227–256.
Scherer, K. R., Banse, R., Wallbott, H. G. and Goldbeck, T. (1991). Vocal cues in emotion encoding and decoding. *Motivation and Emotion* **15**(2): 123–148.
Scherer, K. R. and Bänziger, T. (2004). Emotional expression in prosody: A review and an agenda for future research. In *Proceedings of Speech Prosody 2004*, Nara, Japan, pp. 359–366.
Schlosberg, H. (1954). Three dimensions of emotion. *Psychological Review* **61**(2): 81.
Schuh, R. G. (1978). Tone rules. In *Tone: A linguistic survey*. V. A. Fromkin. New York: Academic Press, pp. 221–256.
Selkirk, E. O. (1980). *On prosodic structure and its relation to syntactic structure*. Bloomington: Indiana University Linguistics Club.
Selkirk, E. O. (1986). On derived domains in sentence phonology. *Phonology Yearbook* **3**: 371–405.
Shattuck-Hufnagel, S. and Turk, A. E. (1996). A prosody tutorial for investigators of auditory sentence processing. *Journal of Psycholinguistic Research* **25**(2): 193–247.
Siemund, P. (2001). Interrogative constructions. In *Language typology and language universals*. M. Haspelmath, E. König, W. Oesterreicher and W. Raible. Berlin: Walter de Gruyter, Vol. 2, pp. 1010–1028.
Sityaev, D. and House, J. (2003). Phonetic and phonological correlates of broad, narrow and contrastive focus in English. In *Proceedings of the 15th International Congress of Phonetic Sciences*, Barcelona, pp. 1819–1822.
Speer, S. R., Kjelgaard, M. M. and Dobroth, K. M. (1996). The influence of prosodic structure on the resolution of temporary syntactic closure ambiguities. *Journal of Psycholinguistic Research* **25**: 249–271.
Steedman, M. (2000). Information structure and the syntax-phonology interface. *Linguistic Inquiry* **31**: 649–689.
Steever, S. B. (1987). Tamil and the Dravidian languages. *The World's Major Languages*, 725–746.

Sugahara, M. (2005). Post-focus prosodic phrase boundaries in Tokyo Japanese: Asymmetric behavior of an f0 cue and domain-final lengthening*. *Studia Linguistica* **59**(2–3): 144–173.

Svec, J. G., Schutte, H. K. and Miller, D. G. (1999). On pitch jumps between chest and falsetto registers in voice: Data from living and excised human larynges. *The Journal of the Acoustical Society of America* **106**: 1523–1531.

Swerts, M. (1997). Prosodic features at discourse boundaries of different length. *The Journal of the Acoustical Society of America* **101**: 514–521.

Swerts, M. and Zerbian, S. (2010). Prosodic transfer in black South African English. In *Proceedings of Speech Prosody 2010*, Chicago.

Taheri-Ardali, M. and Xu, Y. (2012). Phonetic realization of prosodic focus in Persian. In *Proceedings of Speech Prosody 2012*, Shanghai, pp. 326–329.

Terken, J. and Hirschberg, J. (1994). Deaccentuation of words representing 'given' information: Effects of persistence of grammatical function and surface position. *Language and Speech* **37**(2): 125–145.

Thorsen, N. G. (1980). A study of the perception of sentence intonation – evidence from Danish. *The Journal of the Acoustical Society of America* **67**: 1014–1030.

Tiffany, W. R. (1980). The effects of syllable structure on diadochokinetic and reading rates. *Journal of Speech and Hearing Research* **23**: 894–908.

Titze, I. R. (1994). *Principles of voice production*. Englewood Cliffs, NJ: Prentice Hall.

Tsay, J. and Myers, J. (1996). Taiwanese tone sandhi as allomorph selection. In *Proceedings of 22nd Meeting of the Berkeley Linguistics Society*, Berkeley, pp. 394–405.

Umeda, N. (1975). Vowel duration in American English. *The Journal of the Acoustical Society of America* **58**(2): 434–445.

Vainio, M., Mixdorff, H., Järvikivi, J. and Werner, S. (2003). The production and perception of focus in Finnish. In *Proceedings of 15th International Congress of Phonetic Sciences (ICPhS) 2003*, Barcelona, pp. 1831–1834.

van Heuven, V. J. and de Jonge, M. (2011). Spectral and temporal reduction as stress cues in Dutch. *Phonetica* **68**(3): 120–132.

van Heuven, V. J. and Haan, J. (2000). Phonetic correlates of statement versus question intonation in Dutch. In *Intonation*. Dordrecht: Springer, pp. 119–143.

van Santen, J. P. H., Kain, A., Klabbers, E. and Mishra, T. (2005). Synthesis of prosody using multi-level unit sequences. *Speech Communication* **46**: 365–375.

van Santen, J. P. H. and Shih, C. (2000). Suprasegmental and segmental timing models in Mandarin Chinese and American English. *The Journal of the Acoustical Society of America* **107**: 1012–1026.

Wagner, M. (2005). *Prosody and recursion*. Ph.D. Dissertation, Massachusetts Institute of Technology.

Wang, B., Wang, L. and Qadir, T. (2011). Prosodic encoding of focus in six languages in China. In *Proceedings of the 17th International Congress of Phonetic Sciences*, Hong Kong, pp. 144–147.

Wang, B., Xu, Y. and Ding, Q. (2018). Interactive prosodic marking of focus, boundary and newness in Mandarin. *Phonetica* **75**(1): 24–56.

Wang, L., Wang, B. and Xu, Y. (2012). Prosodic encoding and perception of focus in Tibetan (Anduo Dialect). In *Proceedings of Speech Prosody 2012*, Shanghai, pp. 286–289.

Wang, W. S. Y. and Li, K. P. (1967). Tone 3 in Pekinese. *Journal of Speech and Hearing Research* **10**: 629–636.

Warner, N. and Arai, T. (2001). Japanese mora-timing: A review. *Phonetica* **58**: 1–25.

Wightman, C. W., Shattuck-Hufnagel, S., Ostendorf, M. and Price, P. J. (1992). Segmental durations in the vicinity of prosodic phrase boundaries. *The Journal of the Acoustical Society of America* **91**(3): 1707–1717.

Williams, C. E. and Stevens, K. N. (1972). Emotion and speech: Some acoustical correlates. *The Journal of the Acoustical Society of America* **52**: 1238–1250.

Wong, Y. W. (2006a). Contextual tonal variations and pitch targets in Cantonese. In *Proceedings of Speech Prosody 2006*, Dresden, Germany, PS3–13–199.

Wong, Y. W. (2006b). Realization of Cantonese rising tones under different speaking rates. In *Proceedings of Speech Prosody 2006*, Dresden, Germany, PS3–14–198.

Wu, W. L. and Chung, L. (2011). Post-focus compression in English-Cantonese bilingual speakers. In *Proceedings of the 17th International Congress of Phonetic Sciences*, Hong Kong, pp. 148–151.

Wu, W. L. and Xu, Y. (2010). Prosodic focus in Hong Kong Cantonese without post-focus compression. In *Proceedings of Speech Prosody 2010*, Chicago.

Xu, C. X. and Xu, Y. (2003). Effects of consonant aspiration on Mandarin tones. *Journal of the International Phonetic Association* **33**: 165–181.

Xu, Y. (1997). Contextual tonal variations in Mandarin. *Journal of Phonetics* **25**: 61–83.

Xu, Y. (1998). Consistency of tone-syllable alignment across different syllable structures and speaking rates. *Phonetica* **55**: 179–203.

Xu, Y. (1999). Effects of tone and focus on the formation and alignment of F0 contours. *Journal of Phonetics* **27**: 55–105.

Xu, Y. (2001). Fundamental frequency peak delay in Mandarin. *Phonetica* **58**: 26–52.

Xu, Y. (2005). Speech melody as articulatorily implemented communicative functions. *Speech Communication* **46**: 220–251.

Xu, Y. (2009). Timing and coordination in tone and intonation – an articulatory-functional perspective. *Lingua* **119**(6): 906–927.

Xu, Y. (2011). Post-focus compression: Cross-linguistic distribution and historical origin. In *Proceedings of the 17th International Congress of Phonetic Sciences*, Hong Kong, pp. 152–155.

Xu, Y. and Kelly, A. (2010). Perception of anger and happiness from resynthesized speech with size-related manipulations. In *Proceedings of Speech Prosody 2010*, Chicago.

Xu, Y., Kelly, A. and Smillie, C. (2013a). Emotional expressions as communicative signals. In *Prosody and iconicity*. S. Hancil and D. Hirst. Philadelphia: John Benjamins Publishing Co., pp. 33–60.

Xu, Y., Lee, A., Wu, W. L., Liu, X. and Birkholz, P. (2013b). Human vocal attractiveness as signaled by body size projection. *PLoS One* **8**(4): e62397.

Xu, Y. and Prom-on, S. (2014). Toward invariant functional representations of variable surface fundamental frequency contours: Synthesizing speech melody via model-based stochastic learning. *Speech Communication* **57**: 181–208.

Xu, Y. and Sun, X. (2002). Maximum speed of pitch change and how it may relate to speech. *The Journal of the Acoustical Society of America* **111**: 1399–1413.

Xu, Y. and Wallace, A. (2004). Multiple effects of consonant manner of articulation and intonation type on F0 in English. *The Journal of the Acoustical Society of America* **115**(Pt. 2): 2397.

Xu, Y. and Wang, M. (2009). Organizing syllables into groups – evidence from F0 and duration patterns in Mandarin. *Journal of Phonetics* **37**: 502–520.

Xu, Y. and Wang, Q. E. (2001). Pitch targets and their realization: Evidence from Mandarin Chinese. *Speech Communication* **33**: 319–337.

Xu, Y. and Xu, C. X. (2005). Phonetic realization of focus in English declarative intonation. *Journal of Phonetics* **33**: 159–197.

Yang, Y. and Wang, B. (2002). Acoustic correlates of hierarchical prosodic boundary in Mandarin. In *Proceedings of Speech Prosody 2002*, Aix-en-Provence, France, pp. 707–710.

Yip, M. (1989). Contour tones. *Phonology* **6**: 149–174.

Yip, M. (2002). *Tone*. Cambridge: Cambridge University Press.

Yip, M. (2004). Phonological markedness and allomorph selection in Zahao. *Language and Linguistics* **5**: 969–1001.

Zemlin, W. R. (1998). *Speech and hearing science: Anatomy and physiology* (4th edition). Needham Heights, MA: Allyn & Bacon.

Zerbian, S. (2010). Developments in the study of intonational typology. *Language and Linguistics Compass* **4**(9): 874–889.

Zerbian, S., Genzel, S. and Kügler, F. (2010). Experimental work on prosodically-marked information structure in selected African languages (Afroasiatic and Niger-Congo). In *Proceedings of Speech Prosody 2010*, Chicago, pp. 1–4.

Zhang, J. (2014). Tones, tonal phonology, and tone sandhi. *The Handbook of Chinese Linguistics*, 443–464.

Zheng, X. (2006). Voice quality variation with tone and focus in Mandarin. In *Proceedings of the 2nd International Symposium on Tonal Aspects of Languages*, La Rochelle, France, pp. 139–143.

Zsiga, E. and Nitisaroj, R. (2007). Tone features, tone perception, and peak alignment in Thai. *Language and Speech* **50**(3): 343–383.

Part IV
Linguistic/perceptual phonetics

13

The interface between phonetics and phonology

John Kingston

Introduction

An easy place to begin a discussion of the interface between phonetics and phonology is with the *speech chain*, a phrase introduced by Denes and Pinson (1963) to describe the series of transformations a spoken message undergoes from its origin in the mind of the speaker to its destination in the mind of the listener. There appear to be at least two interfaces in this chain, the first between the phonological representation of the speaker's intended message and its realization in their articulations, and the second between the auditory qualities evoked by the speech signal's acoustics and the phonological representation that the listener recognizes. One might imagine that there are also two others, between the articulations and the acoustics of the speech signal and between the acoustics and the auditory qualities they evoke, but they are more properly *transductions* than interfaces because the natures of these transformations are entirely predictable from the physics, physiology, and psychology of the vocal and auditory apparatus. Figure 13.1 shows three representations of the most accessible link in this chain, the acoustic speech signal itself, its phonetic transcription (Figure 13.1a), the waveform (Figure 13.1b), and the spectrogram (Figure 13.1c). The phonetic transcription includes some more detail than the phonological representation (Figure 13.1d), but clearly corresponds more closely to it than to either representation of the utterance's acoustics (Figure 13.1b,c).

Indeed, if one were to compare this rather detailed phonetic transcription of this rather hyperarticulated one-syllable word with the corresponding waveform or spectrogram, one would be immediately struck with how difficult it is to identify the correspondences between the discrete units of the transcription and the intervals and continuous acoustic properties of the waveform or spectrogram. The features and their values in the phonological representation of that word (Figure 13.1d) correspond even less well to the waveform's or spectrogram's intervals and acoustic properties. Correspondences between phonetic transcriptions or phonological representations would be equally hard to detect in a record of the articulatory movements that produced the acoustic signal displayed in the waveform and spectrogram, or in a record of the neural responses to the acoustic properties of that signal in the auditory system. And even though the processes that operate on or the constraints that

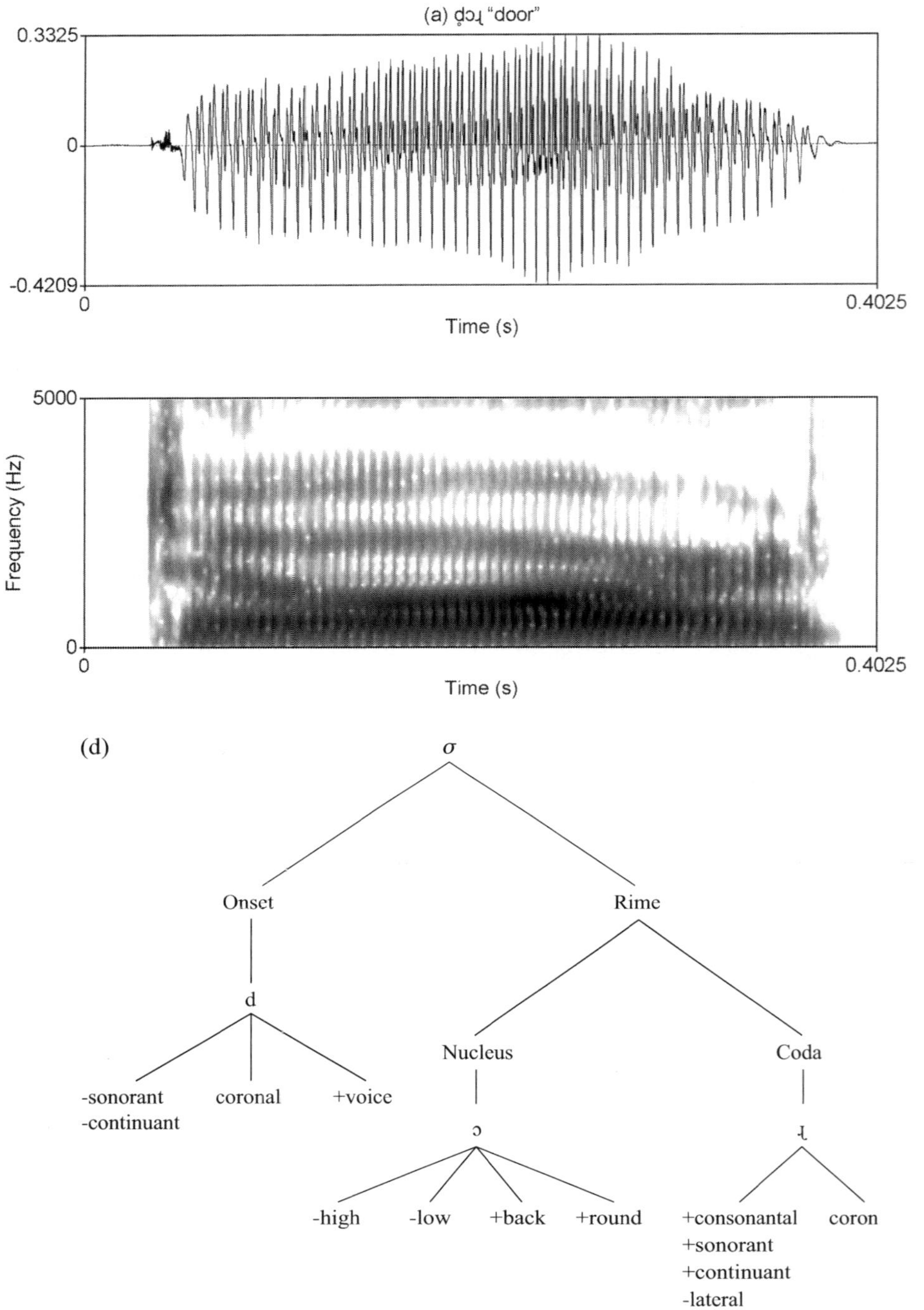

Figure 13.1 (a) Narrow phonetic transcription of *door* as pronounced by the author, the corresponding waveform (b) and spectrogram (c), and its phonological representation (d).

regulate the contents of phonological representations may be motivated by the continuous articulatory, acoustic, or auditory properties of speech, those processes or constraints refer to their constituent segments and features as discrete units.[1] If phonological and phonetic representations nonetheless differ in kind like this, then mechanisms are needed to accomplish two translations. The first translation is from the categories of the speaker's message to the utterance's articulatory continuum, and the second is from the auditory continuum to the categories of the listener's recognition of the message's phonological content. At a minimum, the actual translation mechanism(s) would serve as or mark the interface(s) between the phonology of an utterance and its phonetics.

This description of possible differences between phonological and phonetic representations is amplified in Pierrehumbert's (1990) catalogue. Phonological representations are in the mind, where they constitute a part of speakers' and listeners' implicit linguistic knowledge, differences between them are qualitative, and the rules and constraints that specify phonological well-formedness are syntactic, in specifying combinations and structural arrangements of discrete, symbolic categories. Phonetic representations are events in the world, differences between them are quantitative, and the gradient relationships between their constituents are expressed in calculus.[2] The difference is also often characterized as one of knowing versus doing, where the phonology of a language represents what its speakers and listeners know about its sounds and the patterns they enter into, and its phonetics represents the behaviors of those speakers and listeners when actually producing or perceiving speech. Both this distinction between knowledge and behavior and this equation of phonology with knowledge and phonetics with behavior are, however, challenged by a number of scholars whose proposals are discussed in the following.

If the phonetic representations of utterances whose phonological representations differ in their values for just one distinctive feature were instead compared, then it would be possible to observe phonetic correspondences to phonological contrasts, at least within individual languages in specified contexts. For example, the spectrograms of *tore* and *bore* in Figures 13.2a,b differ from that of *door* in Figure 13.1c in ways that correspond systematically to their different specifications for voicing and place of articulation contrasts, e.g., the long delay between the stop burst and the onset of voicing in *tore* compared to the negligible delay in "door," and the far lower onset of the second formant in *bore* compared to the noticeably higher onset in *door*. These correspondences can, however, be produced by a mechanism that translates the categorical differences between minimally contrasting phonological representations into the phonetic realization of these contrasts as systematically different articulatory movements and one that translates systematically different auditory qualities back into categorical contrasts.[3]

Before presenting evidence in 4 "There is an interface between phonetics and phonology" for a more substantive interface between phonology and phonetics than (a) mere translation mechanism(s), I will first sketch three rather different arguments against there being any substantive interface between phonology and phonetics in the following section.

Three arguments that there is no interface between phonology and phonetics

Here, I present and evaluate three proposals that there is no interface between phonetics and phonology. The first such proposal integrates the direct realist theory of speech perception

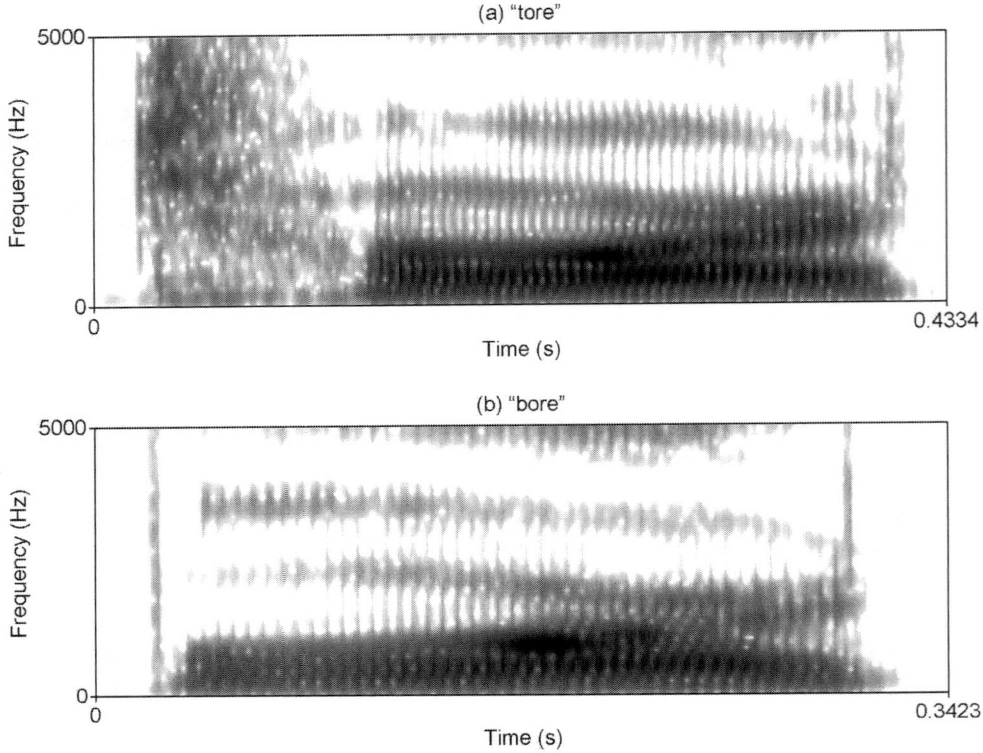

Figure 13.2 Spectrograms of (a) *tore* and (b) *bore*.

(Fowler, 1986a, 1986b) with articulatory phonology (Browman & Goldstein, 1986, 1989, 1992, 1995a; Gafos & Goldstein, 2012; Goldstein & Fowler, 2003), in which the constituents of phonological representations in both the speaker's and listener's minds are articulatory gestures, specifying the location and degree of vocal tract constrictions and their relative coordination or timing. The second consists of an argument that phonological representations have no phonetic substance, nor do the rules or constraints that operate on or regulate them refer to any phonetic substance (Hale & Reiss, 2000, 2008). This argument has two parts. First, the constituents of phonological representations must be purely formal objects, and the rules and constraints that refer to them must be strictly syntactic, as Pierrehumbert (1990) proposed earlier. Second, independent theories of speakers', listeners', and learners' behavior are needed anyway, so it is theoretically extravagant to incorporate phonetics into phonology. The third proposal turns this second argument on its head by insisting that the phonology is so thoroughly entwined with the physiology, physics, and psychology of movement, aerodynamics, acoustics, and audition that it cannot be separated from the phonetics. Phonological patterns and phonetic behavior also cannot be accounted for without appealing to general theories of pattern recognition, memory, and learning (Ohala, 1990, 2005). More modestly, perhaps, phonetic continua may be incorporated directly into phonological grammars (Flemming, 2001). The first of these arguments against any interface between phonetics and phonology asserts that only the world exists, while the last two arguments either deny any connection between phonology and the world or insist that phonology cannot be taken out of the world.

No interface is needed (or possible)

The first argument that there is no interface between phonology and phonetics rests on a perhaps unfamiliar and certainly underappreciated approach to theorizing about speech production and perception. This approach is motivated by the idea that both speakers' and listeners' behavior can be understood entirely by observing what they do in and receive from the world, and that it is therefore unnecessary to hypothesize that what speakers do as speakers is implement a representation whose constituents differ in kind from their actualization as acts of speaking or that listeners map the acoustic properties of the speech signal unto such representations. This idea in turn motivates arguments in Fowler (1986a, 1986b) that there can be no interface between phonology and phonetics, because, if there is a phonology, it cannot be distinguished from the phonetics. Her argument is laid out programmatically in these two quotes:

> The essential modification is to our conceptualization of the relation between knowing and doing. First, phonetic segments as we know them can only have properties that can be realized in articulation. Indeed, from an event perspective, the primary reality of a phonetic segment is its public realization as vocal-tract activity. What we know of segments, we know from hearing them produced by other talkers or by producing them ourselves. Secondly, the idea that speech production involves a translation from a mental domain into a physical, non-mental domain such as the vocal tract must be discarded.
>
> *(Fowler, 1986a, pp. 9–10)*

> In a "bottom-up" account of perceiving speech, a listener has to reconstruct the talker's mental intent from hints that the physical acoustic signal provides. In a "top-down" account, that bottom-up effort is aided by cognitive mediation. In a top-down account of talking, talkers use a mental plan to guide physical gestures of the vocal tract. In all three accounts (i.e., the bottom-up and top-down accounts of speech perception and the top-down account of speech production) there is a causal process transforming input or outputs into or out of a mental domain from or to a physical domain. This is an impossible kind of process. Theories of speech production use a conceptual slight of hand known as the "motor command" to make the translation (Fowler, 1983). It is a sleight of hand because commands are clearly mental kinds of things that a mind can formulate, but the "commands" are obeyed by motor neurons that are physical kinds of things responsive to release of a transmitter substance, not to commands. A workable theory of production and perception has to avoid translation across domains like this.
>
> *(Fowler, 1986b, pp. 168–169)*

Knowing does not differ from doing, or alternatively, what's in the mind is what's in the world, for speakers or listeners. While making clear that Fowler rejects any translation between mental and physical representations, these quotes also appear to convey that she is concerned only with the phonetics of speech. They might, therefore, reasonably prompt the question: where is the phonology in either of these pronouncements?

This appearance is misleading. To see this, we must distinguish between two kinds of information: information about the content of the speaker's message versus information about the articulatory gestures that the speaker produces to convey the message's content. In more familiar conceptions of a phonological representation, the information about the content of the speaker's message is encoded in the phonological representation, in its constituent phonemes or their constituent features and in their arrangement with respect to one another. And the speaker's articulatory gestures are intended to convey that information to the listener, who has to decode it from the acoustic properties of the speech signal produced by those articulatory gestures. In this conception, the information changes form or is represented differently at each stage in the speech chain between the speaker and listener until its original form in the speaker's phonological representation is reconstituted in the listener's phonological representation. But despite its formal differences, it is nonetheless the same information at all stages in the speech chain. Fowler (1986a, pp. 23–24) instead argues, following Gibson (1982), that information about the speaker's articulatory gestures is different from information about the contents of the speaker's message, because information about articulatory gestures is perceived *directly* from the acoustic properties of the speech signal, while information about the contents of the speaker's message is instead perceived *indirectly*, as a product of the direct perception of those gestures.

It's worth noting that distinguishing between two kinds of information in this way is entirely compatible with the consensus that the meaning of a linguistic utterance is arbitrarily related to its form. In the view of Fowler (1986a, 1986b), theories of speech production and perception, as theories of these behaviors, are responsible for explaining how speakers produce forms that listeners recognize as forms, and not for how speech production and perception contribute to conveying the content of the speaker's message to the listener.

Contemporaneous work by Browman and Goldstein (1986) can be viewed as taking up the task of developing an account of phonological representations that is compatible with this view. Browman and Goldstein (1986, et seq.) proposed that the articulatory gestures that speakers produce, and that, according to Fowler (1986a, 1986b), listeners perceive, are also the constituents of the utterance's phonological representation – their proposal is known as "articulatory phonology." As such, articulatory gestures represent as well as convey the speaker's message in just the same, arbitrary way as do the abstract features of a phonological representation like that in Figure 13.1d (see Gafos & Goldstein, 2012; Goldstein & Fowler, 2003, for an explicit argument that representations composed of articulatory gestures are functionally and combinatorically equivalent to representations composed of features). Browman and Goldstein's (1986) proposal thus takes Fowler's argument one essential step further, in also spelling out the relationship between the form of a linguistic message and the meaning that it conveys, i.e., what is indirectly perceived as well as what is directly perceived.

Browman and Goldstein's (1986) proposal nonetheless raises a further question: are the constituents of the phonological representation of an utterance detectable in and identifiable from a record of the speaker's articulatory movements after all, and are they equally detectable in and identifiable from a record of the acoustic properties produced by those movements, as displayed, e.g., in Figures 13.1b,c and 13.2a,b? For Fowler (1986a, 1986b), these are the wrong questions; the right one is instead: can listeners find information in the acoustic signal produced by these articulations that reliably identifies the articulatory gestures which produced those properties? The pervasiveness of coarticulation, which can extend beyond immediately adjacent segments, and reduction, which can in the limit make it impossible to detect an intended segment's occurrence, encourages a skeptical if not an outright negative answer to this question. Fowler nonetheless answers it in the affirmative, and in doing so appears to reject Hockett's (1955) famous description of the phonetic realization of an utterance as the uninterpretable destruction its phonological representation:

> Imagine a row of Easter eggs traveling along a moving belt; the eggs are of various sizes, and variously colored, but not boiled. At a certain point, the belt carries the row of eggs between the two rollers of a wringer, which quite effectively smash them

> and rub them more or less into each other. The flow of eggs before the wringer represents the series of impulses from the phoneme source; the mess that emerges from the wringer represents the output of the speech transmitter. At a subsequent point, we have an inspector whose task it is to examine the passing mess and decide, on the basis of the broken and unbroken yolks, the variously spread-out albumen, and the variously colored bits of shell, the nature of the flow of eggs which previously arrived at the wringer. Note that he does not have to put the eggs together again – a manifest physical impossibility – but only to identify.
>
> *(Hockett, 1955, p. 210)*

This passage's implied pessimism about the likelihood of the inspector – acknowledged as the hearer in the following passage – successfully identifying the phonemic sources of the phonetic mess is actually misleading. Hockett goes on to propose that the inspector/hearer may succeed after all if they treat the allophones of successive phonemes as overlapping in time, and parse each phoneme's contribution to the signal's acoustic properties during the interval when they overlap (see Fowler & Smith, 1986, for a very similar account). As Hockett ultimately does, Fowler (1986a, 1986b) argues that the phonetic realization does not destroy the phonological representation, despite the overlap of the articulations of successive speech sounds.

The argument in Fowler (1986a, 1986b) that representations in the mind are not translated into a different kind of representation in the world appears to rule out any interface, and any need for one. However, some sort of interface is still needed after all to handle the overlap and context-specific variation of articulations and their acoustic products. For that interface between the phonological representation and its phonetic realization to be nondestructive, the articulatory gestures must still be detectable and identifiable in the acoustic signal, at least by the listener, even if not so easily by the phonetician. An interface that is supposed to preserve the detection and identification of articulatory gestures is the task dynamics (Kelso, Saltzman, & Tuller, 1986a, 1986b; Saltzman, 1995; Saltzman & Kelso, 1987; Saltzman & Munhall, 1989). The following description relies principally on Saltzman and Munhall (1989).

To understand how the task dynamics serves as an interface between discrete articulatory gestures and continuous articulatory movements, we must first describe articulatory gestures more precisely. An articulatory gesture is itself a dynamical system, one defined by the goal that it is intended to achieve, for example, to close the lips. These goals don't vary across contexts nor depending on what other goals must be achieved at the same time, rather the articulatory movements that achieve them do. Thus, closing the lips may require more jaw raising following the open vowel in /æp, æb, æm/ than following the closed vowel in /ip, ib, im/. Goals are specified as values for context-independent dynamical parameters that specify the gesture's target, the speed of approach to and away from the target, and the extent to which the gesture controls articulations moment-by-moment over the course of its realization. Individual speech sounds – the "phonetic segments" referred to by Fowler (1986a, 1986b) – consist of gestures whose beginnings and ends are sufficiently contemporaneous that they shape the vocal tract and its acoustic products more or less simultaneously, while successive speech sounds consist of gestures and thus articulations and acoustic products that overlap less in time.

Regardless of how extensive the overlap is, the movements of the various articulators that could contribute to realizing the targets of contemporaneously active gestures must be coordinated and their relative contributions adjusted so that each gesture's target is reached. The kinematics of articulatory movements will thus differ within individual speech sounds and between successive speech sounds, depending on what demands temporally overlapping gestures make on articulators at any moment in time. An example of such variation between contrasting speech sounds is differences between voiced and voiceless stops in the articulatory adjustments needed to manage their contrasting aerodynamic regimes: the oral cavity must be expanded during the closure of a voiced stop to keep oral air pressure from building up so fast that air no longer flows up through the glottis, but greater force is required to maintain the closure of a voiceless stop because the open glottis causes intraoral air pressure to build up more behind it. An example of such variation between successive speech sounds is differences between vowels before voiceless stops compared to before voiced stops or sonorants, where the mouth may not open as far during the vowel in /æp/ as it does in /æb/ or /æm/, because the following lip-closing gesture overlaps more with the vowel and requires that the jaw be raised earlier (but cf. Summers, 1987, for evidence of faster and larger jaw opening before a voiceless than a voiced stop), and the velum may be lowered more or earlier in /æm/ than it is in /im/ to ensure that the open vowel is nasalized enough for that property to be detected (Kingston & Macmillan, 1995; Macmillan, Kingston, Thorburn, Walsh Dickey, & Bartels, 1999).[4] The task dynamics ensures that the gestures' dynamics remain invariant, and the gestures themselves thus remain detectable and identifiable, while permitting the articulators' kinematics to vary within individual speech sounds and between successive speech sounds.

The task dynamics is a genuine interface between a phonological representation consisting of goal-directed articulatory gestures and its phonetic realization as articulatory movements, which takes the time- and context-invariant dynamic parameters' values of the gestures as inputs and outputs the time- and context-varying kinematic properties of actual articulatory movements. But the task dynamics is not an interface that *translates* between one kind of representation and another, but instead one that *transduces* the continuous quantities represented by those dynamic parameters as continuous movements with temporal and spatial kinematics.

This discussion has focused so far on getting from articulatory gestures to movements of articulators. Before closing, it is worthwhile to recognize subsequent developments of the proposal that phonological representations are composed of articulatory gestures that specify goals, not articulator movements, and to note that representing the constituents of speech sounds phonologically as gestures does not differ as much as one might expect from representing them as autosegments. Developments in articulatory phonology show that it accounts very differently for at least: (a) fast speech phenomena – gestures are overlapped and their acoustics obscured by or mixed with those of neighboring sounds rather than sounds deleting or assimilating to neighboring sounds (Browman & Goldstein, 1990), (b) incomplete neutralization of contrasts – the input consists of the articulatory gestures for both the neutralized and unneutralized goals, with the former greater in strength than the latter in neutralizing contexts (Gafos, 2006, see also Smolensky and Goldrick (2016) for a generalization of this approach to any case where more than one phonological element is activated simultaneously during phonetic implementation),[5] (c) syllable structure – the gestures of the consonants in onsets can be coordinated with those of the nuclear vowel differently than the gestures of consonants in codas (Browman & Goldstein, 1988), and languages can differ in how consonants in onsets or codas are coordinated with one another (Hosung, Goldstein, & Saltzman, 2009; Shaw, Gafos,

Hoole, & Zeroual, 2009, 2011), and (d) speech errors – errors are coproductions of the intended gesture and an intruded one rather than whole segment intrusions (Goldstein, Pouplier, Chen, Saltzman, & Byrd, 2007; Pouplier & Goldstein, 2010). Phonological representations composed of articulatory gestures differ from those composed of autosegments in lacking any correspondent to a timing unit or superordinate prosodic unit. But time remained as abstract as in autosegmental representations, until the recent development of more explicit dynamical models incorporating time explicitly (Roon & Gafos, 2016).

Do phonological representations have any phonetic substance?

Instead of arguing that there is no interface between phonology and phonetics because phonological representations cannot and must not be distinguished from their phonetic realizations, Hale and Reiss (2000, 2008), Morén (2007), and Reiss (2017) argue that there is no interface other than translation or transduction from phonological categories to phonetic continua. In their view, neither the form of phonological representations nor the processes operating on them are regulated by the phonetic substance of the speech sounds that realize those representations and processes. The argument has two parts. In the first, these authors argue that what appears to be evidence of phonetic regulation of phonological representations and processes must instead be interpreted as evidence that phonetic substance influences language learning and/or language change. There is thus no need to duplicate the account of that diachronic or ontogenetic influence in the synchronic phonological grammar, nor should such duplication be permitted by phonological theory. In the second part, they argue that phonological theory is responsible only for defining "the set of *computationally possible* human grammars" (Hale & Reiss, 2000, p. 162, emphasis in the original), because that definition would be a step toward explaining the phonological competence that exists in the mind of the speaker.[6] The two parts of this argument turn out to be inseparable at present because there is debate about whether computationally possible grammars must include constraints or other formal devices that are motivated by the phonetic substance of speech and/or by the learning of a language's phonology (for discussion, see Bermúdez-Otero & Börjars, 2006, and see the discussion of Beguš (2017); Hayes (1999) later in this chapter). Nonetheless, the discussion that follows addresses only the first part of this argument, as developed in Hale and Reiss (2000), because only it addresses the nature or existence of any interface between phonology and phonetics.

Hale and Reiss (2000) begin their argument for eliminating phonetic substance from phonological representations and the rules and constraints that refer to those representations by attributing contextually constrained contrasts to acquisition and language change. Beckman (1997) accounted for some of these phenomena as instances of positional faithfulness.[7] Sounds contrast for a feature in some but not all contexts in a language when an identity constraint (IDENT[FEATURE]$_{\text{SPECIFIC}}$) requiring faithful preservation of input feature values in specific contexts outranks a markedness constraint (*FEATURE) that would rule out that specification, which in turn outranks a more general faithfulness constraint preserving that specification everywhere: IDENT[FEATURE]$_{\text{SPECIFIC}}$ >> *FEATURE >> IDENT[FEATURE]$_{\text{GENERAL}}$.

If the language permits the contrast everywhere, IDENT[FEATURE]$_{\text{GENERAL}}$ >> *FEATURE and IDENT[FEATURE]$_{\text{SPECIFIC}}$ can be ranked anywhere, and if it permits it nowhere, *FEATURE >> IDENT[FEATURE]$_{\text{GENERAL}}$, IDENT[FEATURE]$_{\text{SPECIFIC}}$. The distribution of the [voice] contrast in Thai,

English, and Creek represent the three possibilities: in Thai, /b, d/ con-trast with /p, t/ in syllable onsets but not codas, in English, they contrast in codas as well as onsets, and in Creek, there is no [voice] contrast in any position:

1 Language-specific distributions of the [voice] contrast:

a. Thai: IDENT[VOICE]$_{ONSET}$ >> *VOICE >> IDENT[VOICE]
b. English: (IDENT[VOICE]$_{ONSET}$), IDENT[VOICE] >> *VOICE, (IDENT[VOICE]$_{ONSET}$)
c. Creek: *VOICE >> IDENT[VOICE]$_{ONSET}$, IDENT[VOICE]

Beckman's (1997) account explicitly appeals to the substance of the utterance because the possible specific contexts are psycholinguistically prominent and/or phonetically salient, e.g., at the beginning of a word or syllable or in a stressed syllable. Hale and Reiss (2000) observe that the psycholinguistically prominent or phonetically salient contexts in which a contrast is preserved are those where its phonetic correlates are either more likely to be attended to, e.g., in the first syllables of words or the onsets of syllables, or easier to detect because their values are more extreme, e.g., in stressed syllables. Attention and detection are less likely and/or harder in other contexts. A child learning the language might therefore fail to attend to or detect a contrast's correlates in those other contexts. If these failures become general, the language would change into one where the contrast is preserved only in contexts where its correlates are reliably attended to or detected, and the contrast would be restricted synchronically to those contexts. This restriction would be explained by the merger in other contexts resulting from earlier generations' failure to learn the yet earlier language where this contrast appeared in all contexts, not by encoding the restriction as an active constraint in the synchronic phonological grammar (see Blevins, 2004, for a generalization of this proposal regarding the division of explanatory labor between psycholinguistically or phonetically motivated sound change and the contents of the synchronic grammars of individual languages).[8]

On these grounds, Hale and Reiss (2000) argue that there is no practical difference between the experience of a child learning a language like German in which the voicing contrast is restricted to onsets and one learning a language like English in which this contrast is not restricted to any position in the syllable. The child learning German will never encounter voiced obstruents in syllable codas, while the one learning English will encounter numerous examples of voiced obstruents in codas.[9] Both children will receive far more than enough positive evidence regarding the distribution of voiced obstruents for them to successfully learn the contextual distribution of the voicing contrast in their respective languages (again, see Blevins, 2004, for a more general argument that positive evidence is more than enough to inform the learner about what sounds a language has, and how they behave, without requiring that the resulting synchronic grammar consist of anything more than a description of those sounds and their behavior).

This and other similar arguments lead Hale and Reiss (2000) to conclude that,

> Phonology is not and should not be grounded in phonetics since the facts that phonetic grounding is meant to explain can be derived without reference to *phonology*. Duplication of the principles of acoustics and acquisition inside the grammar violates Occam's razor and thus must be avoided. Only in this way will we be able to correctly characterize the univeral aspects of phonological computation.
>
> *(p. 162, emphasis in the original)*

and a bit later,

> The goal of phonological theory, as a branch of cognitive science, is to categorize what is a computationally possible phonology, given the computational nature of the phonological component of UG.
>
> *(p. 163)*

where "computationally possible" is to be contrasted with "diachronically possible" and "ontogenetically possible." The latter are the (much smaller?) set of phonological grammars that can develop over time and that are learnable given psycholinguistic and phonetic constraints. The following two, surprisingly similar cases serve as illustrations (see Browman & Goldstein, 1995b, for further discussion of their similarity). Krakow (1989, 1999) shows that soft palate lowering begins earlier than the oral constriction in a syllable-final nasal like that in *seam E*,[10] and as a result the preceding vowel is nasalized. In a syllable-initial nasal like that in *see me*, soft palate lowering and the oral constriction begin and end more or less at the same time, and neither preceding nor following vowels are nasalized. Sproat and Fujimura (1993) show that the raising of the tongue tip toward the alveolar ridge in a syllable-final lateral like that in *Mr. Beel Hikkovsky* is delayed relative to the dorsal constriction at the uvula, and as a result the rime is a diphthong with an ɰ-like offglide. In a syllable-initial lateral like that in *Mr. B. Likkovsky*, the tongue tip raising and the dorsal constriction begin and end more or less at the same time. The results reported in both studies come entirely from English speakers, but if these timing patterns are shared with other languages, then distinctive vowel nasalization is more likely to develop before syllable-final than syllable-initial nasals, and a syllable-final lateral is more likely to develop into the offglide of a diphthong than a syllable-initial lateral. Both likelihood differences appear to be borne out in what language changes are observed versus unobserved.

But there is no computational reason why a speech community or language learner could not ignore these psycholinguistic and phonetic facts and nasalize a vowel after a syllable-initial nasal or turn a syllable-initial lateral into a velar glide. de Lacy and Kingston (2013) make an analogous argument, that a theory of phonology *sensu strictu* is not responsible for accounting for how often particular sounds or sound patterns occur, as both may be accounted for more perspicuously by an appropriate account of language learning or learnability (see also Staubs, 2014). Blanket appeals to greater learnability must be made cautiously, however, as there is experimental evidence that other criteria may outweigh ease of learning. For example, Rafferty, Griffiths, and Ettlinger (2013) show that an artificial language exhibiting vowel harmony is more successfully learned than one that does not, but that vowel harmony disappears when the language is transmitted across generations of learners.

Once again, the essential difference here is between computationally possible and diachronically or ontogenetically probable languages. The computationally possible languages include those that have entirely arbitrary phonological rules (AKA "crazy" rules (Bach & Harms, 1972); see also (Blust, 2005)). Such rules are diachronically or ontogenetically improbable. Hale and Reiss (2000, 2008) and Reiss (2017) see the learnability of arbitrary rules as a feature rather than a bug, in that arbitrary rules or constraints are computationally possible. On the one hand, this argument is supported by the fact the languages spoken today, and the much smaller subset of which we have adequate descriptions, are surely only a subset of what's a possible human language and thus of what are computationally possible phonological grammars. On the other hand, it hasn't been demonstrated yet that the set of possible languages is equal to the set of those that are computationally possible, nor what are the limits on computational possibility. One needs to know what the primitives may be, and how they may be operated on, and how the patterns they enter into may be constrained. For recent useful discussions of and commentary on a range of possibilities, see Heinz and Idsardi's (2017) introduction to a special issue of *Phonology* on computational phonology and the other papers in that special issue. Their introduction and that special issue show that the computational approaches to phonology are still refreshingly diverse in the computational tools used, the standards of evidence and argument applied, and in the data considered. Heinz (to appear) and related work consist of tests of the formal limits of possible phonological constraints and operations, and thus on determining what the set of possible phonologies are within limits of greater or lesser strictness. In trying to determine how strict these limits are, this work proceeds by examining the range of E-languages rather than assuming that the possible formal contents of I-languages can be decided *a priori*. Moreover, the possible representations and operations are of quite general types, and thus the limits considered are based on entirely different criteria than those imposed by Hale and Reiss (2000, 2008) or Reiss (2017).

Hasty decisions about how to analyze a particular set of facts and the lack of caution they entail can also lead to error. A telling example is the one that Hale and Reiss cite, intervocalic /r/-insertion in Massachusetts English, as an case of an arbitrary rule. It was described as such in McCarthy's (1993) original account of its behavior, but findings reported by Gick (2002) suggest that it's instead well-motivated phonetically. Gick shows that /r/, or more precisely its English approximant pronunciation [ɹ], is the expected glide after the vowels where it's inserted, /a, ɔ, ɘ/, because it resembles those vowels in being produced with a pharyngeal constriction. Inserting /r/ after these vowels is thus just as expected on phonetic grounds as inserting /j/ and /w/ after /i,e/ and /u,o/, respectively. While this case shows that rules which have been supposed to be arbitrary can turn out to phonetically motivated after all, and therefore motivate reexamination of other supposedly arbitrary rules, it does not rule out the possibility that a residue of genuinely arbitrary rules may remain (see, once again, Bach & Harms, 1972, for possible examples).

There is no phonology without phonetics nor phonetics without phonology

Rather than arguing that phonetics must be kept out of phonology, Ohala (1990) argues that it cannot be kept out. He also argues that there can be no interface between phonetics and phonology, because describing their relationship as or via an interface incorrectly assumes that they are two "domains." In one conception of the interface, one domain is phonology, the other phonetics, which meet "where phonological representations become implemented physically." In another conception, phonology and phonetics are "largely autonomous disciplines whose subject matters may be similar . . . but which [are studied] in different ways; there is an area in between [the interface: JK] where the two can cooperate" (p. 153). In place of an interface, Ohala proposes instead a thorough integration of phonetics and phonology, first as a superior account of their actual relationship,

> it will be impossible to characterize either discipline as autonomous or independent. If it boils down to a kind of "phonology = knowing" vs. "phonetics = doing" dichotomy, the knowledge – of units, distinctive features, etc. – is acquired and updated by complex phonetic analysis. . . . There is a growing literature showing that phonological units and processes are what they are largely due to the physical and physiological structure of the speech mechanism. . . . It is equally impossible to imagine a "phonetic"

> component working largely independently of the phonological knowledge or competence of a speaker . . . there has never been any question that the movements in speech are implementations of phonologically-specified word shapes.
>
> *(p. 155)*

Second, he argues that integrating research on phonology and phonetics is a more fruitful method of investigating phonological and phonetic phenomena. Ohala (1990), as well as Ohala (1981, 1983, 2005) and Ohala and Jaeger (1986) and the references cited therein explain a variety of sound patterns and changes as products of the phonetic behavior of speakers and/or listeners.

Ohala (1990, 2005) in particular also contrasts the character and quality of these phonetic explanations with those that cast them in terms of phonological representations. Two examples of such explanations suffice as illustrations. First, the contents of vowel inventories are explained very differently by Lindblom's dispersion model (Liljencrants & Lindblom, 1972; Lindblom, 1986) than by Chomsky and Halle's (1968) markedness conventions (2a–d) as follows. In Lindblom's model, vowels are dispersed sufficiently within a space defined by the ranges of first and second formant frequencies (F_1, F_2) that can be produced by a human vocal tract. The expression of these formants' frequencies in auditory units (Bark rather than Hz) emphasizes that it is the listener who needs the vowels to be sufficiently dispersed. Schwartz, Boë, Valleé, and Abry (1997a, 1997b) added a preference for *focal* vowels; that is, those vowels in which adjacent formants are close enough together (in Bark) to produce a single prominent and presumably perceptually salient spectral peak.[11] Simulations presented in de Boer (2000); Lindblom (1986); Schwartz et al. (1997b) show that dispersion and focalization successfully capture the contents and structure of cross-linguistically common vowel inventories (but see Kingston, 2007, for remaining shortcomings). de Boer's (2000) simulations also showed that sufficiently dispersed vowel inventories could evolve from the interactions between agents trying to learn each other's pronunciations without explicitly invoking a dispersion requirement.

Chomsky and Halle's (1968) marking conventions for vowels in (2a,b) represent the contents of the minimal three-vowel inventory, /i, u, a/, which has more non-low than low vowels, and where the non-low vowels are high. (2a) also represents the fact that larger inventories than /i, u, a/ usually have more non-low than low vowels, while (2b) also represents the fact that high vowels usually occur in these larger inventories, too. (2c,d) represent the common agreement between rounding and backness in non-low vowels, and the common absence of rounding in low vowels.

2 Markedness conventions for vowels:[12]

a. [*u* low] → [−low]
b. [*u* high] → [+high]
c. [*u* round] → [*α*round]/ $[\overline{_{\alpha\text{back}, -\text{low}}}]$
d. [*u* round] → [−round]/ $[\overline{_{+\text{low}}}]$

Despite Chomsky and Halle's (1968) stated goal of trying to capture the contribution of features' phonetic correlates to phonological inventories and patterns by these means, markedness conventions remain no more than descriptively adequate, because they don't explain why high vowels should outnumber low ones nor why a back vowel is more likely to be rounded, and a front vowel unrounded.

The dispersion plus focalization model achieves explanatory adequacy by appealing directly to the limits and liberties on transforming the articulations of vowels into their acoustics and on transforming vowels' acoustics into auditory qualities. The auditory system is more sensitive to frequency differences in the lower part of the spectrum where F_1 varies as a function of tongue body height/closeness. Because vowels differing in F_1 are thus inherently more dispersed than those differing in their frequencies for higher formants as a function of tongue body backness and lip rounding, languages can reliably make finer distinctions in height than backness and rounding – Chomsky and Halle's (1968) markedness conventions don't even describe the greater number of height than backness and rounding distinctions. Differences in tongue body backness also produce a larger range of possible F_2 values when the body constricts the oral cavity along the palate, as it does in high vowels, than when it constricts the oral cavity in the pharynx, as it does in low vowels. Thus, non-low, especially high vowels can be more dispersed than low vowels. The dispersion of high vowels can also be enhanced more than that of low vowels by rounding the lips when the tongue body is backed, and spreading them when it's fronted (see Linker, 1982, for articulatory evidence of more extreme lip positions in higher vowels, and see Kaun (1995, 2004) and Pasquereau (2018) for phonological consequences of these height-determined differences in the degree of lip rounding). The corner vowels are also more likely to be focal, in that F_1 and F_2 are close together in /u, a/ and F_2 and F_3 are close together in /i/.

A second comparison of phonetic with phonological explanations concerns the intrusive stops that appear between nasals and laterals and adjacent fricatives for some English speakers, e.g., in *warmth* [wɔɹm*p*θ] and *false* [fɔl*t*s]. Clements (1987) accounts for the intrusive [p] in *warm[p]th* as a product of the nasal's [−continuant] and place values spreading onto the following fricative's timing slot, where their overlap with the fricative's [−voice] value produces a voiceless, oral bilabial closure. According to Ohala (1990, 2005), the intrusive stop is instead produced in *warm[p]th* when the velum is raised and the glottis is abducted early in anticipation of the fricative's states for these articulators, before the complete oral closure is replaced by the fricative's narrow constriction. On this account, the intrusive stop results from a timing error rather than from spreading two of the fricatives' phonological feature values. Ohala argues, moreover, that the intrusive stops between laterals and fricatives cannot be explained as a product of spreading the feature values from the lateral to the fricative, because both sounds are [+continuant]. Instead, in the transition from air flow around the sides of the tongue in the lateral to air flow down the center of the tongue in the fricative, the sides of the tongue might be raised before the lateral's central constriction is released. The result would be a brief interval when air neither flows around the sides nor down the center of the tongue, i.e., a complete oral closure like that of a stop. The stop would be voiceless if the /s/'s large glottal abduction begins earlier than the lowering of the center of the tongue. Because a timing error can explain intrusive stops in between laterals and fricatives as well as between nasals and fricatives, it is a more general and parsimonious explanation than feature spreading.[13]

This explanation is, however, incomplete, in not accounting completely for the facts. A timing error is no more than a phonetic event without phonological consequences unless and until it becomes systematic. Ohala (1990, 2005) cites examples from English and other languages where the intrusive stop has become part of words' lexical entries. Citing Fourakis and Port (1986), Clements (1987) also proposes that stop intrusion has become systematic between nasals and fricatives in some English dialects, while remaining absent in others. Can a timing error still be responsible for cases where a stop systematically intrudes in particular words or in all eligible words in a particular dialect? Or is the stop's occurrence no longer dependent on its original phonetic cause? (I return to these questions later in sections "Distinguishing between phonology and phonetics" and "Phonetic implementation.") The same question can be raised regarding the role of dispersion and focalization as regulating the contents of vowel inventories. Both may have originally influenced the locations of vowels in the vowel space when a particular vowel inventory emerged in a language, and both may influence any shifts in those locations as vowels are added to or subtracted from that space as a result of sound changes. But do dispersion and focalization continue to regulate vowels' locations in the vowel space during periods, often quite lengthy ones, in a language's history when its vowel inventory remains unchanged? Putting this question more generally, must lexicalized or phonologized sound patterns remain dependent on their phonetic causes?

There appears to be a contradiction here, but one that proves resolvable. On the one hand, it appears that the answer to this question must be "yes," because the phonetic constraints on articulations, their transformation to acoustic properties, and the transformation of those properties to auditory qualities don't go away once they've shaped a language's phonology. They could therefore continue to regulate each of these links in the speech chain between the speaker and listener. On the other hand, it appears that the answer to this question must instead be "no," because subsequent sound changes often obscure or remove entirely a sound pattern's original phonetic motivation, interactions with the language's lexicon or morphology can limit or extend the pattern's scope analogically, and the accumulation of changes can create foci or environments for phonological processes which consist of arbitrary disjunctive sets of features (Garrett, 2015; Mielke, 2008, 2011, and references cited therein). The end results in each kind of subsequent development are synchronic sound patterns that would otherwise be phonetically unlikely if not altogether impossible.

Ohala (2005) argues from the evidence that phonologized sound patterns both do and do not remain dependent on their phonetic causes that it is a mistake to incorporate phonetic naturalness requirements into phonological grammars. The phonetic constraints will regulate what speakers and listeners do without their having to know them. They will thus determine not only how speakers of a language will behave contemporaneously, but also what is likely to happen during a language's history, as well as what are common typological patterns. Phonetic constraints will not, however, determine what must happen; that is, what the sound patterns are of particular languages. Ohala also suggests that what speakers and listeners actually do know will most likely be revealed by psycholinguistic studies of production and perception of speech.

A case that has been much discussed in the literature recently supports Ohala's assessment of both the extent and limitations of phonetic explanations, as well as his suggestion that what speakers and listeners know can best be discovered by studying acts of production and perception. This case is the devoicing of stops and affricates after nasals in two closely related Southern Bantu languages, Tswana (Beguš, 2017; Coetzee & Pretorius, 2010; Gouskova, Zsiga & Boyer, 2011; Hyman, 2001) and Shekgalagari (Solé, Hyman & Monaka, 2010). Hyman (2001) first presented the Tswana case as a challenge to the proposal that there is a phonetically well-motivated constraint *against* the occurrence of voiceless stops and affricates after nasals, *NT (Hayes, 1999; Hayes & Stivers, 1995; Pater, 1999). If *NT is itself as phonetically motivated as these studies suggest, if a possible, indeed frequent repair is to voice the stop, and *if markedness constraints must be phonetically grounded*, then there can in principle be no complementary constraint, *ND, against voiced stops and affricates after nasals.[14] The last condition is essential, as otherwise the observed facts could be obtained so long as *ND remains lower-ranked, and repairs to *NT other than voicing are ruled out by higher ranked faithfulness constraints. For example, *NT,

ID[NASAL], MAX >> IDENT[VOICE], *ND maps /nt nd/ onto [nd nd].[15] Examples of synchronic devoicing, as a possible repair to violation of *ND, after the first person object clitic *N-* from Tswana and Shekgalagari are given on the right in (3, 4) (Hyman, 2001; Solé et al., 2010):

(3)	Tswana:			
	a. "see!"	bón-á	m-pón-á	"see me!"
	b. "watch!"	dís-á	n-tís-á	"watch me!"
	c. "answer!"	áráb-á	ŋ-káráb-á	"watch me!" (< *-gáráb-)
(4)	Shekgalagari:			
	a. "to see"	χʊ-bɔ́n-á	χʊ-m-pɔ́n-á	"to see me"
	b. "to annoint"	χʊ-dʊʒ-a	χʊ-n-tʊʒ-a	"to annoint me"
	c. "to feed"	χʊ-ɟís-a	χʊ-ɲ-cís-a	"to feed me"
	d. "to like"	χʊ-at-a	χʊ-ŋ-kat-a	"to like me" (< -gat-)

There is some debate in this literature about the facts of Tswana, in particular about whether stops only devoice after nasals. This debate can in part be attributed to individual and possibly also dialectal differences between the speakers who provided the data for the various studies (Coetzee & Pretorius, 2010; Gouskova et al., 2011), but instrumental analyses show that at least some speakers consistently devoice voiced stops after nasals and not elsewhere. An instrumental analysis by Solé et al. (2010) produced similar results for the speech of a single speaker of Shekgalagari. So how can voiced stops devoice after nasals when this change is not only *not* phonetically motivated, but voicing after nasals is instead?

Hyman (2001) proposes that at the first relevant stage in Tswana's history (5a), voiced stops that didn't follow nasals lenited to homorganic continuants.[16] Subsequently at the second stage (5b), all stops that remained stops devoiced. Stop devoicing was context-free; that voiced stops only occurred after nasals following their earlier lenition elsewhere was irrelevant (see Beguš, 2017, for a generalization of this account to stop devoicing after nasals in other languages). At the final stage (5c), the voiced fricatives produced by lenition at the first stage became stops once more:

(5) Sequence of sound changes in Tswana:

a. Lenition: b > β, d > l ~ ɽ, g > ɣ; unchanged: mb > mb, nd > nd, ŋg > ŋg
b. Devoicing: b > p, d > t, g > k[17]
c. Stopping: β > b, l > d, (ɣ > 0)

Once the third change turned continuants back into stops, reversing the first change, voiced stops elsewhere were expected to alternate with their voiceless counterparts after nasals.

As noted by Coetzee and Pretorius (2010), the underlying forms of labial stops in the first column in Table 13.1 should therefore have been realized with the surface forms in the second column at this stage in Tswana's history.[18]

Two characteristics of the pronunciation of stops in Tswana (and Shekgalagari) support Ohala's (2005) argument against incorporating a requirement for phonetic naturalness into phonological grammars.

The first and most obvious is the synchronic alternation in both languages between voiceless stops after nasals and voiced stops elsewhere. Post-nasal voicing is phonetically motivated, but post-nasal devoicing is not and cannot be phonetically motivated.[19] Voicing is

Table 13.1 Underlying forms and expected and observed surface forms of labial stops in Tswana I and II. "?" represents consonants in word-initial contexts that Coetzee and Pretorius (2010) did not examine.

Underlying	*Expected*	*Tswana I*	*Tswana II*
bV	bV	?	?
pV	pV	?	?
VbV	VbV	VbV ~ VβV	VbV ~ VβV
VpV	VpV	VpV	VpV ~ VbV
mbV	mpV	mpV	mbV ~ mpV
mpV	mpV	mpV	mbV ~ mpV

likely to continue from the nasal into the oral interval of a nasal-oral stop sequence because the leak through the velopharyngeal port prevents any appreciable rise in intraoral air pressure during the nasal interval. That oral interval is also typically quite brief, as the soft palate is raised just in time to ensure that at least but no more than the release is oral rather than nasal (Beddor & Onsuwan, 2003; Hubbard, 1995; Maddieson, 1989; Maddieson & Ladefoged, 1993). The soft palate is also not raised until late in the closure interval of an oral stop following a contrastively nasalized vowel (Huffman, 1993). Because the entire oral interval is so brief, much or all of it may be voiced even if voicing continues only for a short time itself after the soft palate is raised and air no longer leaks out through the velopharyngeal port. Devoicing would therefore not be expected if it occurred only after nasals.

Beguš (2017) argues, however, that stops are expected to devoice because intraoral air pressure will rise fast enough behind a stop closure to eliminate the pressure drop across the glottis unless the oral cavity is expanded to slow its rise. On his account, it's necessarily irrelevant that the only voiced stops that remain in either Tswana or Shekgalagari after lenition occur after nasals, a context where the aerodynamics not only don't threaten but actually encourage the maintenance of voicing. That is, devoicing has to be context-free in a strict sense, or more precisely, it has to occur without regard to the phonetic conditions in which voiced stops occur after lenition. Beguš makes this point somewhat differently, in emphasizing the continuation of the complementary distribution between stop pronunciations after nasals versus fricative pronunciations elsewhere following the first stage. The competition between one phonetically natural process, stop devoicing, and another, post-nasal voicing, is resolved in favor of the former because it's more general, applying to stops wherever they occur, even if the only context they occur in is one that should inhibit this sound change phonetically (see Hayes, 1999; Moreton & Pater, 2012a, 2012b, for further argument that simpler processes are favored). Devoicing is and must be indifferent to the fact that stops only occur after nasals. This argument implies that a preference for formal generality can determine which of two opposing phonetically motivated outcomes is chosen, and not the relative strengths of the phonetic motivations.

The second piece of evidence supporting Ohala's argument against directly incorporating phonetic naturalness into phonological grammars can be found in Coetzee and Pretorius's (2010) detailed description of individual difference between Tswana speakers' pronunciations. That description demonstrates the push and pull between phonetic naturalness and other pressures (third and fourth columns in Table 13.1). The seven speakers they label as "Tswana I," devoice stops after nasals in 90% or more of tokens, and all but one pronounce

/b/ as a voiced stop [b] rather than a fricative /β/ after vowels in more than 80% of tokens; the exceptional speaker does so in about 50% of tokens. Tswana I speakers pronounce /b/ as a stop [b] rather than a fricative [β] after vowels most often when a clitic boundary falls between the vowel and /b/, less often when a prefix boundary does, and least often inside a morpheme. Voiceless stops remain voiceless stops in nearly all instances and contexts. The five speakers in Tswana II pronounce /b/ as [b] after nasals with variable frequency, one in less than half the tokens, three in more than half, and one in roughly 80% of tokens. Unlike the Tswana I speakers, these speakers appear to be reverting to the phonetically natural pattern of voicing rather than devoicing after nasals. However, the speakers in this group resemble those in Tswana I in producing /b/ as a stop [b] or fricative /β/ with the same sensitivity to the presence and nature of the morphological boundary between the preceding vowel and the consonant. Four of the five Tswana II speakers pronounce /p/ as voiced [b] after vowels in a noticeable minority of tokens, but the voiceless pronunciation is more common for all five speakers in this context. The speakers in these two groups thus differ from one another in how they pronounce voiced stops after nasals, but resemble one another in how they pronounce them after vowels, and how their pronunciations in the latter contexts depend on the sound's morphological context. These facts show that sound patterns are not solely governed by their phonetic realizations, and therefore that phonological grammars should not incorporate a requirement that the patterns they're responsible for be just those that are phonetically natural.

The purpose of the extended discussion of this example has been to support Ohala's (2005) argument that phonological grammars need not be limited to phonetically natural processes or constraints, nor are phonetically natural processes or constraints free from regulation by other components of the grammar. Instead phonetically unexpected patterns, like stop devoicing after nasals, can be incorporated into synchronic grammars as the product of a series of sound changes, each of which may themselves be phonetically motivated. And phonetically expected patterns, like post-vocalic spirantization, can come to be grammatically conditioned. Nonetheless, Ohala's conception of the contents of a phonological grammars remains distinct from Hale and Reiss's (2000) conception, in permitting phonetics to motivate its symbolic content and operations directly, and thereby limiting its content and operation far more narrowly than what can be computed by manipulating symbols.

Like Ohala (2005), Flemming (2001) argues that the phonetics and phonology overlap so thoroughly that there is no interface between them whose purpose is to translate between the categories of phonological representations and the continua of their phonetic realizations. But unlike Ohala, Flemming argues that grammars incorporate naturalness in the form of constraints that are not only phonetically or substantively grounded but that also refer directly to phonetic continua (see also Boersma, 1998, 2011; Boersma & Hamann, 2009, for proposals that grammars refer directly to phonetic continua and that differ formally but not substantively from Flemming's proposals). Flemming motivates his argument by pointing to a variety of cases where phonetic and phonological processes closely resemble one another. More generally, he argues that,

> Phonetics and phonology are not obviously distinguished by the nature of the representations involved, or in terms of the phenomena they encompass. As far as representation is concerned, most of the primitives of the phonological representation remain phonetically based, in the sense that features and timing units are provided with broadly phonetic definitions. This has the peculiar consequence that sound is represented twice in the grammar, once at a coarse level of detail in the phonology and then again at a finer

grain in the phonetics. Perhaps more significant is the fact that there are also substantial similarities between many phenomena which are conventionally classified as phonetic and those which are conventionally classified as phonological; for example coarticulation is similar in many respects to assimilation.

(pp. 9–10)

Before continuing, it's worth noting that Ohala (2005) would see no need to formalize the phonetic motivations for phonological patterns as rules or constraints in the phonological grammar; quite the contrary, it would instead be enough for him to identify those motivations and construct a phonetic *explanation* of those patterns from those motivations.

The rest of this discussion of Flemming's proposal is limited to his central illustration of the last of these observations, namely, the fronting of back vowels by coarticulation with neighboring coronal consonants and the assimilation of back to front vowels in such contexts in languages such as Cantonese. As Flemming notes, coarticulation with a neighboring coronal consonant raises the frequency of the second formant (F_2) in back vowels such as /u/ and /o/. In Cantonese, this phonetic effect of coarticulation is phonologized when coronal consonants occur on both sides of /u/ or /o/, where the contrast between back rounded vowels /u/ and /o/, *tʰok* "to support," *put* "to wipe out," *kot* "to cut," and the corresponding front rounded vowels /y/ and /ø/, *kʰyt* "to decide," *søŋ* "wish," neutralizes to the front vowels, *tyt* "to take off," *jyt* "moon," *jøt* "weak," *tøn* "a shield" – neither **tut* nor **ton* are possible words in Cantonese.

Flemming (2001) accounts for coarticulation via a markedness-like constraint that favors shorter movements of articulators. Perfect satisfaction of this constraint would result in no movement of the articulators between a consonant and a neighboring vowel, and thus no change in the value between the consonant's acoustic target for the second formant (F_2) and the vowel's. Violations of this constraint are a direct scalar function of the difference between the consonant's and the vowel's F_2 values in a candidate. This effort-minimization constraint competes with faithfulness-like constraints requiring that both the consonant's and the vowel's F_2 targets be reached in a candidate; violations of these constraints are also direct scalar functions of the difference between these targets and the actual F_2 values in a candidate. All these functions are weighted, and the cost (disharmony) of a candidate is the sum of their weighted values. The optimal candidate then is the one with the lowest value for this sum, i.e., the lowest cost.

Neutralization of the contrast between back rounded /u, o/ and front rounded /y, ø/ between coronal consonants is accounted for by a constraint which requires that contrasting categories differ by some minimum amount along the relevant phonetic dimension, here F_2, MinDist. Violations of this constraint, too, are assessed by a direct, weighted scalar function of the F_2 difference between the back rounded vowels and their front counterparts. This constraint competes with one which requires that the number of contrasts be maximized, MaximizeContrast, and that would preserve the contrast between back and front rounded vowels. When both flanking consonants are coronal, effort minimization produces an F_2 value for a back rounded vowel that is too close to the F_2 target of its front counterpart, and neutralizes the back:front contrast to the front category when the cost of maintaining the contrast is greater than the benefit of maintaining it, as specified by the weight of MaximizeContrast.

Assessing violations via scalar functions that refer to distances along continuous phonetic dimensions incorporates sounds' phonetic properties directly into the evaluation of candidates' well-formedness. Moreover, phonological categories themselves are represented by their values along continuous phonetic dimensions, so there is no longer any need to translate between discrete categories and continuous values. Finally, unequivocally phonological outcomes like neutralization of contrasts can be achieved by the interaction of constraints that refer to continuous phonetic dimensions, such as MinDist, with categorical constraints, such as MaximizeContrast, which refer to contrasting sounds as discrete units.

Flemming's (2001) effort to erase the formal difference between phonetics and phonology by these means should not, however, be read as an argument that phonology can be reduced to phonetics. Instead, it is intended to show that operations on continua can produce outcomes that amount to operations on categories (see the discussion in phonetic grounding of alternations below of Steriade, 2001, 2008, for an account that resembles Flemming's and Boersma's in its assumption that the phonetics regulates the phonology, but that does not incorporate direct reference to phonetic continua into grammars).

Summary

Three distinct arguments have been reviewed for eliminating a separate interface between phonetics and phonology: no interface is needed (or possible) the units of phonological representations must be of a kind that can be realized in the act of speaking, namely, articulatory gestures; do phonological representations have any phonetic substance? the apparent psycholinguistic and phonetic grounding of phonological representations, processes, and constraints must instead be attributed to learning and diachrony, and phonology must be restricted to formal computation; or there is no phonology without phonetics nor phonetics without phonology phonology and phonetics are so inextricably and mutually intertwined that there is no border between them, no possibility of fruitfully investigating the one without also investigating the other, and finally no need to keep reference to continua out of the phonology. Given the force of each of these arguments, and their variety, it's reasonable to ask whether it is still possible to argue convincingly for an interface between phonetics and phonology. In the remaining sections of this chapter, I present compelling reasons for responding "yes" to this question.

Distinguishing between phonology and phonetics

As a bridge to section "There *is* an interface between phonetics and phonology," it is useful to discuss the arguments that support a widely accepted alternative to the beginning of the preceding quote from Flemming (2001), repeated here for convenience:

> Phonetics and phonology are not obviously distinguished by the nature of the representations involved, or in terms of the phenomena they encompass.

Cohn (1993, 2007), Myers (2000), and Solé (1992, 1995, 2007) all offer diagnostics for deciding whether a pattern is phonological or phonetic. All these diagnostics derive from a distinction between phonological categories and phonetic gradients: the contents of phonological representations consist of *categories* and the processes that operate on them or the constraints that regulate them refer to these categories, while the contents of phonetic representations are gradients and the procedures that implement them refer to gradients (see Pierrehumbert, Beckman, & Ladd, 2000, for an argument that phonology and phonetics cannot be distinguished as referring to categories versus gradients, and compare Pierrehumbert (1990)). These diagnostics are first discussed with respect to the facts of vowel nasalization, VOT, and vowel duration in English versus Spanish or Catalan, before turning to a more general account of diagnostics that might distinguish phonology from phonetics.

Solé (1992, 1995) show that nasalization extends much further into vowels preceding nasals in English than in Spanish, and that nasalization's extent increases with the rate-determined duration of the vowel in English but not Spanish. She interprets these facts as evidence that an allophonic rule produces the extensive vowel nasalization in English, but that coarticulation produces the modest vowel nasalization in Spanish; that is, vowels become phonologically specified as [+nasal] before nasals in English, but not in Spanish, where the brief interval of coarticulation arises in the phonetics.[20]

It's important to carefully examine the effect of rate on the extent of vowel nasalization in English, because Myers (2000) and Solé (2007) have both argued that rate-determined variation is evidence of gradient phonetic implementation, not a categorical phonological process or constraint. Solé (1992, 1995) shows that the vowel lengthened and the absolute extent of nasalization increased as speech rate slowed down, but the duration of the initial unnasalized portion of the vowel remained constant. Its constancy suggests that English speakers time the onset of soft palate lowering relative to the beginning of the vowel and continue to lower it for the remainder of the vowel, no matter how short or long it lasts. Spanish speakers instead time the onset of soft palate lowering relative the onset of the nasal, and thus only nasalize as much of the vowel as they must, given the mechanics of moving from a closed to an open velopharyngeal port. The sort of rate-determined variation observed in English is not therefore evidence that vowel nasalization is phonetically gradient rather than phonologically categorical in that language.

Solé (2007) shows that VOT in long-lag (voiceless aspirated) stops in English also increases as rate slows, but the VOT of short-lag (voiceless unaspirated) stops in Catalan does not, and that vowel duration differences before voiced versus voiceless obstruents increase as rate slows in English, but remain constant across rates in Catalan.[21] The similarity in the effects of rate on vowel nasalization, VOT, and vowel duration leads Solé to argue that the temporal extents of all three properties are controlled by English speakers so as to scale with rate. On her account, controlled properties are phonological properties; others might attribute them instead to phonetic grammars (see 4.3).

Myers (2000) proposes a number of mutually exclusive criteria for diagnosing whether a process or pattern is phonological or phonetic. On the one hand, any process or pattern that refers to morphosyntatic categories, morphological structure, or specific morphemes can only be phonological. Such processes cannot be phonetic because phonetics can only refer to quantities and such processes refer instead to categories. There is a deeper reason why none of these processes can be phonetic: they all entail restrictions on or exceptions to what would otherwise be completely general processes. Phonetic processes are assumed to be exceptionless because they are automatic byproducts of the physics, physiology, and/or psychology of speaking and listening. Any process or pattern that refers to gradients, speaking rate or style, or to differences between speakers can only be phonetic. Such processes or patterns cannot be phonological because they refer to quantities, and there is no evidence in Myers's view that phonological patterns do (cf. Flemming, 2001).

If such a bright line can be drawn between phonological and phonetic processes and patterns, then it follows that some sort of interface is needed to mediate the interaction between the categorical and gradient characteristics of speech sounds.

There *is* an interface between phonetics and phonology

This section begins with discussions of the phonetic grounding of inventories and alternations, before turning to phonetic implementation. Inventories and alternations are static, synchronic properties or characteristics of languages, so the focus in the first two sections is on how they are motivated by, or *grounded* in the phonetic properties of the affected sounds (for other discussions of grounding, see Archangeli & Pulleyblank, 1994; Flack, 2007; Padgett, 2002; Smith, 2002). Implementation is instead behavior, so the focus of the last section is on the procedures that realize the phonological representation of an utterance phonetically.

Phonetic grounding of inventories

Following Ohala (1983), Hayes (1999) reviews phonetic explanations for the absence of anterior voiceless stops, e.g., /p/ in Arabic, and posterior voiced stops, e.g., /g/ in Dutch. But Hayes also observes that both stops frequently occur in the voiced and voiceless series of stop phonemes, despite the phonetic challenges to reliably producing or perceiving them – indeed either gap, no /p/ or no /g/, occurs significantly less often than would be expected by chance.[22] Hayes also observes that phonotactic constraints more often regulate an entire series rather than just its phonetically more challenged members; for example, all voiced stops are devoiced in syllable codas in German, not just the one most susceptible to devoicing, /g/. Hayes argues that this discrepancy can best be resolved by distinguishing between the particularity of phonetic regulation of speaking and hearing and the systematicity of phonological constraints on the occurrence and distribution of segments.[23] Hayes's argument resembles Beguš's (2017) in giving priority to formal generality over phonetic motivation *tout court*, but differs in that formal generality regulates inventory content rather than the choice between competing phonetic motivations.

If the influences of phonetics and phonology on segment inventories and distributions do differ in this way, then the need for an interface between them re-emerges. That interface cannot, however, be a sharp boundary across which the categories of phonological representations are translated into the quantities of their phonetic realizations, but must instead consist of a negotiation between the finer demands of the phonetics and coarser demands of the phonology. In Hayes's account, that negotiation consists of trading off the phonetic grounding of a phonological constraint with its complexity, where a constraint is less complex than another when its structural description is properly included within the other's structural description.

Hayes (1999) estimates that the specific and therefore more complex constraints against /p/ and /g/ are more phonetically grounded than the more general and thus less complex constraints against voiceless and voiced obstruents, respectively. According to Hayes, if phonetic grounding were the only criterion, then stop inventories like those observed in Dutch and Arabic would be far more common than they are (see also Bermúdez-Otero & Börjars, 2006, for further discussion of this point). Instead, languages tend to have voiceless or voiced stops at all three major places of articulation or to have them at none of these places. This fact suggests that there may be general markedness constraints prohibiting voiceless or voiced stops across places of articulation, i.e., *[−Continuant/−Voice] or *[+Voice/−Continuant], rather than place-specific markedness constraints prohibiting aerodynamically challenging /p/ or /g/, i.e., *[−Continuant/−Voice, labial] or *[+Voice/−Continuant, dorsal] – these constraints are stated in this way, because the most frequent repairs that languages apply to eliminate /p/ or /g/ in outputs are spirantization to /ɸ/ or /f/ and devoicing to /k/, respectively. Apparently, simplicity (or generality) governs the contents of inventories, not phonetic grounding. As Ohala (1979) observed, consonant inventories favor maximal over less than maximal use of available distinctive features, and in this respect, differ from vowel inventories, which are more obviously governed by a requirement that their members be sufficiently dispersed in a space defined by phonetic dimensions.

This discussion has had three purposes. First, it lays bare the uncertainties about how far a phonetic explanation of the contents of an inventory may reach, or perhaps in this example, how short its reach may be. Second, it exposes an essential difference between phonetic and phonological explanations, as they are currently understood. Phonetic explanations refer to individual speech sounds or to their characteristics, and they can thus recognize differences between individual sounds that are otherwise very similar to one another, such as those between voiceless or voiced stops at different places of articulation.

Phonological explanations refer instead to sets of speech sounds, which ideally resemble one another phonetically, but which minimally pattern alike. This distinction between more particular and more general reference resembles what Hayes (1999) refers to as more versus less complex, but those terms apply only to the phonological representations of sounds. For example, the sets consisting of /p/ or /g/ alone are more complex that those consisting of /p, t, k/ or /b, d, g/ because they must refer to place.

The relative simplicity of the more inclusive phonological sets does not carry over, however, to the corresponding phonetic sets, [p, t, k] and [b, d, g], even if the context in which these sounds occur was held constant. It does not carry over because the aerodynamic adjustments required to ensure that each member of the set [p, t, k] is realized as a stop and to ensure that each member of the set [b, d, g] is realized as voiced differ between places of articulation, as do the articulators used to produce the closures at each place.

The simplicity of the sets /p, t, k/ and /b, d, g/ does not therefore follow from the phonetic characteristics of their members, but instead only from the length of their phonological definitions. This point is by now obvious, perhaps even belabored, but it was the only way to bring us to the final point of this discussion, which is this: the fact that phonological inventories consist of sets of sounds with simpler phonological descriptions is something to be explained; it is not itself an explanation. A postscript can be added to this final point, namely, not all sets of phonemes, even of consonants, pattern like stops; for example, languages without gaps at any of the three major places in their stop inventories often still lack a contrastive dorsal nasal /ŋ/. A more comprehensive approach to investigating the possible phonetic grounding of typologically common inventories is needed before any decision can be made as to how to divide the labor of explanation between a particular phonetics and a general phonology, along with a more critical examination of what purport to be phonological explanations.

Phonetic grounding of alternations

Steriade (2001, 2008) proposes that phonological alternations are governed by a requirement that alternants differ minimally from one another, and that minimally different alternants are those that are perceptually most similar to one another, not those that differ minimally in their distinctive feature values. Perceptual similarity estimates are obtained from the distances between alternants in the P-map, a representation of the perceptual correspondents of alternants' context-specific phonetic correlates.

Steriade's (2008) central example is the alternation between obstruents that contrast for [voice] in some contexts, and neutralize that contrast to [−voice] in other contexts. Steriade identifies the contexts where the [voice] contrast is usually maintained as those where a vowel or more open sonorant articulation follows the obstruent, and those where the contrast instead neutralizes to [−voice] as preceding another obstruent or a word boundary. An obstruent may also assimilate in [voice] to a following obstruent. In Steriade (2001, 2008), she argues that the contexts where the contrast is preserved are those where its correlates, or "cues," are best realized or best conveyed to the listener, while those contexts in which the contrast is neutralized are those in which those cues are unrealized, poorly realized, or not conveyed to the listener. So Steriade (2008) first grounds her account of alternations phonetically by observing that whether a contrast is maintained in a context depends on how reliably the listener can detect its identifying cues in that context.

The second way in which Steriade (2008) grounds her account is in her solution to the "too-many solutions" problem. This problem arises in optimality theoretic grammars because markedness constraints don't specify how to repair their violation, yet languages don't avail themselves of all the possible repairs. In the case of interest here, the /b/ in inputs such as /tabza, tab/ where its cues would be poorly conveyed could be repaired by devoicing /tapza, tap/, nasalization /tamza, tam/, spirantization /taβza, taβ/, gliding /tawza, taw/, deletion /taza, ta/, epenthesis /tabəza, tabə/, and by a number of other changes, yet the only repair observed is the first, devoicing.[24]

Steriade (2008) argues that only this repair is chosen because /tapza, tap/ are phonologically the most similar to the unrepaired strings /tabza, tab/ of all the possible output strings produced by the alternative repairs. /tabza, tab/ are more similar phonologically to /tapza, tap/ than they are to /tamza, tam/, /taβza, taβ/, etc., because /b/ and /p/ are perceptually more similar to one another than are /b/ and /m/, /b/ and β/, or /b/ any of the other unobserved repairs in those contexts. And the contrast does not neutralize before a sonorant, e.g., in /bra, ba/, because these strings are even more dissimilar phonologically from /pra, pa/ than are /tabza, tab/ from /tapza, tap/. They are more dissimilar because the cues to the [voice] contrast are more robust before a sonorant or a vowel than before an obstruent or a word boundary.

Phonological similarity must reflect perceptual similarity between sounds rather the number of differences in their feature values, because at least three unobserved repairs, nasalization, spirantization, and gliding, like devoicing, change the value of just one distinctive feature: [−nasal] > [+nasal], [−continuant] > [+continuant], and [−sonorant] > [+sonorant], respectively, cf. [+voice] > [−voice].[25] The /b/ is devoiced in /tabza, tab/ because obstruents contrasting for [voice] before another obstruent or a word boundary are perceptually more similar to one another than those before a sonorant or a vowel. They are perceptually more similar before an obstruent or a word boundary because the number, size, and detectability of the phonetic differences are reduced compared to before a sonorant or a vowel.

The other sound pattern that Steriade (2001) argues reflects perceptual similarity is the progressive assimilation in clusters of apico-alveolars and retroflexes[26] and the neutralization of contrasts between them when not preceded by a vowel. She observes that these sounds differ more acoustically during the transition from a preceding vowel than during the transition to a following vowel. She also cites Anderson's (1997) evidence (Table 13.2) that Western Arrente speakers identify apico-alveolars and retroflexes far less well in CV strings made by removing the preceding V from VCV strings than in the original VCV strings, but identify all but one dental and post-alveolar laminal consonants roughly as well in the CV as the VCV strings – the exception is the dental lateral [l̪]. The values in the Drop column for

Table 13.2 Percent correct identification of dental, apico-alveolar, retroflex, and post-alveolar coronal stops, nasals, and laterals by Arrente speakers in VCV versus CV contexts, including the drop in percent correct between the two contexts (Anderson, 1997).

Apical				*Laminal*			
C	*VCV*	*CV*	*Drop*	*C*	*VCV*	*CV*	*Drop*
t	70	35	−35	t̪	96	83	−13
ʈ	74	19	−55	t̠	99	94	−5
n	62	45	−17	n̪	75	70	−5
ɳ	96	28	−69	n̠	88	87	1
l	62	32	−30	l̪	91	55	−36
ɭ	84	45	−39	l̠	95	92	−3

the apical consonants in Table 13.2 also show that retroflex identification suffers more than apico-alveolar identification when the preceding vowel is removed:

Anderson's (1997) results are compelling evidence in support of the first of Steriade's proposals, that contrasts are kept in contexts where their distinguishing acoustic correlates are present and detectable and lost in contexts where they are not. However, they fail to speak to her second proposal, that preferred or possible alternants must be perceptually similar to one another. They fail to do so because the Western Arrente listeners' task in Anderson's experiment was to identify the consonant in each stimulus with a linguistic category. As the following discussion of consonant confusion studies makes clear, identification tasks in which stimuli are assigned to a category in the listeners' native language do not provide any measure of perceptual similarity distinguishable from a measure of linguistic similarity represented by shared distinctive feature values.

The difficulty with both examples, of course, as Steriade (2008) herself acknowledges, is that we lack the necessary measurements of context-specific perceptual similarity between consonants. One possible source of such assessments is studies of confusions between consonants when mixed with noise or filtered, or when the listener's hearing is impaired. A measure of perceptual similarity could be derived from those studies, on the assumption that more similar consonants would be more confusable. This assumption is made explicit by Dubno and Levitt (1981):

> First, it is postulated that in a recognition task, an incorrect response implies that the available acoustic cues were not sufficient to differentiate a certain consonant from a number of other consonants. Second, it is assumed that the listener's incorrect response would be that consonant which is most similar to the target in terms of the acoustic variables that are important in the recognition process.
>
> *(p. 249)*

However, not all studies of consonant confusions have compared the same consonantal contrasts between contexts where their cues are expected to be more versus less reliably conveyed to listeners; exceptions are Benkí (2003), Dubno and Levitt (1981), Redford and Diehl (1999), Cutler, Weber, Smits, and Cooper (2004), and Wang and Bilger (1973). But it has proven difficult to derive a consistent measure of perceptual similarity from even these studies, because their results differ as a function of how confusions were induced, whether confusions were more numerous after than before vowels or vice versa, what the native language of the listeners was, what responses listeners used, and other factors.

Even more research into perceived similarity using confusion studies is unlikely to be fruitful given an unrelieved uncertainty about whether the confusions documented in these studies reflect the phonetic or phonological features of the stimuli. On the one hand, we have Wang and Bilger's (1973)'s reluctant conclusion that they had not been able to show that the listeners' confusions in their study reflected "natural perceptual features" (p. 1249) instead of the phonological features that represent voice, manner, and place contrasts,

> it is possible to account for a large proportion of transmitted information in terms of articulatory and phonological features . . . if natural perceptual features do exist, then there is little evidence in confusion-matrix data to support their existence.
>
> *(p. 1264)*[27]

On the other hand, Dubno and Levitt (1981) identify a suite of acoustic properties that reliably predict the patterns of consonant confusions produced by the listeners in their study. But Dubno and Levitt also observe that,

> the best predictions of incorrect responses was provided by different groups of variables [acoustic properties: JK] for each nonsense syllable subset and each experimental condition. That is, no one set of acoustic information could accurately predict confusions between all types of syllables.
>
> *(p. 258)*

The subsets they refer to consist of different sets of consonants, preceding or following vowels. Dubno and Levitt's observation that the acoustic properties that predict confusions differ between contexts appears to support Steriade's (2008) assertion that alternations arise because the cues to contrasts differ between, or are not conveyed equally well in all contexts. However, no one has appealed yet to Dubno and Levitt's specific observations in explaining why some phonological alternations are observed and others are not.

As an alternative to the equivocal evidence from studies of consonant confusions, Steriade (2008) turns instead to evidence from partial rhymes, direct judgments of similarity, and judgments of foreign accents, all of which point to [−voice] obstruents being more similar to [+voice] obstruents in the neutralization contexts than the other possible repairs (see her paper for citations to the specific studies). But none of this evidence distinguishes a similarity judgment based on comparing sounds' distinctive feature specifications from one based on the perceptual correspondents of their context-specific phonetic correlates any better than the studies of consonant confusions do. Phonological similarity and its regulation of alternations may indeed be grounded in perceptual similarity, but that remains a hypothesis that has not yet been tested directly.

The account offered by Steriade (2001, 2008) of the restrictions on possible alternations was discussed in this section because it appears to appeal so directly to the phonetic characteristics of the alternating sounds in the contexts in which they do and do not alternate. But as the discussion in the preceding paragraphs emphasizes, it only appears to do so, in the sense that phonological similarity is not yet demonstrably grounded in the phonetics of the sounds. In fact, it's difficult to conceive of a means by which phonetic grounding of similarity, *as phonetic grounding*, could be demonstrated with mature language users, as their perception of the sounds of their native language cannot easily be separated from their phonological representations of them. Perhaps, similarity judgments could be made using non-speech analogues, that is, sounds which preserve the acoustics of the speech sounds of interest but which are not recognized either as those sounds nor as speech. But there remains the necessity of showing that the perceived similarity between the original speech sounds scaled directly with the perceived similarity of the corresponding non-speech analogues.

Phonetic implementation

Given that this chapter began with a reference to Pierrehumbert, perhaps it is fitting that it closes with one, too, specifically, a reference to her work developing a model of the phonetic implementation of intonation in English and Japanese (Pierrehumbert, 1980; Liberman & Pierrehumbert, 1984; Pierrehumbert & Beckman, 1988); see also Bruce (1977) for a fundamentally similar account of Swedish intonation. The way in which the labor of explanation of the observed patterns is divided between the phonology and the phonetics in that model is also instructive about how that labor might be divided more generally.

Briefly, in these accounts of both English and Japanese, the phonological representation of intonation consists of a string of high (H) and low (L) tones which are aligned with the string of segments; that is, a tune consisting of H and L tones is aligned with a text consisting of segments. Japanese differs from English in that some of these tones arise from the lexicon, in morphemes bearing HL pitch accents, as well as from the intonational component, while all English tones arise from the intonational component. The intonational components of the two languages also differ considerably in which tones are aligned with particular locations in the text. However, once the string of Hs and Ls is specified and aligned in the utterance's phonological representation, the two languages resemble one another closely in how those Hs and Ls are mapped onto actual f_0 values: both adjust tones' relative prominence, interpolate between specified f_0 targets, apply downstep (AKA "catathesis") and final lowering, and exhibit declination. The mapping consists of translating Hs and Ls into f_0 targets followed by further transformations of those f_0 targets as a function of their prominence and context. In this account of English and Japanese intonation, the phonetics bears the bulk of the labor in determining how an utterance is pronounced, not the phonology.[28] A similar division of labor may be observed in Bruce's (1977) account of Swedish intonation.

Liberman and Pierrehumbert (1984) briefly discuss the generalization of this division of explanatory labor beyond intonation. Their example is the intrusion of stops between nasals and following fricatives already discussed, e.g., *warm[p]th*, *prin[t]ce*, and *leng[k]th*. These intrusions were previously described as a product of devoicing and soft palate raising occurring before opening the complete closure of the nasal into the fricative's narrow constriction, i.e., as an error in the timing of two of the fricative's articulations relative to a third. The occurrence of intrusive stops between a lateral and a following fricative, e.g., *heal[t]th*, *fal[t]se*, and *wel[t]sh*, was explained similarly, as early raising of the sides of the tongue before lowering its center, producing a brief complete closure. The intrusive vowels that occur between liquids and neighboring consonants in a number of languages, e.g., Chilean Spanish *c[o]ronica* "chronicle," Mono *gąf[ū]rū* "mortar," Dutch *kal[a]m* "quiet," Scots Gaelic *tar[a]v* "bull," may also be explained as byproduct of timing, where the articulation of the liquid overlaps so little with the other consonant in the cluster that a simultaneous vowel articulation becomes briefly audible between them (see Hall, 2006, for extensive documentation and the analysis summarized here).

As already noted, Clements (1987) proposes that the phonology rather than timing is responsible for the stops which intrude between nasals and fricatives. This proposal rests first on the observation that (some) speakers of South African English never pronounce nasal-fricative sequences with intrusive stops, while (some) speakers of American English always do (Fourakis & Port, 1986). According to Clements, if members of a speech community behave systematically, then that behavior is necessarily encoded in the grammar, in this case, the phonological grammar of their language. He would presumably make a similar argument for the intrusive stops between laterals and fricatives in English, because not all English speakers produce them, and for the intrusive vowels documented between liquids and other consonants by Hall (2006), because they're not observed in all languages.

But Liberman and Pierrehumbert (1984) suggest an equally plausible alternative, that dialects or languages could differ systematically in the timing and coordination regimes for the articulations of successive consonants. A telling piece of evidence in support of this alternative is that the stops that intrude between nasals and fricatives are considerably shorter than those that realize a /t/ in the input, i.e., in *prince* compared to *prints* (Fourakis & Port, 1986). The nasal is also shorter when the /t/ arises in the input. Clements (1987) accounts for the difference in the stop's duration in a feature-geometric analysis by spreading an oral cavity node that dominates the [−continuant] and place specifications of the nasal to the following fricative. Because the result is a sequence of [−continuant][+continuant] specification dominated by a single timing slot, i.e., *warm[p͡θ]*, *prin[t͡s]e*, and *len[k͡θ]*, the stop closure is shorter than it would be if it occupied an entire timing slot by itself. Because the stop shares a timing slot with the nasal, this account also explains why the nasal is not shortened as much as would be when the /t/ arises in the input. A genuine cluster would compress all the segments in the rime more.

Clements also argues that the intruded stop must be phonological because it is glottalized in some dialects. In his account, glottalization of voiceless stops in codas, too, is a phonological process because it is produced by the members of some speech communities and not by the members of others. On this logic, if glottalization is a phonological process, then stop intrusion must be, too, because only a phonological process can feed another one. This is unconvincing on two grounds. First, my own pronunciation shows that it is possible for a speaker to consistently glottalize voiceless stops in syllable codas, but to not glottalize those that intrude between nasals and fricatives. If stop intrusion doesn't consistently feed glottalization, perhaps it's not a phonological process. Second and less personally, glottalization itself is plausibly a dialect-specific phonetic implementation process, which could be realized on any voiceless closure in the right prosodic context, regardless of whether that closure originates in the input or as the result of a particular pattern of articulatory timing and coordination. That is, there's no need to presume any ordering of processes of the sort found in phonological derivations; intrusion and glottalization would instead be simultaneous (and independent to account for my speech). More generally still, a common characteristic of intrusive vowels does not lend itself to such an account: they are most often identical in quality to the vowels occurring on the other side of the liquid. Assuming the intrusive vowels constitute a vowel node, achieving identity by autosegmental spreading would entail crossing association lines,[29] whereas a phonetic account in which the liquid is loosely coordinated with the preceding consonant and overlaps with the simultaneous vowel gesture faces no such problem (see Hall, 2006, and references cited therein for further discussion of differences between cases that are handled well with autosegments versus gestures).

Although this discussion implies that the division of explanatory labor between phonetics and phonology can be extended quite readily and confidently from intonation to other sound patterns, these remarks should instead be read as only tentatively suggesting an alternative analysis of a very limited if frequently occurring phenomenon, the intrusive segments produced by particular patterns of articulatory coordination. A more comprehensive effort to test the generality of this division of labor can scarcely be said to have begun, much less progressed to a point where one can indeed confidently assert that phonetic implementation is responsible for most of what is observed in patterns of articulations, acoustics, or perception, and phonology is responsible for relatively little (see Kingston & Diehl, 1994; Stevens & Keyser, 2010, pp. 423–426 and p. 18, respectively). Nor that the reverse is true, and the phonetics cedes the responsibility to the phonology.

This lack of progress can probably be attributed to three obvious facts. First, in most cases, no other elements in a phonological representation correspond to a single phonetic correlate in the way that the tones that represent intonational contrasts correspond to f_0. And f_0 is only the most accessible phonetic correlate, among many, of tonal contrasts.

Second, the phonetic correlates of other contrasts, besides being multiple, vary substantially in their realization across contexts, speakers, and languages, such that it's been difficult to proceed beyond mere descriptions of their variation to generalizable formal statements of their implementation.

The third fact requires more discussion. It is the accumulation of evidence that apparently similar or even identical phonological categories are implemented phonetically in different ways across languages. One such example was already discussed, the differences in the timing of soft palate lowering in vowels preceding nasals between English versus Spanish documented by Solé (1992, 1995). An additional example is the differences between languages in the duration of the delay in the onset of voicing following the release of the stop in voiceless unaspirated and aspirated or short- and long-lag stops (VOT) documented by Cho and Ladefoged (1999). This example illustrates the uncertainty about the extent to which a sound pattern can be explained phonetically particularly well, because it shows that variation can be explained only in part by referring to the physics and physiology of speech production. Cho and Ladefoged set out to describe and explain the finding that across languages, velar stops have longer VOTs than dental or alveolar (henceforth "coronal") and bilabial stops. Cho and Ladefoged document the various purely phonetic factors that could contribute to this difference in VOT between velar and more anterior places of articulation. The first three lead to a slower venting of the air trapped behind a velar than a more anterior closure, a slower drop in intraoral air pressure above the glottis, and a longer delay in producing a large enough pressure drop across the glottis for voicing to begin:

1. Aerodynamics: The cavity behind a velar constriction is smaller, which could result in a higher air pressure behind it. The greater inertia of the mass of air in the larger cavity in front of the constriction may also delay the drop in intraoral air pressure.
2. Mass: The active articulator in velar stops is the tongue body, which has much greater mass and thus much greater inertia than the tongue tip and blade or lower lip. A velar closure may therefore be released slower than a coronal or bilabial closure. The closer proximity of a tongue body constriction to the pivot point of jaw rotation also produces a smaller opening through which air can flow out for a given amount of jaw rotation than do the more distant coronal and bilabial constrictions.
3. Constriction length: The tongue body makes more extensive longitudinal contact with the passive articulator, the palate, than do the tongue tip and blade with the alveolar ridge or teeth or the lower lip with the upper lip. The channel through which air can escape from behind the constriction remains narrower longer when the constriction is longer.

4 The oral closure is shorter in bilabial than coronal or velar stops. If the duration of the glottal opening is the same across places of articulation, the result would be a shorter period of glottal opening, and thus aspiration, after the release of bilabial than coronal or velar stops.

All four of these factors could contribute the longer VOTs observed in velar than bilabial stops.

Because Cho and Ladefoged's (1999) sample includes relatively few languages with voiceless aspirated stops and of those only two have bilabial voiceless aspirated stops, the rest of this discussion is limited to comparisons of voiceless unaspirated stops in the 13 (out of 18) languages that have them at bilabial, coronal, and velar places of articulation. Mean VOTs (*ses*) are 16 ms (1.5), 18 ms (1.6), and 37 ms (3.0). One-sided paired t -tests[30] show that bilabial and coronal VOTs don't differ ($t\,(12) = -1.06$, $p > 0.1$), but bilabial and coronal VOTs are both significantly shorter than velar VOTs ($t\,(12) = -6.95$, $p < 0.001$; $t\,(12) = -6.88$, $p < 0.001$). Thus far, the voiceless unaspirated VOTs differ across places as predicted from the phonetic factors listed above: bilabial ≈ coronal < velar.

But Figure 13.3 shows that there is considerable language-specific variation in how much longer velar VOTs are relative to either bilabial or coronal VOTs. Because velar VOTs were

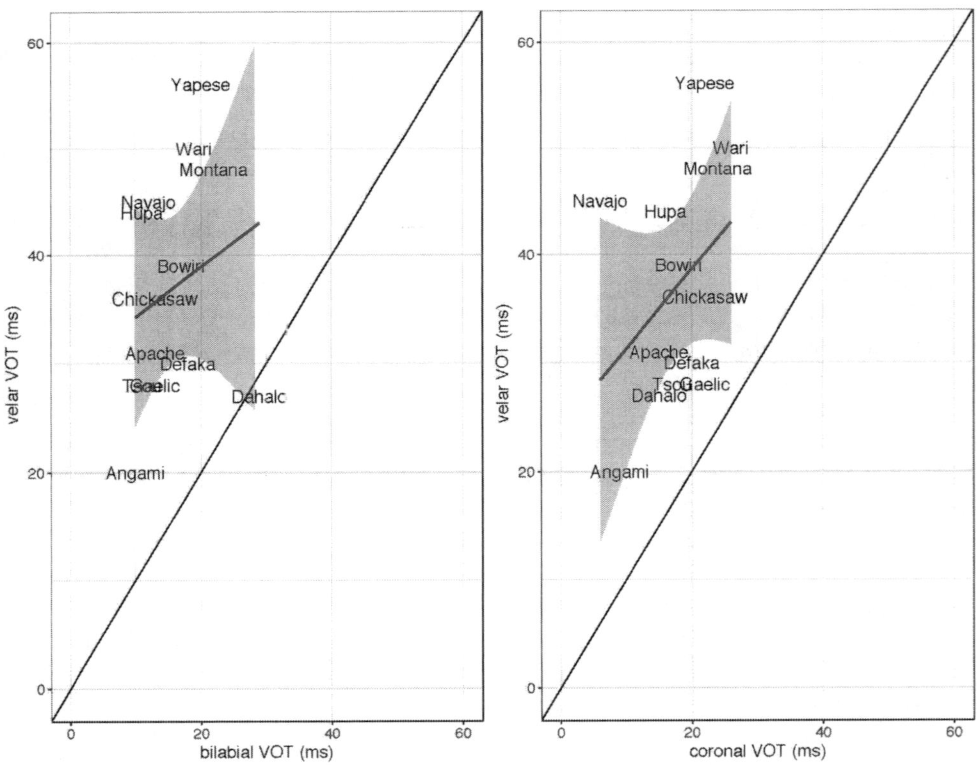

Figure 13.3 (left) Mean velar by bilabial VOTs (right) mean velar by coronal VOTs for voiceless unaspirated stops, with $y = x$ lines and the linear regression fits.

Source: From Cho and Ladefoged (1999).

just shown to be significantly longer than either bilabial or velar VOTs, it's expected that all the points would lie above the $y = x$ line, but the figure also shows that velar VOTs do not scale with either bilabial or coronal VOTs: the lines fit by linear regression to the points both have positive slopes, but these slopes are not significantly different from 0 and the extent of the spread of values around these lines (the gray shading) shows that little in the variation of velar VOTs is predicted from variation in either the bilabial or coronal VOTs. Instead, velar VOTs vary unpredictably between languages from modestly to extremely greater than either bilabial or coronal VOTs. Velar VOTs in some languages, e.g., Yapese, Wari', Montana Salish, Navajo, and Hupa, are long enough to be treated as aspirated in other languages, while others are considerably shorter, e.g., Apache, Defaka, Tsou, Gaelic, Khonoma Angami, and Dahalo. The language with the longest VOT for velar stops, Yapese, doesn't have contrasting voiceless aspirated stops, but two of the languages with long velar VOTs contrast them with voiceless aspirated stops with even longer VOTs, and only one of the languages with shorter VOTs, Apache, contrasts them with voiceless aspirated stops (see Cho & Ladefoged, 1999, themselves for more extensive observations of language-specific differences in VOTs). These differences are not predicted by the physics and physiological differences between velar and more anterior stops listed previously.

Kingston and Diehl (1994) offer two related arguments that speakers' phonetic behavior cannot be entirely predicted by the physical and physiological constraints on articulations and on the transduction of those articulations into the acoustic properties of the speech signal. The first argument was built on a review of explanations for the differences in f_0 in vowels followed stops that contrast for [voice]: f_0 is lower following [+voice] than [−voice] obstruents. These f_0 differences are observed in languages like English, where the [voice] contrast is otherwise realized as a difference between voiceless unaspirated versus voiceless aspirated (or short- versus long-lag) stops at the beginnings of words, and in languages like French, where the contrast is instead realized as a difference between voiced versus voiceless unaspirated (or prevoiced versus short-lag) stops. This review led to us to reject all attempts to explain the covariation of f_0 with VOT as the automatic byproducts of physical or physiological dependencies between the articulations that produce the differences in VOT and those that produce the differences in f_0 (see also Dmitrieva, Llanos, Shultz, & Francis, 2015). In place of such explanations, we next argued that the responsible articulations were controlled independently by speakers in order to combine acoustic properties that would integrate auditorily: a lower f_0 in a following vowel would integrate with an earlier onset of voicing, either in a prevoiced or short-lag stop, to produce a percept of low-frequency energy, while a higher f_0 would instead integrate with a later onset of voicing, either in a short- or a long-lag stop, to produce a percept of the absence of low-frequency energy. Further support for this second argument was reported by Kingston and Diehl (1995) and Kingston, Diehl, Kirk, and Castleman (2008); various challenges are offered by Hanson (2009), Holt, Lotto, and Kluender (2001), and Kirby and Ladd (2016).

If speakers can and do exercise such detailed control over their articulations, then the language-specific differences in VOT documented by Cho and Ladefoged (1999) are entirely unremarkable, even if the specific values observed in each language are still unexplained. These observations also suggest that speakers and listeners have learned a *phonetic* grammar along with their phonological grammar in the course of acquiring competence in their language. A language's phonetic grammar consists of the procedures for implementing the language's phonological representations in ways that characterize the behavior of native speakers and listeners of that language, and that can distinguish their behavior from non-native speakers and listeners.

Concluding remarks

As an *aide-mémoire* for the reader, the principal studies cited in this review are listed as follows, with brief reminders of their arguments:

1 There is no interface between phonetics and phonology

   (a) Fowler (1986a, 1986b) and Browman and Goldstein (1986): Phonological representations are composed of units that occur in the world, articulatory gestures
   (b) Hale and Reiss (2000, 2008) and Reiss (2017): Phonological representations and operations are constrained by what can be computed, not by what can be pronounced, perceived, nor learned
   (c) Ohala (1990, 2005): Phonologies cannot be *explained* without phonetics, nor vice versa
   (d) Flemming (2001): Phonologies refer formally to phonetic continua as well as categories

2 There is an interface between phonetics and phonology

   (a) Beguš (2017) and Hayes (1999): Phonologies refer coarsely to sound's phonetic properties because they favor formal simplicity
   (b) Steriade (2001, 2008): Alternations are governed by perceptual similarity between alternants
   (c) Liberman and Pierrehumbert (1984): Phonetic implementation accounts for much of how sounds pattern and can be formalized

This variety in points of view may dishearten a reader who has gotten this far by leaving them to wonder whether any consensus is possible regarding the nature of the interface between phonology and phonetics. After all, they have read three different arguments denying that there is such interface or any need for one, and the positive proposals also differ dramatically in their account of the interface. This uncertainty and the debates sketched in this chapter show that there is indeed no consensus, but instead at least this multitude of points of view. In fact, this review is certainly not the only attempt to discuss and develop an account of the interface between phonetics and phonology, nor do those other attempts agree with the account developed here. Therefore, the interested reader would also do well to consult at least Keating (1988a, 1988b, 1990), Kingston (2007), and Scobbie (2007) for further discussion and different points of view regarding the interface between phonology and phonetics.

This is of course an entirely unsatisfactory state of affairs. Getting satisfaction will not, however, depend on forcibly reconciling this multitude to a single well-agreed-upon point of view, but instead on a concerted effort to study the interface(s), by developing testable models of the relationship between the speaker's phonological specification of an utterance and its implementation as articulations and their acoustic consequences, and similarly developing testable models of the relationship between an utterance's acoustic properties, their auditory transformation and mapping onto the listener's phonological representation. In this way of putting things, there are at least two interfaces where implementation can be studied, modeled, and formalized, from the speaker to speech and from speech to the listener. This way of putting things also suggests how progress may be made, by focusing on one or another of these two interfaces, and devising proof of concept experiments followed up by more thorough investigation once the proof is obtained. It is because this is only way to get satisfaction that this paper was closed with a discussion of the division of explanatory labor between phonetics and phonology in the account of English, Japanese, and Swedish intonation. As sketched in that discussion, the proposed division of labor was arrived at by developing just such a model of how a tune's phonological representation is implemented in the speaker's production of the corresponding intonation contour in these languages. That division of labor was extended, in favor of a phonetic explanation, to accounting for the occurrence and characteristics of intrusive segments. But this is just potential progress on a small part of the speaker to speech interface; an equally general approach to the speech to listener interface is lacking, largely because of unresolved debates regarding the objects of speech perception (Diehl, Lotto, & Holt, 2004; Fowler, 2006; Lotto & Holt, 2006) and the extent to which the listener's linguistic knowledge interacts with their perception of the signal's acoustic properties (McClelland, Mirman, & Holt, 2006; Norris, McQueen, & Cutler, 2000). This recommendation also implies that developing formal models of phonetic grounding of sound inventories and patterns may best be achieved by first developing such models of phonetic implementation, rather than trying to adjudicate the division of labor on the grounds of *a priori* assumptions of what is properly phonology versus phonetics.

A certain consequence of developing such models of implementation and grounding is sure to be profound and unexpected changes in our conceptions of what phonological representations consist of, as well as the processes and constraints acting on them. It is equally certain that our conceptions of phonetic implementation will change profoundly and unexpectedly, too. But both kinds of changes should be welcome, so long as they are supported by sound empirical work and fully general formal models.

Acknowledgments

I remain very grateful to the editors, William Katz and Peter Assmann, for their invitation to think hard once again about the interface between phonetics and phonology, and even more so for their patience in waiting for me to complete this chapter. I also appreciate the enormous care and interest of three reviewers, Ryan Bennett, Marie Huffman, and Amanda Rysling, whose close readings and clear guidance regarding what needed to be revised, reworked, added, or discarded have not only made this chapter more readable and intelligible than it would have been without their efforts but have also focused and improved my own thinking about the phenomena and theories. Any remaining errors and infelicities are mine alone.

Notes

1 Autosegmental processes or constraints are an apparent exception to this distinction between phonological and phonetic representations of an utterance, but even they refer to the sequence of discrete segments spanned by a feature value rather than to the feature value's temporal extent and its overlap with other phonetic properties. A potentially genuine exception are articulatory phonology's gestural representations; see no interface is needed (or possible) for discussion.

2 There is arguably just one phonological representation for an utterance, which originates in the speaker's mind and hopefully ends up in listener's mind. See Myers (2000, p. 260), for a statement of this premise as the hypothesis that there is one and only one phonological representation for any linguistic expression. But there may be multiple phonetic representations, at least: the motor plans, the articulatory movements that realize them, the acoustic consequences of these movements, and the auditory responses to those acoustic properties. Some might argue that only the first and last of these are representations, in that only they are found in the nervous systems (minds) of the speaker

and listener, respectively. In this narrower interpretation of what can be a representation, these phonetic representations are just as much psychological events in the mind as the phonological representations, and may, therefore, be harder to separate from the speaker's and the listener's implicit knowledge than Pierrehumbert (1990) proposes.

3 As noted already previously, when transduction was distinguished from translation, there is no need to speak of any interface between articulations and acoustic properties nor between acoustic properties and auditory qualities, because these are transformations between one set of continuous events and another, which are fully determined by physics, physiology, and psychology in the speaker or listener. Differences in how their speakers implement the same phonological units, e.g., between retroflexed versus bunched articulations of American English /r/, or how their listeners attend to particular acoustic properties, e.g., between attending to the low third formant of English /r/ as a cue to the contrast between it and /l/, must precede and follow the transduction from articulations to acoustics or from acoustics to auditory qualities, respectively

4 Neither of these examples can be accommodated by the dynamics of the articulatory gestures as currently proposed in the articulatory phonology literature, because all the proposed gestures' goals are too local. However, no insuperable challenges appear to stand in the way of including dynamic parameters that specify more global vocal tract configurations as goals.

5 There are also asymmetries in strength between overlapping gestures such that segments differ in their resistance to coarticulation and its acoustic consequences (Fowler, 2005; Iskarous, Fowler, & Whalen, 2010; Iskarous et al., 2013; Recasens, 1985).

6 Donegan and Stampe (1979, 2009) draw essentially the same line as Hale and Reiss (2000) between what they treat as phonology and what they do not, but Donegan & Stampe apply the label "phonology" to what falls on the opposite side of the line, i.e., the workings of the phonetically purposeful processes that make it possible to recognize and pronounce the contents of the phonological representation, as opposed to the purely formal rules and constraints of the morphophonology.

7 Hale and Reiss's (2000) argument is intended to purge all phonetically motivated constraints from phonology, not just cases of positional faithfulness.

8 To acquire a language in which a contrast is synchronically restricted, say, to first or stressed syllables as a result of the effects of earlier imperfect learning on its diachrony, the learner would have to recognize that a syllable is either first or stressed, and to formally encode the restriction of the contrast to such contexts. Recognizing that a syllable is first in its word or that it's metrically strong could certainly be achieved from the physical properties of strings, appearing at times at the beginning of an utterance or being louder, longer, and/or higher in pitch, but encoding requires generalizing formally across all instances of first or stressed syllables, and they are by no means uniform in their phonetic substance. This variability is, however, a challenge to any account of phonological learning, not just that assumed by Hale and Reiss (2000).

9 Reiss (2017) argues that a string such as Bund [bund] "association" is not absent from the German-learning child's experience because it's banned by any markedness constraint in the phonological grammar of German, but instead because the grammar never generates it. This begs the question: why doesn't the grammar ever generate it? The answer would appear to be that it cannot because no lexical entry includes syllable-final voiced obstruents. The alternation between voiced obstruents, e.g. in Bundes [bun.dəs] "association (gen.)," and voiceless ones, Bund [bunt] "association," does not lead a child learning German to posit a synchronic constraint on the distribution of [+voice] in obstruents, because the [d] occurs syllable initially not finally in the lexical entry for the genitive form.

10 Examples are taken from the sources cited.

11 de Boer (2000) also proposed procedures to weight particular formant frequencies that similarly emphasize their contributions to distinguishing vowels from one another.

12 "*u*" is short for unmarked, and "*α*" is a variable, whose values may be + or −. Thus, (2a) is to be read as that the unmarked value of [low] is [−low], and (2c) is to be read as that the unmarked value of [round] is that which agrees with a non-low vowel's value for [back].

13 Clements (1987) argues instead that stops intrude in lateral-fricative clusters because laterals are [−continuant] like nasals. This proposal predicts, incorrectly, that a stop should intrude between

the lateral and the fricative in words like *gulf*, *shelf*, and *golf*. Because the labio-dental fricative /f/ is not produced by raising the sides of the tongue, no timing error in the transition from the center-up, sides-down position of the tongue in the lateral to the fricative's labio-dental articulation will completely close the oral cavity. A puzzle remains for both accounts: why are intrusive stops much less frequent, if they occur at all, when the fricative is voiced, e.g., in *falls* compared to *false*.

14 I adopt Hyman's (2001) representations, *NT and *ND, for constraints prohibiting voiceless and voiced stops and affricates after nasals, respectively. Unless affricates behave differently from stops, any reference to stops in the rest of this discussion should be interpreted as including affricates, too.

15 I am grateful to Ryan Bennett for pointing this out.

16 In Hyman's (2001) account of Tswana's history, the voiceless stops became aspirated after nasals at this stage, *mp, *nt, *ŋk > mpʰ, ntʰ, ŋkxʰ and lenited to homorganic continuants elsewhere, *p, t, k > ɸ, ɾ̥, x, too.

17 Even though voiced *stops* only occur after nasals following lenition, the preceding nasal has been omitted because devoicing is supposed to be context-free.

18 Coronal stops are expected to pattern similarly, while a voiced velar stop /g/ has been lost except after nasals, where it's expected to merge with its voiceless counterpart /k/.

19 See Hyman (2001) for an argument that devoicing the stop in /mb/ to produce [mp] doesn't improve the contrast of /mb/ and /m/ by increasing their phonetic dispersion.

20 The interpretation offered by Solé (1992, 1995) for the English facts conflicts with that offered by Cohn (1993), who argues that vowel nasalization in English is instead phonetic because it begins at different times in the vowel relative to the onset of the nasal's oral constriction, and it increases gradually once it begins, as though it was interpolating from the vowel's oral target to the nasal's nasal target. There are a number of possible reasons why Solé and Cohn come to opposite conclusions. Perhaps the most likely is that Cohn was comparing the extent of vowel nasalization before nasals in English, with its extent in contrastive nasal vowels in French, where vowels become fully nasalized very early in the vowel. Another is that Solé used a device, the nasograph, that directly measures when the velopharyngeal port begins to open and the relative size of the port over time, while Cohn measured air flow out of the nose. Measurements of the volume of nasal airflow may convey a different estimate of when a vowel becomes nasalized than measurements of velopharyngeal port area, and both may differ from acoustic estimates (Beddor, 2007; Beddor & Krakow, 1999). Finally, the size of the velopharyngeal port opening increased gradually from the moment it started to open in Solé's data, much like the volume of nasal airflow in Cohn's data, so the two measurements are not so dissimilar after all, even if the authors reporting them interpret them differently.

21 Solé's (2007) review shows that these facts are not limited to English and Catalan, and that other factors which increase duration, including stress and intrinsic differences, have similar effects.

22 Using stepwise log-linear modeling of contingency tables representing the co-occurrence frequencies of voiceless stops, /p/, /t/, and /k/, in the 451 languages in UPSID (Maddieson & Precoda, 1992), I found that each stop's occurrence depended positively on each other stop's occurrence. For voiced stops, /b/, /d/, and /g/, an analogous modeling effort showed that /g/'s occurrence depended on /d/'s but not /b/'s occurrence, and /d/'s occurrence depended on /b/'s. For similar conclusions based on X^2 statistics derived from 2x2 contingency tables, see Clements (2003), and see also Ohala (1979) for the observation that consonant inventories tend to use available features maximally.

23 This distinction differs from that made at the beginning of this chapter between a continuous phonetics and a categorical phonology: here, both the phonetics and the phonology refer to categories – the objects being regulated – and to quantities – phonetic grounding values.

24 It is important to emphasize that the too-many solutions problem is not a pathology peculiar to an optimality theoretic account of phonological grammars. It would be just as easy to write a rule that changes a voiced obstruent into a nasal, a fricative, or a glide, that deletes it, or that inserts a vowel after it, as one that changes a voiced obstruent into a voiceless one.

25 The argument that these are each changes in the value of a single feature depends on the assumption that contingent changes in other, redundant feature values, e.g., [−sonorant] > [+sonorant] when [−nasal] > [+nasal], aren't counted because they're predictable.

26 Steriade (2001) cites only one language in which a following retroflex assimilates to preceding apico-alveolar as well as vice versa, Murinbata, and only three in which only a following retroflex assimilates to a preceding apico-alveolar and not vice versa, Kannada, changes from Sanskrit to Middle Indic, and Burarra. In the remaining 12 languages cited, only apico-alveolars assimilate to preceding retroflexes, and not vice versa. The evidence in Table 13.2 that retroflexes are identified better after vowels than apico-alveolars may explain this asymmetry.

Anderson (1997) also shows that with one exception an apico-alveolar is more likely to be misidentified as a retroflex than vice versa, in both VCV and CV strings. The exception is that [ʈ] is more often misidentified as [t] in VCV strings than vice versa.

27 The participants in these experiments might have been forced to use phonological features in place of the "natural perceptual" features because the phonological features are part of what mature speakers of language, like these participants, *know* about the sounds of their language, and that knowledge organizes their perception of the acoustic qualities of the language's sounds.

28 See Clements (1983) and Hyman (1986) for proposals to represent downstep in the phonology as register lowering; and see Ladd (1994) for a similar but more general phonological representation of register shifts, as well as Hayes's (1994) response to Ladd.

29 No association lines would be crossed if vowels are projected on a separate tier from consonants. Then, the intrusive vowel's quality could be made identical to that of the vowel on the other side of the liquid by the same formal means that vowels are caused to agree in their specifications in languages with vowel harmony. I'm indebted to Ryan Bennett for pointing this out.

30 The tests are one-sided because bilabial stops are predicted to have the shortest VOTs, velar stops the longest, with coronal stops falling in between. The larger *se*s for velar than bilabial or coronal stops motivated assuming unequal variances in these tests.

References

Anderson, V. B. (1997). The perception of coronals in Western Arrente. In Proceedings of Eurospeech '97: Fifth European conference on speech communication and technology (Vol. 1, pp. 389–392).

Archangeli, D., & Pulleyblank, D. (1994). *Grounded phonology*. Cambridge, MA: MIT Press.

Bach, E., & Harms, R. (1972). How do languages get crazy rules? In R. Stockwell & R. Macaulay (Eds.), *Linguistic change and generative theory* (pp. 1–21). Bloomington, IN: Indiana University Press.

Beckman, J. (1997). Positional faithfulness, positional neutralization, and Shona vowel harmony. *Phonology*, *14*(1), 1–46.

Beddor, P. S. (2007). Nasals and nasalization: The relationship between segmental and coarticulatory timing. In J. Trouvain & W. J. Barry (Eds.), *Proceedings of the XVIth international congress of phonetic sciences* (pp. 249–254). Saarland University Saarbrücken, Saarbrucken, Germany.

Beddor, P. S., & Krakow, R. A. (1999). Perception of coarticulatory nasalization by speakers of English and Thai: Evidence for partial compensation. *The Journal of the Acoustical Society of America*, *106*, 2868–2887.

Beddor, P. S., & Onsuwan, C. (2003). Perception of prenasalized stops. In M. J. Solé, D. Recasens, & J. Romero (Eds.), *Proceedings of the XVth international congress of phonetic sciences* (pp. 407–410). Causal Productions, Barcelona.

Beguš, G. (2017). *Post-nasal devoicing and a probabilistic model of phonological typology*. Ms.

Benkí, J. R. (2003). Analysis of English nonsense syllable recognition in noise. *Phonetica*, 60, 129–157.

Bermúdez-Otero, R., & Börjars, K. (2006). Markedness in phonology and in syntax: The problem of grounding. *Lingua*, *116*, 710–756.

Blevins, J. (2004). *Evolutionary phonology: The emergence of sound patterns*. Cambridge: Cambridge University Press.
Blust, R. (2005). Must sound change be linguistically motivated? *Diachronica*, *22*, 219–269.
Boersma, P. (1998). *Functional phonology: Formalizing the interaction between articulatory and perceptual drives*. The Hague: Holland Academic Graphics.
Boersma, P. (2011). A programme for bidirectional phonology and phonetics and their acquisition and evolution. In A. Benz & J. Mattausch (Eds.), *Bidirectional optimality theory* (pp. 33–72). Amsterdam: John Benjamins.
Boersma, P., & Hamann, S. (2009). Cue constraints and their interaction in perception and production. In P. Boersma & S. Hamann (Eds.), *Phonology in perception* (pp. 55–110). Berlin: Mouton de Gruyter.
Browman, C. P., & Goldstein, L. M. (1986). Towards an articulatory phonology. *Phonology Yearbook*, *3*, 219–252.
Browman, C. P., & Goldstein, L. M. (1988). Some notes on syllable structure in articulatory phonology. *Phonetica*, *45*, 140–155.
Browman, C. P., & Goldstein, L. M. (1989). Articulatory gestures as phonological units. *Phonology*, *6*, 201–251.
Browman, C. P., & Goldstein, L. M. (1990). Tiers in articulatory phonology, with some implications for casual speech. In J. Kingston & M. E. Beckman (Eds.), *Papers in laboratory phonology I* (pp. 341–376). Cambridge: Cambridge University Press.
Browman, C. P., & Goldstein, L. M. (1992). Articulatory phonology: An overview. *Phonetica*, *49*, 155–180.
Browman, C. P., & Goldstein, L. M. (1995a). Dynamics and articulatory phonology. In R. F. Port & T. V. Gelder (Eds.), *Mind as motion: Explorations in the dynamics of cognition* (pp. 175–193). Cambridge, MA: MIT Press.
Browman, C. P., & Goldstein, L. M. (1995b). Gestural syllable position effects in American English. In F. Bell-Berti & L. J. Raphael (Eds.), *Producing speech: Contemporary issues. For Katherine Harris* (pp. 19–33). New York, NY: AIP Press.
Bruce, G. (1977). *Swedish word accents in sentence perspective*. Lund: Gleerup.
Cho, T., & Ladefoged, P. (1999). Variation and universals in VOT: Evidence from 18 languages. *Journal of Phonetics*, *27*, 207–229.
Chomsky, N., & Halle, M. (1968). *The sound pattern of English*. New York, NY: Harper & Row.
Clements, G. N. (1983). The hierarchical representation of tone features. In I. R. Dihoff (Ed.), *Current approaches to African linguistics* (pp. 145–176). Dordrecht: Foris.
Clements, G. N. (1987). Phonological feature representation and the description of intrusive stops. In A. Bosch, B. Need, & E. Schiller (Eds.), *CLS 23: Parasession on autosegmental and metrical phonology* (pp. 29–50). Chicago, IL: Chicago Linguistic Society.
Clements, G. N. (2003). Feature economy in sound systems. *Phonology*, *20*(3), 287–333.
Coetzee, A. W., & Pretorius, R. (2010). Phonetically grounded phonology and sound change: The case of Tswana labial plosives. *Journal of Phonetics*, *38*, 404–421.
Cohn, A. C. (1993). Nasalisation in English: Phonology or phonetics. *Phonology*, *10*, 43–81.
Cohn, A. C. (2007). Is there gradient phonology? In G. Fanselow, C. Féry, M. Schlesewsky, & R. Vogel (Eds.), *Gradience in grammar: Generative perspectives* (pp. 25–44). Oxford: Oxford University Press.
Cutler, A., Weber, A., Smits, R., & Cooper, N. (2004). Patterns of English phoneme confusions by native and non-native listeners. *The Journal of the Acoustical Society of America*, *116*, 3668–3478.
de Boer, B. (2000). Self-organization in vowel systems. *Journal of Phonetics*, *28*, 441–465.
de Lacy, P., & Kingston, J. (2013). Synchronic explanation. *Natural Language and Linguistic Theory*, *31*, 287–355.
Denes, P. B., & Pinson, E. (1963). *The speech chain*. New York, NY: Bell Telephone Laboratories.
Diehl, R. L., Lotto, A. J., & Holt, L. L. (2004). Speech perception. *Annual Review of Psychology*, *55*, 149–179.

Dmitrieva, O., Llanos, F., Shultz, A. A., & Francis, A. L. (2015). Phonological status, not voice onset time, determines the acoustic realization of onset f0 as a secondary voicing cue in Spanish and English. *Journal of Phonetics*, *49*, 77–95.

Donegan, P. J., & Stampe, D. (1979). The study of natural phonology. In D. A. Dinnsen (Ed.), *Current approaches to phonological theory* (pp. 126–173). Bloomington, IN: Indiana University Press.

Donegan, P. J., & Stampe, D. (2009). Hypotheses of natural phonology. *Poznań Studies in Contemporary Linguistics*, *45*(1), 1–31.

Dubno, J. R., & Levitt, H. (1981). Predicting consonant confusions from acoustic analysis. *The Journal of the Acoustical Society of America*, *69*, 249–261.

Flack, K. (2007). *The sources of phonological markedness* (Ph.D. dissertation). University of Massachusetts, Amherst.

Flemming, E. (2001). Scalar and categorical phenomena in a unified model of phonetics and phonology. *Phonology*, *18.1*, 7–44.

Fourakis, M., & Port, R. (1986). Stop epenthesis in English. *Journal of Phonetics*, *14*, 197–221.

Fowler, C. A. (1983). Converging sources of evidence on spoken and perceived rhythms of speech: Cyclic production of vowels in monosyllabic stress feet. *Journal of Experimental Psychology: General*, *112*(3), 386.

Fowler, C. A. (1986a). An event approach to the study of speech perception from a direct realist perspective. *Journal of Phonetics*, *14*, 3–28.

Fowler, C. A. (1986b). Reply to commentators. *Journal of Phonetics*, *14*, 149–170.

Fowler, C. A. (2005). Parsing coarticulated speech in perception: Effects of coarticulation resistance. *Journal of Phonetics*, *33*, 199–213.

Fowler, C. A. (2006). Compensation for coarticulation reflects gesture perception, not spectral contrast. *Perception and Psychophysics*, *68*, 161–177.

Fowler, C. A., & Smith, M. (1986). Speech perception as vector analysis: An approach to the problems of segmentation and invariance. In J. Perkell & D. H. Klatt (Eds.), *Invariance and variability of speech processes* (pp. 123–136). Hillsdale, NJ: Lawrence Erlbaum Associates.

Gafos, A. I. (2006). Dynamics in grammar: Comment on Ladd and Ernestus & Baayen. In L. M. Goldstein, D. H. Whalen, & C. T. Best (Eds.), *Laboratory phonology 8: Varieties of phonological competence* (pp. 51–79). Berlin: Mouton de Gruyter.

Gafos, A. I., & Goldstein, L. M. (2012). Articulatory representation and organization. In A. C. Cohn, C. Fougeron, & M. K. Huffman (Eds.), *Oxford handbook of laboratory phonology* (pp. 220–231). Oxford: Oxford University Press.

Garrett, A. (2015). Sound change. In *The Routledge handbook of historical linguistics* (pp. 227–248). London: Routledge.

Gibson, J. J. (1982). Notes on affordances. In E. Reed & R. Jones (Eds.), *Reasons for realism: Selected essays of James J. Gibson* (pp. 401–418). Hillsdale, NJ: Lawrence Erlbaum Associates.

Gick, B. (2002). An x-ray investigation of pharyngeal constriction in American English schwa. *Phonetica*, *59*, 38–48.

Goldstein, L. M., & Fowler, C. A. (2003). Articulatory phonology: A phonology for public language use. In N. O. Schiller & A. S. Meyer (Eds.), *Phonetics and phonology in language comprehension and production* (pp. 159–207). Berlin: Mouton de Gruyter.

Goldstein, L. M., Pouplier, M., Chen, L., Saltzman, E., & Byrd, D. (2007). Dynamic action units slip in speech production errors. *Cognition*, *103*(3), 386–412.

Gouskova, M., Zsiga, E., & Boyer, O. T. (2011). Grounded constraints and the consonants of Tswana. *Lingua*, *121*, 2120–2152.

Hale, M. R., & Reiss, C. (2000). Substance abuse and dysfunctionalism: Current trends in phonology. *Linguistic Inquiry*, *31*, 157–169.

Hale, M. R., & Reiss, C. (2008). *The phonological enterprise*. Oxford: Oxford University Press.

Hall, N. (2006). Crosslinguistic patterns of vowel intrusion. *Phonology*, *23*(3), 387–429.

Hanson, H. M. (2009). Effects of obstruent consonants on fundamental frequency at vowel onset in English. *The Journal of the Acoustical Society of America*, *125*, 425–441.

Hayes, B. (1994). "Gesture" in prosody: Comments on the paper by Ladd. In P. A. Keating (Ed.), *Papers in laboratory phonology III: Phonological structure and phonological form* (pp. 64–74). Cambridge: Cambridge University Press.

Hayes, B. (1999). Phonetically-driven phonology: The role of optimality theory and inductive grounding. In M. Darnell, E. Moravscik, M. Noonan, F. Newmeyer, & K. Wheatley (Eds.), *Functionalism and formalism in linguistics* (Vol. 1, pp. 243–285). Amsterdam: John Benjamins.

Hayes, B., & Stivers, T. (1995). *Postnasal voicing*. Ms.

Heinz, J. (to appear). The computational nature of phonological generalizations. In L. M. Hyman & F. Plank (Eds.), *Phonological typology*. Berlin: Mouton de Gruyter.

Heinz, J., & Idsardi, W. J. (2017). Computational phonology today. *Phonology*, *34*, 211–291.

Hockett, C. (1955). A manual of phonology. *International Journal of American Linguistics Monograph Series*, *21*, memoir 11.

Holt, L. L., Lotto, A. J., & Kluender, K. R. (2001). Influence of fundamental frequency on stop consonant voicing perception: A case of learned covariation or auditory enhancement? *The Journal of the Acoustical Society of America*, *109.2*, 764–774.

Hosung, N., Goldstein, L. M., & Saltzman, E. (2009). Self-organization of syllable structure: A coupled oscillator model. In F. Pellegrino, E. Marisco, & I. Chitoran (Eds.), *Approaches to phonological complexity* (pp. 299–328). Berlin and New York, NY: Mouton de Gruyter.

Hubbard, K. (1995). 'Prenasalized consonants' and syllable timing: Evidence from Runyambo and Luganda. *Phonology*, *12*, 235–256.

Huffman, M. K. (1993). Phonetic patterns of nasalization and implications for feature specification. In M. K. Huffman & R. A. Krakow (Eds.), *Nasals, nasalization, and the velum* (pp. 303–327). New York, NY: Academic Press.

Hyman, L. M. (1986). The representation of multiple tone heights. In K. Bogers, H. V. D. Hulst, & M. Mous (Eds.), *The phonological representation of suprasegmentals* (pp. 109–152). Dordrecht: Foris.

Hyman, L. M. (2001). The limits of phonetic determinism in phonology: *NC revisited. In E. Hume & K. Johnson (Eds.), *The role of speech perception in phonology* (pp. 141–185). San Diego: Academic Press.

Iskarous, K., Fowler, C. A., & Whalen, D. H. (2010). Locus equations are an acoustic expression of articulatory synergy. *The Journal of the Acoustical Society of America*, *128*, 2021–2032.

Iskarous, K., Mooshammer, C., Hoole, P., Recasens, D., Shadle, C., Saltzman, E., & Whalen, D. H. (2013). The coarticulation/invariance scale: Mutual information as a measure of coarticulation resistance, motor synergy, and articulatory invariance. *The Journal of the Acoustical Society of America*, *134*, 1271–1282.

Kaun, A. (1995). *The typology of rounding harmony: An optimality theoretic account* (Ph.D. dissertation). University of California, Los Angeles.

Kaun, A. (2004). The typology of rounding harmony. In B. Hayes, R. Kirchner, & D. Steriade (Eds.), *Phonetically based phonology* (pp. 87–116). Cambridge: Cambridge University Press.

Keating, P. (1988a). The phonology-phonetics interface. In F. J. Newmeyer (Ed.), *Linguistics: The Cambridge survey* (Vol. 1, pp. 281–302). Cambridge: Cambridge University Press.

Keating, P. (1988b). Underspecification in phonetics. *Phonology*, *5*, 275–292.

Keating, P. (1990). Phonetic representation in generative grammar. *Journal of Phonetics*, *18*, 321–334.

Kelso, J. A. S., Saltzman, E., & Tuller, B. (1986a). The dynamical theory of speech production: Data and theory. *Journal of Phonetics*, *14*, 29–60.

Kelso, J. A. S., Saltzman, E., & Tuller, B. (1986b). Intentional contents, communicative context, and task dynamics: A reply to the commentators. *Journal of Phonetics*, *14*, 171–196.

Kingston, J. (2007). The phonetics-phonology interface. In P. de Lacy (Ed.), *The Cambridge handbook of phonology* (pp. 435–456). Cambridge: Cambridge University Press.

Kingston, J., & Diehl, R. L. (1994). Phonetic knowledge. *Language*, *70*, 419–454.

Kingston, J., & Diehl, R. L. (1995). Intermediate properties in the perception of distinctive feature values. In B. Connell & A. Arvaniti (Eds.), *Phonology and phonetics: Papers in laboratory phonology* (Vol. IV, pp. 7–27). Cambridge: Cambridge University Press.

Kingston, J., Diehl, R. L., Kirk, C. J., & Castleman, W. A. (2008). On the internal perceptual structure of distinctive features: The [voice] contrast. *Journal of Phonetics*, *36*(1), 28–54.

Kingston, J., & Macmillan, N. (1995). Integrality of nasalization and F1 in vowels in isolation and before oral and nasal consonants: A detection-theoretic application of the garner paradigm. *Journal of Acoustical Society of America*, *97*, 1261–1285.

Kirby, J. P., & Ladd, D. R. (2016). Effects of obstruent voicing on vowel f0: Evidence from true "voicing" languages. *The Journal of the Acoustical Society of America*, *140*, 2400–2411.

Krakow, R. A. (1989). *The articulatory organization of syllables: A kinematic analysis of labial and velar gestures* (Ph.D. dissertation). Yale University.

Krakow, R. A. (1999). Physiological organization of syllables: A review. *Journal of Phonetics*, *27*, 23–54.

Ladd, D. R. (1994). Constraints on the gradient variability of pitch range, or, Pitch level 4 lives! In P. A. Keating (Ed.), *Papers in laboratory phonology III: Phonological structure and phonological form* (pp. 43–63). Cambridge: Cambridge University Press.

Liberman, M., & Pierrehumbert, J. B. (1984). Intonational invariance under changes in pitch range and length. In M. Aronoff & R. T. Oehrle (Eds.), *Language sound structure* (pp. 157–233). Cambridge, MA: MIT Press.

Liljencrants, J., & Lindblom, B. (1972). Numerical simulation of vowel quality systems: The role of perceptual contrast. *Language*, *48*, 839–862.

Lindblom, B. (1986). Phonetic universals in vowel systems. In J. J. Ohala & J. J. Jaeger (Eds.), *Experimental phonology* (pp. 13–44). Orlando: Academic Press.

Linker, W. (1982). Articulatory and acoustic correlates of labial activity in vowels: A cross-linguistic study. *UCLA Working Papers in Phonetics*, *56*.

Lotto, A. J., & Holt, L. L. (2006). Putting phonetic context effects into context: A commentary on Fowler (2006). *Perception and Psychophysics*, *68*, 178–183.

Macmillan, N., Kingston, J., Thorburn, R., Walsh Dickey, L., & Bartels, C. (1999). Integrality of nasalization and F1 II. Basic sensitivity and phonetic labeling measure distinct sensory and decision-rule interactions. *Journal of Acoustical Society of America*, *106*, 2913–2932.

Maddieson, I. (1989). Prenasalized stops and speech timing. *Journal of the International Phonetic Association*, *19*, 57–66.

Maddieson, I., & Ladefoged, P. (1993). Phonetics of partially nasalized consonants. In M. K. Huffman & R. A. Krakow (Eds.), *Nasals, nasalization, and the velum* (pp. 251–301). New York, NY: Academic Press.

Maddieson, I., & Precoda, K. (1992). Syllable structure and phonetic models. *Phonology*, *9*, 45–60.

McCarthy, J. J. (1993). A case of surface rule inversion. *Canadian Journal of Linguistics*, *38*, 169–195.

McClelland, J., Mirman, D., & Holt, L. (2006). Are there interactive processes in speech perception? *TRENDS in Cognitive Sciences*, *10*, 363–369.

Mielke, J. (2008). *The emergence of distinctive features*. Oxford: Oxford University Press.

Mielke, J. (2011). The nature of distinctive features and the issue of natural classes. In A. C. Cohn, C. Fougeron, & M. K. Huffman (Eds.), *Handbook of laboratory phonology* (pp. 185–196). Oxford: Oxford University Press.

Morén, B. (2007). The division of labor between segment-internal structure and violable constraints. In S. Blaho, P. Bye, & M. Krämer (Eds.), *Freedom of analysis?* (pp. 313–344). Berlin: Mouton de Gruyter.

Moreton, E., & Pater, J. (2012a). Structure and substance in artificial-phonology learning. Part 1: Structure. *Language and Linguistics Compass*, *6*, 686–701.

Moreton, E., & Pater, J. (2012b). Structure and substance in artificial-phonology learning. Part 2: Substance. *Language and Linguistics Compass*, *6*, 702–718.

Myers, S. (2000). Boundary disputes: The distinction between phonetic and phonological sound patterns. In N. Burton-Roberts, P. Carr, & G. Docherty (Eds.), *Phonological knowledge: Conceptual and empirical issues* (pp. 245–272). Oxford: Oxford University Press.

Norris, D., McQueen, J. M., & Cutler, A. (2000). Merging information in speech recognition: Feedback is never necessary. *Behavioral and Brain Sciences*, *23*, 299–370.

Ohala, J. J. (1979). Phonetic universals in phonological systems and their explanation. In *Proceedings of the 9th international congress of phonetic sciences* (pp. 5–8).

Ohala, J. J. (1981). The listener as a source of sound change. In *Proceedings of Chicago linguistic society: Papers from the parasession on language and behavior* (p. 178–203). Chicago, IL: Chicago Linguistic Society.

Ohala, J. J. (1983). The phonological end justifies any means. In S. Hattori & K. Inoue (Eds.), *Proceedings of the 13th international congress of linguists* (pp. 232–243). Tokyo, 29 August-4 September 1982: [Distributed by Sanseido Shoten.].

Ohala, J. J. (1990). There is no interface between phonology and phonetics: A personal view. *Journal of Phonetics*, *18*, 153–171.

Ohala, J. J. (2005). Phonetic explanations for sound patterns. Implications for grammars of competence. In W. J. Hardcastle & J. M. Beck (Eds.), *A figure of speech, a festschrift for John Laver* (pp. 23–38). London: Lawrence Erlbaum Associates.

Ohala, J. J., & Jaeger, J. J. (1986). *Experimental phonology*. Orlando: Academic Press.

Padgett, J. (2002). *Constraint conjunction versus grounded constraint subhierarchies in optimality theory*. Santa Cruz: University of California.

Pasquereau, J. (2018). Phonological degrees of labiality. *Language*, *94*(4), e216–e265.

Pater, J. (1999). Austronesian nasal substitution and other NC effects. In R. Kager, H. van der Hulst, & W. Zonneveld (Eds.), *The prosody-morphology interface* (pp. 310–343). Cambridge: Cambridge University Press.

Pierrehumbert, J. B. (1980). *The phonetics and phonology of English intonation* (Doctoral dissertation). Massachusetts Institute of Technology.

Pierrehumbert, J. B. (1990). Phonological and phonetic representation. *Journal of Phonetics*, *18*, 375–394.

Pierrehumbert, J. B., & Beckman, M. E. (1988). *Japanese tone structure*. Cambridge, MA: MIT Press.

Pierrehumbert, J. B., Beckman, M. E., & Ladd, D. R. (2000). Conceptual foundations of phonology as a laboratory science. In N. Burton-Roberts, P. Carr, & G. Docherty (Eds.), *Phonological knowledge: Conceptual and empirical issues* (pp. 273–303). Oxford: Oxford University Press.

Pouplier, M., & Goldstein, L. M. (2010). Intention in articulation: Articulatory timing in alternating consonant sequences and its implications for models of speech production. *Language and Cognitive Processes*, *25*(5), 616–649.

Rafferty, A. N., Griffiths, T. L., & Ettlinger, M. (2013). Greater learnability is not sufficient to produce cultural universals. *Cognition*, *129*(1), 70–87.

Recasens, D. (1985). Coarticulatory patterns and degrees of coarticulatory resistance in Catalan CV sequences. *Language and Speech*, *28.2*, 97–114.

Redford, M. A., & Diehl, R. L. (1999). The relative perceptual distinctiveness of initial and final consonants in CVC syllables. *The Journal of the Acoustical Society of America*, *106*, 1555–1565.

Reiss, C. (2017). Substance free phonology. In S. J. Hannahs & A. Bosch (Eds.), *Routledge handbook of phonological theory*. Abingdon, OX: Routledge.

Roon, K. D., & Gafos, A. I. (2016). Perceiving while producing: Modeling the dynamics of phonological planning. *Journal of Memory and Language*, *89*, 222–243.

Saltzman, E. (1995). Dynamics and coordinate systems in skilled sensorimotor activity. In R. F. Port & T. van Gelder (Eds.), *Mind as motion: Explorations in the dynamics of cognition* (pp. 149–173). Cambridge, MA: MIT Press.

Saltzman, E., & Kelso, J. A. S. (1987). Skilled actions: A task dynamic approach. *Psychological Review*, *94*, 84–106.

Saltzman, E., & Munhall, K. (1989). A dynamical approach to gestural modeling in speech production. *Ecological Psychology*, *1*, 333–382.

Schwartz, J. L., Boë, L. J., Valleé, N., & Abry, C. (1997a). Major trends in vowel system inventories. *Journal of Phonetics*, *25*, 233–253.

Schwartz, J. L., Boë, L. J., Valleé, N., & Abry, C. (1997b). The dispersion focalization theory of vowel systems. *Journal of Phonetics*, *25*, 255–286.

Scobbie, J. (2007). Interface and overlap in phonetics and phonology. In G. Ramchand & C. Reiss (Eds.), *The Oxford handbook of linguistic interfaces* (pp. 17–52). Oxford: Oxford University Press.

Shaw, J. A., Gafos, A. I., Hoole, P., & Zeroual, C. (2009). Syllabification in Moroccan Arabic: Evidence from patterns of stability in articulation. *Phonology*, *26*, 187–215.

Shaw, J. A., Gafos, A. I., Hoole, P., & Zeroual, C. (2011). Dynamic invariance in the phonetic expression of syllable structure: A case study of Moroccan Arabic consonant clusters. *Phonology*, *28*(03), 455–490.

Smith, J. (2002). *Phonological augmentation in prominent positions* (Ph. D. Dissertation). University of Massachusetts, Amherst.

Smolensky, P., & Goldrick, M. (2016). *Gradient symbolic representations in grammar: The case of French liaison*. Rutgers Optimality Archive, 1552.

Solé, M. J. (1992). Phonetic and phonological processes: The case of nasalization. *Language and Speech*, *35*, 29–43.

Solé, M. J. (1995). Spatio-temporal patterns of velopharyngeal action in phonetic and phonological nasalization. *Language and Speech*, *38*, 1–23.

Solé, M. J. (2007). Controlled and mechanical properties of speech: A review of the literature. In M. J. Sole, P. S. Beddor, & J. J. Ohala (Eds.), *Experimental approaches to phonology* (pp. 302–321). Oxford: Oxford University Press.

Solé, M. J., Hyman, L. M., & Monaka, K. C. (2010). More on post-nasal devoicing: The case of Shekgalagari. *Journal of Phonetics*, *38*, 604–615.

Sproat, R., & Fujimura, O. (1993). Allophonic variation in English /l/ and its implications for phonetic implementation. *Journal of Phonetics*, *21*, 291–311.

Staubs, R. (2014). *Computational modeling of learning biases in stress typology* (Unpublished doctoral dissertation). University of Massachusetts, Amherst.

Steriade, D. (2001). Directional asymmetries in place assimilation: A perceptual account. In E. Hume & K. Johnson (Eds.), *The role of speech perception in phonology* (pp. 219–250). New York, NY: Academic Press.

Steriade, D. (2008). The phonology of perceptibility effects: The P-map and its consequences for constraint organization. In K. Hanson & S. Inkelas (Eds.), *The nature of the word: Studies in honor of Paul Kiparsky* (pp. 151–180). Cambridge, MA: MIT Press.

Stevens, K. N., & Keyser, S. J. (2010). Quantal theory, enhancement and overlap. *Journal of Phonetics*, *38*, 10–19.

Summers, W. V. (1987). Effects of stress and final-consonant voicing on vowel production: Articulatory and acoustic analyses. *Journal of Acoustical Society of America*, *82*, 847–863.

Wang, M. D., & Bilger, R. C. (1973). Consonant confusions in noise: A study of perceptual features. *Journal of Acoustical Society of America*, *54*, 1248–1266.

14

The phonetic basis of the origin and spread of sound change

Jonathan Harrington, Felicitas Kleber, Ulrich Reubold, Florian Schiel, and Mary Stevens

Introduction

The city of Munich where the authors of this chapter all live was known after it was founded in the 10th–11th centuries as *apud Munichen*, which means "by/near the monks." Some of the sound changes that have led to the present-day form /mynçən/ (*München*) from the Old High German stem /munic/ "monk" (from Greek μοναχός: Grimm & Grimm, 1854) can be linked to well-known effects of phonetic variation. The high front rounded vowel in present-day *München* has evolved historically from umlaut that can be associated synchronically with trans-consonantal vowel coarticulation (Hoole & Pouplier, 2017; Öhman, 1966) which in this case caused /u/ to front to /y/ under the influence of /i/ in the following syllable of *Munichen*. The loss of this /i/ is likely to have come about because it occurs in a weak, unstressed syllable which is often prone to reduction or deletion in continuous speech.

The present-day German for "monk" is *Mönch*, /mœnç/ in which the vowel has been lowered relative to the High German form with /u/ or the /y/ of *München*. There are several examples in English of diachronic /u/-lowering in proximity to a nasal consonant such as "come" (Old English: *cuman*), "honey" (Old English: *hunig*), "some" (Old English: *sum*), "hound" (cf. Dutch *hond*: /ɦɔnt/, German *Hund*: /hʊnt/), and "storm" (cf. German, *Sturm*: /ʃtʊɐm/). Some (Denham & Lobeck, 2010, p. 447) have suggested that the origin of such alternations is a scribe's substitution of "u" for "o" in order to differentiate the vowel in the orthography more clearly from the following letters "m," "n," or "r." But perhaps there is instead a phonetic explanation. Vowels are often nasalized in nasal contexts. This leads acoustically to the introduction of a low frequency nasal formant which in turn has the perceptual effect of high vowel lowering, the same form of lowering that is responsible for the inflections in French for "one" between the masculine *un* /œ̃/ with a phonetically mid-low and nasalized vowel and feminine *une* /yn/, which has an oral high vowel (Kawasaki, 1986; Krakow et al., 1988).

The *München* example can begin to provide a framework for many of the issues to be discussed in this chapter. There are obviously categorical changes over time (e.g., the substitution of /u/ for /y/; the deletion of consonants and vowels) – possibly also involving the creation of new phonemic oppositions (development of front rounded /y, œ/ contrasting with front unrounded /i, e/) that can be related to everyday synchronic continuous variation in how sounds overlap with and influence each other. The task at hand is not just to show associations between diachronic and synchronic observations as sketched above, but to explain sound change using a model of human speech processing. Thus, the central question is, "What is it about the assembly of words out of their constituent sounds in speech production and their transmission to a listener that can occasionally result in sound change?" The focus is on words, rather than on how words are built into larger phrases because, as argued in Ohala (1993), the domain of sound change is in almost all cases the word or clitic phrases (Kiparsky, 2015) that have been lexicalized.

The chapter is organized as follows: the first section explains how sound change originates in non-contrastive phonetic variation. The following section addresses phonologization, i.e., how such phonetic variation can come to carry the cues for a phonological contrast. Subsequently, a section examines production and perception dynamics at the level of the individual and the group as sound changes progress. The next section presents an overview of the relevance of variations in hyper- and hypoarticulated speech for understanding sound change. A final section outlines how cognitive-computational agent-based models of sound change that combine theories of system dynamics and exemplar models of speech might enable the origin and spread of sound change to be brought together. Throughout the chapter, and consistent with prominent sound change studies (e.g., Beddor, 2009), we use the term "effect" to refer to contextual influences on a speech sound and "source" to refer to the speech sound that gives rise to them.

Sound change and coarticulation

One of the very important insights from the framework of articulatory phonology (Browman & Goldstein, 1992) and its forerunner action theory (Fowler, 1983; Fowler, 1984) is that speech production can be modeled as a constellation of orchestrated gestures that overlap with each other in time. Contextual vowel nasalization that occurs in English words like *ban* comes about according to this theory because of overlap between the independently controlled gestures of tongue and soft-palate movement. Although this overlap causes dramatic changes to the acoustic signal's formant structure during the interval marked by vowel voicing, there is experimental evidence to show that listeners typically hear acoustically nasalized vowels as oral, when they occur in the context of nasal consonants (Kawasaki, 1986; Krakow et al., 1988). This is presumed to be so according to articulatory phonology because there is a parity between the modalities of production and perception: listeners hear not a blending of orality and nasality but instead the interleaving of the independently controlled gestures in speech production (Fowler & Smith, 1986; Fowler & Thompson, 2010). Thus, the onset of (coarticulatory) nasality is not blended in human speech processing with the vowel (as the acoustic record would suggest) but perceptually associated or parsed with the source of coarticulation, i.e., with the following nasal consonant. From another perspective, the gestures of the oral vowel and the nasal consonant with which it overlaps are both produced and perceived in parallel and independently of each other.

According to Ohala (1993, 2012), sound change is but a drop in the ocean of synchronic phonetic variation precisely because listeners have become so adept at normalizing for context (Fujisaki & Kunisaki, 1976; Mann & Repp, 1980). As long as listeners associate or parse the coarticulatory effect – such as vowel nasalization in English – with the source (the following consonant) that gave rise to it, then no sound change can occur. But if such parsing should fail, then (for this example) some of the nasalization will be perceptually attached to the vowel. There is then a perceptual switch between the listener's interpretation of the vowel as oral (if coarticulatory nasalization is parsed with the following consonant) to an interpretation as inherently nasal (if it is not). The term "inherently nasal" means that nasalization has become a phonological distinctive property of the vowel and has the potential to become lexically contrastive (as in, e.g., French), just as a contact between the tip of the tongue and alveolar ridge is a distinctive property of /t/ and contrastive in most languages. For Ohala, such a switch in perceptual re-interpretation is both abrupt and categorical, and can be likened to the illusion created by a Necker cube. Thus, just as a Necker cube creates uncertainty for the viewer due to a repeated switch between two plausibly (and categorically) different ways of interpreting shape, so, too, do ambiguities in the acoustic signal suggest two categorically different ways to the listener of parsing the signal into the gestures that produced it. The sound change is therefore in speech perception: notice that no change to speech production has actually taken place. Indeed, such a change would only have the potential to occur if the perceptually confused listener subsequently produced a nasalized vowel in their own speech. It is because the probability of sound change actually occurring is so low – requiring the listener not to normalize for context and to carry this over to speech production and then for this behavior to spread throughout the community – that the typical, and far more probable, state in Ohala's model is one of extensive phonetic variation but with scarcely any sound change. Such scarcity raises the question of why phonetic variation should turn into sound change in any one language (or variety of a language) but not in another (e.g., why /k/ was lost around the 17th–18th centuries in English "knight" and "knot," but not in German *Knecht* and *Knoten* that still have initial /kn/). This intriguing question, known as sound change actuation (Weinreich et al., 1968) is in Ohala's model not due to phonetic principles but is instead simply a matter of chance (see also Sóskuthy, 2015; Stevens & Harrington, 2014 for recent reviews).

The well-known sound changes that have been found in many of the world's languages, such as vowel nasalization (Beddor, 2012), tonogenesis (Hombert et al., 1979), domain-final voicing neutralization (Charles-Luce, 1985; Kleber et al., 2010), velar palatalization (Guion, 1998), nasal deletion or insertion before obstruents (Ohala, 1975, 1997), and /u/-fronting (Ohala & Feder, 1994; Harrington et al., 2011) are all examples in which there can be perceptual ambiguity in the extent to which a coarticulatory effect can be attributed to the source that caused it. These sound changes have two main other commonalities. First, most show an asymmetry in that $x \rightarrow y$ does not imply $y \rightarrow x$: for example, while there are several instances in which velars have historically palatalized before front vowels, there are perhaps none in the other direction. Such asymmetries are typically matched by an asymmetry in phonetic variation. Thus, there is some evidence that listeners are much more likely to confuse /k/ with anterior consonants such as /t/ before front vowels than the other way round (Winitz et al., 1972), principally because when the mid-frequency peak that characterizes acoustically fronted velars is obscured, the signal bears a close acoustic resemblance to that of an alveolar (Chang et al., 2001). Because in spontaneous speech there is a much greater likelihood for a mid-frequency peak to be obscured than for it to be inserted, the perceptual confusion is asymmetric. Second, all these sound changes originate – at least in terms of Ohala's model – from the different ways that a speaker and a listener associate phonological categories with the acoustic signal. A listener must have inserted perceptually a /p/ into the surname "Thompson" (see also "glimpse" from Old English *glimsian* related to "gleam") which was originally derived from "the son of Thom" (and importantly, not from "the son of Thomp"). Thus, there is a mismatch between the modalities: in production the surname originally had the categories /ms/ and the acoustic silence [p] arose because the velum was raised before the lips were opened for /m/; in perception, this acoustic silence was reinterpreted as /mps/.

All of the types of sound change sketched so far come about in terms of Ohala's (1993) model because a listener does not parse coarticulation with its source. A much rarer type of sound change is dissimilation in which in Ohala's (1993) model listeners over-normalize for the contextual effects of coarticulation. Grassman's law is an example of dissimilation in which an initial aspirated consonant came to be deleted in ancient Greek preceding another aspirated consonant in the same word. Thus, the nominative and genitive singular for "hair" in ancient Greek are/t^{h}riks/ and /trik^{h}os/, respectively, suggesting that the latter was originally derived from /t^{h}rik^{h}os/ in which the first aspirated segment came to be deleted under the influence of the second. The interpretation in Ohala's model is that aspiration spreads throughout the entire first syllable due to the coarticulatory effect of the second stop. Listeners then factor out this coarticulatory influence but erroneously also factor out the initial aspirated segment. Thus, dissimilation happens because coarticulation perceptually camouflages the initial aspiration: since listeners are unable to distinguish between the two, all the aspiration including that which is an inherent distinctive property of the first segment is filtered out perceptually. This filtering uses the same mechanisms that listeners routinely apply to filtering out the effects of coarticulation, such as coarticulatory vowel nasalization as discussed above. One of the differences in the output between sound change due to under-normalizing (e.g., tonogenesis, development of phonological vowel nasalization) and over-normalizing (dissimilation) for coarticulation is that the former can create new sets of phonological contrasts that were not previously in the language (e.g., tonal contrasts in vowels as a consequence of tonogenesis). Another is that dissimilation typically applies to speech sounds that have a long time window (Alderete & Frisch, 2006), i.e., whose influence extends through several consonants and vowels (e.g., West, 2000 for liquids). Although Ohala's theory is elegant in linking a range of sound changes within the same mechanism of listener parsing errors, it has so far been difficult to demonstrate in the laboratory that dissimilation comes about as a consequence of over-normalization for coarticulation (Abrego-Collier, 2013; Harrington et al., 2016).

Metathesis is a sound change in which speech sounds swap serial position, e.g., English "burnt" versus German *brennt*. Blevins and Garrett (2004) suggest that the origin of perceptual metathesis is quite similar to that of dissimilation: in both cases the source is a sound that has a long time window. Whereas in dissimilation the long time window can mask another sound, in perceptual metathesis it causes confusion in their serial order. Thus, Blevins and Garrett (2004) note that a sound change in which a breathy voice and a vowel swap position i.e., CVɦC → CɦVC, comes about because the post-vocalic breathy voice causes breathiness throughout the vowel which obscures their serial order. Ruch and Harrington (2014) use this type of argument to explain the results of their apparent-time study of production data of a sound change in progress in Andalusian Spanish, in which older speakers have *pre*-aspirated stops derived originally from /s/ in words like pasta, /pa^{h}ta/, which younger speakers increasingly produce as *post*-aspirated /pat^{h}a/.

Sound change and phonologization

Phonologization in sound change is usually concerned with explaining how a phonological contrast is lost or attenuated from a source or conditioning environment and transposed to a coarticulatory effect. Thus, with regard to tonogenesis, the aim is to understand how a phonological stop voicing contrast /pa, ba/ (the source) is obliterated as higher and lower pitch in the vowel following a voiceless and voiced stop, respectively (the coarticulatory effect) develops into the rising vs. falling tonal contrast in the vowel /pá, pà/.

In Kiparsky's (2015) model based on stratal optimality theory (Bermúdez-Otero & Hogg, 2003), new contrasts can be added to a language when constraints percolate upwards from the autonomous levels of post-lexical phonology, to word phonology, to stem phonology. The first stage of Kiparsky's three-stage model of phonologization involves a constraint operating at the post-lexical level. Post-lexical constraints can then become perceptually salient as they enter the superordinate level of word phonology as so-called quasi-phonemes, which differ from phonemes only in that they are not contrastive (i.e., they are allophonic). The third stage involves a change in phonological status from quasi-phonemes to phonemes, which comes about when the conditioning environment is reduced or deleted. In the development of umlaut in German (see chapter Introduction), the initial stages of sound change were in the earliest forms of Old High German in which, according to Kiparsky (2015), trans-consonantal vowel coarticulation was post-lexical. Umlaut could therefore apply across word boundaries to forms such as *mag iz* → *meg iz* ("may it") in which the /a/ → /e/ change was induced by trans-consonantal vowel coarticulation with /i/ in the next word. At a later stage in time, umlaut occurred only word-internally and not across word boundaries: this is the stage at which the phonetic variants due to umlaut, including presumably the front rounded vowels /ø, y/, would have entered the lexicon as quasi-phonemes. Their subsequent change in status from quasi-phonemes to phonemes comes about when the source is lost: that is when /i/ reduces to /ə/ to give present-day *Füße*, /fysə/ "feet" from Old High German /fotiz/.

Various studies by Solé (1992, 1995, 2007) have been concerned with establishing diagnostics to determine whether or not a coarticulatory effect has been phonologized. Solé reasons that the temporal proportion over which coarticulation extends should show fewer changes due to variation in speech rate if the coarticulation is (or is in the process of) being phonologized. In American English, there are reasons to suppose that vowel nasalization has been phonologized (Beddor et al., 2007) so that the main feature distinguishing pairs like "bent"/"bet" or "bend"/"bed" is not so much the presence of the nasal consonant in "bent" and "bend" but rather the temporal extent of nasalization in the vowel. In Spanish, there may well be coarticulatory nasalization in the vowel in VN sequences, but in contrast to American English nasalization has not been phonologized. Solé shows, using physiological techniques, that in American English, the temporal proportion of the vowel that is nasalized remains about the same, irrespective of whether the vowel shortens or lengthens due to rate changes. This is exactly what is to be expected if nasalization has become an inherent property of the vowel, i.e., has been phonologized. In Spanish, by contrast, the temporal extent of nasalization does not vary in proportion to vowel duration, as it does for American English, but instead begins at a fixed time prior to the onset of the nasal consonant irrespective of rate-induced changes to vowel duration: this suggests that nasalization is for Spanish (in contrast to American English) a property of the nasal consonant and not of the vowel.

Studies by Beddor (2009, 2012, 2015) confront more directly the association between the destruction of the source that causes the coarticulatory effect and the latter's phonologization. One of the main paths towards sound change for Beddor is that listeners typically do not parse all of the coarticulation with its source. Thus, if there is total normalization for the effects of context, then listeners should hear a nasalized vowel in an NVN context as oral (if they parse all of the coarticulatory nasalization in the vowel with the surrounding nasal consonants). However, the results in Beddor and Krakow (1999) suggest that for some listeners at least, normalization is only partial. If so, then only some (but not all) of the nasalization will have been parsed with the N and the rest remains attached to the vowel: that is, listeners in their experiments associated *some* of the contextual nasalization with the vowel, even though the source (the N) was clearly present. If some of the coarticulatory nasalization is parsed with the vowel, then the vowel must sound partially nasal, and it is this partial compensation for a coarticulatory effect that makes sound change possible in Beddor's model (although sound change does not *necessarily* take place under such conditions).

One of the first stages of sound change for Beddor is when the coarticulatory effect and source enter into a trading-relationship, i.e., start to covary. When cues to a phonological contrast covary, then there is a coherent and systematic relationship between them, such that if one happens to be not especially salient in the speech signal, then listeners can direct their attention to the other cue with which it trades and so still identify the phonological contrast. For example, the more listeners rely on voice-onset-time as a cue to obstruent voicing, the less they rely on fundamental frequency (Repp, 1982). (Fundamental frequency is often higher following voiceless stops because of the greater laryngeal tension in order to suppress voicing: Löfqvist et al., 1989). Beddor showed that a perceptual trading relationship exists between the duration of anticipatory coarticulatory nasalization in the vowel and the duration of following nasal consonant in American English VNC_{voice} sequences in words like *send*. The empirical evidence for such a trading relationship was that listeners had difficulty hearing the difference between $\tilde{V}_S N_L$ and $\tilde{V}_L N_S$ where the subscript denotes Short or Long and where $\tilde{V}$ is the portion of the vowel that is nasalized: that is, a short nasalized vowel followed by a long nasal consonant was shown to be perceptually indistinguishable for many listeners from a long nasal vowel followed by a short nasal consonant. Just this is to be expected if the temporal extent of coarticulatory vowel nasalization and the duration of the final nasal consonant trade perceptually.

In American English $VNC_{voiceless}$ sequences in words like *sent*, the sound change by which nasalization is phonologized is at a more advanced stage than in VNC_{voice} sequences. This implies that vowel nasalization is likely to be more critical to listeners for distinguishing pairs like "set"/"sent" than "said"/"send," just as it is (but perhaps not quite to the same extent) for French listeners when they distinguish between *vais* vs. *vingt*, /vɛ, vɛ̃/ (1st pers. sing. "go" vs. "twenty"). Accordingly, listeners in Beddor et al. (2007) were shown to be especially sensitive to the beginning of nasalization in the vowel in "sent" irrespective of the duration of the following nasal consonant. Thus, the importance of Beddor's studies is that the path to phonologization may well initially develop out of a trading relationship between coarticulatory effect (vowel nasalization) and source (the following nasal consonant) which then gives way to perceptual attention being focused on the coarticulatory effect *irrespective of whether or not the source is present*.

Sound change and the association between perception and production

In Ohala's (1993) model, the conversion of phonetic variation to sound change happens via two separate stages. The first is perceptual, in which phonetic variation can be phonologized for the listener, often as a result of under- or (more exceptionally) over-normalizing for coarticulation. In the second stage, the listener may or may not carry over this perceptual shift to speech production. The implication of this model is therefore that, when a sound change develops, changes to the perceptual processing of coarticulation should in general precede those that take place in speech production.

Harrington et al. (2008) tested this idea by analyzing the production and perception of coarticulation for tense /u/-fronting (lexical set GOOSE) in Standard Southern British in which a sound change has been in progress since the 1960s. This was an apparent time study (Bailey et al. 1991) in which the extent of sound change was inferred by comparing younger and older speakers of this accent on the production and perception of coarticulation. The reason for analyzing coarticulation was that there is other evidence indicating that /u/-fronting in Standard Southern British was a coarticulation-induced sound change, i.e., that it originated in contexts in which /u/ is fronted synchronically (Harrington, 2007).

The results in Harrington et al. (2008) showed that coarticulation was matched across the modalities. This is because older speakers had a retracted /u/ and extensive coarticulation in production, and they also normalized i.e., compensated for these effects in perception. By contrast younger speakers' production was characterized by a fronted /u/ in all contexts (i.e., a minimal change due to coarticulation) and they normalized much less for coarticulation than older speakers.

The study in Harrington et al. (2008) does therefore not provide any evidence that changes to the perception of coarticulatory relationships precede those in production during an ongoing sound change in progress, as predicted by Ohala's (1993) model. But there is some evidence for this in Kleber et al.'s (2012) apparent-time study of the sound change in progress to lax /ʊ/-fronting (lexical set FOOT) in the same variety. Their results showed that, whereas the magnitude of coarticulation in /ʊ/ was about the same for both age groups in production, the degree to which listeners normalized for this coarticulatory effect was much less for younger than for older subjects. This finding can be interpreted in favor of a mismatch between the modalities in which perceptual normalization for coarticulation in younger subjects has waned ahead of a reduction in the size of coarticulation in production. This finding is therefore to a certain extent consistent with Ohala's (1993) model that changes to coarticulation in perception precede those in production. A more recent apparent-time study by Kuang and Cui (2016) provides evidence for a sound change in progress in the Tibeto-Burman language of Southern Yi in which tongue root differences are taking over from phonation as the primary cues to a tense/lax distinction. Compatibly with the results in Kleber et al. (2012), they also showed that this change is occurring in perception ahead of production.

Based on analyses of perception and production within the same individuals in two different types of sound change in American English and Afrikaans, Beddor's (2015) results are consistent with an alignment between the modalities during sound change. For nasalization in American English, Beddor shows that some individuals who were highly sensitive to vowel nasalization as a cue to the distinction between e.g., "sent"/"set" also showed extensive nasalization in "sent" words in their production. Similarly, for a sound change in progress in Afrikaans, in which fundamental frequency is taking over from voice onset time (VOT) as the primary cue to the stop voicing contrast, those older listeners who produced the contrast with voicing differences were also sensitive (and more so than younger listeners) to VOT as a cue in perception. Compatibly with Beddor (2015), a study of coarticulatory nasalization in 39 American English participants by Zellou (2017) showed a relationship between subjects' perceptual sensitivity to nasalization and the magnitude with which nasalization occurred in their own speech production. There is therefore no evidence from any of these studies on sound change in progress within the individual to suggest that changes to coarticulation in perception lead those in production during a sound change in progress.

The results of the un-merging of a phonological contrast in both Müller et al. (2011) and Bukmaier et al. (2014) are equivocal about whether production and perception are aligned during a sound change in progress. Both of these studies were concerned with neutralizations that are common at least amongst older speakers in two German dialects: in Müller et al. (2011), the concern was with post-vocalic voicing neutralization such that standard German word pairs like *baden*/*baten* ("bathe"/"bid") are homophonous (both with lenis /d/) in Franconian; the focus of the analysis in Bukmaier et al. (2014) was on neutralization of the post-vocalic sibilant place of articulation such that the standard German /s, ʃ/ contrast (e.g., *wisst*/*wischt*, /wɪst, wɪʃt/, "knows"/"wipes") is neutralized as /ʃ/ in Swabian German. The apparent-time study by Müller et al. (2011) showed that younger Franconian participants produced and perceived the post-vocalic /t, d/ contrast to a much greater extent than did older Franconians but not as sharply as Standard German participants. Thus, the modalities for all three subject groups were matched (between no contrast, partial contrast, and complete contrast in older Franconians, younger Franconians, and Standard German participants respectively). In Bukmaier et al. (2014), there was some evidence that the magnitude of the distinction was greater in perception than in production for older participants. They showed that older Swabians < younger Swabians < standard German participants, where < denotes the degree to which participants distinguished between /s, ʃ/ in production. But concerning the magnitude of the /s, ʃ/ contrast in perception, the results showed older Swabians = younger Swabians < standard German participants. Thus, older Swabians perceived the /s, ʃ/ contrast at least as sharply as younger Swabians even though they scarcely distinguished between the sibilants in production.

A merger is a sound change in the other direction in which a phonological contrast collapses. There is some evidence that mergers take place in perception before production, i.e., that individuals report not being able to hear a contrast, even though they consistently show differences on the contrast in production (Kiparsky, 2016; Labov et al., 1991; Yu, 2007). On the other hand, the results of a series of studies on the near-merger in New Zealand English /iə, eə/ (lexical sets NEAR, SQUARE) toward /iə/ show a more complex picture. In one study, Warren et al. (2007) found a strong linear correlation between the extent to which New Zealanders distinguished these falling diphthongs in their own production and their ability to identify NEAR and SQUARE type words perceptually. But Hay et al. (2010) found that the degree to which such near-merged items were perceived to be distinct depended on a number of other factors including whether the perceptual task tapped lexical or phonological knowledge. The extent to which participants perceived the contrast in a speaker was also found to be influenced by their judgment of the speaker's age and social class (Hay et al., 2006): this finding also shows that phonological categorization in perception is influenced by memory and social information (see also Jannedy & Weirich, 2014). In a more recent study of the /e, a/ merger in "Ellen"/"Allen" words in New Zealand English and of the vowels in lexical sets LOT and THOUGHT in American English using both real and nonwords, Hay et al. (2013) note that they were not able to find any systematic relationship between an individual's production and perception.

Based on the findings reviewed in this section, it is not yet clear how perception changes with respect to production during a sound change in progress *within* the individual. As far as coarticulation is concerned, the equivocal results may derive from the considerable variation in processing coarticulation within and between individuals in both production and perception (Grosvald & Corina, 2012; Yu, 2010; Yu et al., 2013). The variable nature of the results concerning how the modalities are related within individuals may also be due to the nature of the experimental task that is conducted. Zellou (2017) suggests that rating the presence of a phonetic feature (e.g., the degree to which a vowel is nasalized) may tap into community-level phonetic norms to a greater extent than in discrimination tasks.

Regarding changes at the group level – which can be assessed by comparing the alignment of modalities between e.g., younger and older participants – the review of the previously mentioned studies provides some evidence that perception can lead production during a sound change in progress. This greater influence of sound change on perception may come about because of the increased need for the perceptual processing of speech to remain flexibly adaptable given the considerable variation across the different types of speakers, speaking styles, and accents to which a listener is constantly exposed (Beddor, 2015). Research is yet to identify the mechanisms by which speech production does eventually catch up with the faster changes in speech perception associated with a sound change in progress.

Finally, it is of course well-known from the quantal theory of speech (Stevens, 1972, 1989) that the relationship between speech production and perception is non-linear: incremental articulatory changes can lead to discrete differences in the acoustic output. A question that has not been sufficiently addressed is whether this nonlinear relationship is a factor that contributes to incremental phonetic variation becoming a categorical change. Perhaps during a sound change in progress, incremental articulatory change leads to an abrupt and marked change in acoustics and perception as a quantal boundary is crossed. This would be another instance in which perception and production are out of step with each other, at least during a sound change in progress, since perceptual changes at the boundary between quantal regions would be more marked than those in production. For example, it is well known that there is just such a quantal change between /u/ and /y/ produced respectively with back and front tongue dorsum positions (Stevens, 1972, 1989). Suppose a sound change in progress initially involves incremental tongue-dorsum fronting in a tongue-backed /u/. Then at some point in this gradual fronting, there will be a sudden acoustic (and perceptual) change at the quantal boundary (Figure 14.1): that is, as a quantal boundary is crossed, F_2 increases

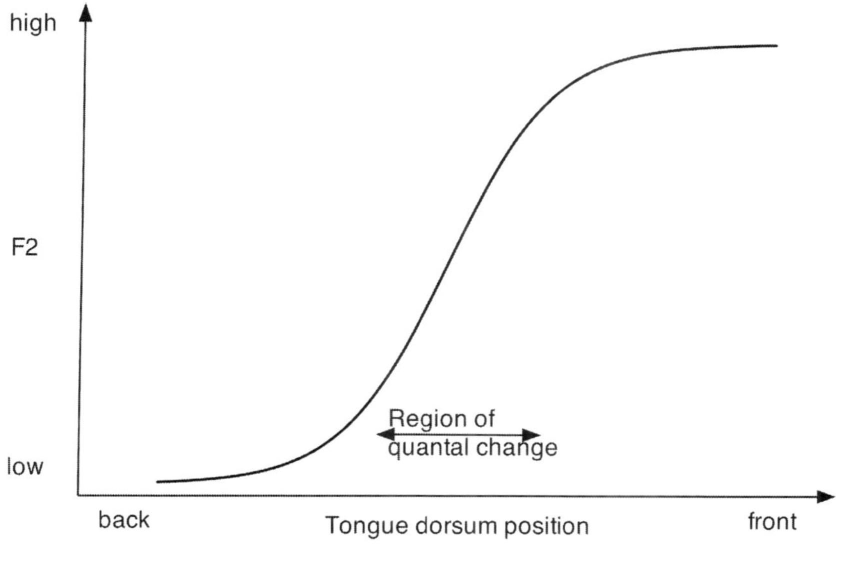

Figure 14.1 A schematic outline showing the quantal relationship (Stevens, 1972, 1989) between the tongue dorsum position (horizontal axis) and the second formant frequency (vertical axis) over the interval between a tongue back position for /u/ and tongue front position for /y/.

dramatically in relation to production. Sound change that is initially phonetic and gradient might become a category change (from /u/ to /ʉ/ or to /y/) once the incrementally gradual sound change has pushed the tongue dorsum sufficiently far forward into this quantal region so that the acoustic and perceptual change are suddenly quite marked.

This idea is largely untested. However, there is some evidence compatible with this hypothesis from the combined ultrasound and acoustic analysis of /l/-vocalization in American English in labial and lateral contexts in Lin et al. (2014). In /l/-vocalization, the tongue dorsum remains high but the tongue tip is lenited. But in this study, very small tongue-tip lenitions of just 1–2 mm were enough to cause quite a dramatic reduction in F_2 towards F_1. Perhaps it is this small articulatory but large acoustic change that is the key to understanding /l/-vocalization as a sound change resulting in e.g., French *autre* from Latin *alter* (cf. also English "false," French /fo/, *faux* < Latin *falsus*).

Sound change and hypoarticulation

Whereas Ohala sees the origin of many kinds of sound change in coarticulation, the main type of phonetic variation that causes sound change in Lindblom et al. (1995) is due to hyper- and hypoarticulation (H&H). According to the highly influential H&H theory (Lindblom, 1990), a speaker adapts speech production to the predicted needs of the listener for understanding what is being said. A word tends to be hypoarticulated – i.e., produced with minimal articulatory effort and lenited/reduced – if the speaker calculates that the listener will be able to predict the word from context; but it is hyperarticulated when the semantic and situational contexts provide only very limited clues to its meaning. In hypoarticulated speech, the attention of the listener is typically not directed at the signal both because it is an impoverished acoustic representation of its phonological structure and because there is no need to, if the word can be predicted from context. Sound change in Lindblom et al. (1995) exceptionally comes about if (for whatever reason) the listener's attention is focused on the signal, i.e., on the phonetic content during hypoarticulated speech. In this case, the hypoarticulated form can be added to the listener's lexicon. The model of Lindblom et al. (1995) is therefore a forerunner to some of the important ideas in episodic models of speech (Pierrehumbert, 2003, 2006), namely that a lexical item can be associated with multiple phonetic forms. It seems as if the theory of Lindblom et al. (1995) is restricted to predicting that only weak constituents of lexical items would be prone to change. However, this is not so since any word including its prominent syllables with full vowels can be hypoarticulated (if they are semantically predictable) and thereby subject to sound change in this model.

Both Lindblom and Ohala consider therefore that sound change comes about when the listener *decontextualizes* speech. In Ohala, the decontextualization is because coarticulation is interpreted independently of its source; in Lindblom et al. (1995), the decontextualization is because a mode of listening is engaged in hypoarticulated speech that is usually reserved for perceiving semantically unpredictable aspects of pronunciation. A prediction of both models is that less experienced listeners – perhaps children or second language learners – should be amongst the primary drivers of sound change if they have less ability to normalize perceptually for the effects of coarticulation and/or to vary listening strategies in response to the semantic predictability of the utterance. Both models also have answers to the following paradox raised by Kiparsky (2003). On the one hand, sound change according to the Neogrammarians (Osthoff & Brugman, 1878; Paul, 1886) proceeds largely imperceptibly, incrementally, and without the guidance of top-down processing from contrasts in the lexicon; but on the other hand, phonological systems across the known languages of the world nevertheless fall into patterns (such that, as far as is known, most languages have some form of /i, u, a/ before complexifying the vowel system further). The paradox is that if the sounds of languages change imperceptibly and without regard to linguistic knowledge, then the types of phonological contrasts should be much more varied and unpredictable than the ones that are actually observed. That they are not is because the pool of phonetic variation is not infinite: in Lindblom's model there is a compromise between factors such as articulatory effort and perceptual distinctiveness, while in Ohala's model the possible sound changes are constrained by the types of coarticulatory overlap that the vocal tract is able to produce and that the listener is most likely to misperceive (i.e., phonological contrasts are unlikely to develop if they could not have developed from the synchronic way in which speech sounds overlap and influence each other).

The two models also differ in important ways that are illuminating for understanding sound change. For Ohala, the mismatch between the speaker and listener is in how phonological categories are associated with signal dynamics, whereas for Lindblom the mismatch relates to speaking style (hypoarticulated for the speaker, but hyperarticulated for the listener). Another difference is that Ohala's model is not concerned with how sound change spreads beyond an individual's grammar, whereas for Lindblom (1998) "it may be unnecessary to limit the phonetic contribution to sound change to the initiation stage" (p. 245). Yet another difference is that in Ohala's model, just as in the Neogrammarian view, sound change applies across the board to the words that are affected by it. In Lindblom on the other hand, sound change is word-specific because hypoarticulated forms of a particular word may be added to the lexicon. Lindblom et al. (1995) are somewhat vague about how sound change might then carry over to other words, but suggest that this will be a compromise between articulatory efficiency, perceptual distinctiveness, and evaluation by society for its social acceptability. Compatibly with some other studies (Bybee, 2002; Chen & Wang, 1975; Hay & Foulkes, 2016; Phillips, 2006), Lindblom et al.'s model contains the idea that sound change should initially take place in lexically frequent words. This is because lexically frequent words tend to be more predictable from context and therefore more likely to be hypoarticulated (which provides the conditions for sound change to occur in Lindblom et al., 1995). On the other hand, there is no association between sound change and lexical statistics in the model of Ohala (1993). Finally, Lindblom (1988) reasons that there are parallels between sound change and biological evolution. This is because in this model, sound change arises out of the variation caused by the flexible adaptations of the speaker to the needs of the listener or audience. On the other hand, Ohala (1988) provides several compelling reasons why sound change is not the same as biological evolution. One fundamental difference is that in Darwin's theory of evolution it is the individuals that are optimally adapted to their environment that are most likely to survive, whereas there is no evidence that there is competition between different pronunciation forms of words, nor that those variants that survive are the ones that are optimally adapted to their communication environment (Ohala, 1988, p. 177).

There is an interesting overlap between some of the predictions made from sociolinguistic typology in Trudgill (2011) and those of Lindblom's model. For Trudgill (2011), sound change that is internal to a community – i.e., which develops without any external contact from other varieties – is likely over a very long timespan to lead to greater complexity in phonological inventories in remote (i.e., with low contact), small, and socially tightly knit societies. This is because interlocutors are likely to be known to each other in such societies and because the range of topics is also to a large extent predictable. As a consequence, speakers should be able to deploy hypoarticulated speech extensively which, according to the model of Lindblom et al. (1995), would then provide ample opportunity for radically hypoarticulated forms – that is, pronunciations which, if presented in isolation, would in all likelihood be unintelligible – to be added to the lexicon. Phonological complexification – which can take various forms, including the incorporation of typologically unusual contrasts – is in Trudgill's (2011) framework of sociolinguistic typology a direct consequence of the uptake over a long timespan of hypoarticulated speech in such remote, socially tightly knit communities. A challenge for future research will be, perhaps with the aid of computational modeling (see next section), to delimit more precisely the cognitive mechanisms by which phonological complexification emerges from hypoarticulated speech in low-contact, remote communities.

An unresolved issue is how hypoarticulation in semantically predictable parts of utterances might be related to phonologization. Recall that one of the major puzzles in phonologization is to explain how a coarticulatory effect becomes disassociated from its source: that is how vowel nasalization can become phonologized (i.e., function to distinguish between word meanings) with the loss of the following nasal consonant in some languages; or how umlaut develops from VCV coarticulation in words like *Gäste* ("guests") in present-day standard German from Old High German /gasti/ when the final /i/ (the source) that causes the vowel to be raised from /a/ to /ɛ/ (the effect) is bleached, resulting in present-day standard German /gɛstə/. In Kiparsky's (2015) model of sound change based on stratal OT mentioned earlier, phonologization comes about when the coarticulatory effect is promoted to quasi-phonemic and lexical status and is in a different stratum from the coarticulatory source that is post-lexical. Reductive processes (such as due to hypoarticulation) might then apply predominantly *post-lexically*, as a result of which the source would be eroded while the quasi-phonemic status of the coarticulatory effect at the superordinate *lexical* stratum would be unaffected.

A problem for this analysis is, however, more recent research showing that the attrition of the source interacts with lexical frequency. In their apparent-time study of coarticulatory nasalization in American English, Zellou and Tamminga (2014) found that lexically more frequent words tended to show the pattern like "sent" in Beddor's studies in which vowels were strongly nasalized coupled with an attrition of the source, the following nasal consonant. Similarly, the study by Lin et al. (2014) referred to earlier found that lenition of the tongue tip but maintenance of the tongue dorsum raising gesture as a path towards the sound change of /l/-vocalization is more likely in lexically frequent words such as "milk" than infrequent ones like "whelp." But lexical frequency is inherently lexical: consequently, the disassociation of the coarticulatory effect (which is preserved or enhanced) from the coarticulatory source (which is eroded) must refer to lexical information and cannot be explained by a post-lexical operation which has no access to lexical information, as in stratal OT phonology.

The explanation for the preservation or even enhancement (Hyman, 2013) of the coarticulatory effect but attrition of the source is likely to be phonetic rather than couched in terms of relegating the two to different lexical strata. More specifically, the phonologization of sound change may come about when hypoarticulation breaks the integrity of a consonant or vowel by leaving unaffected or even enhancing one set of cues and attenuating others. In many cases, the cues that are unaffected/enhanced are those due to the coarticulatory effect and the ones that are attenuated are associated with the coarticulatory source. This is so for the development of umlaut in /gasti/ → /gɛstə/ mentioned earlier. Trans-consonantal vowel coarticulation has the effect of shifting the first vowel (V_1) from /a/ to /ɛ/. Hypoarticulation also tends to shift /a/ in the direction of /ɛ/. This is because in a hypoarticulated speaking-style – such as when the word is in an unaccented position or produced in a faster speaking style – vowel shortening is often accompanied by jaw raising (Beckman et al., 1992; Harrington et al., 1995) i.e., the vowel quality shifts in the direction of a phonetically raised vowel. *Thus, both coarticulation and hypoarticulation are additive* because they both cause phonetic V_1 raising. They are also additive in V_1 in Old High German /futiz/ → Standard German /fysə/ (*Füße*, "feet") because they both cause phonetic fronting: coarticulation because V_2 = /i/; and hypoarticulation because the high back vowel position is typically undershot in more casual speaking styles, which is manifested acoustically as F_2-raising (Moon & Lindblom, 1994; Harrington et al., 2011). Finally, while enhancing coarticulation in V_1, hypoarticulation simultaneously causes reduction and centralization of V_2 (= /i/) in both these cases: this is because V_2 is unstressed, i.e., occurs in a prosodically weak constituent.

Hypoarticulation also dismantles the integrity of the coda alveolar in the sound changes leading to vowel nasalization in *send* and to *l*-vocalization in *milk*. This is because once again there is one set of cues that, while not necessarily enhanced, is largely unaffected by hypoarticulation; and another set of cues whose effectiveness is compromised in a hypoarticulated speaking style. In *send*, coarticulatory vowel nasalization is unlikely to be affected by hypoarticulation. As Zellou and Tamminga (2014) show, the vowels in lexically more frequent words, which are more often hypoarticulated than their less frequent counterparts (Aylett & Turk, 2004; Wright, 2003), were found to be just as nasalized as vowels in words of low lexical frequency. In *l*-vocalization, the degree of tongue dorsum lowering is also largely unaffected by lexical frequency (and by extension hypoarticulation), as the previously mentioned study by Lin et al. (2014) demonstrates. On the other hand, as numerous studies have shown (Guy, 1980; Mitterer & Ernestus, 2006; Raymond et al., 2006; Zimmerer et al., 2014) alveolar consonants in coda position in words like *send* or *milk* are very often lenited or reduced.

The commonality across these different types of sound change is therefore that phonologization is brought about by the forces of hypoarticulation which enhances or leaves unaffected one set of cues while simultaneously destroying others, therefore dismantling the integrity of a phonological unit. The more general conclusion is that pragmatic variation drives sound change given that variations along an H&H continuum are very often made in response to the degree to which an utterance is semantically predictable from the dialogue and situational context in which it occurs. This idea therefore brings together pragmatics, phonologization, coarticulation, and hypoarticulation within a model of sound change.

The final question to be considered is whether sound change is more likely to be driven by normalizing or compensating for coarticulation in perception as in Ohala (1981, 1993) or – as suggested here and based on Lindblom et al. (1995) – by the forces of hypoarticulation. The different predictions of the two models can be assessed with respect to Figure 14.2 which shows schematic psychometric curves when listeners provide categorical responses of either (high front) /y/ or (high back) /u/ to a synthetic continuum between these two vowels that has been embedded in a fronting t_t and non-fronting p_p contexts. As various studies have shown (e.g., Ohala & Feder, 1994; Lindblom & Studdert-Kennedy, 1967), there is a greater probability of hearing /u/ in a fronting consonantal context because listeners attribute some of the vowel fronting to the coarticulatory influence of the anterior consonant(s) and factor this out, i.e., they bias their responses towards /u/. According to Ohala (1981, 1993), the path to sound change is when listeners exceptionally do not compensate for coarticulation. In terms of the model in Figure 14.2, this would mean the following change to perception in a t_t context within the interval marked "normalize" in Figure 14.2: instead

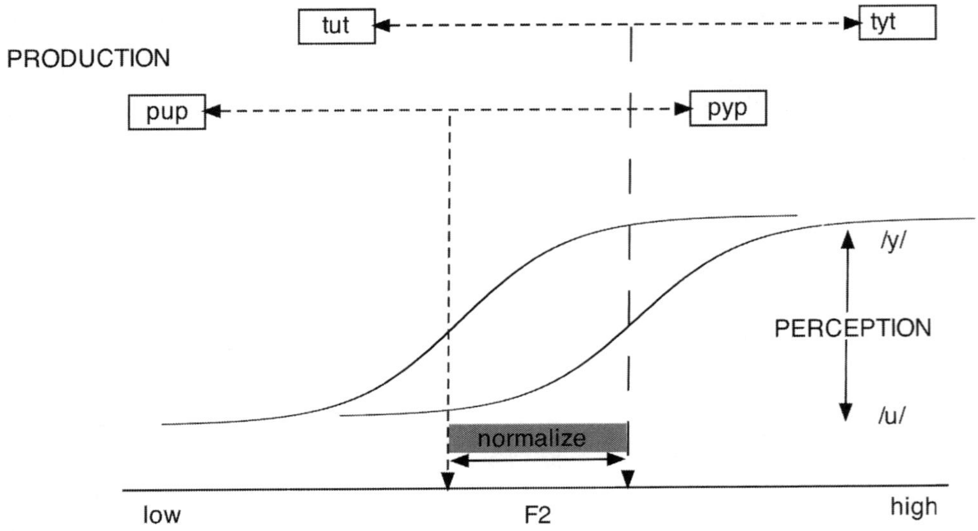

Figure 14.2 A schematic outline of the relationship between the production and perception of coarticulation. The upper part of the display illustrates the hypothetical positions of /pup, tut/ with low F_2 and with /pyp, tyt/ with high F_2. Because of the fronting effects of context, the positions in the t_t context are shifted towards higher F_2 values than for p_p. The lower panel shows the distribution of the corresponding perceptual responses under the assumption that the production and perception of coarticulation are exactly aligned. The degree to which listeners normalize for coarticulation in this model is shown by the gray shaded area marked "normalize" which extends between the two sigmoids' cross-over boundaries at which the probability of perceiving /u/ or /y/ are both 50%. Within this interval of ambiguity, a vowel is perceived as /y/ in a p_p context and as /u/ in a t_t context.

Adapted from Harrington et al. (2016).

of hearing /u/ within this interval in a t_t context, they would perceive /y/ if they no longer compensated for coarticulation. This is because perceptual responses would no longer be adjusted for (and biased towards /u/) to compensate for the coarticulatory fronting effects of the consonantal context.

Notice that in terms of this model, giving up compensating for coarticulation implies that the psychometric curve in the t_t context must shift to the left, i.e., towards the psychometric curve in the p_p context, if listeners ignore the fronting influence of the t_t context in making their judgments about vowel quality.

If, on the other hand, the sound change is driven by hypoarticulation, then listeners would notice high F_2 values in hypoarticulated speech but would not attribute them to the effects of this particular speaking style on vowel quality. Thus, high F_2 values, which may have been interpreted as /y/ are instead interpreted as /u/: that is, the range of what is considered to be an acceptable /u/ extends progressively towards higher F_2 values in a sound change led by hypoarticulation. In this case, it is the left boundary in Figure 14.2 that is shifted to the right as variants in non-fronting contexts that originally had low F_2 values catch up with the higher F_2 values of their coarticulated variants.

The issue that must be considered, then, is which of these alternatives is more plausible: whether it is the right boundary in Figure 14.1 that shifts to the left as listeners increasingly judge vowels with a low F_2 in a t_t context to be /y/; or whether it is the left boundary that shifts to the right as listeners increasingly judge vowels with a high F_2 in a p_p context to be /u/. Two studies shed some light on this issue. In Standard Southern British, /u/ has fronted in the last 50 years or so (Henton, 1983; Hawkins & Midgley, 2005). Compatibly, the apparent-time study in Harrington et al. (2008) showed that participants from a younger age group typically had a fronted /u/ in production and that their cross-over boundary in perception between /u/ and /i/ was shifted toward the front so that on an /u–i/ continuum, younger listeners heard more /u/ than older listeners. But these age differences were confined to the non-fronting context. That is, the main difference in perception between the age groups was in the non-fronting *sweep-swoop* context, which was much more front for younger listeners. This result suggests therefore that in the last 50 years, the /u-i/ cross-over boundary in the non-fronting context has shifted from the back (as for older listeners) towards the front (as for younger listeners), just as would be expected in a model of diachronic /u/-fronting driven synchronically by hypoarticulation. In Harrington et al. (2016), first language child and adult speakers of German labeled /u-y/ continua (in which the difference in vowel fronting is phonologically contrastive) in precisely the contexts shown in Figure 14.2. The results showed that children's psychometric curves were closer together than for adults. If the children had normalized less for coarticulation, then this should have been manifested as response differences between the age groups in the fronting t_t context. Consistent with the apparent-time analysis in Harrington et al. (2008), the difference was present in the p_p context which was substantially fronted (towards t_t) for children compared with adults. This suggests that if children's lack of phonetic experience is in some way related to sound change, as Ohala (1993) suggests, then it is not because they have greater difficulty in compensating for coarticulation, but instead because they might over-estimate the extent of hypoarticulation in citation-form contexts of the kind presented in the experiment in Harrington et al. (2016). This over-estimation may come about because children and adults alike typically hear words in spontaneous speech in a hypoarticulated speaking style and rarely in this laboratory-style isolated word presentation; and so, children may not yet have learned sufficiently how to associate shifts in hyper- and hypoarticulation with speaking-style variation. The conclusion based on these results is the same as earlier: if children drive sound change then it is more likely to be because they have not yet had sufficient experience of the mapping between pragmatic meaning and spontaneous speech (e.g., Redford, 2009) that allows them to identify how a particular speaking style is positioned along the H&H continuum. Once again this result (based this time on language acquisition) points to the importance of the mapping between pragmatics and spontaneous speech as one of the drivers of sound change.

Sound change and agent-based modeling

In the last 50–60 years, there has been a fairly clear division between models concerned with the phonetic conditions that give rise to sound change (e.g., Ohala, 1993) as opposed to the social factors that cause the spread of sound change around a community of speakers (e.g., Eckert, 2012; Labov, 2001; Milroy, 1992). The general consensus has been that while phonetic factors in particular due to coarticulation and reduction provide the conditions by which sound change may take place, the spread of sound change is determined by social factors (Janda & Joseph, 2003). Thus, speakers might have knowledge of a social factor such as class as well as of certain spoken attributes that might characterize it (e.g., that London Cockney English has more *l*-vocalization than the standard accent of England). According to this view of sound change, speakers preferentially copy the speaking style of the social category that they want to belong to. This view is characteristic of models of sound change in both Baker et al. (2011) and Garrett and Johnson (2013). Thus, Baker et al. (2011) in their analysis of /s/-retraction note that sound change may be started by speakers with extreme i.e., outlier forms of coarticulation; but that sound change becomes possible if the variation is conditioned by "social factors" in which there is a leader of linguistic change such as from upwardly mobile female speakers of the highest status social group. One of the computer simulations in Garrett and Johnson (2013) is built on the idea that "imitation is socially constrained" (p. 89) and that "a group that is aware of some social distance from another group may attend to phonetic deviations from the norm as marks of social differentiation" (p. 94).

There is, however, no reason to presume that the spread of sound change must be socially conditioned in this way. An alternative is that the propagation of sound change around a community of speakers derives from the principle of communication density (Bloomfield, 1933) and depends on which speakers talk to each other and how often (see also Labov, 2001, p. 24 for a similar view). Communication density is considered by Trudgill (2008a, 2008b) to be the main factor (at least in the earlier stages) that shaped the phonetic characteristics of New Zealand English, which bears a predictable relationship to the relative proportions of the different spoken accents of the first settlers to New Zealand in the 19th century. Similarly, the results of the longitudinal analysis of the annual Christmas broadcasts produced by Queen Elizabeth II in Harrington et al. (2000) suggest that the shift from her aristocratic accent in the direction of (but without attaining) a more middle-class accent came about, not because the Queen preferentially wanted to sound like one of the people, but instead because the Queen increasingly came into contact with persons of a middle-class accent during the decades (1960s, 1970s) in which a social revolution was taking place in England (Cannadine, 1998).

In other approaches derived rather more directly from communication density than either Baker et al. (2011) or Garrett and Johnson (2013), the spread of sound change at least in its initial stages is not a consequence of social factors but emerges instead from the propagation of different types of phonetic variation around a population of speakers and how these are modified during communication. According to a view based on communication density, sound change emerges from the often very slightly different ways in which speakers put their vocal organs and speech perception apparatus to use during speech communication. Thus, speakers constantly update their pronunciation during conversation without necessarily being socially selective about which aspects to imitate and which to ignore. Compatibly, while there is some evidence that phonetic imitation is socially selective (Babel, 2012; Babel et al., 2014), there are also studies showing that this need not be so (Delvaux & Soquet, 2007; Nielsen, 2011, 2014; Pardo et al., 2012) and that phonetic imitation may derive from the same mechanisms that cause non-speech alignments in posture, body movements, and sway (Fowler et al., 2008; Sebanz et al., 2006). Seen from this perspective, the issue to be modeled is how these types of inevitable phonetic modifications that arise at a microscopic level when individuals converse are related at a macroscopic level to community level, categorical change.

The problem of how microscopic phonetic variation and macroscopic sound change are connected cannot be solved from analyses of speech production or perception alone because it would require identifying sound changes before they have occurred as well as sampling from a large cross-section of the community longitudinally over a long time period. Partly for this reason, an alternative approach is to view language and language change in terms of the theory of systems dynamics: a theory often applied using computational simulation in a variety of fields – biology, the economy, the environment (Meadows, 2015) to mention but a few. In systems dynamics, a system, as the famous parable of the Blind Men and the Elephant shows, cannot be understood just from the components out of which it is made: it requires a coherent model of the elements, their interconnections and how these are related to the overall purpose of the system. A characteristic feature of a system is that it is self-organizing (and often self-repairing) which means that an organizing structure emerges flexibly as a consequence of interacting elements (Oudeyer, 2006; Shockley et al., 2009). This idea is central to theories of emergent phonology in which macroscopic phonological categories emerge but are variably sustained as a consequence of microscopic interactions between the elements, in this case between the speakers of the community (Blevins & Wedel, 2009; de Boer, 2001; Lindblom et al., 1984; Studdert-Kennedy, 1998). Given that the speakers, the conversations that they have and how frequently they interact necessarily vary unpredictably, it follows that the association between phonological categories and the speech signals that sustain them is both stochastic and in constant flux. These stochastic variations occur because the system is inherently bi-directional with feedback (Wedel, 2007). It is bi-directional because, from a top-down point of view, phonology obviously shapes speech production output as well as judgments in speech perception (e.g., Hay et al., 2004); and because from a bottom-up point of view, speech output and perceived speech in this type of model shape phonological categories.

The phonetic variation might be small and category-internal, but under certain conditions the system self (re)organizes such that there is a phonological category change, i.e., sound change occurs at the level of the community. Establishing the conditions under which this type of change takes place – how for example top-down processing interacts with bottom-up changes to phonetic variation that might be caused by variations in the population – is of fundamental concern to research in this area.

The computational approach for solving this problem is typically agent-based modeling which is used to understand how the interaction between individuals that are represented by agents connected together in a network can bring about global (community) changes (Castellano et al., 2009). In research on sound change, the agent-based models draw upon many of the insights into human speech processing from usage (Bybee, 2002) and experienced-based (exemplar or episodic) models of speech (Pierrehumbert, 2003, 2006), precisely because such models are bi-directional in which phonological categories are updated by individuals' experiences in speech communication (Pierrehumbert, 2001; Blevins, 2004; Wedel, 2007).

In many agent-based models of sound change, the population might consist of a number of agents representing individuals. Each agent is typically equipped with a rudimentary lexicon, phonology, and parameterizations (e.g., formant frequencies, fundamental frequency etc.) of several stored speech signals per word. There is also usually some form of statistical, often Gaussian association between categories and parametric representations of the stored signals. Thus, a phonological category might be defined as a multidimensional Gaussian distribution (whose axes are the parameters) over the stored signals with which it is associated. Communication is often between an agent-talker and an agent-listener. One of the ways in which the agent talks is by generating a random sample from the statistical distributions of whichever categories are to be produced. The agent-listener may or may not add the perceived item (consisting of the generated sample and associated category labels) to memory depending on certain filtering conditions: in some models (Blevins & Wedel, 2009; Harrington & Schiel, 2017; Sóskuthy, 2015; Wedel, 2006), the item is not added if it is potentially confusable with another of the agent listener's categories (if for example, an agent-talker's /i/ is probabilistically closest to the agent listener's /u/). Models sometimes also make use of some parameterized form of memory decay in order to remove items from the listener's memory. This can be important not just to offset the increase of items in memory that occur following a large number of interactions, but also to counteract the potentially infinite broadening, i.e., increase in the variance in the signals that make up a category with an increasing number of interactions.

The preceding is intended as a generic overview of agent-based modeling in sound change. The details vary quite considerably between studies. Thus, whereas in Blevins and Wedel (2009) and Sóskuthy (2015) there is only one agent that talks to itself, in Harrington and Schiel (2017) there are multiple agents based on real talkers, and in Kirby (2014) communication is from 100 learner to 100 teacher agents. Most models use artificially generated, static acoustic data as starting conditions (analogous to, e.g., formant values obtained at a single time slice from a theoretically derived, lossless model of the vocal tract); in Harrington and Schiel (2017) the starting conditions are dynamically changing parameters from real speakers. A Gaussian model is used in most studies to define the association between categories and signals, but in Ettlinger (2007) the statistical model is based on exemplar strength. In Harrington and Schiel (2017), the oldest exemplar is removed from memory each time an agent-listener adds a new one; in Ettlinger (2007), memory decay comes about by decrementing the strength of each exemplar exponentially over time (see also Pierrehumbert, 2001).

Agent-based models are typically designed to analyze specific aspects of sound change. In Ettlinger (2007), the main aim is to show that vowel chain shifting emerges as a natural consequence of stored and updated exemplars. The agent-based model in Kirby (2014) simulates a sound change by which fundamental frequency has taken over from duration as the main cue in distinguishing initial singleton stops vs. stop clusters with /r/ in the Phnom Penh variety of Khmer. Kirby's (2014) agent-based model is used to show that this type of change is driven by functional considerations, i.e., by a combination of the acoustic effectiveness of the cue for distinguishing between phonological categories combined with the extent to which the category distinguishes between lexical items. The purpose of the computational model in Blevins and Wedel (2009) is to explain why sound change often does not create homophones, especially if a pair of words that is about to merge acoustically cannot be further disambiguated by pragmatic information. They show how two phonological categories that are closely positioned in an acoustic space repel each other on the assumption that no update takes place from exemplars that are acoustically ambiguous between the categories. The agent-based model in Harrington and Schiel (2017) tested whether the phonetic approximation between two groups of speakers of Standard Southern British with retracted /u/ and fronted /ʉ/ was influenced by how these variants were oriented with respect to each in an acoustic space. They showed that, because older speakers' retracted /u/ was oriented toward that of younger speakers' fronted /ʉ/ (but not the other way round), the influence was correspondingly asymmetric, with a large shift following interaction in the older speaker's retracted variant towards the front of the vowel space. Stanford and Kenny (2013) used their agent-based model to test various aspects of Labov's (2007) theory of sound change by transmission, incrementation (brought about when children increment sound change from one generation to the next), and diffusion (brought about principally by contact between adults). Their model includes agents that represent adults (with stored speech knowledge) and children (without such knowledge) from two North American cities: from Chicago, in which a sound change, the Northern Cities vowel shift, is taking place; and from St. Louis where it is not. The model was set up to simulate travel (and therefore contact) between agents from the two cities. Only agents that were in close proximity could converse with each other (and therefore influence each other's speech characteristics). Incrementation came about in their simulations because the agent children had fewer exemplars and so were less resistant to change. Diffusion arose because the St. Louis agent listeners learned the vowel chain shift from Chicago speakers imperfectly. Contrary to Labov (2007), the conclusion in Stanford and Kenny (2013) is that incrementation and diffusion are not due to different kinds of language learning, but instead both derive from exemplar learning (as outlined previously) and communication density, i.e., the frequency with which talkers represented by agents happen to communicate with each other.

Finally, there is the potential in an agent-based model to test the influence on sound change of different types of social network structures. Such research takes up the idea, explored predominantly within the sociolinguistics literature, that sound change might be differently affected depending on whether individuals are centrally or peripherally connected in the community (Borgatti et al., 2013; Mühlenbernd & Quinley, 2013; Stoessel, 2002; Wasserman & Faust, 1994). The computational simulation in Fagyal et al. (2010) suggests that leaders, i.e., those connected to many others, are drivers of sound change. On the other hand, Milroy and Milroy's (1985) study of Belfast English showed that sound change was less likely to occur in centrally connected members of a community (i.e., those with connections to many others); sound change was instead often caused by individuals with weaker ties to the community who introduced innovations from other communities with which they were associated. Compatibly, the computational model of Pierrehumbert et al. (2014) showed that highly connected individuals tended not to be instigators of sound change because their output was modulated by the very large number of connections to others (who might resist change). They suggest instead that linguistic change originates in tightly knit communities amongst individuals with only average connections but who tend to share innovations.

Concluding remarks

The sharp separation between the origin and the spread of sound change that was mentioned in the preceding section is to a certain extent a consequence of excluding social factors from cognitive models of speech processing, an approach that has typified speech research in much of the 20th century (see also Docherty & Mendoza-Denton, 2012; Docherty & Foulkes, 2014). The architecture suggested by episodic models in which there is a bi-directional, probabilistic association between phonological categories and speech signals that is incrementally updated through interaction provides the cognitive and computational architecture for bringing these strands of research together. This type of architecture can also begin to provide testable hypotheses concerning the actuation of sound change (Weinreich et al., 1968) that was mentioned in the section on sound change and coarticulation. This mercurial aspect of sound change is to be expected given a language model in which categories and signals are stochastically related and mutually updated by random interactions between individuals who, because they increment their phonological knowledge through experience, are also phonetically necessarily idiosyncratic (Laver, 1994, p. 66).

As Trudgill (2012) notes, sound change can cause what were once mutually intelligible spoken accents of a single language to evolve over a long time scale into separate languages. A somewhat neglected area of research lies in explaining quite how speech processing is incremented to produce this divergence in spoken accents that originally had a shared or at least quite similar phonology and marginally different phonetic characteristics. There is a gap in this area of research because most studies model the relationship between synchronic variation and diachronic change in terms of quite broad phonological features: how phonetic variation leads to categorical changes in e.g., lenition, voicing, nasalization, palatalization, vowel height – and typically with an emphasis on patterns of change that are found across languages. But this type of analysis – mapping signals directly to distinctive phonological features – is too coarse-grained to explain spoken accent diversification. This is because spoken accents differ from one another at a much finer level of phonetic detail, especially when comparing sociolects of the same dialect (e.g., Docherty & Mendoza-Denton, 2012; Mendoza-Denton, 2008). Because this remarkable level of fine phonetic detail is nearly impossible to imitate in adulthood, spoken accent may in evolutionary terms have functioned as a tag for identifying imposters (Cohen, 2012). With databases of sufficiently large numbers of speakers and word items, it may be possible to model the steps by which sound change causes accents to diversify by using a cognitive-computational architecture based on episodes, incrementation, and feedback of the kind reviewed earlier. This is because this type of model provides and indeed predicts a stochastic link between phonological categories and precisely this very fine and nuanced level of phonetic detail that characterizes spoken accent and language differences (Pierrehumbert et al., 2000).

This review of the literature on sound change also suggests that this type of architecture needs to be extended in two ways. The first is by incorporating a model of hyper- and hypoarticulation in relation to pragmatic meaning, given the arguments presented in the section on sound change and hypoarticulation that it may well be this type of mapping that can shed new light on phonologization. The second is to incorporate associations between perception and production based more directly on the nonlinear mapping between speech physiology and acoustics (Stevens, 1989) possibly by incorporating the mathematics of nonlinear dynamics in associating phonological categories with speech output (e.g., Roon & Gafos, 2016). This will make it easier to test connections between the emergence of sound change from phonetic variation on the one hand and quantal jumps in acoustics due to incrementation in speech production on the other.

Acknowledgments

This research was supported by the European Research Council Advanced Grant no 742289 “Human interaction and the evolution of spoken accent” (2017–2022). Our thanks to Pam Beddor and to the editors for very many helpful comments on an earlier draft of this paper.

References

Abrego-Collier, C. (2013). Liquid dissimilation as listener hypocorrection. *Proceedings of the 37th annual meeting of the Berkeley linguistics society*, pp. 3–17.

Alderete, J., & Frisch, S. (2006). Dissimilation in grammar and the lexicon. In P. de Lacy (Ed.) *The Cambridge Handbook of Phonology*. Cambridge University Press: Cambridge.

Aylett, M., & Turk, A. (2004). The smooth signal redundancy hypothesis: A functional explanation for relationships between redundancy, prosodic prominence, and duration in spontaneous speech. *Language and Speech*, 47, 31–56.

Babel, M. (2012). Evidence for phonetic and social selectivity in spontaneous phonetic imitation. *Journal of Phonetics*, 40, 177–189.

Babel, M., McGuire, G., Walters, S., & Nicholls, A. (2014). Novelty and social preference in phonetic accommodation. *Laboratory Phonology*, 5, 123–150.

Bailey, G., Wikle, T., Tillery, J., & Sand, L. (1991). The apparent time construct. *Language Variation and Change*, 3, 241–264.

Baker, A., Archangeli, D., & Mielke, J. (2011). Variability in American English s-retraction suggests a solution to the actuation problem. *Language Variation and Change*, 23, 347–374.

Beckman, M., Edwards, J., & Fletcher, J. (1992). Prosodic structure and tempo in a sonority model of articulatory dynamics. In G. Docherty & R. Ladd (Eds.) *Papers in Laboratory Phonology II: Gesture, Segment, Prosody*. Cambridge University Press: Cambridge, pp. 68–86.

Beddor, P. (2009). A coarticulatory path to sound change. *Language*, 85, 785–821.

Beddor, P. (2012). Perception grammars and sound change. In M. J. Solé & D. Recasens (Eds.) *The Initiation of Sound Change: Perception, Production, and Social factors*. John Benjamin: Amsterdam, pp. 37–55.

Beddor, P. (2015). The relation between language users' perception and production repertoires. *Proceedings of the 18th international congress of phonetic sciences*, Glasgow, UK.

Beddor, P., Brasher, A., & Narayan, C. (2007). Applying perceptual methodsto phonetic variation and sound change. In M. J. Solé, et al. (Eds.) *Experimental Approaches to Phonology*. Oxford University Press: Oxford, pp. 127–143.

Beddor, P., & Krakow, R. A. (1999). Perception of coarticulatory nasalization by speakers of English and Thai: Evidence for partial compensation. *The Journal of the Acoustical Society of America*, 106, 2868–2887.

Bermúdez-Otero, R., & Hogg, R. (2003). The actuation problem in optimality theory: Phonologization, rule inversion, and rule loss. In D. Eric Holt (Ed.) *Optimality Theory and Language Change*. Kluwer: Dordrecht.

Blevins, J. (2004). *Evolutionary Phonology: The Emergence of Sound Patterns*. Cambridge University Press: Cambridge.

Blevins, J., & Garrett, A. (2004). The evolution of metathesis. In B. Hayes, R. Kirchner, & D. Steriade (Eds.) *Phonetically-Based Phonology*. Cambridge University Press: Cambridge, pp. 117–156.

Blevins, J., & Wedel, A. (2009). Inhibited sound change: An evolutionary approach to lexical competition. *Diachronica*, 26, 143–183.

Bloomfield, L. (1933). *Language*. Holt: New York.

Borgatti, S., Everett, M., & Johnson, J. (2013). *Analyzing Social Networks*. Sage Publications: London.

Browman, C., & Goldstein, L. (1992). Articulatory phonology: An overview. *Phonetica*, 49, 155–180.

Bukmaier, V., Harrington, J., & Kleber, F. (2014). An analysis of post-vocalic /s-ʃ/ neutralization in Augsburg German: Evidence for a gradient sound change. *Frontiers in Psychology*, 5, 1–12.

Bybee, J. (2002). Word frequency and context of use in the lexical diffusion of phonetically conditioned sound change. *Language Variation and Change*, 14, 261–290.

Cannadine, D. (1998). *Class in Britain*. Yale University Press: New Haven.

Castellano, C., Fortunato, S., & Loreto, V. (2009). Statistical physics of social dynamics. *Reviews of Modern Physics*, 81, 591–646.

Chang, S., Plauché, M., & Ohala, J. (2001). Markedness and consonant confusion asymmetries In E. Hume & K. Johnson (Eds.) *The Role of Speech Perception in Phonology*. Academic Press: San Diego, CA, pp. 79–101.

Charles-Luce, J. (1985). Word-final devoicing in German: Effects of phonetic and sentential contexts. *Journal of Phonetics*, 13, 309–324.

Chen, M., & Wang, W. (1975). Sound change: Actuation and implementation. *Language*, 51, 255–281.

Cohen, E. (2012). The evolution of tag-based cooperation in humans: The case for accent. *Current Anthropology*, 53, 588–616.

de Boer, B. (2001). *The Origins of Vowel Systems*. Oxford University Press: Oxford.

Delvaux, V., & Soquet, A. (2007). The influence of ambient speech on adult speech productions through unintentional imitation. *Phonetica*, 64, 145–173.

Denham, K., & Lobeck, A. (2010). *Linguistics for Everyone: An Introduction* (2nd edition). Wadsworth: Boston.

Docherty, G., & Foulkes, P. (2014). An evaluation of usage-based approaches to the modeling of sociophonetic variability. *Lingua*, 142, 42–56.

Docherty, G., & Mendoza-Denton, N. (2012). Speaker-related variation – sociophonetic factors. In A. Cohn, C. Fougeron, & M. Huffman (Eds.) *The Oxford Handbook of Laboratory Phonology*. Oxford University Press: Oxford, pp. 44–60.

Eckert, P. (2012). Three waves of variation study: The emergence of meaning in the study of sociolinguistic variation. *Annual Review of Anthropology*, 41, 87–100.

Ettlinger, M. (2007). An exemplar-based model of chain shifts. *Proceedings of the 16th international congress of the phonetic science*, pp. 685–688.

Fagyal, Z., Escobar, A., Swarup, S., Gasser, L., & Lakkaraju, K. (2010). Centers and peripheries: Network roles in language change. *Lingua*, 120, 2061–2079.

Fowler, C. (1983). Converging sources of evidence on spoken and perceived rhythms of speech: Cyclic production of vowels in monosyllabic stress feet. *Journal of Experimental Psychology General*, 112, 386–412.

Fowler, C. (1984). Segmentation of coarticulated speech in perception. *Perception and Psychophysics*, 36, 359–368.

Fowler, C., Richardson, M., Marsh, K., & Shockley, K. (2008). Language use, coordination, and the emergence of cooperative action. In A. Fuchs & V. Jirsa (Eds.) *Understanding Complex Systems*. Springer: Berlin, pp. 261–279.

Fowler, C., & Smith, M. (1986). Speech perception as "vector analysis": An approach to the problems of segmentation and invariance. In J. Perkell & D. Klatt (Eds.) *Invariance and Variability in Speech Processes*. Erlbaum: Hillsdale, NJ, pp. 123–139.

Fowler, C., & Thompson, J. (2010). Listeners' perception of compensatory shortening. *Attention, Perception & Psychophysics*, 72, 481–491.

Fujisaki, H., & Kunisaki, O. (1976). Analysis, recognition and perception of voiceless fricative consonants in Japanese. *Annual Bulletin Research Institute of Logopedics and Phoniatrics*, 10, 145–156.

Garrett, A., & Johnson, K. (2013). Phonetic bias in sound change. In A. Yu (Ed.) *Origins of Sound Change*. Oxford University Press: Oxford, pp. 51–97.

Grimm, J., & Grimm, W. (1854). *Das Deutsche Wörterbuch*. Online dictionary at: http://dwb.uni-trier.de/de/

Grosvald, M., & Corina, D. (2012). The production and perception of sub-phonemic vowel contrasts and the role of the listener in sound change. In M. J. Solé & D. Recasens (Eds.) *The initiation of sound change: Production, perception, and social factors*. John Benjamins: Amsterdam, pp. 77–100.

Guion, S. (1998). The role of perception in the sound change of velar palatalization. *Phonetica*, 55, 18–52.

Guy, G. (1980). Variation in the group and the individual: The case of final stop deletion. In: W. Labov (Ed.) *Locating Language in Time and Space*. Academic Press: New York, pp. 1–36.

Harrington, J. (2007). Evidence for a relationship between synchronic variability and diachronic change in the Queen's annual Christmas broadcasts. In: J. Cole and J. Hualde (Eds.) *Laboratory Phonology 9*. Mouton: Berlin, pp. 125–143.

Harrington, J., Fletcher, J., & Roberts, C. (1995). Coarticulation and the accented/unaccented distinction: Evidence from jaw movement data. *Journal of Phonetics*, 23, 305–322.

Harrington, J., Hoole, P., Kleber, F., & Reubold, U. (2011). The physiological, acoustic, and perceptual basis of high back vowel fronting: Evidence from German tense and lax vowels. *Journal of Phonetics*, 39, 121–131.

Harrington, J., Kleber, F., & Reubold, U. (2008). Compensation for coarticulation, /u/-fronting, and sound change in Standard Southern British: An acoustic and perceptual study. *The Journal of the Acoustical Society of America*, 123, 2825–2835.

Harrington, J., Kleber, F., & Stevens, M. (2016). The relationship between the (mis)-parsing of coarticulation in perception and sound change: Evidence from dissimilation and language acquisition. In A. Esposito & M. Faundez-Zany (Eds.) *Recent Advances in Nonlinear Speech Processing*. Springer Verlag: Berlin, pp. 15–34.

Harrington, J., Palethorpe, S., & Watson, C. (2000). Does the queen speak the queen's English? *Nature*, 408, 927–928.

Harrington, J., & Schiel, F. (2017). /u/-fronting and agent-based modeling: The relationship between the origin and spread of sound change. *Language*, 93(2), 414–445.

Hawkins, S., & Midgley, J. (2005). Formant frequencies of RP monophthongs in four age groups of speakers. *Journal of the International Phonetic Association*, 35, 183–199.

Hay, J., Drager, K., & Thomas, B. (2013). Using nonsense words to investigate vowel merger. *English Language and Linguistics*, 17, 241–269.

Hay, J., Drager, K., & Warren, P. (2010). Short-term exposure to one dialect affects processing of another. *Language & Speech*, 53, 447–471.

Hay, J., & Foulkes, P. (2016). The evolution of medial /t/ over real and remembered time. *Language*, 92(2), 298–330.

Hay, J., Nolan, A., & Drager, K. (2006). From fush to feesh: Exemplar priming in speech perception. *The Linguistic Review*, 23, 351–379.

Hay, J., Pierrehumbert, J., & Beckman, M. (2004). Speech perception, well-formedness, and the statistics of the lexicon. In *Papers in Laboratory Phonology VI*. Cambridge University Press: Cambridge, pp. 58–74.

Henton, C. (1983). Changes in the vowels of received pronunciation. *Journal of Phonetics*, 11, 353–371.

Hombert, J. M., Ohala, J., & Ewan, G. (1979). Phonetic explanations for the development of tones. *Language*, 55, 37–58.

Hoole, P., & Pouplier, M. (2017). Öhman returns: New horizons in the collection and analysis of articulatory imaging data. *Computer Speech and Language*, 45, 253–277.

Hyman, L. M. (2013). Enlarging the scope of phonologization. In A. Yu (Ed.) *Origins of Sound Change: Approaches to Phonologization*. Oxford University Press: Oxford, pp. 3–28.

Janda, R., & Joseph, B. (2003). Reconsidering the canons of sound-change: Towards a "big bang" theory. In B. Blake & K. Burridge (Eds.) *Selected Papers from the 15th International Conference on Historical Linguistics*. John Benjamins: Amsterdam, pp. 205–219.

Jannedy, S., & Weirich, M. (2014). Sound change in an urban setting: Category instability of the palatal fricative in Berlin. *Laboratory Phonology*, 5, 91–122.

Kawasaki, H. (1986). Phonetic explanation for phonological universals: The case of distinctive vowel nasalization. In J. Ohala & J. Jaeger (Eds.) *Experimental Phonology*. Academic Press: Orlando, FL, pp. 81–103.

Kiparsky, P. (2003). The phonological basis of sound change. In B. Joseph & R. Janda (Eds.) *The Handbook of Historical Linguistics*. Blackwell: Oxford.

Kiparsky, P. (2015). Phonologization. In P. Honeybone & J. Salmons (Eds.) *Handbook of Historical Phonology*. Oxford University Press: Oxford.

Kiparsky, P. (2016). Labov, sound change, and phonological theory. *Journal of Sociolinguistics*, 20, 464–488.

Kirby, J. (2014). Incipient tonogenesis in Phnom Penh Khmer: Computational studies. *Laboratory Phonology*, 5, 195–230.

Kleber, F., John, T., & Harrington, J. (2010). The implications for speech perception of incomplete neutralization of final devoicing in German. *Journal of Phonetics*, 38, 185–196.

Kleber, F., Harrington, J., & Reubold, U. (2012). The relationship between the perception and production of coarticulation during a sound change in progress. *Language & Speech*, 55, 383–405.

Krakow, R., Beddor, P., Goldstein, L., & Fowler, C. (1988). Coarticulatory influences on the perceived height of nasal vowels. *The Journal of the Acoustical Society of America*, 83, 1146–1158.

Kuang, J., & Cui, A. (2016). Relative cue weighting in perception and production of a sound change in progress. In *Proceedings of the 15th laboratory phonology conference*, Ithaca. Online dictionary at: https://labphon.org/labphon15/long_abstracts/LabPhon15_Revised_abstract_237.pdf

Labov, W. (2001). *Principles of Linguistic Change. Vol. 2: Social Factors*. Blackwell: Oxford.

Labov, W. (2007). Transmission and diffusion. *Language*, 83, 344–387.

Labov, W., Mark, K., & Corey, M. (1991). Near-mergers and the suspension of phonemic contrast. *Language Variation and Change*, 3, 33–74.

Laver, J. (1994). *Principles of Phonetics*. Cambridge University Press: Cambridge.

Lin, S., Beddor, P., & Coetzee, A. (2014). Gestural reduction, lexical frequency, and sound change: A study of post-vocalic /l/. *Laboratory Phonology*, 5, 9–36.

Lindblom, B. (1988). Phonetic invariance and the adaptive nature of speech. In B. A. G. Elsendoorn & H. Bouma (Eds.) *Working Models of Human Perception*. Academic Press: London, pp. 139–173.

Lindblom, B. (1990). Explaining phonetic variation: A sketch of the H & H theory. In W. Hardcastle & A. Marchal (Eds.) *Speech Production and Speech Modeling*. Kluwer: Dordrecht, pp. 403–439.

Lindblom, B. (1998). Systemic constraints and adaptive change in the formation of sound structure. In J. Hurford, M. Studdert-Kennedy, & C. Knight (Eds.) *Approaches to the Evolution of Language*. Cambridge University Press: Cambridge, pp. 242–264.

Lindblom, B., Guion, S., Hura, S., Moon, S. J., & Willerman, R. (1995). Is sound change adaptive? *Rivista di Linguistica*, 7, 5–36.

Lindblom, B., MacNeilage P., & Studdert-Kennedy, M. (1984). Self-organizing processes and the explanation of phonological universals. In B. Butterworth, B. Comrie, & O. Dahl (Eds.) *Explanation for Language Universals*. Mouton: Berlin, pp. 181–203.

Lindblom, B., & Studdert-Kennedy, M. (1967). On the role of formant transitions in vowel recognition. *The Journal of the Acoustical Society of America*, 42, 830–843.

Löfqvist, A., Baer, T., McGarr, N., & Story, R. (1989). The cricothyroid muscle in voicing control. *The Journal of the Acoustical Society of America*, 85, 1314–1321.

Mann, V., & Repp, B. (1980). Influence of vocalic context on the perception of [ʃ]-[s] distinction: I. Temporal factors. *Perception & Psychophysics*, 28, 213–228.

Meadows, D. (2015). *Thinking in Systems: A Primer*. Earthscan: London.

Mendoza-Denton, N. (2008). *Homegirls: Language and Cultural Practice Among Latina Youth Gangs*. Blackwell: Malden, MA.

Milroy, J. (1992). Social network and prestige arguments in sociolinguistics. In K. Bolton & H. Kwok (Eds.) *Sociolinguistics Today: International Pers*pectives. Routledge: London, pp. 146–162.

Milroy, J., & Milroy, L. (1985). Linguistic change, social network, and speaker innovation. *Journal of Linguistics*, 21, 339–384.

Mitterer, H., & Ernestus, M. (2006). Listeners recover /t/s that speakers reduce: Evidence from /t/-lenition in Dutch. *Journal of Phonetics*, 34, 73–103.

Moon, S. J., & Lindblom, B. (1994). Interaction between duration, context, and speaking style in English stressed vowels. *The Journal of the Acoustical Society of America*, 96, 40–55.

Mühlenbernd, R., & Quinley, J. (2013). Signaling and simulations in sociolinguistics. *University of Pennsylvania Working Papers in Linguistics*, Vol. 19, Article 16. Online dictionary at: http://repository.upenn.edu/pwpl/vol19/iss1/16

Müller, V., Harrington, J., Kleber, F., & Reubold, U. (2011). *Age-Dependent Differences in the Neutralization of the Intervocalic Voicing Contrast: Evidence from an Apparent-Time Study on East Franconian*. Interspeech: Florence.

Nielsen, K. (2011). Specificity and abstractness of VOT imitation. *Journal of Phonetics*, 39, 132–142.

Nielsen, K. (2014). Phonetic imitation by young children and its developmental changes. *Journal of Speech Language and Hearing Research*, 57, 2065–2075.

Ohala, J. (1975). Phonetic explanations for nasal sound patterns. In C. Ferguson, L. Hyman, & J. Ohala (Eds.) *Nasálfest: Papers from a Symposium on Nasals and Nasalization*. Language Universals Project: Stanford, pp. 289–316.

Ohala, J. (1981). The listener as a source of sound change. In C. S. Masek, R. A. Hendrick, & M. F. Miller (Eds.) *Papers from the Parasession on Language and Behavior*. Chicago Linguistic Society: Chicago, pp. 178–203.

Ohala, J. (1988). Discussion of Lindblom's 'Phonetic invariance and the adaptive nature of speech'. In B. A. G. Elsendoorn & H. Bouma (Eds.) *Working Models of Human Perception*. Academic Press: London, pp. 175–183.

Ohala, J. (1993). The phonetics of sound change. In C. Jones (Ed.) *Historical Linguistics: Problems and Perspectives*. Longman: London, pp. 237–278.

Ohala, J. (1997). Aerodynamics of phonology. In *Proceedings of the 4th Seoul International Conference on Linguistics [SICOL]*, pp. 92–97.

Ohala, J. (2012). The listener as a source of sound change: An update. In In M. J. Solé & D. Recasens (Eds.) *The Initiation of Sound Change. Perception, Production, and Social factors*. John Benjamins: Amsterdam, pp. 21–36.

Ohala, J., & Feder, D. (1994). Listeners' identification of speech sounds is influenced by adjacent "restored" phonemes. *Phonetica*, 51, 111–118.

Öhman, S. (1966). Coarticulation in VCV utterances: Spectrographic measurements. *The Journal of the Acoustical Society of America*, 39, 151–168.

Osthoff, H., & Brugmann, K. (1878). *Morphologische Untersuchungen auf dem Gebiete der indogermanischen Sprachen, Band I*. Verlag von S. Hirzel: Leipzig.

Oudeyer, P. Y. (2006). *Self-Organization in the Evolution of Speech*. Oxford University Press: Oxford.

Pardo, J., Gibbons, R., Suppes, A., & Krauss, R. (2012). Phonetic convergence in college roommates. *Journal of Phonetics*, 40, 190–197.

Paul, H. (1886). *Prinzipien der Sprachgeschichte* (2nd edition). Niemeyer: Halle.

Phillips, B. (2006). *Word Frequency and Lexical Diffusion*. Palgrave Macmillan: Basingstoke.

Pierrehumbert, J. (2001). Exemplar dynamics: Word frequency, lenition, and contrast. In J. Bybee & P. Hopper (Eds.) *Frequency Effects and the Emergence of Lexical Structure*. John Benjamins: Amsterdam, pp. 137–157.

Pierrehumbert, J. (2003). Phonetic diversity, statistical learning, and acquisition of phonology. *Language and Speech*, 46, 115–154.

Pierrehumbert, J. (2006). The next toolkit. *Journal of Phonetics*, 34, 516–530.

Pierrehumbert, J., Beckman, M., & Ladd, D. R. (2000). Conceptual foundations of phonology as a laboratory science. In N. Burton-Roberts, P. Carr, & G. Docherty (Eds.) *Phonological Knowledge*. Oxford University Press: Oxford, pp. 273–303.

Pierrehumbert, J., Stonedahl, F., & Dalaud, R. (2014). A model of grassroots changes in linguistic systems. arXiv:1408.1985v1.

Raymond, W., Dautricourt, R., & Hume, E. (2006). Word internal /t, d/ deletion in spontaneous speech: Modeling the effects of extra-linguistic, lexical, and phonological factors. *Language Variation and Change*, 18, 55–97.

Redford, M. A. (2009). The development of distinct speaking styles in preschool children. *Journal of Speech, Language, and Hearing Research*, 52, 1434–1448.

Repp, B. H. (1982). Phonetic trading relations and context effects: New experimental evidence for a speech mode of perception. *Psychological Bulletin*, 92, 81–110.

Roon, K., & Gafos, A. (2016). Perceiving while producing: Modeling the dynamics of phonological planning. *Journal of Memory and Language*, 89, 222–243.

Ruch, H., & Harrington, J. (2014). Synchronic and diachronic factors in the change from pre-aspiration to post-aspiration in Andalusian Spanish. *Journal of Phonetics*, 45, 12–25.

Shockley, K., Richardson, D., & Dale, R. (2009). Conversation and coordinative structures. *Topics in Cognitive Science*, 1, 305–319.

Sebanz, N., Bekkering, H., & Knoblich, G. (2006). Joint action: Bodies and minds moving together. *Trends in Cognitive Sciences*, 10, 70–76.

Solé, M. (1992). Phonetic and phonological processes: The case of nasalization. *Language and Speech*, 35, 29–43.

Solé, M. (1995). Spatio-temporal patterns of velo-pharyngeal action in phonetic and phonological nasalization. *Language and Speech*, 38, 1–23.

Solé, M. (2007). Controlled and mechanical properties in speech: A review of the literature. In M. J. Solé, P. Beddor, & M. Ohala (Eds.) *Experimental Approaches to Phonology*. Oxford University Press: Oxford, pp. 302–321.

Sóskuthy, M. (2015). Understanding change through stability: A computational study of sound change actuation. *Lingua*, 163, 40–60.

Stanford, J., & Kenny, L. (2013). Revisiting transmission and diffusion: An agent-based model of vowel chain shifts across large communities. *Language Variation and Change*, 25, 119–153.

Stevens, K. (1972). The quantal nature of speech: Evidence from articulatory-acoustic data. In E. David & P. Denes (Eds.) *Human Communication: A Unified View*. McGraw-Hill: New York, pp. 51–66.

Stevens, K. (1989). On the quantal nature of speech. *Journal of Phonetics*, 17, 3–45.

Stevens, M., & Harrington, J. (2014). The individual and the actuation of sound change. *Loquens* 1(1), e003. http://dx.doi.org/10.3989/loquens.2014.003

Stoessel, S. (2002) Investigating the role of social networks in language maintenance and shift. *International Journal of the Sociology of Language*, 153, 93–131.

Studdert-Kennedy, M. (1998). Introduction: The emergence of phonology. In J. Hurford, M. Studdert-Kennedy, & C. Knight (Eds.) *Approaches to the Evolution of Language*. Cambridge University Press: Cambridge, pp. 169–176.

Trudgill, P. (2008a). Colonial dialect contact in the history of European languages: On the irrelevance of identity to new-dialect formation. *Language in Society*, 37, 241–254.

Trudgill, P. (2008b). On the role of children, and the mechanical view: A rejoinder. *Language in Society*, 37, 277–280.

Trudgill, P. (2011). *Sociolinguistic Typology*. Oxford University Press: Oxford.

Trudgill, P. (2012). On the functionality of linguistic change. *Current Anthropology*, 53, 609–610.

Warren, P., Hay, J., & Thomas, B. (2007). The loci of sound change effects in recognition and perception. In J. Cole & J. I. Hualde (Eds.) *Laboratory phonology 9*. Mouton de Gruyter: Berlin, pp. 87–112.

Wasserman, S., & Faust, K. (1994). *Social Network Analysis: Methods and Applications*. Cambridge University Press: Cambridge.

Wedel, A. (2006). Exemplar models, evolution and language change. *The Linguistic Review*, 23, 247–274.

Wedel, A. (2007). Feedback and regularity in the lexicon. *Phonology*, 24, 147–185.

Weinreich, U., Labov, W., & Herzog, M. (1968). Empirical foundations for a theory of language change. In W. Lehmann & Y. Malkiel (Ed.) *Directions for Historical Linguistics*, University of Texas Press: Austin, pp. 95–195.

West, P. (2000). Long-distance coarticulatory effects of British English /l/ and /r/: an EMA, EPG, and acoustic study. In *Proceedings of the 5th seminar on speech production: Models and data*. Online dictionary at: www.phonetik.uni-muenchen.de/institut/veranstaltungen/SPS5/abstracts/68_abs.html

Winitz, H., Scheib, M., & Reeds, J. (1972). Identification of stops and vowels for the burst portion of /p, t, k/ isolated from conversational speech. *The Journal of the Acoustical Society of America*, 51, 1309–1317.

Wright, R. (2003). Factors of lexical competition in vowel articulation. In J. Local, R. Ogden, & R. Temple (Eds.) *Papers in Laboratory Phonology VI*. Cambridge University Press: Cambridge, pp. 75–87.

Yu, A. (2007). Understanding near mergers: The case of morphological tone in Cantonese. *Phonology*, 24, 187–214.

Yu, A. (2010). Perceptual compensation is correlated with individuals' "autistic" traits: Implications for models of sound change. *PLoS One*, 5(8), e11950.

Yu, A., Abrego-Collier, C., & Sonderegger, M. (2013). Phonetic imitation from an individual-difference perspective: Subjective attitude, personality, and 'autistic' traits. *PLoS One*, 8(9), e74746.

Zellou, G. (2017). Individual differences in the production of nasal coarticulation and perceptual compensation. *Journal of Phonetics*, 61, 13–29.

Zellou, G., & Tamminga, M. (2014). Nasal coarticulation changes over time in Philadelphia English. *Journal of Phonetics*, 47, 18–35.

Zimmerer, F., Scharinger, M., & Reetz, H. (2014). Phonological and morphological constraints on German /t/-deletions. *Journal of Phonetics*, 45, 64–75.

15

The phonetics of second language learning and bilingualism

Charles B. Chang

Introduction

How are speech sounds and patterns mastered in a second language (L2), especially when the L2 is learned later in life? This question is at the heart of research in L2 speech learning, an interdisciplinary field at the nexus of phonetics, phonology, cognitive psychology, L2 acquisition, and applied linguistics. The broad goal of L2 speech research is to understand the mechanisms and processes underlying L2 speech development, with a view toward applications in language learning and language pedagogy. This chapter provides an overview of the major theories and findings in the field of L2 speech learning. For reasons of space, the discussion focuses primarily on four main conceptual frameworks, among the most detailed and widely tested in the field: the Perceptual Assimilation Model – L2, the Native Language Magnet Theory, the Automatic Selective Perception Model, and the Speech Learning Model. These frameworks differ in terms of empirical focus, including the type of learner (e.g., beginner vs. advanced) and target modality (e.g., perception vs. production), and in terms of theoretical assumptions, such as the basic unit or window of analysis that is relevant (e.g., articulatory gestures, position-specific allophones).

To evaluate the predictive differences among these theories, this chapter discusses a number of empirical studies that have investigated L2 speech primarily at a segmental level. However, it should be pointed out that research on L2 speech learning addresses many different aspects of speech, including overall accent (e.g., Yeni-Komshian, Flege, and Liu, 2000), segment sequences (i.e., phonotactics; Dupoux, Hirose, Kakehi, Pallier, and Mehler, 1999; Altenberg, 2005a; Davidson, 2006; Hallé and Best, 2007), and higher-level prosodic structure (e.g., word boundaries and cross-word sandhi phenomena; Altenberg, 2005b; Zsiga, 2011; Schwartz, 2016). Further, because other recent publications in L2 phonetics and phonology already provide extensive reviews of empirical findings in this area (e.g., Eckman, 2012; Broselow and Kang, 2013; Colantoni, Steele, and Escudero, 2015; Simonet, 2016; Davidson, 2017; Bohn, 2017), the current contribution is oriented instead toward presenting a synthesis of theoretical approaches to the study of L2 speech. Thus, although several empirical studies are covered in a fair amount of detail, we will concentrate primarily on exploring the points of convergence and divergence, as well as the complementarities, among theories of L2 speech.

Despite the ways in which theories of L2 speech differ from one another, three recurring themes emerge from the L2 speech literature. First, the learning of a target L2 structure (segment, feature, phonotactic constraint, prosodic pattern, etc.) is influenced by phonetic and/or phonological similarity to structures in the native language (L1). In particular, L1-L2 similarity exists at multiple levels and does not necessarily benefit L2 outcomes. Second, the role played by certain factors, such as acoustic-phonetic similarity between close L1 and L2 sounds, changes over the course of learning, such that advanced learners may differ from novice learners with respect to the effect of a given variable on observed L2 behavior. Third, the connection between L2 perception and production (insofar as the two are hypothesized to be linked) differs significantly from the perception-production links observed in L1 acquisition. Each of these themes is addressed in more detail in the rest of the chapter.

As an interdisciplinary area of inquiry, L2 speech research is intrinsically linked not only to experimental advances in phonetics and laboratory phonology, but also to theoretical views of the process and outcomes of L2 acquisition. Crucially, the view of L2 acquisition adopted in this chapter is one that identifies the start of L2 acquisition with the onset of bilingualism. That is, the chapter considers L2 learners both as acquirers of a new language and as individuals with two languages, for two reasons. First, many individuals exposed to an L2 will eventually become proficient bilinguals, and there is no clear dividing line between "L2 learner" and "bilingual." Second, given that the majority of the world can be described as bilingual or multilingual (Tucker, 2001), bilingualism, rather than monolingualism, may be the most appropriate point of departure for considering interlanguage phenomena in L2 learning. As such, this chapter situates the study of L2 speech within the long tradition of bilingualism research on bidirectional cross-linguistic interactions. Under this view, it benefits L2 speech research to consider not only L2 outcomes, but also the manner in which learners' developing L2 knowledge may influence their knowledge and use of the L1 (e.g., Cook, 2003). Thus, it should be noted that, although not covered here in detail, the burgeoning literature on L1 phonetic and phonological change in L2 learners (for reviews, see Celata, in press; Chang, in press; de Leeuw, in press) is relevant to the study of L2 speech because it can provide unique insights into learners' observed trajectory of L2 development.

In the rest of this chapter, we review the principles of the four selected conceptual frameworks for the study of L2 speech and discuss two topics that remain areas of active research in L2 phonetic learning and bilingualism: (a) the role of the L1 – in particular, the type and degree of similarity between the L1 and L2 – in L2 phonetic development, and (b) links between L2 perception and L2 production.

Theoretical frameworks

The theoretical review first examines frameworks focusing on L2 perception, and then proceeds to the main framework addressing L2 production. We begin with arguably the most widely tested theory of nonnative and L2 speech perception, the Perceptual Assimilation Model – L2.

The Perceptual Assimilation Model – L2

One of the most influential theories of L2 speech perception, the Perceptual Assimilation Model – L2 (PAM-L2) was proposed by Best and Tyler (2007), expanding upon an earlier theory of nonnative speech perception focused on naive listeners, the Perceptual

Table 15.1 Types of perceptual (non)assimilation posited in PAM-L2. TC: Two Category, CG: Category Goodness, SC: Single Category, UC: Uncategorized-Categorized, UU: Uncategorized-Uncategorized, NA: Non-Assimilable. Accuracy scale: 1 = poor, 2 = fair, 3 = good, 4 = excellent.

	TC	*CG*	*SC*	*UC*	*UU*	*NA*
L2 sounds perceived as speech?	yes	yes	yes	yes	yes	no
L2 sounds both assimilated to L1?	yes	yes	yes	no	no	no
Difference in goodness-of-fit to L1?	no	yes	no	yes	–	–
Discrimination accuracy (1–4 scale)	4	2–3	1	4	1–2	3–4

Assimilation Model (PAM; Best, 1994). PAM-L2 expands upon PAM by incorporating a role for the additional knowledge that L2 learners, but not naive monolinguals, have about the target language (e.g., phonological knowledge). However, the two models are similar in their assumption of articulatory gestures as the basic phonetic unit (a view following from the direct realist approach to speech perception; for further discussion, see Best, 1995, pp. 172–175), in their focus on perception, and in their account of L2 perceptual patterns in terms of *perceptual assimilations* to L1 sounds.

The core logic of PAM-L2 is that sounds of an L2 are differentially discriminable according to how they are perceptually assimilated to (i.e., interpreted in terms of) L1 sounds. The theory sets out a typology of diverse ways in which two L2 sounds *x* and *y* can be assimilated to L1 sounds, which lead to different degrees of success discriminating *x* and *y* (see Table 15.1). In the case of Two Category (TC) assimilation, *x* and *y* are assimilated to two different L1 sound categories and, given that there is no pressure from the L1 toward perceptual conflation of *x* and *y*, L2 learners are able to discriminate them with a high degree of accuracy. On the other hand, in Single Category (SC) assimilation, *x* and *y* are assimilated to the same L1 sound category, each with a similarly high goodness-of-fit (i.e., *x* and *y* are both phonetically close to the L1 attractor); in this case, there is strong pressure from the L1 toward perceptual conflation of *x* and *y*, and consequently L2 learners discriminate them poorly. Finally, in Category Goodness (CG) assimilation, *x* and *y* are assimilated to the same L1 sound category, but with different degrees of fit (i.e., *x* and *y* are unequally close to the L1 attractor), leading to discrimination performance that is intermediate between the TC and SC cases (ranging from fair to good). For example, for L1 English listeners, the Zulu contrasts between lateral fricatives /ɬ/ and /ɮ/, bilabial stops /b/ and /ɓ/, and velar stops /kʰ/ and /k'/ were predicted, respectively, to undergo TC assimilation (to a voiceless English fricative such as /ʃ/ and a voiced English fricative such as /ʒ/), CG assimilation (both to English /b/, with different degrees of fit), and SC assimilation (both to English /k/, with similar degrees of fit), and indeed English listeners' discrimination of these contrasts was, respectively, good, somewhat less good, and poor (Best, McRoberts, and Goodell, 2001).

In addition to the TC, SC, and CG types of perceptual assimilation, which all involve both members of the L2 sound contrast being assimilated to L1 sounds, it is possible for one or both members of an L2 contrast not to be assimilated to L1 sounds. In Uncategorized-Categorized (UC) assimilation, only one of the L2 sounds is identified with an L1 sound, while the other is perceived as unlike any L1 sound. Because here the L2 contrast reduces to an opposition between L1-like and non-L1-like sounds, L2 learners are able to discriminate the sounds well (e.g., Thai back unrounded vowels /ɯ/ and /ɤ/ for L1 English listeners; Tyler, Best, Faber, and Levitt, 2014). However, in Uncategorized-Uncategorized

(UU) assimilation, neither of the L2 sounds is perceived as similar to an L1 sound. In this case, therefore, there is no possibility of using a framework of "L1-like" vs. "non-L1-like," and discrimination accuracy ranges from poor to intermediate, depending on the degree to which the members of the contrast (partially) resemble the same L1 sound or different L1 sounds.

Finally, it is possible for L2 sounds not only to resist identification with an L1 sound, but also to be perceived as non-linguistic. In the rare Non-Assimilable (NA) case of L2 sounds, the L2 sounds are so divergent from any member of the L1 sound inventory that they are effectively treated as non-speech. In this case, discrimination of the L2 contrast may benefit from a non-speech mode of auditory processing that has not been warped by linguistic categories (see next section, *The Native Language Magnet Theory*). This possibility was elegantly demonstrated in a series of studies on nonnative click perception (Best, McRoberts, and Sithole, 1988; Best, Traill, Carter, Harrison, and Faber, 2003). Contrary to the hypothesis that nonnative clicks would be most easily discriminated by speakers already familiar with clicks from their L1, speakers with L1 clicks tended to do relatively poorly on nonnative click discrimination; by contrast, L1 English speakers who had no experience with clicks performed relatively well. The explanation for this result lies in the fact that click-language speakers are subject, at least some of the time, to SC assimilation due to L1 click categories that serve as perceptual attractors for nonnative clicks. Non-click-language speakers such as L1 English speakers, however, are unencumbered by L1 click categories and, furthermore, have nothing in their L1 inventory that remotely resembles clicks auditorily. Therefore, they are free to discriminate the nonnative click contrasts purely in terms of their acoustic characteristics.

As for the basis of perceptual assimilation of L2 sounds to L1 sounds, PAM-L2 posits that L2-to-L1 mapping may occur due to cross-linguistic similarity at a gestural level as well as at a phonological level. Indeed, for L2 learners (as opposed to non-learners) abstract phonological knowledge of the L2 is likely to play an important role in establishing equivalences between L1 and L2 sounds; we will return to this topic later in the chapter. Broadly speaking, however, the basis for perceptual assimilation can be viewed as proximity between L2 sounds and L1 attractors. In the next section, we introduce a theory which, like PAM-L2, formalizes the role of L1 attractors in speech perception, but with respect to the internal structure of L1 phonological categories and the acoustic perceptual space.

The Native Language Magnet Theory

Developed originally to account for L1 perceptual development in infants, Kuhl's Native Language Magnet (NLM) Theory has been applied to the study of L2 speech as well (Kuhl and Iverson, 1995; Ellis, 2006). In particular, the revised and expanded Native Language Magnet Theory (NLM-e) enumerates a number of basic principles, several of which help account for aspects of L2 perception (Kuhl et al., 2008). First, the L1 learner progresses from perceiving speech in a universal manner (i.e., not specialized for the L1) to perceiving it in an L1-specific manner, a transition that is driven both by the detection of distributional patterns in the ambient L1 input and by the enhanced acoustic properties of infant-directed speech. Second, exposure to the L1 leads to a *neural commitment* to L1 speech patterns, which biases future speech learning (cf. the "selective perception routine" of the Automatic Selective Perception Model, discussed in the next section). Third, L1 phonetic learning is influenced by social interaction. Fourth, L1 acquisition involves forming links between speech perception and speech production (i.e., perception-production links are developed through experience rather than being innate).[1] Fifth, early perceptual abilities for, as well as neural responses to, native and nonnative sound contrasts are predictors of L1 development. In particular, better perceptual abilities (e.g., better discrimination performance) for the L1 predict faster L1 development, whereas better perceptual abilities for nonnative speech predict slower L1 development.

The first and second of the preceding principles relate to two core concepts relevant for the study of L2 speech: *perceptual warping* and the *perceptual magnet*. Perceptual warping refers to the way in which the acoustic perceptual space related to a given type of speech sound (e.g., a multidimensional formant space in the case of vowels) is transformed with the accumulation of linguistic (i.e., L1) experience, while a perceptual magnet is a specific part of that modified perceptual space – namely, the prototype of a contrastive sound category. L1 learners develop such prototypes for speech sounds early in life during their distributional analysis of L1 input, and these prototypes act as attractors for newly perceived speech tokens, leading to the observation of a so-called "perceptual magnet effect" in humans only (Kuhl, 1991). The perceptual magnet effect describes essentially the same type of phenomenon as perceptual assimilation (as in PAM-L2), except that the perceptual magnet effect does not refer to cross-linguistic assimilation per se; rather, the idea is that, once there are phonological categories in place, listeners are biased to perceive incoming speech input in terms of these categories as opposed to objectively, without reference to categories. This effect thus underlies both the "categorical perception" of L1 speech (Liberman, Harris, Hoffman, and Griffith, 1957) as well as the perceptual assimilation of L2 sounds to L1 categories.

Crucially, however, the strength of the perceptual magnet effect differs according to proximity to a category prototype (i.e., the magnet). That is to say, a speech token, regardless of its source language, is more likely to be perceived in terms of an L1 category the closer it is to the category prototype. This pattern relates back to the notion of perceptual warping: with L1 experience and the development of prototypes, the acoustic perceptual space becomes "warped," with the result that a given phonetic distance is perceived as smaller when close to a prototype than when far from a prototype. The reason for this phenomenon is the nature of a prototype's "gravitational pull," which diminishes in strength as one moves further away from the prototype.

Applied to L2 speech perception, the perceptual warping involved in L1 development provides a converging, yet slightly different, account for many of the same findings as PAM-L2, such as the lower discriminability of SC contrasts compared to CG contrasts (recall from previous discussion the Zulu contrasts /kʰ/-/k'/ and /b/-/ɓ/, respectively SC and CG for L1 English listeners). In the case of an SC contrast and a CG contrast whose members are equally far apart phonetically, the SC contrast, by virtue of the fact that both members are by definition very close to the L1 category to which they are assimilated, will necessarily be closer overall to the L1 category prototype than the CG contrast. Therefore, the phonetic distance represented in the SC contrast will be harder to perceive than the (equal) phonetic distance represented in the CG contrast, because the former is more strongly pulled into the L1 category.

In short, the NLM(-e) view of L1 development in terms of prototype formation and perceptual warping formalizes crucial outcomes of L1 experience that have consequences for L2 perception. In the next section, we review a theory of L2 perception which is similar to NLM in terms of formalizing outcomes of L1 experience and additionally draws an explicit link to L2 perception.

The Automatic Selective Perception Model

Like NLM, the Automatic Selective Perception (ASP) Model of L2 speech perception (Strange, 2011) understands L1 biases in L2 perception as the outcome of a process of perceptual specialization for the L1. According to ASP, perceptual specialization involves establishing *selective perception routines* (SPRs) that allow perception to be targeted, automatic, and robust in adverse conditions. Consistent with the NLM view of perceptual specialization for the L1 as a central component of L1 perceptual ability, ASP views the development of L1-appropriate SPRs as critical to becoming a skilled L1 listener. However, these L1 SPRs also lead to L1 interference in perception of an L2, because the L2 will often require learners to attend to different properties of the speech signal than the ones relevant in their L1, and/or to integrate these cues differently.

Crucially, in ASP (consistent with the SLM and theories of L1 phonological development such as the Processing Rich Information from Multidimensional Interactive Representations framework; Werker and Curtin, 2005), the unspecialized (i.e., language-general) processing abilities evident in childhood remain available throughout life (and, therefore, in adulthood as well). However, when the cognitive demands of a language task are high (e.g., in processing a syntactically complex L2 utterance), L2 learners' access to these abilities may be blocked, resulting in a default to automatized L1 SPRs. Thus, the effect of task demands on processing L2 speech is a core consideration of ASP, which distinguishes this theory from NLM.

Another aspect of ASP that distinguishes it from NLM is the explicit link it draws between stage of L2 acquisition and manner of L2 perceptual processing. ASP identifies L2 experience as a factor influencing L2 perception, consistent with studies suggesting that advanced L2 learners tend to perceive the L2 significantly differently from novice L2 learners – namely, in a more "phonologized" manner. This process of phonologization was apparent, for example, in Levy and Strange's (2008) study of experienced and inexperienced L2 listeners of French, both from an L1 English background. These L2 listeners were tested on discrimination of several French vowel contrasts, including front rounded vowels that do not occur in English (/y/, /œ/) and vowels occurring in both bilabial and alveolar contexts. Results showed two systematic disparities between the experienced and inexperienced groups. First, with the exception of /u/-/y/, the experienced listeners outperformed the inexperienced listeners overall on most of the vowel contrasts. Second, there was a significant context effect for inexperienced listeners, but not for experienced listeners: inexperienced listeners performed differently on certain vowel contrasts across coarticulatory contexts (e.g., higher error rate on /u/-/y/ in an alveolar context than in a bilabial context). These findings are consistent with the view that L2 speech learning involves developing distinct representations for new L2 sounds (e.g., /y/ and /œ/ for L1 English speakers) as well as familiarity with rule-governed coarticulatory patterns in the L2, which allows learners to abstract over phonemically non-contrastive coarticulatory variation, such as the vowel fronting effect associated with alveolars.

Findings in studies such as Levy and Strange (2008) converge with the results of many other studies (e.g., Bradlow, Pisoni, Akahane-Yamada, and Tohkura, 1997; Wang, Spence, Jongman, and Sereno, 1999; Aoyama, Flege, Guion, Akahane-Yamada, and Yamada, 2004; Tajima, Kato, Rothwell, Akahane-Yamada, and Munhall, 2008) in suggesting that L2 experience generally helps the L2 learner to become more skilled at perceiving the L2 (though see Holliday, 2016 for an interesting counterexample from L1 Mandarin learners of Korean). This positive correlation between L2 experience and L2 perceptual performance can be attributed to two beneficial, and related, outcomes of L2 speech learning: (a) development of mental representations for the contrastive sounds of the L2, particularly those which do not occur in the L1, and (b) development of SPRs for the L2. Both of these developments allow L2 perception to be more targeted, automatic, and robust, resulting in a significant advantage for experienced L2 listeners compared to naive or inexperienced listeners.

Thus, ASP accounts for L1 biases in L2 perception, as well as for L2 perceptual learning over time, in terms of the same fundamental construct: SPRs, which direct a listener's attention to a proper subset of the numerous acoustic properties that a listener could potentially attend to in the speech signal. ASP differs from PAM-L2 and NLM in focusing more on cue weighting than on cross-linguistic mapping or category prototypes; this focus helps to account for perceptual variation observed among L2 learners with similar L1 phonological constraints (see, e.g., Chang, 2018). However, all three of these theories are similar in that they are theories of L2 perception, not theories of L2 production. Next, we discuss a theory of L2 speech that addresses aspects of both perception and production.

The Speech Learning Model

Unlike the theories discussed above, Flege's (1995, 1996, 2002) Speech Learning Model (SLM) is a theory of both L2 perception and L2 production. Its account of L2 speech consists of six main tenets, the first three being that (a) language learners maintain continuous access to the same basic learning mechanisms over the lifespan (i.e., adult learners are not fundamentally different from child learners in this respect), (b) L1 and L2 sounds exist in a "common phonological space" (Flege, 1995, p. 239), and learners are generally motivated to maintain cross-linguistic contrast between them, and (c) there is a tendency for *equivalence classification* of L2 sounds with close L1 counterparts. This mechanism of equivalence classification is not specific to L2 learning, but rather is used in the L1 to abstract appropriately over phonetic variability in L1 speech. The inappropriate operation of equivalence classification in L2 speech learning, however, may result in problems with perception and/or production of target L2 sounds.

A fourth, and central, claim of the SLM is that L2 sounds are differentially difficult to learn, depending on their phonetic proximity to L1 sounds (see Figure 15.1). In particular, the SLM posits three types of L2 sounds – *identical*, *new*, and *similar* – which form a hierarchy of learning difficulty as follows (from least to most difficult): identical < new < similar. Identical sounds are the least difficult to learn because in all relevant aspects they are exactly the same as their closest L1 sound; therefore, straight transfer of the L1 sound to the L2 will result in high accuracy with the L2 sound immediately. New sounds, by contrast, are more difficult to learn because, although they resist equivalence classification with L1 sounds due to a high degree of disparity along one or more dimensions, this cross-linguistic disparity also requires some novel aspects of the L2 sound to be learned to approximate target-like performance. These novel aspects, however, are hypothesized to be learnable in the long term. On the other hand, similar sounds are the most difficult to learn because they are close enough to L1 sounds to undergo equivalence classification with them, yet far enough from L1 sounds that simple transfer of the L1 sounds is not sufficient for target-like performance. In other words, similar sounds exist in an intermediate space of cross-linguistic similarity (as shown in Figure 15.1), which introduces the possibility of inappropriate influence from properties of close L1 sounds.

The nature of L1 influence for the three types of L2 sounds is captured in the fifth tenet of the SLM: L2 sounds may either approximate (i.e., assimilate properties of) or dissimilate

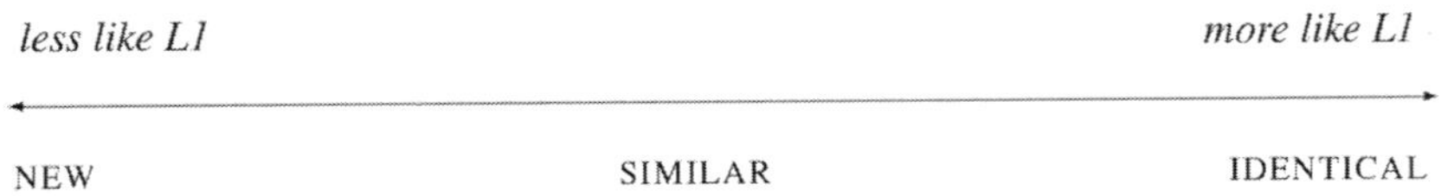

Figure 15.1 Continuum of similarity of L2 sounds to L1 sounds. NEW sounds are the least similar to L1 sounds; IDENTICAL sounds, the most similar; and SIMILAR sounds, intermediate in similarity.

from L1 sounds. In particular, when an L2 sound undergoes equivalence classification with a close L1 sound (as in the case of identical and similar sounds), the L1 and L2 sounds become "diaphones," sounds that are *perceptually linked* in the mind of the L2 learner. In the case of a similar L2 sound, this perceptual linkage (i.e., partial or total co-representation of the L2 sound with the L1 sound) eventually leads to the L1 and L2 sounds approximating each other in production (e.g., Williams, 1979; Major, 1992). On the other hand, when an L2 sound avoids equivalence classification with L1 sounds (as in the case of new sounds), the L2 sound is represented distinctly from L1 sounds. This distinct representation allows the L2 sound to be produced eventually in a target-like manner (e.g., Williams, 1977; Antoniou, Best, Tyler, and Kroos, 2010). Alternatively, however, L2 sounds represented distinctly from the closest L1 categories may dissimilate from them so as to maximize cross-linguistic contrast within the shared L1-L2 phonological space; such dissimilation may also result in L2 sounds diverging from native (monolingual) norms. For example, whereas early L1 Korean-L2 English bilinguals were found to produce native-like voice onset time (VOT) in their L2 voiceless stops (Kang and Guion, 2006), an early L1 French-L2 English bilingual produced L2 VOTs that were longer than native (i.e., past the English monolingual norm), in an apparent attempt to differentiate the L2 stops from the L1 stops (Mack, 1990).

Although assimilation and dissimilation result in opposite directions of movement relative to an L1 sound, crucially they may affect sounds of both the L1 and the L2, in line with the sixth tenet of the SLM: cross-linguistic influence (CLI) is, in principle, bidirectional. Thus, CLI is not limited to L1 sounds influencing L2 sounds (i.e., "forward transfer"), but may also result in L2 sounds influencing L1 sounds (i.e., "backward transfer"). Bidirectionality of CLI at the phonetic level was shown in a seminal study of English-French bilinguals, L1 English late learners of French and L1 French late learners of English (Flege, 1987). This study focused on two acoustic properties of learners' speech in both the L1 and the L2: the VOT of /t/ (canonically short-lag in French, but long-lag in English) and the second formant (F_2) frequency of /u/ (canonically low in French, but high in English) as well as /y/, a vowel phoneme that occurs only in French. Results provided evidence for bidirectional CLI. On the one hand, many (but not all) L1 English learners of French produced French /t/ with too-long VOTs (i.e., as English-influenced) and English /t/ with too-short VOTs (i.e., as French-influenced); a similar pattern was found with the VOTs of L1 French learners of English. As for F_2, both L1 English learners of French and L1 French learners of English produced French /u/ with too-high F_2 values (i.e., as English-influenced), although only the L1 French learners of English also produced English /u/ with too-low F_2 values. Notably, the L1 English learners additionally managed to produce the French /y/ with native-like F_2 values. Thus, overall, the pattern of results in this study was consistent with the SLM in two main respects: (a) showing a disparity between "similar" sounds (e.g., English and French /t/), which evince CLI due to equivalence classification, and "new" sounds (e.g., French /y/ for L1 English learners), which avoid CLI, and (b) showing bidirectional CLI.

Two aspects of the SLM that distinguish it from other influential theoretical frameworks for L2 speech research are its explicit application to production (as opposed to a focus on perception) and its prediction of bidirectional CLI (as opposed to unidirectional CLI, specifically L1 influence on the L2). These aspects of the framework make it especially appropriate for studies of L2 production (as in Flege, 1987) and studies of L1 change in L2 learners, both in production (e.g., Major, 1992, 1996; Chang, 2011, 2012b, 2013; de Leeuw, Schmid, and Mennen, 2010; Dmitrieva, Jongman, and Sereno, 2010) and perception (e.g., Tice and Woodley, 2012; Ahn, Chang, DeKeyser, and Lee-Ellis, 2017).

Summary and synthesis

In short, while the theories discussed at the beginning of this chapter often make convergent predictions in regard to L2 phonetic development, they differ in a number of ways. The primary dimensions of difference among these theoretical frameworks are summarized in Table 15.2, including the L2 experience or proficiency level of the learner described by the theory, the basic unit of analysis, the L2 domain(s) covered, and the foundation of the theory's explanation of CLI in either direction (L1-to-L2, L2-to-L1).

As discussed above, CLI at the phonetic level has been of special concern in the study of L2 speech and bilingualism, spawning a wealth of findings on L1-L2 phonetic interaction in L2 learners of various backgrounds (for further reviews, see Mack, 2003 and Kartushina, Frauenfelder, and Golestani, 2016). Apart from showing L1 influence in their L2 production (e.g., Port and Mitleb, 1983; Gass, 1984), learners may produce neither the L1 nor the L2 as native-like (Flege and Eefting, 1987b); they may also show little to no phonetic differentiation between the two languages (e.g., Williams, 1979; Major, 1992), leading to "compromise" values between L1 and L2 norms (e.g., Flege, 1987). On the other hand, learners' production of the L2, as well as of the L1, may also be native-like (e.g., Fokes, Bond, and Steinberg, 1985; Mack, 1989), and especially for early bilinguals, close approximation of monolingual norms for both languages is clearly possible (e.g., Caramazza, Yeni-Komshian, Zurif, and Carbone, 1973; Williams, 1977; Flege and Eefting, 1987a; Kang and Guion, 2006; Antoniou et al., 2010). All of the theories discussed in this chapter address CLI in the

Table 15.2 Comparison of selected frameworks for L2 speech research. PAM-L2: Perceptual Assimilation Model-L2, SLM: Speech Learning Model, NLM: Native Language Magnet Theory, ASP: Automatic Selective Perception Model. CLI: cross-linguistic influence. NA: not applicable.

	PAM-L2	*NLM*	*ASP*	*SLM*
Learner level	novice to advanced	advanced	novice to advanced	advanced
Basic unit	articulatory gesture	phonological category	auditory cue	position-specific allophone
About perception?	yes	yes	yes	yes
About production?	no	no	no	yes
Account of L1 → L2 CLI?	perceptual assimilation	perceptual warping	perceptual attunement	L1-L2 diaphones
Account of L1 ← L2 CLI?	NA	NA	NA	L1-L2 diaphones

L1-to-L2 direction, but not necessarily in the L2-to-L1 direction. In this regard, the SLM is unique in providing an account of bidirectional CLI.

To close this section, it is worth noting that the diversity of L1 and L2 outcomes in L2 learners has been approached analytically in additional ways, including systems typology and computational modeling. In regard to typology, Laeufer (1996) presents an attempt to schematize the different possible bilingual phonological systems, which each lead to a specific pattern of L1 and L2 speech production. Combining aspects of the bilingual lexical/conceptual model of Weinreich (1953) with the tripartite speech production model of Keating (1984), Laeufer distinguishes among three types of bilingual phonological system (coexistent, merged, and super-subordinate) in terms of the conflation of the L1 and L2 at various levels of representation (for further discussion, see Chang, 2010a, pp. 49–54). In regard to modeling, Tobin, Nam and Fowler (2017) provide an example of a formal computational account of shifts in bilingual speech through variation in the ambient language environment. This computational account assumes a dynamical systems framework, increasingly common in research on language development and change (see, e.g., de Bot, Lowie, and Verspoor, 2007; de Leeuw, Mennen, and Scobbie, 2013), and is also consistent with exemplar approaches to phonology and L2 acquisition incorporating a role for episodic memory (Johnson, 1997; Pierrehumbert, 2001; Hazan, 2007).

The role of L1-L2 similarity

Although the theories of L2 speech discussed in this chapter differ in a number of ways, what they have in common is the acknowledgment and incorporation of a role for the L1 in L2 development. Whether described as perceptual assimilation to the L1, equivalence classification with the L1, or simply transfer of an L1 category space or L1 selective perception routines, aspects of the L1 are taken to exert a powerful influence on L2 speech. The SLM and PAM-L2 in particular are based on cross-linguistic mapping of L2 sounds to L1 sounds, which raises the question of how L2 learners identify the L1 correspondents of L2 sounds. In other words, assuming that the main criterion for establishing L1-L2 correspondence is linguistic similarity, how do L2 learners make judgments of similarity between L1 and L2 sounds?

At the heart of this question is a crucial feature of L2 learners that distinguishes them from naive listeners: abstract knowledge of the target language. As acknowledged in PAM-L2, unlike naive listeners (who, by definition, are not familiar with the L2), L2 learners may have a considerable amount of higher-level knowledge of the L2, including knowledge of the phonemic inventory, phonotactic constraints, allophonic alternations, and/or the orthographic system used to visually represent the sounds of the language (cf. Polka, 1991, 1992; Best and Tyler, 2007; Boomershine, Hall, Hume, and Johnson, 2008; Davidson, 2011). Consequently, there are several sources of information about L2 sounds that L2 learners may take into account in forming a judgment of L1-L2 similarity that go beyond the raw phonetic data available to both L2 learners and naive listeners (which is generally taken to be gestural in PAM-L2 and acoustic in the SLM).

For L2 learners, the availability of multiple sources of information about L2 sounds introduces the possibility of conflict between those sources (Chang, 2015). To take one example pointed out by Chang, Yao, Haynes, and Rhodes (2011), which parallels the situation in Flege (1987), high rounded vowels in Mandarin Chinese (i.e., /y/ and /u/) resemble American English vowels at two levels: (a) an acoustic level (e.g., F_2 frequency, formant trajectories), and (b) a phonemic level (e.g., being a high back rounded vowel, /u/). In terms of acoustic proximity in $F_1 \times F_2$ space, Mandarin /y/ is closer to English /u/ than is Mandarin /u/, due to the fact that (American) English /u/ tends to be relatively front and, in certain dialects such as Southern Californian English, phonetically unrounded as well (Hagiwara, 1997; Ladefoged, 1999).[2] However, in terms of phonemic correspondence, Mandarin /u/ is the closer match to English /u/, because Mandarin /u/ (and not /y/) is a high back rounded vowel like English /u/; this is reflected, for example, in similar phonotactic patterning in the two languages (e.g., nonoccurrence of onset C/wu/).

Thus, in the case of L1 English learners of Mandarin, production of the L2 Mandarin vowels /y/ and /u/ could be influenced by the properties of English /u/ in at least two different ways, depending on whether acoustic or phonemic considerations take precedence in cross-linguistic mapping. First, Mandarin /y/ could be mapped to English /u/, with Mandarin /u/ avoiding equivalence classification with an English vowel; this would lead to too-low F_2 values for Mandarin /y/ (as English /u/ is characterized by a lower F_2 than Mandarin /y/) and target-like production of Mandarin /u/ (a "new" sound in SLM terms). Alternatively, Mandarin /u/ could be mapped to English /u/, with Mandarin /y/ avoiding equivalence classification with an English vowel; this would lead to too-high F_2 values for Mandarin /u/ (as English /u/ is characterized by a higher F_2 than Mandarin /u/) and a target-like production of Mandarin /y/. What Chang et al. (2011) found was the latter: relatively experienced L1 English learners of Mandarin produced Mandarin /u/ with F_2 values that were higher than those of L1 Mandarin speakers, but Mandarin /y/ with F_2 values not significantly different from those of L1 Mandarin speakers, replicating the pattern reported in Flege (1987) for advanced L1 English learners of French.

Together with a range of other results from L2 perception (Polka and Bohn, 1996; Strange, Levy, and Lehnholf, 2004), loanword adaptation (Kang, 2008; Chang, 2009, 2012a), and phonetic drift (Chang, 2012b, 2013), findings such as in Flege (1987) and Chang et al. (2011) contribute to a picture in which cross-linguistic mapping (i.e., relating an L2 sound to an L1 sound) often follows the phonemic route over the acoustic route. To take one other example from loanword adaptation, high lax vowels in English loanwords are adapted by French-English bilinguals not with the acoustically closest mid vowels of French, but with the phonemically parallel (and acoustically more distant) high vowels of French (LaCharité and Paradis, 2005). The fact that this happens with both of the English vowels at issue (/ɪ/ and /ʊ/), not just with one or the other, suggests that cross-linguistic mapping on a phonemic basis is systematic rather than idiosyncratic. Thus, at least for advanced L2 learners, there may be a privileged status of abstract (higher-level) information about L1 and L2 sounds in making judgments of cross-linguistic similarity. However, the specific dynamics of interaction between phonetic and phonological types of cross-linguistic similarity, the manner in which these dynamics may change over the course of L2 learning, and the influence of a changing construct of perceived (dis)similarity in shaping L2 outcomes (cf. Aoyama et al., 2004) remain open questions.

Linking L2 perception and L2 production

Although theories of L2 speech such as the SLM are often concerned with fundamental similarities between child and adult learners, there are some important differences between L1 learning and L2 learning of a target language, and one area in which such differences are observed is the link between perception and production. According to NLM-e, perception and production are closely linked in L1 acquisition, and these links are understood to form during L1 acquisition, due in part to the articulatory-auditory loop associated with an infant hearing the consequences of her own vocalizations. Further, the timing of perception and production milestones in L1 development, which typically shows children reliably perceiving speech sounds well before they can produce them, suggests that perception generally precedes production when it comes to the L1 (although, given the aforementioned role of production in perceptual development, this should be regarded as a gross view of perception-production ordering in L1 development).

In L2 speech learning, the relationship between perception and production is less clear than in L1 development. One body of findings that bears on this issue comes from research on phonetic training – in particular, transfer of training gains from the trained modality to the untrained modality. In brief, although some studies report perception-production correlations and/or carryover of training gains across modalities (e.g., Catford and Pisoni, 1970; Leather, 1996; Wang, Jongman, and Sereno, 2003; Kartushina, Hervais-Adelman, Frauenfelder, and Golestani, 2015), much of this literature evinces little to no relationship between perception and production for L2 speech. For example, Kartushina and Frauenfelder (2014) tested a sample of L1 Spanish learners of French on their perception and production of French front mid vowel contrasts and found no correlation between learners' performance in perception and production (see also Peperkamp and Bouchon, 2011). Of course, failure to find a statistically significant correlation between the two modalities does not constitute evidence that there is no relationship between them; however, when correlations have been found across modalities, the effect size has often been small (Bradlow et al., 1997; Akahane-Yamada, McDermott, Adachi, Kawahara, and Pruitt, 1998; Flege, MacKay, and Meador, 1999). Furthermore, L2 production accuracy does not seem to depend on high L2 perceptual ability (Sheldon and Strange, 1982). These findings suggest that transfer of perceptual learning to production, and vice versa, may be complicated by a variety of intervening factors (for recent reviews, see Kartushina, 2015; Kartushina et al., 2015).

The complex relationship between L2 developments in perception and production invites the question of whether L2 outcomes might generally benefit from training involving more than one modality (see Chapter 19, this volume, discussing multichannel training of the L2). If L2 training in one modality tends to improve mainly the trained modality and not necessarily the untrained modality, could L2 speech development be enhanced or accelerated with multimodal training involving more than one stimulus channel (e.g., auditory and articulatory, auditory and visual)? The logic of "more is better" would predict yes, and some findings show a significant benefit of visual feedback on learners' production combined with auditory exposure to a native model (e.g., Kartushina, 2015). However, two recent studies suggest that multimodal L2 engagement does not necessarily improve L2 outcomes, and in certain cases can actually be detrimental to L2 speech development. In one study of L1 English speakers being trained on Mandarin tones (Godfroid, Lin, and Ryu, 2017), several types of multimodal perceptual training were systematically compared to each other, including three "single-cue" types of training (involving exposure to only one visual cue alongside auditory stimuli: number, pitch contour, or color) and two "dual-cue" types of training (involving exposure to two visual cues: color and number, or color and pitch contour). Although test results showed perceptual gains with all training types, single-cue exposure to numbers or pitch contours was more beneficial than single-cue exposure to colors, while neither dual-cue exposure was more beneficial than single-cue exposure. In another study of L1 Spanish learners of Basque (Baese-Berk and Samuel, 2016), both inexperienced and experienced learners were trained on L2 Basque sounds in two conditions: (a) perception only and (b) perception and production (where an oral repetition task was interleaved with auditory exposure and perceptual judgments). Results showed a detrimental effect of producing speech during the perceptual training, which was mitigated (but not eliminated) by previous experience with the L2 (see also Leach and Samuel, 2007; Baese-Berk, 2010, for similar findings).

Why would multimodal L2 exposure not necessarily facilitate L2 learning outcomes? There are at least three possible, and not mutually exclusive, explanations. Baese-Berk and Samuel (2016) allude to the role of cognitive (over)load in this type of multimodal setting (see, e.g., van Merriënboer and Sweller, 2005), while Godfroid et al. (2017) additionally consider the potentially detrimental effect of extraneous processing of redundant or irrelevant information. Either or both of these factors may be responsible for the observed interference associated with varying task-irrelevant phonetic features in L2 speech training (Antoniou and Wong, 2016). Godfroid et al. (2017), however, are careful to point out that performance in their dual-cue condition was never *worse* than in the single-cue condition, which is not entirely consistent with an account of their results in terms of cognitive load or extraneous processing. Consequently, they explain the lack of benefit associated with adding a second cue in terms of an implementation issue: given the way in which color was incorporated into the stimuli, participants may have perceptually backgrounded the color cue, such that "color might have played a more peripheral role than intended" (Godfroid et al., 2017, p. 846).

Thus, the findings of L2 speech research present a mixed picture regarding the relationship of perception and production in L2 development. On the one hand, studies such as Bradlow et al. (1997) and Baese-Berk and Samuel (2016), which show facilitation or interference across modalities, provide evidence that perception and production processes must draw on mental representations that are at least partly shared between the two modalities. On the other hand, studies such as Kartushina and Frauenfelder (2014), which fail to find a close correlation between perception and production performance in an L2, suggest some degree of dissociation between perception and production representations as well. The degree to which L2 perception and L2 production processes overlap, the nature of this overlap, and the manner in which the perception-production relationship differs between L1 and L2 learning remain some of the basic questions in research on L2 speech learning and phonetic development more generally.

Concluding remarks

This chapter has attempted to synthesize core insights and claims of influential theories in the field of L2 speech learning. The four selected frameworks discussed here (PAM-L2, NLM, ASP, SLM) are some of the most detailed and widely tested theories in the field. However, it should be noted that other frameworks, such as Eckman's Markedness Differential Hypothesis and Structural Conformity Hypothesis (Eckman, 1977, 1991, 2008), Brown's featural model of L2 perception (Brown, 2000), the Ontogeny Phylogeny Model (Major, 2001), the Second Language Linguistic Perception Model (Escudero, 2009; van Leussen and Escudero, 2015), and additional Optimality Theoretic approaches (cf. Hancin-Bhatt, 2008), also address aspects of L2 speech learning with different emphases, such as the role of language-universal factors (Markedness Differential Hypothesis) and developmental changes over the course of learning (Ontogeny Phylogeny Model). Furthermore, the burgeoning field of L2 prosody has led to new developments and theories focusing on suprasegmental features of the L2, such as rhythm and intonation (e.g., Li and Post, 2014; Mennen and de Leeuw, 2014; Mennen, 2015).

In closing, although the focus of this chapter has been phonetic development in typical late-onset L2 learners, it is worth drawing the reader's attention to some related areas of research activity that, for reasons of space, have not been given extensive discussion here. First, CLI is being understood in new ways, not just in terms of "negative" or "positive" transfer from the L1 (Lado, 1957; Goto, 1971; Odlin, 1989; Cutler, 2001) but also in terms of native-language transfer benefits for L2 learning (Bohn and Best, 2012; Chang and Mishler, 2012; Chang, 2016). Moreover, the variables of age and profile of acquisition have long spurred, and continue to spur, research on differences between early and late L2 learners (Yeni-Komshian et al., 2000; Guion, 2003; Kang and Guion, 2006; Oh et al., 2011) and between typical L2 learners and heritage speakers or L1 (re)learners (Knightly, Jun, Oh, and Au, 2003; Chang, 2011; Chang and Yao, 2016). Additional work has been examining the effect of other properties of the individual learner, such as language aptitude and basic perceptual ability, in order to better understand the wide range in L2 outcomes observed across learners of the same L1 background (e.g., Chang, 2010b; Perrachione, Lee, Ha, and Wong, 2011; Bowles, Chang, and Karuzis, 2016). Input and linguistic factors such as talker variability and phonological context are also being investigated as contributors to variation in L2 outcomes (e.g., Bradlow et al., 1997; Kingston, 2003; Perrachione et al., 2011; Chang and Bowles, 2015).

In light of transnational migration and multilingualism across the world, these and other lines of inquiry are poised to shape practices and policy affecting the linguistic lives of many people. For example, research examining the linguistic knowledge of heritage speakers in relation to late L2 learners is helping to inform language course design so as to better serve the unique needs of heritage language learners. Studies of third language (L3) learners are investigating what factors influence speech learning in multilingual situations (Gallardo del Puerto, 2007), how L3 learning resembles and differs from L2 learning (Onishi, 2013; Wrembel, 2014), and how L3 learning may influence the phonological representations and processes associated with previously learned languages (Cabrelli Amaro, 2017), in line with the multicompetence view of language development over the lifespan (Cook, 1991, 1992, 2003). Finally, it would be remiss not to mention the work of scholars who are connecting L2 speech research to L2 instructional practices and strategies (see, e.g., Mora and Levkina, 2017). Far from declining, research in L2 speech learning is thriving. We can look forward to many new discoveries in the years to come, with practically relevant implications we cannot yet imagine.

Notes

1 This contrasts with the direct realist view of PAM(-L2), which assumes that perception-production links do not have to be learned. Under this view, both perception and production are based in articulatory gestures, so "no translation is needed between perception and production because they are informationally compatible" (Best, 1994, p. 180).

2 Thanks to Geoffrey Schwartz for pointing out that different outcomes for acoustic proximity could result from examining alternative metrics of vowel quality (e.g., distances between adjacent formants such as F_2 and F_3; cf. Syrdal and Gopal, 1986, on the role of formant convergences in vowel perception). In the case of measuring vowel frontness/backness in terms of F_3–F_2 (rather than F_2), this metric, when applied to the production data from the speakers in Chang et al. (2011), is consistent with the view that native English /u/ (M_{F3-F2} = 3.617 Bark) is phonetically closer to native Mandarin /y/ (M_{F3-F2} = 1.367 Bark) than to native Mandarin /u/ (M_{F3-F2} = 8.588 Bark).

References

Ahn, S., Chang, C. B., DeKeyser, R., and Lee-Ellis, S. (2017). Age effects in first language attrition: Speech perception by Korean-English bilinguals. *Language Learning*, *67*(3), 694–733.

Akahane-Yamada, R., McDermott, E., Adachi, T., Kawahara, H., and Pruitt, J. S. (1998). Computer-based second language production training by using spectrographic representation and HMM-based speech recognition scores. In *Proceedings of the 5th International Conference on Spoken Language Processing (ICSLP-1998)* (paper 0429). Sydney, Australia: International Speech Communication Association.

Altenberg, E. P. (2005a). The judgment, perception, and production of consonant clusters in a second language. *International Review of Applied Linguistics in Language Teaching*, *43*(1), 53–80.

Altenberg, E. P. (2005b). The perception of word boundaries in a second language. *Second Language Research*, *21*(4), 325–358.

Antoniou, M., Best, C. T., Tyler, M. D., and Kroos, C. (2010). Language context elicits native-like stop voicing in early bilinguals' productions in both L1 and L2. *Journal of Phonetics*, *38*(4), 640–653.

Antoniou, M., and Wong, P. C. M. (2016). Varying irrelevant phonetic features hinders learning of the feature being trained. *The Journal of the Acoustical Society of America*, *139*(1), 271–278.

Aoyama, K., Flege, J. E., Guion, S. G., Akahane-Yamada, R., and Yamada, T. (2004). Perceived phonetic dissimilarity and L2 speech learning: The case of Japanese /r/ and English /l/ and /r/. *Journal of Phonetics*, *32*(2), 233–250.

Baese-Berk, M. M. (2010). *The relationship between perception and production when learning novel phonological categories*. Ph.D. thesis, Northwestern University.

Baese-Berk, M. M., and Samuel, A. G. (2016). Listeners beware: Speech production may be bad for learning speech sounds. *Journal of Memory and Language*, *89*, 23–36.

Best, C. T. (1994). The emergence of native-language phonological influences in infants: A perceptual assimilation model. In J. C. Goodman and H. C. Nusbaum (Eds.), *The development of speech perception: The transition from speech sounds to spoken words* (pp. 167–224). Cambridge, MA: MIT Press.

Best, C. T. (1995). A direct realist view of cross-language speech perception. In W. Strange (Ed.), *Speech perception and linguistic experience: Issues in cross-language research* (pp. 171–204). Baltimore, MD: York Press.

Best, C. T., McRoberts, G. W., and Goodell, E. (2001). Discrimination of non-native consonant contrasts varying in perceptual assimilation to the listener's native phonological system. *The Journal of the Acoustical Society of America*, *109*(2), 775–794.

Best, C. T., McRoberts, G. W., and Sithole, N. M. (1988). Examination of perceptual reorganization for nonnative speech contrasts: Zulu click discrimination by English-speaking adults and infants. *Journal of Experimental Psychology: Human Perception and Performance*, *14*(3), 345–360.

Best, C. T., Traill, A., Carter, A., Harrison, K. D., and Faber, A. (2003). !Xóõ click perception by English, Isizulu, and Sesotho listeners. In M. J. Solé, D. Recasens, and J. Romero (Eds.), *Proceedings of the 15th international congress of phonetic sciences* (pp. 853–856). Barcelona, Spain: Causal Productions.

Best, C. T., and Tyler, M. D. (2007). Nonnative and second-language speech perception: Commonalities and complementarities. In O. S. Bohn and M. J. Munro (Eds.), *Language experience in second language speech learning: In honor of James Emil Flege* (pp. 13–34). Amsterdam, The Netherlands: John Benjamins Publishing.

Bohn, O. S. (2017). Cross-language and second language speech perception. In E. M. Fernández and H. S. Cairns (Eds.), *The handbook of psycholinguistics* (pp. 213–239). Hoboken, NJ: John Wiley & Sons.

Bohn, O. S., and Best, C. T. (2012). Native-language phonetic and phonological influences on perception of American English approximants by Danish and German listeners. *Journal of Phonetics*, *40*(1), 109–128.

Boomershine, A., Hall, K. C., Hume, E., and Johnson, K. (2008). The impact of allophony versus contrast on speech perception. In P. Avery, E. Dresher, and K. Rice (Eds.), *Contrast in phonology* (pp. 143–172). Berlin, Germany: Mouton de Gruyter.
Bowles, A. R., Chang, C. B., and Karuzis, V. P. (2016). Pitch ability as an aptitude for tone learning. *Language Learning*, *66*(4), 774–808.
Bradlow, A. R., Pisoni, D. B., Akahane-Yamada, R., and Tohkura, Y. (1997). Training Japanese listeners to identify English /r/ and /l/, IV: Some effects of perceptual learning on speech production. *The Journal of the Acoustical Society of America*, *101*(4), 2299–2310.
Broselow, E., and Kang, Y. (2013). Phonology and speech. In J. Herschensohn and M. Young-Scholten (Eds.), *The Cambridge handbook of second language acquisition* (pp. 529–554). Cambridge: Cambridge University Press.
Brown, C. (2000). The interrelation between speech perception and phonological acquisition from infant to adult. In J. Archibald (Ed.), *Second language acquisition and linguistic theory* (pp. 4–63). Malden, MA: Blackwell Publishers.
Cabrelli Amaro, J. (2017). Testing the phonological permeability hypothesis: L3 phonological effects on L1 versus L2 systems. *International Journal of Bilingualism*, *21*(6), 698–717.
Caramazza, A., Yeni-Komshian, G. H., Zurif, E. B., and Carbone, E. (1973). The acquisition of a new phonological contrast: The case of stop consonants in French-English bilinguals. *The Journal of the Acoustical Society of America*, *54*(2), 421–428.
Catford, J. C., and Pisoni, D. B. (1970). Auditory vs. Articulatory training in exotic sounds. *The Modern Language Journal*, *54*(7), 477–481.
Celata, C. (in press). Phonological L1 attrition. In M. S. Schmid and B. Köpke (Eds.), *The Oxford handbook of language attrition*. Oxford: Oxford University Press.
Chang, C. B. (2009). English loanword adaptation in Burmese. *Journal of the Southeast Asian Linguistics Society*, *1*, 77–94.
Chang, C. B. (2010a). *First language phonetic drift during second language acquisition*. Ph.D. thesis, University of California, Berkeley, CA.
Chang, C. B. (2010b). The implementation of laryngeal contrast in Korean as a second language. *Harvard Studies in Korean Linguistics*, *13*, 91–104.
Chang, C. B. (2011). Systemic drift of L1 vowels in novice L2 learners. In W. S. Lee and E. Zee (Eds.), *Proceedings of the 17th international congress of phonetic sciences* (pp. 428–431). Hong Kong, China: City University of Hong Kong.
Chang, C. B. (2012a). Phonetics vs. Phonology in loanword adaptation: Revisiting the role of the bilingual. In S. Berson, A. Bratkievich, D. Bruhn, A. Campbell, R. Escamilla, A. Giovine, L. Newbold, M. Perez, M. Piqueras-Brunet, and R. Rhomieux (Eds.), *Proceedings of the 34th annual meeting of the Berkeley Linguistics Society: General session and parasession on information structure* (pp. 61–72). Berkeley, CA: Berkeley Linguistics Society.
Chang, C. B. (2012b). Rapid and multifaceted effects of second-language learning on first-language speech production. *Journal of Phonetics*, *40*(2), 249–268.
Chang, C. B. (2013). A novelty effect in phonetic drift of the native language. *Journal of Phonetics*, *41*(6), 491–504.
Chang, C. B. (2015). Determining cross-linguistic phonological similarity between segments: The primacy of abstract aspects of similarity. In E. Raimy and C. E. Cairns (Eds.), *The segment in phonetics and phonology* (pp. 199–217). Chichester: John Wiley & Sons.
Chang, C. B. (2016). Bilingual perceptual benefits of experience with a heritage language. *Bilingualism: Language and Cognition*, *19*(4), 791–809.
Chang, C. B. (2018). Perceptual attention as the locus of transfer to nonnative speech perception. *Journal of Phonetics*, *68*, 85–102.
Chang, C. B. (in press). Phonetic drift. In M. S. Schmid and B. Köpke (Eds.), *The Oxford handbook of language attrition*. Oxford: Oxford University Press.
Chang, C. B., and Bowles, A. R. (2015). Context effects on second-language learning of tonal contrasts. *The Journal of the Acoustical Society of America*, *138*(6), 3703–3716.

Chang, C. B., and Mishler, A. (2012). Evidence for language transfer leading to a perceptual advantage for non-native listeners. *The Journal of the Acoustical Society of America*, *132*(4), 2700–2710.

Chang, C. B., and Yao, Y. (2016). Toward an understanding of heritage prosody: Acoustic and perceptual properties of tone produced by heritage, native, and second language speakers of Mandarin. *Heritage Language Journal*, *13*(2), 134–160.

Chang, C. B., Yao, Y., Haynes, E. F., and Rhodes, R. (2011). Production of phonetic and phonological contrast by heritage speakers of Mandarin. *The Journal of the Acoustical Society of America*, *129*(6), 3964–3980.

Colantoni, L., Steele, J., and Escudero, P. (2015). *Second language speech: Theory and practice*. Cambridge: Cambridge University Press.

Cook, V. J. (1991). The poverty-of-the-stimulus argument and multicompetence. *Second Language Research*, *7*(2), 103–117.

Cook, V. J. (1992). Evidence for multicompetence. *Language Learning*, *42*(4), 557–591.

Cook, V. J. (2003). The changing L1 in the L2 user's mind. In V. Cook (Ed.), *Effects of the second language on the first* (pp. 1–18). Clevedon: Multilingual Matters.

Cutler, A. (2001). Listening to a second language through the ears of a first. *Interpreting*, *5*(1), 1–23.

Davidson, L. (2006). Phonology, phonetics, or frequency: Influences on the production of non-native sequences. *Journal of Phonetics*, *34*(1), 104–137.

Davidson, L. (2011). Phonetic, phonemic, and phonological factors in cross-language discrimination of phonotactic contrasts. *Journal of Experimental Psychology: Human Perception and Performance*, *37*(1), 270–282.

Davidson, L. (2017). Cross-language speech perception and production. In M. Aronoff (Ed.), *Oxford bibliographies in linguistics*. Oxford: Oxford University Press.

de Bot, K., Lowie, W., and Verspoor, M. (2007). A dynamic systems theory approach to second language acquisition. *Bilingualism: Language and Cognition*, *10*(1), 7–21.

de Leeuw, E. (in press). Phonetic L1 attrition. In M. S. Schmid and B. Köpke (Eds.), *The Oxford handbook of language attrition*. Oxford: Oxford University Press.

de Leeuw, E., Mennen, I., and Scobbie, J. M. (2013). Dynamic systems, maturational constraints and L1 phonetic attrition. *International Journal of Bilingualism*, *17*(6), 683–700.

de Leeuw, E., Schmid, M. S., and Mennen, I. (2010). The effects of contact on native language pronunciation in an L2 migrant setting. *Bilingualism: Language and Cognition*, *13*(1), 33–40.

Dmitrieva, O., Jongman, A., and Sereno, J. (2010). Phonological neutralization by native and non-native speakers: The case of Russian final devoicing. *Journal of Phonetics*, *38*(3), 483–492.

Dupoux, E., Hirose, Y., Kakehi, K., Pallier, C., and Mehler, J. (1999). Epenthetic vowels in Japanese: A perceptual illusion? *Journal of Experimental Psychology: Human Perception and Performance*, *25*(6), 1568–1578.

Eckman, F. R. (1977). Markedness and the contrastive analysis hypothesis. *Language Learning*, *27*(2), 315–330.

Eckman, F. R. (1991). The structural conformity hypothesis and the acquisition of consonant clusters in the interlanguage of ESL learners. *Studies in Second Language Acquisition*, *13*(1), 23–41.

Eckman, F. R. (2008). Typological markedness and second language phonology. In J. G. Hansen Edwards and M. L. Zampini (Eds.), *Phonology and second language acquisition* (pp. 95–115). Amsterdam, The Netherlands: John Benjamins Publishing.

Eckman, F. R. (2012). Second language phonology. In S. M. Gass and A. Mackey (Eds.), *The Routledge handbook of second language acquisition* (pp. 91–105). New York, NY: Routledge.

Ellis, N. C. (2006). Selective attention and transfer phenomena in L2 acquisition: Contingency, cue competition, salience, interference, overshadowing, blocking, and perceptual learning. *Applied Linguistics*, *27*(2), 164–194.

Escudero, P. (2009). Linguistic perception of "similar" L2 sounds. In P. Boersma and S. Hamann (Eds.), *Phonology in perception* (pp. 151–190). Berlin, Germany: Mouton de Gruyter.

Flege, J. E. (1987). The production of "new" and "similar" phones in a foreign language: Evidence for the effect of equivalence classification. *Journal of Phonetics*, *15*(1), 47–65.

Flege, J. E. (1995). Second language speech learning: Theory, findings, and problems. In W. Strange (Ed.), *Speech perception and linguistic experience: Issues in cross-language research* (pp. 233–272). Baltimore, MD: York Press.

Flege, J. E. (1996). English vowel productions by Dutch talkers: More evidence for the "similar" vs "new" distinction. In A. James and J. Leather (Eds.), *Second-language speech: Structure and process* (pp. 11–52). Berlin, Germany: Mouton de Gruyter.

Flege, J. E. (2002). Interactions between the native and second-language phonetic systems. In P. Burmeister, T. Piske, and A. Rohde (Eds.), *An integrated view of language development: Papers in honor of Henning Wode* (pp. 217–244). Trier, Germany: Wissenschaftlicher Verlag.

Flege, J. E., and Eefting, W. (1987a). Cross-language switching in stop consonant perception and production by Dutch speakers of English. *Speech Communication*, *6*(3), 185–202.

Flege, J. E., and Eefting, W. (1987b). Production and perception of English stops by native Spanish speakers. *Journal of Phonetics*, *15*(1), 67–83.

Flege, J. E., MacKay, I. R. A., and Meador, D. (1999). Native Italian speakers' perception and production of English vowels. *The Journal of the Acoustical Society of America*, *106*(5), 2973–2987.

Fokes, J., Bond, Z. S., and Steinberg, M. (1985). Acquisition of the English voicing contrast by Arab children. *Language and Speech*, *28*(1), 81–92.

Gallardo del Puerto, F. (2007). Is L3 phonological competence affected by the learner's level of bilingualism? *International Journal of Multilingualism*, *4*(1), 1–16.

Gass, S. (1984). Development of speech perception and speech production in adult second language learners. *Applied Psycholinguistics*, *5*(1), 51–74.

Godfroid, A., Lin, C. H., and Ryu, C. (2017). Hearing and seeing tone through color: An efficacy study of web-based, multimodal Chinese tone perception training. *Language Learning*, *67*(4), 819–857.

Goto, H. (1971). Auditory perception by normal Japanese adults of the sounds "L" and "R." *Neuropsychologia*, *9*(3), 317–323.

Guion, S. G. (2003). The vowel systems of Quichua-Spanish bilinguals: Age of acquisition effects on the mutual influence of the first and second languages. *Phonetica*, *60*(2), 98–128.

Hagiwara, R. (1997). Dialect variation and formant frequency: The American English vowels revisited. *The Journal of the Acoustical Society of America*, *102*(1), 655–658.

Hallé, P. A., and Best, C. T. (2007). Dental-to-velar perceptual assimilation: A cross-linguistic study of the perception of dental stop+/l/ clusters. *The Journal of the Acoustical Society of America*, *121*(5), 2899–2914.

Hancin-Bhatt, B. (2008). Second language phonology in optimality theory. In J. G. Hansen Edwards and M. L. Zampini (Eds.), *Phonology and second language acquisition* (pp. 117–146). Amsterdam, The Netherlands: John Benjamins Publishing.

Hazan, V. (2007). Second language acquisition and exemplar theory. In J. Trouvain and W. J. Barry (Eds.), *Proceedings of the 16th international congress of phonetic sciences* (pp. 39–42). Dudweiler, Germany: Pirrot.

Holliday, J. J. (2016). Second language experience can hinder the discrimination of nonnative phonological contrasts. *Phonetica*, *73*(1), 33–51.

Johnson, K. (1997). Speech perception without speaker normalization: An exemplar model. In K. Johnson and J. W. Mullennix (Eds.), *Talker variability in speech processing* (pp. 145–165). San Diego, CA: Academic Press.

Kang, K. H., and Guion, S. G. (2006). Phonological systems in bilinguals: Age of learning effects on the stop consonant systems of Korean-English bilinguals. *The Journal of the Acoustical Society of America*, *119*(3), 1672–1683.

Kang, Y. (2008). Interlanguage segmental mapping as evidence for the nature of lexical representation. *Language and Linguistics Compass*, *2*(1), 103–118.

Kartushina, N. (2015). *Second language phonological acquisition in adults*. Ph.D. thesis, University of Geneva.

Kartushina, N., and Frauenfelder, U. H. (2014). On the effects of L2 perception and of individual differences in L1 production on L2 pronunciation. *Frontiers in Psychology*, *5*, 1246.

Kartushina, N., Frauenfelder, U. H., and Golestani, N. (2016). How and when does the second language influence the production of native speech sounds: A literature review. *Language Learning, 66*(S2), 155–186.

Kartushina, N., Hervais-Adelman, A., Frauenfelder, U. H., and Golestani, N. (2015). The effect of phonetic production training with visual feedback on the perception and production of foreign speech sounds. *The Journal of the Acoustical Society of America, 138*(2), 817–832.

Keating, P. A. (1984). Phonetic and phonological representation of stop consonant voicing. *Language, 60*(2), 286–319.

Kingston, J. (2003). Learning foreign vowels. *Language and Speech, 46*(2–3), 295–349.

Knightly, L. M., Jun, S. A., Oh, J. S., and Au, T. K. (2003). Production benefits of childhood overhearing. *The Journal of the Acoustical Society of America, 114*(1), 465–474.

Kuhl, P. K. (1991). Human adults and human infants show a "perceptual magnet effect" for the prototypes of speech categories, monkeys do not. *Perception and Psychophysics, 50*(2), 93–107.

Kuhl, P. K, Conboy, B. T., Coffey-Corina, S., Padden, D., Rivera-Gaxiola, M., and Nelson, T. (2008). Phonetic learning as a pathway to language: New data and native language magnet theory expanded (NLM-e). *Philosophical Transactions of the Royal Society B, 363*, 979–1000.

Kuhl, P. K., and Iverson, P. (1995). Linguistic experience and the "Perceptual Magnet Effect." In W. Strange (Ed.), *Speech perception and linguistic experience: Issues in cross-language research* (pp. 121–154). Baltimore, MD: York Press.

LaCharité, D., and Paradis, C. (2005). Category preservation and proximity versus phonetic approximation in loanword adaptation. *Linguistic Inquiry, 36*(2), 223–258.

Ladefoged, P. (1999). American English. In The International Phonetic Association (Ed.), *Handbook of the international phonetic association: A guide to the use of the international phonetic alphabet* (pp. 41–44). Cambridge: Cambridge University Press.

Lado, R. (1957). *Linguistics across cultures: Applied linguistics for language teachers*. Ann Arbor, MI: University of Michigan Press.

Laeufer, C. (1996). Towards a typology of bilingual phonological systems. In A. James and J. Leather (Eds.), *Second-language speech: Structure and process* (pp. 325–342). Berlin, Germany: Mouton de Gruyter.

Leach, L., and Samuel, A. G. (2007). Lexical configuration and lexical engagement: When adults learn new words. *Cognitive Psychology, 55*(4), 306–353.

Leather, J. (1996). Interrelation of perceptual and productive learning in the initial acquisition of second-language tone. In A. James and J. Leather (Eds.), *Second-language speech: Structure and process* (pp. 75–101). Berlin, Germany: Mouton de Gruyter.

Levy, E. S., and Strange, W. (2008). Perception of French vowels by American English adults with and without French language experience. *Journal of Phonetics, 36*(1), 141–157.

Li, A., and Post, B. (2014). L2 acquisition of prosodic properties of speech rhythm: Evidence from L1 Mandarin and German learners of English. *Studies in Second Language Acquisition, 36*(2), 223–255.

Liberman, A. M., Harris, K. S., Hoffman, H. S., and Griffith, B. C. (1957). The discrimination of speech sounds within and across phoneme boundaries. *Journal of Experimental Psychology, 54*(5), 358–368.

Mack, M. (1989). Consonant and vowel perception and production: Early English-French bilinguals and English monolinguals. *Perception and Psychophysics, 46*(2), 187–200.

Mack, M. (1990). Phonetic transfer in a French-English bilingual child. In P. H. Nelde (Ed.), *Language attitudes and language conflict* (pp. 107–124). Bonn, Germany: Dümmler.

Mack, M. (2003). The phonetic systems of bilinguals. In M. T. Banich and M. Mack (Eds.), *Mind, brain, and language: Multidisciplinary perspectives* (pp. 309–349). Mahwah, NJ: Lawrence Erlbaum Press.

Major, R. C. (1992). Losing English as a first language. *The Modern Language Journal, 76*(2), 190–208.

Major, R. C. (1996). L2 acquisition, L1 loss, and the critical period hypothesis. In A. James and J. Leather (Eds.), *Second-language speech: Structure and process* (pp. 147–159). Berlin, Germany: Mouton de Gruyter.

Major, R. C. (2001). *Foreign accent: The ontogeny and phylogeny of second language phonology*. Mahwah, NJ: Lawrence Erlbaum Associates.

Mennen, I. (2015). Beyond segments: Towards a L2 intonation learning theory. In E. Delais-Roussarie, M. Avanzi, and S. Herment (Eds.), *Prosody and language in contact: L2 acquisition, attrition and languages in multilingual situations* (pp. 171–188). Berlin, Germany: Springer Verlag.

Mennen, I., and de Leeuw, E. (2014). Beyond segments: Prosody in SLA. *Studies in Second Language Acquisition, 36*(2), 183–194.

Mora, J. C., and Levkina, M. (2017). Task-based pronunciation teaching and research: Key issues and future directions. *Studies in Second Language Acquisition, 39*(2), 381–399.

Odlin, T. (1989). *Language transfer: Cross-linguistic influence in language learning*. Cambridge: Cambridge University Press.

Oh, G. E., Guion-Anderson, S., Aoyama, K., Flege, J. E., Akahane-Yamada, R., and Yamada, T. (2011). A one-year longitudinal study of English and Japanese vowel production by Japanese adults and children in an English-speaking setting. *Journal of Phonetics, 39*(2), 156–167.

Onishi, H. (2013). *Cross-linguistic influence in third language perception: L2 and L3 perception of Japanese contrasts*. Ph.D. thesis, University of Arizona.

Peperkamp, S., and Bouchon, C. (2011). The relation between perception and production in L2 phonological processing. In *Proceedings of the 12th international conference on spoken language processing (Interspeech-2011)* (pp. 168–171). Florence, Italy: International Speech Communication Association.

Perrachione, T. K., Lee, J., Ha, L. Y. Y., and Wong, P. C. M. (2011). Learning a novel phonological contrast depends on interactions between individual differences and training paradigm design. *The Journal of the Acoustical Society of America, 130*(1), 461–472.

Pierrehumbert, J. (2001). Exemplar dynamics: Word frequency, lenition, and contrast. In J. Bybee and P. Hopper (Eds.), *Frequency effects and the emergence of lexical structure* (pp. 137–157). Amsterdam, The Netherlands: John Benjamins Publishing.

Polka, L. (1991). Cross-language speech perception in adults: Phonemic, phonetic and acoustic contributions. *The Journal of the Acoustical Society of America, 89*(6), 2961–2977.

Polka, L. (1992). Characterizing the influence of native language experience on adult speech perception. *Perception and Psychophysics, 52*(1), 37–52.

Polka, L., and Bohn, O. S. (1996). A cross-language comparison of vowel perception in English-learning and German-learning infants. *The Journal of the Acoustical Society of America, 100*(1), 577–592.

Port, R. F., and Mitleb, F. M. (1983). Segmental features and implementation in acquisition of English by Arabic speakers. *Journal of Phonetics, 11*(3), 219–229.

Schwartz, G. (2016). Word boundaries in L2 speech: Evidence from Polish learners of English. *Second Language Research, 32*(3), 397–426.

Sheldon, A., and Strange, W. (1982). The acquisition of /r/ and /l/ by Japanese learners of English: Evidence that speech production can precede speech perception. *Applied Psycholinguistics, 3*(3), 243–261.

Simonet, M. (2016). The phonetics and phonology of bilingualism. In *Oxford handbooks online* (pp. 1–25). Oxford: Oxford University Press.

Strange, W. (2011). Automatic Selective Perception (ASP) of first and second language speech: A working model. *Journal of Phonetics, 39*(4), 456–466.

Strange, W., Levy, E., and Lehnholf, R., Jr. (2004). Perceptual assimilation of French and German vowels by American English monolinguals: Acoustic similarity does not predict perceptual similarity. *The Journal of the Acoustical Society of America, 115*(5), 2606.

Syrdal, A. K., and Gopal, H. S. (1986). A perceptual model of vowel recognition based on the auditory representation of American English vowels. *The Journal of the Acoustical Society of America, 79*(4), 1086–1100.

Tajima, K., Kato, H., Rothwell, A., Akahane-Yamada, R., and Munhall, K. G. (2008). Training English listeners to perceive phonemic length contrasts in Japanese. *The Journal of the Acoustical Society of America, 123*(1), 397–413.

Tice, M., and Woodley, M. (2012). Paguettes and bastries: Novice French learners show shifts in native phoneme boundaries. *UC Berkeley Phonology Lab Annual Report*, 72–75.

Tobin, S. J., Nam, H., and Fowler, C. A. (2017). Phonetic drift in Spanish-English bilinguals: Experiment and a self-organizing model. *Journal of Phonetics, 65*, 45–59.

Tucker, G. R. (2001). A global perspective on bilingualism and bilingual education. In J. E. Alatis and A. H. Tan (Eds.), *Language in our time: Bilingual education and official English, Ebonics and standard English, immigration and the Unz initiative* (pp. 332–340). Washington, DC: Georgetown University Press.

Tyler, M. D., Best, C. T., Faber, A., and Levitt, A. G. (2014). Perceptual assimilation and discrimination of non-native vowel contrasts. *Phonetica, 71*(1), 4–21.

van Leussen, J. W., and Escudero, P. (2015). Learning to perceive and recognize a second language: The L2LP model revised. *Frontiers in Psychology, 6*, 1000.

van Merriënboer, J. J. G., and Sweller, J. (2005). Cognitive load theory and complex learning: Recent developments and future directions. *Educational Psychology Review, 17*(2), 147–177.

Wang, Y., Jongman, A., and Sereno, J. A. (2003). Acoustic and perceptual evaluation of Mandarin tone productions before and after perceptual training. *The Journal of the Acoustical Society of America, 113*(2), 1033–1043.

Wang, Y., Spence, M. M., Jongman, A., and Sereno, J. A. (1999). Training American listeners to perceive Mandarin tones. *The Journal of the Acoustical Society of America, 106*(6), 3649–3658.

Weinreich, U. (1953). *Languages in contact: Findings and problems*. The Hague, The Netherlands: Mouton de Gruyter.

Werker, J. F., and Curtin, S. (2005). PRIMIR: A developmental framework of infant speech processing. *Language Learning and Development, 1*(2), 197–234.

Williams, L. (1977). The perception of stop consonant voicing by Spanish-English bilinguals. *Perception and Psychophysics, 21*(4), 289–297.

Williams, L. (1979). The modification of speech perception and production in second-language learning. *Perception and Psychophysics, 26*(2), 95–104.

Wrembel, M. (2014). VOT patterns in the acquisition of third language phonology. *Concordia Working Papers in Applied Linguistics, 5*, 750–770.

Yeni-Komshian, G. H., Flege, J. E., and Liu, S. (2000). Pronunciation proficiency in the first and second languages of Korean-English bilinguals. *Bilingualism: Language and Cognition, 3*(2), 131–149.

Zsiga, E. (2011). External sandhi in a second language: The phonetics and phonology of obstruent nasalization in Korean and Korean-accented English. *Language, 87*(2), 289–345.

16

Innovations in sociophonetics

Erik R. Thomas

Defining sociophonetics

The term *sociophonetics* has experienced a steady growth in its use over the past few decades. According to Foulkes and Docherty (2006), it was apparently coined by Deschaies-Lafontaine (1974). During the 1970s and 1980s it was used primarily as an occasional title for sessions at phonetics conferences, encompassing studies that examined some sort of dialectal difference in a phonetic property. During the 1990s, however, its usage grew, particularly after sociolinguists began using it for studies of linguistic variation that utilized modern phonetic analyses – i.e., acoustic, articulatory, and perceptual investigations. The term is now commonplace. There are currently two textbooks on it (Di Paolo and Yaeger-Dror 2011; Thomas 2011) and at least two collections of studies (Preston and Niedzielski 2010; Celata and Calamai 2014) with *sociophonetics* in the title, as well as a special issue of the *Journal of Phonetics* in 2006 and one of *Lingua* in 2012 dedicated to it. A number of articles (Hay and Drager 2007; Thomas 2007, 2013; Foulkes, Scobbie, and Watt 2010) have reviewed it. The International Congress of Phonetic Sciences (ICPhS) regularly holds multiple sessions devoted to it, and the annual conference on New Ways of Analyzing Variation (NWAV) has held a workshop on it for several years running. Clearly, *sociophonetics* has become an essential component of contemporary linguistics.

What, however, is sociophonetics besides a nebulous area in which phonetics and linguistic variation overlap? Phoneticians have tended to apply the term to descriptive studies on dialectal variation in any phonetic property. This descriptive focus can be seen in early papers from the *Journal of Phonetics* (e.g., Caramazza and Yeni-Komshian 1974; Kvavik 1974) and the *Journal of the International Phonetic Association* (e.g., Nally 1971; Johnson 1971). The descriptive focus is still seen in recent papers in the latter journal (e.g., Wikström 2013; Kirtley et al. 2016), as well as in a large fraction of presentations in sessions at the International Congress of Phonetic Sciences with "sociophonetics" in their title (see the ICPhS archive at www.internationalphoneticassociation.org/content/icphs). There have been ample exceptions, such as Szakay and Torgersen's (2015) study of gender/ethnicity interaction and Nguyen et al.'s (2015) perception experiment linking affective attitudes toward an ethnic group with accuracy in speech recognition. Conspicuously absent from studies by phoneticians that have been labeled as sociophonetics, however, are papers addressing such historically important phonetic issues as quantal theory, motor theory, locus equation theory, and invariance.

Studies by sociolinguists that fall within the ambit of sociophonetics have their descriptive tradition as well (e.g., Thomas 2001). However, most have some other goal. Much of William Labov's work with vowels (e.g., Labov, Yaeger, and Steiner 1972; Labov 1991, 1994, 2001) has aimed to determine general tendencies in how vowels shift diachronically. The mechanisms behind phonological mergers have been another key focus (e.g., Labov, Karan, and Miller 1991; Rae and Warren 2002; Johnson 2010). Another crucial issue has been language contact (e.g., Purnell, Salmons, and Tepeli 2005a, 2005b; Kerswill, Torgersen, and Fox 2008; Sharbawi and Deterding 2010; Queen 2012). A key aim has been to determine the social meaning – the second-order indexicality – of particular variants; that is, how people use phonetic forms to signal or interpret identity for a community or smaller networks of people (indexicality being the identification by a word of some quality of its referent or speaker). Two studies of how vowel variants signify opposing social groups in high schools – Habick's (1980) investigation of a rural Illinois school and Fought's (1999) study of a mostly Latino school in Los Angeles – exemplify this focus.

A third source of input to sociophonetics, one that largely involves perception experiments, has roots in social psychology. This tradition extends back at least to Mason's (1946) experiment on identification of dialects by military personnel. A watershed moment came when Lambert et al. (1960) introduced the matched guise experiment, which in that study involved having listeners respond to recordings of the same speakers using French in one excerpt and English in another. Subjects rated the same voices more highly on various aptitude scales when the person was speaking English than when the individual was speaking French. Another innovation came when Brown, Strong, and Rencher (1972) introduced speech synthesis to subjective reaction experimentation. Sociolinguists eventually adopted the methods – e.g., in Frazer's (1987) and van Bezooijen's (1988) use of excerpts of different dialects to elicit subjective reactions – and they applied them to various other problems as well.

At this point, one might ask whether sociophonetics has a true focus. While many, though not all, phoneticians have confined *sociophonetic* to descriptive studies of individual features, sociolinguists have enthusiastically applied it to studies of issues such as the use of linguistic variants for projecting identity, the mechanisms of sound change, and the relationship between language and societal inequality. The remaining sections will illustrate the diversity of studies that fall under the label *sociophonetic* and then suggest that there is more to sociophonetics than merely the interface of phonetics and sociolinguistics: in fact, studies of phonetic variation can shed light on some of the most basic questions in linguistics. These questions include the nature of sound change and the nature of cognition of language. For the latter, sociophonetic investigations are vital for dissecting problems such as the relationship between structural and metalinguistic aspects of language and between abstract and episodic representations of linguistic cognition.

Socio-production

Segmental variation

Vocalic variation

Perhaps the most robust enterprise in sociophonetics has been inquiry into vowel shifting. This line of research, which relies on acoustic analysis of vowel formant frequencies, began with Labov, Yaeger, and Steiner (1972), who analyzed vowel configurations in various dialects of English, mostly in the United States. Formant analysis revealed sound shifts that previous auditory analyses had largely or entirely overlooked. The primary aim was to identify principles governing how vowels shifted, and the principles they proposed continued to appear, with small modifications, in Labov's later work (especially Labov 1991, 1994, 2001). For example, they proposed that long or tense vowels tend to rise along the periphery of the vowel envelope (i.e., the plotted F_1/F_2 space occupied by vowels) and that short or lax vowels tend to fall in the interior of the vowel envelope. Labov and his students exploited the methods for various sociolinguistic studies (e.g., Hindle 1980; Labov 1980; Veatch 1991), and, until the 1990s, they conducted nearly all of the sociophonetic work on vowels.

Another issue besides principles of vowel shifting that acoustic studies have explored is the geographical extent of vocalic variants and their diffusion. The largest-scale studies have been most successful. Labov et al. (2006) was able to demarcate the extent of nearly every known vowel shift in North American English and to delineate boundaries of dialects, which for the most part matched those of older studies. It also turned up some previously unknown shifts. Another recent large-scale project is SweDia (Eriksson 2004), a survey of regional variation in Swedish in which balanced samples of older and younger and male and female speakers were interviewed across the Swedish-speaking area. Leinonen (2010) conducted an analysis of vocalic variation in SweDia using a novel acoustic analysis involving sampling intensity at multiple frequencies, followed by three layers of statistical analysis. She determined that some dialect leveling was occurring within regions and change was occurring most rapidly in the region around Stockholm, but no sharp dialectal boundaries emerged.

Numerous smaller-scale acoustic vowel studies have appeared in recent decades, with a variety of aims. Some have examined the configuration of all the vowels or those involved in vowel rotation patterns in specific communities, usually correlating them with sex or social networks and/or tracking change across generations (e.g., Ito and Preston 1998; Fridland 2001; Baranowski 2007; Durian 2012; Labov, Rosenfelder, and Fruehwald 2013). Others have focused on allophony or splits of individual vowels (e.g., Zeller 1997; Boberg and Strassel 2000, Ash 2002; Blake and Josey 2003; Moreton and Thomas 2007; Fruehwald 2016). A few (e.g., Evanini 2008; Thomas 2010) have explored how geographical dialect boundaries change over time. There are also descriptive studies intended to provide phoneticians with information about dialectal variation (Hagiwara 1997; Clopper, Pisoni, and de Jong 2005). Another important sociophonetic application of vowel analysis has been to ethnic variation. Studies of African American English (AAE) have shed light on the traditional controversies surrounding AAE: how it originated (Thomas and Bailey 1998), its ongoing relationship with white vernaculars (e.g., Wolfram and Thomas 2002; Fridland 2003a, 2003b; Fridland and Bartlett 2006; Labov 2014), and its degree of geographical and other internal variation (e.g., Deser 1990; Yaeger-Dror and Thomas 2010; Kohn 2013). Vowel formant analysis for other ethnic groups has largely concerned language contact and its aftereffects. Studies of Latino English in the United States have yielded descriptive studies (e.g., Godinez 1984; Godinez and Maddieson 1985; Thomas 2001), studies of accommodation to matrix speech when the community social ecology allows it (e.g., Ocumpaugh 2010; Roeder 2010), and studies of how social identity leads to Latino (sub)dialects (Fought 1999; Thomas 2019). Other language contact situations in which vowels have been studied instrumentally include immigrant communities in London (Evans, Mistry, and Moreiras 2007; Kerswill, Torgerson, and Fox 2008) and the Chinese American community of San Francisco (Hall-Lew 2009).

Vocalic mergers have been the subject of considerable sociophonetic research. In English, the merger of the /ɑ/ and /ɔ/ vowels, making pairs such as *cot/caught* and *hock/hawk* homophonous, has generated numerous papers (e.g., Irons 2007; Johnson 2010; Benson, Fox, and Balkman 2011). Other authors, however, have reported that the contrast may be maintained subtly in some regions (Di Paolo 1992; Fridland, Kendall, and Farrington 2014), the former study reporting phonation differences and the latter durational differences, and Di Paolo and Faber (1990) found that phonation can maintain distinctions between certain classes of pre-/l/ vowels as well. Elsewhere, other mergers, such as the *fear/fair* merger in New Zealand English (Hay et al. 2006) and the merger of long and short vowels in Seoul Korean (Kang, Yoon, and Han 2015) have been examined. For formant values, measures of overlap such as Pillai scores (Hay, Nolan, and Drager 2006) and Bhattacharyya's affinity (Johnson 2015) have been useful. Nevertheless, overlap measures can fail to register a distinction if the distinction is maintained by factors such as duration, dynamics, or phonation instead of by static formant values. They can also imply that a nonexistent distinction is present if mismatched segmental or prosodic contexts in the tokens that are measured create a spurious differentiation in the formant values.

Recent methodological innovations have expanded vocalic studies in new directions. One innovation has been the examination of vowel trajectories, for which readings are taken at multiple time points through a vowel instead of just one or two points. Various studies (e.g., Fox and Jacewicz 2009; Jacewicz, Fox, and Salmons 2011; Jacewicz and Fox 2012; Leinonen 2010; Hoffman 2011; Kirtley et al. 2016) have used this technique profitably for the notoriously dynamic English vowels. Another innovation is the use of automatic formant extraction routines, which permit the collection of large amounts of data quickly (see, e.g., Labov, Rosenfelder and Fruehwald 2013; Reddy and Stanford 2015; Fruehwald 2016). One potentially game-changing development is the advent of ultrasound for examining tongue configuration. This innovation has so far barely infiltrated vocalic variation studies (see Bauer and Parker 2008; De Decker and Nycz 2012; Mielke, Carignan, and Thomas 2017). Its impact has been stronger for consonantal studies.

The North American bias of the vocalic research should be obvious. Varieties of English outside North America have received much less sociophonetic work on their vowels: see Cox (1999) on Australian English; Torgersen and Kerswill (2004) and Baranowski (2017) on England English; McClure (1995) and Schützler (2011) on Scottish English; Maclagan (1982) and Maclagan and Hay (2007) on New Zealand English. Vowels of "New Englishes" in Asia and Africa have also been analyzed acoustically, largely for descriptive purposes (Deterding 2003, 2005; Deterding, Wong, and Kirkpatrick 2008; Sarmah, Gogoi, and Wiltshire 2009; Tan and Low 2010; Hoffman 2011). Outside of English, acoustic analysis of vowel variation has remained quite limited. There have been a few studies tracing regional variation and change in Dutch (van Heuven, Edelman, and van Bezooijen 2002; Adank et al. 2007; Van der Harst, Van de Velde, and Van Hout 2014), but aside from work on SweDia described earlier, very few on other languages (e.g., Willis 2007b, 2008 for Spanish, Moosmüller and Granser 2006 for Albanian; Liu and Liang 2016 for Xinyang Mandarin; and Schoormann, Heeringa, and Peters 2017 for Saterland Frisian).

Consonantal variation

Sociophonetic analysis of consonantal variation, though not as extensive as that of vowels, has been active. Approximants have garnered considerable attention. Among laterals, most research has examined "dark /l/," the velarization of alveolar laterals. Studies have examined this development in Catalan (Recasens and Espinosa 2005), British English (Carter and Local 2007), Spanish-influenced forms of American English (Van Hofwegen 2009; Newman 2010), and, with ultrasound technology, dialects of British English (Turton 2014). Another variable is the vocalization of /l/, examined acoustically in American English by Dodsworth and Hazen (2012).

Rhotics have provided more fodder for sociophonetic work than laterals. In English and Dutch, an important issue is whether /r/ is produced with a retroflex or a "bunched" articulation. Both involve two constrictions, one of which is pharyngeal, but the other constriction is retro-apical for the retroflex form and dorso-palatal for the "bunched" one. Because the two forms sound almost identical, ultrasound has become the preferred analysis method. Mielke, Baker, and Archangeli (2010) discussed contextual constraints of the variants, also finding the "bunched" form more common, in American English. Scobbie and Sebregts (2011) and Sebregts (2014) showed that both forms occur in Netherlandic Dutch, mainly in syllable codas. Work in Scotland, including ultrasound analyses of Edinburgh speech (Lawson, Scobbie, and Stuart-Smith 2011, 2013) and acoustic analyses of Glasgow speech (Stuart-Smith 2007) have revealed a class-based schism in which middle-class speakers prefer "bunched" /r/, whereas working-class speakers tend toward apical realizations that can undergo weakening or elision. The uvularization of /r/ that is widespread in European languages has been investigated extensively by auditory means, but the main instrumental studies are those by Scobbie and Sebregts (2011) and Sebregts (2014) on Dutch. They found uvular forms to be widespread, especially in syllable onsets, but more common in some locales than others.

Another widespread process affecting rhotics is assibilation. In Spanish, both trilled and tapped rhotics, which contrast only intervocalically, may become a fricative such as [z̞] or may be reduced to aspiration, depending on dialect. Studies have used acoustic analysis to demonstrate dialect-specific assibilation of intervocalic trills (Willis and Bradley 2008; Henriksen and Willis 2010) and word-initial rhotics (Colantoni 2006). Willis (2007a) documented the presence in Dominican Spanish of breathiness preceding medial rhotics, sometimes with loss of the lingual maneuver, leaving only voiced aspiration. Rafat (2010) examined rhotics in Farsi acoustically and noted a strong tendency toward assibilation in some contexts, especially for female subjects.

Fricatives have generally been analyzed using either spectral center of gravity (COG) or the frequency of the highest-amplitude spectral peak. Weakening of /s/ to [h] or deletion has been analyzed using COG for Dominican (Erker 2010) and Columbian (File-Muriel and Brown 2011) Spanish. [s] normally exhibits considerable energy in the 4–10 kHz range and drastic changes in COG can signify non-sibilant realizations. Another Spanish variable, fortition of /j/ to [ʒ~ʃ], was analyzed by Colantoni (2006) in two Argentinian dialects. In English, variation in [s] variants, such as laminal and apical forms, has been explored (e.g., Stuart-Smith 2007; Podesva and Van Hofwegen 2016; Zamman 2017) as a marker of social identity. Another English variable is the retraction of [s] in /str/ clusters toward [ʃ] (e.g., Rutter 2011; Baker, Archangeli, and Mielke 2011). The preceding two shifts are identifiable from a moderate lowering of COG values.

Several stop variables have been examined instrumentally. Although place of articulation has been coded auditorily in most variation studies, Purnell (2008) used x-ray data to show that /g/ had a fronter articulation than /k/ in Wisconsin English, and ultrasound holds promise for further work on any number of place variables. Wisconsin English furnished another key variable involving the cues used to signal the voicing distinction for Purnell,

Salmons, and Tepeli (2005a, 2005b). These studies showed that the shift of German Americans from German, in which voicing is neutralized word-finally, to English led to an unusual situation in which vowels were longer before voiceless stops than before voiced stops. This configuration was compensated for by exaggeration of the duration distinction for voiced and voiceless occlusions.

A different sort of stop variable, pre-aspiration, in which vowels become breathy or voiceless before a voiceless stop, occurs in some northwestern European languages. Lectal variation in the amount of pre-aspiration, both geographical and by gender, has been examined for Swedish (Wretling, Strangert, and Schaeffler 2002, using SweDia data; Stölten and Engstrand 2002; Tronnier 2002) and Welsh English (Hejna 2015). The mere presence of pre-aspiration sets Newcastle upon Tyne apart from other parts of England (Docherty and Foulkes 1999; Foulkes and Docherty 2006).

Other stop variables include glottalization and voice-onset time (VOT). Glottalization, common in British English dialects, involves replacement of medial /t/ with [ʔ]. Though it is usually evaluated auditorily, Docherty and Foulkes (1999) and Foulkes and Docherty (2006) have shown that it occurs in multiple forms, including glottal reinforcement of [t], [ʔ] without coronal occlusion, and a period of creakiness between vowels. Some studies, e.g., Straw and Patrick's (2007) examination of ethnic differences in London, have incorporated inspection of spectrograms into coding of glottalization. VOT is often analyzed when dialects emerge from language contact situations, e.g., Punjabi/English by Heselwood and McChrystal (1999), Māori/English by Maclagan et al. (2009), and Yucatec Mayan/Spanish by Michnowicz and Carpenter (2013). In such cases, the stop series of the languages in contact do not coincide in VOT properties. However, there are studies of VOT variation in non-contact situations (e.g., Japanese in Takada and Tomimori 2006; Scots in Scobbie 2006). An unusual case is Korean, in which a VOT distinction between two stop series is being replaced with a tonal distinction (e.g., Choi 2002).

Epenthetic stops, as occur between the /n/ and /s/ in *dense*, are the subject of Fourakis and Port (1986). The finding that dialects differed in whether they had the stops, even while the epenthetic stops averaged shorter than underlying stops as in *dents*, defied traditional notions about the respective realms of phonology and phonetics. It was an important demonstration of how language variation can provide insights into the cognitive organization of speech.

A few studies have investigated lenition or loss of stops. Syrika, Kong, and Edwards (2011) analyzed the softening of Greek /k/ before front vowels from [kʲ] to [tɕ~tʃ] in certain dialects. Two cases involving language contact are Mansfield (2015), who showed how a speaker's linguistic background affected the degree to which the speaker elided initial stops in the indigenous Australian language Murrinh Patha, and Sadowski and Aninao (2019), who analyzed various lenition products of /p/ in Mapudungan-influenced Chilean Spanish.

Although sociophoneticians have focused on these previously mentioned variables, those processes certainly do not exhaust the consonantal possibilities. For example, Rohena-Madrazo (2015) analyzed vocal pulsing to show that Argentine Spanish /j/, as in *ya* "already," which is well-known to have shifted earlier to [ʒ~ʝ], is now undergoing devoicing to [ʃ]. Other such studies will undoubtedly materialize in the future. In addition, the automatic extraction routines that increasingly have been used for vowel measurement are now becoming applicable to analysis of some consonantal properties as well (e.g., Baranowski and Turton, forthcoming).

Suprasegmental variation

Prosody has attracted far less attention from sociophoneticians than segmental properties, though intonation is accumulating a sizable sociophonetic literature. Prosodic rhythm has garnered a moderate amount of work. Rate of speech and lexical tone lag far behind.

Prosodic rhythm

Prosodic rhythm is thought of as consisting of a grade from syllable-timing to stress-timing; in syllable-timing, syllables (or the vowels within them) are supposed to have approximately the same durations, whereas in stress-timing, rhythmic feet have roughly equal durations but syllables may differ widely. Although the notion of strict isochrony in "syllable-timed" languages has been disproved (e.g., Wenk and Wiolland 1982) and numerous questions remain about whether prosodic rhythm is a feature in its own right or merely an artifact of other processes and about the best method of measuring it (Turk and Shattuck-Hufnagel 2013), a small body of work has addressed how it is manifested as a sociolinguistic variable. Most of these studies involve language contact situations or sites of former language contact. Furthermore, even though prosodic rhythm has been applied to numerous languages, most studies that examine intra-language variation in it have focused on English. In all cases, heritage English speakers have proved to exhibit relatively stress-timed speech compared to speakers of "New Englishes," in some cases even after the group that shifted to English had become English-dominant. Cases examined include Singapore English, with Malay and Chinese substrates (Low, Grabe, and Nolan 2000; Deterding 2001), Latino English (Carter 2005), Welsh English (White and Mattys 2007), Cherokee English (Coggshall 2008), Māori English (Szakay 2008), Thai English (Sarmah, Gogoi, and Wiltshire 2009), and Multicultural London English (Torgerson and Szakay 2012). In fact, rhythm that is less stress-timed than heritage English has even been attributed to substrate effects from languages that were abandoned long ago in the cases of Shetland and Orkney English (White and Mattys 2007) and earlier African American English (Thomas and Carter 2006). Dialectal variation in rhythm that is not explicable from substrate influences has been found for Bristol English compared to standard British English (White and Mattys 2007) and across US regions (Clopper and Smiljanic 2015), but far more variation of that type undoubtedly exists and awaits investigation. Three exceptions to the English focus are Frota and Vigário (2001), who found some rhythmic differences between European and Brazilian Portuguese; Gazali, Hamdi, and Barkat (2002), who noted some differences across Arabic; and O'Rourke (2008), who compared prosodic rhythm of Spanish monolinguals and Quichua/Spanish bilinguals in Peru.

Intonation

Contemporary intonation analyses are necessarily acoustic because they involve reference to f_0 tracks. A great deal of dialectal description of intonational variation consists of this sort of analysis, in which the analyst performs a combination of reading f_0 tracks and making auditory judgments. In contrast to vocalic and rhythmic studies, languages besides English have dominated these analyses. For example, studies have covered various national varieties of Spanish, as well as contact situations involving Spanish (see O'Rourke 2014 for a review). Examples of comparative dialectal studies of additional languages are Dalton and Ní Chasaide (2003) for Irish, Grabe (2004) for English, and Grice et al. (2005) for Italian. In English, the most heavily studied feature has been the "high rising terminal" (HRT), popularly called "uptalk," an innovative development in which statements terminate in a rise in f_0 instead of a fall (for a review, see Warren 2005). The 2016 Speech Prosody conference (http://sites.bu.edu/speechprosody2016/) had two full sessions on HRT. One exemplary instrumental analysis of HRT is Szakay's (2008) comparison of white and Māori New Zealanders' prosody.

Nevertheless, numerous other intonational studies have gone beyond simply interpreting f_0 tracks to conducting quantitative analyses of the acoustics. Various kinds of analyses have been used. Some metrics target timing, ordinarily examining f_0 peaks and troughs. One of the more commonly used metrics is peak delay, which compares the position of the highest f_0 value associated with a pitch accent with some landmark in the host vowel or host syllable, such as the lowest f_0 value or the offset of the vowel/syllable. Atterer and Ladd (2004) and Mücke et al. (2009) demonstrated that southern German tends to show later peaks and troughs than northern German. Aufterbeck (2004) and Ladd et al. (2009) each compared a variety of Scottish English to Southern British English (SBE), and both found that peaks averaged later in the Scottish varieties than in SBE when prosodic context was controlled for. Another study, Arvaniti and Garding (2007), showed that the f_0 maximum for L*+H pitch accents averages later in California English than in Minnesota English. Other examples of studies examining dialectal variation in the temporal placement of peaks include van Heuven and van Leyden (2003) for Shetland and Orkney English and O'Rourke (2012) for Peruvian Spanish varieties with and without influence from Quechua. Peters, Hanssen, and Gussenhoven (2015) tested a related phenomenon, that of how a peak moves when a nuclear word or foot is lengthened, with speakers from five locations in The Netherlands and one in Germany. They found variation among the dialects, depending on prosodic context, in whether the peak was aligned with the onset or offset of the word/foot or with both.

Intonational metrics can also involve measurements of f_0 frequencies of the peak of a pitch accent or edge tone, often converted to ERB units and sometimes examining the pitch excursion – i.e., the difference in Hz or ERB between the peak and a corresponding trough. Some inquiries (e.g., Colantoni and Gurlekian 2004; Willis 2007c; O'Rourke 2014) have shown how excursion patterns of different kinds of utterances define certain dialects of Spanish. Another use of frequency was developed by Grabe et al. (2000), who showed that various English dialects in the British Isles differ in whether they maintain the amount of excursion (compression) or reduce the excursion (truncation) when the duration of a foot is reduced. The shape of a peak – pointed or flat-topped – is an additional factor for which f_0 frequency could be assessed (see Niebuhr and Hoekstra 2015).

Most intonation work is descriptive, examining the structure of a dialect or comparing intonational structures across dialects, or is designed to investigate phonetic questions such as how peak placement is affected as metrical feet grow longer. Some, such as Queen (2001, 2006, 2012), Elordieta (2003), Colantoni and Gurlekian (2004), and O'Rourke (2014), tie intonational features of specific dialects to language contact. Few studies have examined how intonation is used for social indexicality. One exception is Podesva (2011), who showed how gay men manipulated the f_0 and duration of intonational contours to project different personas.

Lexical tone

Because sociophoneticians have predominantly set their sights on Western languages, it is unsurprising that little instrumental work has been conducted on variation in lexical tone. There are a few exceptions. Bauer, Kwan-Hin, and Pak-Man (2003) and Mok, Zuo, and

Wong (2013) examined tonal merger in Hong Kong Cantonese, and Zhang (2014) performed comparisons of regional, age group, and stylistic variation in Wu tones. Two studies analyzed threatened languages in southern China, Stanford (2008) on how tone in Sui is affected by dialect contact and Yang, Stanford, and Yang (2015) on a tonal split in Lalo. Nevertheless, most work on tonal variation continues to rely on auditory transcription, and acoustic work on lexical tone is clearly a wide-open field.

Rate of speech

Rate of speech has not been explored extensively from the perspective of social variation. Much of the existing literature focuses on differences in overall rate of speech among different groups (e.g., Ray and Zahn 1990; Robb, Maclagan, and Chen 2004; Quené 2008). Kendall (2013), however, offers a demonstration of other methods for approaching it, such as analyzing pause durations, taking conversations apart into different sections, and correlating rate of speech with other variables. Some of these suggestions are incorporated into Clopper and Smiljanic (2015), who found complex interactions between gender and region within the US for rate and duration of pauses. The latter study also reported modest regional differences in articulation rates, with the slowest from Midland and Southern speakers and the fastest from New England and Mid-Atlantic subjects.

Voice quality

Voice quality has rarely been explored in instrumental sociophonetic studies. A few studies have examined differences in overall f_0, showing that some groups produce higher or lower average f_0 values than others (e.g., Walton and Orlikoff 1994; Szakay and Torgersen 2015). Yuasa (2008) went a step further, showing that Japanese and American men and women employ pitch range differently according to cultural and gender norms for particular pragmatic functions. Yuasa (2010) showed that American women use creaky voicing extensively, whereas Japanese women do not (see also Wolk, Abdelli-Beruh, and Slavin 2011 and a subjective reaction experiment in Anderson et al. 2014). A study of performed speech by entertainers (Moisik 2012) suggested that harsh voice quality is stereotypically associated with African Americans. Soskuthy et al. (2017) suggested a possible connection between changes in voice quality and /r/ production in Glasgow English. Plichta (2002) employed both acoustic and articulatory measures to show that differing levels of nasality characterize a particular vowel in different sections of Michigan, and Ikuta (2013) showed that nasality characterizes the speech of clerks in shops with a young clientele in Japan, but otherwise nasality has attracted little sociophonetic study.

The state of socio-production studies

As can be seen in the preceding sections, sociophonetic studies of speech production have been extensive insofar as they have covered virtually every genre of phonetic variable. This research has illuminated both fine details of phonetic structures and structural properties of variation and change in language. A great deal of information has been uncovered on such issues as how phonological contrasts can be maintained, how language transfer can affect sound systems, what kinds of transitional forms occur in particular sound changes, and how broad the span of features for which apparently similar dialects can differ is.

Nevertheless, the indexicality of variants is not always examined, and when it is, it tends to be limited to gross demographic factors, such as geographical dialects, gender, or ethnic groups. Relatively few studies, such as Fought (1999), Lawson, Scobbie, and Stuart-Smith (2011, 2013) and Podesva (2011), have used instrumental techniques to examine the indexicality of forms with networks of people or for projecting one's identity in various settings. Most sociolinguistic projects that have dealt in depth with the construction of identity (e.g., Mendoza-Denton 2008; Hoffman and Walker 2010; Meyerhoff and Schleef 2012) have not exploited instrumental phonetic techniques to any great extent.

What is needed is inquiry that combines advanced instrumental methods with careful attention to the indexical properties of linguistic variants. Research that successfully amalgamates these two areas will be useful for explaining how sound changes can take on social meanings and then how this metalinguistic information passes through social networks. Moreover, it can also help sociophoneticians to address cognitive aspects of language. Indexicality is often lodged in phonetic subtleties and its extraction requires instrumental analysis (Docherty and Foulkes 1999). The cognitive links between forms and social meaning are essential to language. Exploration of these connections is commonly relegated to perception studies, the topic of the next section, but more attention should be given to them in production studies as well. Greater study of style shifting would be particularly useful in that regard, as would studies of second dialect acquisition (e.g., Nycz 2013) and accommodation (e.g., Pardo et al. 2012).

Socio-perception

Speech perception has always played an important role in sociophonetics, even though much of the perception research has had a low profile. The experimental problems addressed have been diverse, which has made socio-perception seem more difficult than production work to summarize in a succinct narrative. Nevertheless, perception experiments, along with functional neural imaging, represent the most direct routes for exploring cognition of language variation.

Certain types of experiments are designed to test whether a listener has two phonological categories merged or distinct. One such design is a commutation experiment, in which listeners are played recordings of words containing the sounds in question, uttered by speakers of their own dialect or other dialects, and are asked to identify each word (see Labov 1994 for examples). Another design, used by Janson and Schulman (1983), involves creation of a synthetic continuum of sounds within a frame representing a word and asking listeners to identify which word they hear for each stimulus. Labov, Karan, and Miller (1991) pointed out a limitation in that design – it depends on conscious knowledge of the language and thus can be affected by factors such as standardization – and created a functional test in which listeners heard a story for which the interpretation hinged on a single word that could contain either of the potentially merged sounds. More recently, some brain scanning work using event-related potentials (ERP) has been conducted on how listeners with and without a phonological merger process the affected sounds (Conrey, Potts, and Niedzielski 2005; Brunelliére et al. 2009).

A similar experimental design is to present listeners with stimuli and to ask them to identify the phone they hear. Earlier examples (Willis 1972; Janson 1983, 1986; Thomas 2000) examined how dialectal differences and ongoing sound change created differences in perceptual boundaries between sounds among different speakers. More recent experiments have shown that these perceptual boundaries can be surprisingly malleable. Rakerd and Plichta (2010) demonstrated that listeners from a dialect in which a vowel shift had occurred adjusted a perceptual boundary according to whether the carrier sentence of a stimulus was spoken in their dialect or not. Evans and Iverson (2004) reported similar shifts for British listeners when they heard different English accents. Other experiments have shown that being told that a speaker is from one dialect or another (Niedzielski 1999) or even seeing items suggestive of one region or another (Hay, Nolan, and Drager 2006; Hay and Drager 2010) can induce listeners to shift their perceptual boundaries. Maye, Aslin, and Tanenhaus (2008) had subjects listen to an artificial dialect and then to identify stimuli, and the results showed that the listeners' perceptual boundaries had shifted. In contrast, however, Evans and Iverson (2007) found that natives of northern England who had moved to southern England exhibited shifting of their perceptual norms only if their production norms had also shifted.

A third kind of experiment involves having listeners identify characteristics of speakers whose voices they hear in stimuli. One sort of identification task is to have listeners identify each speaker's dialect. Numerous such experiments have been carried out with American regional dialects (e.g., Preston 1993; Clopper, Levi, and Pisoni 2006; Clopper and Pisoni 2007; Clopper and Bradlow 2009; Baker, Eddington and Nay 2009), but other varieties of English (Bush 1967; van Bezooijen and Gooskens 1999; Williams, Garrett, and Coupland 1999) and Dutch dialects (van Bezooijen and Gooskens 1999) have also been tested. Moreover, dozens of experiments on the distinguishability of European American and African American voices have been conducted; see Thomas and Reaser (2004, 2015) for reviews. These experiments have examined not just whether listeners can identify dialects but also what features they rely on, whether some dialects are more perceptually similar than others, whether more prototypical or stereotypical speakers are easier to identify than others, and whether some listeners are better at identification (usually based on level of exposure) than others. In addition to dialect identification, however, listeners may also be asked to name personal attributes of speakers, such as intelligence, friendliness, or trustworthiness, in a subjective reaction experiment. The matched-guise experiment of Lambert et al. (1960) falls into this category. An extensive review of early subjective reaction experiments appears in Giles and Powesland (1975); see also the review in Thomas (2002). The aim of such experiments is to lay bare the listeners' stereotypical attitudes or, as in such recent studies as Labov et al. (2011), Levon and Fox (2014), and Bekker and Levon (2017), the social indexicality of variants. Some recent experiments, notably Hay, Warren, and Drager (2006), have gone a step further in showing that listeners cognitively tie forms with specific subgroups within a community. All of these identification experiments target what Kristiansen (2008) terms listeners' "receptive competence," their often subconscious association of linguistic forms with groups of speakers and stereotypes about those groups.

Finally, many experiments have tested the intelligibility of particular voices according to their dialect. Some experiments (e.g., Mason 1946; Arahill 1970; van Bezooijen and Gooskens 1999; van Bezooijen and van den Berg 1999), simply test the general intelligibility of different dialects. Nguyen et al. (2015) showed that listeners' affective attitudes about speakers influenced their accuracy in identifying vowels. Other experiments have introduced timing of responses (e.g., Floccia et al. 2006; Impe, Geeraerts, and Speelman 2008; Adank et al. 2009), finding that dialects have some processing cost for listeners, especially if they are unfamiliar to the listeners, but not as much as foreign accents, and that listeners adapt to the dialects. An ERP study by Goslin, Duffy, and Floccia (2012) also found that regional dialects are processed more quickly and by a different cognitive mechanism than foreign accents. Sumner and Samuel (2009) constructed a prime/target experiment with response timing and corroborated the importance of familiarity, though they also suggested that listeners familiar with a dialect might differ in whether they store only one or both competing forms in memory.

The cognitive perspective afforded by socio-perceptual work has allowed researchers to address more general issues of linguistic representation. Since Johnson (1997) proposed an exemplar model of linguistic processing, in which linguistic forms are stored and accessed as statistically stored memories of heard utterances instead of as abstractions, there has been considerable debate about episodic vs. abstract models of language. The feature of episodic models that makes them attractive for sociolinguists, as Foulkes and Docherty (2006) argued, is that memories of the context and speaker are retained along with the linguistic form, and all of this information is cognitively linked together. Thus, the indexicality of social information becomes firmly rooted within one's linguistic competence. Since then, "hybrid models" that incorporate both episodic and abstract aspects (Connine and Pinnow 2006; Pierrehumbert 2006; Sumner et al. 2014) have come into vogue. Such models parallel current neurolinguistic models (e.g., Paradis 2000) that recognize both implicit (related to abstract competence) and explicit (related to episodic processing) aspects of language processing in the brain. A hybrid model is outlined in Figure 16.1. Information flows from the exemplars – shown scattered across a hypothetical phonetic space – to the lexical representations, either via phonological coding or directly. The

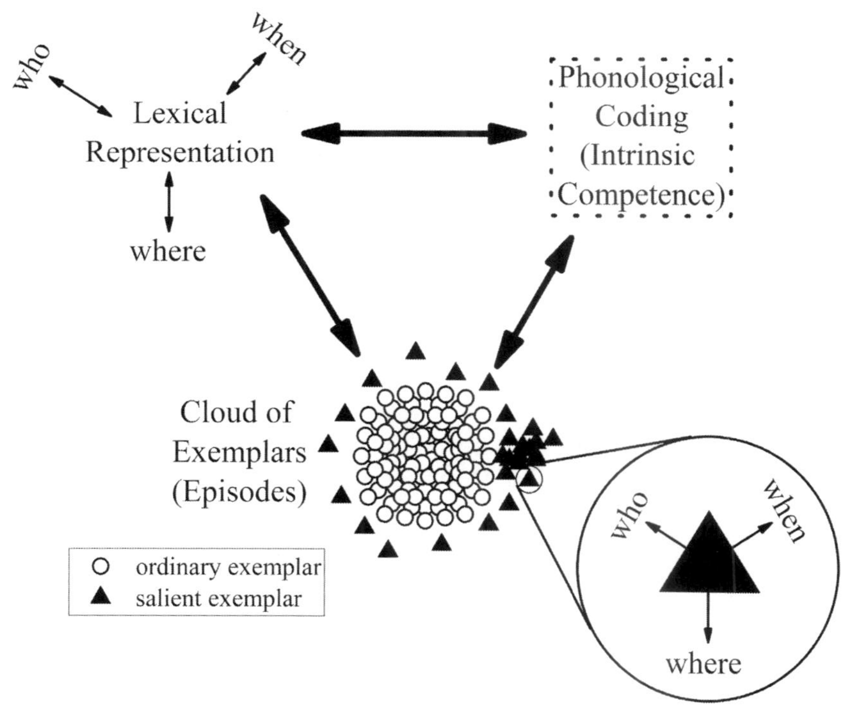

Figure 16.1 A "hybrid" model of the processing of phonetic signals, with both a direct route between the exemplar cloud and a route via phonological coding. The cluster of salient exemplars on the right side of the exemplar cloud represents input from an overtly or covertly prestigious dialect differing from the speaker's own. The exemplars are arranged on hypothetical perceptual dimensions as processed by the auditory system. The dashed lines around the Phonological Coding represent some degree of modularity for that component of the system.

phonological coding component explains why speech shows categorical effects – e.g., heard sounds are immediately interpreted as one phonological category (a phoneme or allophone) or another, but not as some intermediate form. However, perceptual boundaries between those categories are capable of shifting over time as a person is exposed to input from different dialects, or the listener can develop customized perception norms for different dialects. The person's production norms can also shift subtly, especially if he or she is immersed in a new dialectal setting. Episodic effects explain this flexibility. Memories of exemplars, especially the most salient ones – which are typically the phonetically most atypical ones – exhibit neural connections to memories of who said them, when they were said, and in what situation they were uttered, aiding the perception of speech uttered by diverse people. Production forms are selected to match remembered exemplars and they may be tailored to match the audience based on the remembered store of exemplars. Older episodic models appeared similar except that they lacked the phonological coding stage.

Further socio-production work has suggested that episodic representations can be sufficient for explaining how the "same" word may be realized differently according to social situation (Drager 2011) and for explaining lexical effects in sound change (Hay et al. 2015). Details about the social associations remain to be worked out. The statistical understanding that Johnson (1997) contended to be important for constructing phonetic forms might also be applied to other remembered aspects of exemplars; as Clark and Trousdale (2010) suggest, people may construct associations with social contexts, not just particular events, and link them cognitively with phonetic forms. Another such detail is that of why some exemplars are more salient than others. Sumner et al. (2014) argue that the simultaneous storage of linguistic and social information about exemplars is accompanied by social weighting so that some forms, such as certain hyperstandard forms – in their example, released, unglottalized final [t] as opposed to the glottalized, unreleased forms that are more common in conversational American English – receive more cognitive activation. A similar memory bias might be associated with forms uttered by people the listener wishes to emulate.

General assessment

Sociophonetics has grown to become an essential element of phonetics, sociolinguistics, and laboratory phonology. In the process, it has become the favored paradigm for studies of variation in phonetic properties of languages. The major difficulty limiting its further growth is that practitioners frequently see it as just a methodological approach (especially in sociolinguistics) or as a convenient label for studies that involve dialectal variation (particularly in phonetics). It should be recognized that sociophonetics has a theoretical side that can serve as an avenue for exploration of major linguistic questions. One of these major issues is that of how linguistic change occurs. As discussed in earlier sections, a large proportion of sociophonetic work has been devoted to examining sound change, and these studies not only have permeated all types of phonetic factors but also have shown how pervasive variation is, how it operates in languages, and how communities can transition from one form to another. The next step is to explore the cognition of variation. Perception studies have begun to do that, but among production studies a disconnect has emerged between those that have focused on metalinguistic knowledge and those that have taken advantage of modern phonetic methods. That is, much sociolinguistic work on production in recent years has dealt with such issues as theories of identity construction, but these studies often rely on old methods such as auditory transcription; conversely, sociolinguistic studies that employ cutting-edge acoustic techniques seldom address the most current sociolinguistic theories.

A cognitive approach to sociophonetics must emphasize the indexicality of variants: what do people "know" about who uses a variant and the contexts in which people use it? This sort of work often focuses on social networks in asking which networks use a form, how a form can become an identity marker for a network, and how knowledge about usage and identity is disseminated through communities. Sociolinguists concerned with those issues can become preoccupied with the networks themselves, which certainly are sociologically important. However, linguists need to look toward how this metalinguistic information is cognitively linked to linguistic structures. For linguists, the ultimate goal is to discover how language is mentally encoded. Episodic accounts of language (along with hybrid models that include episodic components) suggest that all linguistic forms come with contextual information, and sociolinguistic research has shown that contextual knowledge directs linguistic choices at every level. As a result, understanding mental connections, not just between strictly linguistic levels such as lexical and post-lexical or implicit and explicit but between metalinguistic knowledge and linguistic structures, is what makes sociophonetics relevant for the larger enterprises in linguistics.

References

Adank, Patti, Bronwen G. Evans, Jane Stuart-Smith, and Sophie K. Scott. 2009. Comprehension of familiar and unfamiliar native accents under adverse listening conditions. *Journal of Experimental Psychology: Human Perception and Performance* 35:520–529.

Adank, Patti, Roeland van Hout, and Hans van de Velde. 2007. An acoustic description of the vowels of northern and southern standard Dutch II: Regional varieties. *The Journal of the Acoustical Society of America* 121:1130–1141.

Anderson, Rindy C., Casey A. Klofstad, William J. Mayew, and Mohan Venkatachalam. 2014. Vocal fry may undermine the success of young women in the labor market. *PLoS One* 9.5:1–8.

Arahill, Edward Joseph. 1970. The effect of differing dialects upon the comprehension and attitude of eighth grade children. Ph.D. diss., University of Florida.

Arvaniti, Amalia, and Gina Garding. 2007. Dialectal variation in the rising accents of American English. In Jennifer Cole and José Ignacio Hualde, eds., *Laboratory Phonology 9*, pp. 547–575. Berlin/New York: Mouton de Gruyter.

Ash, Sharon. 2002. The distribution of a phonemic split in the Mid-Atlantic region: Yet more on short *a*. *University of Pennsylvania Working Papers in Linguistics* 8:1–15.

Atterer, Michaela, and D. Robert Ladd. 2004. On the phonetics and phonology of "segmental anchoring" of f_0: Evidence from German. *Journal of Phonetics* 32:177–197.

Aufterbeck, Margit. 2004. Identifying sociolinguistic variables in intonation: The onset onglide in Anstruther Scottish English. In Gilles and Peters, *Regional Variation in Intonation*. Linguistische Arbeiten, Band 492, eds., pp. 33–48. Tübingen: Max Niemeyer Verlag.

Baker, Adam, Diana Archangeli, and Jeff Mielke. 2011. Variability in American English *s*-retraction suggests a solution to the actuation problem. *Language Variation and Change* 23:347–374.

Baker, Wendy, David Eddington, and Lyndsey Nay. 2009. Dialect identification: The effects of region of origin and amount of experience. *American Speech* 84:48–71.

Baranowski, Maciej. 2007. *Phonological Variation and Change in the Dialect of Charleston, South Carolina*. Publication of the American Dialect Society, Vol. 82. Durham, NC: Duke University Press.

Baranowski, Maciej. 2017. Class matters: The sociolinguistics of GOOSE and GOAT in Manchester English. *Language Variation and Change* 29:301–339.

Baranowski, Maciej, and Danielle Turton. Forthcoming. TD-deletion in British English: New evidence for the long lost morphological effect. *Language Variation and Change*.

Bauer, Matt, and Frank Parker. 2008. /æ/-raising in Wisconsin English. *American Speech* 83:403–431.

Bauer, Robert S., Cheung Kwan-Hin, and Cheung Pak-Man. 2003. Variation and merger of the rising tones in Hong Kong Cantonese. *Language Variation and Change* 15:211–225.

Bekker, Ian, and Erez Levon. 2017. The embedded indexical value of /s/-fronting in Afrikaans and South African English. *Linguistics* 55:1109–1139.

Benson, Erica J., Michael J. Fox, and Jared Balkman. 2011. *The bag that Scott bought*: The low vowels in northwest Wisconsin. *American Speech* 86:271–311.

Bezooijen, Renée van. 1988. The relative importance of pronunciation, prosody and voice quality for the attribution of social status and personality characteristics. In Roeland van Hout and Uus Knops, eds., *Language Attitudes in the Dutch Language Area*, pp. 85–103. Dordrecht: Foris.

Blake, Renée, and Meredith Josey. 2003. The /ay/ diphthong in a Martha's Vineyard community: What can we say 40 years after Labov? *Language in Society* 32:451–485.

Boberg, Charles, and Stephanie M. Strassel. 2000. Short-a in Cincinnati. *Journal of English Linguistics* 28:108–126.

Brown, Bruce L., William J. Strong, and Alvin C. Rencher. 1972. Acoustic determinants of perceptions of personality from speech. *International Journal of the Sociology of Language* 6:11–32.

Brunelliére, Angéle, Sophie Dufour, Noël Nguyen, and Ulrich Hans Frauenfelder. 2009. Behavioral and electrophysiological evidence for the impact of regional variation on phoneme perception. *Cognition* 111:390–396.

Bush, Clara N. 1967. Some acoustic parameters of speech and their relationships to the perception of dialect differences. *TESOL Quarterly* 1.3:20–30.

Caramazza, Alfonso, and Grace H. Yeni-Komshian. 1974. Voice onset time in two French dialects. *Journal of Phonetics* 2:239–245.

Carter, Paul, and John Local. 2007. F_2 variation in Newcastle and Leeds English liquid systems. *Journal of the International Phonetic Association* 37:183–199.

Carter, Phillip M. 2005. Quantifying rhythmic differences between Spanish, English, and Hispanic English. In Randall Gess, ed., *Theoretical and Experimental Approaches to Romance Linguistics: Selected Papers from the 34th Linguistic Symposium on Romance Languages*, pp. 63–75. Amsterdam/Philadelphia: John Benjamins.

Celata, Chiara, and Silvia Calamai, eds. 2014. *Advances in Sociophonetics*. Studies in language variation, 15. Amsterdam/Philadelphia: John Benjamins.

Choi, H. 2002. Acoustic cues for the Korean stop contrast – dialectal variation. *ZAS Papers in Linguistics* 28:1–12.

Clark, Lynn, and Graeme Trousdale. 2010. A cognitive approach to quantitative sociolinguistic variation: Evidence from th-fronting in central Scotland. In Dirk Geeraerts, Gitte Kristiansen, and Yves Peirsman, eds., *Advances in Cognitive Sociolinguistics*, pp. 291–321. Cognitive linguistics research, no. 45. Berlin/New York: Mouton de Gruyter.

Clopper, Cynthia G., and Ann R. Bradlow. 2009. Free classification of American English dialects by native and non-native listeners. *Journal of Phonetics* 37:436–451.

Clopper, Cynthia G., Susannah V. Levi, and David B. Pisoni. 2006. Perceptual similarity of regional dialects of American English. *The Journal of the Acoustical Society of America* 119:566–574.

Clopper, Cynthia G., and David B. Pisoni. 2007. Free classification of regional dialects of American English. *Journal of Phonetics* 35:421–438.

Clopper, Cynthia G., David B. Pisoni, and Kenneth de Jong. 2005. Acoustic characteristics of the vowel systems of six regional varieties of American English. *The Journal of the Acoustical Society of America* 118:1661–1676.

Clopper, Cynthia G., and Rajka Smiljanic. 2015. Regional variation in temporal organization in American English. *Journal of Phonetics* 49:1–15.

Coggshall, Elizabeth L. 2008. The prosodic rhythm of two varieties of Native American English. *University of Pennsylvania Working Papers in Linguistics* 14:1–9.

Colantoni, Laura. 2006. Micro and macro sound variation and change in Argentine Spanish. In Nuria Sagarra and Almeida Jacqueline Toribio, eds., *Selected Proceedings of the 9th Hispanic Linguistics Symposium*, pp. 91–102. Somerville, MA: Cascadilla.

Colantoni, Laura, and Gorge Gurlekian. 2004. Convergence and intonation: Historical evidence from Buenos Aires Spanish. *Bilingualism: Language and Cognition* 7:107–119.

Connine, Cynthia M., and Eleni Pinnow. 2006. Phonological variation in spoken word recognition: Episodes and abstractions. *The Linguistic Review* 23:235–245.

Conrey, Brianna, Geoffrey F. Potts, and Nancy A. Niedzielski. 2005. Effects of dialect on merger perception: ERP and behavioral correlates. *Brain and Language* 95:435–449.

Cox, Felicity. 1999. Vowel change in Australian English. *Phonetica* 56:1–27.

Dalton, Martha, and Ailbhe Ní Chasaide. 2003. Modelling intonation in three Irish dialects. In *Proceedings of the 15th International Congress of Phonetic Sciences, Barcelona*. www.internationalphoneticassociation.org/icphs/icphs2003

De Decker, Paul, and Jennifer R. Nycz. 2012. Are tense [æ]s really tense? The mapping between articulation and acoustics. *Lingua* 122:810–821.

Deschaies-Lafontaine, Denise. 1974. A socio-phonetic study of a Québec French community: Trois-Riviéres. Ph.D. diss., University College London.

Deser, Toni. 1990. Dialect transmission and variation: An acoustic analysis of vowels in six urban Detroit families. Ph.D. diss., Boston University.

Deterding, David. 2001. The measurement of rhythm: A comparison of Singapore and British English. *Journal of Phonetics* 29:217–230.

Deterding, David. 2003. An instrumental study of the monophthong vowels of Singapore English. *English World-Wide* 24:1–16.

Deterding, David. 2005. Emergent patterns in the vowels of Singapore English. *English World-Wide* 26:179–197.

Deterding, David, Jennie Wong, and Andy Kirkpatrick. 2008. The pronunciation of Hong Kong English. *English World-Wide* 29:148–175.

Di Paolo, Marianna. 1992. Hypercorrection in response to the apparent merger of (ɔ) and (ɑ) in Utah English. *Language and Communication* 12:267–292.

Di Paolo, Marianna, and Alice Faber. 1990. Phonation differences and the phonetic content of the tense-lax contrast in Utah English. *Language Variation and Change* 2:155–204.

Di Paolo, Marianna, and Malcah Yaeger-Dror. 2011. *Sociophonetics: A Student's Guide*. London: Routledge.

Docherty, Gerard J., and Paul Foulkes. 1999. Derby and Newcastle: Instrumental phonetics and variationist studies. In Paul Foulkes and Gerard J. Docherty, eds., *Urban Voices: Accent Studies in the British Isles*, pp. 47–71. London: Arnold.

Dodsworth, Robin, and Kirk A. Hazen. 2012. Going to L in Appalachia: Language change for L-vocalization in the Mountain State. *Presented at the 86th Annual Meeting of the Linguistic Society of America,* Portland, OR, January.

Drager, Katie K. 2011. Sociophonetic variation and the lemma. *Journal of Phonetics* 39:694–707.

Durian, David. 2012. A new perspective on vowel variation across the 19th and 20th centuries in Columbus. Ph.D. diss., The Ohio State University, OH.

Elordieta, Gorka. 2003. The Spanish intonation of speakers of a Basque pitch-accent dialect. *Catalan Journal of Linguistics* 2:67–95.

Eriksson, Anders. 2004. Swedia-Projektet: Dialektforskning i ett jämförande perspektiv. *Folkmålsstudier* 43:11–31.

Erker, Daniel G. 2010. A subsegmental approach to coda /s/ weakening in Dominican Spanish. *International Journal of the Sociology of Language* 201:9–26.

Evanini, Keelan. 2008. A shift of allegiance: The case of Erie and the North/Midland boundary. *University of Pennsylvania Working Papers in Linguistics* 14:72–82.

Evans, Bronwen G., and Paul Iverson. 2004. Vowel normalization for accent: An investigation of best exemplar locations in northern and southern British English sentences. *The Journal of the Acoustical Society of America* 115:352–361.

Evans, Bronwen G., and Paul Iverson. 2007. Plasticity in vowel perception and production: A study of accent change in young adults. *The Journal of the Acoustical Society of America* 121:3814–3826.

Evans, Bronwen G., Ajay Mistry, and Caroline Moreiras. 2007. An acoustic study of first- and second-generation Gujarati immigrants in Wembley: Evidence for accent convergence? In *Proceedings of the 16th International Conference on Phonetic Sciences, Saarbrücken, 6–10 August*, pp. 1741–1744.

File-Muriel, Richard J., and Earl K. Brown. 2011. The gradient nature of s-lenition in Caleño Spanish. *Language Variation and Change* 23:223–243.

Floccia, Caroline, Jeremy Goslin, Frédérique Girard, and Gabriel Konopczynski. 2006. Does a regional accent perturb speech processing? *Journal of Experimental Psychology: Human Perception and Performance* 32:1276–1293.

Fought, Carmen. 1999. A majority sound change in a minority community: /u/-fronting in Chicano English. *Journal of Sociolinguistics* 3:5–23.

Foulkes, Paul, and Gerard J. Docherty. 2006. The social life of phonetics and phonology. *Journal of Phonetics* 34:409–438.

Foulkes, Paul, James M. Scobbie, and Dominic J. L. Watt. 2010. Sociophonetics. In William J. Hardcastle and John Laver, eds., *Handbook of Phonetic Sciences*, pp. 703–754. 2nd ed. Oxford: Wiley-Blackwell.

Fourakis, Marios, and Robert Port. 1986. Stop epenthesis in English. *Journal of Phonetics* 14:197–221.

Fox, Robert A., and Ewa Jacewicz. 2009. Cross-dialectal variation in formant dynamics of American English vowels. *The Journal of the Acoustical Society of America* 126:2603–2618.

Frazer, Timothy C. 1987. Attitudes toward regional pronunciation. *Journal of English Linguistics* 20:89–100.

Fridland, Valerie. 2001. The social dimension of the southern vowel shift: Gender, age and class. *Journal of Sociolinguistics* 5:233–253.

Fridland, Valerie. 2003a. Network strength and the realization of the southern shift among African Americans in Memphis, Tennessee. *American Speech* 78:3–30.

Fridland, Valerie. 2003b. 'Tie, tied and tight': The expansion of /ai/ monophthongization in African-American and European-American speech in Memphis, Tennessee. *Journal of Sociolinguistics* 7:279–298.

Fridland, Valerie, and Kathy Bartlett. 2006. The social and linguistic conditioning of back vowel fronting across ethnic groups in Memphis, Tennessee. *English Language and Linguistics* 10:1–22.

Fridland, Valerie, Tyler Kendall, and Charlie Farrington. 2014. Durational and spectral differences in American English vowels: Dialect variation within and across regions. *The Journal of the Acoustical Society of America* 136:341–349.

Frota, Sónia, and Marina Vigário. 2001. On the correlates of rhythmic distinctions: The European/Brazilian Portuguese case. *Probus* 13:247–275.

Fruehwald, Josef. 2016. The early influence of phonology on a phonetic change. *Language* 92:376–410.

Ghazali, Salem, Rym Hamdi, and Melissa Barkat. 2002. Speech rhythm variation in Arabic dialects. In *Proceedings of Speech Prosody*, pp. 331–334. Aix-en-Provence: Laboratorie Parole et Langage. http://aune.lpl.univ-aix.fr/sp2002/

Giles, Howard, and Peter F. Powesland. 1975. *Speech Style and Social Evaluation*. New York: Academic.

Gilles, Peter, and Jörg Peters, eds. 2004. *Regional Variation in Intonation*. Linguistische Arbeiten 492. Tübingen: Max Niemeyer Verlag.

Godinez, Manuel, Jr. 1984. Chicano English phonology: Norms vs. interference phenomena. In Ornstein-Galicia, Jacob, ed., *Form and Function in Chicano English*, pp. 42–47. Rowley, MA: Newberry.

Godinez, Manuel, Jr., and Ian Maddieson. 1985. Vowel differences between Chicano and general Californian English? *International Journal of the Sociology of Language* 53:43–58.

Goslin, Jeremy, Hester Duffy, and Caroline Floccia. 2012. An ERP investigation of regional and foreign accent processing. *Brain and Language* 122:92–102.

Grabe, Esther. 2004. Intonational variation in urban dialects of English spoken in the British Isles. In Gilles, Peter and Jörg, Peters, eds., *Regional Variation in Intonation*. Linguistische Arbeiten 492, pp. 9–31. Tübingen: Max Niemeyer Verlag.

Grabe, Esther, Brechtje Post, Francis Nolan, and Kimberley Farrar. 2000. Pitch accent realization in four varieties of British English. *Journal of Phonetics* 28:161–185.

Grice, Martine, Mariapaola D'Imperio, Michelina Savino, and Cinzia Avesani. 2005. Strategies for intonation labelling across varieties of Italian. In Sun-Ah Jun, ed., *Prosodic Typology: The Phonology of Intonation and Phrasing*, pp. 362–389. Oxford: Oxford University Press.

Habick, Timothy. 1980. Sound change in Farmer City: A sociolinguistic study based on acoustic data. Ph.D. diss., University of Illinois at Urbana-Champaign.

Hagiwara, Robert. 1997. Dialect variation and formant frequency: The American English vowels revisited. *The Journal of the Acoustical Society of America* 102:655–658.

Hall-Lew, Lauren. 2009. Ethnicity and phonetic variation in a San Francisco neighborhood. Ph.D. diss., Stanford University.

Hay, Jennifer, and Katie Drager. 2007. Sociophonetics. *Annual Review of Anthropology* 36:89–103.

Hay, Jennifer, and Katie Drager. 2010. Stuffed toys and speech perception. *Linguistics* 48:865–892.

Hay, Jennifer, Aaron Nolan, and Katie Drager. 2006. From *fush* to *feesh*: Exemplar priming in speech production. *The Linguistic Review* 23:351–379.

Hay, Jennifer B., Janet B. Pierrehumbert, Abby J. Walker, and Patrick LaShell. 2015. Tracking word frequency effects through 130 years of sound change. *Cognition* 139:83–91.

Hay, Jennifer B., Paul Warren, and Katie Drager. 2006. Factors influencing speech perception in the context of a merger-in-progress. *Journal of Phonetics* 34:458–484.

Hejna, Michaela. 2015. Pre-aspiration in Welsh English: A case study of Aberystwyth. Ph.D. thesis, University of Manchester.

Henriksen, Nicholas C., and Erik W. Willis. 2010. Acoustic characterization of phonemic trill production in Jerezano Andalusian Spanish. In Marta Ortega-Llebaria, ed., *Selected Proceedings of the 4th Conference on Laboratory Approaches to Spanish Phonology*, pp. 115–127. Somerville, MA: Cascadilla.

Heselwood, Barry, and Louise McChrystal. 1999. The effect of age-group and place of L1 acquisition on the realisation of Panjabi stop consonants in Bradford: An acoustic sociophonetic study. *Leeds Working Papers in Linguistics and Phonetics* 7:49–69.

Hindle, Donald. 1980. The social and structural conditioning of vowel variation. Ph.D. diss., University of Pennsylvania.

Hoffman, Michol F., and James A. Walker. 2010. Ethnolects and the city: Ethnic orientation and linguistic variation in Toronto English. *Language Variation and Change* 22:37–67.

Hoffman, Thomas. 2011. The black Kenyan English vowel system. *English World-Wide* 32:147–173.

Ikuta, Shoko. 2013. Nasality as a social identity marker in urban Japanese. *Journal of English & American Literature and Linguistics* 128:61–74.

Impe, Leen, Dirk Geeraerts, and Dirk Speelman. 2008. Mutual intelligibility of standard and regional Dutch varieties. *International Journal of Humanities and Arts Computing* 2:101–117.

Irons, Terry Lynn. 2007. On the status of low back vowels in Kentucky English: More evidence of merger. *Language Variation and Change* 19:137–180.

Ito, Rika, and Dennis R. Preston. 1998. Identity, discourse, and language variation. *Journal of Language and Social Psychology* 17:465–483.

Jacewicz, Ewa, and Robert A. Fox. 2012. The effects of cross-generational and cross-dialectal variation on vowel identification and classification. *The Journal of the Acoustical Society of America* 131:1413–1433.

Jacewicz, Ewa, Robert A. Fox, and Joseph Salmons. 2011. Vowel change across three age groups of speakers in three regional varieties of American English. *Journal of Phonetics* 39:683–693.

Janson, Tore. 1983. Sound change in perception and production. *Language* 59:18–34.

Janson, Tore. 1986. Sound change in perception: An experiment. In John J. Ohala and Jeri J. Jaeger, eds., *Experimental Phonology*, pp. 253–260. Orlando: Academic.

Janson, Tore, and Richard Schulman. 1983. Non-distinctive features and their use. *Journal of Linguistics* 19:321–336.

Johnson, Bruce Lee. 1971. The western Pennsylvania dialect of American English. *Journal of the International Phonetic Association* 1:69–73.

Johnson, Daniel Ezra. 2010. *Stability and Change along a Dialect Boundary*. Publication of the American Dialect Society, 85. Durham, NC: Duke University Press.

Johnson, Daniel Ezra. 2015. Quantifying overlap with Bhattacharyya's affinity and other measures! *Paper presented at the 44th conference on New Ways of Analyzing Variation, Toronto, 25 October*.

Johnson, Keith. 1997. Speech perception without speaker normalization: An exemplar model. In Keith Johnson and John W. Mullennix, eds., *Talker Variability in Speech Processing*, pp. 145–165. San Diego: Academic.

Kang, Yoonjung, Tae-Jin Yoon, and Sungwoo Han. 2015. Frequency effects on the vowel length contrast merger in Seoul Korean. *Laboratory Phonology* 6:469–503.

Kendall, Tyler. 2013. *Speech Rate, Pause, and Sociolinguistic Variation: Studies in Corpus Linguistics*. Basingstoke: Palgrave Macmillan.

Kerswill, Paul, Eivind Nessa Torgersen, and Susan Fox. 2008. Reversing "drift:" Innovation and diffusion in the London diphthong system. *Language Variation and Change* 20:451–491.

Kirtley, M. Joelle, James Grama, Katie Drager, and Sean Simpson. 2016. An acoustic analysis of the vowels of Hawai'i English. *Journal of the International Phonetic Association* 46:79–97.

Kohn, Mary. 2013. Adolescent ethnolinguistic stability and change: A longitudinal study. Ph.D. diss., University of North Carolina at Chapel Hill.

Kristiansen, Gitte. 2008. Style-shifting and shifting styles: A socio-cognitive approach to lectal variation. In Gitte Kristiansen and René Dirven, eds., *Cognitive Sociolinguistics: Language Variation, Cultural Models, Social Systems*, pp. 45–88. Berlin/New York: Mouton de Gruyter.

Kvavik, Karen H. 1974. An analysis of sentence-initial and final intonational data in two Spanish dialects. *Journal of Phonetics* 2:351–361.

Labov, William. 1980. The social origins of sound change. In William Labov, ed., *Locating Language in Time and Space*, pp. 251–265. New York: Academic.

Labov, William. 1991. The three dialects of English. In Penelope Eckert, ed., *NewWays of Analyzing Sound Change*, pp. 1–44. New York: Academic.

Labov, William. 1994. *Principles of Linguistic Change. Volume 1: Internal Factors*. Language in Society, 20. Oxford/Malden, MA: Wiley-Blackwell.

Labov, William. 2001. *Principles of Linguistic Change. Volume 2: Social Factors*. Language in Society, 29. Oxford/Malden, MA: Wiley-Blackwell.

Labov, William. 2014. The role of African Americans in Philadelphia sound change. *Language Variation and Change* 26:1–19.

Labov, William, Sharon Ash, and Charles Boberg. 2006. *The Atlas of North American English: Phonetics, Phonology and Sound Change. A Multimedia Reference Tool*. Berlin: Mouton de Gruyter.

Labov, William, Sharon Ash, Maya Ravindranath, Tracey Weldon, Maciej Baranowski, and Naomi Nagy. 2011. Properties of the sociolinguistic monitor. *Journal of Sociolinguistics* 15:431–463.

Labov, William, Mark Karan, and Corey Miller. 1991. Near-mergers and the suspension of phonemic contrast. *Language Variation and Change* 3:33–74.

Labov, William, Ingrid Rosenfelder, and Josef Fruehwald. 2013. One hundred years of sound change in Philadelphia: Linear incrementation, reversal, and reanalysis. *Language* 89:30–65.

Labov, William, Malcah Yaeger, and Richard Steiner. 1972. *A Quantitative Study of Sound Change in Progress*. Philadelphia: U.S. Regional Survey.

Ladd, D. Robert, Astrid Schepman, Laurence White, Louise May Quarmby, and Rebekah Stackhouse. 2009. Structural and dialectal effects on pitch peak alignment in two varieties of British English. *Journal of Phonetics* 37:145–161.

Lambert, W[allace] E., Richard C. Hodgson, Robert C. Gardner, and Stanley Fillenbaum. 1960. Evaluational reaction to spoken language. *Journal of Abnormal and Social Psychology* 60:44–51.

Lawson, Eleanor, James M. Scobbie, and Jane Stuart-Smith. 2011. The social stratification of tongue shape for postvocalic /ɹ/ in Scottish English. *Journal of Sociolinguistics* 15:256–268.

Lawson, Eleanor, James M. Scobbie, and Jane Stuart-Smith. 2013. Bunched /r/ promotes vowel merger to schwar: An ultrasound tongue imaging study of Scottish sociophonetic variation. *Journal of Phonetics* 41:198–210.

Leinonen, Therese Nanette. 2010. An acoustic analysis of vowel pronunciation in Swedish dialects. Ph.D. diss., Rijksuniversiteit Groningen.

Levon, Erez, and Sue Fox. 2014. Social salience and the sociolinguistic monitor: A case study of ING and TH-fronting in Britain. *Journal of English Linguistics* 42:185–217.

Liu, Huangmei, and Jie Liang. 2016. VISC as acoustic cues for sub-dialect identification in Chinese. In *Proceedings of the 2016 Conference of the Oriental Chapter of the International Committee for Coordination and Standardization of Speech Databases and Assessment Techniques (O-COCOSDA)*, pp. 132–136. https://ieeexplore.ieee.org/stamp/stamp.jsp?tp=&arnumber=7918998

Low, Ee Ling, Esther Grabe, and Francis Nolan. 2000. Quantitative characterizations of speech rhythm: Syllable-timing in Singapore English. *Language and Speech* 43:377–401.

Maclagan, Margaret A. 1982. An acoustic study of New Zealand English vowels. *New Zealand Speech Therapists' Journal* 37:20–26.

Maclagan, Margaret A, and Jennifer Hay. 2007. Getting *fed* up with our *feet*: Contrast maintenance and the New Zealand "short" front vowel shift. *Language Variation and Change* 19:1–25.

Maclagan, Margaret A., Catherine I. Watson, Ray Harlow, Jeanette King, and Peter Keegan. 2009. /u/ fronting and /t/ aspiration in Māori and New Zealand English. *Language Variation and Change* 21:175–192.

Mansfield, John Basil. 2015. Consonant lenition as a sociophonetic variable in Murrinh Patha (Australia). *Language Variation and Change* 27:203–225.

Mason, Harry M. 1946. Understandability of speech in noise as affected by region of origin of speaker and listener. *Speech Monographs* 13.2:54–58.

Maye, Jessica, Richard N. Aslin, and Michael K. Tanenhaus. 2008. The weckud wetch of the wast: Lexical adaptation to a novel accent. *Cognitive Science* 32:543–562.

McClure, J. Derrick. 1995. The vowels of Scottish English – formants and features. In Jack Windsor Lewis, ed., *Studies in General and English Phonetics: Essays in Honour of Professor J. D. O'Connor*, pp. 367–378. London/New York: Routledge.

Mendoza-Denton, Norma. 2008. *Homegirls: Language and Cultural Practice among Latina Youth Gangs*. New directions in ethnography, no. 2. Malden, MA: Wiley-Blackwell.

Meyerhoff, Miriam, and Erik Schleef. 2012. Variation, contact and social indexicality in the acquisition of (ing) by teenage migrants. *Journal of Sociolinguistics* 16:398–416.

Michnowicz, Jim, and Lindsay Carpenter. 2013. Voiceless stop aspiration in Yucatan Spanish. *Spanish in Context* 10:410–437.

Mielke, Jeff, Adam Baker, and Diana Archangeli. 2010. Variability and homogeneity in American English /ɹ/ allophony and /s/ retraction. In Cécile Fougeron, Barbara Kühnert, Mariapaola D'Imperio, and Nathalie Vallée, ed., *Variation, Detail, and Representation (LabPhon10)*, pp. 699–719. Berlin: Mouton de Gruyter.

Mielke, Jeff, Christopher Carignan, and Erik R. Thomas. 2017. The articulatory dynamics of pre-velar and pre-nasal /æ/-raising in English: An ultrasound study. *The Journal of the Acoustical Society of America* 142:332–349.

Moisik, Scott Reid. 2012. Harsh voice quality and its association with Blackness in popular American media. *Phonetica* 69:193–215.

Mok, Peggy P. K., Donghui Zuo, and Peggy W. Y. Wong. 2013. Production and perception of a sound change in progress: Tone merging in Hong Kong Cantonese. *Language Variation and Change* 3:341–370.

Moosmüller, Sylvia, and Theodor Granser. 2006. The spread of standard Albanian: An illustration based on an analysis of vowels. *Language Variation and Change* 18:121–140.

Moreton, Elliott, and Erik Thomas. 2007. Origins of Canadian Raising in voiceless-coda effects: A case study in phonologization. In Jennifer Cole and José Ignacio Hualde, eds., *Papers in Laboratory Phonology 9*, pp. 36–74. Berlin: Mouton de Gruyter.

Mücke, Doris, Martine Grice, Johannes Becker, and Anne Hermes. 2009. Sources of variation in tonal alignment: Evidence from acoustic and kinematic data. *Journal of Phonetics* 37:321–338.

Nally, E. V. 1971. Notes on a Westmeath dialect. *Journal of the International Phonetic Association* 1:33–38.

Newman, Michael. 2010. Focusing, implicational scaling, and the dialect status of New York Latino English. *Journal of Sociolinguistics* 14:207–239.

Nguyen, Nhung, Jason A. Shaw, Michael D. Tyler, Rebecca T. Pinkus, and Catherine T. Best. 2015. Affective attitudes towards Asians influence perception of Asian-accented vowels. In *Proceedings of the 18th International Congress of Phonetic Sciences*. Glasgow, UK. www.internationalphoneticassociation.org/icphs/icphs2015

Niebuhr, Oliver, and Jarich Hoekstra. 2015. Pointed and plateau-shaped pitch accents in North Frisian. *Laboratory Phonology* 6:433–468.

Niedzielski, Nancy. 1999. The effect of social information on the perception of sociolinguistic variables. *Journal of Language and Social Psychology* 18:62–85.

Nycz, Jennifer. 2013. Changing words or changing rules? Second dialect acquisition and phonological representation. *Journal of Pragmatics* 52:49–62.

Ocumpaugh, Jaclyn Lorraine. 2010. Regional variation in Chicano English: Incipient dialect formation among L1 and L2 speakers in Benton Harbor. Ph.D. diss., Michigan State University, MI.

O'Rourke, Erin. 2008. Speech rhythm variation in dialects of Spanish: Applying the pairwise variability index and variation coefficients to Peruvian Spanish. *Paper presented at Speech Prosody 2008: Fourth Conference on Speech Prosody, May 6–9, 2008, Campinas, Brazil*. http://isle.illinois.edu/sprosig/sp2008/index.html

O'Rourke, Erin. 2012. The realization of contrastive focus in Peruvian Spanish intonation. *Lingua* 122:494–510.

O'Rourke, Erin. 2014. Intonation in Spanish. In José Ignacio Hualde, Antxon Olarrea, and Erin O'Rourke, eds., *The Handbook of Hispanic Linguistics*, pp. 173–191. Malden, MA: Wiley-Blackwell.

Paradis, Michel. 2000. Generalizable outcomes of bilingual aphasia research. *Folia Phoniatrica et Logopaedica* 52:54–64.

Pardo, Jennifer S., Rachel Gibbons, Alexandra Suppes, and Robert M. Krauss. 2012. Phonetic convergence in college roommates. *Journal of Phonetics* 40:190–197.

Peters, Jörg, Judith Hanssen, and Carlos Gussenhoven. 2015. The timing of nuclear falls: Evidence from Dutch, West Frisian, Dutch Low Saxon, German Low Saxon, and High German. *Laboratory Phonology* 6:1–52.

Pierrehumbert, Janet B. 2006. The next toolkit. *Journal of Phonetics* 34:516–530.

Plichta, Bartlomiej. 2002. Vowel nasalization and the Northern Cities Shift in Michigan. Unpublished typescript.

Podesva, Robert J. 2011. Salence and the social meaning of declarative contours: Three case studies of gay professionals. *Journal of English Linguistics* 39:233–264.

Podesva, Robert J., and Janneke Van Hofwegen. 2016. /s/exuality in small-town California: Gender normativity and the acoustic realization of /s/. In Erez Levon and Ronald Beline Mendes, eds., *Language, Sexuality, and Power: Studies in Intersectional Sociolinguistics*, pp. 168–188. Oxford: Oxford University Press.

Preston, Dennis R. 1993. Folk Dialectology. In Dennis R. Preston, ed., *American Dialect Research*, pp. 333–377. Amsterdam/Philadelphia: John Benjamins.

Preston, Dennis R., and Nancy Niedzielski, eds. 2010. *A Reader in Sociophonetics*. Trends in linguistics: Studies and monographs 219. New York: De Gruyter Mouton.

Purnell, Thomas C. 2008. Prevelar raising and phonetic conditioning: Role of labial and anterior tongue gestures. *American Speech* 83:373–402.

Purnell, Thomas C, Joseph Salmons, and Dilara Tepeli. 2005a. German substrate effects in Wisconsin English: Evidence for final fortition. *American Speech* 80:135–164.

Purnell, Thomas C, Joseph Salmons, Dilara Tepeli, and Jennifer Mercer. 2005b. Structured heterogeneity and change in laryngeal phonetics: Upper Midwestern final obstruents. *Journal of English Linguistics* 33:307–338.

Queen, Robin. 2001. Bilingual intonation patterns: Evidence of language change from Turkish-German bilingual children. *Language in Society* 30:55–80.

Queen, Robin. 2006. Phrase-final intonation in narratives told by Turkish-German bilinguals. *International Journal of Bilingualism* 10:153–178.

Queen, Robin. 2012. Turkish-German bilinguals and their intonation: Triangulating evidence about contact-induced language change. *Language* 88:791–816.

Quené, Hugo. 2008. Multilevel modeling of between-speaker and within-speaker variation in spontaneous speech tempo. *The Journal of the Acoustical Society of America* 123:1104–1113.

Rae, Megan, and Paul Warren. 2002. Goldilocks and the three beers: Sound merger and word recognition in NZE. *New Zealand English Journal* 16:33–41.

Rafat, Yasaman. 2010. A socio-phonetic investigation of rhotics in Persian. *Iranian Studies* 43:667–682.

Rakerd, Brad, and Bartłomiej Plichta. 2010. More on Michigan listeners' perceptions of /ɑ/ fronting. *American Speech* 85:431–449.

Ray, George B., and Christopher J. Zahn. 1990. Regional speech rates in the United States: A preliminary analysis. *Communication Speech Reports* 7:34–37.

Recasens, Daniel, and Aina Espinosa. 2005. Articulatory, positional and coarticulatory characteristics for clear /l/ and dark /l/: Evidence from two Catalan dialects. *Journal of the International Phonetic Association* 35:1–25.

Reddy, Sravana and James N. Stanford. 2015. Toward completely automated vowel extraction: Introducing DARLA. *Linguistics Vanguard: A Multimodal Journal for the Language Sciences* 1:15–28.

Robb, Michael P., Margaret A. Maclagan, and Yang Chen. 2004. Speaking rates of American and New Zealand varieties of English. *Clinical Linguistics & Phonetics* 18:1–15.

Roeder, Rebecca. 2010. Northern cities Mexican American English: Vowel production and perception. *American Speech* 85:163–184.

Rohena-Madrazo, Marcos. 2015. Diagnosing the completion of a sound change: Phonetic and phonological evidence for /ʃ/ in Buenos Aires Spanish. *Language Variation and Change* 27:287–317.

Rutter, Ben. 2011. Acoustic analysis of a sound change in progress: The consonant cluster /stɹ/ in English. *Journal of the International Phonetic Association* 41:27–40.

Sadowski, Scott, and María José Aninao. 2019. Spanish in Santiago, Chile: Globalization, internal migration and ethnicity. In Andrew Lynch, ed., *The Routledge Handbook of Spanish in the Global City*. London: Routledge.

Sarmah, Prijankoo, Divya Verma Gogoi, and Caroline Wiltshire. 2009. Thai English: Rhythm and vowels. *English World-Wide* 30:196–217.

Schoormann, Heike E., Wilbert J. Heeringa, and Jörg Peters. 2017. A cross-dialectal acoustic study of Saterland Frisian vowels. *The Journal of the Acoustical Society of America* 141:2893–2908.

Schützler, Ole. 2011. Charting vowel spaces in Edinburgh middle-class speech. *English World-Wide* 32:24–45.

Scobbie, James M. 2006. Flexibility in the face of incompatible English VOT systems. In Louis Goldstein, D. H. Whalen, and Catherine T. Best, eds., *Laboratory Phonology 8. Phonology and Phonetics,* pp. 4–2. Berlin/New York: Mouton de Gruyter.

Scobbie, James M., and Koen D. C. J. Sebregts. 2011. Acoustic, articulatory and phonological perspectives on rhoticity and /r/ in Dutch. In Rafaella Folli and Christiane Ulbrich, eds., *Interfaces in Linguistics: New Research Perspectives*, pp. 257–277. Oxford: Oxford University Press.

Sebregts, Koen D. C. J. 2014. *The Sociophonetics and Phonology of Dutch* r. Utrecht: Landelijke Onderzoekschool Taalwetenschap.

Sharbawi, Salbrina, and David Deterding. 2010. Rhoticity in Brunei English. *English World-Wide* 31:121–137.

Soskuthy, Marton, Jane Stuart-Smith, Rachel Macdonald, Robert Lennon, and Farhana Alam. 2017. When is sound change more than segmental change? Coda /r/ and voice quality shifts in Glasgow since 1890. *Paper presented at the 11th U.K. Language Variation and Change conference, Cardiff, 31 August.*

Stanford, James N. 2008. A sociotonetic analysis of Sui dialect contact. *Language Variation and Change* 20:409–450.

Stölten, Katrin, and Olle Engstrand. 2002. Effects of sex and age in the Arjeplog dialect: A listening test and measurements of preaspiration and VOT. *Proceedings of Fonetik, TMH-QPSR* 44:29–32. www.speech.kth.se/qpsr

Straw, Michelle, and Peter L. Patrick. 2007. Dialect acquisition of glottal variation in /t/: Barbadians in Ipswich. *Language Sciences* 29:385–407.

Stuart-Smith, Jane. 2007. Empirical evidence for gendered speech production: /s/ in Glaswegian. In Jennifer Cole and José Ignacio Hualde, eds., *Laboratory Phonology 9*, pp. 65–86. Berlin/New York: Mouton de Gruyter.

Sumner, Meghan, Seung Kyung Kim, Ed King, and Kevin B. McGowan. 2014. The socially weighted encoding of spoken words: A dual-route approach to speech perception. *Frontiers in Psychology* 4:1–13.

Sumner, Meghan, and Arthur G. Samuel. 2009. The effect of experience on the perception and representation of dialect variants. *Journal of Memory and Language* 60:487–501.

Syrika, Asimina, Eun Jong Kong, and Jan Edwards. 2011. Velar softening: An acoustic study in Modern Greek. In W. S. Lee and E. Zee, eds., *Proceedings of the 17th International Conference of Phonetic Sciences*, pp. 1926–1929. Hong Kong: City University of Hong Kong.

Szakay, Anita. 2008. Ethnic dialect identification in New Zealand: The role of prosodic cues. Ph.D. diss., University of Canterbury.

Szakay, Anita, and Eivind Torgersen. 2015. An acoustic analysis of voice quality in London English: The effect of gender, ethnicity and f_0. In *Proceedings of the 18th International Congress of Phonetic Sciences,* Glasgow, UK. www.internationalphoneticassociation.org/icphs/icphs2015

Takada, Mieko, and Nobuo Tomimori. 2006. The relationship between VOT in initial voiced plosives and the phenomenon of word-medial plosives in Nigata and Shikoku. In Yuji Kawaguchi, Susumu Zaima, and Toshihiro Takagaki, eds., *Spoken Language Corpus and Linguistic Informatics*, pp. 365–379. Usage-based linguistic informatics 5. Amsterdam/Philadelphia: John Benjamins.

Tan, Rachel Siew Kuang, and Ee-Ling Low. 2010. How different are the monophthongs of Malay speakers of Malaysian and Singapore English? *English World-Wide* 31:162–189.

Thomas, Erik R. 2000. Spectral differences in /ai/ offsets conditioned by voicing of the following consonant. *Journal of Phonetics* 28:1–25.

Thomas, Erik R. 2001. *An Acoustic Analysis of Vowel Variation in New World English.* Publication of the American Dialect Society, 85. Durham, NC: Duke University Press.

Thomas, Erik R. 2002. Sociophonetic applications of speech perception experiments. *American Speech* 77:115–147.

Thomas, Erik R. 2007. Sociophonetics. In Robert Bayley and Ceil Lucas, eds., *Sociolinguistic Variation: Theories, Methods, and Analysis*, pp. 215–233. Cambridge: Cambridge University Press.

Thomas, Erik R. 2010. A longitudinal analysis of the durability of the Northern/Midland dialect boundary in Ohio. *American Speech* 85:375–430.

Thomas, Erik R. 2011. *Sociophonetics: An Introduction.* Basingstoke, UK: Palgrave Macmillan.

Thomas, Erik R. 2013. Sociophonetics. In J. K. Chambers and Natalie Schilling-Estes, eds., *The Handbook of Language Variation and Change.* 2nd edn, pp. 108–127. Oxford/Malden, MA: Wiley-Blackwell.

Thomas, Erik R., ed. 2019. *Mexican American English: Substrate Influence and the Birth of an Ethnolect.* Cambridge: Cambridge University Press.

Thomas, Erik R., and Guy Bailey. 1998. Parallels between vowel subsystems of African American Vernacular English and Caribbean creoles. *Journal of Pidgin and Creole Languages* 13:267–296.

Thomas, Erik R., and Phillip M. Carter. 2006. Rhythm and African American English. *English World-Wide* 27:331–355.

Thomas, Erik R., and Jeffrey Reaser. 2004. Delimiting perceptual cues used for the ethnic labeling of African American and European American voices. *Journal of Sociolinguistics* 8:54–86.

Thomas, Erik R., and Jeffrey Reaser. 2015. An experiment on cues used for identification of voices as African American or European American. In Michael D. Picone and Catherine Evans Davies, eds., *New Perspectives on Language Variety in the South: Historical and Contemporary Perspectives*, pp. 507–522. Tuscaloosa, AL: University of Alabama Press.

Torgerson, Eivind Nessa, and Anita Szakay. 2012. An investigation of speech rhythm in London English. *Lingua* 122:822–840.

Torgersen, Eivind, and Paul Kerswill. 2004. Internal and external motivation in phonetic change: Dialect levelling outcomes for an English vowel shift. *Journal of Sociolinguistics* 8:23–53.

Tronnier, Mechtild. 2002. Preaspiration in southern Swedish dialects. *Proceedings of Fonetik, TMH-QPSR* 44:33–36. www.speech.kth.se/qpsr

Turk, Alice, and Stefanie Shattuck-Hufnagel. 2013. What is speech rhythm? A commentary on Arvaniti and Rodriquez, Krivokapić, and Goswami and Leong. *Laboratory Phonology* 4:93–118.

Turton Danielle. 2014. Some /l/s are darker than others: Accounting for variation in English /l/ with ultrasound tongue imaging. *University of Pennsylvania Working Papers in Linguistics* 20:189–198.

van Bezooijen, Renee, and Charlotte Gooskens. 1999. Identification of language varieties: The contribution of different linguistic levels. *Journal of Language and Social Psychology* 18:31–48.

van Bezooijen, Renée, and Rob van den Berg. 1999. Word intelligibility of language varieties in the Netherlands and Flanders under minimal conditions. In René Kager and Renée van Bezooijen, eds., *Linguistics in the Netherlands 1999*, pp. 1–12. Amsterdam: John Benjamins.

Van der Harst, Sander, Hans Van de Velde, and Roeland Van Hout. 2014. Variation in Standard Dutch vowels: The impact of formant measurement methods on identifying the speaker's regional origin. *Language Variation and Change* 26:247–272.

van Heuven, Vincent J., Loulou Edelman, and Renée van Bezooijen. 2002. The pronunciation of /ɛi/ by male and female speakers of avant-garde Dutch. In Hans Broekhuis and Paula Fikkert, eds., *Linguistics in the Netherlands*, pp. 61–72. Amsterdam/Philadelphia: John Benjamins.

van Heuven, Vincent J., and Klaske van Leyden. 2003. A contrastive acoustical investigation of Orkney and Shetland intonation. In *Proceedings of the 15th International Congress of Phonetic Sciences, Barcelona*. www.internationalphoneticassociation.org/icphs/icphs2003

Van Hofwegen, Janneke. 2009. Cross-generational change in /l/ in Chicano English. *English World-Wide* 30:302–325.

Veatch, Thomas Clark. 1991. English vowels: Their surface phonology and phonetic implementation in vernacular dialects. Ph.D. diss., University of Pennsylvania.

Walton, Julie H., and Robert F. Orlikoff. 1994. Speaker race identification from acoustic cues in the vocal signal. *Journal of Speech and Hearing Research* 37:738–745.

Warren, Paul. 2005. Patterns of late rising in New Zealand English: Intonational variation or intonational change? *Language Variation and Change* 17:209–230.

Wenk, Brian J., and François Wiolland. 1982. Is French really syllable-timed? *Journal of Phonetics* 10:193–216.

White, Laurence, and Sven L. Mattys. 2007. Rhythmic typology and variation in first and second languages. In Pilar Prieto, Joan Mascaró, and Maria-Josep Solé, eds., *Segmental and Prosodic Issues in Romance Phonology*, pp. 237–257. Current issues in linguistic theory series. Amsterdam/Philadelphia: John Benjamins.

Wikström, Jussi. 2013. An acoustic study of the RP English LOT and THOUGHT vowels. *Journal of the International Phonetic Association* 43:37–47.

Williams, Angie, Peter Garrett, and Nikolas Coupland. 1999. Dialect Recognition. In Dennis R. Preston, *Handbook of Perceptual Dialectology*. Vol. 1, pp. 345–358. Philadelphia/Amsterdam: John Benjamins.

Willis, Clodius. 1972. Perception of Vowel Phonemes in Fort Erie, Ontario, Canada, and Buffalo, New York: An Application of Synthetic Vowel Categorization Tests to Dialectology. *Journal of Speech and Hearing Research* 15:246–255.

Willis, Erik W. 2007a. An acoustic study of the "pre-aspirated trill" in narrative Cibaeño Spanish. *Journal of the International Phonetic Association* 37:33–49.
Willis, Erik W. 2007b. An initial examination of Southwest Spanish vowels. *Southwest Journal of Linguistics* 24:185–18198.
Willis, Erik W. 2007c. Utterance signaling and tonal levels in Dominican Spanish declaratives and interrogatives. *Journal of Portuguese Linguistics* 5.6:179–202.
Willis, Erik W. 2008. No se comen, pero sí se mascan: Variación de las vocales plenas en el español dominicano. In *Las Actas de la Asociación de Lingüística y Filología de Latino-América, Montevideo, Uruguay*. www.mundoalfal.org/indexe.htm
Willis, Erik W., and Travis G. Bradley. 2008. Contrast maintenance of taps and trills in Dominican Spanish: Data and analysis. In Laura Colantoni and Jeffrey Steele, eds., *Selected Proceedings of the 3rd Conference on Laboratory Approaches to Spanish Phonology*, pp. 87–100. Somerville, MA: Cascadilla.
Wolfram, Walt, and Erik R. Thomas. 2002. *The Development of African American English*. Language in Society. Vol. 31. Oxford: Wiley-Blackwell.
Wolk, Lesley, Nassima B. Abdelli-Beruh, and Dianne Slavin. 2011. Habitual use of vocal fry in young adult female speakers. *Journal of Voice* 26:e111–e116.
Wretling, Pär, E. Strangert, and F. Schaeffler. 2002. Quantity and preaspiration in northern Swedish dialects. In B. Bel and I. Marlien, eds., *Proceedings of Speech Prosody 2002: An International Conference*. Aix-en-Provence, France: Laboratorie de Parole et Langue, CNRS/University of Provence.
Yaeger-Dror, Malcah, and Erik R. Thomas, eds. 2010. *African American English Speakers and Their Participation in Local Sound Changes: A Comparative Study*. Publication of the American Dialect Society 94. Durham, NC: Duke University Press.
Yang, Cathryn, James N. Stanford, and Zhengyu Yang. 2015. A sociotonetic study of Lalo tone split in progress. *Asia-Pacific Language Variation* 1:52–77.
Yuasa, Ikuko Patricia. 2008. *Culture and Gender of Voice Pitch: A Sociophonetic Comparison of the Japanese and Americans*. London: Equinox.
Yuasa, Ikuko Patricia. 2010. Creaky voice: A new feminine voice quality for young urban-oriented upwardly mobile American women? *American Speech* 85:315–337.
Zamman, Lal. 2017. Variability in /s/ among transgender speakers: Evidence for a socially grounded account of gender and sibilants. *Linguistics* 55:993–1019.
Zeller, Christine. 1997. The investigation of a sound change in progress: /æ/ to /e/ in Midwestern American English. *Journal of English Linguistics* 25:142–155.
Zhang, Jingwei. 2014. A sociophonetic study on tonal variation of the Wúxī and Shànghǎi dialects. Ph.D. diss., Utrecht University.

17

Phonetics and second language teaching research

Murray J. Munro and Tracey M. Derwing

Introduction

Broadly speaking, *applied phonetics* can be assumed to cover a range of practical implementations of phonetic expertise, including forensic speech science, speech-language pathology, dialect coaching for actors, and pronunciation teaching. The last of these has had an especially long and successful engagement with the field of phonetics, as evidenced by an extensive research literature, as well as centuries of close attention from prominent speech researchers and theorists. The following discussion surveys the historical use of phonetics in second language (L2) pronunciation, summarizes research bearing on current teaching practices, and previews probable future trends in the field. Because so much of the recent research literature has been motivated by issues in English language teaching, it is inevitable that any such review would draw heavily on examples from English. Many of the observations made here are applicable to diverse language teaching contexts; however, a fuller understanding of pronunciation teaching and learning will require more studies involving other languages. This chapter's focus on adult phonetic learning is well-justified on linguistic grounds, since children typically acquire L2 pronunciation mainly through naturalistic, as opposed to instructed, learning.

Historical overview

The speech sciences have enjoyed a long and fruitful relationship with the field of language pedagogy. Although the first scholarly discussions of the uses of phonetics in teaching cannot be pinpointed, English pronunciation specialists had taken a deep interest in practical questions well before Henry Sweet and the era of modern speech research (Subbiondo, 1978). Some of the earliest phonetic descriptions of English, such as Hart's (1569) *An orthographie*, were motivated by the push for English spelling reform, while others, like Robinson's (1617) *Art of pronunciation*, focused on the development of a systematic phonetic alphabet. One of the first volumes to feature an explicitly pedagogical orientation was *The vocal organ*, by the Welsh schoolmaster, Owen Price (1665). Intended for an audience comprising both "outlanders" and native English speakers wishing to enhance their social status through speech "improvement," it featured some of the earliest-published diagrams of the articulators, along with articulatory descriptions of English speech sounds. Still another work from the same era was William Holder's (1669) *Elements of Speech*, which carried the subtitle, "A study of applied English phonetics and speech therapy." Holder's development of a detailed and influential theory of segmental phonetics was a byproduct of his desire to promote the teaching of speech to the deaf.

The issues motivating these works – systematic phonetic transcription, pronunciation instruction (PI) for language learners, and the teaching of elocution – were revisited many times afterward by scholars committed to teaching. The elocutionist Alexander Melville Bell, for instance, developed *Visible Speech* (1867), an iconic transcription system, as a tool for teaching the deaf to articulate accurately, while his son, Alexander Graham Bell, invented the telephone while searching for ways to automatically represent spoken utterances on the printed page. The younger Bell also devoted much of his career to teaching the deaf. Remarkably, one of the most important achievements of the field of phonetics, the IPA, owes its existence to the work of language teachers, particularly Paul Passy, a specialist in French pronunciation and founder of the International Phonetic Association, which had been an organization of teachers in an earlier incarnation.

One of the giants of phonetics, Henry Sweet, was deeply interested in language teaching, as is reflected in his handbook (1900), *The practical study of languages; a guide for teachers and learners*. Sweet saw pronunciation as the central aspect of second language (L2) learning, and offered extensive advice to learners on how to acquire the sounds of a new language. Key to his perspective was the view that phonetic expertise was essential for teachers:

> Phonetics makes us independent of native teachers. It is certain that a phonetically trained Englishman who has a clear knowledge of the relations between French and English sounds can teach French sounds to English people better than an unphonetic Frenchman who is unable to communicate his pronunciation to his pupils, and perhaps speaks a dialectal or vulgar form of French
>
> *(p. 48).*

Although we view his "certainty" on this point with considerable skepticism, Sweet's appraisal of the goals of language teaching seems to have been rooted in a realistic understanding of the capabilities of L2 learners. He did not, for instance, advocate attempting to acquire the L2 with perfectly native-like accuracy, but instead identified a suitable goal as "moderate fluency and sufficient accuracy of pronunciation to insure intelligibility" (Sweet, 1900, p. 152). His work thus presaged subsequent discussions of the merits of the "nativeness" and "intelligibility" principles (Levis, 2005) covered later in this chapter.

By the mid-20th century, a burgeoning interest in foreign language instruction in North America led to the development of a behaviorist approach to teaching known as the Audiolingual (AL) method. Based on the notion of "language-as-habit," AL instruction had its roots in techniques developed for language training in the US military. It focused heavily on aural and oral skills, with near-native pronunciation as one of its aims. Languages were taught directly (i.e., without translation into the native language), and learners mimicked utterances after recorded native-speaker models, with the expectation that their productions would become increasingly accurate as a function of practice. The post-WWII availability of classroom technologies such as the tape recorder and the language laboratory was even thought to obviate the need for teachers to have proficiency in the languages they taught.

Although AL methodology was often derided because of its reliance on tedious repetition and rote memorization, its impact on teaching was both powerful and long-lasting (Richards & Rodgers, 2014).

The advent of AL instruction in grade-school curricula coincided with a flurry of scholarly work on pronunciation pedagogy that began to appear in teaching-oriented journals in both the USA and the UK. Among these was Abercrombie's (1949) paper in the British journal *English Language Teaching*. A professor and luminary at the University of Edinburgh, Abercrombie had impeccable credentials in phonetics, having studied under Daniel Jones. Abercrombie's *Elements of General Phonetics*, originally published in 1967, is still in print and is recognized as one of the most important works in the field.

Like Sweet (1900), Abercrombie (1949) promoted intelligibility over nativeness, arguing that while aspiring secret agents might need to develop perfect L2 accents, such a goal was not only unnecessary for most language learners, but very unlikely to be achieved. He also argued a number of other points that remain contentious. For instance, he took the view that a detailed technical knowledge of phonetics should not be expected of pronunciation teachers and that phonetic transcription, though potentially helpful, was not a requirement in language classrooms. His work also reflected an awareness of large individual differences in pronunciation learning success. Furthermore, he observed that an array of social factors may lead some learners to choose to pronounce their L2 less accurately than they are actually able. The latter point has resurfaced frequently in 21st-century discussions of the relationship between pronunciation and learner identity (Moyer, 2009), though contemporary writers are often unaware that this issue was first identified many decades ago.

While many, if not most, of Abercrombie's (1949) recommendations on pronunciation teaching continue to be pertinent, they represent an orientation towards pedagogy that might be characterized as "phonetics applied" rather than "applied phonetics." The former refers to the general use by teaching specialists of knowledge derived from phonetics, even though such knowledge was not obtained with the goal of addressing teaching practices. In contrast, "applied phonetics" is a sub-focus within the field of phonetics that specifically aims to answer questions of pedagogical importance, such as what to teach, how to teach, and when to do so. Abercrombie's proposals were rooted in a detailed understanding of general phonetics and were further informed by his own observations of language learning in his students and colleagues. The same was true of the work of several other prominent phoneticians of the era, such as Pierre Delattre, who, in addition to his role as a leading researcher of speech synthesis at Haskins Laboratories, also had a reputation in the USA as a master teacher of French (Eddy, 1974).

Neither Abercrombie nor Delattre used empirical research to test their ideas about teaching; nor did they have the benefit of an extensive pedagogically focused research literature to draw upon. However, with the rise of the AL method, an interest in empirical investigations of teaching *per se* began to emerge. Mid-20th-century research in such journals as *Language Learning*, the *Revue de phonétique appliquée*, and even *Language* often took the form of pedagogical intervention studies in which investigators explored such issues as the general effects of instruction on learning, the benefits of particular pedagogical techniques, and the nature of perception and production difficulties experienced by learners. Observing that "controlled experimentation is perhaps the largest remaining frontier in the field of Teaching English as a Foreign Language" (p. 217), Strain (1963) conducted experimental work intended to pinpoint the pronunciation difficulties of Japanese learners of English both with and without instruction. Despite concluding that his study was largely unsuccessful in addressing his research question, he argued that his findings were useful in highlighting some of the difficulties of carrying out L2 pronunciation research. Strain's work, in fact, exemplifies an orientation of the field that contrasts with the "phonetics applied" perspective mentioned earlier. Instead, it belongs to a research stream designed specifically to focus on pedagogical questions. This type of "applied phonetics" has its own raison d'être, which is distinct from that of general experimental phonetics; it is motivated by its own research questions, executed with its own methods, and communicated to audiences through its own terminological conventions. To help clarify the distinction, one might compare a pedagogically relevant inference drawn from general knowledge of phonetics with the results of an instructional study. From basic articulatory phonetics, for instance, we can describe the typical configurations of the tongue during the articulation of English plosives using sagittal diagrams, along with appropriate terminology. One might consider providing such articulatory descriptions to a learner of English as a means of teaching accurate articulation. Doing so illustrates "phonetics applied," in the sense that particular pieces of knowledge from the field of phonetics are exploited in teaching. However, the fact that one can explain to a learner how plosives are produced says nothing about whether and to what degree the learner can actually exploit such knowledge when it is gained through such instruction. In fact, a central issue in PI has long been the observation that explicit instruction is sometimes ineffective. Brière (1966), for instance, successfully trained native English speakers to articulate certain exotic sounds such as /x/ and a dental unaspirated initial /t̪/, but had little success with /ɯ/ and /ɦ/. Similarly, explicit suprasegmental instruction can be both successful and ineffectual (Pennington & Ellis, 2000). But even when instruction succeeds there is no guarantee that the learners' new skill will offer any true communicative benefit. Many English pronunciation specialists, for instance, argue that some segmentals, such as interdental fricatives, do not merit detailed attention because the time required does not justify the minimal intelligibility gains (if any) the learner is likely to experience (see Derwing & Munro, 2015). We expand on this issue in the discussion of functional load below.

Error prediction

It has often been claimed that L2 teachers can benefit from knowing in advance the phonological difficulties that particular groups of learners will experience. However, ample evidence indicates that linguistically based error prediction is too fraught with problems to be more than minimally applicable in teaching (Munro, 2018b). One of the theoretical offshoots of behaviorist language teaching was the proposal that linguistic comparisons of L1 and L2 can yield predictions of learners' areas of difficulty. The *Contrastive Analysis Hypothesis (CAH)* motivated extensive discussions of error hierarchies in the learning of sounds and grammar (Lado, 1957; Stockwell & Bowen, 1983). A key assumption of the phonological component of CAH was that structural differences between L1 and L2, described in terms of taxonomic phonemics, served as the basis for pronunciation errors. The purpose of error hierarchies was to predict relative degrees of difficulty of particular L2 sounds or sound pairs. For instance, a *phonemic split*, in which a single L1 phoneme corresponds to two separate phonemes in L2, was expected to be extremely challenging. The case of the Japanese flap category apparently subsuming the English /ɹ/ – /l/ distinction illustrates such a split, which would be predicted to make acquisition of that opposition difficult for Japanese learners of English. In contrast, a mere *distributional difference* between languages, such as the occurrence of word-final voiced consonants in English, but not in German, should offer only minimal difficulty to German learners of English.

Clearly, a contrastive approach can offer some insights into pronunciation difficulties. Japanese learners' common difficulties with the perception and production of /ɹ/ – /l/ for instance, have been well documented. Nonetheless, empirical work in the 1960s demonstrated that the original conception of CAH was untenable, and the proposal received harsh criticism (Wardaugh, 1970). A rigorously executed intervention study by Brière (1966) yielded important counter-evidence to the assumed phonological error hierarchies. After teaching English speakers a contrived phonological inventory from a fictional language, he found that the predicted degrees of difficulty did not match the learners' performance. The reasons for the failure of CAH in this case and in others are manifold. As Brière himself observed, most taxonomic phonemic comparisons are too crude to capture the perceptual and articulatory nuances that come into play in phonetic learning. However, a more general problem with CAH is the "language-as-object" fallacy that underlies it. Wardaugh (1970) recognized this problem when he pointed out that an ideal CAH analysis could supposedly be carried out entirely on the basis of previously published linguistic descriptions, with no need for any further observations of language learners. This expectation is at odds with the well-established finding that inter-speaker variability in L2 phonetic learning is large (Smith & Hayes-Harb, 2011), even when a wide range of outside influences are held constant. In a multi-year longitudinal study of English L2 vowel acquisition, for example, Munro and Derwing (2008) found that learners with identical L1 backgrounds, equivalent levels of formal education, and very similar starting proficiency levels, exhibited diverse learning trajectories in production performance. While a great deal of individual variation may be accounted for by the age at which learning begins and by differences in the amount and quality of L2 experience, other influences tied to motivation and aptitude almost certainly played a role (Derwing, 2018b; Flege, Frieda, & Nozawa, 1997; Trofimovich, Kennedy, & Foote, 2015).

On the one hand, one might argue that an exhaustive knowledge both of the phonetic details of the L1 and L2, and of individual learning circumstances, could account for the performance of a particular learner in acquiring the L2 sound system. However, even if it is true, such a proposal has few useful implications for classroom practice. Effective pedagogy entails determining students' actual needs and addressing them as efficiently as possible. Given that learners differ widely in their pronunciation difficulties, even when they share the same L1 background, the most promising strategy for teaching is to carry out individual learner assessments prior to the beginning of instruction to pinpoint the specific problems that each learner experiences (Derwing, 2018a; Munro, Derwing, & Thomson, 2015).

Disenchantment with Audiolingual instruction eventually led to its abandonment in favor of so-called "designer methods" in the mid-1970s, which emphasized pronunciation to varying degrees (e.g., The Silent Way; Suggestopedia; Community-Counselling Learning) (Brown, 2014). Communicative Language Teaching (CLT) eventually came to dominate North American L2 classrooms in the 1980s, and is still the most popular approach with the addition of a task-based focus. CLT was informed by Canale and Swain's (1980) seminal model of communicative competence and by Krashen's (1981) Input Hypothesis, which claimed that with sufficient input, L2 pronunciation could be acquired without explicit instruction. At about the same time, Purcell and Suter (1980) published a correlational study in which they failed to find an effect of PI on learners' L2 pronunciation, understood by them to refer to native-like production. That finding, interpreted in the context of CLT and the popularity of Krashen's research, contributed to a radical decline in PI. Although a few expert practitioners insisted on PI's importance for communicative purposes (e.g., Judy Gilbert, Wayne Dickerson, Joan Morley), it nearly disappeared from language classrooms.

During this period, researchers were actively investigating aspects of pronunciation, but they were not pedagogically driven (Leather, 1983).

By the 1970s, an important new line of work on non-native speech perception emerged. For example, an influential study by Miyawaki et al. (1975) revealed differences between Japanese and American listeners' discrimination of a synthetic /ɹɑ/–/lɑ/ continuum. The poorer performance of the Japanese group was accounted for in terms of language experience, and in the decades since then, countless studies have probed both perception and production of this English liquid distinction. The focus has also expanded to include research on other consonant and vowel distinctions, and to evaluate theoretical proposals, such as Best's Perceptual Assimilation Model (PAM) (Best, McRoberts, & Sithole, 1988; Best & Tyler, 2007) and Flege's Speech Learning Model (SLM) (1995).

These models are also described in Chapter 16 of this volume. The now vast body of research carried out by Winifred Strange, Catherine Best, and James Flege, along with their many students and colleagues, is not pedagogically oriented either in terms of its objectives or its dissemination. However, it has relevance to teaching in terms of what it has revealed about phonetic learning, particularly in adults. One especially important aspect of their work is its emphasis on the role of perceptual processes in L2 acquisition. PAM and SLM both assume that the perception of non-native categories entails activation and engagement of previously well-established L1 representations. To acquire the L2 phonological inventory, learners must somehow escape the confining effects of this previously acquired knowledge. Studies of English liquid perception have shown that such learning is at least partially possible in adults, with numerous feedback studies confirming that perceptual accuracy increases with modest amounts of systematic training (Lively, Pisoni, Yamada, Tohkura, & Yamada, 1994; Logan, Lively, & Pisoni, 1991). Perhaps more intriguing is the fact that production accuracy can improve as a result of the same perceptual feedback, even when no explicit instruction on production is given (Bradlow, Pisoni, Akahane-Yamada, & Tohkura, 1997). Although the original feedback research was motivated primarily by interest in psycholinguistic issues, the implications for teaching are obvious. However, the transfer of findings from the laboratory to the classroom is not automatic. Speech scientists do not normally read or publish their work in education journals, and pedagogical specialists frequently find the research that appears in speech journals to be inaccessible due to its technical detail.

Current issues and research

Dimensions of L2 speech

Over the past few decades, pronunciation experts have made explicit the distinction between the Nativeness Principle, which emphasizes accuracy in L2 speakers' pronunciation, versus the Intelligibility Principle, which underscores the importance of producing speech that listeners can readily understand, even if it diverges from a native norm. As observed by Levis (2005), much of the twentieth century research on pronunciation focused on nativeness, despite calls from Abercrombie (1949), Gimson (1962), and others for an intelligibility-oriented approach. Not until the late 1990s, however, did empirical studies involving the assessment of intelligibility, comprehensibility, and accent establish the quasi-independence of these dimensions of L2 speech (Derwing & Munro, 1997; Derwing, Munro, & Wiebe, 1998; Munro & Derwing, 1995a, 1995b). Since then, it has become apparent that instruction may influence one of these dimensions without necessarily changing the others. In other words, it is possible to improve intelligibility without a noticeable change in accentedness, and an improvement in accentedness does not necessarily entail any intelligibility benefit, and may even be detrimental (Winters & O'Brien, 2013).

Phoneticians have long been interested in the construct of *intelligibility*, whether in connection with speech that is normal, disordered, synthetic, or foreign-accented. Schiavetti (1992) defined it as "the match between the intention of the speaker and the response of the listener to speech passed through the transmission system" (p. 13). Intelligibility is the most vital of the pronunciation dimensions, because it underlies the success of virtually all spoken communication. Operationalization of this construct includes a variety of approaches, the most common of which employs orthographic transcription by listeners followed by a word match analysis between the transcription and the intended message (Schiavetti, 1992). Other approaches have included responses to True/False utterances (Munro & Derwing, 1995b); comprehension questions (Hahn, 2004); summaries (Perlmutter, 1989); and segment identification (Munro et al., 2015).

Importantly, intelligibility is distinct from foreign *accentedness*, another dimension that has been probed extensively in the speech literature, and which is usually understood as the perceived degree of difference between an individual speaker's production patterns and some particular variety. Listeners' extraordinary sensitivity to accented features was documented in Flege (1984), who observed successful accent detection in excerpts of speech as short as 30 ms. Munro, Derwing, and Burgess (2010), in extending this line of research, found reliable accent detection for utterances played backwards and severely degraded through random splicing and pitch monotonization. Brennan, Ryan, and Dawson (1975) confirmed the reliability and validity of listener judgments of accentedness by utilizing magnitude estimation and sensory modality matching (squeezing a handheld device to indicate strength of accent). More recently, degree of accent has been typically measured using quasi-continuous or Likert-type scales. In the former, listeners indicate the accentedness of utterances with respect to two anchor points (e.g., "no foreign accent," "very strong foreign accent") by positioning a lever (Flege, Munro & MacKay, 1995) or clicking on a particular point on a screen (Saito, Trofimovich, & Isaacs, 2017). Likert assessments use a numbered scale; although there is debate regarding the appropriate scale resolution, a scale of at least nine points is known to yield highly reliable results (Isaacs & Thomson, 2013; Munro, 2018a). Degree of accentedness correlates with both segmental and suprasegmental accuracy, as described by Brennan et al. (1975) and Anderson-Hsieh, Johnson, and Koehler (1992). In short, more errors lead to stronger accentedness ratings. However, accentedness is partially independent of intelligibility, in that some (often very salient) accent features do not interfere with understanding or do so only minimally, while others are highly detrimental. As Munro and Derwing (1995a) demonstrated, heavily accented speech is often perfectly understood.

Comprehensibility, a third dimension of L2 speech, has been defined in several different ways (Gass & Varonis, 1984; Munro & Derwing, 1995a; Smith & Nelson, 1985); however, the prevailing sense in the pedagogical literature is Varonis and Gass' (1982) definition: "how easy it is to interpret the message" (p. 125). Although this speech dimension has received less attention than intelligibility, Munro and Derwing (1995a) recognized the need to distinguish the two, because utterances that are equally well understood may nonetheless require significantly different degrees of effort on the part of the listener. This conceptualization is very similar to the notion in cognitive psychology of "processing fluency" (Alter & Oppenheimer, 2009), which refers to the amount of effort required for a particular cognitive task. Measurement of comprehensibility has relied upon the same types of scaling as accentedness. The reliability of nine-point scalar ratings is well-attested, and the validity of the construct is supported by evidence that listeners' judgments correlate with response time measures (Munro & Derwing, 1995b; Bürki-Cohen, Miller, & Eimas, 2001; Clarke & Garrett, 2004; Floccia, Butler, Goslin, & Ellis, 2009). Even when speech is fully intelligible, limited comprehensibility has potentially negative consequences for interactions. If listeners have to expend a great deal of effort to understand an interlocutor, they may be disinclined to carry out further interactions (Dragojevic & Giles, 2016). For this reason, comprehensibility is more important to successful communication than is accentedness.

Although *fluency* is sometimes used to refer to proficiency, we restrict our discussion to Segalowitz's (2010) tripartite conceptualization of cognitive, utterance, and perceived fluency. The first of these refers to "the speaker's ability to efficiently mobilize and integrate the underlying cognitive processes responsible for producing utterances with the characteristics that they have" (p. 48). Utterance fluency is generally addressed by measuring speech and articulation rates, pausing, repairs and other temporal phenomena. The third type of fluency is typically measured through listeners' scalar ratings. Perceived and utterance fluency correlate well (Derwing, Rossiter, Munro, & Thomson, 2004) and are assumed to be a reflection of cognitive fluency (Derwing, 2017). Derwing et al. (2004) observed moderate to high correlations between perceived fluency and comprehensibility, as did Thomson (2015), whereas the relationship between fluency and accentedness was weaker. Speech rate, a component of utterance fluency, is typically slower in L2 speakers than in native speakers (MacKay & Flege, 2004; Munro & Derwing, 2001). Rate manipulations have shown that computer accelerated L2 speech tends to be judged as less accented and more comprehensible than unmodified speech in all but very fast L2 talkers (Munro & Derwing, 2001). Although L2 speakers may often be advised to slow their speech down to make it more comprehensible, the available evidence does not support such a recommendation. As Derwing and Munro (1997) concluded, a seemingly fast speaking rate may be a scapegoat for other aspects of an L2 accent that necessitate additional cognitive processing on the part of the listener. For instance, when listeners find L2 speech difficult to understand because of unexpected differences in segments and prosody, they may incorrectly attribute their processing difficulty to a fast rate. There is no reason to assume that instructing such L2 speakers to slow their speech will address the root cause of their lack of comprehensibility. In fact, deliberately slowed L2 speech has been shown to have deleterious effects on communication, at least in some circumstances (Munro & Derwing, 1998).

How L2 speech research informs pedagogical practice

As noted previously, throughout most of the 20th century, pronunciation instruction relied heavily on intuition, anecdotal observations, and untested theoretical proposals. It is increasingly recognized, however, that evidence-based pronunciation instruction is both possible and necessary (Munro & Derwing, 2015). In intuition-guided practice, instructors can be misled into placing emphasis on highly salient accent features that are only minimally relevant to intelligibility. For instance, mispronunciations of the English interdental fricatives are both common and noticeable, but there is no evidence that they detract significantly from comprehensibility and intelligibility (Munro & Derwing, 2006). In light of previous practice in which accent features alone guided instructional choices, leading to PI that is not motivated by the Intelligibility Principle, we argue that empirical data should be used to determine pedagogical priorities.

We propose a model of the relationship between research and pronunciation teaching as depicted in Figure 17.1. Although research and teaching need not be theory-driven, theory, both formal and informal, may influence each aspect of the model.

The first balloon in Figure 17.1 represents the knowledge and attitudes regarding pronunciation that underlie effective pedagogy. Questions that can be addressed through research include the following:

- How well can we reasonably expect learners to acquire L2 pronunciation?
- How does phonological knowledge of the L1 influence speech in the L2?
- How does pronunciation learning proceed *without* instruction?
- Which cognitive mechanisms underlie L2 pronunciation learning?

To illustrate potentially useful research findings within this domain, we might consider the numerous studies of the relationship between age of second language learning and accentedness. Research evidence shows that the two are closely related and that the likelihood of acquiring unaccented L2 speech becomes vanishingly small as adulthood approaches (Abrahamsson & Hyltenstam, 2009; Munro & Mann, 2005). While the underlying reasons for the relationship remain controversial, an obvious implication is that teachers cannot reasonably expect adult language learners to acquire fully native-sounding speech, suggesting that the Nativeness Principle (Levis, 2005) should not guide their practice.

The second balloon in Figure 17.1, Pedagogical Goals, points to several questions for researchers to address:

- What can we reasonably expect L2 learners to achieve through pronunciation instruction?
- Which aspects of the L2 sound system are learnable?
- Which aspects of the L2 sound system are teachable?
- What must be taught, rather than learned naturalistically?

An example of how research can address such questions comes from a pedagogical intervention study by Derwing et al. (1998), who compared the production performance of a control group with learners in two instructional conditions. In a blind listening task, judges rated comprehensibility and accentedness pre- and post-instruction of an extemporaneous speaking passage. Learners who received prosodically focused instruction showed

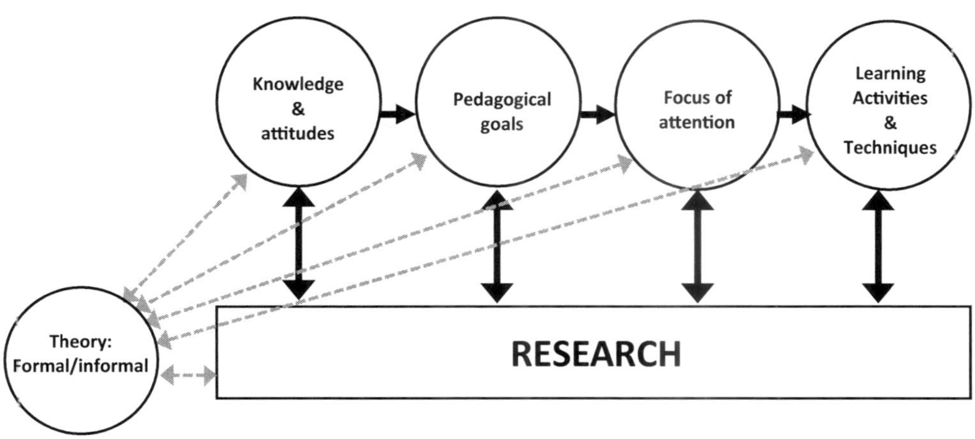

Figure 17.1 A proposed model of evidence-based applied phonetics.

improved comprehensibility, whereas neither the control group nor the group who received exclusively segmental instruction improved on this dimension. This finding provides evidence that improvements in comprehensibility can be achieved through instruction over a relatively short period of time, though this particular study did not address long-term retention, a matter that has so far received only limited consideration. At least two research studies have confirmed lasting effects of PI for three months (Couper, 2006) and seven months (Derwing, Foote & Munro, forthcoming), but far more work in this area with a larger sample of learners and different pronunciation features is necessary.

Although a meta-analysis of 86 instructional studies (Lee, Jang, & Plonsky, 2015) indicated that most showed a significant improvement in accentedness, further analysis by Thomson and Derwing (2015) demonstrated that only 9% of 75 studies (all of which also appeared in Lee et al., 2015) measured either comprehensibility or intelligibility (Thomson & Derwing, 2015). As awareness of the Intelligibility Principle grows, researchers will presumably focus less on the accentedness dimension because of its limited importance for communication.

The next balloon depicts Focus of Attention, which relates to the following issues:

- Which phonetic details (individual segments, lexical stress, prosodic features) should teachers prioritize in order to achieve their pedagogical goals?
- How should individual and shared needs be assessed?
- Which non-linguistic matters need attention during instruction (e.g., attitudes, expectations)?

An example of a study that partially addressed the first question with regard to segments is Munro and Derwing's (2006) exploration of the functional load of minimal pairs. Defined as the "amount of work" done by a particular phonemic distinction within the language (Catford, 1987), it takes into account the number of minimal pairs exhibiting the distinction, word frequencies, and contextual distributions. Functional load has the potential to predict problematic substitutions that may result in comprehensibility breakdowns. For example, a high functional load pair of segments, /n/ and /l/, are often interchanged in Cantonese-accented English. Learners from the same background also commonly fail to distinguish the low functional load pair, /d/ and /ð/. When Cantonese-accented utterances were presented to native English listeners for comprehensibility judgments, high functional load errors resulted in a greater comprehensibility decrement than did the low functional load errors. Moreover, the effect of the high functional load errors was additive, whereas that of the low functional load errors was not. Although these results were preliminary, the authors proposed that instructors of English should consider functional load when choosing segments for a teaching focus. Although Catford (1987) proposed a hierarchy of minimal pairs based on functional load, its accuracy remained untested for two decades. Munro and Derwing's (2006) empirical study exemplifies how a theoretically based pedagogical recommendation can be assessed. For a more recent critical overview of this concept, see Sewell (2017).

The last balloon in Figure 17.1, Learning Activities and Techniques, raises several questions as well:

- What specific learning activities will bring about desired changes?
- How much time must be devoted to a particular pronunciation issue for lasting improvement to be realized?

- How can the transfer of learning to situations outside the classroom be ensured?
- How can backsliding be minimized?

Among the still sparse research evaluating specific ways of teaching, a handful of studies have demonstrated that perceptual learning alone by L2 speakers can lead to improved productions (Bradlow et al., 1997; Lambacher, Martens, Kakehi, Marasinghe, & Molholt, 2005; Thomson, 2011; Thomson & Derwing, 2016). In an implementation designed for Computer-Assisted Pronunciation Teaching (CAPT), Thomson (2011) evaluated the effects of High Variability Phonetic Training (HVPT) on L2 vowel intelligibility. The listeners identified random presentations of ten target vowels in monosyllables produced by 20 native speakers. They received both auditory and visual feedback over the course of the eight-session intervention. Not only did their perception of vowels improve, but their own vowel productions were also more intelligible after the intervention, as assessed in a blind listener identification task. Although HVPT has been studied extensively in phonetics, it is practically unheard of in pedagogical circles, despite its effectiveness (Thomson, 2018b). This is just one learning activity that warrants more empirical study, but this entire category of research questions, like the others, merits further interdisciplinary research.

In Figure 17.1, research is depicted as the foundation for addressing the areas identified in the balloons. While some of this research takes the form of intervention studies (as cited previously), other, non-pedagogical investigations can inform these areas, as well. For instance, Tajima, Port, and Dalby's (1997) study of the effects of resynthesizing L2 speech to correct temporal errors demonstrated a significant improvement in intelligibility. Their findings are therefore indicative of the potential benefit of including a focus on the same temporal features in instructional contexts. Unfortunately, many phonetics studies that could have beneficial applications in pedagogical contexts, such as the preceding HVPT example, are almost entirely unknown to teachers or teacher trainers. An attempt to bridge this gap is now emerging with the advent of the *Journal of Second Language Pronunciation*, and conferences and workshops such as *Pronunciation in Second Language Learning and Teaching* (PSLLT) (North America), *Accents* (Poland), *New Sounds* (various countries), *English Pronunciation: Issues and Practices* (EPIP) (various countries), and *Speech and Language Technology in Education* (SLaTE) (various countries).

Social evaluation of accented speech

In spite of the clear importance of intelligibility and comprehensibility in pronunciation teaching, the broader social ramifications of an L2 accent are also worthy of study because of their impact on communication. A line of research dating back many decades has probed the effects of accent on listeners' judgments of a variety of speaker traits, such as employability, competence, and intelligence (Anisfeld, Bogo, & Lambert, 1962; Kalin & Rayko, 1978; Reisler, 1976). Together, these and other studies demonstrate that listeners make social judgments about speakers on the basis of accent, even though these may be entirely unwarranted. Lambert, Hodgson, Gardner, and Fillenbaum (1960) pioneered the matched guise test, an approach for detecting biases based on accent. In matched guise, a single individual speaks in two conditions differing in accent alone, e.g., Canadian English and Canadian French. By controlling for speaker, content, and physical appearance (if an image is used), the technique uncovers the listener's accent-related biases. Typically, the speech samples are rated by listeners on a scale for characteristics such as friendliness, intelligence, competence, honesty, and laziness, among others. In general, this type of task has demonstrated that listeners sometimes judge speakers negatively simply because of the way they speak. Other evidence indicates that some members of the public act on their prejudices (e.g., Dávila, Bohara, & Saenz, 1993; Munro, 2003); however, researchers' understanding of the way in which accent relates to social evaluation has become more nuanced in recent years. McGowan (2015), for instance, found that listeners' expectations based on physical appearance influence access to existing knowledge in such a way as to facilitate or compromise comprehension. When presented with congruent accents and faces, e.g., Chinese accent/Chinese face, American accent/Caucasian face, listeners transcribed speech samples more accurately than in incongruent conditions. Thus, what might appear to be social stereotyping when an American accent is paired with a Chinese face is actually a more complex cognitive processing issue.

Another influence on the willingness of individuals to interact with L2 speakers is familiarity with their accent. While it might be expected that familiarity should improve comprehension of a particular accent, the existing research has yielded inconsistent results. Gass and Varonis (1984) manipulated familiarity with content, foreign accent in general, a specific foreign accent, and a specific speaker and found a familiarity benefit for the listeners in all cases. Bent and Bradlow (2003) identified an intelligibility benefit for listeners of shared L1s when speech samples were presented (in noise) in the L2. Munro, Derwing, and Morton (2006), however, found inconsistent benefits of a shared L1 background in the intelligibility of extemporaneously produced L2 speech. They concluded, as did Major, Fitzmaurice, Bunta, and Balasubramanian (2002) that L2 speech in one's own L1 accent is sometimes understood better, but not always.

Both speakers and listeners have responsibility for the success of an interaction. While pronunciation instruction may improve low comprehensibility speech, sometimes a focus on the listener may also be useful. From a practical perspective, increasing people's familiarity with L2 accents may enhance their inclination to interact with L2 speakers, as was found by Derwing, Rossiter, and Munro (2002), who provided explicit training to listeners. Students in a social work program were given eight weekly intercultural awareness sessions with Vietnamese-accented examples relevant to their social work content. Furthermore, they were taught aspects of a Vietnamese accent, such as final consonant deletions, reduction of consonant clusters, use of implosive stops, substitution of initial /f/ for /p/, substitution of final /s/ for any other final C, and inaccurate stress placement. The students reported much higher confidence in their own abilities to communicate with an L2 speaker at the end of the program. In a different awareness-raising activity, Weyant (2007) played a passage narrated by a female L2 speaker. One group of listeners who wrote a paragraph depicting a typical day from her point of view (using the first person pronoun) later registered more positive impressions of the speaker than did another group who wrote a similar paragraph but from a third person stance. This short intervention illustrates how attitudinal changes may be altered through a relatively simple task. Lindemann, Campbell, Litzenberg, and Subtirelu (2016) compared implicit and explicit accent training with native speakers of English. One group transcribed sentences after having practiced transcribing Korean-accented speech, while the other group did so after instruction comparing Korean- and American-accented English. Both groups improved. The same participants answered comprehension questions on a Korean-accented, TOEFL-based lecture but neither group showed significant improvement. In both the Lindemann et al. and the Derwing et al. (2002) studies, the interventions were very short. More research is necessary to determine whether this type of instruction can positively influence comprehension as well as attitudes.

Longstanding issues

Segments vs. prosody

A question often asked by teachers is "which matters more – segments or prosody?" to which the only sensible answer is "it depends." It depends on the phonetic inventories of the L1 and the L2 and on the individual learner's errors: students who share the same L1 exhibit tremendous variability (Munro et al., 2015). It also depends on the location of a segmental error in a word – an initial consonant error can have more serious implications for intelligibility than an error elsewhere (Bent, Bradlow, & Smith, 2007; Zielinski, 2008). In addition, it depends on the nature of both the segmental and prosodic errors. It is clear that both segments and prosody can affect intelligibility and comprehensibility (Derwing et al., 1998). More research on concepts such as functional load and studies similar to that of Hahn (2004) may elucidate which segments and aspects of prosody matter most, but more research is also needed to examine the combined effects of errors (Derwing, 2008).

Phonetic transcription in the language classroom

Teachers often ask whether phonetic transcription should be used in pronunciation classes. Abercrombie (1949) argued that pronunciation instructors can be effective without using transcription, and certainly, if they are not fully conversant and comfortable with transcription, they should not use it. Moreover, if learners have limited literacy skills, introducing another writing system is likely to confuse them. However, if the instructor has a good grasp of transcription, and the students are literate, then some use of IPA symbols may be advantageous, at least in languages such as English, which has a nontransparent orthography. Transcription is generally unnecessary for languages such as Finnish or Spanish, because their orthographic systems correspond very closely to their sound systems, at least at the phonemic level.

Which variety to teach?

In countries where English is not the language of the majority, teachers commonly raise the question of which variety to teach. Usually the debate is whether to employ British or American English in the classroom, as if these two descriptors were monolithic. In fact, much of the instruction is likely to be in the accent of the teacher, regardless of program directives (Derwing & Munro, 2015). However, technology allows choices. Recordings of multiple dialects of English (and other languages) are now readily available, some of which are designed expressly for pronunciation teaching, and others, such as YouTube videos and TED Talks, have been produced for other reasons but can easily be repurposed. Introducing students to multiple varieties of the L2 may have benefits for their own comprehension.

Teaching ELF

With the increasing attention on English as a Lingua Franca (ELF) over the past 15 years, it has been argued that learners should not be expected to emulate a native model of English, but should instead strive for mutual intelligibility using a core set of pronunciation features (Jenkins, 2002). Adherents of ELF make the case that most nonnative speakers will interact primarily with other nonnative speakers; therefore, their pronunciation model should not be a native speaker variety (Walker, 2011). This notion has been criticized on several grounds. Isaacs (2014) for instance, indicated that

> the inclusion criteria for speech samples in the English as a lingua franca corpus that Jenkins and her colleagues frequently cite have not been clarified. Therefore, substantially more empirical evidence is needed before the lingua franca core can be generalized across instructional contexts or adopted as a standard for assessment.
>
> *(p. 8)*

Szpyra-Kozłowska (2015) argues that implementation of an ELF curriculum is extremely difficult, indicating also that since "the majority of English learners in the Expanding Circle already use English pronunciation based on some native model, EFL users might have problems not only communicating with native speakers, but also with non-native speakers" (p. 21). Given the diversity of English varieties, it seems prudent to expose learners to several, taking into consideration where they live and with whom they are likely to interact. In immigrant-receiving countries such as Australia, Canada, New Zealand, the UK, and the USA, the local varieties should receive the main focus of attention, but regardless of location, all learners would likely benefit from having access to several dialects.

Should reduction of English forms be taught?

Another frequently raised question is whether teachers should instruct their learners on speech reduction features. Given that L2 perception and production are closely linked, one of the goals of pronunciation instruction should be improved perception on the part of the learners. It is likely that students can implement knowledge about reduction processes to enhance their understanding of their interlocutors. For instance, the reduced form of "going to" (i.e., /ˈɡʌnə/) differs dramatically from its citation pronunciation, and may be unrecognizable to a learner who has not been explicitly taught what to listen for. Because full forms are probably at least as comprehensible to listeners of L2 speech as reduced forms, we surmise that students should not be required to produce reductions. If so, class time would be better spent on enhancing aspects of speech that typically interfere with comprehensibility.

When is the best time to learn a language for optimal pronunciation?

A long-standing question is "when is the best time to learn a second language for optimal pronunciation?" Studies indicate that near-native accents in the L2 are tied to early childhood learning (Abrahamsson & Hyltenstam, 2009; Flege et al., 1995). Furthermore, infants begin losing their ability to distinguish sound contrasts that are not in their own L1 within the first year of birth (Werker & Tees, 2002), presumably making L1 acquisition more efficient. Flege et al.'s (1995) study examined accentedness in Italian immigrants who came to Canada at different ages; arrivals as young as four years of age showed evidence of an L2 accent in adulthood. However, many people, especially immigrants, cannot choose when they have to learn an L2. The age question is thus of limited practical relevance. An L2 accent is a completely normal phenomenon and should not be considered "a problem" unless a speaker has issues of intelligibility and/or comprehensibility (Derwing & Munro, 2015).

Emerging issues

The role of technology

Various forms of technology have become prominent in pronunciation instruction, and are likely to take on a larger role in the years to come. Audio recording devices have been widely available since the mid-20th century, but with the advent of smartphones, students can easily send sound files back and forth to their instructors. CAPT is often employed to enhance learners' perceptual skills. In addition, evidence-based pedagogical tools, such as the *English Accent Coach* (Thomson, 2018a), provide training that can be individualized to the needs of the students. This software, which employs HVPT for ten vowels and 24 consonants, has been shown to significantly improve L2 students' perception and production (Thomson, 2018b).

In Lee et al.'s (2015) meta-analysis of pronunciation instruction research, CAPT studies were less effective than teacher-led activities, but since many language teachers are hesitant to offer any pronunciation instruction, CAPT on its own can still play a role. The clear advantages of CAPT include the amount of practice time it affords and the option for individualization catering to the needs of each user. In addition, as Ferrier, Reid, and Chenausky (1999) discovered, students whose progress was closely monitored by a teacher outperformed those left to their own devices. More gamified software targeting L2 pronunciation is being developed regularly; however, with a few notable exceptions, the publishers have tended to focus on aspects of the technology, without enough attention to important linguistic issues and best pedagogical practices (Foote & Smith, 2013). Visual feedback on speech for CAPT has been studied for some time and may offer new directions for PI (see Chapter 19 in this volume).

Technological advances over recent decades have influenced PI, and future innovations are certain to continue the trend. The wide availability of digital audio, for example, has made spoken utterance models, including dialectal variants, easily accessible to learners, and audio dictionaries have, to some degree, obviated the need for phonetic transcription as a guide to pronunciation at the lexical level. Text-to-speech applications also offer promise as a source of aural input during instruction (Bione, Grimshaw, & Cardoso, 2016). Of particular interest are the significant advances in the implementation of automatic speech recognition (ASR) for teaching purposes. As noted earlier, a recurrent finding in pronunciation research is inter-speaker variability, which points to the need for individual assessment and instruction tailored to each learner's needs. It is widely recognized that a general benefit of computer-based instruction is individualization; high-quality ASR, in particular, offers the possibility of immediate pronunciation feedback to learners that can assist them in modifying their productions (Cucchiarini & Strik, 2018). Research on ASR-based feedback using a CAPT system designed for learning Dutch (Cucchiarini, Neri, & Strik, 2009) indicated relatively high error-detection rates along with positive feedback from users. The overall benefits of ASR feedback for learners, however, ultimately depend on how well the CAPT system addresses individual needs so as to highlight pronunciation difficulties that compromise intelligibility and comprehensibility (O'Brien et al., 2018). In addition, adaptive systems offer much promise, yet remain largely under-developed.

Ethical practices and L2 accent

The rapidly growing field of accent reduction raises ethical issues regarding the qualifications of those offering PI and the claims they make regarding the value and extent of their services. Entrepreneurs with little or no training have opened businesses as accent coaches. Some of these enterprises are small, with a single individual offering services over Skype, while others are large companies, catering to other organizations (Derwing & Munro, 2015; Thomson, 2014). In many cases, advertising presents highly inaccurate statements about the English phonological system, betraying a lack of knowledge on the part of the providers. The obvious factual errors on many websites suggest that learners might receive little or no value for their money, and worse, they could be seriously misled to the point that they become less intelligible. Among the documented false and unsubstantiated claims are the following: English has no syllables; a syllabic /n/ is the same as a "long" /n/; practicing speech with a marshmallow between the lips is effective for accent reduction (for a detailed review, see Derwing & Munro, 2015).

In addition to falsehoods promoted by many accent reductionists, it is commonly claimed that accents can be "eliminated" in short periods of time. In fact, we know of no empirical evidence indicating that typical adult L2 learners can achieve such a goal (Derwing & Munro, 2015). It is understandable that some L2 speakers are concerned about the social consequences of their accents and may wish to sound native-like, even when they are already highly intelligible and easy to understand. Their fears are a response to societal bias including discriminatory practices against immigrants. Moreover, the advertising on accent reduction websites seems to exploit those fears and conveys the message that accent reduction can somehow reduce discrimination. We know of no research supporting such a conclusion. On the one hand, there is no reason to deny L2 learners whatever instruction they wish, including so-called accent reduction; on the other, there is no reason to give credence to the message that accents can be eliminated or that reducing an accent is effective in improving social status or opening employment options.

Currently there are no regulatory bodies for practitioners of accent reduction. As Lippi-Green (2012) observed, anyone can claim to be an accent coach, just as anyone can claim to "have developed a miracle diet and charge money for it" (p. 229). A consequence of this absence of regulation is a proliferation of predatory websites, which at best simply waste people's money, but may actually cause them to be less intelligible (Derwing & Munro, 2015). This growing problem is exacerbated by the fact that so many ethical instructors of English feel inadequately trained to teach pronunciation (Foote, Holtby, & Derwing, 2011).

Other practitioners who sometimes offer "L2 accent modification" are speech-language pathologists (SLPs). As Thomson (2014) has pointed out, SLP credentials alone do not guarantee adequate background for teaching pronunciation to L2 learners, and indeed, most SLPs lack training in this area (Müller, Ball, & Guendouzi, 2000; Schmidt & Sullivan, 2003; Thomson, 2013). Unless they engage with the applied phonetics literature and second language acquisition research, they have little foundation for providing learners with a focus on comprehensibility and may even entertain ill-informed perspectives on accent. On its website, the American Speech-Language-Hearing Association (2018) emphasizes "that accents are NOT a communication disorder" and that "SLPs who serve this population should be appropriately trained to do so." However, Thomson (2013) indicates that some SLPs do treat accent as a clinical disorder, a perception documented by Schmidt and Sullivan (2003) in a national American survey of SLP attitudes. Thus, some practitioners do not necessarily adhere to ASHA's recommendations on this issue.

An alternative to "accent reduction" and "accent modification" is "pronunciation teaching," the term typically employed by applied linguists. Language teachers, however, as indicated previously, often have limited access to training, because university teacher education programs rarely include coursework on how to teach pronunciation. In a survey of Canadian language programs, Foote et al. (2011) found that teachers generally recognize the importance of pronunciation, but often feel they have inadequate skills. In light of the recent explosion of applied phonetics research, more teacher training opportunities are likely to emerge in the future.

Future directions

The current momentum in pronunciation research will lead to advancements in a variety of subdomains. Areas of particular need can be identified through an examination of Figure 17.1. *Knowledge and Attitudes* represents a subdomain in which a great deal of valuable work has already been carried out. Remaining avenues to explore include the benefits of intensive PI during the first massive exposure to the L2, referred to as the "Window of Maximal Opportunity" (WMO) (Derwing & Munro, 2015). Nevertheless, this area of work, along with *Pedagogical Goals*, represents the least urgent needs of the field. Such is not the case for *Focus of Attention*, which requires considerably more investigation. Teachers need guidance on where to focus their priorities in the pursuit of intelligibility and comprehensibility goals. Suitable issues for empirical inquiry include functional load, error gravity, and combinatory effects of pronunciation errors.

Of the four areas identified in Figure 17.1, though, *Learning Activities and Techniques* is the one most in need of attention. Whether learners receive the PI they need depends on how new knowledge of evidence-based practices finds its way to the classroom. Not only must research findings be incorporated into materials and software, but they must be communicated to teachers through appropriate training. Teachers must be able to identify students' individual comprehensibility needs, and to implement the learning activities necessary to bring about positive changes. Given that teachers often have insights into the complexities of their students' communication needs and the constraints inherent in the language classroom, the best results for students will be realized if researchers and teachers collaborate to a greater degree.

With respect to the design of learning tasks, the emphasis in research must be placed on identifying activities that are both engaging and demonstrably effective. Exploratory studies such as Lee and Lyster's (2016) and Saito and Lyster's (2012) comparison of the effects of types of classroom feedback on speech perception offer a promising direction for replication and extension. On a micro level, Couper (2011) and Fraser (2006) have discussed the importance of using socially constructed feedback: "metalanguage developed by students working together with the teacher using already understood first language (L1) concepts to help in the formation of target language phonological concepts" (Couper, 2011, p. 159). Another potentially useful avenue of investigation is that of Galante and Thomson (2017), who compared two oral classroom activities to determine which had the best outcomes on dimensions such as fluency and comprehensibility. Expansion of this research to encompass a range of activities would be valuable.

As noted earlier, technology has always held promise for advances in PI, but its impact has been attenuated by insufficient balance of linguistically accurate, pedagogically sound and technologically sophisticated considerations. Specialist teams, including phoneticians, L2 pedagogical experts, engineers, and computing experts can produce work together that takes into account the multifaceted needs of individual learners. While such collaboration is taking place in The Netherlands (e.g., Cucchiarini & Strik, 2018), it has yet to expand internationally.

Finally, as the importance of "big data" emerges, PI research would benefit from new or revised methodology. Corpus-based approaches (see, e.g., Yoon et al. 2009), larger scale studies, delayed post-tests (carried out months or even years after interventions), longitudinal studies with different populations, and investigations of the acquisition of pronunciation in a wider range of L2s could all lead to better insights, provided that the ultimate goal of applied phonetics research is understood to be enhanced communication skills for L2 speakers.

Further reading

Derwing, T. M., & Munro, M. J. (2015). *Pronunciation fundamentals: Evidence-based perspectives for L2 teaching and research*. Amsterdam, NL: John Benjamins.

Levis, J. M., & Munro, M. J. (2017). *Pronunciation, Vols. 1–4*. London & New York, NY: Routledge.

Related topics

Applied linguistics, L2 pronunciation, speech perception, speech production, second language teaching

References

Abercrombie, D. (1949). Teaching pronunciation. *ELT Journal*, *3*, 113–122.

Abrahamsson, N., & Hyltenstam, K. (2009). Age of onset and nativelikeness in a second language: Listener perception versus linguistic scrutiny. *Language Learning*, *59*, 249–306.

Alter, A. L., & Oppenheimer, D. M. (2009). Uniting the tribes of fluency to form a metacognitive nation. *Personality and Social Psychology Review*, *13*, 219–235.

American Speech-Language-Hearing Association. (2018). *Document*. Retrieved March 9, 2018 from www.asha.org/Practice-Portal/Professional-Issues/Accent-Modification/

Anderson-Hsieh, J., Johnson, R., & Koehler, K. (1992). The relationship between native speaker judgments of nonnative pronunciation and deviance in segmentals, prosody, and syllable structure. *Language Learning*, *42*, 529–555.

Anisfeld, M., Bogo, N., & Lambert, W. (1962). Evaluational reactions to accented English speech. *Journal Abnormal Psychology*, *65*, 223–231.

Bell, A. M. (1867). *Visible speech*. London: Simpkin Marshall & Co.

Bent, T., & Bradlow, A. R. (2003). The interlanguage speech intelligibility benefit. *The Journal of the Acoustical Society of America*, *114*, 1600–1610.

Bent, T., Bradlow, A. R., & Smith, B. L. (2007). Segmental errors in different word positions and their effects on intelligibility of non-native speech. In O. S. Bohn & M. J. Munro (Eds.), *Language experience in second language speech learning: In honor of James Emil Flege* (pp. 331–347). Amsterdam, NL: John Benjamins.

Best, C. T., McRoberts, G. W., & Sithole, N. M. (1988). Examination of perceptual reorganization for nonnative speech contrasts: Zulu click discrimination by English speaking adults and infants. *Journal of Experimental Psychology: Human Perception and Performance*, *14*, 345–360.

Best, C. T., & Tyler, M. D. (2007). Nonnative and second-language speech perception: Commonalities and complementarities. In O. S. Bohn & M. J. Munro (Eds.), *Language experience in second language speech learning* (pp. 13–34). Amsterdam, NL: John Benjamins.

Bione, T., Grimshaw, J., & Cardoso, W. (2016). An evaluation of text-to-speech synthesizers in the foreign language classroom: Learners' perceptions In S. Papadima-Sophocleous, L. Bradley, & S. Thouësny (Eds.), *CALL communities and culture – Short papers from Eurocall 2016* (pp. 50–54). Dublin, Ireland: Research-Publishing.net.

Bradlow, A. R., Pisoni, D. B., Akahane-Yamada, R., & Tohkura, Y. I. (1997). Training Japanese listeners to identify English/ɪ/and/l/: IV. Some effects of perceptual learning on speech production. *The Journal of the Acoustical Society of America*, *101*, 2299–2310.

Brennan, E. M., Ryan, E. B., & Dawson, W. E. (1975). Scaling of apparent accentedness by magnitude estimation and sensory modality matching. *Journal of Psycholinguistic Research, 4*, 27–36.

Brière, E. (1966). An investigation of phonological interference. *Language, 42*, 769–796.

Brown, H. D. (2014). *Principles of language learning and teaching* (6th ed.). New York, NY: Pearson Education.

Bürki-Cohen, J., Miller, J. L., & Eimas, P. D. (2001). Perceiving non-native speech. *Language and Speech, 44*, 149–169.

Canale, M., & Swain, M. (1980). Theoretical bases of communicative approaches to second language teaching and testing. *Applied Linguistics, 1*(1), 1–47.

Catford, J. C. (1987). Phonetics and the teaching of pronunciation: A systemic description of the teaching of English phonology. In J. Morley (Ed.), *Current perspectives on pronunciation: Practices anchored in theory* (pp. 83–100). Washington, DC: TESOL.

Clarke, C. M., & Garrett, M. F. (2004). Rapid adaptation to foreign-accented English. *The Journal of the Acoustical Society of America, 116*, 3647–3658.

Couper, G. (2006). The short and long-term effects of pronunciation instruction. *Prospect, 21* (1), 46–66.

Couper, G. (2011). What makes pronunciation teaching work? Testing for the effect of two variables: Socially constructed metalanguage and critical listening. *Language Awareness, 20*, 159–182.

Cucchiarini, C., Neri, A., & Strik, H. (2009). Oral proficiency training in Dutch L2: The contribution of ASR-based corrective feedback. *Speech Communication, 51*, 853–863.

Cucchiarini, C., & Strik, H. (2018). Automatic speech recognition for second language pronunciation assessment and training. In O. Kang, R. I. Thomson, & J. M. Murphy (Eds.), *The Routledge handbook of English pronunciation* (pp. 556–569). New York, NY: Routledge.

Dávila, A., Bohara, A. K., & Saenz, R. (1993). Accent penalties and the earnings of Mexican Americans. *Social Science Quarterly, 74*, 902–916.

Derwing, T. M. (2008). Curriculum issues in teaching pronunciation to second language learners. In J. Hansen Edwards & M. Zampini (Eds.), *Phonology and second language acquisition* (pp. 347–369). Amsterdam: John Benjamins.

Derwing, T. M. (2017). L2 fluency. In S. Louwen & M. Sato (Eds.), *The Routledge handbook of instructed second language acquisition* (pp. 246–259). New York, NY: Taylor & Francis.

Derwing, T. M. (2018a). The efficacy of pronunciation instruction. In O. Kang, R. I. Thomson, & J. M. Murphy (Eds.), *The Routledge handbook of contemporary English pronunciation* (pp. 320–334). New York, NY: Routledge.

Derwing, T. M. (2018b). The role of phonological awareness in language learning. In P. Garrett & J. M. Cots (Eds.), *Routledge handbook of language awareness* (pp. 339–353). New York, NY: Routledge.

Derwing, T. M., Foote, J. A., & Munro, M. J. (forthcoming). *Long-term benefits of pronunciation instruction in the workplace*.

Derwing, T. M., & Munro, M. J. (1997). Accent, intelligibility, and comprehensibility. *Studies in Second Language Acquisition, 19*, 1–16.

Derwing, T. M., & Munro, M. J. (2015). *Pronunciation fundamentals: Evidence-based perspectives for L2 teaching and research*. Amsterdam, NL: John Benjamins.

Derwing, T. M., Munro, M. J., & Wiebe, G. (1998). Evidence in favor of a broad framework for pronunciation instruction. *Language Learning, 48*, 393–410.

Derwing, T. M., Rossiter, M. J., & Munro, M. J. (2002). Teaching native speakers to listen to foreign-accented speech. *Journal of Multilingualism and Multicultural Development, 23*, 245–259.

Derwing, T. M., Rossiter, M. J., Munro, M. J., & Thomson, R. I. (2004). Second language fluency: Judgments on different tasks. *Language Learning, 54*, 655–679.

Dragojevic, M., & Giles, H. (2016). I don't like you because you're hard to understand: The role of processing fluency in the language attitudes process. *Human Communication Research, 42*, 396–420.

Eddy, F. D. (1974). Pierre Delattre, teacher of French. *The French Review, 47*, 513–517.

Ferrier, L. J., Reid, L. N., & Chenausky, K. (1999). Computer-assisted accent modification: A report on practice effects. *Topics in Language Disorders*, *19*(4), 35–48.

Flege, J. E. (1984). The detection of French accent by American listeners. *The Journal of the Acoustical Society of America*, *76*, 692–707.

Flege, J. E. (1995). Second-language speech learning: Theory, findings, and problems. In W. Strange (Ed.), *Speech perception and linguistic experience: Theoretical and methodological issues* (pp. 233–277). Timonium, MD: York Press.

Flege, J. E., Frieda, E. M., & Nozawa, T. (1997). Amount of native-language (L1) use affects the pronunciation of an L2. *Journal of Phonetics*, *25*, 169–186.

Flege, J. E., Munro, M. J., & MacKay, I. R. A. (1995). Factors affecting strength of perceived foreign accent in a second language. *The Journal of the Acoustical Society of America*, *97*, 3125–3134.

Floccia, C., Butler, J., Goslin, J., & Ellis, L. (2009). Regional and foreign accent processing in English: Can listeners adapt? *The Journal of Psycholinguistic Research*, *38*, 379–412.

Foote, J. A., Holtby, A. K., & Derwing, T. M. (2011). Survey of the teaching of pronunciation in adult ESL programs in Canada, 2010. *TESL Canada Journal*, *29*(1), 1–22.

Foote, J., & Smith, G. (2013, September). *Is there an app for that?* Paper presented at the 5th Pronunciation in Second Language Learning and Teaching Conference, Ames, Iowa.

Fraser, H. (2006). Helping teachers help students with pronunciation: A cognitive approach. *Prospect*, *21*(1), 80–96.

Galante, A., & Thomson, R. I. (2017). The effectiveness of drama as an instructional approach for the development of second language oral fluency, comprehensibility, and accentedness. *TESOL Quarterly*, *51*, 115–142.

Gass, S., & Varonis, E. M. (1984). The effect of familiarity on the comprehensibility of nonnative speech. *Language Learning*, *34*, 65–89.

Gimson, Alfred C. (1962). *Introduction to the Pronunciation of English*. London: Edward Arnold.

Hahn, L. D. (2004). Primary stress and intelligibility: Research to motivate the teaching of suprasegmentals. *TESOL Quarterly*, *38*(2), 201–223.

Hart, J. (1569). *An orthographie*. London: William Seres.

Holder, W. (1669). *Elements of speech*. London: T. N. for J. Martyn. Reprinted (1967), R. C. Alston (Ed.). Menston: Scolar Press.

Isaacs, T. (2014). Assessing pronunciation. In A. J. Kunnan (Ed.), *The companion to language assessment* (pp. 140–155). Hoboken, NJ: Wiley-Blackwell.

Isaacs, T., & Thomson, R. I. (2013). Rater experience, rating scale length, and judgments of L2 pronunciation: Revisiting research conventions. *Language Assessment Quarterly*, *10*, 135–159.

Jenkins, J. (2002). A sociolinguistically based, empirically researched pronunciation syllabus for English as an international language. *Applied Linguistics*, *23*(1), 83–103.

Kalin, R., & Rayko, D. S. (1978) Discrimination in evaluative judgments against foreign-accented job candidates. *Psychological Reports*, *43*, 1203–1209.

Krashen, S. D. (1981). *Second language acquisition and second language learning*. Oxford: Pergamon.

Lado, R. (1957). *Linguistics across cultures*. Ann Arbor, MI: University of Michigan Press.

Lambacher, S., Martens, W., Kakehi, K., Marasinghe, C., & Molholt, G. (2005). The effects of identification training on the identification and production of American English vowels by native speakers of Japanese. *Applied Psycholinguistics*, *26*, 227–247.

Lambert, W. E., Hodgson, R. C., Gardner, R. C., & Fillenbaum, S. (1960). Evaluational reactions to spoken language. *Journal of Abnormal and Social Psychology*, *60*, 44–51.

Leather, J. (1983). Second-language pronunciation learning and teaching. *Language Teaching*, *16*(3), 198–219.

Lee, A. H., & Lyster, R. (2016). Effects of different types of corrective feedback on receptive skills in a second language: A speech perception training study. *Language Learning*, *66*, 809–833.

Lee, J., Jang, J., & Plonsky, L. (2015). The effectiveness of second language pronunciation instruction: A meta-analysis. *Applied Linguistics*, *36*, 345–366.

Levis, J. M. (2005). Changing contexts and shifting paradigms in pronunciation teaching. *TESOL Quarterly*, *39*, 369–377.

Lindemann, S., Campbell, M. A., Litzenberg, J., & Subtirelu, N. C. (2016). Explicit and implicit training methods for improving native English speakers' comprehension of nonnative speech. *Journal of Second Language Pronunciation*, *2*, 93–108.

Lippi-Green, R. (2012). *English with an accent: Language, ideology, and discrimination in the United States* (2nd ed.). New York, NY: Routledge.

Lively, S. E., Pisoni, D. B., Yamada, R. A., Tohkura, Y. I., & Yamada, T. (1994). Training Japanese listeners to identify English/r/and/l/. III. Long-term retention of new phonetic categories. *The Journal of the Acoustical Society of America*, *96*, 2076–2087.

Logan, J. S., Lively, S. E., & Pisoni, D. B. (1991). Training Japanese listeners to identify English /r/ and/l/: A first report. *The Journal of the Acoustical Society of America*, *89*, 874–886.

MacKay, I. R. A., & Flege, J. E. (2004). Effects of the age of second-language learning on the duration of first-language and second-language sentences: The role of suppression. *Applied Psycholinguistics*, *25*, 373–396.

Major, R. C., Fitzmaurice, S. F., Bunta, F., & Balasubramanian, C. (2002). The effects of nonnative accents on listening comprehension: Implications for ESL assessment. *TESOL Quarterly*, *36*, 173–190.

McGowan, K. B. (2015). Social expectation improves speech perception in noise. *Language and Speech*, *58*, 502–521.

Miyawaki, K., Jenkins, J. J., Strange, W., Liberman, A. M., Verbrugge, R., & Fujimura, O. (1975). An effect of linguistic experience: The discrimination of [r] and [l] by native speakers of Japanese and English. *Perception & Psychophysics*, *18*(5), 331–340.

Moyer, A. (2009). Input as a critical means to an end: Quantity and quality of experience in L2 phonological attainment. In T. Piske & M. Young-Scholten (Eds.), *Input matters in SLA* (pp. 159–174). Bristol: Multilingual Matters.

Müller, N., Ball, M. J., & Guendouzi, J. (2000). Accent reduction programs: Not a role for speech-language pathologists? *Advances in Speech-Language Pathology*, *2*, 119–129.

Munro, M. J. (2003). A primer on accent discrimination in the Canadian context. *TESL Canada Journal*, *20*(2), 38–51.

Munro, M. J. (2018a). Dimensions of pronunciation. In O. Kang, R. I. Thomson, & J. M. Murphy (Eds.), *Routledge handbook of contemporary English pronunciation* (pp. 413–431). New York, NY: Routledge.

Munro, M. J. (2018b). How well can we predict L2 learners' pronunciation difficulties. *The CATESOL Journal*, *30*, 267–281.

Munro, M. J., & Derwing, T. M. (1995a). Foreign accent, comprehensibility, and intelligibility in the speech of second language learners. *Language Learning*, *45*, 73–97.

Munro, M. J., & Derwing, T. M. (1995b). Processing time, accent, and comprehensibility in the perception of native and foreign-accented speech. *Language and Speech*, *38*, 289–306.

Munro, M. J., & Derwing, T. M. (1998). The effects of speech rate on the comprehensibility of native and foreign accented speech. *Language Learning*, *48*, 159–182.

Munro, M. J., & Derwing, T. M. (2001). Modelling perceptions of the comprehensibility and accentedness of L2 speech: The role of speaking rate. *Studies in Second Language Acquisition*, *23*, 451–468.

Munro, M. J., & Derwing, T. M. (2006). The functional load principle in ESL pronunciation instruction: An exploratory study. *System*, *34*, 520–531.

Munro, M. J., & Derwing, T. M. (2008). Segmental acquisition in adult ESL learners: A longitudinal study of vowel production. *Language Learning*, *58*, 479–502.

Munro, M. J., & Derwing, T. M. (2015). A prospectus for pronunciation research methods in the 21st century: A point of view. *Journal of Second Language Pronunciation*, *1*, 11–42.

Munro, M. J., Derwing, T. M., & Burgess, C. S. (2010). Detection of nonnative speaker status from content-masked speech. *Speech Communication*, *52*, 626–637.

Munro, M. J., Derwing, T. M., & Morton, S. L. (2006). The mutual intelligibility of L2 speech. *Studies in Second Language Acquisition*, *28*, 111–131.

Munro, M. J., Derwing, T. M., & Thomson, R. I. (2015). Setting segmental priorities for English learners: Evidence from a longitudinal study. *International Review of Applied Linguistics in Language Teaching*, *53*(1), 39–60.

Munro, M., & Mann, V. (2005). Age of immersion as a predictor of foreign accent. *Applied Psycholinguistics*, *26*, 311–341.

O'Brien, M. G., Derwing, T. M., Cucchiarini, C., Hardison, D. M., Mixdorff, H., Thomson, R. I., Strik, H., Levis, J. M., Munro, M. J., Foote, J. A., & Levis, G. M. (2018). Directions for the future of technology in pronunciation research and teaching. *Journal of Second Language Pronunciation*, *4*, 182–206.

Pennington, M. C., & Ellis, N. C. (2000). Cantonese speakers' memory for English sentences with prosodic cues. *The Modern Language Journal*, *84*, 372–389.

Perlmutter, M. (1989). Intelligibility rating of L2 speech pre-and post-intervention. *Perceptual and Motor Skills*, *68*, 515–521.

Price, O. (1665). *The vocal organ*. Menston, Yorkshire: Scolar Press, A Scolar Press Facsimile.

Purcell, E. T., & Suter, R. W. (1980). Predictors of pronunciation accuracy: A re-examination. *Language Learning*, *30*, 271–287.

Reisler, M. (1976). Always the laborer, never the citizen: Anglo perceptions of the Mexican immigrant during the 1920s. *Pacific Historical Review*, *45*, 231–254.

Richards, J. C., & Rodgers, T. S. (2014). *Approaches and methods in language teaching*. Cambridge: Cambridge University Press.

Robinson, R. (1617). *The art of pronunciation*. London: Nicholas Oakes. Reprinted in 1969 by Menston, England: The Scolar Press.

Saito, K., & Lyster, R. (2012). Effects of form-focused instruction and corrective feedback on L2 pronunciation development of /ɹ/ by Japanese learners of English. *Language Learning*, *62*, 595–633.

Saito, K., Trofimovich, P., & Isaacs, T. (2017). Using listener judgements to investigate linguistic influences on L2 comprehensibility and accentedness: A validation and generalization study. *Applied Linguistics*, *38*, 439–462.

Schiavetti, N. (1992). Scaling procedures for the measurement of speech intelligibility. In R. D. Kent (Ed.), *Intelligibility in speech disorders* (pp. 11–34). Philadelphia, PA: John Benjamins.

Schmidt, A. M., & Sullivan, S. (2003). Clinical training in foreign accent modification: A national survey. *Contemporary Issues in Communication Science and Disorders*, *30*, 127–135.

Segalowitz, N. (2010). *Cognitive bases of second language fluency*. New York, NY: Routledge.

Sewell, A. (2017). Functional load revisited. *Journal of Second Language Pronunciation*, *3*(1), 57–79.

Smith, B. L., & Hayes-Harb, R. (2011). Individual differences in the perception of final consonant voicing among native and non-native speakers of English. *Journal of Phonetics*, *39*, 115–120.

Smith, L. E., & Nelson, C. L. (1985). International intelligibility of English: Directions and resources. *World Englishes*, *4*, 333–342.

Stockwell, R., & Bowen, J. (1983). Sound systems in conflict: A hierarchy of difficulty. In B. J. Robinett & J. Schacter (Eds.), *Second language learning: Contrastive analysis, error analysis, and related aspects* (pp. 20–31), Ann Arbor, MI: University of Michigan Press.

Strain, J. E. (1963). Difficulties in measuring pronunciation improvement. *Language Learning*, *13*(3–4), 217–224.

Subbiondo, J. L. (1978). William Holder's 'elements of speech (1669)': A study of applied English phonetics and speech therapy. *Lingua*, *46*(2–3), 169–184.

Sweet, H. (1900). *The practical study of languages: A guide for teachers and learners*. New York, NY: Henry Holt & Co.

Szpyra-Kozłowska, J. (2015). *Pronunciation in EFL instruction: A research-based approach*. Bristol: Multilingual Matters.

Tajima, K., Port, R., & Dalby, J. (1997). Effects of temporal correction on intelligibility of foreign-accented English. *Journal of Phonetics*, *25*, 1–24.

Thomson, R. I. (2011). Computer assisted pronunciation training: Targeting second language vowel perception improves pronunciation. *Calico Journal*, *28*, 744–765.

Thomson, R. I. (2013). Accent reduction. In Chappelle, C. A. (Ed.), *The encyclopedia of applied linguistics* (pp. 8–11). Hoboken, NJ: Wiley-Blackwell.

Thomson, R. I. (2014). Myth: Accent reduction and pronunciation instruction are the same thing. In L. Grant (Ed.), *Pronunciation myths: Applying second language research to classroom teaching* (pp. 160–187). Ann Arbor, MI: University of Michigan Press.

Thomson, R. I. (2015). Fluency. In M. Reed & J. M. Levis (Eds.), *The handbook of English pronunciation* (pp. 209–226). Hoboken, NJ: Wiley.

Thomson, R. I. (2018a). *English Accent Coach* [Online resource]. Retrieved from www.englishaccentcoach.com

Thomson, R. I. (2018b). High variability [pronunciation] training (HVPT): A proven technique about which every language teacher and learner ought to know. *Journal of Second Language Pronunciation, 4,* 207–230.

Thomson, R. I., & Derwing, T. M. (2015). The effectiveness of L2 pronunciation instruction: A narrative review. *Applied Linguistics*, *36*, 326–344.

Thomson, R. I., & Derwing, T. M. (2016). Is phonemic training using nonsense or real words more effective? In J. Levis, H. Le, I. Lucic, E. Simpson, & S. Vo (Eds.), *Proceedings of the 7th Pronunciation in Second Language Learning and Teaching Conference*, October 2015 (pp. 88–97). Ames, IA: Iowa State University.

Trofimovich, P., Kennedy, S., & Foote, J. A. (2015). Variables affecting L2 pronunciation development. In M. Reed & J. M. Levis (Eds.), *The handbook of English pronunciation* (pp. 353–373). Chichester, West Sussex: Wiley-Blackwell.

Varonis, E. M., & Gass, S. (1982). The comprehensibility of non-native speech. *Studies in Second Language Acquisition*, *4*, 114–136.

Walker, R. (2011). *Teaching the pronunciation of English as a Lingua Franca*. Oxford: Oxford University Press.

Wardaugh, R. (1970). The contrastive analysis hypothesis. *TESOL Quarterly*, *4*, 123–130.

Werker, J. F., & Tees, R. C. (2002). Cross-language speech perception: Evidence for perceptual reorganization during the first year of life. *Infant Behavior and Development*, *25*(1), 121–133.

Weyant, J. M. (2007). Perspective taking as a means of reducing negative stereotyping of individuals who speak English as a second language. *Journal of Applied Social Psychology*, *37*, 703–716.

Winters, S., & O'Brien, M. G. (2013). Perceived accentedness and intelligibility: The relative contributions of f_0 and duration. *Speech Communication*, *55*, 486–507.

Yoon, S. Y., Pierce, L., Huensch, A., Juul, E., Perkins, S., Sproat, R., & Hasegawa-Johnson, M. (2009). Construction of a rated speech corpus of L2 learners' spontaneous speech. *CALICO Journal*, *26*, 662–673.

Zielinski, B. W. (2008). The listener: No longer the silent partner in reduced intelligibility. *System*, *36*, 69–84.

Part V
Applications and extensions

18

The phonetics of sex and gender

Benjamin Munson and Molly Babel

Defining the question

The late Peter Ladefoged was fond of telling stories about his days on the set of the 1964 film version of *My Fair Lady*. He loved to regale the UCLA students of the day (tempered with appropriate British reserve) with the story of the day that Audrey Hepburn brought cookies to the set. The lunch room at UCLA had a picture of him on set, coaching Rex Harrison on how to understand the visible speech symbols that were prominently featured in many scenes in that film. That anecdote comes to mind in writing this chapter because of a line that Mr. Harrison's character Henry Higgins utters in that film: "Why can't a woman be more like a man?" More to the point of this chapter, why can't a man *sound* more like a woman? Why do men and women speak differently? What consequences do male-female differences in speech have for our understanding of the nature of human language? How are these differences rooted in our biology, our evolutionary path since diverging from our last common species, and our participation in different social and cultural activities?

Variation in the spoken form of language is pervasive. Consider Figure 18.1. This shows four plots of phonetic characteristics of a set of single-word productions by 22 men and 22 women. These are the men and women described in Munson, McDonald, DeBoe, and White (2006). Briefly, Munson et al. (2006) was an exploratory study of the acoustic characteristics of heterosexual and gay speech from young adult men and women from a uniform dialect region (see Munson 2007a, 2007b for additional analyses of this corpus of talkers). The recordings from that study are used to illustrate various phenomena in this chapter. For a description of the general methods used to make the recordings and the measures, please see Munson et al. (2006). The parameters plotted in Figure 18.1 are temporal and spectral characteristics of consonants and vowels. These parameters were chosen at random from Munson et al.'s exploratory study. Values for men are plotted with crosses, and values for women are plotted with an open circle. As these visualizations show, there is considerable variation in all eight parameters. There are clear clusters of talkers in Figure 18.1a in both dimensions, and clear clusters along one of the two dimensions in Figures 18.1b and 18.1c. These clusters correspond to whether the talkers self-reported as men or women. There is no clear cluster in either dimension of Figure 18.1d. If one didn't know anything about the speakers, and were to subject their acoustic data to an unsupervised clustering algorithm, one of the main divisions in the stimuli would likely correspond to whether the participant identified as male or female when asked to report either sex or gender. Hierarchical clustering applied to these four plots resulted in a perfect classification for Figure 18.1a, near-perfect classification for Figures 1b and 1c (in these cases, one man was classified into a group that included the 22 women), and poor classification for Figure 18.1d (where there were two clusters, one comprising six women and one man, and the other comprising the remaining individuals). Together, these figures show that men and women don't differ in all possible acoustic parameters. However, they do differ in enough parameters that they pattern differently in many cases, even when the acoustic parameters are chosen at random.

Given how strongly men and women's speech cluster together, it is not surprising that a handbook on phonetics would dedicate a chapter to this topic. What is surprising, however,

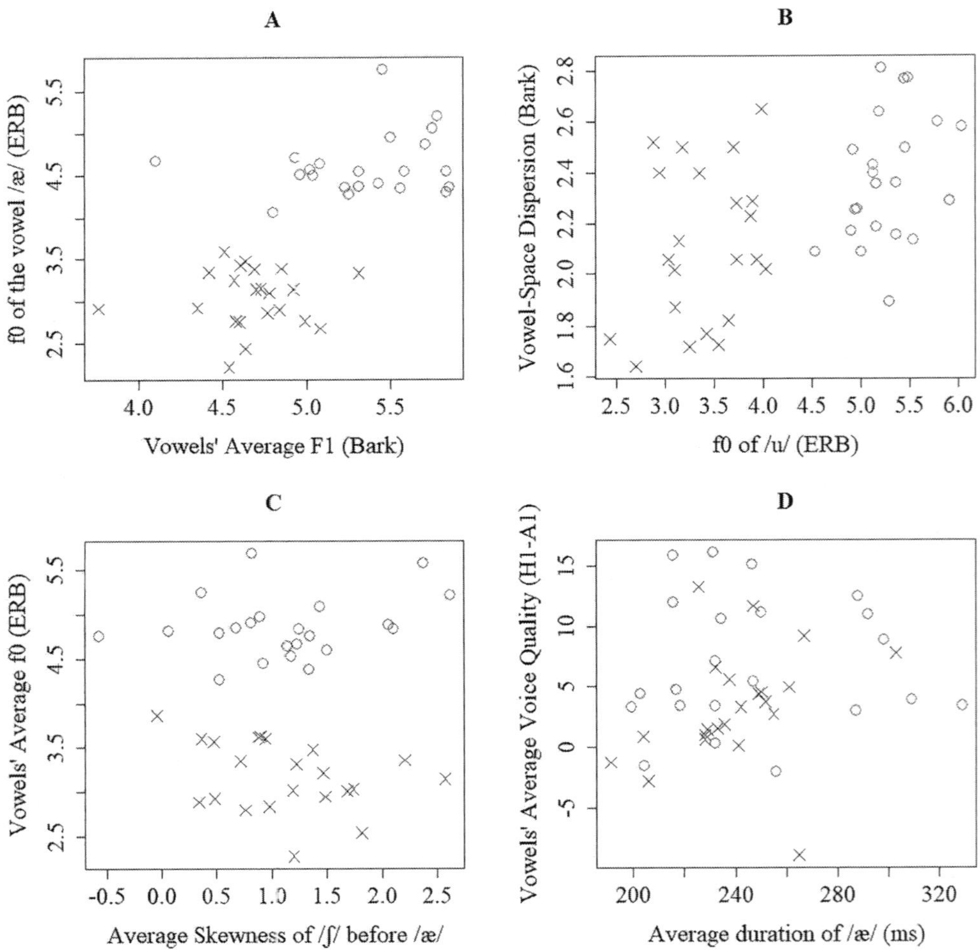

Figure 18.1 Scatterplots of eight phonetic parameters for 22 men and 22 women. The talkers are taken from Munson et al. (2006). The phonetic measures represent a random subset of a variety of spectral and temporal measures of consonants and vowels produced in single words. The men's values are plotted in crosses, and the women's are plotted in circles.

is how complicated the explanation is for these differences. Understanding why men and women differ so strongly involves understanding anatomy (including its development over the lifespan), acoustics, and social dynamics. It requires understanding the full range of variation that occurs in different languages, in different cultural contexts, and at different points in development. We argue that it is a question of deep importance. Given their status as two of the most pervasive sources of variation, understanding the mechanisms through which sex and gender affect speech has the potential to help us better understand how to model the production of variation more generally, an argument we make in greater detail elsewhere (Babel & Munson, 2014).

The phrase "sex and gender" in the title of this paper immediately invites a definition of each of these terms. Most of the quick definitions of these concepts can be summarized simply as "sex is biological, while gender is either socially or culturally determined." This definition has a strong core of truth to it, but its brevity belies the complexity associated with defining and understanding both sex and gender. Regardless, this definitional split is greatly preferable to simply using the terms interchangeably, or to using "gender" simply because it sounds more polite than "sex," which also has the meaning "sexual intercourse." Neither sex nor gender is completely binary. Biological sex in complex multicellular organisms like birds and mammals encompasses numerous traits, such as chromosomal composition, genitals, hormone levels, and secondary sex characteristics. While there are statistical patterns of co-occurrence among these variables, these correlations are not inevitable. The presence of a Y chromosome is correlated at far greater-than-chance levels with the existence of a penis and testicles, a particular level of testosterone, and a large larynx that descends at puberty. However, counterexamples can be found: individuals can be born with ambiguous genitals, or can have a Y chromosome but female genitals. Individuals can opt to take hormone therapy, or to undergo genital reassignment surgery. Both of these interventions would lead an individual to have some canonically male and some female biological attributes at a moment in time. Consequently, individuals can demonstrate characteristics intermediate between the canonical male and female presentations. That is, while there are strong clusters of characteristics that imply the existence of two predominant categories of biological sex, male and female, by no means do these do not describe all individuals.

The existence of sexual dimorphism (i.e., anatomical differences between sexes) is pervasive in the animal kingdom, and the human animal is no exception to this. Many of men and women's speech production mechanisms – from the capacity of the lungs, to the size and position of the larynx, to the size and shape of the vocal tract – create phonetic properties that form statistical distributions whose means differ greatly (but across large population samples, show some degree of overlap). Not surprisingly, then, a recurring theme in this chapter is that many of the sex differences in the speech of men and women are grounded in sexual dimorphism. These speech differences are either direct consequences of the sexual dimorphism of the speech-production mechanism, or are intentional exaggerations or attenuations of the effects of sexual dimorphism.

Still other differences between men and women appear, however, to be completely arbitrary. The apparent arbitrary nature of those differences implies that they are learned behaviors. Another theme in this chapter is that these learned behaviors might reflect an individual's expression of their gender. What, then, is gender? Just as biological sex is complex, so is gender. For the purposes of this chapter, we consider very broadly the notion that gender is a set of practices that individuals engage in that reinforce a social division between men and women. A summary of this as it relates to language variation is given by Eckert and Wenger (2005). In this sense, gender is highly dimensional. As an example, consider the act of expressing emotional vulnerability. According to a survey study conducted in Amsterdam, some experimental evidence suggests that individuals identify this as a "female" trait (Timmers, Fischer, & Manstead, 2003). While the origin and existence of sex differences in emotional expression are a matter of debate (Eagly & Wood, 1999; Chaplin, 2015), the data collected thus far on the topic of gender suggest that when a woman practices vulnerability, and when a man fails to practice vulnerability, they are reinforcing this gender association. Failing to conform to these stereotypes may have consequences: When a man expresses vulnerability, he may face the potential consequence of being thought of as feminine, at least in the Western cultures that have been the subject of most of the research on this topic. In these cultures, these gender differences evolve over generations, are culturally specific, and are potentially fluid over one's lifetime. As reviewed by Eagly and Wood, some of these gender differences are grounded in sex differences in anatomy or physiology, or in the roles that men and women are expected to take in different cultures, like caregiving or money-earning.

As the reader of this chapter will see, our understanding of sex and gender differences in speech is richest when we consider those differences in speech acoustics that can be traced directly to anatomical and physiological differences between the sexes. These differences have parallels in the vocalizations of nonhuman animals, and hence we can speculate on how they arose over the course of human evolution. Our understanding of gender and speech is considerably more tenuous. This is because it is only recently that studies have begun to use equally sophisticated methods for measuring speech and for coding social categories and social meanings. Indeed, only very recently have experimental phoneticians begun to exploit the scholarship on coding gender and sex as something other than as a self-report as either "male" or "female." See, for example, Eckert (2014) for recommendations on improving the coding of these constructs in research. However, there is a small but robust literature in sociocultural linguistics that we can draw on to begin to understand the ways that the many components of gender are coded phonetically.

This chapter is structured as follows: We begin by talking about sex differences between men and women's speech production mechanisms, and describing the speech differences that arise because of these. We then describe those differences in speech that do not have a plausible basis in anatomical or physiological differences between the sexes. We then discuss how sex- and gender-based differences in speech are perceived, and how they develop over the lifespan. We end the chapter with suggestions for ongoing research in this area.

Larynxes

Any discussion of speech acoustics should follow the most influential theory of speech production, the acoustic source-filter theory (Chiba & Kajiyama, 1941; Fant, 1970). This theory posits that the acoustic characteristics of speech sounds reflect the combined influences of a sound source and a filter through which it is passed. The first set of speech features that we consider are those related to the sound source for voiced sounds, namely, the vibration of the vocal folds. Women tend to have smaller and lighter vocal folds than men. By virtue of this difference in morphology, women's vocal folds vibrate at a faster rate than men's (Titze, 1989). Acoustically, this produces a higher fundamental frequency (henceforth f_0). As listeners, we perceive this increased rate of vibration and higher f_0 as an increase in pitch. The source spectrum generated at the glottis is a complex signal, composed of the fundamental frequency and harmonics, which are positive, whole-number multiples of the fundamental frequency. With harmonics as multiples of the fundamental, this means that men have harmonically more dense voices than women.

Consider the following example to make this important distinction between male and female voices more concrete. Figure 18.2 presents power spectra from the midpoint of the vowel /æ/ for a woman (dashed line) and a man (solid line). These are two speakers from the corpus of 44 talkers described by Munson et al. (2006). They represent the extremes of f_0 in that sample. The female who produced this token has a mean f_0 of 223 Hz, and, therefore, has harmonics occurring at 223 Hz, 446 Hz, 669 Hz, and all other positive whole-number multiples of the f_0. The male who produced this token has a mean f_0 of 96 Hz, with harmonics occurring regularly every 96 Hz: 96 Hz, 192 Hz, 288 Hz, etc. So, from 0 to 1000 Hertz, this male has ten harmonics, while this female only has four. While a direct laryngoscopic examination of these individuals was not performed, we can presume that these differences are due, at least in part, to physiological and anatomical differences between these two people's vocal folds.

Given the sex differences illustrated by Figure 18.2, one sensible assumption is that the habitual rate of vibration of the vocal folds can be calculated, and used as an estimate of the mass and thickness of an individual's vocal folds. Perhaps this is true, given that the samples of speech used to estimate f_0 are long enough to average over all of the many other sources of f_0 variation. Over shorter samples, there are likely to be substantial differences. This is illustrated by Sandage, Plexico, and Schiwitz's (2015) assessment of f_0 estimates taken from a variety of speech samples that are often used in clinical assessments of voice. Sandage et al. showed that the estimates for women's f_0 can vary considerably across different speech genres (i.e., counting, sentence reading, and narrative readings). A simple illustration of the effect that one variable can have on f_0 measures is given in the two pitch tracks shown in

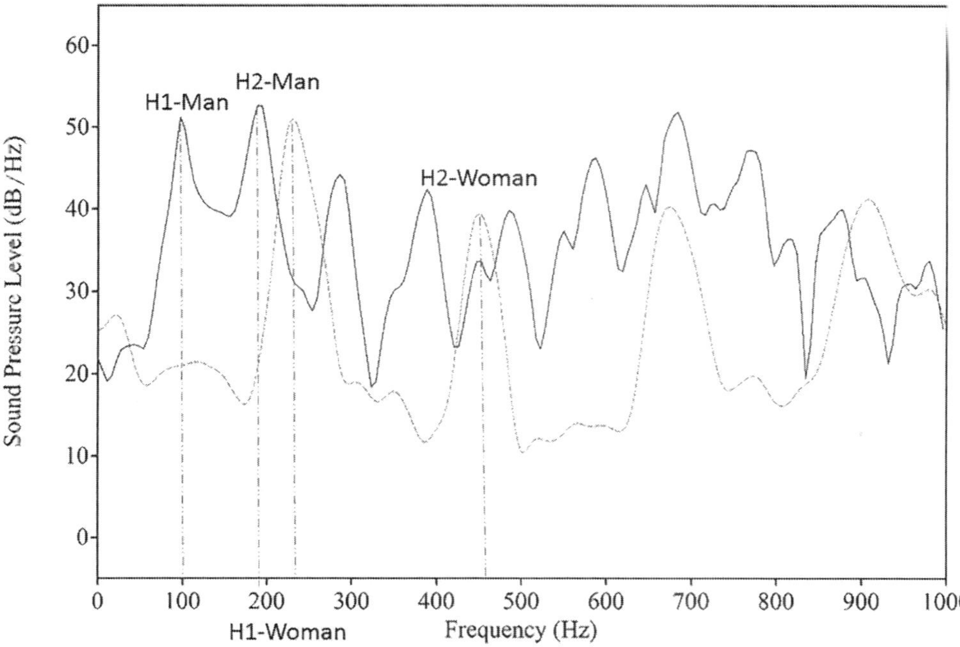

Figure 18.2 LPC-smoothed spectra of 50 ms slices of the midpoint of a token of the vowel /æ/ from the word "pack" produced by one woman (dashed line) and one man (solid line). The first and second harmonics are marked with text and vertical dashed-dotted lines.

Figure 18.3. These are estimates of f_0 over the course of two readings of the sentence *the red bus that you get in the city center takes forever*.

The first of these, shown in the top f_0 trace, was produced with a single intonational phrase, in which the words *red, bus, city, center, takes*, and *forever* were given intonational accents, followed by a fall in pitch at the end of the utterance. The typed words represent the approximate location of each of the words, as determined from a spectrogram. In the second reading of the sentence, there were three intonational phrases, with an intonational phrase boundary after the words *bus* and *center*. This is shown in the bottom pitch trace. The medial intonational phrase was produced as a parenthetical comment, and hence had a lower overall pitch than the first and third intonational phrases (Dehé, 2014). The net result of these differences is that the average f_0 for the first reading is 130 Hz, and 120 Hz for the second reading. This difference reflects the meaningful linguistic difference between the two utterances. The information status of the phrase *which you get in the city center* is different in the two utterances, and the f_0 range is one of the salient cues to this difference. This difference does not, however, have anything to do with the mass or thickness of the vocal folds. Hence, caution must be exercised when interpreting f_0 estimates of individuals' voices, as they reflect the combined influence of many factors.

Sex differences in the mass of the vocal folds also contribute to a typical *voice quality* difference between male and female speakers. Voice quality is a complex phenomenon. Readers are referred to Chapter 4 in this volume for a more detailed treatment of this topic. One relevant parameter for understanding voice quality variation is the *open quotient*, i.e., the amount the glottis is unobstructed during the opening-and-closing gesture of the vocal folds within each cycle of vibration during voicing. Modal voicing occurs when the open quotient is 0.5, that is, when the open and closed phases of the vibratory cycle are approximately equally long. Higher open quotient values indicate that the glottis is more open than it is closed, resulting in a voice quality that is termed *breathy*. Lower open quotient values indicate the glottis is more closed than open, generating a *creaky* voice quality. Many studies have documented breathy voice qualities for women's voices (Klatt & Klatt, 1990), and computational modeling demonstrates that women's thinner vocal folds are less likely

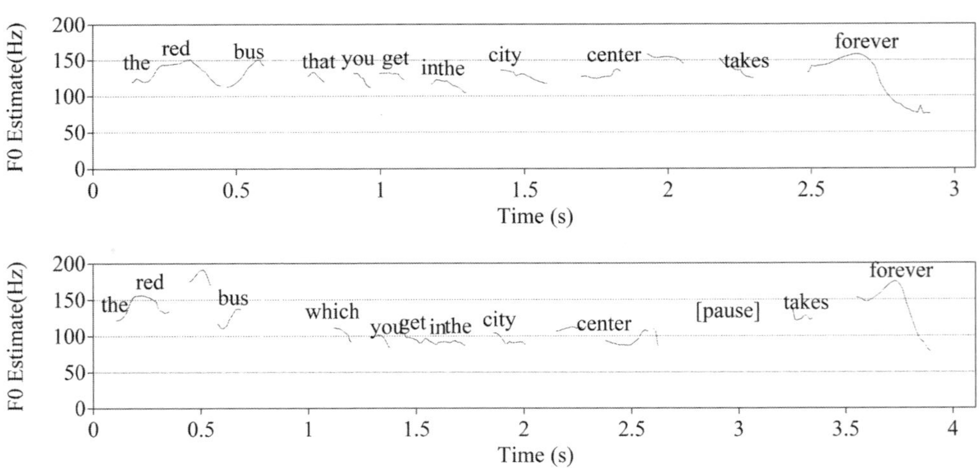

Figure 18.3 Estimates of the f_0 of two sentences produced by the first author. Text represents the approximate locations of the words comprising the sentences, as judged from a spectrogram.

to achieve complete closure when voicing (Titze, 1989), thus producing a breathier voice quality.

A commonly used measure of voice quality is H1-H2, which is calculated subtracting the amplitude of the second harmonic from that of the first. The two individuals whose productions are plotted in Figure 18.2 show a difference in H1-H2. The woman's production has a much larger difference between H1 and H2 than does the man's. This may be due to her producing the word with a breathier voice quality than the man. Indeed, that is the perceptual impression that these two speakers give (at least to the first author, who was trained in the assessment of voice disorders): the man sounds considerably less breathy than the woman. In Figure 18.2, the H1 and H2 frequencies are far away from the nearest formant frequency; hence, their amplitudes can be assumed to largely reflect voice quality, and to reflect vocal-tract resonance properties only minimally. This would not be the case, for example, if the vowel were /i/ or /u/, which have F_1 frequencies that are much closer to the frequencies of H1 and H2. In those cases, the amplitudes of H1 and H2 reflect a combination of voice quality and vocal-tract resonance. In these cases and other instances where the estimation of F_1 can be a challenge, H1-H2 is a less-useful measure of voice quality. A complex correction needs to be made for the potential effects of vocal-tract resonances, such as that described by Iseli, Shue, and Alwan (2007).

Even when corrections are made for vocal-tract characteristics, this measure is still potentially problematic. Simpson (2012) strongly advises against the use of this measure for voice quality, particularly to compare across male and female speakers. The specific problem relates to the fact that the difference between H1 and H2 amplitude can also be affected by the degree of nasality in a person's speech. The reasoning is important to our understanding of sex differences in speech because issues arise when an acoustic parameter that has no global sex difference (e.g., nasal formants) is superimposed on known sex differences (e.g., oral formants), thus obscuring the mechanism behind the measurement. The acoustics of nasals are difficult to predict because of individual differences in nasal anatomy. To create a nasal stop or a nasalized oral sound (e.g., nasalized vowels), a speaker lowers his/her velum. This lowers the amplitude and increases the F_1 bandwidth of the resulting sound (Chen, 1997). This also creates a nasal formant around 200–300 Hertz (Chen, 1997), for *both* male and female speakers. The individual differences in nasal anatomy outweigh any global sex-based differences in the location of the nasal formant. However, this amplification in the lower-frequency spectrum generally serves to increase the amplitude of H1 for female speakers and H2 or H3 for male speakers. So, while the acoustics of this nasal formant that does not have a sex-specific component itself, it amplifies different harmonics in the female and male spectra, based on sex- or gender-specific f_0 patterns. This confounds the use of H1-H2 as a measurement for voice quality, a phonetic feature we know to have sex-specific patterns based in part on physiology. In sum, laryngeal differences can result in male-female differences in speech. However, great care must be applied to the interpretation of these measures.

Vocal tracts: formants

In the source-filter model of speech production, the source spectrum generated at the glottis for voiced sounds is filtered by the vocal tract. This filtering process amplifies the harmonic frequencies that fall at or near the resonant peaks of the vocal tract. Those resonant peaks are determined by the size and shape of the vocal tract, that is, the articulatory configuration of the speech organs. Hence, the next set of male-female differences that we discuss is plausibly related to differences in anatomy. This discussion begins with one basic fact: On average, men have longer vocal tracts than women (Fitch & Giedd, 1999). The resonant frequencies of sounds produced with a relatively open vocal tract are inversely proportional to the length of the vocal tract. Hence, it is not surprising that the formant frequencies of women's vowels are, on average, higher than those of men's. This was first illustrated in Peterson and Barney (1952), a large-scale study on individual differences in vowel production in English, and by Fant (1970), which was a smaller-scale study of speakers of Swedish. They have been confirmed in every large-scale study on vowel production that has been conducted subsequently, including Hillenbrand, Getty, Clark, and Wheeler's (1995) follow-up to Peterson and Barney.

One somewhat surprising finding from these studies is that the differences between men and women's formant frequencies are not equivalent for all of the vowels of English or Swedish. This appears to be due to the fact that the size of the ratio of the size of the oral and pharyngeal cavities is sex-specific. It is approximately equal in women. However, men have disproportionately lower larynxes than women (Fant, 1966; Fitch & Giedd, 1999). This means that they have larger pharyngeal cavities than oral cavities. This leads to especially low F_2 frequencies for men's productions of low-back vowels, when compared to women's productions. Nonetheless, these vowel-specific sex differences can still be explained in strictly anatomical terms, following the source-filter theory of speech production (Chiba & Kajiyama, 1941; Fant, 1970).

The fact that men and women's formant frequencies are scaled differently shows that listeners' perception of vowels cannot involve a simple mapping between ranges of formant frequencies and particular vowel categories. This problem of *acoustic invariance* is one of the longest-standing questions in speech perception: How do listeners map a seemingly infinitely variable acoustic signal onto invariant perceptual representation? The finding that men and women's formant frequencies differ in ways that appear to be related to the overall length of their vocal tracts implies that listeners can account for this source of variability by making inferences about speakers' overall vocal-tract size, and then factoring out the effect of vocal-tract length on formant frequencies. This possibility has been explored at great length in experimental and computational work by Patterson and colleagues (e.g., Irino & Patterson, 2002; Patterson, Smith, van Dinther, & Walters, 2008; Smith & Patterson, 2005; Smith, Patterson, Turner, Kawahara, & Irino, 2005). That work suggests that speakers' overall stature can be estimated from formant frequencies, and that listeners make these estimates at a relatively early stage of speech processing. Indeed, overall height and vocal-tract length are correlated (Cherng, Wong, Hsu, & Ho, 2002). Once an estimate of size is made, subsequent formants can be interpreted relative to that scaling factor. This explanation is appealing not only because of its mathematical elegance, but also because it is observed across numerous species. Reby et al. (2005) argue that male red deer (*cervus elaphus*) make inferences about an antagonist's body size during antagonistic interactions from formant frequencies. Rendall, Owren, Weerts, and Hienz (2004) showed that baboons (*Papio hamadryas*) can also discriminate caller size from call acoustics.

There are, however, data that seem to contradict the strong claim that human male-female formant-frequency differences can be reduced to differences in overall size. Much of this research focuses on within-sex relationships between talker size and resonant frequencies. The first of these pieces of evidence is that the correlation between talker height and formants is much weaker than anticipated if the scaling of the entire ensemble of vowels in the F_1/F_2 space were due only to overall size. Moreover, the correlation is stratified by sex: it is stronger in females than males (Gonzalez, 2004). The lower correlation in males might indicate that men make more maneuvers than women to mask their true body size (i.e., to sound bigger or smaller). The composition of the stimuli used to assess this relationship are likely of great importance. Barreda (2017) found that listener judgments of speaker heights were more accurate when based on productions of certain vowels. Barreda's finding suggests that a comparison of relationships between height and acoustics must consider stimulus composition carefully.

As an illustration of the correlation between height and speech acoustics, consider Figure 18.4, which plots of the relationship between height and both the average F_1 and the average F_2 for the 22 adults in Munson et al. (2006). These are the same adults whose data are presented in Figures 18.1 and 18. 2, using the same symbols for men and women. These

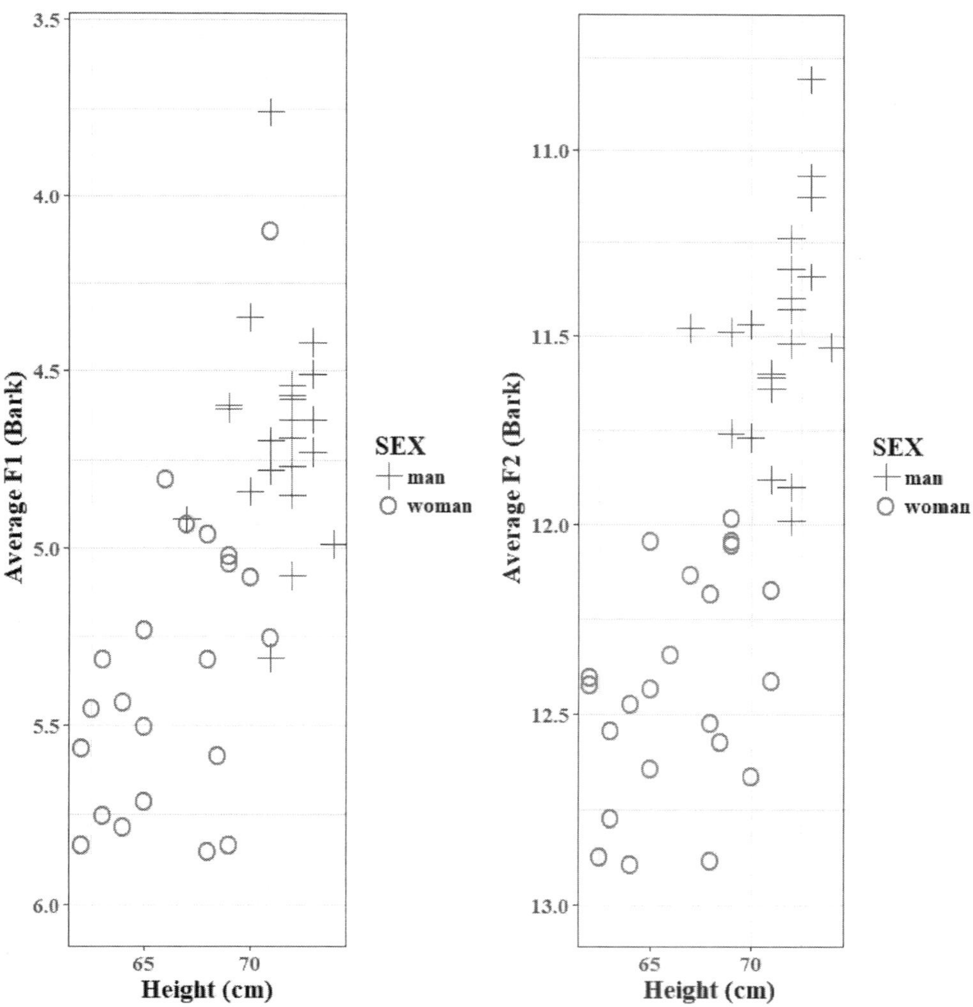

Figure 18.4 Scatterplots of 44 talkers' height (in cm) against the average F_1 (top figure) and average F_2 (bottom figure) of a variety of monophthongal vowels, taken at midpoint. The men's values are plotted in crosses, and the women's are plotted in circles. Details concerning the words and the measurement methods can be found in Munson et al. (2006).

data show the correlation between height and average F_1 (top) and average F_2 (bottom) for a variety of monophthongal vowels. These averages are simply the linear mean of the F_1 and F_2 of many dozens of productions of different vowels, taken at the vowel midpoint. They were the same vowels and the same words for all speakers. When both sexes are included, these correlations are very robust ($r = -0.68$ for F_1, $r = -.76$, $p < 0.001$ for both F_1 and F_2 correlations). Indeed, they are much larger than those noted by Gonzalez. However, they do follow the sex differences shown by Gonzalez: the correlations are stronger for women than for men (for F_1: $r = -0.51$, $p = 0.02$ for women, $r = -0.01$, $p = 0.97$ for men; for F_2: $r = -0.39$, $p = 0.07$ for women, $r = -0.37$, $p = 0.09$ for men). These patterns hold when the logs of formant frequencies are used, as is discussed by Neary (1989). Simply put, while average formant frequencies are affected by speaker size, the weak correlations with size suggest that other factors are at play in determining these values. The general dearth of research in this area, and the small, age-limited sample sizes that have been used, leave this a very open area for future research.

The second, somewhat striking counterexample to the relationship between height and formant frequencies comes from Johnson's (2006) survey of available formant frequency data for men and women's productions of the five vowels /i e a o u/ by speakers of 17 languages. (Johnson's data came from published sources, a full list of which can be found in the Appendix accompanying his article.) While the languages were overwhelmingly Indo-European (and within Indo-European, overwhelmingly Germanic), the set does have some typological diversity (i.e., it includes Hebrew and Korean). Within these data, the degree of gender difference varied widely across languages. One possibility is that these differences are simply related to population differences in vocal-tract length, which we can estimate from differences in overall height (as in Cherng et al., 2002). To explore this possibility, Johnson compared Bark-scaled formant-frequency data to height data within each language population, correlating the gender difference in formant values for a given language to the gender difference in height within that same population. The relationship that Johnson found does not support the hypothesis that the language-specificity of sex differences is due to the population-specific differences in men and women's height: there was a weak relationship between population differences in height and differences in formant frequencies. Johnson concluded that these differences reinforce the idea that there are socially, culturally, and linguistically conventional ways of expressing gender through speech, and that these can mitigate or enhance sex differences in speech communities.

There are many ways to interpret and test Johnson's hypothesis, and we return to it later in this chapter. Here, we discuss one related hypothesis that Johnson's data inspires. This is the idea that the mitigation or enhancement of sex differences that Johnson noted is the result of people modifying the length of their vocal tract. The notion that people's vocal-tract length can be manipulated is supported by a great deal of research (Sachs, Lieberman, & Erikson, 1972). Vocal-tract length can be increased by lowering the larynx or protruding the lips, and, conversely, can be shortened by raising the larynx or spreading the lips. Articulatory studies show that individuals can perform both maneuvers. For example, French- and Mandarin-speaking individuals lower their larynx when producing the round vowels /u/ and /y/ with an articulatory perturbation that prevents them from rounding their lips (Riordan, 1977). Further evidence for the malleability of vocal-tract length comes from experimental studies of the acoustic characteristics of the speech produced by individuals who were instructed to change the impression of their overall body size. K. Pisanski et al. (2016) examined the speech of men and women who were instructed to make themselves sound larger or smaller.

They found that, across a variety of languages and cultures, individuals made modifications to the formant frequencies that are consistent with an overall stretching or compression of the vocal tract. Similar findings are reported in studies of imitated masculinity and femininity in speech. Individuals modify all of the lowest four-formant frequencies when instructed to speak in a more masculine style, and increase them when asked to speak in a more feminine style (Cartei, Cowels, & Reby, 2012). While Cartei et al. and K. Pisanski et al. did not conduct articulatory measures to ascertain how individuals changed their formant frequencies, the consistency with which they did so (across vowels and different speaking tasks) makes it very plausible that they did so by lengthening and shortening their vocal tracts, respectively.

The relationship between body size and formant frequencies can be seen in other animal species that communicate vocally and are characterized by variation in body size. For example, Budka and Osiejuk (2013) show that formant frequencies are related to body size in male corncrakes (*Crex crex*). As described by Fitch and Hauser (2002) and Rendall and Owren (2010), there are numerous cases of deceptive vocalizations in nonhuman animals that give the illusion of being larger or smaller than one actually is. Indeed, one of the motivations of the studies by Cartei and colleagues and by K. Pisanski and colleagues is to understand the extent to which vocal signals communicate information that might be consistent across a diverse group of animal species, rather than specific to human language.

In sum, there is ample evidence that men and women's different-sized vocal tracts lead to acoustic differences in their production of vowels. There is also evidence that male-female differences in vocal-tract size cannot account for all of the differences in vowels between men and women.

Fricatives and stops

This next section considers sex differences in the production of consonants. As the reader will see, there are relatively fewer of these studies than there are studies of sex differences in vowels. We interpret this asymmetry in the research as stemming from two factors. The first of these is that the articulatory-acoustic relationships for consonants are more poorly understood than are those for vowels. Second, the acoustic measures that are generally used to characterize stops and fricatives are less transparently related to their articulatory characteristics than are those for vowels.

Fricatives are characterized by turbulent airflow, which can be produced by forcing air through a narrow constriction, one that is narrow enough that given a particular volume velocity, the flow is turbulent in nature or by forcing air against an obstacle, such as the vocal tract walls or the front teeth. The turbulent noise is then shaped or filtered by the vocal tract cavity in front of the noise source. The result of this filtering is that different places of articulation for fricatives have different frequency-amplitude distributions. The size of the channel constriction, the articulatory configuration (especially involving the tongue), and the distance between channel and obstacle turbulence sources are some of the many factors at play in determining the acoustic qualities of a fricative (Catford, 1977; Shadle, 1991; Stevens, 2000). For our purposes, we focus on articulatory positions that are potentially related to sex differences. For example, given the sexual-dimorphic differences between males and females, we can predict that at a particular oral constriction, the front cavity for a male speaker will be larger than the equivalent for a female speaker's vocal tract, resulting in lower resonant frequencies. Just as with vowels, this cavity size can also be easily manipulated. Speakers can, for example, round their lips, effectively extending the length of the front cavity and, thus, lowering the frequencies that will be amplified. Speakers can also subtly retract the constriction location to create a larger front cavity.

Jongman, Wayland, and Wong (2000) provide a detailed acoustic analysis of the voiced and voiceless fricatives in American English /f v θ ð s z ʃ ʒ/ for 20 speakers. They document higher spectral peaks for female speakers, but not uniformly across fricative place of articulation. While female speakers have higher spectral peak frequencies in the sibilant fricatives, the pattern is less robust in non-sibilant fricatives, where perceptually listeners seem to rely rather heavily on adjacent formant transitions (Babel & McGuire, 2013). Acoustically, English fricatives produced by males have lower spectral means, lower variance, lower kurtosis, and higher skewness than the same fricatives produced by females. It is important to note, however, that these effect sizes are tiny, and vary across the different acoustic measures and the different fricative place of articulations (Jongman et al., 2000).

Stuart-Smith (2007) investigated gendered productions of /s/ in Glaswegian English in males and females from social groups that varied in terms of their prescribed gender norms. While the number of participants in this study was relatively small (n = 32), it is an example of research that is rich in the sophistication of its acoustic measurements, analyses, and social theory. Hence, it is a useful illustration of research on the phonetics of sex and gender. According to Stuart-Smith, middle-class Glaswegian concepts of gender involve more differentiation between men and women than do working-class gender norms. For example, female behavior in the middle class involves more explicit discussion of the domestic realm, compared to the gendered norms for working-class females. In Stuart-Smith's study, younger (aged 13–14) and older (aged 40–60) males and females from middle class and working class socioeconomic backgrounds were recorded reading a wordlist that included /s/ words and one /ʃ/ word. These /s/ and /ʃ/ words were predicted not to show social variation between the groups of speakers. Indeed, they were originally conceived of as control words in a study that focused on sounds whose variation had been studied previously. Stuart-Smith reasoned that, if fricative acoustics were not influenced by socially constructed class-prescribed norms, we would expect that age and sex would both affect fricative acoustics, as speakers developmentally changed in size throughout the lifespan. Effects and interactions of age and gender with social class and a lack of age and gender effects, however, would provide evidence that /s/ production is shaped by the social conventions of the working- and middle-class cultures.

Across a range of acoustic measurements, Stuart-Smith found that young-working class girls have /s/ whose acoustics pattern with the male speakers, despite the lack of evidence of anatomical similarities between these speaker groups. Boys and men from both working and middle class backgrounds clustered together in the analyses, providing evidence of a socially structured "male" style that is exploited by male speakers regardless of age and class. Hence, Stuart-Smith provided some of the first evidence that variation in /s/ was not due to anatomical influences alone in women, as /s/ differed across groups of women for whom there were no obvious differences in anatomy.

Further data on the social mediation of sex differences in /s/ is provided by Podesva and Van Hofwegen (2014), who studied variation in a rural Northern California community. They found greater /s/ differentiation between men and women in that community than had been found previously in people living in urban centers. The authors speculated that this related to the people in this community adhering to more traditional male and female variants, while those in urban centers were freer to use a variety of /s/ variants. Like Stuart-Smith, Podesva and Von Hofwegen provide strong evidence that an apparent sex difference can be mediated by a number of other social factors, like age, social class, and whether one is rural or urban.

There are many opportunities for talker sex to conceivably affect the acoustic-phonetic realization of oral stops. One commonly investigated feature is voice onset time. With their larger vocal tract volumes, males may have an easier time setting up the specific aerodynamic configurations to generate voicing of the vocal folds, leading to lower voice onset time values in voiceless unaspirated stops (e.g., Whiteside & Irving, 1998). Across languages, however, we see considerable variation in terms of whether males or female exhibit longer or shorter voice onset time values, strongly suggesting that temporal patterns of stop articulation are subject to language-specific learned patterns of gender performance (Oh, 2011).

Foulkes and Docherty (2005) examined variants of /t/ in English speakers in and around Newcastle, England. There are at least two variants of word-medial /t/ in this dialect: a plain variant, and a variant that is produced with a very constricted glottis. The glottal variant is produced at high rates by men, regardless of age or social class. For women, the rate of production of the glottal variant differs systematically across age (older women produce fewer glottal tokens than younger women) and social class (middle-class women produce fewer glottal tokens than working-class women).

The fact that sex differences in /s/ and /t/ production in the studies reviewed in the preceding are so strongly mediated by other social variables calls into question whether an explanation for them based on strictly biological factors is even plausible. There is no reason to believe that vocal tract size and shape should differ systematically between, for example, rural and urban individuals. However, research directly examining the relative influence of vocal-tract variables and potentially social influences on consonant variation is sparse. One example of such a study is presented by Fuchs and Toda (2010), who examined whether a variety of anatomical measures of palate shape and size could predict the magnitude of male-female differences in /s/ production. They found no evidence that anatomical factors can explain the sex differences in /s/ production. Given this lack of a relationship, they reasoned that sex differences in /s/ must reflect learned factors.

"Potentially social" variation

The cases of /s/ in Glaswegian and /t/ in Newcastle are cases of what are arguably socially driven cases of differences in speech. Given that these are stratified by self-reported biological sex, it is not inaccurate to label them as sex differences. However, the fact that they are mediated by social factors like age and socioeconomic status suggests that they are cases of socially driven variation. In the remainder of this chapter, will refer to these as cases of *potentially socially driven* variation. By this, we mean that the variation does not have any basis in anatomical differences between the sexes. The word *potentially* is key, because we regard it as unwise to attribute a social origin or social meaning to a pattern of variation simply because one can think of no other source of the variation. We believe that something cannot be deemed to be socially meaningful variation unless there are rigorous, methodologically appropriate studies both of its origin and of the consequences of this variation on social functioning and social evaluation.

With that proviso in mind, consider again the finding described earlier that men's and women's formant frequencies differ across languages. What would a social explanation for those patterns involve? One possibility, discussed earlier, is that it might involve language-specific maneuvers to lengthen or shorten the vocal tract. One reasonable hypothesis is that such behaviors developed because a culture placed high value on sounding a particular way. Such an explanation would need to be verified by rigorous examination of this hypothesis. One model study of a method for a hypothesis like this is presented by Van Bezooijen

(1995). This study examined f_0 differences across languages, rather than formant differences, but the methodology is one that we feel is ideally suited to introduce the reader to a method for studying socially motivated variation of any phonetic variable.

Van Bezooijen investigated why there appears to be more sex differentiation in f_0 in Japanese speakers than in Dutch speakers, a finding previously documented by Yamazawa and Hollien (1992). She hypothesized that these language-specific tendencies relate to culture-specific value ascribed to f_0 variation. She reasoned that Japanese culture would place a higher value on having an f_0 that matches one's biological sex than would Dutch culture. A series of rating experiments found evidence for this: Japanese-speaking listeners evaluated women as being less attractive when their speech had been altered to have a low f_0. They rated men to be less attractive when the speech was altered to have a high f_0. The effect of f_0 on Dutch listeners' evaluation was smaller. Moreover, Japanese-speaking listeners indicated that the attributes of what they believed to be an ideal woman were those associated with higher pitch across both Dutch and Japanese subjects, and the attributes for an ideal man were those associated with lower pitch. Dutch listeners' attributes of an ideal man and woman were more similar, and not as clearly linked to having a high or low f_0. Van Bezooijen's study is an example of an investigation that seeks to ground differences in observed male-female speech in differences in values and expectations across cultures.

Identifying and understanding phonetic differences between men and women is challenging in any context, but researchers' ability to delineate physiological or anatomically induced variation from potentially social variation is further diminished when the community is undergoing sound changes. Let us take as an example GOOSE-fronting, a sound change affecting many varieties of English including varieties spoken in the United Kingdom (Harrington, Kleber, & Reubold, 2008) and North America (Hagiwara, 1997; Hall-Lew, 2011). GOOSE-fronting affects the second formant frequency of a high-, non-front vowel. The historically older vowel is a true high-back vowel, with a characteristically low F_2. The more contemporary production involves a generally more front tongue body position. The smaller front cavity of the new production results in a higher F_2. Sound changes that affect resonant properties, like GOOSE-fronting, can masquerade as sex-based differences if viewed from a narrow lens. That is, if women show a higher second formant frequency in GOOSE than men, one may incorrectly conclude that this is due to women making an articulatory maneuver to shorten their vocal tract. However, an equally plausible explanation is simply that women engage in the sound change more frequently than men, or to a greater extent than men.

A recent and impressive example of potentially social variation is described in Labov, Rosenfelder, and Fruehwald (2013). Labov et al. describe sound changes in the speech of 379 White Philadelphians born between 1888 and 1991, who were recorded across a nearly 40-year period. Labov et al. describe several sound changes in progress in the Philadelphian English vowel system. For many of these sound changes, women were more likely to engage in the sound change at its inception than were men. For example, women and men born around the beginning of the 20th century did not differ in the position of the GOAT vowel, symbolized with /oʊ/ in many American dialects, in their vowel space. As the century progressed, women begin fronting their GOAT vowel, as evidenced by its F_2 frequencies. That is, there is a correlation between when women were born, and the F_2 of their GOAT vowel. The F_2 in GOAT reaches its peak for those who were born around 1940, and women born after this date have progressively lower F_2 frequencies in GOAT. This is a strong example of potentially social variation. There is no evidence that women born in Philadelphia around the middle of the 20th century are markedly different anatomically from women born in the earlier and later parts of the century. There is no epidemiological evidence to suggest, for example, that there was a spike in a particular craniofacial malformation, or in a distinctive pattern of dentition that might affect the front-back movement of the tongue. A reasonable hypothesis, then, is that women in different time periods were simply engaging in different social trends that affect the pronunciation of the GOAT vowels.

Further evidence of social variation comes from studies using ethnographic methods. Ethnography involves careful observation of behaviors occurring in natural environments. One example of a detailed ethnographic study that examined (among other things) phonetic variation is given by Mendoza-Denton (2008). Mendoza-Denton examined a variety of markers of gang affiliation in girls in a high school in East Palo Alto, CA. Her study was noteworthy in many ways, two of which are relevant to this chapter. First, she sampled data very densely over a long period of time. Hence, the observations are very rich, and show how individuals' behaviors changed as a function of their affiliation with different groups in this high school. The ethnographic method allowed Mendoza-Denton to assess the various meanings that the people she observed ascribed to different behaviors, including the use of different phonetic variants. Second, she used acoustic analysis to examine speech. One salient social category that emerged from her study is an identity of "having an attitude" (Mendoza-Denton, 2008: 251). Acoustic analysis showed that individuals who projected this particular identity were more likely to produce the KIT vowel with a more peripheral articulation, resulting in a vowel that is raised in the vowel space with a lower F_1 and a higher F_2. This more FLEECE-like pronunciation is not related to anatomical differences in these individuals, but is an example of potentially social variation, where a speaker's production reflects the identity they wish to project.

One example of a study using a mix of ethnographic and experimental methods to examine gendered speech is given by Zimman's research on the speech of transgender men (some of whom self-identify with the terms trans man or transmasculine man). The speech of trans men is a particularly interesting area of research, because it provides a potential to study how speech changes as an individual's gender identity (e.g., one's experience with their gender, which may or may not correspond to one's sex assigned at birth) and gender presentation (i.e., visible markers of gender, like hair length and clothes) change. In a series of observational, acoustic, and perceptual studies (e.g., Zimman, 2013, 2017), Zimman has shown that there is considerable variation in the acoustic characteristics of the speech of transmasculine men – individuals who are born female, but identify with masculine practices more than female practices. These appear to correlate with a variety of characteristics, such as their gender presentation, and participation in gendered roles and communities. For example, Zimman (2017) shows how these different factors predict variation in /s/ among a group of 15 transmasculine men.

The papers reviewed thus far in this section show convincingly that there are cases where anatomical information can potentially explain phonetic variation, and cases where it cannot. The latter cases include ones in which there is clear evidence, either from demographic patterns or from ethnographic observation, that social factors are a driving force in the variation. The last discussion in this section highlights a particular problem for this research, and that is the cases in which there are multiple, potential explanations for a given sex difference. The specific case is that of the size of the vowel space in men and women. If we are to plot the peripheral vowels of English in the first formant (F_1) by second formant (F_2) space, we would likely find that the size of the F_1/F_2 space is larger for women than it is for men (e.g., Hillenbrand et al., 1995). Why is this? Is this a case of anatomical variation, of potentially social variation, or something else altogether that we haven't yet considered? The answer is "yes," which is to say that there are many potential explanations for this finding. These explanations are not meant to be exhaustive, nor are they necessarily mutually exclusive. But, they are presented in this chapter for two reasons. The first is simply pedagogical. As this is a review chapter, we feel that it is important to give the reader a sense of the myriad explanations that might exist for a particular pattern of variation. The second, however, is to emphasize that there are often multiple plausible explanations for patterns of variation that come from very different academic fields. The norms for research methods and sources of evidence can differ widely across fields, and these differences can then limit researchers' willingness to read research that uses methods that are different from their own. Ultimately, all of these accounts have great merit and potential explanatory value. Let us now consider these explanations in turn. The discussion in this section follows similar explanations given by Simpson (2009).

The first explanation for these differences is anatomical. Women have smaller-sized vocal tracts than men. Hence, equivalent articulatory movements will have different consequences for men and women. A tongue movement of 7 mm by a woman might result in a more extreme articulation than would the same 7 mm movement by a man, given her smaller-sized vocal tract. This more-extreme movement would presumably translate to more-extreme acoustic values. Hence, we might posit that this sex difference is due in large part to an anatomical difference between the sexes. This argument is elaborated upon in Simpson (2002).

The second set of explanations can be called potentially social. These explanations appeal to the sociolinguistic literature on the use of standard and nonstandard forms of language, such as *isn't* vs. *ain't*. As reviewed by Coates (2016), there is a long history of research showing that women are less likely than men to use nonstandard forms like *ain't*. There are numerous purely social explanations for this. For example, because women are involved in child-rearing roles, they perhaps have an onus to preserve the standard forms of the language in their speech to children, which is frequently described as hyperarticulated (Kuhl et al., 1997). Alternatively, women's historical status as subordinate to men might prompt them to use more standard language as a way of sounding polite or educated, as this would potentially regain some of the ground lost due to social inequities. These purely social explanations assume that larger-sized vowel spaces are more standard than smaller-sized ones. Indeed, this is likely to be so, as larger-sized vowel spaces are associated with more intelligible speech (Bradlow, Torretta, & Pisoni, 1996).

The third explanation concerns the perceptibility of male and female voices. Consider again Figure 18.2. The higher fundamental frequency for the woman in Figure 18.2 leads her to have more widely spaced harmonics than the man. This is sometimes referred to as sparser sampling of harmonics. The F_1 and F_2 frequencies that determine the size of the vowel space are based on the resonant frequencies of the vocal tract. These formant frequencies are used to identify vowels, and to discriminate vowels from one another. The sparser sampling of women's harmonics means that their harmonics are less likely to align with a formant frequency than are men's harmonics. The larger-sized vowel spaces produced by women might reflect their tacit knowledge that their high f_0 makes their speech vulnerable to misperception, and that producing an exaggerated acoustic difference between pairs of vowels might remedy this (Diehl, Lindblom, Hoemeke, & Fahey, 1996). The hypothesis that sex differences in vowel-space size are affected by ease of perception is further supported by Munson (2007b). Munson showed that the differences between men and women's vowel-space sizes are biggest for words that are predicted to be easy to perceive based on their frequency of use and their inherent confusability with other real words, suggesting that significant social phonetic variation manifests in words where that variation may be more likely to be noticed.

As noted at the outset of this section, these explanations for why the F_1/F_2 vowel spaces are larger for females than males are neither exhaustive nor are they mutually exclusive. Here, they serve to illustrate the wide variety of methods used to assess and understand sex and gender differences in speech.

Perceiving sex and gender through speech

The discussion of speech perception at the end of the previous section segues into talking about how sex and gender differences in speech are perceived. This section summarizes the literature on the consequence of sex- and gender-based phonetic variation for speech perception. First, we consider individuals' perception of speaker sex through patterns of phonetic variation. Given how pervasively sex affects phonetic characteristics, it is not surprising that statistical discrimination functions can readily identify sex from even brief stretches of content-neutral speech (Bachorowski & Owren, 1999). Listener identification is similarly robust. Only four of the 44 talkers in Munson et al. (2006) were identified as their biological sex less than 95% of the time by a group of naïve listeners who were presented with single words and asked to judge sex. Moreover, all 44 talkers were identified accurately at greater-than-chance levels. This is noteworthy because the group varied considerably in other measures of sex typicality, including ratings of the masculinity and femininity of their speech (Munson, 2007a). Cases of the opposite can be found: Matar, Portes, Lancia, Legou, and Baider (2016) examined the acoustic and perceptual characteristics of the speech of women with Reinke's edema (RE). RE is a condition that affects the health of the vocal folds, and which leads to a dramatic decrease in f_0. Matar et al. report that Lebanese Arabic-speaking women with RE are often mistaken for men, and that they find this very troubling.

What do people listen for when they identify a talker as male or female? Readers of the chapter thus far should not be surprised to know that the answer is: many things. First, consider the relative contribution of characteristics of the voicing source and the vocal-tract filter to the identification of sex. This was the subject of a recent series of studies (Skuk & Schweinberger, 2014; Skuk, Dammann, & Schweinberger, 2015). Skuk and Schweinberger (2014) created sets of male to female voice morphs that independently morphed f_0 trajectories or spectral properties related to vocal tract resonance, and asked listeners to categorize the voices as male or female. The identification of certain voice morphs as androgynous-sounding then allowed them to combine, for example, and androgynous f_0 trajectory with female-sounding vocal tract resonance properties. Their results demonstrate that while f_0 may be the most important single parameter, such a conclusion stems from the outsized role of f_0 on the perception of voices for those with the lowest of f_0 values. For all other voice types – which is most voice types – f_0 and vocal tract resonances both substantially contribute to the perception of voices as male or female. Using similar morphing techniques in the context of a selective adaptation paradigm, Skuk et al. (2015) find that timbre (operationalized by the authors as the acoustic characteristics that distinguish voices with the same perceived pitch and loudness) induces larger aftereffects than f_0 manipulations, suggesting timbre affects the identification of voice gender more strongly than fundamental frequency.

The interaction between source and filter characteristics in perceiving sex was also explored by Bishop and Keating (2012). Speakers were asked to produce their maximal f_0 ranges, eliciting steady-state vowels in nine roughly equally spaced steps across their f_0 range for the vowel /a/. Listeners then evaluated where they felt that production landed within the speakers' ranges. In a second experiment, they asked listeners to categorize the gender of the speakers. They found that f_0 position-within-range was interpreted with respect to the speaker's gender, indicating that listeners have clear expectations about f_0 distributions across genders and interpret variable f_0 accordingly. Listeners seem to compare a given f_0 to a gender-based population sample, which indicates that gender categorization is necessary in interpreting absolute f_0 values.

Listeners have pervasive stereotypes of how men and women speak. Indeed, these stereotypes are so strong that they are the subject of frequent debate in the media. Rigorous instrumental investigation of these stereotypes shows that they are often deceptive. One common stereotype that is apparent through internet searches and pop science books (e.g., Brizendine, 2006) is that women speak faster than men. Acoustic-phonetic analyses suggest otherwise: Byrd (1994) provided some early evidence that the contrary is true: women speak more *slowly* than men. Following from the fact that more complex phonetic events are perceived as being longer (Lehiste, 1976; Cumming, 2011), Weirich and Simpson (2014) reasoned that the perception that women speak more quickly than men relates to the increased vowel space typically produced by women (cite): "a speaker traversing a larger acoustic space in the same time as a speaker traversing a small acoustic space might be perceived as speaking faster" (Weirich & Simpson, 2014: 2). Weirich and Simpson synthetically controlled the f_0 contours and durations of 40 male and female speakers, who naturally varied in the size of their vowel space. Indeed, listeners judged speakers with a larger acoustic vowel space as speaking faster, resulting in women being judged as faster talkers, despite the lack of actual duration differences in the speech samples.

The descriptive norms for men's and women's voices sometimes appear to translate into listeners having prescriptive expectations for how men and women *should* speak. That is, listeners' preferences for male and female voices often reflect a preference for voices that fit typical gendered speech patterns. Listeners' expectations and stereotypes about voices appear to be stronger for female speakers, at least in American English, with correlations between judgments about what's vocally attractive and what is vocally typical for female voices being stronger than male voices (Babel & McGuire, 2015).

Vocal preferences have been most frequently explored in the literature from the perspective of vocal attractiveness, given the evolutionary interest in voices as a sign of Darwinian fitness and a guiding force in mate selection. This line of research typically finds that listeners have a preference for vocal patterns that provide acoustic evidence for sexual dimorphism, conveying evidence for gender-stereotypical vowel acoustics. That is, listeners tend to find average or slightly higher-than-average pitch preferable for female voices and average or slightly lower-than-average pitch more vocally attractive for male voices (Zuckerman & Miyake, 1993; Riding, Lonsdale, & Brown, 2006; Saxton, Caryl, & Roberts, 2006; Feinberg, Jones, Little, Burt, & Perrett, 2005; Feinberg, DeBruine, Jones, & Perrett, 2008). Previous research on vocal preferences has approached the speech signal as though humans are robots programmed to vocalize based on the constraints imposed by their hardware (e.g., unpliable vocal tracts and articulators). While providing important basic insights on the apparent roles of perceived pitch on voice preferences, this work often uses linguistically impoverished stimuli, such as vowels produced in isolation, which tend to then be produced in a sing-song quality with artificially high f_0. The cultural and social variations on spoken language, however, highlight that speakers have some agency in shaping the outputs of their vocal tracts. In this spirit, Babel, McGuire, and King (2014) attempted a step forward in our understanding of vocal preferences, assessing listeners' judgments of vocal attractiveness from a perspective of speaker agency and malleability, making acoustic measurements that go beyond f_0 and apparent vocal tract size. While still using non-ideal speech data – single words produced in isolation – they showed that (specifically Californian) listeners' vocal preferences were based on suite of acoustic-phonetic features that related to sexual dimorphism, as previously well documented, in addition to apparent health and youth and a speaker's engagement with community-level sound changes. These results suggest that vocal preferences cannot be reduced to signals listeners use to infer a speaker's physical stature.

To better understand social meanings, experimental phoneticians must be mindful not to fall into the trap of over-interpreting the results of perception experiments. Consider, for example, a hypothetical experiment examining how a sentence's average f_0 affects judgments of how masculine a man's speech is. Imagine that the two sentences shown in Figure 18.3 were used as stimuli, and that they elicited different judgments of vocal masculinity. It might be tempting to interpret this finding as evidence that pitch influences masculinity. However, given that the pitch differences are due to the presence of a parenthetical comment in the sentence, this interpretation is likely to be an oversimplification. The association between pitch and masculinity in this hypothetical experiment is just as likely to reflect knowledge of the extent to which men and women use parenthetical comments in discourse.

Indeed, the literature on the perception of speaker attributes is replete with examples of cases where listeners identify a speaker as having an attribute that is different from what they might be trying to express. In Matar et al.'s research on women with RE, described earlier, the source of the mismatch is biomechanical. Other, more complex cases might be due to listeners' behavior when asked to judge a social category about which they know little. For example, Smith, Hall, and Munson (2010) showed that different variants of /æ/ elicited judgments of different states of health (i.e., weight, and whether or not a person smoked). Questions about speaker health were included in Smith et al.'s study as filler items. The main focus of that study was on sexual orientation and /æ/ variation. There is no evidence that a person's health affects the type of /æ/ they produce. A more likely explanation is that listeners developed a complex logic over the course of the experiment that led to these judgments. For example, listeners might have associated /æ/ variants with different geographic regions (rightly so, as /æ/ does vary according to region), and then applied stereotypes about people who live in those regions. Another example of this is given by Zimman (2013), who showed that many transmasculine men are rated by listeners as sounding gay, despite the fact that they do not identify as gay men. This may be due to listeners having only weak stereotypes about how gay men talk, or due to the lack of response categories that reflected what the listeners actually perceived. One potential solution to this problem comes from D'Onofrio (2015), who showed that listeners perceive speech more quickly when primed with an authentic social category than when provided with one that is overly general.

Gendered speech development

Another fruitful source of information about the nature of gendered speech comes from its development. The evidence presented thus far shows the sex differences in the speech production mechanism explain many acoustic differences between men and women, and that potentially social explanations explain other differences. The potentially social variation would have to be learned. This invites an investigation of when sex differences in the vocal-tract mechanism develop, and when and how the learned differences between men and women are acquired.

Evidence for the early emergence of sex-specific articulatory behavior is given by Perry, Ohde, and Ashmead (2001). Perry et al. examined listeners' perception of hVd words produced by 4-, 8-, 12-, and 16-year-old boys and girls. Listeners rated their production on a six-point scale, ranging from "definitely a male" to "definitely a female." There were significant differences in the ratings for all four groups. The ratings for the youngest three groups clustered around the two middle values, which represented "unsure, may have been a male," and "unsure, may have been a female." The ratings were predicted by measures of vowels' formant frequencies. Not surprisingly, the largest differences were found for the oldest group. This includes speakers who have undergone puberty. At puberty, the male larynx descends dramatically. This change in the size of the vocal tract is the primary factor driving sex differentiation in formant frequencies.

Other studies have examined the acoustic characteristics of boys' and girls' speech. The formant frequencies of children aged 7–8 show gender differences that vary in size across the vowel space, with part of this difference attributable to sex differences physical size (Bennett, 1981). Bennett also reasons that some of the differences are due to "sex-specific articulatory behaviors" (p. 238). Similar results are reported by Whiteside (2001) where the differences in resonant frequencies for males and females across the lifespan cannot be wholly attributed to vocal tract morphology, but must have some footing in learned, gendered ways of pronunciation.

Part of the seemingly contradictory evidence in the studies reviewed in the previous paragraph is because they did not have access to anatomical data from their participants. Recent research by Vorperian and colleagues has considered the question of the development of sex differentiation in vocal tracts. Vorperian et al. (2011) made a large suite of measurements to MRI and CT images of 605 individuals aged birth to 19 (broken down into four cohorts, as follows: Cohort 1, birth to 4;11; Cohort 2, 5 to 9;11; Cohort 3, 10 to 14;11; Cohort 4, 15 to 19;11) to identify and quantify developmental changes in vocal tract morphology. These included the following measures: vocal tract length, vocal tract vertical (distance from the glottis to the palatal plane), posterior cavity length, nasopharyngeal length, vocal tract horizontal (distance from lips to the pharyngeal wall), lip thickness, anterior cavity length, oropharyngeal width, and vocal tract oral (vocal tract horizontal minus lip thickness). They find that there are pre-puberty differences in the size of the vocal tract's horizontal length and vocal tract's oral size, with the gender differences increasing in the puberty and post-puberty age groups in the pharynx (vocal tract vertical and posterior cavity length increases). There are no differences in the nasopharyngeal length. Crucially, Vorperian et al. document that sex differences in vocal tract anatomy are not stable across development. Rather, the sex differences wax and wane at different developmental time points. However, Barbier et al. (2015) were unable to replicate the finding of gender differences before puberty in growth curves fit to measurements taken from midsagittal X-rays recorded in longitudinal studies of the development of dentition, and argued that the early sex differences found in Vorperian et al. (2009) were an artifact of imbalanced sampling of sexes and ages within the large moving window used in their statistical model. The very question of the robustness of the differences in early vocal-tract size is an open one. This, in turn, invites the question of the extent to which these vocal-tract differences might explain any observed differences in the speech of boys and girls.

Still other cases provided evidence for the learning of potentially social variation. One such case involves the variants of medial /t/ in Newcastle English, described earlier. Foulkes, Docherty, and Watt (2005) examined productions of medial /t/ by children acquiring that dialect. They found that boys and girls began to produce variants of medial /t/ between three and four years of age that mirrored those spoken by adult men and women, respectively. This is a very striking finding, as it suggests very early learning of this feature. Even more striking was the finding that mothers' use of different variants of /t/ in child-directed speech differed depending on whether they were speaking to a boy or to a girl. Mothers used more male-typed variants when speaking to boys than when speaking to girls. This suggests that child-directed speech may be one mechanism through which linguistic variation is taught.

Still other evidence of the learning of gendered speech comes from studies of the relationship between social preferences and speech in children. Two recent studies found an association between the extent to which children's interests and self-presentation aligned with those that are expected of their biological sex, and how sex-typical their voices were. Munson, Crocker, Pierrehumbert, Owen-Anderson, and Zucker (2015) examined acoustic and perceptual characteristics of 30 North American English-speaking boys diagnosed with gender identity disorder (GID). A label of GID (a now-obsolete diagnostic category, replaced by the label Gender Dysphoria) indicates that the child has social preferences and, potentially, a gender identity that does not align with her or his biological sex. Munson et al. found that boys with GID were rated by a group of naïve listeners to sound less prototypically boy-like than boys without GID. However, the acoustic differences between the groups were subtle, and did not suggest that they differed in ways that would suggest differences in vocal-tract size or vocal-fold morphology. That is, the differences suggested that listeners were attending to subtle, learned differences between the groups. Li et al. (2016) examined correlations between the spectral characteristics of /s/ and measures of children's gender identity taken from a parent questionnaire about children's behavior. Li et al. found significant correlations between the acoustic characteristics of boys' productions of /s/ and performance on the questionnaire. Together, Li et al. and Munson et al.'s findings support the hypothesis that children learn gendered speech variants, and that the learning of these variants correlates with social preferences.

A research agenda

The literature reviewed in this chapter is merely a subset of the existing literature on the phonetics of sex and gender. However, even if the literature had been reviewed comprehensively, the message would be the same: previous work has raised more questions about the nature of gender and sex effects on speech than they have answered. Indeed, we regard this fact as one appealing aspect of the science of phonetics: much work is left to be done. Many sex and gender differences in speech are, in truth, under-documented, understudied, and have origins that can remain unknown. Hence, there is much room for new research. This section outlines three areas of research that we believe to be very important, at least at the time that this chapter was written in late 2018.

The first item on the future agenda is to better understand the potential anatomical grounding of sex differences in consonant production. There are numerous benefits to studying sex differences in sounds produced with a relatively open vocal tract: their acoustic modeling is readily accessible to individuals with relatively modest training in mathematics, and they comprise a large portion of the speech stream. However, as detailed acoustic-phonetic investigations of social differences progress, it has become increasingly clear that there are many cases of consonant variation, such as the variation in /s/ and /t/ described above. While these are seemingly unrelated to vocal-tract features, that conclusion is limited by the fact that our understanding of the articulatory-acoustic relationships for consonants is less developed than our understanding for vowels. One useful set of techniques to address this shortcoming is analysis by synthesis. By this, we mean using speech synthesis to infer the articulatory configurations that might have produced specific vocalizations. There now exist a variety of speech synthesizers based on articulatory models of the vocal tract that use simple interfaces (e.g., Plummer & Beckman, 2016). Individuals can manipulate articulatory variables and compare acoustic output with that observed in laboratory and field studies. The result of this is a step toward understanding the articulatory bases of the sex and gender differences that exist in acoustic signals.

A second agenda moving forward concerns the availability of corpora to study sex and gender differences. It is here that there is perhaps the biggest mismatch between research on gender differences in speech that have been conducted using methods from sociolinguistics and ones that have been conducted using methods from experimental phonetics. Consider the corpus studies of Peterson and Barney (1952) and Hillenbrand et al. (1995) These studies examine productions of words that minimize linguistic sources of variation (i.e., they minimize coarticulatory effects by using words with phonetic contexts that are as neutral as possible). Moreover, the use of read speech, produced without an interlocutor present, minimizes any motivation to produce speech with socially meaningful variation. Indeed, the task of producing speech in such a context may suppress the production of socially meaningful variation.

In contrast, consider sociolinguistic studies of gender, such as those described by Stuart-Smith, Zimman, and others. Those studies use methods that maximize the likelihood of eliciting socially significant variation, by making recordings in socially meaningful environments, and with specific interlocutors. These are sensible choices when the goal is to elicit socially meaningful variation. However, these same choices increase the likelihood that recordings will include background noise that will obscure acoustic measures, or that sounds will be elicited in a small number of words, and that the characteristics of words will obscure or enhance sex differences, or that the speech will reflect accommodation to particular interlocutors.

There is no easy solution to this conundrum. One solution is to be careful to interpret male-female differences cautiously, given the limitations of the methods used to collect the corpus in question. Consider, for example, the finding that there are some differences in speech that appear not to be due to vocal-tract length differences. This conclusion does not compromise the fact that vocal-tract length influences are nonetheless present in speech signals: individuals do not have the capacity to shorten or lengthen their vocal tracts infinitely. A naïve listener who assumes that all speaker differences are due to individual vocal-tract sizes will be right more often than they are wrong. Such a finding invites the question of whether children's learning of sex and gender differences first involves attending to these gross speech features, before attending to finer-grained features like the phonetic detail of a medial /t/ or the spectral characteristics of an /s/.

The third item on our future research agenda is to collect data on more languages. The advent of affordable, high-quality recording equipment and free acoustic analysis software means that there are more opportunities than ever to analyze data on under-documented languages. We make the strong argument that no language documentation should be conducted without considering carefully the demographic characteristics of speakers. Having access to more carefully balanced samples can lead to testing hypotheses about the universality of some of the male-female differences that we summarized in this paper. The charge to collect data on more languages includes data on development.

The final item in our research agenda relates to mindset. Many readers will have noticed that throughout this article, we have presented our argument as if the male pronunciation was the standard, and the female pronunciation was the aberrant one, requiring an explanation. This was done in part out of habit. However, once we realized that we were writing this way, we decided to remain consistent, and to close the chapter by encouraging readers to break out of this mindset when studying gender and speech. We hope that the work we have reviewed convinces the reader that sex and gender differences are best understood as cases of linguistic variation, not as cases of deviation from a standard. We encourage the reader to continue to pursue this topic with a mindset of understanding the roots and consequences of this variation, rather than carrying on Henry Higgins' lament that women don't speak like men.

Acknowledgments

The authors would like to thank their collaborators for helping them develop the ideas presented in this article, especially Mary E. Beckman, Jan Edwards, Keith Johnson, Grant McGuire, and Andrew Plummer. All remaining errors are ours alone.

References

Babel, M., & McGuire, G. (2013). Listener expectations and gender bias in nonsibilant fricative perception. *Phonetica*, *70*(1–2), pp. 117–151.

Babel, M., & McGuire, G. (2015). Perceptual fluency and judgments of vocal aesthetics and stereotypicality. *Cognitive Science*, *39*(4), pp. 766–787.

Babel, M., McGuire, G., & King, J. (2014). Towards a more nuanced view of vocal attractiveness. *PLoS One*, *9*(2), p. e88616.

Babel, M., & Munson, B. (2014). Producing Socially Meaningful Variation. In M. Goldrick, V. Ferreira, & M. Miozzo (Eds.), *The Oxford handbook of language production* (pp. 308–328). Oxford: Oxford University Press.

Bachorowski, J., & Owren, M. (1999). Acoustic correlates of talker sex and individual talker identity are present in a short vowel segment produced in running speech. *The Journal of the Acoustical Society of America*, *106*(2), pp. 1054–1063.

Barbier, G., Boë, L., Captier, G., & Laboissière, R. (2015). Human vocal tract growth: A longitudinal study of the development of various anatomical structures. *Interspeech-2015*, pp. 364–368.

Barreda, S. (2017). Listeners respond to phoneme-specific spectral information when assessing speaker size from speech. *Journal of Phonetics*, *63*, pp. 1–18.

Bennett, S. (1981). Vowel formant frequency characteristics of preadolescent males and females. *The Journal of the Acoustical Society of America*, *69*(1), pp. 321–328.

Bishop, J., & Keating, P. (2012). Perception of pitch location within a speaker's range: Fundamental frequency, voice quality and speaker sex. *The Journal of the Acoustical Society of America*, *132*(2), pp. 1100–1112.

Bradlow, A., Torretta, G., & Pisoni, D. (1996). Intelligibility of normal speech I: Global and fine-grained acoustic-phonetic talker characteristics. *Speech Communication*, *20*(3–4), pp. 255–272.

Brizendine, L. (2006). *The female brain*. New York, NY: Broadway Books.

Budka, M., & Osiejuk, T. (2013). Formant frequencies are acoustic cues to caller discrimination and are a weak indicator of the body size of corncrake males. *Ethology*, *119*(11), pp. 1–10.

Byrd, D. (1994). Relations of sex and dialect to reduction. *Speech Communication*, *15*(1–2), pp. 39–54.

Cartei, V., Cowles, H., & Reby, D. (2012) Spontaneous voice gender imitation abilities in adult speakers. *PLoS One*, *7*(2), p. e31353

Catford, J. C. (1977). *Fundamental problems in phonetics*. Bloomington, IN: Indiana University Press.

Chaplin, T.M., 2015. Gender and emotion expression: A developmental contextual perspective. *Emotion Review*, *7*(1), pp. 14–21

Chen, M. Y. (1997). Acoustic correlates of English and French nasalized vowels. *The Journal of the Acoustical Society of America*, *102*(4), pp. 2360–2370.

Cherng, C. H., Wong, C. S., Hsu, C. H., & Ho, S.T. (2002). Airway length in adults: Estimation of the optimal endotracheal tube length for orotracheal intubation. *Journal of Clinical Anesthesia, 14*(4), pp. 271–274.

Chiba, T., & Kajiyama, M. (1941). *The vowel: Its nature and structure*. Tokyo: Kaiseikan.

Coates, J. (2016). *Women, men, and language: A sociolinguistic account of gender differences in language* (3rd ed.). New York, NY: Routledge.

Cumming, R. (2011). The effect of dynamic fundamental frequency on the perception of duration. *Journal of Phonetics, 39*(3), pp. 375–387.

Dehé, N. (2014). *Parentheticals in spoken English: The syntax-prosody relation*. New York, NY: Cambridge University Press.

Diehl, R., Lindblom, B., Hoemeke, K., & Fahey, P. (1996). On explaining certain male-female differences in the phonetic realization of vowel categories. *Journal of Phonetics, 24*(2), pp. 187–208.

Docherty, G. J., & Foulkes, P. (2005). Glottal variants of/t/in the Tyneside variety of English. In Hardcastle, W. J., & Beck, J. M. (Eds.), *A Figure of Speech: A Festschrift for John Laver* (pp. 173–197). New York: Routledge.

D'Onofrio, A. (2015). Persona-based information shapes linguistic perception: Valley Girls and California vowels. *Journal of Sociolinguistics, 19*(2), pp. 241–256.

Eagly, A. H., & Wood, W. (1999). The origins of sex differences in human behavior: Evolved dispositions versus social roles. *American Psychologist, 5*(6), pp. 408–423.

Eckert, P. (2014). The Problem with binaries: Coding for gender and sexuality. *Language and Linguistics Compass, 8*(11), pp. 529–535.

Eckert, P., & Wenger, E. (2005). Communities of practice in sociolinguistics. *Journal of Sociolinguistics, 9*(4), pp. 582–589.

Fant, G. (1966). A note on vocal tract size factors and nonuniform F-pattern scalings. *Speech Transactions Laboratory Quarterly Progress and Status Report, 7*(44), pp. 22–30.

Fant, G. (1970). *Acoustic theory of speech production* (2nd ed.). Paris: Mouton de Gruyter.

Feinberg, D. R., DeBruine, L. M., Jones, B. C., & Perrett, D. I. (2008). The role of femininity and averageness of voice pitch in aesthetic judgments of women's voices. *Perception, 37*(4), pp. 615–623.

Feinberg, D. R., Jones, B. C., Little, A. C., Burt, D. M., & Perrett, D. I. (2005). Manipulations of fundamental and formant frequencies influence the attractiveness of human male voices. *Animal Behaviour, 69*(3), pp. 561–568.

Fitch, W. T., & Giedd, J. (1999). Morphology and development of the human vocal tract: A study using magnetic resonance imaging. *The Journal of the Acoustical Society of America, 106*(3), pp. 1511–1522.

Fitch, W. T., & Hauser, M. (2002). Unpacking" Honesty": Vertebrate vocal production and the evolution of acoustic signals. In A. Simmons, R., Fay, & A. Popper (Eds), *Acoustic communication* (pp. 65–137). New York, NY: Springer.

Foulkes, P., Docherty, G., & Watt, D. (2005). Phonological variation in child-directed speech. *Language, 81*(1), pp. 177–206.

Fuchs, S., & Toda, M. (2010). Do differences in male versus female /s/ reflect biological or sociophonetic factors? In S. Fuchs, M. Toda, & M. Zygis (Eds.), *Turbulent sounds: An interdisciplinary guide* (pp. 281–302). Berlin: Mouton de Gruyter.

González, J. (2004). Formant frequencies and body size of speaker: A weak relationship in adult humans. *Journal of Phonetics, 32*(2), pp. 277–287.

Hagiwara, R. (1997). Dialect variation and formant frequency: The American English vowels revisited. *The Journal of the Acoustical Society of America, 102*(1), pp. 655–658.

Hall-Lew, L. (2011). The completion of a sound change in California English. *Proceedings of the International Congress of Phonetic Sciences, 17*, pp. 807–810.

Harrington, J., Kleber, F., & Reubold, U. (2008). Compensation for coarticulation,/u/-fronting, and sound change in standard southern British: An acoustic and perceptual study. *The Journal of the Acoustical Society of America, 123*(5), pp. 2825–2835.

Hillenbrand, J., Getty, L. A., Clark, M. J., & Wheeler, K. (1995). Acoustic characteristics of American English vowels. *The Journal of the Acoustical Society of America*, *97*(5), pp. 3099–3111.

Irino, T., & Patterson, R. D. (2002). Segregating information about the size and shape of the vocal tract using a time-domain auditory model: The stabilised wavelet-mellin transform. *Speech Communication*, *36*(3–4), pp. 181–203.

Iseli, M., Shue, Y. L., & Alwan, A. (2007). Age, sex, and vowel dependencies of acoustic measures related to the voice source. *The Journal of the Acoustical Society of America*, *121*(4), pp. 2283–2295.

Johnson, K. (2006). Resonance in an exemplar-based lexicon: The emergence of social identity and phonology. *Journal of Phonetics*, *34*(4), pp. 485–499.

Jongman, A., Wayland, R., & Wong, S. (2000). Acoustic characteristics of English fricatives. *The Journal of the Acoustical Society of America*, *108*(3), pp. 1252–1263.

Klatt, D. H., & Klatt, L. C. (1990). Analysis, synthesis, and perception of voice quality variations among female and male talkers. *The Journal of the Acoustical Society of America*, *87*(2), pp. 820–857.

Kuhl, P. K., Andruski, J. E., Chistovich, I. A., Chistovich, L. A., Kozhevnikova, E. V., Ryskina, V. L., . . . Lacerda, F. 1997. Cross-language analysis of phonetic units in language addressed to infants. *Science*, *277*(5326), pp. 684–686.

Labov, W., Rosenfelder, I., & Fruehwald, J. (2013). One hundred years of sound change in Philadelphia: Linear incrementation, reversal, and reanalysis. *Language*, *89*(1), pp. 30–65.

Lehiste, I. (1976). Influence of fundamental frequency pattern on the perception of duration. *Journal of Phonetics*, *4*(2), pp. 113–117.

Li, F., Rendall, D., Vasey, P. L., Kinsman, M., Ward-Sutherland, A., & Diano, G. (2016). The development of sex/gender-specific /s/ and its relationship to gender identity in children and adolescents. *Journal of Phonetics, 57*, 59–70.

Matar, N., Portes,. C., Lancia, L., Legou, T., & Baider, F. (2016). Voice quality and gender stereotypes: A study on Lebanese women with Reinke's edema. *Journal of Speech Language and Hearing Research*, *59*(6), pp. S1608–S1617.

Mendoza-Denton, N. (2008). *Homegirls: Symbolic practices in the making of Latina Youth styles*. Maiden, MA: Wiley-Blackwell.

Munson, B. (2007a). The acoustic correlates of perceived masculinity, perceived femininity, and perceived sexual orientation. *Language and Speech*, *50*(1), pp. 125–142.

Munson, B. (2007b). Lexical characteristics mediate the influence of talker sex and sex typicality on vowel-space size. In J. Trouvain & W. Barry (Eds.), *Proceedings of the International Congress on Phonetic Sciences* (pp. 885–888). Saarbrucken, Germany: University of Saarland.

Munson, B., Crocker, L., Pierrehumbert, J., Owen-Anderson, A., & Zucker, K. (2015). Gender typicality in children's speech: A comparison of the speech of boys with and without gender identity disorder. *The Journal of the Acoustical Society of America*, *137*(4), pp. 1995–2003.

Munson, B., McDonald, E. C., DeBoe, N. L., & White, A. R. (2006). Acoustic and perceptual bases of judgments of women and men's sexual orientation from read speech. *Journal of Phonetics*, *34*(2), pp. 202–240.

Neary, T. M. (1989). Static, dynamic, and relational properties in vowel perception. *The Journal of the Acoustical Society of America*, *85*(5), pp. 2088–2113.

Oh, E. (2011). Effects of speaker gender on voice onset time in Korean stops. *Journal of Phonetics*, *39*(1), pp. 59–67.

Patterson, R. D., Smith, D. R. R., van Dinther, R., & Walters, T. C. (2008). Size information in the production and perception of communication sounds. In W. A. Yost, A. N. Popper, & R. R. Fay (Eds.), *Auditory perception of sound sources* (pp. 43–75). New York, NY: Springer.

Perry, T. L., Ohde, R. N., & Ashmead, D. H. (2001). The acoustic bases for gender identification from children's voices. *The Journal of the Acoustical Society of America*, *109*(6), pp. 2988–2998.

Peterson, G. E., & Barney, H. L. (1952). Control methods used in a study of the vowels. *The Journal of the Acoustical Society of America*, *24*(2), pp. 175–184.

Pisanski, K., Mora, E., Pisanski, A., Reby, D., Sorokowski, P., Frackowiak, T., & Feinberg, D. (2016). Volitional exaggeration of body size through fundamental and formant frequency modulation in humans. *Scientific Reports*, *6*, p. 34389.

Plummer, A., & Beckman, M. (2016). Sharing speech synthesis software for research and education within low-tech and low-resource communities. *Proceedings of INTERSPEECH* (pp. 1618–1622). San Francisco, CA: International Speech Communication Association.

Podesva, R., & Van Hofwegen, J. (2014). How conservatism and normative gender constrain variation in inland California: The case of /s/. *University of Pennsylvania Working Papers in Linguistics*, *20*(2), pp. 129–137.

Reby, D., McComb, K., Cargnelutti, B., Darwin, C., Fitch, W. T., et al. (2005) Red deer stags use formants as assessment cues during intrasexual agonistic interactions. *Proceedings of the Royal Society B*, *272*(1566), pp. 941–947.

Rendall, D., & Owren, J. (2010). Vocalizations as tools for influencing the affect and behavior of others. In Brudzynski, S. (Ed.), *Handbook of mammalian vocalization: An integrative neuroscience approach* (pp. 177–185). Oxford: Academic Press.

Rendall, D., Owren, M., Weerts, E., & Hienz, R. (2004). Sex differences in the acoustic structure of vowel-like vocalizations in baboons and their perceptual discrimination by baboon listeners. *The Journal of the Acoustical Society of America*, *115*(1), pp. 411–421.

Riding, D., Lonsdale, D., & Brown, B. (2006). The effects of average fundamental frequency and variance of fundamental frequency on male vocal attractiveness to women. *Journal of Nonverbal Behaviour*, *30*(2), pp. 55–61.

Riordan, C. (1977). Control of vocal-tract length in speech. *The Journal of the Acoustical Society of America*, *62*(4), pp. 998–1002.

Sachs, J., Lieberman, P., & Erikson, D. (1972). Anatomical and cultural determinants of male and female speech. In R. W. Shuy & R. W. Fasold (Eds.), *Language attitudes: Current trends and prospects* (pp. 74–84). Washington, DC: Georgetown University Press.

Sandage, M., Plexico, L., & Schiwitz, A. (2015). Clinical utility of CAPE-V sentences for determination of speaking fundamental frequency. *Journal of Voice*, *29*(4), pp. 441–445.

Saxton, T., Caryl, P., & Roberts, S. C. (2006). Vocal and facial attractiveness judgments of children, adolescents and adults: The ontogeny of mate choice. *Ethology*, *112*(12), pp. 1179–1185.

Shadle, C. H. (1991). The effect of geometry on source mechanisms of fricative consonants. *Journal of Phonetics*, *19*(4), pp. 409–424.

Simpson, A. P. (2002). Gender-specific articulatory – acoustic relations in vowel sequences. *Journal of Phonetics*, *30*(3), pp. 417–435.

Simpson, A. P. (2009). Phonetic differences between male and female speech. *Language and Linguistics Compass*, *3*(2), pp. 621–640.

Simpson, A. P. (2012). The first and second harmonics should not be used to measure breathiness in male and female voices. *Journal of Phonetics*, *40*(3), pp. 477–490.

Skuk, V., Dammann, L., & Schweinberger, S. (2015). Role of timbre and fundamental frequency in voice gender adaptation. *The Journal of the Acoustical Society of America*, *138*(2), pp. 1180–1193.

Skuk, V., & Schweinberger, S. (2014). Influences of fundamental frequency, formant frequencies, aperiodicity, and spectrum level on the perception of voice gender. *Journal of Speech, Language, and Hearing Research*, *57*(1), pp. 285–296.

Smith, D., & Patterson, R. (2005). The interaction of glottal-pulse rate and vocal-tract length in judgements of speaker size, sex and age. *The Journal of the Acoustical Society of America*, *118*(5), pp. 3177–3186.

Smith, D., Patterson, R., Turner, R., Kawahara, H., & Irino, T. (2005). The processing and perception of size information in speech sounds. *The Journal of the Acoustical Society of America*, *117*(1), pp. 305–318.

Smith, E. A., Hall, K. C., & Munson, B. (2010). Bringing semantics to sociophonetics: Social variables and secondary entailments. *Laboratory Phonology*, *1*(1), pp. 121–155.

Stevens, K. N. (2000). *Acoustic phonetics*. Boston, MA: MIT Press.

Stuart-Smith, J. (2007). Empirical evidence for gendered speech production: /s/ in Glaswegian. In J. Cole & J. Hualde (Eds.), *Laboratory phonology 9* (pp. 65–86). Berlin: Mouton de Gruyter.

Timmers, M., Fischer, A., & Manstead, A. (2003). Ability versus vulnerability: Beliefs about men and women's emotional behavior. *Cognition and Emotion*, *17*(1), pp. 41–63.

Titze, I. (1989). Physiologic and acoustic differences between male and female voices. *The Journal of the Acoustical Society of America*, *85*(4), pp. 1699–1707.

van Bezooijen, R. (1995). Sociocultural aspects of pitch differences between Japanese and Dutch women. *Language and Speech*, *38*(3), pp. 253–265.

Vorperian, H. K., Wang, S., Chung, M. K., Schimek, E. M., Durtschi, R. B., Kent, R. D., . . . Gentry, L. R. (2009). Anatomic development of the oral and pharyngeal portions of the vocal tract: An imaging study. *The Journal of the Acoustical Society of America*, *125*(3), pp. 1666–1678.

Vorperian, H. K., Wang, S., Schimek, E. M., Durtschi, R. B., Kent, R. D., Gentry, L. R., & Chung, M. K. (2011). Developmental sexual dimorphism of the oral and pharyngeal portions of the vocal tract: An imaging study. *Journal of Speech, Language, and Hearing Research*, *54*(4), pp. 995–1010.

Weirich, M., & Simpson, A. P. (2014). Differences in acoustic vowel space and the perception of speech tempo. *Journal of Phonetics*, *43*, pp. 1–10.

Whiteside, S. P. (2001). Sex-specific fundamental and formant frequency patterns in a cross-sectional study. *The Journal of the Acoustical Society of America*, *110*(10), pp. 464–478.

Whiteside, S. P., & Irving, C. J. (1998). Speakers' sex differences in voice onset time: A study of isolated word production. *Perceptual and Motor Skills*, *86*(2), pp. 651–654.

Yamazawa, H., & Hollien, H. (1992). Speaking fundamental frequency patterns of Japanese women. *Phonetica*, *49*(2), pp. 128–140.

Zimman, L. (2013). Hegemonic masculinity and the variability of gay-sounding speech: The perceived sexuality of transgender men. *Journal of Language & Sexuality*, *2*(1), pp. 1–39.

Zimman, L. (2017). Variability in /s/ among transgender speakers: Evidence for a socially-grounded account of gender and sibilants. *Linguistics*, *55*(5), pp. 993–1019.

Zuckerman, M., & Driver, R. (1989). What sounds beautiful is good: The vocal attractiveness stereotype. *Journal of Nonverbal Behavior*, *13*(2), pp. 67–82.

Zuckerman, M., & Miyake, K. (1993). The attractive voice: What makes it so? *Journal of Nonverbal Behavior*, *17*(2), pp. 119–135.

19

New horizons in clinical phonetics

William F. Katz

Introduction

Clinical phonetics is a field concerned with speech sound description and analysis applied to people with communication disorders (Crystal, 1980, 1981, 1984; Powell and Ball, 2010; Shriberg et al., 2013). Analyses of recent publication patterns show that clinical phonetic research constitutes a major portion of clinical linguistics, the parent field (Perkins et al., 2011; Crystal, 2013). However, despite the growing popularity of clinical phonetics, the history of phonetics does not reflect a longstanding priority to describe speech and language disorders. The creators of the International Phonetic Alphabet (IPA) (e.g., Passy, 1884; Sweet, 1902; Jones, 1928) were chiefly concerned with language teaching, pronunciation, and translation. As a result, the IPA has primarily evolved to describe sound details pertaining to world language differences, and not variability typical of pathology (see discussion by Howard and Heselwood, 2002). In this sense, the field resembles sociophonetics, which has traditionally also had impoverished tools for describing language variation (see chapter by Thomas, this volume). For years phoneticians have noted this shortcoming, as illustrated by Trim's (1953) comment that the IPA "is still inadequately furnished with tools for the use of speech therapists" (p. 24).

Nonetheless, certain key founders of phonetics did express an interest in the physiology of speech perception and production, for both healthy and disordered individuals. Perhaps the strongest early advocates for this viewpoint were those Ohala (2004) described as taking a "*scientific*" (or "positivist," more physically based) phonetic approach, as opposed to a "*taxonomic*" approach (chiefly concerned with naming, classifying, and transcribing speech sounds). Examples may be observed in 17th-century attempts to get the deaf to speak, such as Amman (1694, 1700), van Helmont (1667), Holder (1669), and Wallis (1969). Other historians offer John Thelwall (1794–1834) as an important bridge figure in the later 19th-century period. This British elocutionist formed the first school for pupils with "impediments of speech," incorporating therapies based on prosody and articulatory phonetics (Rockey, 1977; Thelwall, 1981; Duchan, 2006). Additional prominent examples include Alexander Melville Bell (1867) and Alexander Graham Bell (1872) working to promote visible speech for the deaf.

Both scientific and taxonomic approaches remain crucial to the current field of clinical phonetics. These approaches are ultimately interrelated, since taxonomy cannot exist without an underlying theoretical framework, and scientific advancement requires precise nomenclature.[1] As the writings of Jespersen (1910) and Jakobson (1968) indicate, some linguists who made prominent taxonomic contributions were inspired to address the speech and language of healthy and disordered individuals.

From 1940s to 1960s, many important breakthroughs in linguistics served as fertile ground for the eventual genesis of clinical phonetics as a field. This included the *Fundamentals of Language* (Jakobson and Halle, 1956) and the concepts of distinctive features, markedness, and language universals. In addition, new generative paradigms in linguistics and their potential cognitive implications also had the effect of broadening perspectives from individual case studies and/or treatment plans to more extensive theoretical issues.

The field of clinical linguistics began to emerge into a recognized specialty area around 1976 and continued into the early 1980s, at least in the USA and Britain (Powell and Ball, 2010). A pivotal development was the 1981 publication of the book *Clinical Linguistics* by David Crystal, who defined clinical linguistics as "the application of linguistic science to the study of communication disability, as encountered in clinical situations" (p. 1). Crystal and colleagues provided initial frameworks for the analysis of healthy and disordered segmental phonology, syntax, morphology, and semantics. Subsequently Crystal (1984, p. 31) and several other researchers (e.g., Code and Ball, 1984) stressed the importance of phonetics to the field.

As Muller and Ball (2013) note, clinical linguistics research can be uni- or bi-directional with respect to the relation between clinical populations and linguistic/neurological theory. That is, some researchers emphasize applying linguistic theory for the benefit of patients (a clinical approach), others use data from clinical populations to gain insight into linguistic or neurological theory (a neurolinguistic approach),[2] while many now assume a bi-directional flow of information between clinical data and theory. As an example of the clinical approach, Dinnsen et al. (2014) employed Optimality Theory (OT; Prince and Smolensky, 1993) to better understand the sound system of a child with a phonological delay and to propose some clinical recommendations. In contrast, a classic neurolinguistic approach is found in Jakobson's consideration of child language and the language of individuals with aphasia in order to elaborate phonetic feature theory (Jakobson, 1968).

As clinical phonetics has progressed, numerous studies have addressed the shortcomings of IPA description with respect to clinical populations (see e.g., Howard and Heselwood, 2002; Muller and Ball, 2013, for detailed reviews). For instance, Shriberg and Kent (1982) provided important examples of procedures useful for examining clinical populations, including perceptual analyses and suggestions for transcription. Shriberg and colleagues also worked on improving transcription by investigating consensus methodologies (Shriberg et al., 1984) and comparing reliability across different techniques (Shriberg and Lof, 1991). Other researchers developed transcription methods specifically for disordered output (e.g., Ball et al., 2009; Rutter et al., 2010), including cleft palate speech (Trost, 1981) and prosodic changes in the speech of hearing impaired (e.g., Ball et al., 1994) and cochlear-implanted (Teoh and Chin, 2009) patients.

A systematic effort to develop symbol sets designed for use with individuals having speech and language disorders began when a King's Fund working party developed the Phonetic Representation of Disordered Speech (PRDS, 1983). These symbols were considered at the 1989 IPA meeting (Kiel), resulting in a recommended set of Extensions to the International Phonetic Alphabet (ExtIPA), designed for clinical use (Duckworth et al.,

1990). The ExtIPA has since been updated (2008) to encompass description of the airstream mechanism, phonation, nasalization, articulatory strength, articulatory timing, and prosodic features of disordered speech (see Appendix 1).

For the most part, the ExtIPA consists of letters and diacritics not used for healthy speech. For example, "nareal fricative" (as found in a nasal lisp) would not occur in healthy adult speech. In contrast, some articulatory descriptions, such as the diacritics for "alveolar" and "linguolabial", use IPA symbols that can also be applied to healthy speech. For disordered prosody, musical notation is borrowed to describe phenomena such as abnormally loud [*f*] or fast speech [*allegro*], as may be found in disorders such as cluttering or "press for speech" associated with mania.

The Voice Quality Symbols (VoQS) were developed by Ball et al. (1995; updated 2015) to provide a systematic means of transcribing unusual or disordered voice quality by specifying airstream types and phonation types, larynx height, and supralaryngeal settings (see Appendix 2). Similar to the ExtIPA, some symbols pertain to disordered conditions (e.g., trachea-oesophageal speech, [{IO}], or spasmodic dysphonia, [{ꟿ}]), while many symbols can also represent the voice of a healthy talker during unusual speaking conditions, e.g., whisper, [{W}], faucalized ("yawning") voice, [{Vᐥ}], or open-jaw voice, [{J̞}]. Overall, the ExtIPA and VoQs add symbolic capacity to the IPA for describing the features and voice quality of healthy talkers (Heselwood, 2013, p. 122; Esling, 2010, p. 694).

As this short history suggests, the field of clinical phonetics has evolved in response to both scientific and clinical needs. It is common for researchers in the brain and cognitive sciences to question how speech and language processing is involved when modeling or measuring behavior. Thus, clinical phonetics is frequently at the center of cutting-edge investigations in the behavioral and brain sciences. Clinical phonetics' ongoing priority of developing symbol sets and descriptors for disordered speech provides practical benefits for clinicians. In a related sense, situations arguably arise in which traditional phonetic transcription may have significant limitations, e.g., for describing "covert contrasts," where sound distinctions may be perceptually unreliable but acoustically and/or kinematically distinct (Hewlett, 1988). The field has therefore seen an increasing use of acoustic and kinematic measures to help describe healthy and disordered speech.

The next section briefly reviews multisensory information in speech processing; a topic that has long been ignored within the broader framework of clinical phonetics but that I believe should be emphasized for at least three reasons: First, a growing literature indicates that multisensory speech processing in healthy adults and children is crucial for everyday language function. Thus, in order to understand the phonetics of disordered language acquisition and breakdown, a multisensory approach may be essential. Second, audiovisual (face-to-face) speech communication is increasingly facilitated via new electronic systems (e.g., cell phones, videoconferencing, telemedicine) and this may well have clinical import for populations with speech and language disorders. Third, technological advances in measuring speech kinematics have permitted researchers to more easily describe and model the movement of speech articulators than was previously possible. Here, I emphasize recent studies of AV speech properties, including motion of the head, face, lips, jaw and tongue, in order to further our understanding of the speech of individuals presenting with speech and language problems.[3]

The multisensory nature of speech

It is common to portray speech as necessarily involving the auditory modality, comprising the link between talker and listener (e.g., Denes and Pinson, 1993; Raphael et al., 2007).

Nonetheless, researchers widely recognize that speech communication involves multisensory processing, noted for instance in a recent, explicit addition of multisensory streams to the "speech chain" (Gick et al., 2012, p. 272). What follows is a brief overview of this issue.

"Multisensory" commonly refers to audiovisual (AV) processing, such as when facing others in conversation (or watching TV or movies). Although the multisensory processing of speech includes proprioceptive and somatosensory (e.g., haptic, and aero-tactile) information (discussed later), we shall begin with AV processing, as study of this topic began at least as early as Alexander Melville Bell (*Visible Speech*, 1867). Seminal work by Sumby and Pollack (1954) contrasted listeners' perception of English spondees in auditory and audiovisual conditions, across different size word sets, and at different levels of noise masking. A key finding is that the relative contribution of vision to AV perception is constant across a wide range of signal-to-noise ratios. This suggests that the AV processing of speech is a natural mode of attention and is relatively indifferent to purely auditory phonetic processes (Remez, 2012). Research by Summerfield and colleagues (e.g., Summerfield, 1979, 1983, 1992; Brooke and Summerfield, 1983) has provided valuable information concerning the AV processing involved in lip-reading, including the permissible amounts of AV asynchrony, which cognitive skills are recruited for this ability, and which regions of synthetic faces and lips (including teeth) are required for heightened intelligibility. These issues are further described in the next section of this chapter.

Other critical information on AV perception has derived from research into the McGurk effect (McGurk and MacDonald, 1976), in which a visual stimulus (e.g., /ga/) alters the perception of an auditory stimulus (e.g., /ba/) that is perfectly audible on its own (Alsius et al., 2017). Listeners commonly report hearing a fusion of both modalities (e.g., /da/). This effect has been noted for different types of stimuli (e.g., Walker et al., 1995; Quinto et al. 2010), across different perceiver ages (e.g., Rosenblum et al., 1997; Burnham and Dodd, 2004; Sekiyama et al., 2014) and languages (Sekiyama and Tohkura, 1991; Burnham and Dodd, 1996), and under different temporal constraints (Munhall et al., 1996) and attentional demands (e.g., Alsius et al., 2005). Several questions and controversies remain concerning the large degree of inter-subject variability observed (e.g., Mallick et al., 2015) and the exact mechanisms involved (see e.g., Tiippana, 2014; Alsius et al., 2017) in the McGurk effect. Despite these controversies, there is consensus that the effect is quite robust, occurs whether one has knowledge of it or not, and likely has theoretical and clinical relevance for people with communication disorders. For instance, reduced McGurk effects have been reported for individuals with dyslexia (Bastien-Toniazzo et al., 2010), children with specific language impairment (Norrix et al., 2007; Kaganovich et al., 2015), autism spectrum disorders (Williams et al., 2004; Mongillo et al., 2008; Taylor et al., 2010), and language learning disabilities (Norrix et al., 2006), and for adults with Alzheimer's disease (Delbeuck et al. 2007) and aphasia (Youse et al., 2004; Hessler et al., 2012).

In addition to using noise masking and incongruent stimuli (McGurk) paradigms to assay AV integration (as described previously), new versions of the "phonemic restoration" paradigm have provided some intriguing results and may hold promise for studying clinical populations. Jerger et al. (2014) examined children aged 4–14 years old in an experiment in which congruent audio and visual speech syllables were presented, and in which for some conditions the auditory token (/ba/) had weakened acoustic cues (here, flattened formant frequency transitions for the /b/, such that only "a" is heard). When this weakened acoustic stimulus was paired with a visual whole syllable /ba/, the weakened auditory cue was effectively restored. The authors concluded that the children use visual speech to compensate for non-intact auditory speech. Other researchers are developing this paradigm to study AV perception in healthy individuals and in clinical populations (e.g., Irwin et al., 2014; Irwin and DiBlasi, 2017).

Proprioception refers to sensing of the body position in space, while somatosensory refers to sensations such as pressure, pain or temperature, superficial or deep to the organism. Sensing one's position in space enables orienting the head toward a sound, which in turn assists localization and identification by vision of the sound source (e.g., Lewald and Ehrenstein, 1998; Lewald et al., 2000). Anecdotal evidence supporting the importance of proprioception in speech comes from the testimony of astronauts experiencing "earth sickness" after returning to gravity after weightlessness. For instance, Canadian astronaut Chris Hadfield, of International Space Station Expedition 35, stated, "Right after I landed, I could feel the weight of my lips and tongue and I had to change how I was talking. I didn't realize I had learned to talk with a weightless tongue" (Hadfield, 2013). Experimental support may be found in dual-processing tasks, such as requiring subjects to speak while walking. Plummer D-Amato et al. (2011) tested a series of cognitively demanding tasks on gait in a dual-task interference paradigm and found that speech produced the greatest interference of all tasks tested. These results suggest that speech and body positioning (i.e., involving proprioception) use common regulatory mechanisms. Speaking tasks can particularly affect the posture and gait of certain populations, including slow walkers, the elderly, and individuals recovering from stroke.

Evidence of a role for proprioception in speech also comes from study of individuals with focal damage to the nervous system, including the cerebellum and basal ganglia. Kronenbuerger et al. (2009) studied individuals with essential tremor (ET), including those with and without cerebellar involvement. They observed syllable production, gait, and posture. Results indicated increased postural instability and increased syllable duration, particularly for individuals with ET resulting from cerebellar disorders. The results suggest that deficits in balance and dysarthria arise with an impairment to the cerebellum. Similarly, Cantiniaux et al. (2010) observed rhythmic problems in the speech and gait of individuals with Parkinson's disease (PD), suggesting a linked pathophysiological process for these individuals having cerebellar/basal ganglia disorders. In summary, studies of gait, posture, and focally disordered speech processing support proprioceptive links to speech by means of shared neural bases, including the cerebellum.

To investigate speech-related somatosensory information, Nasir and Ostry (2006) conducted a series of speaking experiments in which participants were required to talk with unexpected loads applied to the lower lip and jaw. The results indicated that precise somatosensory specification was required for speech production, in addition to presumed auditory targets. A subsequent study by Ito et al. (2009) used a robotic device to create patterns of skin deformation that would normally be involved in speech production. Listeners heard computer-generated productions of CVC stimuli ranging from "head" to "had." Listeners' skin-stretched (perturbed) responses varied systematically from their non-perturbed responses, suggesting a role of the somatosensory system in speech perception.

Early studies of haptic speech (e.g., gestures felt from manual tactile contact with the speaker's face) were conducted to develop effective communication methods for deaf-blind individuals, the Tadoma method (Alcorn, 1932; Norton, 1977). More recently, investigations have established that auditory information can influence haptic sensation ("the parchment skin illusion"; Jousmaki and Hari, 1998) and that haptic information can benefit speech perception in healthy individuals. These (latter) studies include cross-modal perception and production tasks (Fowler and Dekle, 1991), cross-modal perception with degraded acoustic information (Sato et al., 2010), tests of speech intelligibility in noise (Gick et al., 2008), and neural processing (evoked potentials) in live dyadic interactions (Treille et al., 2014). Considered together with the somatosensory perturbation experiments described earlier (Nasir and Ostry, 2006; Ito et al., 2009), this literature suggests that listeners integrate auditory and haptic information, perhaps occurring relatively early during the speech perception process (Treille et al., 2014, p. 75).

A more specific form of the tactile modality, aero-tactile stimulation, is under active investigation. Gick and Derrick (2009) gave listeners a slight, inaudible puff of air to the hand or neck while they heard noise-masked CV syllables differing in initial-consonant voicing ("pa"/"ba," "ta"/"da"). Syllables heard with simultaneous air puffs were more likely to be perceived as voiceless, suggesting that tactile information (timed to correspond with articulatory aspiration events) is integrated with auditory information during speech perception. Subsequent work showed that such aero-tactile effects also improve listeners' ability to differentiate stop-fricative pairs ("fa"/"ba" and "da"/"sha") in a forced-choice task (Derrick et al., 2014).

In summary, ample evidence indicates that the multisensory processing of speech is a vital part of the everyday language experience for healthy individuals. We may therefore reason that the field of clinical phonetics can benefit by considering the multisensory nature of speech in developing theories, clinical applications, and phonetic description. For instance, as will be described further in later sections of this chapter, researchers using visual feedback of articulatory motion report success for treating speech errors in individuals with apraxia of speech (see McNeil et al., 2010 for review), and dysarthria (Vick et al., 2014, 2017), raising questions about the nature of speech representation and the locus of breakdown with different types of brain damage. The next section describes AV information processing for speech, including data for healthy adults and children, as well as individuals having speech and language disorders. Co-verbal motion of the head is considered first, followed by orofacial motion.

Audiovisual speech processing: Healthy individuals, clinical populations

Rigid head movement

Healthy talkers accompany their everyday speech with head motion. However, determining exactly which types of linguistic and paralinguistic information are relayed by head motion, how this behavior develops, and how it is interpreted by perceivers has posed a challenge to researchers. This section briefly reviews studies of head motion in speech production and perception by adults, the development of co-verbal head motion in infants and children, and how head AV processing may be impacted by disease processes.

Healthy adults

Early investigations of adult head movement during conversation provide information indicating a role in signaling phrasing (juncture) and contrastive stress (e.g., Hadar et al., 1983). These studies also provide evidence for the semantic or narrative discourse functions of head gestures (McNeill, 1985; McClave, 2000). For example, McClave (2000) describes side-to-side head shakes (rotation) correlating with expressions of inclusivity and intensification, head nods (flexion/extension) serving as backchannel requests, and lateral movements correlating with uncertain statements and lexical repairs.

At a phonetic level, Yehia et al. (2002) examined the relation between head motion (kinematics) and fundamental frequency (f_0) during speech production. An LED-tracking system measured face and rigid head motion while Japanese- and English-speaking talkers produced short sentences. Correlation analysis showed that with rising f_0, talkers' heads tilt upward and away from the chest, while the head tips downward (towards the chest) with falling f_0. The authors suggest this is a primarily functional linkage, as most talkers can volitionally override these effects, such as by placing the chin low while making a higher pitch (Yehia et al., 2002, p. 568). A similar functional linkage between the amplitude of the speech signal and head motion was noted by Yehia et al. (2002). Other evidence of head movement affecting speech can be found from cases in which individuals speak while temporarily placed in head restraints, such as subjects in early speech experiments or singers/actors during certain types of stage training (Vatikiotis-Bateson and Kuratate, 2012; Roon et al., 2016). In such cases, people tend to talk much more quietly than usual and report feeling unnatural.

Studies of adults' perception of co-verbal head motion have provided a wealth of information over the past few decades, and the findings raise many intriguing new questions (Vatikiotis-Bateson and Munhall, 2015). Initial research suggested that listeners are able to decipher head and eyebrow movements to detect differences in emphatic stress (e.g., Thompson, 1934; Risberg and Lubker, 1978; Bernstein et al. 1989) and in sentence-level intonation (Fisher, 1969; Bernstein et al., 1989; Nicholson et al., 2002). Other research has found that the timing of head motion is consistent with prosodic structure, suggesting that head motion may be valuable for segmenting spoken content (Graf et al., 2002). The notion that head motion plays a role in "visual prosody" was promoted in a study by Munhall et al. (2004) in which Japanese subjects viewed a talking-head animation during a speech-in-noise task. The participants correctly identified more syllables with natural head motion than without it, suggesting that head motion helps people synchronize their perception to speech rhythm, and thereby retrieve phonetic information.

Head motion also conveys paralinguistic information in speech, including emotional prosody. For instance, Busso et al. (2007) derived statistical measures from an AV database and found that head motion patterns of activation, range, and velocity provide discriminating information about sadness, happiness, anger, and neutral emotional states. The researchers then used these statistically derived features to drive facial animations, which raters perceived as more natural than the original head motion sequences. Critically, head motion played a major role enhancing the emotional content of the animations. Similar results were observed in a study of vocalists singing and speaking semantically neutral statements produced with different emotional intentions (Livingstone and Palmer, 2016). Observers could identify the intended emotions of these vocalists well above chance levels solely by their head movements, at similar levels of accuracy for both speech and song.

Indeed, viewing rigid motion of only *part* of the head can still assist listeners with speech perception. Davis and Kim (2006) found that showing listeners a talker's moving upper head produced a small but reliable improvement in speech intelligibility for expressive sentences made with major head movements. Cvejic et al. (2010) conducted a cross-modal AV priming task under a variety of conditions including video conditions with outlines only (rigid motion). They found that top of the head movements produced by the speakers were sufficient to convey information about the prosodic nature of an utterance.

To summarize, adult head motion is correlated with voice pitch (and to a lesser degree, amplitude), both of which are used for linguistic and paralinguistic purposes during speech. Study of the timing and coordination of co-verbal head movement suggests a complex relationship with speech. More research, including work with annotative systems originally designed for the analysis and synthesis of speech and gesture (e.g., Kong et al., 2015; Johnston, 2017), may help clarify these issues. It would also be important to investigate the strength of any language- and culture-specific factors in these effects, in order to establish the extent to which this behavior is universal or language-particular.

Development

Head shakes and nods, like hand pointing gestures, are early emerging forms of preverbal communication. Fenson et al. (1994) found that a large sample of American children produce head shakes (12 mos.) and nods (14 mos.) approximately three to five months earlier than their corresponding verbal forms, "no" and "yes." Studies suggest that young children quickly recruit these early head gestures for purposes of communicative competence. Examples include using head nods to clarify the intent of vocalizations (e.g., Yont et al., 2001) and employing head gestures to facilitate turn-taking exchanges (Fusaro, 2012). Overall, these data imply that head motion plays a role in developing discourse-relevant skills as children's speech and language skills map in.

With respect to speech perception, researchers have asked whether infants are able to extract suprasegmental phonetic information from head movement during infant-directed (ID) exchanges. To address this question, researchers must consider the many factors known to be involved in contingent mother-infant interactions. Thus, cross-modal and cross-talker factors, as well as linguistic and social goals all come into play during the mother-child dyad (see Leclere et al., 2014; Viaux-Savelon, 2016). Kitamura et al. (2014, experiment 2) had 8-month-old infants hear a short sentence while watching two silent, line-joined, point-light displays: One depicted rigid (head only) verbal motion and the other non-rigid (face only) verbal motion. The researchers were interested in determining whether the infants were sensitive to the match between audio and visual correlates of ID speech prosody. Results indicate that infants look longer to a visual match in the rigid condition than to a visual mismatch in the non-rigid condition. The researchers concluded that 8-month-old infants can extract information about speech prosody from head movement and from voice (i.e., are sensitive to their match), and were less sensitive to lip movement and voice information. They speculate that head signals are prioritized in order to track the slower rate of global prosody (e.g., as would be found in sentence-level intonation) over local rhythm (e.g., as found in lexical stress). To determine whether mothers produce special head motion during ID speech, Smith and Strader (2014) conducted an eye-tracking study contrasting mothers talking under ID and AD (adult directed) conditions. The results suggest that mothers exaggerate their head movement as a form of visual prosody, in a manner analogous to the acoustical exaggerations in their speech (e.g., Fernald, 1989).

Taken together, studies of children's production and perception of head motion, as well as head motion produced in ID speech, suggest that an association of head movement with speech is a fundamental attribute of children's speech and language development. Future studies should consider studying languages other than English, as this would help substantiate some recent claims advanced, such as whether head motion signals "universals in discourse and communicative function" (Smith and Strader, 2014) or whether head motion indicates "global prosody over local prosody" (Kitamura et al., 2014). In addition, dyadic studies that track synchronized (contingent) aspects of AV co-verbal head motion during mother-infant interactions would be very useful.

Clinical populations

Limitations or exaggerations in head movement occurring from a variety of medical causes (e.g., inherited genetic factors, injury, stroke, or neurological disorders) can affect speech production. Such problems may be direct or indirect. The patient's speech production may be directly affected, particularly in the case of an erratically moving head (e.g., in cerebral palsy or Huntington's disease) by interfering with rigid head movement cues normally associated with speech. That is, assuming a conversation partner is used to attending to a healthy talker's moving head, viewing an erratically moving head (or an abnormally still head, as in the case of paralysis) may degrade perception by interfering with rigid motion cues. Head movement problems during speaking may also produce indirect effects by reducing visible facial cues otherwise available for prosody and discourse information. Simply put, if the talker's head is turned away during conversation, his/her face cannot be easily viewed. Unfortunately, these issues have not been systematically addressed in the literature.

Individuals with neurological disorders that result in speech dysarthria (e.g., cerebral palsy, Huntington's disease, amyotrophic lateral sclerosis, Parkinson's disease) also present with postural and motor control deficits (including tremor), issues that in themselves can potentially affect speech production. To illustrate how such motor control disorders can affect head positioning and ultimately impair speech processing, it will be useful to consider cerebral palsy (CP), a mixed group of early-onset, non-progressive, neuromotor disorders that affect the developing nervous system (Rosenbaum et al., 2007). CP results in changes in movement, posture, and muscle tone. The speech characteristics of this population may include respiratory anomalies, strained-strangled voice, pitch/loudness fluctuations, imprecise articulation, rate and timing problems, and hypernasality (Scholderle et al., 2014). Notably, head stability issues are common in children with even with mild-to-moderate CP (Saavedra et al., 2010). Research using head-mounted inertial sensors suggests that these stability deficits are predominantly due to "negative motor signs," including postural problems resulting from insufficient muscle activity and/or neural motor control (Velasco et al., 2016).

Although there appears to be a link between the severities of gross motor impairment and speech disorders in CP (Himmelmann and Uvebrant, 2011; Nordberg et al., 2013) scant data exist concerning the specific role of head movement in the communication difficulties experienced by individuals with CP. Research in this area might also examine whether the family and caretakers of individuals with CP learn to adapt (compensate) for reduced head motion by attending to other information (secondary cues) present in the auditory or visual streams.

Orofacial movement

Healthy adults

Orofacial movement for speech involves ensembles of articulatory movements, including non-rigid movement of the lips and face (via the combined action of the facial and perioral muscles), rigid jaw movement, and effects due to regulation of intraoral air pressure (Vatikiotis-Bateson, 1998). Extensive research on the kinematics of the oral region has focused on lip movement (e.g., opening/closing gestures), lip shape (e.g., protrusion, inversion, spread), and the oral aperture during speech (e.g., Linker, 1982; Ramsay et al., 1996). Overall, the lips have a comparatively small movement range but can reach relatively high speeds, while the jaw has a larger range but slower speeds. Considering displacement, the lips' range of motion is approximately 6 mm for the upper lip and 12 mm for the lower lip (Sussman et al., 1973; Smith, 1992). Jaw motion for speech mainly involves midsagittal movements of up to 10 mm of translation and 10–15 degrees of rotation (Vatikiotis-Bateson, 1998). In terms of velocity, early reports of lip movement fundamental frequencies were <10 Hz (Muller and MacLeod, 1982), whereas more recent reports describe speeds ranging up to ~20 Hz, varying as a function of the gesture/consonant produced (Gracco, 1994; Lofqvist and Gracco, 1997) and voicing quality (Higashikawa et al., 2003). Jaw movement velocities during oral reading are reported to have a fundamental frequency of ~4 Hz (Ohala, 1975) and show averaged rates falling roughly in the same range (e.g., Ostry and Flanagan, 1989).

Orofacial movements have been linked to vocal tract and acoustic regularities. Based on a series of experiments evaluating English and Japanese sentence production using flesh-point tracking systems and acoustic analysis, Vatikiotis-Bateson and Munhall (2015) describe a "tight, causal coupling between kinematic (vocal tract and face) and acoustic data" (p. 179). Using multivariate correlations, over 80% of facial motion was estimated from vocal tract articulations. In addition, 65% of the speech acoustics examined were estimated from the vocal tract articulation. Lastly, approximately 95% of the 3D facial motion could be predicted from the acoustic signal if small movements of the cheeks (corresponding to structured changes of intraoral air pressure) were considered. (p. 180). The researchers suggest that perceivers could in principle take advantage of these kinematic/acoustic linkages, although they also advise caution in such an interpretation as many questions remain to be answered (see next section, "Viewing the tongue during speech").

Speech perception studies emphasize that the mouth is the most important visible region of the face for extracting visual features pertaining to speech (e.g., Hassanat, 2014). For instance, seeing only the mouth area is sufficient for speech reading and for eliciting McGurk effects (Hietanen et al., 2001; Rosenblum et al., 2000; Thomas and Jordan 2004). However, studies have shown that oral kinematic patterns are highly correlated with movements produced in the outer regions of the face, including the side of the jaw and cheeks (Vatikiotis-Bateson and Munhall, 2015). The fact that oral movements are linked to those of the jaw and cheeks suggests that such extra-oral information is available to perceivers, such as when simple occlusions block vision of the mouth of a talker (Jordan and Thomas, 2011).

Advances in understanding co-verbal facial perception have also come from the fields of face perception and face recognition. Face perception is known to depend on attending to features (e.g., mouth, eyes, and nose) and, more importantly, on featural configuration (e.g., the fact that the eyes are above the nose, and that Joe's eyes may be wider apart than Jim's) (Valentine, 1988; Farah et al., 1998). Analysis of the well-known "Thatcher illusion" (Thompson, 1980) shows that configuration information is less effective when the face is presented upside down (Bartlett and Searcy, 1993; Carbon et al., 2005; Bruce and Young, 2012). The Thatcher illusion occurs when viewers note that a face with inverted eyes and mouth looks grotesque when a face is upright, but not inverted. A "Thatcherized" face can greatly reduce the strength of the McGurk illusion (described previously), but only when the face is upright (Rosenblum et al., 2000; Rosenblum, 2001). Thus, a head with an inverted mouth producing "va" heard synchronously with auditory /ba/ is usually perceived as "ba" when the face is upright (no McGurk effect), but shifts to "va" when the face is inverted. However, this effect does not rely solely on inversion of the mouth segment, as it does not occur when the mouth segment is shown in isolation. These findings, named the "McThatcher" effect (Rosenblum, 2001) suggest that configuration information is important for visual and AV speech perception. Subsequent work has also related the

McThatcher effect to a physiological index of brain processing, the McGurk mismatch negativity (Eskelund et al., 2015).

In summary, adults produce facial movement correlated with speech sufficient for perceivers to boost intelligibility in situations such as speech reading or speech intelligibility in noise. Facial movement also contributes to perceptual illusions (e.g., McGurk and McThatcher) suggesting features and configuration information are processed to derive co-verbal facial cues. While these facts support the general importance of facial AV information in speech processing, many aspects of AV facial processing remain poorly understood. For example, AV gating studies using phoneme identification tasks indicate that the salience and time course of audio and visual information streams differ for various sounds tested (Jesse and Massaro, 2010; Sánchez-García et al., 2018). That is, some sounds cannot be neatly classified in terms of their time course or modality. Thus, in hearing an upcoming /f/ in a VC syllable presented under AV conditions, perceivers show earlier identification in visual and audiovisual presentation (compared to audio), suggesting a visual-dominated phoneme (Sánchez-García et al., 2018). Conversely, in cases of an upcoming /g/ sound under AV conditions, perceivers show no earlier identification when compared with a purely auditory presentation, implying an auditory-dominated phoneme. Finally, some phonemes (e.g., /s/) appear to have more complex time-courses and AV contributions that are not clearly classifiable as "auditory" or "visual" dominant (Sánchez-García et al., 2018). These considerations potentially complicate current models of AV processing.

In addition, some co-verbal facial patterns are quantifiable during production but not discernible to perceivers. For example, the labial stops (/p/, /b/, /m/) are not visually distinguishable by people (Fisher, 1968), but can be classified using optic flow techniques and machine recognition systems using visual features (Abel et al., 2011). While good news for machine recognition systems, these data suggest some AV contrasts are not relevant for clinical linguistic purposes.

Development

Babies pay exquisite attention to the faces of their caretakers, and data suggest infants have early sensitivity to AV speech. Kuhl and Meltzoff (1984) conducted a preferential looking paradigm and found that 4-month-old infants favor looking at faces that match heard vowels (/ɑ/ and /i/). Infants also use multimodal information when imitating speech sounds (Legerstee, 1990) and this use of AV information extends to influences from their own lip positions (spread or puckered) during vowel perception (Yeung and Werker, 2013). As infants enter the canonical babbling phase at about seven months of age, they deploy selective attention to the mouth of a talking face when learning speech (e.g., Haith et al., 1977; Lewkowicz and Hansen-Tift, 2012). Other studies have proposed more precise timelines for this process, in consideration of infants' exposure to AV synchronization issues and linguistic experience. For example, Hillairet de Boisferon et al. (2017) tested infants (aged 4-, 6-, 8-, 10-, and 12-mo.) in an eye-gaze study with synchronized and desynchronized speech presented in their native and non-native languages. They found that, regardless of language, desynchronization interrupted the usual pattern of relatively more attention to mouth than eyes found in synchronized speech for the 10 month olds, but not at any other age. The authors concluded that prior to the emergence of language, temporal asynchrony mediates attentional responsiveness to a talker's mouth, after which attention to temporal synchrony declines in importance. As this research continues, we may expect a better understanding of the AV speech acquisition process.

Infants show multimodal effects for discordant AV stimuli in the McGurk paradigm (Rosenblum et al., 1997; Burnham and Dodd, 2004). Although some inconsistencies have been pointed out in these studies due to results being dependent on testing and stimulus conditions (Desjardins and Werker, 2004), the data nonetheless suggest that infants obtain important information from facial cues in learning the phonological structure of language. In summary, a varied literature suggests that young infants pay attention to face (mouth and eyes) during the first year of speech perception.

In contrast to the general importance of visual facial information in speech perception by adults and infants, these influences appear to have less effect on the speech processing of young children (Massaro, 1984; Massaro et al., 1986; Hockley and Polka, 1994; Desjardins et al., 1997; Sekiyama and Burnham, 2004; Dupont et al., 2005; Wightman et al., 2006). Rather, many studies support the overall concept that young children show an *auditory* input bias (Sloutsky and Napolitano, 2003).

As children mature, visual speech processing improves, although the reasons for this improvement remain poorly understood. Possibilities include gaining speech production experience, shifts in perceptual weighting and emphasis (developmental cue-trading), and age-related changes in speech reading and/or language resulting from formal education (Desjardins et al., 1997; Green, 1998; Massaro et al., 1986; Sekiyama and Burnham, 2004). Jerger et al. (2009) report a "U shaped" pattern, with a significant influence of visual speech in 4-year-olds and in 10- to 14-year-olds, but not in 5- to 9-year-olds, perhaps indicating reorganization of phonology in response to formal literacy instruction. Many factors potentially complicate children's progression from less to more visually perceived speech. One complication is that observed effects may not reflect actual age-related effects but may instead result from different task demands imposed by the tests used at different ages (see Jerger et al., 2009, for discussion). Another issue is that children's information processing ability changes with age. For younger children, visual speech may act as an "alerting" or "motivational" signal (Arnold and Hill, 2001; Campbell, 2006), boosting attention, and thus broadly affecting information processing. Also, children may have particular issues processing faces, due to gaze aversion, in which individuals reduce environmental stimulation in an attempt to reduce cognitive load and enhance processing (Glenberg et al., 1998). Indeed, children's face-to-face communication is relatively poor on certain types of tasks (Doherty-Sneddon et al., 2000; Doherty-Sneddon et al., 2001). In summary, while it is generally agreed that children improve visual speech processing with maturation, studies that carefully control for task demands and age-dependent cognitive capabilities are needed to make further progress on this complex issue.

As researchers compile databases to study children's speech development (e.g., Beckman et al., 2017), it would be useful to consider measures of AV speech in order to improve our knowledge of how these speech capabilities mature. While a growing literature is addressing the development of speech motor control in children (see e.g., reviews by Goffman et al., 2010; Smith, 2010; Green and Nip, 2010), most studies focus on the auditory modality, and the development of AV speech motor control is less described. That is, there are relatively few data addressing how young children's facial movements contribute to their AV speech quality. Additionally, with respect to children's speech perception, little is known about how children interpret orofacial movements for speech, how these capabilities develop over time, or how children's co-verbal orofacial movements are perceived by others during face-to-face conversation.

One promising direction in this research addresses children's audio-temporal binding, which refers to the determination that stimuli presented in close spatial and temporal correspondence are more likely to be "bound" into a single perceptual entity. Recent findings suggest that these capabilities coalesce slowly by early childhood (e.g., age four) and continue to refine through adolescence (Hillock-Dunn and Wallace, 2012; Lewkowicz and Flom, 2014). These data imply that children have a perceptual basis for adult-like AV speech perception at a young age and refine these skills with maturation. Extensions of this type of research to examine children of younger ages and to encompass speech and language disorders would seem promising.

Clinical populations

Orofacial movement disorders can result from many causes, including neurological conditions (e.g., dystonias, apraxias, ataxias, and tremor), facial nerve disease and/or damage, primary muscle disorders, and medication side effects. Parkinson's disease (PD) is a prime example, a progressive neurological disorder affecting approximately 2% of the world population over 65 years old. Individuals with PD present with gait difficulties, tremor, rigidity, balance, slowed movement (bradykinesia), and speech and swallowing problems (see Sveinbjornsdottir, 2016, for review). Approximately 70–75% of individuals with PD present with hypokinetic dysarthria, including reduced amplitude and irregularly timed speech (Hartelius and Svensson, 1994; Tjaden, 2008). Individuals with PD also commonly have a condition called "masked facies" (or hypomimia), in which there is a marked loss of facial expressiveness. Studies using facial rating scales have shown that individuals with PD produce less frequent facial expressions (Katsikitis and Pilowsky, 1988, 1991), recruit fewer muscles when reacting to certain stimuli (Simons et al., 2003), and generate lower-amplitude facial movements compared to healthy controls (Bologna et al., 2012).

Impaired orofacial movements affect how well talkers with PD are able to portray emotions (Borod et al., 1990; Tickle-Degnen and Lyons, 2004), including emotions in spoken language. For example, acoustic analyses suggest there is diminished emotional prosody in the productions of individuals with PD (Borod et al., 1990; Buck and Duffy, 1980; Hertrich and Ackermann, 1993), and perceptual analyses propose this reduced information corresponds with less successful detection of emotional qualities on the part of listeners (Pell et al., 2006). Data also indicate that individuals with PD have a deficit in the perception of emotions (e.g., Paulmann and Pell, 2010), including both the voice and the face (Gray and Tickle-Degnen, 2010), and this perceptual deficit may contribute to their inability to portray emotion in their expressions (see also Pell and Monetta, 2008; Ricciardi et al., 2015). In summary, it is likely that orofacial movement restrictions of talkers with PD contribute to their reduced capacity for expressing emotion, but the strength of this contribution has not been systematically tested.

Although studies have examined global aspects of speech prosody in PD in order to gauge speech intelligibility (e.g., Logemann et al., 1978; Klopfenstein, 2009; Ma et al., 2015), little is known about the extent to which PD orofacial impairments (e.g., hypomimia) affect their AV speech processes. One interesting approach to studying this issue may come from comparing individuals with PD to patients having Moebius Syndrome, a rare congenital disease that commonly causes facial paralysis. Nelson and Hodge (2000) conducted acoustic (F_2 locus equations) and perceptual analyses (identification in V and AV modes) of /bV/ and /dV/ syllables produced by a 7 year, 11 month old girl with Moebius Syndrome. Her productions were compared with those of an age-matched healthy talker. The main results indicate the girl with facial paralysis produced conflicting cues for stop place for the /bV/ syllables and this influenced listeners' perceptions, especially in the AV mode. Thus, the more visible phoneme showed greater perceptual deficits. It may be fruitful to investigate these issues in talkers with PD, as similar patterns would be predicted for individuals with masked facies. For such research, using an expanded inventory of speech sounds (e.g., requiring lip shape, oral aperture, and jaw position changes) would be helpful.

Orofacial movement problems may also be involved in communication difficulties affecting the mother-child dyad (see previous section on Development). Maternal depression has been consistently associated with a variety of adverse childhood developmental outcomes, including poor cognitive functioning, insecure attachment, and difficulties in behavioral and emotional adjustment (see reviews by Rutter, 1997; Murray and Cooper, 2003; Murray et al., 2015). Exposure to maternal depressive symptoms, whether during the prenatal period, postpartum period, or chronically, increases children's risk for later cognitive and language difficulties (Sohr-Preston and Scaramella, 2006). For severely depressed mothers, reduced facial expressiveness is part of the problem: their infants are less responsive to faces and voices, as early as the neonatal period (Field et al., 2009). Newborns of mothers with high-adversity depressive symptoms are less expressive (Lundy et al., 1996) and these children show high rates of distress and avoidance of social interaction with their mothers (Murray et al., 2015, p. 140). Thus, among other problems, infants of depressed mothers may not receive normal AV (facial) cues for speech, either at the segmental or suprasegmental (prosodic) level. Further study of these topics can provide evidence about the role of AV information in infant development and potentially contribute to improved speech and language outcomes for at-risk children.

Viewing the tongue during speech: Ongoing and new approaches

> By localizing sensory feedback signals of speech motor response so that the S has a clear and immediate sensory indication of his movements, tracking tasks can be utilized as part of a rehabilitative program for those with sensorimotor impairments of the articulation apparatus. In addition to providing a simplified task that children could easily perform, auxiliary feedback channels can be used, such as visual feedback, to take the place of malfunctioning or missing feedback modes. Such an approach represents a fruitful area of study on both normal and abnormal populations to help ascertain the cortical control functions underlying speech and language.
>
> – *Harvey M. Sussman (1970, pp. 318–319)*

As Sussman notes in the preceding quote from an article on tongue movement control, there is a healthy tradition of studying the tongue[4] in experimental phonetics. This tradition is seen in early kymograms (Rousselot, 1897), palatograms, and linguograms (e.g., Jones, 1922; Firth, 1948; Abercrombie, 1957; Ladefoged, 1957), x-ray cinematography films (Moll, 1960; Munhall et al., 1995), and x-ray microbeam images (Kiritani et al., 1975; Westbury et al., 1990). Current imaging techniques (including MRI, Ultrasound, EPG, and EMA) are described in Chapter 2 of this volume and in reviews by Scott et al. (2014), Whalen and McDonough (2015), Cleland et al. (2016), Sorensen et al. (2016), Wang et al. (2016), Gibbon and Lee (2017), and Preston et al. (2017a). Using these imaging techniques, the speech-related motion of the tongue can be studied and related to acoustic and perceptual data. Another means of understanding the tongue is to model its biomechanics in order to better understand muscle forces and activation patterns (e.g., Perkell, 1974; Gerard et al., 2006; Stavness et al., 2012; Woo et al. 2016; Anderson et al., 2017; Hermant et al., 2017; Yu et al., 2017; Tang et al., 2017). Taking a rather different approach, this section focuses on the tongue's visual properties, one of its lesser-studied aspects, in order to further understand

AV speech processing and to introduce techniques that appear useful in training pronunciation in healthy individuals as well as persons with speech and language disorders.

Some important data addressing visual aspects of tongue movement have come from the speech technology literature, including the fields of automated speech recognition (ASR) and visual animated speech (VAS). In the development of early ASR systems, researchers working with acoustic-based speech processing systems found that results could be made more robust by adding visual information concerning articulatory movement (Potamianos et al., 2004). Critical to this effort is the notion of a *viseme*, the basic unit of mouth movements (Fisher, 1968; Chen and Rao, 1998). Visemes chiefly involve lip movement and mouth opening, and share a many-to-one mapping with phonemes. Visemes are classified by systems that are roughly articulatory (e.g., /p/, /b/, and /m/ belonging to one viseme group involving "bilabial" closure). However, the resulting visual under-specification can result in notorious lip-reading equivalents, such as the phrases "*I love you*" and "*Elephant juice*" involving similar visemes. In the rapidly developing field of ASR, approaches have changed dramatically since their inception in the 1960s/70s (see Huang et al., 2014; Singh et al., 2017 for review), and deep neural net (DNN) systems currently surpass performance of previous systems in both audio and AV speech recognition (e.g., Son Chung, 2017). Critically, as research has proceeded on audiovisual automatic speech recognition (AVASR) systems, data have shown that large performance gains result from the addition of visual information, both for noisy audio conditions and for clean speech (Potamianos et al., 2003; Mroueh et al., 2015; Potamianos et al., 2017).

Study of visual animated speech (VAS), such as lip synch models or text-to-AV-speech systems, also point to the usefulness of visually displayed tongue information. Facial animation, a branch of computer-generated imagery (CGI), has become increasingly sophisticated in the approaches used to simulate talking faces and heads (e.g., Theobald, 2007; Mattheyses and Verhelst, 2015). From the early development of these systems, researchers have noted that depicting the anterior part of the tongue (e.g., for such sounds as /a/ and /l/) increases speech animation quality, both in terms of subjective ratings of naturalness and improved intelligibility (e.g., Beskow, 1995; King and Parent, 2001, 2005). Work in this area continues to model tongue movement in order to increase accuracy and naturalness (e.g., Rathinavelu et al., 2006; Musti et al., 2014; Yu, 2017).

A related issue concerns the extent to which individuals can benefit from viewing the tongue's internal motion, motion that is ordinarily inaccessible in face-to-face conversation and can only be viewed using speech instrumentation. Researchers are investigating this topic to develop applications for L2 pronunciation training and speech correction in clinical populations. As will be described in the next section, the data potentially bear on a number of questions relevant to clinical phonetics, including (a) the role of audio and visual streams in speech processing, (b) feedback and feedforward mechanisms in speech and their breakdown in disease, and (c) the relation between speech and non-speech oral motor processing.

Visual articulatory feedback: Second language (L2) training applications

Animated images of tongue movement have been included in computer-assisted pronunciation training (CAPT) systems, such as "Baldi" (Massaro and Cohen, 1998; Massaro, 2003; Massaro et al., 2006), "ARTUR" (Engwall et al., 2004; Engwall and Bälter, 2007; Engwall, 2008), "ATH" (Badin et al., 2008), "Vivian" (Fagel and Madany, 2008), and "Speech Tutor" (Kröger et al., 2010). These systems employ animated talking heads, most of which optionally display transparent vocal tracts showing (training) tongue movement. "Tongue reading" studies based on these systems have shown small but consistent perceptual improvement when tongue movement information is added to the visual display. Such effects are noted in word retrieval for acoustically degraded sentences (Wik and Engwall, 2008) and in a forced-choice consonant identification task (Badin et al., 2010).

Whereas the visual effects of these CAPT systems on speech perception are fairly well established, the effects on speech production are less well understood. Massaro and Light (2003) investigated the effectiveness of Baldi in teaching non-native phonetic contrasts (/r/-/l/) to Japanese learners of English. Both external and internal views (i.e., showing images of the speech articulators) of Baldi were found to be effective, with no added benefit noted for the internal articulatory view. A subsequent, rather preliminary report on English-speaking students learning Chinese and Arabic phonetic contrasts reported similar negative results for the addition of visual, articulatory information (Massaro et al., 2008). In this study, training with the Baldi avatar showing face (Mandarin) or internal articulatory processes (Arabic) provided no significant improvement in a small group of students' productions, as rated by native listeners. In contrast, Liu et al. (2007) observed potentially positive effects of visual feedback on speech production for 101 English-speaking students learning Mandarin. This investigation contrasted three feedback conditions: Audio only, human AV, and a Baldi avatar showing visible articulators. A key finding was that for the training of Chinese final rimes, the stimuli that most involved viewing tongue motion, both the human AV and Baldi condition scores were higher than audio-only, with the Baldi condition significantly higher than the audio condition. This pattern is compatible with the view that information concerning the internal articulators assists in L2 production.

Researchers have further addressed these issues by adapting speech instrumentation systems in order to provide real-time visual feedback of tongue motion. An electropalatography (EPG) system was used to provide visual feedback for accent reduction in the training of two Japanese students learning English /r/ and /l/ distinctions (Gibbon et al., 1991). Positive findings for EPG feedback were also noted for three Thai-speaking subjects learning English/r/-/l/, /s/-/ʃ/, and /t/-/θ/ distinctions (Schmidt and Beamer, 1998). According to these authors, "EPG makes possible exploration of the details of sound production by L2 speakers, as well as possible effects on L1 sound production related to the learning of new or modified articulations" (p. 402).

More recently, Hacking et al. (2017) used EPG to train palatalized consonant productions to native American English learners of Russian. Acoustic analysis (second formant of the pre-consonantal vowel, and final consonant release "noise") suggested significant improvement with this phonological contrast. However, perceptual tests with three native Russian listeners showed only a modest increase in identification accuracy. The authors concluded that such short-term EPG training may nevertheless be effective for adult L2 learners.

Studies conducted in our laboratory have used electromagnetic articulography (EMA) as a means of investigating visual feedback in training non-native consonants and vowels for healthy talkers. Levitt and Katz (2008) trained two groups of American English speakers to produce Japanese /r/ (apico-postalveolar flap). One group received traditional L2 instruction alone and the other group received traditional L2 instruction plus visual feedback for tongue movement provided by a 2D EMA system (Carstens AG100). Acoustic (consonant duration) and perceptual (on/off target judgments by Japanese native listeners) results indicated improved acquisition and maintenance by the participants who received traditional instruction plus EMA training. These findings suggest that visual information regarding consonant place of articulation can assist L2 learners with accent modification.

Recent studies from our lab have utilized real-time software designed to interface with 3D EMA-based input (Opti-Speech, Katz et al., 2014). This system is designed to provide talkers with online visual feedback of their tongue and jaw movement, with virtual articulatory targets that can be set by the operator during speaking practice (Figure 19.1). In an initial study, four monolingual English speakers produced stop CV syllables that alternated in initial consonant place of articulation (e.g., /pɑ/-/kɑ/-/tɑ/-/jɑ/). One talker was given articulatory visual feedback of his tongue movement and requested to "hit the target" during production. The target region was a 1 cm virtual sphere (placed at the alveolar ridge), that changed color when the tongue tip sensor entered. Results showed that subjects in the no-feedback condition performed less accurately than the subject given visual feedback. These findings suggest that real-time tongue tracking may be useful for phonetic training purposes, including L2 learning applications concerning consonantal place of articulation (Katz et al., 2014).

Katz and Mehta (2015) used the Opti-Speech system to investigate the accuracy with which American English talkers can produce a novel, non-English speech sound (a voiced, coronal, palatal stop) and whether learning can benefit from short-term training with visual feedback. Five talkers' productions were evaluated based on kinematic (EMA/tongue-tip spatial positioning) and acoustic (burst spectra) measures. The kinematic results indicated a rapid gain in accuracy associated with visual feedback training for all talkers, which corresponded with acoustic shifts in the predicted direction for three of the five talkers. In summary, although the data from these small-scale studies remain preliminary, the findings

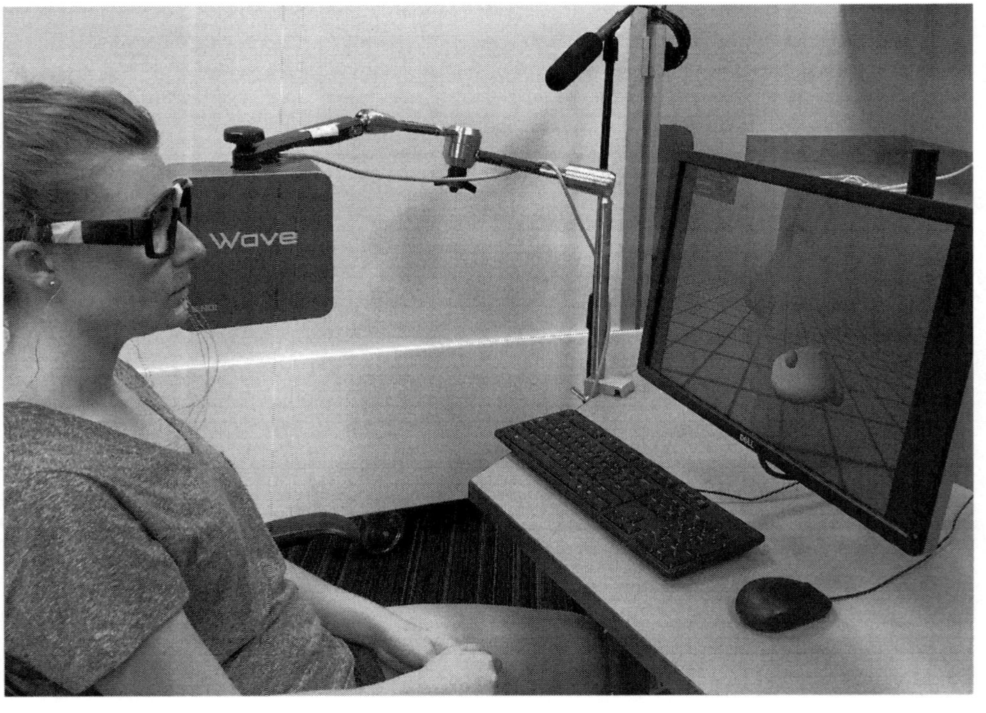

Figure 19.1 Illustration of the Opti-Speech system, with participant wearing EMA sensors and (head position-aligning) orientation glasses. She faces a computer screen showing the real-time movement of her tongue toward a virtual target sphere placed at the alveolar ridge. When the virtual target is "hit" with the tongue sensor, the target color changes from red to green, providing visual feedback for a spoken goal.

suggest that augmented visual information concerning one's own tongue movement can assist skill acquisition when learning consonant place of articulation.

Studies are investigating vowel production under real-time tongue visual feedback conditions. Suemitsu et al. (2015) provided real-time EMA-based articulatory feedback to facilitate production of an unfamiliar English vowel (/æ/) by five native speakers of Japanese. Learner-specific vowel target positions were computed for each participant (using a model estimated from American English vowels) and feedback was provided in the form of a multiple-sensor, mid-sagittal display. Acoustic analysis of subjects' productions indicated that acoustic and articulatory training resulted in significantly improved /æ/ productions.

A related approach to tongue-based visual feedback is to devise speech training games that incorporate consonant and vowel targets. Tilsen et al. (2015) describe preliminary findings with an EMA real-time feedback system that uses input from a WAVE magnetometer system for a series of articulatory training games. Tasks included hitting a target line positioned along the palate with the tongue tip while saying "ta," bilabial closure and release ("QuickLips"), and a rapid tongue targeting task ("QuickTongue"). Overall, it was suggested that articulatory biofeedback systems can provide useful methods for investigating speech motor control, conducting therapy, and improving phonetic performance by increasing motivation.

Ultrasound offers portability and cost advantages over other speech imaging systems and its use in visual feedback applications is being actively pursued. For instance, Gick et al. (2008) describe the use of ultrasound to train English /l/ and /r/ for three Japanese students with persistent difficulties producing these sounds in certain phonetic environments. After an initial assessment, the participants were shown ultrasound video-recordings of their "best and most troublesome productions" in a brief training session. Post-training assessment indicated that all participants showed improvement, including stimulus generalization to other lexical items. The authors suggested that ultrasound visual feedback has important potential in L2 pronunciation instruction. Positive training results for ultrasound in L2 applications have also been reported for Japanese students learning the vowels /y/ and /u/ in French (Pillot-Loiseau et al., 2013), and for Italian talkers learning the American English /ɑ/-/ʌ/ distinction (Sisinni et al., 2016). These data suggest that, at least for certain consonants and vowels, ultrasound visual feedback of tongue motion is beneficial for L2 learning applications.

In summary, studies based on instructional avatars and on real-time imaging systems (EPG, EMA and ultrasound) suggest that visual real-time articulatory feedback is helpful for improving L2 learning of consonant and vowel contrasts in healthy children and adults. More research is needed to expand our knowledge of the motor principles involved in this type of training and the types of sounds amenable to training by different methodologies.

Visual articulatory feedback: Clinical applications

Of the many recent speech imaging technologies, EPG has perhaps seen the widest use in providing visual feedback for various clinical populations. This includes assessment and treatment of children with speech sound disorders (e.g., Morgan Barry and Hardcastle, 1987; Hickey, 1992; Dagenais, 1995; Gibbon et al., 1999; Gibbon and Wood, 2010), cleft palate (e.g., Abe et al., 1977; Dent et al., 1992; Gibbon et al., 2007; Scobbie et al., 2004; Lohmander et al., 2010; Maine and Serry, 2011), Down's syndrome (e.g., Wrench et al., 2002; Cleland et al., 2009), hearing impairment (e.g., Fletcher and Hasagawa, 1983; Dagenais, 1992; Crawford,

1995; Martin et al., 2007; Pratt, 2007; Bacsfalvi et al., 2007; Bacsfalvi and Bernhardt, 2011), and acquired neurological disorders (e.g., Morgan Barry, 1995; Gibbon and Wood, 2003; Lundeborg and McAllister, 2007; Morgan et al., 2007; Nordberg et al., 2011).

A recent study illustrates some of the strengths of EPG therapy in working with children, while also showing the complexity of working with different sound classes. Hitchcock et al. (2017) provided EPG feedback therapy for five English-speaking, school-aged children who misarticulated /r/ in words. The results indicated that 4/5 participants were able to accurately produce /r/ during treatment (as judged perceptually and acoustically), while two participants generalized these patterns to non-treated targets (as judged by blinded listeners). It was concluded that EPG therapy can help some children with rhotic errors, but its utility appears to vary across individuals (perhaps because /r/ can be realized in so many more ways than were illustrated by the EPG targets in this experiment).

EPG feedback studies of adult clinical populations have investigated glossectomy (Suzuki, 1989; Wakumoto, 1996) and neurological disorders (Hartelius et al., 2001; Howard and Varley, 1995; McAuliffe and Ward, 2006; Mauszycki et al., 2016). Overall, this literature overwhelmingly suggests that providing child and adult patients with visual information concerning tongue-palate contact improves the accuracy of consonant production. Nevertheless, a recent study by Mauszycki and colleagues (2016) illustrate some of the potential complexities with this type of translational research and highlight some important directions for future research. These investigators treated five individuals with Broca's aphasia and apraxia of speech (AOS) on a series of target sounds (treated and untreated) in two-word phrases. Participants received articulatory-kinematic treatment in combination with EPG visual feedback. Results indicated improved accuracy for the majority of treated sounds, with generalization for most trained sounds (including better long-term maintenance of treated sounds in trained and untrained stimuli for two of the participants). The authors concluded that EPG may be a potential treatment tool for individuals with AOS, pending several considerations: Many treatment steps were taken in the study (and in other recent visual feedback studies) that could lead to participant improvement, including pairing visual feedback with verbal feedback, progressing from simple to more complex speech tasks, gradually reducing clinician feedback, and using a large number of treatment trials within a session. Thus, teasing out the exact effects of visual feedback in these studies is important to determine whether providing such therapy for clinical populations offers advantages over more traditional types of therapy.

Electromagnetic articulography (EMA) has been increasingly used to investigate clinical populations, as current systems offer the ability to record both consonant and vowel articulation in 3D. Because EMA systems require the attachment of sensors to the speech articulators, it is somewhat more invasive than EPG and therefore study populations have tended to involve adults rather than children (cf. Katz and Bharadwaj, 2001). However, as researchers devise better methods of sensor placement, more EMA studies involving children are being reported (e.g., Vick et al., 2014, 2017). Feedback studies of adult clinical populations have included individuals with Broca's aphasia and apraxia of speech (Katz et al., 1999, 2002, 2007, 2010; McNeil et al., 2007, 2010), dysarthria (Watkins, 2015) and hearing impairment (Bock, 2009). Across a series of studies completed in our laboratory using midsagittal EMA displays, we found that lingual visual feedback generally helped individuals with AOS improve the accuracy of consonant place of articulation (see Katz and McNeil, 2010, for review). All the same, as described in the previous discussion of EPG training studies, more work must be done to better understand the exact contribution that visual training provides over associated intervention procedures. The variable strength of effects noted for different sounds and for different participants remains a challenge to our current understanding.

Other new challenges and opportunities are noted for real-time EMA feedback experimentation. For instance, our early work was limited to showing patients midsagittal images of their articulatory trajectories, together with spatial "targets" representing regions that the EMA sensors must hit in order to receive real-time augmented visual feedback. Using newer systems (e.g., Carstens AG500, Carstens Medezinelektronik, GmbH), one can present high-resolution, spherical targets and consider a greater range of articulatory motion, including diagonal and loop-like patterns that may be more typical of speech. One can also devise pursuit tracking experiments to determine the precision with which the tongue can follow oscillating targets at different speeds and at either predictable or unpredictable frequencies (e.g., Fazel and Katz, 2016). These experimental capabilities permit study of issues such as whether there are shared (or disparate) motor bases for speech and non-speech motor control (e.g., by making targets more speech-like or less speech-like) and the extent to which participants recruit feedforward and feedback processes in voluntary oral motor control.

Other researchers have suggested ways to make 3D EMA feedback systems more user-friendly and affordable for clinical and teaching settings (Shtern et al., 2012; Haworth et al., 2014; Tilsen et al., 2015). For instance, Shtern and colleagues (2012) describe a game system based on an interactive EMA system (WAVE, Northern Digital Inc, Waterloo, Canada) that represents participant tongue position as either a simulated wooden plank that can be maneuvered up and down, or as a honeybee that can be guided to a target flower. Further data are needed to determine whether different types of interactive displays are better suited for particular clinical populations, whether particular views are preferred, and whether certain types of game training scenarios (e.g., competitive versus cooperative) are optimal. These parameters will likely interact with the type of speech sounds being trained.

With developments in ultrasound technology, visual feedback research has greatly accelerated, particularly for children with speech and language disorders. Ultrasound intervention studies have been conducted for children with developmental speech sound disorders (e.g., Shawker and Sonies, 1985; Adler-Bock et al., 2007; Byun et al., 2014; Cleland et al., 2015; Bressmann et al., 2016; Preston et al., 2017b), hearing impairment (Bernhardt et al., 2003, 2005; Bacsfalvi et al., 2007; Bacsfalvi, 2010; Bacsfalvi and Bernhardt, 2011), cleft lip and palate (Roxburgh et al., 2016), and childhood apraxia of speech, or CAS (Preston et al., 2016, 2017c). For adults, Down's syndrome (Fawcett et al., 2008), glossectomy (Blyth et al., 2016), AOS (Preston and Leaman, 2014), and nonfluent aphasia (Haldin et al., 2017) have recently been investigated.

Similar to EPG visual feedback, a preponderance of ultrasound studies suggest positive results for intervention paradigms conducted with clinical populations. A potential difference from EPG is that ultrasound can be used to provide an image of the tongue ("ultrasound tongue imaging") which is arguably less abstract and more intuitive than the palate-contact image displayed by EPG. In addition, researchers can use ultrasound to image the tongue shape of vowels in an accurate and relatively non-invasive manner. Nonetheless, this research is also in an early stage and many challenges remain. For example, a recent study compared the ability of adults to interpret slow motion EPG and ultrasound (silent) movies and reported some surprising results (Cleland et al., 2013). As predicted, participants scored above chance for consonants using both techniques, suggesting that most participants can "tongue-read" these sounds. However, EPG was preferred by subjects and showed higher overall accuracy rates for both consonants and vowels, while participants performed at chance level for vowels shown in the ultrasound condition. These latter findings suggest that feedback quality may play a role: Many participants described the ultrasound images being "unclear" or "fuzzy," while those preferring ultrasound described benefit from an "actual tongue" (p. 308). The authors further suggest that the success of using ultrasound in therapy is likely not only due to tongue-reading, but also the training and support of a clinician (p. 309).

To summarize, studies using real-time visual feedback (based on EPG, EMA, or ultrasound) suggest that viewing normally invisible movement of the tongue can assist in pronunciation training for individuals with speech/language disorders. However, most of these studies have examined small subject groups and more data are needed. Future investigations should continue to examine how articulatory training draws on principles of motor learning, including the type, frequency, and scheduling of feedback (Ballard et al., 2012). In addition, studies should further address the functional and neural underpinnings of the visual feedback gains shown by participants.

Implications for computational neural models

An intriguing question concerns whether special processing routes may be involved when accessing (normally) invisible articulators during the use of feedback systems (e.g., with Opti-Speech or Vizart3D, Hueber et al., 2012). This issue may be relevant when interpreting other data, such as the results of a discordant, cross-modal feedback paradigm (e.g., McGurk effect). Real-time visual feedback of the articulators may plausibly engage slightly different behavioral mechanisms and cortical pathways than those pathways involved in more traditional learning (e.g., "watch me, memorize, repeat").

One way to address this issue is to consider recent visual feedback findings in light of current neurocomputational models of speech production (e.g., "Directions Into Velocities of Articulators" (DIVA) (Guenther and Perkell, 2004; Guenther, 2006; Guenther et al., 2006; Guenther and Vladusich, 2012) and "ACTion" (ACT) (Kröger et al., 2009). These models seek to provide an integrated explanation for speech processing, incorporated in testable artificial neural networks. Both DIVA and ACT assume as input an abstract speech sound unit (a phoneme, syllable, or word), and generate as output both articulatory and auditory representations of speech. The systems operate by computing neural layers (or "maps") as distributed activation patterns. Producing an utterance involves fine-tuning between speech sound maps, sensory maps, and motor maps, guided by feedforward (predictive) processes and concurrent feedback from the periphery. Learning in these models critically relies on forward and inverse processes, with the internal speech model iteratively strengthened by the interaction of feedback information. This feedback may include simple mirroring of the lips and jaw, or instrumentally augmented visualizations of the tongue (via EMA, ultrasound, MRI, or articulatory inversion systems that convert sound signals to visual images of the articulators; e.g., Hueber et al., 2012). The remaining audio and visual preprocessing and mapping stages are similar between this internal route and the external (modeled) pathways.

Findings of L2 learning under conditions of visual (self) feedback training supports this internal route and the role of body sensing and motor familiarity (shaded region at bottom of Figure 19.2). This internal route also accounts for the fact that talkers can discern between natural and unnatural tongue movements displayed by an avatar (Engwall and Wik, 2009), and that training systems based on a talkers' own speech may be especially beneficial for L2 learners (see Felps et al., 2009 for discussion).

The neural processing of visual feedback for speech learning is an interesting topic for future research. Data on this topic are few. A recent ultrasound training study examined individuals with Broca's type aphasia and included fMRI imaging before and after tongue-image "sensory motor feedback" in order to investigate potential neural correlates

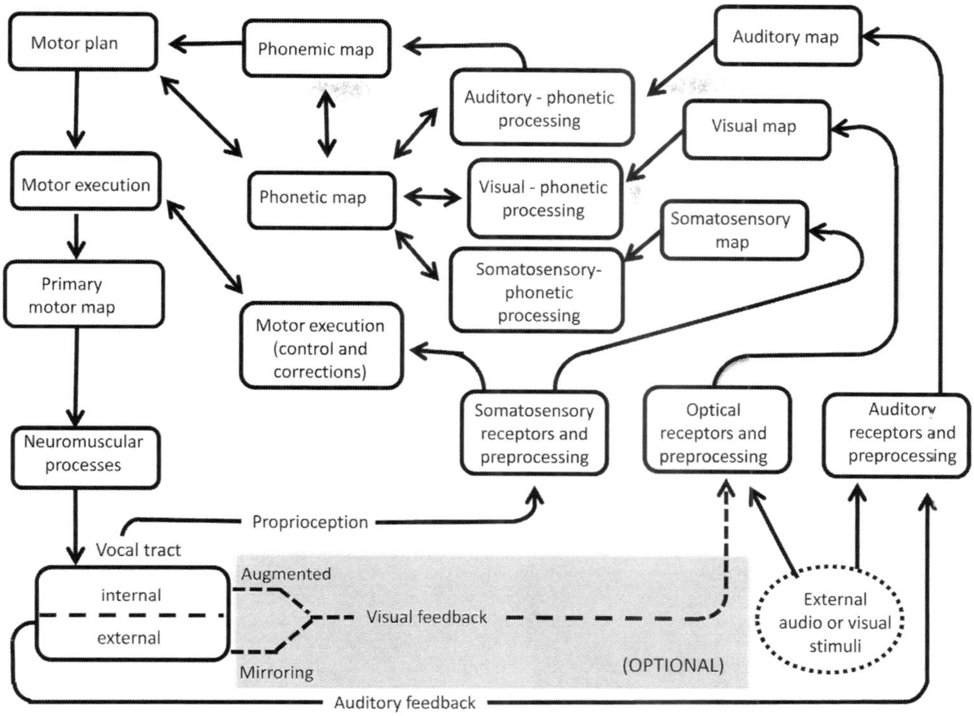

Figure 19.2 A simplified neurocomputational model of speech based on ACT (Kröger et al., 2009) highlighting input pathways for external AV stimuli (oval at bottom right) and optional feedback circuits to the vocal tract, including internal "invisible" articulators.

of training (Haldin et al., 2017). For both rhyme detection and syllable repetition tasks, the post-training results indicated cerebral activation for brain regions related to articulatory, auditory and somatosensory processes. These included changes in left superior-medial frontal and left precentral gyrus, right frontal middle and superior and superior temporal gyri, and right cerebellum for rhyme detection. The authors interpreted these cerebral changes as evidence of strengthened production and perception networks, while the cerebellar data changes were considered possible sources of improved attention, memory, or internal model factors associated with speech gains. For syllable repetition, feedback training corresponded with increased activation of the left inferior frontal gyrus and left insula. Activation in these regions were claimed to relate to improved sensorimotor interaction and articulatory coordination.

In addition to brain systems associated with articulatory, auditory, and somatosensory processes, visual feedback tasks require a participant to sense one's own body in motion. As described in Daprati et al. (2010), this involves both corporeal identity (the feeling of one's own body) and sense of agency (experiencing oneself as the cause of an action). Substantial data implicate parietal and insular cortex supporting these processes awareness (e.g., Farrer et al., 2003, 2008; Berlucchi and Aglioti, 2010), including specialized roles of the two parietal lobes to generate and supervise the internal model (left parietal) while the right parietal maintains spatial (egocentric) reference. Based on these findings, one might predict contributions from parietal and insular circuitry to support visual articulatory feedback. With respect to the specific task of visual feedback and speech learning, Berthier and Moreno-Torres (2016) discuss two specific structures that may be expected to participate: anterior insular cortex and anterior cingulate cortex. These structures are noted to be part of larger systems that can be voluntarily self-controlled (Ninaus et al. 2013), process multimodal information (Moreno-Torres et al., 2013), and relate to speech initiation (Goldberg, 1985). Additional brain structures that may play a role are those associated with reward dependence during behavioral performance, including lateral prefrontal cortex and the striatum (Pochon et al., 2002; Ullsperger and von Cramon, 2003; Liu et al., 2011; Dayan et al., 2014; Widmer et al., 2016).

Katz and Mehta (2015) speculate that speech visual feedback for normally invisible articulators (such as the tongue) rely in part on oral self-touch mechanism (particularly for consonant production) by visually guiding participants to the correct place of articulation, at which point somatosensory processes take over. This mechanism may prove particularly important for consonants, which are produced with more articulatory contact than vowels (see also Ladefoged, 2005). As data accrue with respect to both external (mirroring) and internal ("tongue reading") visual speech feedback, it will be important to continue study of the relevant neural control structures, in order to develop more complete models of speech production. Future studies should focus on extending the range of speech sounds, features, and articulatory structures trained with real-time feedback, with a focus on vowels as well as consonants. It will also be important to examine the extent and nature of individual variation across talkers.

Conclusion

This chapter has briefly reviewed the history of clinical phonetics, emphasizing its prominence within the larger field of clinical linguistics and noting rapid developments in light of innovations in medicine, linguistics, and speech science. Two important goals of clinical phonetics are to (1) develop scientific and clinical knowledge based on two-way information flow between clinical practice and linguistic/cognitive theory, and (2) perfect symbol systems useful in describing healthy and disordered speech. These goals are considered in light of recent evidence concerning the audiovisual (AV) nature of speech processing. Evidence is reviewed from speech produced and perceived by adults, children, and individuals with speech/language disorders. We find that because healthy speech production and perception is strongly audiovisual in nature, our understanding of speech- and language-disordered populations should include a similar emphasis. This will entail scrutiny of speech-related head and orofacial motion when considering the speech and language difficulties of individuals with communication disorders, as well as their families. Such research may also involve new ways of thinking about the articulators most commonly associated with speech (lips, jaw, tongue and velum); for instance, by considering the role played by normally invisible articulators, such as the tongue, when made visible by means of real-time instrumentation.

In the course of this chapter, many examples of AV properties related to speech and language have been described, including instances of impairment resulting from the misprocessing of such information. We may draw examples for the first current goal of clinical phonetics, namely two-way information flow between theory and practice. Researchers have used neurocomputational frameworks to gain important insights about speech and language disorders, including apraxia of speech (AOS) in adults (Kröger et al., 2011; Hickok et al., 2014; Maas et al., 2015), childhood apraxia of speech (Terband et al., 2009; Terband

and Maassen, 2010), developmental speech sound disorders (Terband et al., 2014), and stuttering (Max et al., 2004; Civier et al., 2010). For example, DIVA and ACT simulations have been used to test the claim that apraxic disorders result from relatively preserved feedback (and impaired feedforward) speech motor processes (Civier et al., 2010; Maas et al., 2015) or from defective neural motor speech mappings leading to types of AOS of varying severity (Kröger et al., 2011). These neurocomputational modeling-based findings correspond with largely positive results from visual augmented feedback intervention studies for individuals with AOS (see Katz and McNeil, 2010 for review; also, Preston and Leaman, 2014). Overall, recent intervention findings have suggested that visual augmented feedback of tongue movement can help remediate speech errors in individuals with AOS, presumably by strengthening the internal model. Other clinical studies have reported that visual feedback can positively influence the speech of individuals with a variety of speech and language problems in children and adults, including articulation/phonological disorders, residual sound errors, and dysarthria. This research has included training with electropalatography (EPG), ultrasound, and strain gauge transducer systems (Shirahige et al., 2012; Yano et al., 2015).

The findings concerning AV processing also potentially relate to the second goal of clinical phonetics, perfecting symbol systems. Over the years, some researchers have mentioned the concept of "optical phonetics," either in relation to the visual perception of prosody (e.g., Scarborough et al., 2009) or for lip-reading (e.g., Jiang et al., 2007; Bernstein and Jiang, 2009). Understandably, these considerations have not affected the International Phonetic Alphabet, which is based on features that express either articulatory or acoustic characteristics. However, assuming our understanding of AV speech processing continues to support the importance of AV speech processing (and deficits with impairment), I would think it reasonable that phonetic features such as "decreased head motion," "excessive head motion," and "masked facies" (problems of AV speech noted in clinical populations) should be considered for the ExtIPA. Here, I leave this as a friendly suggestion for future consideration.

Acknowledgments

The author gratefully acknowledges support from the University of Texas at Dallas Office of Sponsored Projects, the UTD Callier Center Excellence in Education Fund, and a grant awarded by NIH/NIDCD (R43 DC013467) for portions of this work. I greatly appreciate Carstens Medezinelektronik GmbH for material support towards this research. I would also like to thank Peter F. Assmann, Martin J. Ball, Susan Behrens, Bryan Gick, Lisa Goffman, Sonya Mehta, and Patrick Reidy for helpful comments on previous versions of this manuscript. All remaining errors are mine alone.

Notes

1 Rather similar to the "taxonomic" versus "scientific" approaches to phonetics described by Ohala (2004), "notebook" versus "experimental" linguistic approaches to phonology are discussed by Coleman (2011). Coleman proposes that both types are useful, but more abstract, subjective (notebook) description will eventually be supplanted by empirical evidence.

2 Whereas the term "neurolinguistics" is used here to describe extrapolating from clinical data to linguistic theory, this term can also be more broadly used to designate whenever neurologists and linguists collaborate for joint research (e.g., Lesser, 1989, pg. 160).

3 In terms of the source-filter theory (Fant, 1971), this review is "filter-centric" in that feedback of the vocal source is not considered, as well as "oral-centric," omitting discussion of visual feedback

for nasal sounds. For more information on visual feedback for control of nasalization, see Witzel et al., 1988; Ysunza et al., 1997; Anderson et al., 2014; Murray et al., 2016.

4 Different cultures may define "the tongue" using dissimilar anatomical boundaries, raising potential caveats about artificially compartmentalizing body parts in phonetics (see Chapter 5, this volume, for discussion). Yet despite these flexible definitions, it is clear the tongue is essential for shaping the vocal tract in order to produce intelligible speech (Hiiemae and Palmer, 2003). Although some speakers can produce remarkable compensation for restriction to lingual movement, such as in rare cases of aglossia or hypoglossia (e.g., Toutios et al., 2017), the tongue ordinarily plays a crucial role in shaping the sound quality of most consonants and vowels.

References

Abe, M., Fukusako, Y. and Sawashima, M., 1977. Results of articulation training on 60 cleft palate patients. *The Japan Journal of Logopedics and Phoniatrics*, *18*(2), pp. 67–73.

Abel, J., Barbosa, A.V., Black, A., Mayer, C. and Vatikiotis-Bateson, E., 2011. The labial viseme reconsidered: Evidence from production and perception. *The Journal of the Acoustical Society of America*, *129*(4), p. 2456.

Abercrombie, D., 1957. Direct palatography. *STUF-Language Typology and Universals*, *10*(1–4), pp. 21–25.

Adler-Bock, M., Bernhardt, B.M., Gick, B. and Bacsfalvi, P., 2007. The use of ultrasound in remediation of North American English /r/ in 2 adolescents. *American Journal of Speech-Language Pathology*, *16*(2), pp. 128–139.

Alcorn, S., 1932. The Tadoma method. *Volta Review*, *34*, pp. 195–198.

Alsius, A., Navarra, J., Campbell, R. and Soto-Faraco, S., 2005. Audiovisual integration of speech falters under high attention demands. *Current Biology*, *15*(9), pp. 839–843.

Alsius, A., Paré, M. and Munhall, K.G., 2017. Forty years after Hearing lips and seeing voices: The McGurk effect revisited. *Multisensory Research*, *31*(1–2), pp. 111–144.

Amman, J.C., 1700. *Dissertatio de loquela, qua non solum vox humana, et loquendi artificium ex originibus suis eruuntur: Sed et traduntur media, quibus ii, qui ab incunabulis surdi et muti fuerunt, loquelam adipisci . . . possint* (Vol. 1). Amsterdam: Apud Joannem Wolters.

Amman, J.C., 1694. *The Talking Deaf Man: Or, a Method Proposed Whereby He Who Is Born Deaf May Learn to Speak*. London: Tho. Howkins

Anderson, P., Fels, S., Harandi, N.M., Ho, A., Moisik, S., Sánchez, C.A., Stavness, I. and Tang, K., 2017. FRANK: A hybrid 3D biomechanical model of the head and neck. *Biomechanics of Living Organs*, pp. 413–447.

Anderson, S.R., Keating, P.A., Huffman, M.K. and Krakow, R.A., 2014. *Nasals, Nasalization, and the Velum* (Vol. 5). Amsterdam: Elsevier.

Arnold, P. and Hill, F., 2001. Bisensory augmentation: A speechreading advantage when speech is clearly audible and intact. *British Journal of Psychology*, *92*(2), pp. 339–355.

Bacsfalvi, P., 2010. Attaining the lingual components of /r/ with ultrasound for three adolescents with cochlear implants. *Canadian Journal of Speech-Language Pathology & Audiology*, *34*(3).

Bacsfalvi, P. and Bernhardt, B.M., 2011. Long-term outcomes of speech therapy for seven adolescents with visual feedback technologies: Ultrasound and electropalatography. *Clinical Linguistics & Phonetics*, *25*(11–12), pp. 1034–1043.

Bacsfalvi, P., Bernhardt, B.M. and Gick, B., 2007. Electropalatography and ultrasound in vowel remediation for adolescents with hearing impairment. *Advances in Speech Language Pathology*, *9*(1), pp. 36–45.

Badin, P., Elisei, F., Bailly, G. and Tarabalka, Y., 2008, July. An audiovisual talking head for augmented speech generation: Models and animations based on a real speaker's articulatory data. In *International Conference on Articulated Motion and Deformable Objects* (pp. 132–143). Springer, Berlin, Heidelberg.

Badin, P., Tarabalka, Y., Elisei, F. and Bailly, G., 2010. Can you 'read' tongue movements? Evaluation of the contribution of tongue display to speech understanding. *Speech Communication*, *52*(6), pp. 493–503.

Ball, M.J., Code, C., Rahilly, J. and Hazlett, D., 1994. Non-segmental aspects of disordered speech: Developments in transcription. *Clinical linguistics & phonetics*, *8*(1), pp. 67–83.

Ball, M.J., Esling, J. and Dickson, C., 1995. The VoQS system for the transcription of voice quality. *Journal of the International Phonetic Association*, *25*(2), pp. 71–80.

Ball, M., Müller, N., Klopfenstein, M. and Rutter, B., 2009. The importance of narrow phonetic transcription for highly unintelligible speech: Some examples. *Logopedics Phoniatrics Vocology*, *34*(2), pp. 84–90.

Ballard, K.J., Smith, H.D., Paramatmuni, D., McCabe, P., Theodoros, D.G. and Murdoch, B.E., 2012. Amount of kinematic feedback affects learning of speech motor skills. *Motor Control*, *16*, pp. 106–119.

Bartlett, J.C. and Searcy, J., 1993. Inversion and configuration of faces. *Cognitive Psychology*, *25*(3), pp. 281–316.

Bastien-Toniazzo, M., Stroumza, A. and Cavé, C., 2010. Audio-visual perception and integration in developmental dyslexia: An exploratory study using the McGurk effect. *Current Psychology Letters. Behaviour, Brain & Cognition*, *25*(3, 2009).

Beckman, M.E., Plummer, A.R., Munson, B. and Reidy, P.F., 2017. Methods for eliciting, annotating, and analyzing databases for child speech development. *Computer Speech & Language*, *45*, pp. 278–299.

Bell, A.G., 1872. *Establishment for the Study of Vocal Physiology: For the Correction of Stammering, and Other Defects of Utterance: And for Practical Instruction in "Visible Speech."* [Boston: AG Bell], 1872 (Boston: Rand, Avery).

Bell, Alexander Melville (Visible Speech, 1867).

Berlucchi, G. and Aglioti, S.M., 2010. The body in the brain revisited. *Experimental Brain Research*, *200*(1), p. 25.

Bernhardt, B., Gick, B., Bacsfalvi, P. and Adler-Bock, M., 2005. Ultrasound in speech therapy with adolescents and adults. *Clinical Linguistics & Phonetics*, *19*(6–7), pp. 605–617.

Bernhardt, B., Gick, B., Bacsfalvi, P. and Ashdown, J., 2003. Speech habilitation of hard of hearing adolescents using electropalatography and ultrasound as evaluated by trained listeners. *Clinical Linguistics & Phonetics*, *17*(3), pp. 199–216.

Bernstein, L.E., Eberhardt, S.P. and Demorest, M.E., 1989. Single-channel vibrotactile supplements to visual perception of intonation and stress. *The Journal of the Acoustical Society of America*, *85*(1), pp. 397–405.

Bernstein, L.E. and Jiang, J., 2009. Visual Speech Perception, Optical Phonetics, and Synthetic Speech. In *Visual Speech Recognition: Lip Segmentation and Mapping* (pp. 439–461).IGI Global, Hershey, PA.

Berthier, M.L. and Moreno-Torres, I., 2016. Commentary: Visual feedback of tongue movement for novel speech sound learning. *Frontiers in Human Neuroscience*, *10*, p. 662.

Beskow, J., 1995. Rule-based visual speech synthesis. In *EUROSPEECH '95. 4th European Conference on Speech Communication and Technology* (pp. 299–302).

Blyth, K.M., Mccabe, P., Madill, C. and Ballard, K.J., 2016. Ultrasound visual feedback in articulation therapy following partial glossectomy. *Journal of Communication Disorders*, *61*, pp. 1–15.

Bock, R., 2009. Effectiveness of visual feedback provided by an electromagnetic articulograph (EMA) system: training vowel production in individuals with hearing impairment. Independent Studies and Capstones. *Paper 206. Program in Audiology and Communication Sciences*, Washington University School of Medicine.

Bologna, M., Fabbrini, G., Marsili, L., Defazio, G., Thompson, P.D. and Berardelli, A., 2012. Facial bradykinesia. *Journal of Neurology, Neurosurgery, and Psychiatry*, pp. 1–5.

Borod, J.C., Welkowitz, J., Alpert, M., Brozgold, A.Z., Martin, C., Peselow, E. and Diller, L., 1990. Parameters of emotional processing in neuropsychiatric disorders: Conceptual issues and a battery of tests. *Journal of Communication Disorders*, *23*(4–5), pp. 247–271.

Bressmann, T., Harper, S., Zhylich, I. and Kulkarni, G.V., 2016. Perceptual, durational and tongue displacement measures following articulation therapy for rhotic sound errors. *Clinical Linguistics & Phonetics*, *30*(3–5), pp. 345–362.

Brooke, N.M. and Summerfield, Q., 1983. Analysis, synthesis, and perception of visible articulatory movements. *Journal of Phonetics*, *11*(1), pp. 63–76.

Bruce, V. and Young, A.W., 2012. *Face Perception*. New York, NY: Psychology Press.

Buck, R. and Duffy, R.J., 1980. Nonverbal communication of affect in brain-damaged patients. *Cortex*, *16*(3), pp. 351–362.

Burnham, D. and Dodd, B., 1996. Auditory-visual speech perception as a direct process: The McGurk effect in infants and across languages. In *Speechreading by Humans and Machines* (pp. 103–114). Berlin, Heidelberg: Springer.

Burnham, D. and Dodd, B., 2004. Auditory-visual speech integration by pre-linguistic infants: Perception of an emergent consonant in the McGurk effect. *Developmental Psychobiology*, *44*, pp. 209–220.

Busso, C., Deng, Z., Grimm, M., Neumann, U. and Narayanan, S., 2007. Rigid head motion in expressive speech animation: Analysis and synthesis. *IEEE Transactions on Audio, Speech, and Language Processing*, *15*(3), pp. 1075–1086.

Byun, T.M., Hitchcock, E.R. and Swartz, M.T., 2014. Retroflex versus bunched in treatment for rhotic misarticulation: Evidence from ultrasound biofeedback intervention. *Journal of Speech, Language, and Hearing Research*, *57*(6), pp. 2116–2130.

Campbell, R., 2006. Audio-visual speech processing. *The Encyclopedia of Language and Linguistics*, pp. 562–569.

Cantiniaux, S., Vaugoyeau, M., Robert, D., Horrelou-Pitek, C., Mancini, J., Witjas, T. and Azulay, J.P., 2010. Comparative analysis of gait and speech in Parkinson's disease: Hypokinetic or dysrhythmic disorders? *Journal of Neurology, Neurosurgery & Psychiat*ry, *81*(2), pp. 177–184.

Carbon, C.C., Grüter, T., Weber, J.E. and Lueschow, A., 2007. Faces as objects of non-expertise: Processing of thatcherised faces in congenital prosopagnosia. *Perception*, *36*(11), pp. 1635–1645.

Carbon, C.C., Schweinberger, S.R., Kaufmann, J.M. and Leder, H., 2005. The Thatcher illusion seen by the brain: An event-related brain potentials study. *Cognitive Brain Research*, *24*(3), pp. 544–555.

Chen, T. and Rao, R., 1998. Audio-visual integration in multimodal communication. *Proceedings of the IEEE*, *86*(5), pp. 837–852.

Son Chung, J., Senior, A., Vinyals, O. and Zisserman, A., 2017. Lip reading sentences in the wild. In *Proceedings of the IEEE Conference on Computer Vision and Pattern Recognition* (pp. 6447–6456).

Civier, O., Tasko, S.M. and Guenther, F.H., 2010. Overreliance on auditory feedback may lead to sound/syllable repetitions: Simulations of stuttering and fluency-inducing conditions with a neural model of speech production. *Journal of Fluency Disorders*, *35*(3), pp. 246–279.

Cleland, J., McCron, C. and Scobbie, J.M., 2013. Tongue reading: Comparing the interpretation of visual information from inside the mouth, from electropalatographic and ultrasound displays of speech sounds. *Clinical Linguistics & Phonetics*, *27*(4), pp. 299–311.

Cleland, J., Scobbie, J.M. and Wrench, A.A., 2015. Using ultrasound visual biofeedback to treat persistent primary speech sound disorders. *Clinical Linguistics & Phonetics*, *29*(8–10), pp. 575–597.

Cleland, J., Scobbie, J.M. and Zharkova, N., 2016. Insights from ultrasound: Enhancing our understanding of clinical phonetics. *Clinical Linguistics and Phonetics*, *30*, pp. 171–173.

Cleland, J., Timmins, C., Wood, S.E., Hardcastle, W.J. and Wishart, J.G., 2009. Electropalatographic therapy for children and young people with Down's syndrome. *Clinical Linguistics & Phonetics*, *23*, pp. 926–939.

Code, C. and Ball, M.J., 1984. *Experimental Clinical Phonetics: Investigatory Techniques in Speech Pathology and Therapeutics*. Worcester: Billing & Sons Limited.

Coleman, J., 2011. A history maker. *Journal of Linguistics*, *47*, pp. 201–217.

Crawford, R., 1995. Teaching voiced velar stops to profoundly deaf children using EPG, two case studies. *Clinical Linguistics and Phonetics*, *9*, pp. 255–270.

Crystal, D., 1980. *An Introduction to Language Pathology*. London: Edward Arnold.

Crystal, D., 1981. *Clinical Linguistics: Disorders of Human Communication vol. 3*. Wien: Sprinter.

Crystal, D., 1984. *Linguistic Encounters with Language Handicap*. Oxford: Wiley-Blackwell.

Crystal, D., 2002. Clinical linguistics and phonetics' first 15 years: An introductory comment. *Clinical Linguistics & Phonetics*, *16*(7), pp. 487–489.

Crystal, D., 2013. Clinical linguistics: Conversational reflections. *Clinical Linguistics Phonetics*, *27*(4), pp. 236–243.

Cvejic, E., Kim, J. and Davis, C., 2010. Prosody off the top of the head: Prosodic contrasts can be discriminated by head motion. *Speech Communication*, *52*(6), pp. 555–564.

Dagenais, P.A., 1992. Speech training with glossometry and palatometry for profoundly hearing-impaired children. *Volta Review*, *94*, pp. 261–282.

Dagenais, P.A., 1995. Electropalatography in the treatment of articulation/phonological disorders. *Journal of Communication Disorders*, *28*, pp. 303–329.

Daprati, E., Sirigu, A. and Nico, D., 2010. Body and movement: Consciousness in the parietal lobes. *Neuropsychologia*, *48*(3), pp. 756–762.

Davis, C. and Kim, J., 2006. Audio-visual speech perception off the top of the head. *Cognition*, *100*(3), pp. B21–B31.

Dayan, E., Hamann, J.M., Averbeck, B.B. and Cohen, L.G., 2014. Brain structural substrates of reward dependence during behavioral performance. *Journal of Neuroscience*, *34*, 16433–16441.

Delbeuck, X., Collette, F. and Van der Linden, M., 2007. Is Alzheimer's disease a disconnection syndrome? Evidence from a crossmodal audio-visual illusory experiment. *Neuropsychologia*, *45*(14), pp. 3315–3323.

Denes, P.B. and Pinson, E., 1993. *The Speech Chain*. London: Macmillan.

Dent, H., Gibbon, F. and Hardcastle, W., 1992. Inhibiting an abnormal lingual pattern in a cleft palate child using electropalatography. In M.M. Leahy and J.L. Kallen (Eds.) *Interdisciplinary Perspectives in Speech and Language Pathology* (pp. 211–221). Dublin: School of Clinical Speech and Language Studies.

Derrick, D., O'Beirne, G.A., Rybel, T.D. and Hay, J., 2014. Aero-tactile integration in fricatives: Converting audio to air flow information for speech perception enhancement. In *Fifteenth Annual Conference of the International Speech Communication Association* (pp. 2580–2284). International Speech Communication Association, Baixas.

Desjardins, R.N., Rogers, J. and Werker, J.F., 1997. An exploration of why preschoolers perform differently than do adults in audiovisual speech perception tasks. *Journal of Experimental Child Psychology*, *66*(1), pp. 85–110.

Desjardins, R.N. and Werker, J.F., 2004. Is the integration of heard and seen speech mandatory for infants? *Developmental Psychobiology*, *45*(4), pp. 187–203.

Dinnsen, D.A., Gierut, J.A., Morrisette, M.L. and Rose, D.E., 2014. Unraveling phonological conspiracies: A case study. *Clinical Linguistics & Phonetics*, *28*(7–8), pp. 463–476.

Doherty-Sneddon, G., Bonner, L. and Bruce, V., 2001. Cognitive demands of face monitoring: Evidence for visuospatial overload. *Memory & Cognition*, *29*(7), pp. 909–919.

Doherty-Sneddon, G., McAuley, S., Bruce, V., Langton, S., Blokland, A. and Anderson, A.H., 2000. Visual signals and children's communication: Negative effects on task outcome. *British Journal of Developmental Psychology*, *18*(4), pp. 595–608.

Duchan, J.F., 2006. How conceptual frameworks influence clinical practice: Evidence from the writings of John Thelwall, a 19th-century speech therapist. *International Journal of Language & Communication Disorders*, *41*(6), pp. 735–744.

Duckworth, M., Allen, G., Hardcastle, W. and Ball, M., 1990. Extensions to the International Phonetic Alphabet for the transcription of atypical speech. *Clinical Linguistics & Phonetics*, *4*(4), pp. 273–280.

Dupont, S., Aubin, J. and Ménard, L., 2005. A Study of the McGurk Effect in 4 and 5-Year-Old French Canadian Children. *Leibniz Center for General Linguistics (ZAS) Papers in Linguistics*, *40*, pp. 1–17.

Engwall, O., 2008. Can audio-visual instructions help learners improve their articulation?-An ultrasound study of short term changes. *Interspeech*, pp. 2631–2634.

Engwall, O. and Bälter, O., 2007. Pronunciation feedback from real and virtual language teachers. *Computer Assisted Language Learning*, *20*(3), pp. 235–262.

Engwall, O. and Wik, P., 2009. Can you tell if tongue movements are real or synthesized? *AVSP*, pp. 96–101.

Engwall, O., Wik, P., Beskow, J., Granstrom, G., 2004. Design strategies for a virtual language tutor. *Proceedings of International Conference on Spoken Language Processing*, *3*, pp. 1693–1696.

Eskelund, K., MacDonald, E.N. and Andersen, T.S., 2015. Face configuration affects speech perception: Evidence from a McGurk mismatch negativity study. *Neuropsychologia*, *66*, pp. 48–54.

Esling, J.H., 2010. Phonetic notation. In *The Handbook of Phonetic Sciences, Second Edition* (pp. 678–702). Oxford: Wiley–Blackwell.

Fagel, S. and Madany, K., 2008. A 3-D virtual head as a tool for speech therapy for children. *Proceedings of Interspeech 2008* (pp. 2643–2646). ISCA, Brisbane, Australia.

Fant, G., 1971. *Acoustic Theory of Speech Production: With Calculations Based on X-Ray Studies of Russian Articulations* (Vol. 2). Berlin: Walter de Gruyter.

Farah, M.J., Wilson, K.D., Drain, M. and Tanaka, J.N., 1998. What is "special" about face perception? *Psychological Review*, *105*(3), p. 482.

Farrer, C., Franck, N., Georgieff, N., Frith, C.D., Decety, J. and Jeannerod, M., 2003. Modulating the experience of agency: A positron emission tomography study. *Neuroimage*, *18*(2), pp. 324–333.

Farrer, C., Frey, S.H., Van Horn, J.D., Tunik, E., Turk, D., Inati, S. and Grafton, S.T., 2008. The angular gyrus computes action awareness representations. *Cerebral Cortex*, *18*(2), pp. 254–261.

Fawcett, S., Bacsfalvi, P. and Bernhardt, B.M., 2008. Ultrasound as visual feedback in speech therapy for /r /with adults with Down Syndrome. *Down Syndrome Quarterly*, *10*(1), pp. 4–12.

Fazel, V. and Katz, W., 2016. Visuomotor pursuit tracking accuracy for intraoral tongue movement. *The Journal of the Acoustical Society of America*, *140*(4), pp. 3224–3224.

Felps, D., Bortfeld, H. and Gutierrez-Osuna, R., 2009. Foreign accent conversion in computer assisted pronunciation training. *Speechan Communication*, *51*(10), pp. 920–932.

Fenson, L., Dale, P.S., Reznick, J.S., Bates, E., Thal, D.J., Pethick, S.J., Tomasello, M., Mervis, C.B. and Stiles, J., 1994. Variability in early communicative development. *Monographs of the Society for Research in Child Development*, pp. 1–185.

Fernald, A., 1989. Intonation and communicative intent in mothers' speech to infants: Is the melody the message? *Child Development*, pp. 1497–1510.

Field, T., Diego, M. and Hernandez-Reif, M., 2009. Depressed mothers' infants are less responsive to faces and voices. *Infant Behavior and Development*, *32*(3), pp. 239–244.

Firth, J.E., 1948. Word-palatograms and articulation. *Bulletin of the School of Oriental and African Studies*, *12*(3–4), pp. 857–864.

Fisher, C.G., 1968. Confusions among visually perceived consonants. *Journal of Speech, Language, and Hearing Research*, *11*(4), pp. 796–804.

Fisher, C.G., 1969. The visibility of terminal pitch contour. *Journal of Speech, Language, and Hearing Research*, *12*(2), pp. 379–382.

Fletcher, S. and Hasagawa, A., 1983. Speech modification by a deaf child through dynamic orometric modelling and feedback. *Journal of Speech and Hearing Disorders*, *48*, pp. 178–185.

Fowler, C.A. and Dekle, D.J., 1991. Listening with eye and hand: Cross-modal contributions to speech perception. *Journal of Experimental Psychology: Human Perception and Performance*, *17*(3), p. 816.

Fusaro, M., Harris, P.L. and Pan, B.A., 2012. Head nodding and head shaking gestures in children's early communication. *First Language*, *32*(4), pp. 439–458.

Gerard, J.M., Perrier, P. and Payan, Y., 2006. *3D Biomechanical Tongue Modeling to Study Speech Production*. New York: Psychology Press.

Gibbon, F., Hardcastle, B. and Suzuki, H., 1991. An electropalatographic study of the /r/, /l/ distinction for Japanese learners of English. *Computer Assisted Language Learning*, *4*(3), pp. 153–171.

Gibbon, F., Law, J. and Lee, A., 2007. Electropalatography for articulation disorders associated with cleft palate (protocol). In *Cochrane Collaboration, The Cochrane Library I*. Hoboken, NJ: Wiley.

Gibbon, F.E. and Lee, A., 2017. Electropalatographic (EPG) evidence of covert contrasts in disordered speech. *Clinical Linguistics & Phonetics*, *31*(1), pp. 4–20.

Gibbon, F., Stewart, F., Hardcastle, W.J. and Crampin, L., 1999. Widening access to electropalatography for children with persistent sound system disorders. *American Journal of Speech-Language Pathology*, *8*, pp. 319–334.

Gibbon, F.E. and Wood, S.E., 2003. Using electropalatography (EPG) to diagnose and treat articulation disorders associated with mild cerebral palsy: A case study. *Clinical Linguistics & Phonetics*, *17*(4–5), pp. 365–374.

Gibbon, F. and Wood, S.E., 2010. Visual feedback therapy with electropalatography (EPG) for speech sound disorders in children. In L. Williams, S. McLeod and R. McCauley (Eds.) *Interventions in Speech Sound Disorders* (pp. 509–536). Baltimore: Brookes.

Gick, B., Bernhardt, B., Bacsfalvi, P., Wilson, I. and Zampini, M.L., 2008. Ultrasound imaging applications in second language acquisition. *Phonology and Second Language Acquisition*, *36*, pp. 315–328.

Gick, B. and Derrick, D., 2009. Aero-tactile integration in speech perception. *Nature*, *462*(7272), pp. 502–504.

Gick, B., Wilson, I. and Derrick, D., 2012. *Articulatory Phonetics* (p. 272). Hoboken, NJ: John Wiley & Sons.

Glenberg, A.M., Schroeder, J.L. and Robertson, D.A., 1998. Averting the gaze disengages the environment and facilitates remembering. *Memory & Cognition*, *26*(4), pp. 651–658.

Goffman, L., Maassen, B. and Van Lieshout, P.H., 2010. Dynamic interaction of motor and language factors in normal and disordered development. *Speech Motor Control: New Developments in Basic and Applied Research*, pp. 137–152.

Goldberg, G., 1985. Supplementary motor area structure and function: Review and hypothesis. *Behavioral and Brain Sciences*, *8*, pp. 567–615.

Gracco, V.L., 1994. Some organizational characteristics of speech movement control. *Journal of Speech, Language, and Hearing Research*, *37*(1), pp. 4–27.

Graf, H.P., Cosatto, E., Strom, V. and Huang, F.J., 2002, May. Visual prosody: Facial movements accompanying speech. In *Automatic Face and Gesture Recognition, 2002. Proceedings: Fifth IEEE International Conference* (pp. 396–401).

Gray, H.M. and Tickle-Degnen, L., 2010. A meta-analysis of performance on emotion recognition tasks in Parkinson's disease. *Neuropsychology*, *24*(2), pp. 176–191.

Green, J.R. and Nip, I.S., 2010. Some organization principles in early speech development. In *Speech Motor Control: New Developments in Basic and Applied Research*, pp. 171–188.

Green, K.P., 1998. The use of auditory and visual information during phonetic processing: Implications for theories of speech perception. *Hearing by Eye II: Advances in the Psychology of Speechreading and Auditory-Visual Speech*, *2*, p. 3.

Guenther, F.H., 2006. Cortical interactions underlying the production of speech sounds. *Journal of Communication Disorders*, *39*(5), pp. 350–365.

Guenther, F.H., Ghosh, S.S. and Tourville, J.A., 2006. Neural modeling and imaging of the cortical interactions underlying syllable production. *Brain and Language*, *96*(3), pp. 280–301.

Guenther, F.H. and Perkell, J.S., 2004. A neural model of speech production and supporting experiments. In *From Sound to Sense Conference: Fifty+ Years of Discoveries in Speech Communication* (pp. 98–106). Cambridge, MA.

Guenther, F.H. and Vladusich, T., 2012. A neural theory of speech acquisition and production. *Journal of Neurolinguistics*, *25*(5), pp. 408–422.

Hacking, J.F., Smith, B.L. and Johnson, E.M., 2017. Utilizing electropalatography to train palatalized versus unpalatalized consonant productions by native speakers of American English learning Russian. *Journal of Second Language Pronunciation*, *3*(1), pp. 9–33.

Hadar, U., Steiner, T.J., Grant, E.C. and Clifford Rose, F., 1983. Head movement correlates of juncture and stress at sentence level. *Language and Speech*, *26*(2), pp. 117–129.

Hadfield, C. (2013). Astronaut Chris Hadfield savors fresh air of Earth. www.cbc.ca/news/technology/astronaut-chris-hadfield-savours-fresh-air-of-earth-1.1304791, Posted May 16th 2013.

Haith, M.M., Bergman, T. and Moore, M.J., 1977. Eye contact and face scanning in early infancy. *Science*, *198*(4319), pp. 853–855.

Haldin, C., Acher, A., Kauffmann, L., Hueber, T., Cousin, E., Badin, P., Perrier, P., Fabre, D., Pérennou, D., Detante, O. and Jaillard, A., 2017. Speech recovery and language plasticity can be facilitated by sensori-motor fusion training in chronic non-fluent aphasia. A case report study. *Clinical Linguistics & Phonetics*, pp. 1–27.

Hartelius, L.L., Mcauliffe, M., Murdoch, B.E. and Theodoros, D.G., 2001, January. The use of electropalatography in the treatment of disordered articulation in traumatic brain injury: A case study. In *4th International Speech Motor Conference* (pp. 192–195).Uitgeverij Vantilt, Nijmegen.

Hartelius, L.L. and Svensson, P., 1994. Speech and swallowing symptoms associated with Parkinson's disease and multiple sclerosis: A survey. *Folia Phoniatrica et Logopaedica*, *46*(1), pp. 9–17.

Hassanat, A., 2014. Visual speech recognition. *Eprint Arxiv*, *32*(3), pp. 2420–2424.

Haworth, B., Kearney, E., Baljko, M., Faloutsos, P. and Yunusova, Y. 2014. *Electromagnetic articulography in the development of 'serious games' for speech rehabilitation*. Paper presented at the Second International Workshop on BioMechanical and Parametric Modelling of Human Anatomy, Vancouver, Canada.

Hermant, N., Perrier, P. and Payan, Y., 2017. Human tongue biomechanical modeling. *Biomechanics of Living Organs*, pp. 395–411.

Hertrich, I. and Ackermann, H., 1993. Acoustic analysis of speech prosody in Huntington's and Parkinson's disease: A preliminary report. *Clinical Linguistics & Phonetics*, *7*(4), pp. 285–297.

Heselwood, B., 2013. *Phonetic Transcription in Theory and Practice*. Edinburgh: Edinburgh University Press.

Hessler, D., Jonkers, R. and Bastiaanse, R., 2012. Processing of audiovisual stimuli in aphasic and non-brain-damaged listeners. *Aphasiology*, *26*(1), pp. 83–102.

Hewlett, N., 1988. Acoustic properties of /k/ and /t/ in normal and phonologically disordered speech. *Clinical Linguistics & Phonetics*, *2*(1), pp. 29–45.

Hickey, J., 1992. The treatment of lateral fricatives and affricates using electropalatography: A case study of a 10 year old girl. *Journal of Clinical Speech and Language Studies*, *1*, pp. 80–87.

Hickok, G., Rogalsky, C., Chen, R., Herskovits, E.H., Townsley, S. and Hillis, A.E., 2014. Partially overlapping sensorimotor networks underlie speech praxis and verbal short-term memory: Evidence from apraxia of speech following acute stroke. *Frontiers in Human Neuroscience*, *8*, p. 649.

Hietanen, J.K., Manninen, P., Sams, M. and Surakka, V., 2001. Does audiovisual speech perception use information about facial configuration? *European Journal of Cognitive Psychology*, *13*(3), pp. 395–407.

Higashikawa, M., Green, J.R., Moore, C.A. and Minifie, F.D., 2003. Lip kinematics for /p/ and /b/ production during whispered and voiced speech. *Folia Phoniatrica et Logopaedica*, *55*(1), pp. 17–27.

Hiiemae, K.M. and Palmer, J.B., 2003. Tongue movements in feeding and speech. *Critical Reviews in Oral Biology & Medicine*, *14*(6), pp. 413–429.

Hillairet de Boisferon, A., Tift, A.H., Minar, N.J. and Lewkowicz, D.J., 2017. Selective attention to a talker's mouth in infancy: Role of audiovisual temporal synchrony and linguistic experience. *Developmental Science*, *20*(3).

Hillock-Dunn, A. and Wallace, M.T., 2012. Developmental changes in the multisensory temporal binding window persist into adolescence. *Developmental Science*, *15*(5), pp. 688–696.

Himmelmann, K. and Uvebrant, P., 2011. Function and neuroimaging in cerebral palsy: A population-based study. *Developmental Medicine & Child Neurology*, *53*(6), pp. 516–521.

Hitchcock, E.R., Byun, T.M., Swartz, M. and Lazarus, R., 2017. Efficacy of Electropalatography for Treating Misarticulation of /r/. *American Journal of Speech-Language Pathology*, *26*(4), pp. 1141–1158.

Hockley, N.S. and Polka, L., 1994. A developmental study of audiovisual speech perception using the McGurk paradigm. *The Journal of the Acoustical Society of America*, *96*(5), pp. 3309–3309.

Holder, W., 1669. *Elements of Speech: An Essay of Inquiry into the Natural Production of Letters: With an Appendix Concerning Persons Deaf & Dumb*. London: John Martyn.

Howard, S.J. and Heselwood, B.C., 2002. Learning and teaching phonetic transcription for clinical purposes. *Clinical Linguistics & Phonetics*, *16*(5), pp. 371–401.

Howard, S. and Varley, R., 1995. III: EPG in therapy using electropalatography to treat severe acquired apraxia of speech. *European Journal of Disorders of Communication*, *30*(2), pp. 246–255.

Huang, X., Baker, J. and Reddy, R., 2014. A historical perspective of speech recognition. *Communications of the ACM*, *57*(1), pp. 94–103.

Hueber, T., Ben-Youssef, A., Badin, P., Bailly, G. and Eliséi, F., 2012. Vizart3D: Retour Articulatoire Visuel pour l'Aide à la Prononciation (Vizart3D: Visual Articulatory Feedack for Computer-Assisted Pronunciation Training) [in French]. In *Proceedings of the Joint Conference JEP-TALN-RECITAL 2012, Volume 5: Software Demonstrations* (pp. 17–18). Grenoble, France.

Irwin, J. and DiBlasi, L., 2017. Audiovisual speech perception: A new approach and implications for clinical populations. *Language and Linguistics Compass*, *11*(3), pp. 77–91.

Irwin, J., Preston, J., Brancazio, L., D'angelo, M. and Turcios, J., 2014. Development of an audiovisual speech perception app for children with autism spectrum disorders. *Clinical Linguistics & Phonetics*, *29*(1), pp. 76–83.

Ito, T., Tiede, M. and Ostry, D.J., 2009. Somatosensory function in speech perception. *Proceedings of the National Academy of Sciences*, *106*(4), pp. 1245–1248.

Jakobson, R., 1968. *Child Language, Aphasia and Phonological Universals* (Vol. 72). The Hague: de Gruyter Mouton.

Jakobson, R. and Halle, M., 1956. *Fundamentals of Language*. The Hague: Mouton & Co.

Jerger, S., Damian, M.F., Spence, M.J., Tye-Murray, N. and Abdi, H., 2009. Developmental shifts in children's sensitivity to visual speech: A new multimodal picture – word task. *Journal of Experimental Child Psychology*, *102*(1), pp. 40–59.

Jerger, S., Damian, M.F., Tye-Murray, N. and Abdi, H., 2014. Children use visual speech to compensate for non-intact auditory speech. *Journal of Experimental Child Psychology*, *126*, pp. 295–312.

Jespersen, O., 1910. What is the use of phonetics? *Educational Review*.

Jesse, A. and Massaro, D.W., 2010. The temporal distribution of information in audiovisual spoken-word identification. *Attention, Perception, & Psychophysics*, *72*(1), pp. 209–225.

Jiang, J., Auer, E.T., Alwan, A., Keating, P.A. and Bernstein, L.E., 2007. Similarity structure in visual speech perception and optical phonetic signals. *Perception & Psychophysics*, *69*(7), pp. 1070–1083.

Johnston, M., 2017. Extensible multimodal annotation for intelligent interactive systems. In *Multimodal Interaction with W3C Standards* (pp. 37–64). Cham: Springer.

Jones, D., 1922. *An Outline of English Phonetics*. Berlin: BG Teubner.

Jones, D., 1928. *Das System der Association Phonétique Internationale (Weltlautschriftverein)*. In Heepe, Martin (Ed.) *Lautzeichen und ihre Anwendung in verschiedenen Sprachgebieten* (pp. 18–27). Berlin: Reichsdruckerei. Reprinted in Le Maître Phonétique 23, July–September 1928. Reprinted in Collins, Beverly and Inger M. Mees, eds., 2003. *Daniel Jones: Selected Works, Volume VII: Selected Papers*. London: Routledge.

Jordan, T.R. and Thomas, S.M., 2011. When half a face is as good as a whole: Effects of simple substantial occlusion on visual and audiovisual speech perception. *Attention, Perception, & Psychophysics*, *73*(7), p. 2270.

Jousmäki, V. and Hari, R., 1998. Parchment-skin illusion: Sound-biased touch. *Current Biology*, *8*(6), pp. R190–R191.

Kaganovich, N., Schumaker, J., Macias, D. and Gustafson, D., 2015. Processing of audiovisually congruent and incongruent speech in school-age children with a history of specific language impairment: A behavioral and event-related potentials study. *Developmental Science*, *18*(5), pp. 751–770.

Katsikitis, M. and Pilowsky, I., 1991. A controlled quantitative study of facial expression in Parkinson's disease and depression. *Journal of Nervous and Mental Disease*, *79*(11), pp. 683–688.

Katsikitis, M. and Pilowsky, I., 1988. A study of facial expression in Parkinson's disease using a novel microcomputer-based method. *Journal of Neurology, Neurosurgery & Psychiatry*, *51*(3), pp. 362–366.

Katz, W.F. and Bharadwaj, S., 2001. Coarticulation in fricative-vowel syllables produced by children and adults: A preliminary report. *Clinical Linguistics & Phonetics*, *15*(1–2), pp. 139–143.

Katz, W.F., Bharadwaj, S.V. and Carstens, B., 1999. Electromagnetic articulography treatment for an adult with Broca's aphasia and apraxia of speech. *Journal of Speech, Language, and Hearing Research*, *42*(6), pp. 1355–1366.

Katz, W.F., Bharadwaj, S.V., Gabbert, G. and Stetler, M., 2002, October. Visual augmented knowledge of performance: Treating place-of-articulation errors in apraxia of speech using EMA. *Brain and Language, 83*(1), pp. 187–189.

Katz, W., Campbell, T.F., Wang, J., Farrar, E., Eubanks, J.C., Balasubramanian, A., Prabhakaran, B. and Rennaker, R., 2014. Opti-speech: A real-time, 3D visual feedback system for speech training. *Proceedings of Interspeech* (pp. 1174–1178).

Katz, W.F., Garst, D.M., Carter, G.S., McNeil, M.R., Fossett, T.R., Doyle, P.J. and Szuminsky, N.J., 2007. Treatment of an individual with aphasia and apraxia of speech using EMA visually-augmented feedback. *Brain and Language*, *103*(1–2), pp. 213–214.

Katz, W.F. and McNeil, M.R., 2010. Studies of articulatory feedback treatment for apraxia of speech based on electromagnetic articulography. *Perspectives on Neurophysiology and Neurogenic Speech and Language Disorders*, *20*(3), pp. 73–80.

Katz, W.F., McNeil, M.R. and Garst, D.M., 2010. Treating apraxia of speech (AOS) with EMA-supplied visual augmented feedback. *Aphasiology*, *24*(6–8), pp. 826–837.

Katz, W.F. and Mehta, S., 2015. Visual feedback of tongue movement for novel speech sound learning. *Frontiers in Human Neuroscience*, *9*, p. 612.

King, S.A. and Parent, R.E., 2001. A 3d parametric tongue model for animated speech. *Computer Animation and Virtual Worlds*, *12*(3), pp. 107–115.

King, S.A. and Parent, R.E., 2005. Creating speech-synchronized animation. *IEEE Transactions on Visualization and Computer Graphics*, *11*(3), pp. 341–352.

Kiritani, S., Itoh, K. and Fujimura, O., 1975. Tongue-pellet tracking by a computer-controlled x-ray microbeam system. *The Journal of the Acoustical Society of America*, *57*(6), pp. 1516–1520.

Kitamura, C., Guellaï, B. and Kim, J., 2014. Motherese by eye and ear: Infants perceive visual prosody in point-line displays of talking heads. *PLoS One*, *9*(10), p. e111467.

Klopfenstein, M., 2009. Interaction between prosody and intelligibility. *International Journal of Speech-Language Pathology*, *11*(4), pp. 326–331.

Kong, A.P.H., Law, S.P., Kwan, C.C.Y., Lai, C. and Lam, V., 2015. A coding system with independent annotations of gesture forms and functions during verbal communication: Development of a database of speech and gesture (DoSaGE). *Journal of Nonverbal Behavior*, *39*(1), pp. 93–111.

Kröger, B.J., Birkholz, P., Hoffmann, R. and Meng, H., 2010. Audiovisual tools for phonetic and articulatory visualization in computer-aided pronunciation training. In *Development of Multimodal Interfaces: Active Listening and Synchrony* (pp. 337–345). Berlin, Heidelberg: Springer.

Kröger, B.J., Kannampuzha, J. and Neuschaefer-Rube, C., 2009. Towards a neurocomputational model of speech production and perception. *Speech Communication*, *51*(9), pp. 793–809.

Kröger, B.J., Miller, N., Lowit, A. and Neuschaefer-Rube, C., 2011. Defective neural motor speech mappings as a source for apraxia of speech: Evidence from a quantitative neural model of speech processing. In A. Lowit and R. Kent (Eds.) *Assessment of Motor Speech Disorders* (pp. 325–346). San Diego, CA: Plural Publishing.

Kronenbuerger, M., Konczak, J., Ziegler, W., Buderath, P., Frank, B., Coenen, V.A., Kiening, K., Reinacher, P., Noth, J. and Timmann, D., 2009. Balance and motor speech impairment in essential tremor. *The Cerebellum*, *8*(3), pp. 389–398.

Kuhl, P.K. and Meltzoff, A.N., 1984. The intermodal representation of speech in infants. *Infant Behavior and Development*, *7*(3), pp. 361–381.

Ladefoged, P., 1957. Use of palatography. *Journal of Speech and Hearing Disorders*, *22*(5), pp. 764–774.

Ladefoged, P., 2005. Speculations on the control of speech. In W.J. Hardcastle and J.M. Beck (Eds.) *A Figure of Speech: A Festschrift for John Laver* (pp. 3–21). Macwah, NJ: Lawrence Erlbaum.

Leclère, C., Viaux, S., Avril, M., Achard, C., Chetouani, M., Missonnier, S. and Cohen, D., 2014. Why synchrony matters during mother-child interactions: A systematic review. *PLoS One*, *9*(12), p. e113571.

Legerstee, M., 1990. Infants use multimodal information to imitate speech sounds. *Infant Behavior and Development*, *13*(3), pp. 343–354.

Lesser, R., 1989. *Linguistic Investigations of Aphasia*. London: Whurr Publishers.

Levitt, J.S. and Katz, W.F., 2008. Augmented visual feedback in second language learning: Training Japanese post-alveolar flaps to American English speakers. *Proceedings of Meetings on Acoustics 154ASA*, *2*(1), p. 060002. ASA.

Lewald, J., Dörrscheidt, G.J. and Ehrenstein, W.H., 2000. Sound localization with eccentric head position. *Behavioural Brain Research*, *108*(2), pp. 105–125.

Lewald, J. and Ehrenstein, W.H., 1998. Influence of head-to-trunk position on sound lateralization. *Experimental Brain Research*, *121*(3), pp. 230–238.

Lewkowicz, D.J. and Flom, R., 2014. The audiovisual temporal binding window narrows in early childhood. *Child Development*, *85*(2), pp. 685–694.

Lewkowicz, D.J. and Hansen-Tift, A.M., 2012. Infants deploy selective attention to the mouth of a talking face when learning speech. *Proceedings of the National Academy of Sciences*, *109*(5), pp. 1431–1436.

Linker, W.J., 1982. *Articulatory and Acoustic Correlates of Labial Activity: A Cross-Linguistic Study*. Ph.D. dissertation, UCLA.

Liu, X., Hairston, J., Schrier, M. and Fan, J., 2011. Common and distinct networks underlying reward valence and processing stages: A meta-analysis of functional neuroimaging studies. *Neuroscience and Biobehavioral Review*, *35*, 1219–1236.

Liu, Y., Massaro, D.W., Chen, T.H., Chan, D. and Perfetti, C., 2007. Using visual speech for training Chinese pronunciation: An in-vivo experiment. In *Proceedings of the International Speech Communication (ISCA)* (pp. 29–32). ITRW SLaTE, Farmington, PA.

Livingstone, S.R. and Palmer, C., 2016. Head movements encode emotions during speech and song. *Emotion*, *16*(3), p. 365.

Lofqvist, A. and Gracco, V.L., 1997. Lip and jaw kinematics in bilabial stop consonant production. *Journal of Speech, Language, and Hearing Research*, *40*(4), pp. 877–893.

Logemann, J.A., Fisher, H.B., Boshes, B. and Blonsky, E.R., 1978. Frequency and cooccurrence of vocal tract dysfunctions in the speech of a large sample of Parkinson patients. *Journal of Speech and Hearing Disorders*, *43*(1), pp. 47–57.

Lohmander, A., Henriksson, C. and Havstam, C., 2010. Electropalatography in home training of retracted articulation in a Swedish child with cleft palate: Effect on articulation pattern and speech. *International Journal of Speech-Language Pathology*, *12*(6), pp. 483–496.

Lundeborg, I. and McAllister, A., 2007. Treatment with a combination of intra-oral sensory stimulation and electropalatography in a child with severe developmental dyspraxia. *Logopedics Phoniatrics Vocology*, *32*(2), pp. 71–79.

Lundy, B., Field, T. and Pickens, J., 1996. Newborns of mothers with depressive symptoms are less expressive. *Infant Behavior and Development*, *19*(4), pp. 419–424.

Ma, J.K.Y., Schneider, C.B., Hoffmann, R. and Storch, A., 2015. Speech prosody across stimulus types for individuals with Parkinson's Disease. *Journal of Parkinson's Disease*, *5*(2), pp. 291–299.

Maas, E., Mailend, M.L. and Guenther, F.H., 2015. Feedforward and feedback control in apraxia of speech: Effects of noise masking on vowel production. *Journal of Speech, Language, and Hearing Research*, *58*(2), pp. 185–200.

Maine, S. and Serry, T., 2011. Treatment of articulation disorders in children with cleft palate. *Journal of Clinical Practice in Speech-Language Pathology*, *13*(1), p. 136.

Mallick, D.B., Magnotti, J.F. and Beauchamp, M.S., 2015. Variability and stability in the McGurk effect: Contributions of participants, stimuli, time, and response type. *Psychonomic Bulletin & Review*, *22*(5), pp. 1299–1307.

Martin, K.L., Hirson, A., Herman, R., Thomas, J. and Pring, T., 2007. The efficacy of speech intervention using electropalatography with an 18-year-old deaf client: A single case study. *Advances in Speech Language Pathology*, *9*(1), pp. 46–56.

Massaro, D.W., 1984. Children's perception of visual and auditory speech. *Child Development*, pp. 1777–1788.

Massaro, D.W., 2003, November. A computer-animated tutor for spoken and written language learning. In *Proceedings of the 5th International Conference on Multimodal Interfaces* (pp. 172–175). ACM, New York.

Massaro, D.W., Bigler, S., Chen, T., Perlman, M. and Ouni, S., 2008. Pronunciation training: The role of eye and ear. In *Interspeech 2008* (pp. 2623–2626). Brisbane, Australia.

Massaro, D.W. and Cohen, M.M., 1998. Visible speech and its potential value for speech training for hearing-impaired perceivers. In *Proceedings of the Speech Technology in Language Learning (STiLL'98)* (pp. 171–174). Marholmen, Sweden.

Massaro, D.W. and Light, J., 2003. Read my tongue movements: Bimodal learning to perceive and produce non-native speech /r/ and /l. In *Eurospeech 2003* (pp. 2249–2252). Geneva, Switzerland.

Massaro, D.W., Liu, Y., Chen, T.H. and Perfetti, C., 2006. A multilingual embodied conversational agent for tutoring speech and language learning. In *Proceedings of the 9th International Conference on Spoken Language Processing (Interspeech 2006 – ICSLP)* (pp. 825–828). Pittsburgh, PA.

Massaro, D.W., Thompson, L.A., Barron, B. and Laren, E., 1986. Developmental changes in visual and auditory contributions to speech perception. *Journal of Experimental Child Psychology*, *41*(1), pp. 93–113.

Mattheyses, W. and Verhelst, W., 2015. Audiovisual speech synthesis: An overview of the state-of-the-art. *Speech Communication*, *66*, pp. 182–217.

Mauszycki, S.C., Wright, S., Dingus, N. and Wambaugh, J.L., 2016. The use of electropalatography in the treatment of acquired apraxia of speech. *American Journal of Speech-Language Pathology*, *25*(4S), pp. S697–S715.

Max, L., Guenther, F.H., Gracco, V.L., Ghosh, S.S. and Wallace, M.E., 2004. Unstable or insufficiently activated internal models and feedback-biased motor control as sources of dysfluency: A theoretical model of stuttering. *Contemporary Issues in Communication Science and Disorders*, *31*(31), pp. 105–122.

McAuliffe, M.J. and Ward, E.C., 2006. The use of electropalatography in the assessment and treatment of acquired motor speech disorders in adults: Current knowledge and future directions. *NeuroRehabilitation*, *21*(3), pp. 189–203.

McClave, E.Z., 2000. Linguistic functions of head movements in the context of speech. *Journal of Pragmatics*, *32*(7), pp. 855–878.

McGurk, H. and MacDonald, J., 1976. Hearing lips and seeing voices. *Nature*, *264*(5588), p. 746.

McNeil, M.R., Fossett, T.R., Katz, W.F., Garst, D., Carter, G., Szuminsky, N. and Doyle, P.J., 2007. Effects of on-line kinematic feedback treatment for apraxia of speech. *Brain and Language*, *1*(103), pp. 223–225.

McNeil, M.R., Katz, W.F., Fossett, T.R.D., Garst, D.M., Szuminsky, N.J., Carter, G. and Lim, K.Y., 2010. Effects of online augmented kinematic and perceptual feedback on treatment of speech movements in apraxia of speech. *Folia Phoniatrica et Logopaedica*, *62*(3), pp. 127–133.

McNeill, D., 1985. So you think gestures are nonverbal?. *Psychological Review*, *92*(3), p. 350.

Moll, K.L., 1960. Cinefluorographic techniques in speech research. *Journal of Speech, Language, and Hearing Research*, *3*(3), pp. 227–241.

Mongillo, E.A., Irwin, J.R., Whalen, D.H., Klaiman, C., Carter, A.S. and Schultz, R.T., 2008. Audiovisual processing in children with and without autism spectrum disorders. *Journal of Autism and Developmental Disorders*, *38*(7), pp. 1349–1358.

Moreno-Torres, I., Berthier, M.L., del Mar Cid, M., Green, C., Gutiérrez, A., García-Casares, N., Walsh, S.F., Nabrozidis, A., Sidorova, J., Dávila, G. and Carnero-Pardo, C., 2013. Foreign accent syndrome: A multimodal evaluation in the search of neuroscience-driven treatments. *Neuropsychologia*, *51*(3), pp. 520–537.

Morgan, A.T., Liegeois, F. and Occomore, L., 2007. Electropalatography treatment for articulation impairment in children with dysarthria post-traumatic brain injury. *Brain Injury*, *21*(11), pp. 1183–1193.

Morgan Barry, R.A., 1995. EPG treatment of a child with the Worster-Drought syndrome. *International Journal of Language & Communication Disorders*, *30*(2), pp. 256–263.

Morgan Barry, R.A. and Hardcastle, W.J., 1987. Some observations on the use of electropalatography as a clinical tool in the diagnosis and treatment of articulation disorders in children. In *Proceedings of the First International Symposium on Specific Speech and Language Disorders in Children* (pp. 208–222). AFASIC, Reading.

Mroueh, Y., Marcheret, E. and Goel, V., 2015, April. Deep multimodal learning for audio-visual speech recognition. In *2015 IEEE International Conference on Acoustics, Speech and Signal Processing (ICASSP)* (pp. 2130–2134). IEEE, Brisbane, Australia.

Müller, E. and MacLeod, G., 1982. Perioral biomechanics and its relation to labial motor control. *The Journal of the Acoustical Society of America*, *71*(S1), pp. S33–S33.

Müller, N. and Ball, M.J., 2013. 1 Linguistics, phonetics, and speech-language Pathology: Clinical linguistics and phonetics. In *Research Methods in Clinical Linguistics and Phonetics: A Practical Guide*. Oxford: Wiley-Blackwell.

Munhall, K.G., Gribble, P., Sacco, L. and Ward, M., 1996. Temporal constraints on the McGurk effect. *Perception & Psychophysics*, *58*(3), pp. 351–362.

Munhall, K.G., Jones, J.A., Callan, D.E., Kuratate, T. and Vatikiotis-Bateson, E., 2004. Visual prosody and speech intelligibility: Head movement improves auditory speech perception. *Psychological Science*, *15*(2), pp. 133–137.

Munhall, K.G., Vatikiotis-Bateson, E. and Tohkura, Y.I., 1995. X-ray film database for speech research. *The Journal of the Acoustical Society of America*, *98*(2), pp. 1222–1224.

Murray, E.S.H., Mendoza, J.O., Gill, S.V., Perkell, J.S. and Stepp, C.E., 2016. Effects of biofeedback on control and generalization of nasalization in typical speakers. *Journal of Speech, Language, and Hearing Research*, *59*(5), pp. 1025–1034.

Murray, L. and Cooper, P., 2003. *Unipolar Depression: A Lifespan Perspective*. New York: Oxford Univesity Press.

Murray, L., Fearon, P. and Cooper, P., 2015. Postnatal depression, mother – infant interactions, and child development. In *Identifying Perinatal Depression and Anxiety: Evidence-Based Practice in Screening, Psychosocial Assessment, and Management* (pp. 139–164). Chichester: John Wiley & Sons Ltd.

Musti, U., Ouni, S., Zhou, Z. and Pietikäinen, M., 2014, December. 3D Visual speech animation from image sequences. In *Proceedings of the 2014 Indian Conference on Computer Vision Graphics and Image Processing* (p. 47).

Nasir, S.M. and Ostry, D.J., 2006. Somatosensory precision in speech production. *Current Biology*, *16*(19), pp. 1918–1923.

Nelson, M.A. and Hodge, M.M., 2000. Effects of facial paralysis and audiovisual information on stop place identification. *Journal of Speech, Language, and Hearing Research*, *43*(1), pp. 158–171.

Nicholson, K.G., Baum, S., Cuddy, L.L. and Munhall, K.G., 2002. A case of impaired auditory and visual speech prosody perception after right hemisphere damage. *Neurocase*, *8*(4), pp. 314–322.

Ninaus, M., Kober, S.E., Witte, M., Koschutnig, K., Stangl, M., Neuper, C. and Wood, G., 2013. Neural substrates of cognitive control under the belief of getting neurofeedback training. *Frontiers in Human Neuroscience*, *7*, p. 914.

Nordberg, A., Carlsson, G. and Lohmander, A., 2011. Electropalatography in the description and treatment of speech disorders in five children with cerebral palsy. *Clinical Linguistics & Phonetics*, *25*(10), pp. 831–852.

Nordberg, A., Miniscalco, C., Lohmander, A. and Himmelmann, K., 2013. Speech problems affect more than one in two children with cerebral palsy: Swedish population-based study. *Acta Paediatrica*, *102*(2), pp. 161–166.

Norrix, L.W., Plante, E. and Vance, R., 2006. Auditory – visual speech integration by adults with and without language-learning disabilities. *Journal of Communication Disorders*, *39*(1), pp. 22–36.

Norrix, L.W., Plante, E., Vance, R. and Boliek, C.A., 2007. Auditory-visual integration for speech by children with and without specific language impairment. *Journal of Speech, Language, and Hearing Research*, *50*(6), pp. 1639–1651.

Norton, S.J., 1977. Analytic study of the Tadoma method: Background and preliminary results. *Journal of Speech & Hearing Research*, *20*, pp. 625–637.

Ohala, J.J., 1975. The temporal regulation of speech. *Auditory Analysis and Perception of Speech*, pp. 431–453.

Ohala, J.J., 2004. Phonetics and phonology: Then, and then, and now. *LOT Occasional Series*, *2*, pp. 133–140.

Ostry, D.J. and Flanagan, J.R., 1989. Human jaw movement in mastication and speech. *Archives of Oral Biology*, *34*(9), pp. 685–693.

Passy, P., 1884. *Premier livre de lecture*. Paris: Firmin-Didot.

Paulmann, S. and Pell, M.D., 2010. Dynamic emotion processing in Parkinson's disease as a function of channel availability. *Journal of Clinical and Experimental Neuropsychology*, *32*(8), pp. 822–835.

Pell, M.D., Cheang, H.S. and Leonard, C.L., 2006. The impact of Parkinson's disease on vocal-prosodic communication from the perspective of listeners. *Brain and Language*, *97*(2), pp. 123–134.

Pell, M.D. and Monetta, L., 2008. How Parkinson's disease affects non-verbal communication and language processing. *Language and Linguistics Compass*, *2*(5), pp. 739–759.

Perkell, J.S., 1974. A physiologically-oriented model of tongue activity in speech production (Doctoral dissertation. Massachusetts Institute of Technology).

Perkins, M.R., 2011. Clinical linguistics: Its past, present and future. *Clinical Linguistics & Phonetics*, *25*(11–12), pp. 922–927.

Perkins, M.R., Howard, S. and Simpson, J., 2011. Clinical linguistics. *The Routledge Handbook of Applied Linguistics*, pp. 112–124.

Phonetic Representation of Disordered Speech Working Party, 1983. *The Phonetic Representation of Disordered Speech: Final Report of the PRDS Project Working Party*. London: King's Fund.

Pillot-Loiseau, C., Antolík, T.K. and Kamiyama, T., 2013, August. Contribution of ultrasound visualisation to improving the production of the French /y/-/u/ contrast by four Japanese learners. In *Proceedings of the PPLC13: Phonetics, Phonology, Languages in Contact Contact: Varieties, Multilingualism, Second Language Learning* (pp. 86–89).

Plummer-D'Amato, P., Altmann, L.J. and Reilly, K., 2011. Dual-task effects of spontaneous speech and executive function on gait in aging: Exaggerated effects in slow walkers. *Gait & Posture*, *33*(2), pp. 233–237.

Pochon, J.B., Levy, R., Fossati, P., Lehericy, S., Poline, J.B., Pillon, B., Le Bihan, D. and Dubois, B., 2002. The neural system that bridges reward and cognition in humans: An fMRI study. *Proceedings of the National Academy of Sciences*, *99*(8), pp. 5669–5674.

Potamianos, G., Neti, C., Gravier, G., Garg, A. and Senior, A.W., 2003. Recent advances in the automatic recognition of audiovisual speech. *Proceedings of the IEEE*, *91*(9), pp. 1306–1326.

Potamianos, G., Neti, C., Luettin, J. and Matthews, I., 2004. Audio-visual automatic speech recognition: An overview. *Issues in Visual and Audio-Visual Speech Processing*, *22*, p. 23.

Potamianos, G., Marcheret, E., Mroueh, Y., Goel, V., Koumbaroulis, A., Vartholomaios, A. and Thermos, S., 2017, April. Audio and visual modality combination in speech processing applications. In *The Handbook of Multimodal-Multisensor Interfaces* (pp. 489–543). Association for Computing Machinery and Morgan & Claypool.

Powell, T.W.P. and Ball, M.J.B. eds., 2010. *Clinical Linguistics: Critical Concepts in Linguistics: Applications of Clinical Linguistics and Phonetics*. London: Routledge.

Pratt, S.R., 2007. Using electropalatographic feedback to treat the speech of a child with severe-to-profound hearing loss. *The Journal of Speech and Language Pathology – Applied Behavior Analysis*, *2*(2), p. 213.

Preston, J.L., Byun, T.M., Boyce, S.E., Hamilton, S., Tiede, M., Phillips, E., Rivera-Campos, A. and Whalen, D.H., 2017a. Ultrasound Images of the Tongue: A Tutorial for Assessment and Remediation of Speech Sound Errors. *Journal of Visualized Experiments: JoVE, 119*.

Preston, J.L. and Leaman, M., 2014. Ultrasound visual feedback for acquired apraxia of speech: A case report. *Aphasiology*, *28*(3), pp. 278–295.

Preston, J.L., Leece, M.C. and Maas, E., 2017b. Motor-based treatment with and without ultrasound feedback for residual speech-sound errors. *International Journal of Language & Communication Disorders*, *52*(1), pp. 80–94.

Preston, J.L., Leece, M.C., McNamara, K. and Maas, E., 2017c. Variable practice to enhance speech learning in ultrasound biofeedback treatment for childhood apraxia of speech: A single case experimental study. *American Journal of Speech-Language Pathology*, *26*(3), pp. 840–852.

Preston, J.L., Maas, E., Whittle, J., Leece, M.C. and McCabe, P., 2016. Limited acquisition and generalisation of rhotics with ultrasound visual feedback in childhood apraxia. *Clinical Linguistics & Phonetics*, *30*(3–5), pp. 363–381.

Prince, A., and Smolensky, P. 1993/2004. *Optimality Theory: Constraint interaction in generative grammar*. Malden, MA:Blackwell..

Quinto, L., Thompson, W.F., Russo, F.A. and Trehub, S.E., 2010. A comparison of the McGurk effect for spoken and sung syllables. *Attention, Perception, & Psychophysics*, *72*(6), pp. 1450–1454.

Ramsay, J.O., Munhall, K.G., Gracco, V.L. and Ostry, D.J., 1996. Functional data analyses of lip motion. *The Journal of the Acoustical Society of America*, *99*(6), pp. 3718–3727.

Raphael, L.J., Borden, G.J. and Harris, K.S., 2007. *Speech Science Primer: Physiology, Acoustics, and Perception of Speech*. Philadelphia, PA: Lippincott Williams & Wilkins.

Rathinavelu, A., Thiagarajan, H. and Savithri, S.R., 2006. Evaluation of a computer aided 3D lip sync instructional model using virtual reality objects. In *International Conference on Disability, Virtual Reality & Associated Technologies* (pp. 67–73). Esbjerg, Denmark.

Remez, R., 2012. Three puzzles of multimodal speech perception. In G. Bailly, P. Perrier and E. Vatikiotis-Bateson (Eds.) *Audiovisual Speech Processing* (pp. 4–20). Cambridge: Cambridge University Press.

Ricciardi, L., Bologna, M., Morgante, F., Ricciardi, D., Morabito, B., Volpe, D., Martino, D., Tessitore, A., Pomponi, M., Bentivoglio, A.R. and Bernabei, R., 2015. Reduced facial expressiveness in Parkinson's disease: A pure motor disorder? *Journal of the Neurological Sciences*, *358*(1), pp. 125–130.

Risberg, A. and Lubker, J., 1978. Prosody and speechreading. *Speech Transmission Laboratory Quarterly Progress Report and Status Report*, *4*, pp. 1–16.

Rockey, D., 1977. The logopaedic thought of John Thelwall, 1764–1834: First British speech therapist. *International Journal of Language & Communication Disorders*, *12*(2), pp. 83–95.

Roon, K.D., Dawson, K.M., Tiede, M.K. and Whalen, D.H., 2016. Indexing head movement during speech production using optical markers. *The Journal of the Acoustical Society of America*, *139*(5), pp. EL167–EL171.

Rosenbaum, P.L., Paneth, N., Leviton, A., Goldstein, M., Bax, M., Damiano, D., Dan, B. and Jacobsson, B., 2007. A report: The definition and classification of cerebral palsy April 2006. *Developmental Medicine & Child Neurology*, *109* (Suppl 109), pp. 8–14.

Rosenblum, L.D., 2001. Reading upside-down lips. www.faculty.ucr.edu/~rosenblu/VSinverted-speech.html

Rosenblum, L.D., Schmuckler, M.A. and Johnson, J.A., 1997. The McGurk effect in infants. *Perception & Psychophysics*, *59*(3), pp. 347–357.

Rosenblum, L.D., Yakel, D.A. and Green, K.P., 2000. Face and mouth inversion effects on visual and audiovisual speech perception. *Journal of Experimental Psychology: Human Perception and Performance*, *26*(2), p. 806.

Rousselot, J-P., 1897. *Principes de Phonétique Expérimentale* (Vols. 1 and 2). Paris, Didier.

Roxburgh, Z., Cleland, J. and Scobbie, J.M., 2016. Multiple phonetically trained-listener comparisons of speech before and after articulatory intervention in two children with repaired submucous cleft palate. *Clinical Linguistics & Phonetics*, *30*(3–5), pp. 398–415.

Rutter, B., Klopfenstein, M., Ball, M.J. and Müller, N., 2010. My client is using non-English sounds! A tutorial in advanced phonetic transcription. Part II: Prosody and unattested sounds. *Contemporary Issues in Communication Science and Disorders*, *37*, pp. 111–122.

Rutter, M., 1997. Maternal depression and infant development: Cause and consequence; sensitivity and specificity. *Postpartum Depression and Child Development*, pp. 295–315.

Saavedra, S., Woollacott, M. and Van Donkelaar, P., 2010. Head stability during quiet sitting in children with cerebral palsy: Effect of vision and trunk support. *Experimental Brain Research*, *201*(1), pp. 13–23.

Sánchez-García, C., Kandel, S., Savariaux, C. and Soto-Faraco, S., 2018. The time course of audio-visual phoneme identification: A high temporal resolution study. *Multisensory Research*, *31*(1–2), pp. 57–78.

Sato, M., Buccino, G., Gentilucci, M. and Cattaneo, L., 2010. On the tip of the tongue: Modulation of the primary motor cortex during audiovisual speech perception. *Speech Communication*, *52*(6), pp. 533–541.

Scarborough, R., Keating, P., Mattys, S.L., Cho, T. and Alwan, A., 2009. Optical phonetics and visual perception of lexical and phrasal stress in English. *Language and Speech*, *52*(2–3), pp. 135–175.

Schmidt, A.M. and Beamer, J., 1998. Electropalatography treatment for training Thai speakers of English. *Clinical Linguistics & Phonetics*, *12*(5), pp. 389–403.

Schölderle, T., Staiger, A., Lampe, R., Strecker, K. and Ziegler, W., 2014. Dysarthria in Adults with Cerebral Palsy: Clinical Presentation, Communication, and Classification. *Neuropediatrics*, *45*(S 01), p. fp012.

Scobbie, J.M., Wood, S.E. and Wrench, A.A., 2004. Advances in EPG for treatment and research: An illustrative case study. *Clinical Linguistics & Phonetics*, *18*(6–8), pp. 373–389.

Scott, A.D., Wylezinska, M., Birch, M.J. and Miquel, M.E., 2014. Speech MRI: Morphology and function. *Physica Medica: European Journal of Medical Physics*, *30*(6), pp. 604–618.

Sekiyama, K. and Burnham, D., 2004. Issues in the development of auditory-visual speech perception: Adults, infants, and children. In S.H. Kim and D.H. Yuon (Eds.) *Proceedings of the Eighth International Conference on Spoken Language Processing* (pp. 1137–1140). Sunjin Printing, Seoul, Korea.

Sekiyama, K., Soshi, T. and Sakamoto, S., 2014. Enhanced audiovisual integration with aging in speech perception: A heightened McGurk effect in older adults. *Frontiers in Psychology*, *5*, p. 323.

Sekiyama, K. and Tohkura, Y.I., 1991. McGurk effect in non-English listeners: Few visual effects for Japanese subjects hearing Japanese syllables of high auditory intelligibility. *The Journal of the Acoustical Society of America*, *90*(4), pp. 1797–1805.

Shawker, T.H. and Sonies, B.C., 1985. Ultrasound biofeedback for speech training. Instrumentation and preliminary results. *Investigative Radiology*, *20*(1), pp. 90–93.

Shirahige, C., Oki, K., Morimoto, Y., Oisaka, N. and Minagi, S., 2012. Dynamics of posterior tongue during pronunciation and voluntary tongue lift movement in young adults. *Journal of Oral Rehabilitation*, *39*(5), pp. 370–376.

Shriberg, L.D. and Kent, R.D., 1982. *Clinical Phonetics*. New York: John Wiley and Sons.

Shriberg, L.D., Kwiatkowski, J. and Hoffmann, K., 1984. A procedure for phonetic transcription by consensus. *Journal of Speech, Language, and Hearing Research*, *27*(3), pp. 456–465.

Shriberg, L.D. and Lof, G.L., 1991. Reliability studies in broad and narrow phonetic transcription. *Clinical Linguistics & Phonetics*, *5*(3), pp. 225–279.

Shtern, M., Haworth, M.B., Yunusova, Y., Baljko, M. and Faloutsos, P., 2012, November. A game system for speech rehabilitation. In *International Conference on Motion in Games* (pp. 43–54). Springer, Berlin, Heidelberg.

Simons, G., Ellgring, H. and Smith Pasqualini, M., 2003. Disturbance of spontaneous and posed facial expressions in Parkinson's disease. *Cognition & Emotion*, *17*(5), pp. 759–778.

Singh, N., Agrawal, A. and Khan, R.A., 2017. Automatic speaker recognition: Current approaches and progress in last six decades. *Global Journal of Enterprise Information System*, *9*(3), pp. 45–52.

Sisinni, B., d'Apolito, S., Fivela, B.G. and Grimaldi, M., 2016. Ultrasound articulatory training for teaching pronunciation of L2 vowels. In *Conference Proceedings. ICT for Language Learning* (p. 265). libreriauniversitaria. it Edizioni, Limena, Italy.

Sloutsky, V.M. and Napolitano, A.C., 2003. Is a picture worth a thousand words? Preference for auditory modality in young children. *Child Development*, *74*(3), pp. 822–833.

Smith, A., 1992. The control of orofacial movements in speech. *Critical Reviews in Oral Biology & Medicine*, *3*(3), pp. 233–267.

Smith, A., 2010. Development of neural control of orofacial movements for speech. In *The Handbook of Phonetic Sciences, Second Edition* (pp. 251–296). Oxford: Wiley–Blackwell.

Smith, N.A. and Strader, H.L., 2014. Infant-directed visual prosody: Mothers' head movements and speech acoustics. *Interaction Studies*, *15*(1), pp. 38–54.

Sohr-Preston, S.L. and Scaramella, L.V., 2006. Implications of timing of maternal depressive symptoms for early cognitive and language development. *Clinical Child and Family Psychology Review*, *9*(1), pp. 65–83.

Sorensen, T., Toutios, A., Goldstein, L. and Narayanan, S.S., 2016. Characterizing vocal tract dynamics across speakers using real-time MRI. *Interspeech*, pp. 465–469.

Stavness, I., Lloyd, J.E. and Fels, S., 2012. Automatic prediction of tongue muscle activations using a finite element model. *Journal of Biomechanics*, *45*(16), pp. 2841–2848.

Suemitsu, A., Dang, J., Ito, T. and Tiede, M., 2015. A real-time articulatory visual feedback approach with target presentation for second language pronunciation learning. *The Journal of the Acoustical Society of America*, *138*(4), pp. EL382–EL387.

Sumby, W.H. and Pollack, I., 1954. Visual contribution to speech intelligibility in noise. *The Journal of the Acoustical Society of America*, *26*(24), pp. 212–215.

Summerfield, Q., 1979. Use of visual information for phonetic perception. *Phonetica*, *36*(4–5), pp. 314–331.

Summerfield, Q., 1983. Audio-visual speech perception, lipreading and artificial stimulation. *Hearing Science and Hearing Disorders,* pp. 131–182.

Summerfield, Q., 1992. Lipreading and audio-visual speech perception. *Philosophical Transactions of the Royal Society B: Biological Sciences*, *335*(1273), pp. 71–78.

Sussman, H.M., 1970. The role of sensory feedback in tongue movement control. *Journal of Auditory Research*, *10*(4), pp. 296–321.

Sussman, H.M., MacNeilage, P.F. and Hanson, R.J., 1973. Labial and mandibular dynamics during the production of bilabial consonants: Preliminary observations. *Journal of Speech, Language, and Hearing Research*, *16*(3), pp. 397–420.

Suzuki, N., 1989. Clinical applications of EPG to Japanese cleft palate and glossectomy patients. *Clinical Linguistics & Phonetics*, *3*(1), pp. 127–136.

Sveinbjornsdottir, S., 2016. The clinical symptoms of Parkinson's disease. *Journal of Neurochemistry*, *139*, pp. 318–324.

Sweet, H., 1902. *A Primer of Phonetics* (2nd ed.). Oxford: Oxford University Press.

Tang, K., Harandi, N.M., Woo, J., El Fakhri, G., Stone, M. and Fels, S., 2017. Speaker-specific biomechanical model-based investigation of a simple speech task based on tagged-MRI. *Proceedings Interspeech*, pp. 2282–2286.

Taylor, N., Isaac, C. and Milne, E., 2010. A comparison of the development of audiovisual integration in children with autism spectrum disorders and typically developing children. *Journal of Autism and Developmental Disorders*, *40*(11), pp. 1403–1411.

Teoh, A.P. and Chin, S.B., 2009. Transcribing the speech of children with cochlear implants: Clinical application of narrow phonetic transcriptions. *American Journal of Speech-Language Pathology*, *18*(4), pp. 388–401.

Terband, H. and Maassen, B., 2010. Speech motor development in childhood apraxia of speech: Generating testable hypotheses by neurocomputational modeling. *Folia Phoniatrica et Logopaedica*, *62*(3), pp. 134–142.

Terband, H., Maassen, B., Guenther, F.H. and Brumberg, J., 2009. Computational neural modeling of speech motor control in childhood apraxia of speech (CAS). *Journal of Speech, Language, and Hearing Research*, *52*(6), pp. 1595–1609.

Terband, H., Maassen, B., Guenther, F.H. and Brumberg, J., 2014. Auditory – motor interactions in pediatric motor speech disorders: Neurocomputational modeling of disordered development. *Journal of Communication Disorders*, *47*, pp. 17–33.

Thelwall, R., 1981. The phonetic theory of John Thelwall (1764–1834). *Towards a History of Phonetics*, pp. 186–203.

Theobald, B., 2007, August. Audiovisual speech synthesis. *International Congress on Phonetic Sciences,* pp. 285–290.

Thomas, S.M. and Jordan, T.R., 2004. Contributions of oral and extraoral facial movement to visual and audiovisual speech perception. *Journal of Experimental Psychology: Human Perception and Performance*, *30*(5), p. 873.

Thompson, D.M., 1934. On the detection of emphasis in spoken sentences by means of visual, tactual, and visual-tactual cues. *The Journal of General Psychology*, *11*(1), pp. 160–172.

Thompson, P., 1980. Margaret Thatcher: A new illusion. *Perception*, *9*, pp. 483–484.

Tickle-Degnen, L. and Lyons, K.D., 2004. Practitioners' impressions of patients with Parkinson's disease: The social ecology of the expressive mask. *Social Science & Medicine*, *58*(3), pp. 603–614.

Tiippana, K., 2014. What is the McGurk effect?. *Frontiers in Psychology*, *5*, p. 725.

Tilsen, S., Das, D. and McKee, B., 2015. Real-time articulatory biofeedback with electromagnetic articulography. *Linguistics Vanguard*, *1*(1), pp. 39–55.

Tjaden, K., 2008. Speech and swallowing in Parkinson's disease. *Topics in Geriatric Rehabilitation*, *24*(2), p. 115.

Toutios, A., Byrd, D., Goldstein, L. and Narayanan, S.S., 2017. Articulatory compensation strategies employed by an aglossic speaker. *The Journal of the Acoustical Society of America*, *142*(4), pp. 2639–2639.

Treille, A., Cordeboeuf, C., Vilain, C. and Sato, M., 2014. Haptic and visual information speed up the neural processing of auditory speech in live dyadic interactions. *Neuropsychologia*, *57*, pp. 71–77.

Trim, J., 1953. Some suggestions for the phonetic notation of sounds in defective speech. *Speech*, *17*, pp. 21–24.

Trost, J.E., 1981. Articulatory additions to the classical description of the speech of persons with cleft palate. *The Cleft Palate Journal*, *18*(3), pp. 193–203.

Ullsperger, M. and Von Cramon, D.Y., 2003. Error monitoring using external feedback: Specific roles of the habenular complex, the reward system, and the cingulate motor area revealed by functional magnetic resonance imaging. *Journal of Neuroscience*, *23*(10), pp. 4308–4314.

Valentine, T., 1988. Upside-down faces: A review of the effect of inversion upon face recognition. *British Journal of Psychology*, *79*(4), pp. 471–491.

van Helmont, F.M., 1667. *Alphabeti Vere Naturalis Hebraici Brevissima Delineatio*. Sulzbach: A. Lichtenthaler.

Vatikiotis-Bateson, E., 1998. The moving face during speech communication. *Hearing by Eye II: Advances in the Psychology of Speechreading and Auditory-Visual Speech*, *2*, p. 123.

Vatikiotis-Bateson, E. and Kuratate, T., 2012. Overview of audiovisual speech processing. *Acoustical Science and Technology*, *33*(3), pp. 135–141.

Vatikiotis-Bateson, E. and Munhall, K.G., 2015. Auditory-visual speech processing. In *The Handbook of Speech Production*, (pp. 178–199). John Wiley & Sons, 2015.

Velasco, M.A., Raya, R., Ceres, R., Clemotte, A., Bedia, A.R., Franco, T.G. and Rocon, E., 2016. Positive and negative motor signs of head motion in cerebral palsy: Assessment of impairment and task performance. *IEEE Systems Journal*, *10*(3), pp. 967–973.

Viaux-Savelon, S., 2016. Establishing parent – infant interactions. In *Joint Care of Parents and Infants in Perinatal Psychiatry* (pp. 25–43). Cham: Springer.

Vick, J., Foye, M., Schreiber, N., Lee, G. and Mental, R., 2014. Tongue motion characteristics during vowel production in older children and adults. *The Journal of the Acoustical Society of America*, *136*(4), pp. 2143–2143.

Vick, J., Mental, R., Carey, H. and Lee, G.S., 2017. Seeing is treating: 3D electromagnetic midsagittal articulography (EMA) visual biofeedback for the remediation of residual speech errors. *The Journal of the Acoustical Society of America*, *141*(5), pp. 3647–3647.

Wakumoto, M., Ohno, K., Imai, S., Yamashita, Y., Akizuki, H. and MICHI, K.I., 1996. Analysis of the articulation after glossectomy. *Journal of Oral Rehabilitation*, *23*(11), pp. 764–770.

Walker, S., Bruce, V. and O'Malley, C., 1995. Facial identity and facial speech processing: Familiar faces and voices in the McGurk effect. *Perception & Psychophysics*, *57*(8), pp. 1124–1133.

Wallis, J., 1969. *Grammatica Linguae Anglicanae 1653*. Menston: Scolar Press.

Wang, J., Samal, A., Rong, P. and Green, J.R., 2016. An optimal set of flesh points on tongue and lips for speech-movement classification. *Journal of Speech, Language, and Hearing Research*, *59*(1), pp. 15–26.

Watkins, C.H., 2015. *Sensor driven realtime animation for feedback during physical therapy*. MS thesis. The University of Texas at Dallas.

Westbury, J., Milenkovic, P., Weismer, G. and Kent, R., 1990. X-ray microbeam speech production database. *The Journal of the Acoustical Society of America*, *88*(S1), pp. S56–S56.

Whalen, D.H. and McDonough, J., 2015. Taking the laboratory into the field. *Annual Review Of Linguistics*, *1*(1), pp. 395–415.

Widmer, M., Ziegler, N., Held, J., Luft, A. and Lutz, K., 2016. Rewarding feedback promotes motor skill consolidation via striatal activity. In *Progress in Brain Research* (Vol. 229, pp. 303–323). Amsterdam: Elsevier.

Wightman, F., Kistler, D. and Brungart, D., 2006. Informational masking of speech in children: Auditory-visual integration. *The Journal of the Acoustical Society of America*, *119*(6), pp. 3940–3949.

Wik, P. and Engwall, O., 2008, June. Looking at tongues – can it help in speech perception?. *Proceedings FONETIK*, pp. 57–61.

Williams, J.H., Massaro, D.W., Peel, N.J., Bosseler, A. and Suddendorf, T., 2004. Visual – auditory integration during speech imitation in autism. *Research in Developmental Disabilities*, *25*(6), pp. 559–575.

Witzel, M.A., Tobe, J. and Salyer, K., 1988. The use of nasopharyngoscopy biofeedback therapy in the correction of inconsistent velopharyngeal closure. *International Journal of Pediatric Otorhinolaryngology*, *15*(2), pp. 137–142.

Woo, J., Xing, F., Lee, J., Stone, M. and Prince, J.L., 2016. A spatio-temporal atlas and statistical model of the tongue during speech from cine-MRI. *Computer Methods in Biomechanics and Biomedical Engineering: Imaging & Visualization*, pp. 1–12.

Wrench, A., Gibbon, F., McNeill, A.M. and Wood, S., 2002. An EPG therapy protocol for remediation and assessment of articulation disorders. In *Seventh International Conference on Spoken Language Processing (ICSLP2002) – INTERSPEECH 2002*. Denver, Colorado, USA, September 16–20, 2002.

Yano, J., Shirahige, C., Oki, K., Oisaka, N., Kumakura, I., Tsubahara, A. and Minagi, S., 2015. Effect of visual biofeedback of posterior tongue movement on articulation rehabilitation in dysarthria patients. *Journal of Oral Rehabilitation*, *42*(8), pp. 571–579.

Yehia, H.C., Kuratate, T. and Vatikiotis-Bateson, E., 2002. Linking facial animation, head motion and speech acoustics. *Journal of Phonetics*, *30*(3), pp. 555–568.

Yeung, H.H. and Werker, J.F., 2013. Lip movements affect infants' audiovisual speech perception. *Psychological Science*, *24*(5), pp. 603–612.

Yont, K.M., Snow, C.E. and Vernon-Feagans, L., 2001. Early communicative intents expressed by 12-month-old children with and without chronic otitis media. *First Language*, *21*(63), pp. 265–287.

Youse, K.M., Cienkowski, K.M. and Coelho, C.A., 2004. Auditory-visual speech perception in an adult with aphasia. *Brain Injury*, *18*(8), pp. 825–834.

Ysunza, A., Pamplona, M., Femat, T., Mayer, I. and García-Velasco, M., 1997. Videonasopharyngoscopy as an instrument for visual biofeedback during speech in cleft palate patients. *International Journal of Pediatric Otorhinolaryngology*, *41*(3), pp. 291–298.

Yu, J., 2017, January. Speech synchronized tongue animation by combining physiology modeling and X-ray image fitting. In *International Conference on Multimedia Modeling* (pp. 726–737). Cham, Switzerland: Springer.

Yu, J., Jiang, C. and Wang, Z., 2017. Creating and simulating a realistic physiological tongue model for speech production. *Multimedia Tools and Applications*, *76*(13), pp. 14673–14689.

Appendix 1

extIPA SYMBOLS FOR DISORDERED SPEECH

(Revised to 2008)

CONSONANTS (other than on the IPA Chart)

	bilabial	labiodental	dentolabial	labioalv.	linguolabial	interdental	bidental	alveolar	velar	velophar.
Plosive		p̪ b̪	p͆ b͆	p͇ b͇	t̼ d̼	t̪͆ d̪͆				
Nasal			m͆	m͇	n̼	n̪͆				
Trill					r̼	r̪͆				
Fricative median			f͆ v͆	f͇ v͇	θ̼ ð̼	θ̪͆ ð̪͆	h̪͆ ɦ̪͆			ʩ
Fricative lateral+median								ʪ ʫ		
Fricative nareal	m͋							n͋	ŋ͋	
Percussive	ʬ						ʭ			
Approximant lateral					l̼	l̪͆				

Where symbols appear in pairs, the one to the right represents a voiced consonant. Shaded areas denote articulations judged impossible.

DIACRITICS

͍	labial spreading	s͍	͈	strong articulation	f͈	͊	denasal	m͊
͆	dentolabial	v͆	͉	weak articulation	v͉	͋	nasal escape	v͋
̪͆	interdental/bidental	n̪͆	\	reiterated articulation	p\p\p	͌	velopharyngeal friction	s͌
͇	alveolar	t͇	͎	whistled articulation	s͎	↓	ingressive airflow	p↓
̼	linguolabial	d̼	͢	sliding articulation	θ͢s	↑	egressive airflow	!↑

CONNECTED SPEECH

(.)	short pause
(..)	medium pause
(...)	long pause
f	loud speech [{$_{f}$ laʊd $_{f}$}]
ff	louder speech [{$_{ff}$ laʊdɚ $_{ff}$}]
p	quiet speech [{$_{p}$ kwaɪət $_{p}$}]
pp	quieter speech [{$_{pp}$ kwaɪətɚ $_{pp}$}]
allegro	fast speech [{$_{allegro}$ fɑst $_{allegro}$}]
lento	slow speech [{$_{lento}$ sloʊ $_{lento}$}]
crescendo, ralentando, etc. may also be used	

VOICING

ˬ	pre-voicing	ˬz
ˬ	post-voicing	zˬ
(̥)	partial devoicing	(z̥)
(̥	initial partial devoicing	(z̥
̥)	final partial devoicing	z̥)
(̬)	partial voicing	(s̬)
(̬	initial partial voicing	(s̬
̬)	final partial voicing	s̬)
⁼	unaspirated	p⁼
ʰ	pre-aspiration	ʰp

OTHERS

◯, (C̲), (V̲)	indeterminate sound, consonant, vowel	ʞ	Velodorsal articulation
(P̲l̲.v̲l̲s̲), (N̲)	indeterminate voiceless plosive, nasal, etc	¡	sublaminal lower alveolar percussive click
( )	silent articulation (ʃ), (m)	!¡	alveolar and sublaminal clicks (cluck-click)
(( ))	extraneous noise, e.g. ((2 sylls))	*	sound with no available symbol

Appendix 2

VoQS: Voice Quality Symbols

Airstream Types

ↀ	buccal airstream	↓	pulmonic ingressive speech
Œ	œsophageal airstream	Ю	tracheo-œsophageal speech

Phonation Types

V	modal voice	F	falsetto	W	whisper	C	creak
Ṿ	whispery voice	V̰	creaky voice	V̤	breathy voice	V!	harsh voice
F̣	whispery falsetto	F̰	creaky falsetto	F!	harsh falsetto	C!	harsh creak
Ṿ!	harsh whispery voice			V̰!	harsh creaky voice		
Ṿ̰	whispery creaky voice			Ṿ̰!	harsh whispery creaky voice		
F̣̰	whispery creaky falsetto			F̣̰!	harsh whispery creaky falsetto		
V͉	slack/lax voice			V͈	pressed phonation / tight voice		
V‼	ventricular phonation			V̬‼	diplophonia		
Ṿ‼	whispery ventricular phonation			Vᴧᴧ	aryepiglottic phonation		
ꟿ	spasmodic dysphonia			И	electrolarynx phonation		

Larynx Height

L̝	raised-larynx voice	L̞	lowered-larynx voice

Supralaryngeal Settings
Labial settings, lingual settings, state of the velum, jaw and tongue settings

Vꟹ	labialized voice (open rounded)	Vʷ	labialized voice (close rounded)
V͍	spread-lip voice	Vᶹ	labio-dentalized voice
V̺	linguo-apicalized voice	V̻	linguo-laminalized voice
Vʵ	retroflex voice	V̪	dentalized voice
V͇	alveolarized voice	V͇ʲ	palato-alveolarized voice
Vʲ	palatalized voice	Vˠ	velarized voice
Vʶ	uvularized voice	Vˤ	pharyngealized voice
V̝ˤ	laryngo-pharyngealized voice	Vᴴ	faucalized voice
Ṽ	nasalized voice	V͊	denasalized voice
J̞	open-jaw voice	J̝	close-jaw voice
J͔	right offset-jaw voice	J͕	left offset-jaw voice
J̟	protruded-jaw voice	Θ	protruded-tongue voice

Labeled braces and numerals mark degree and combinations of voice quality:

[ˈnɔ˞məl ˈvɔɪs {3V! ˈvɛɹi ˈhɑ˞ʃ ˈvɔɪs 3V!} {L̝ 1V! ˈlɛs ˈhɑ˞ʃ ˈvɔɪs wɪð ˈɹeɪzd ˈlæɹɪŋks 1V! L̝}]

20

Vocal-tract models in phonetic teaching and research

Takayuki Arai

Introduction

The series of events involved in speech communication is traditionally called the "Speech Chain" (Denes and Pinson, 1993), and it represents how two people, a speaker and a listener, communicate using speech. First, a message of the speaker at the linguistic level is transformed into an acoustic signal via output at the physiological level. Then, on the listener's side, the acoustic signal is transformed back to the linguistic level via input at the physiological level. Although the speaker's speech organs and the listener's auditory organs are clearly important, the speaker's auditory system also plays a significant role in online monitoring for production. Moreover, current versions of the speech chain describe the importance of multisensory information (e.g., Gick et al., 2013).

In this chapter, we discuss how physical models of the human vocal tract may be used to better understand the speech chain. In particular, we discuss applications of mechanical vocal tract models to the fields of articulatory, acoustic, and auditory phonetics. Such fields are related to other areas of study, such as phonology, speech pathology, psychoacoustics, applied linguistics, and speech technology, where the models may also find application. Because phonetics is related to many fields in speech communication, this chapter will hopefully be beneficial for a wide range of readers.

As described in Chapter 1 of this volume ("History of speech synthesis"), mechanical models of the human vocal tract are not new. In the 18th century, Kratzenstein created mechanical models of five vowels (Korpiun, 2015). In 1791, Wolfgang von Kempelen summarized his work on a manually operated speech synthesizer in a 451-page book entitled, "Mechanismus der menschlichen Sprache und Beschreibung einer sprechenden Machine (The mechanisms of human speech, with a description of a speaking machine)" (von Kempelen, 1791; Arai, 2013a). Dudley and Tarnoczy (1950) reviewed the development of von Kempelen's mechanical synthesizer. They described von Kempelen's synthesizer as having a bellow operated with the forearm, which simulates the lungs. The airflow from the bellow causes a reed to oscillate, and the sound source excites a single, hand-varied resonator to produce voiced sounds. Various small whistles and levers controlled most of the consonants (Gold and Morgan, 2000). Bell and Wheatstone duplicated von Kempelen's machine in the late 19th century (Flanagan, 1965) and it was also recently replicated and discussed by Trouvain and Brackhane (2011).

Lindsay (1997) described Faber's demonstration of his "talking head" in the early 19th century. Flanagan (1965) noted that Willis claimed to have synthesized all the human vowel sounds as a continuum using a uniform diameter tube with varying length in 1830, and that Riesz also designed a mechanical talker. In 1923, Paget successfully simulated artificial vocal folds and also discovered the closest approximation of the shape of an actual vocal tract by conducting a comparative study of sounds emitted by model cavities of various shapes that he constructed (Chiba and Kajiyama, 1941–1942).

In the modern era, *The Vowel* by Chiba and Kajiyama (1941–1942) drew foundational conclusions on the mechanisms of vowel production and laid the groundwork for the modern field of speech science and acoustic phonetics. Subsequently, with a focus not only on vowels but also consonants, the field of acoustic phonetics was systematically and rapidly developed by core founders, such as Fant (1960) and Stevens (1998). Unlike previous two-dimensional measurements, Chiba and Kajiyama (1941–1942) took three-dimensional (3D) measurements of the human vocal tract during vowel production. In the section called, "Artificial Vowels," they made physical models out of clay based on their simplified 3D measurements. Finally, they showed that vowel-like sounds can be produced by introducing different types of sound sources into the glottal end of the tubes or vocal-tract models.

Chiba and Kajiyama further investigated the relationship between 3D configurations of the vocal tract and the spectral characteristics of vowels and showed that differences in vowel quality are caused by the differences in vocal-tract configuration. Later, Fant (1960) established the fundamental principal of vowel production as "the source-filter theory of speech production." Furthermore, speech sounds, including vowels and consonants, are modeled as the result of resonance filtering of one or more of the four sound sources: phonation (glottal source), aspiration, transient, and frication (Stevens, 2005).

After Chiba and Kajiyama published *The Vowel* in 1941–1942, many researchers designed mechanical models for their own research purposes. For example, Umeda and Teranishi (1966) developed a mechanical model to investigate vowel and voice qualities. In Umeda and Teranishi's model, the VTM-UT, a set of plastic bars were inserted on one side to simulate an arbitrary vocal tract shape. The model also had a nasal cavity, enabling nasalized sounds to be produced. By controlling a glottal source signal and vocal-tract configuration – including length – they successfully produced different vowels with male, female and child speaker characteristics. Dang and Honda (1995) designed a mechanical model for measuring the effect of pyriform fossa side branches at the larynx. Honda et al. (2004) designed precise physical models of a human vocal tract using magnetic resonance images. In 1989–1991, Martin Riches has built an intricate, artistic wooden model of Fant's (1960) published area functions and fashioned them into a speaking machine (Riches, 2018). In addition, he built another speaking machine called, "Motor Mouth" in 1994–1999.

Vocal-tract modeling and speech simulation have been conducted in many studies, such as Stevens et al. (1953), Fant (1960), Maeda (1982), Story et al. (1996), Espy-Wilson et al. (2000), and Carre (2004). For example, Maeda (1982) proposed a time-domain simulation method of the vocal tract. Story (2005) proposed a model of the vocal-tract area function by incorporating many aspects of speech production systems (see Chapter 1). Takemoto et al. (2006) reported how the laryngeal cavity affects resonance of the vocal tract by applying computer simulations.

For teaching purposes, some museums have physical models of the human vocal tract. For example, there is a set of vocal tract models at the Exploratorium in San Francisco under the supervision of John J. Ohala. Additionally, Arai (2001) replicated Chiba and Kajiyama's mechanical models of the human vocal tract from transparent materials. The replica models and their extended models are exhibited at the following museums: Shizuoka Science Museum (Japan), Hitachi Civic Center Science Museum (Japan), Okinawa Zoo & Museum (Japan), Händel-Haus (Germany), and Estonian National Museum (Estonia).

Arai (e.g., 2007, 2012a, 2016b) showed that the models are useful as educational tools, and an educational package, including a whole set of physical models and computer-based tools for studying phonetics, will be introduced in the following sections. Because some of the physical models help one gain a more intuitive understanding of basic acoustic concepts in speech production, such as the source-filter theory and the relationship between vocal-tract configurations and vowel quality, we will be referring to the appropriate models in our discussions. Different models are helpful for understanding other acoustic phenomena, theories and mechanisms, as well. Thus, we will refer to particular models from time to time in this chapter, whenever doing so will facilitate understanding.

VTM family

Figure 20.1 shows the vocal-tract model family, hereafter abbreviated VTM, including a set of models, sound sources, and computer- or web-based educational tools. The sound sources are mainly used to excite the VTMs. Combining the physical models with computer-based tools enhances understanding of the concepts. The following sections of this chapter provide a series of explanations of the VTMs. In addition, sound and video demonstrations of some

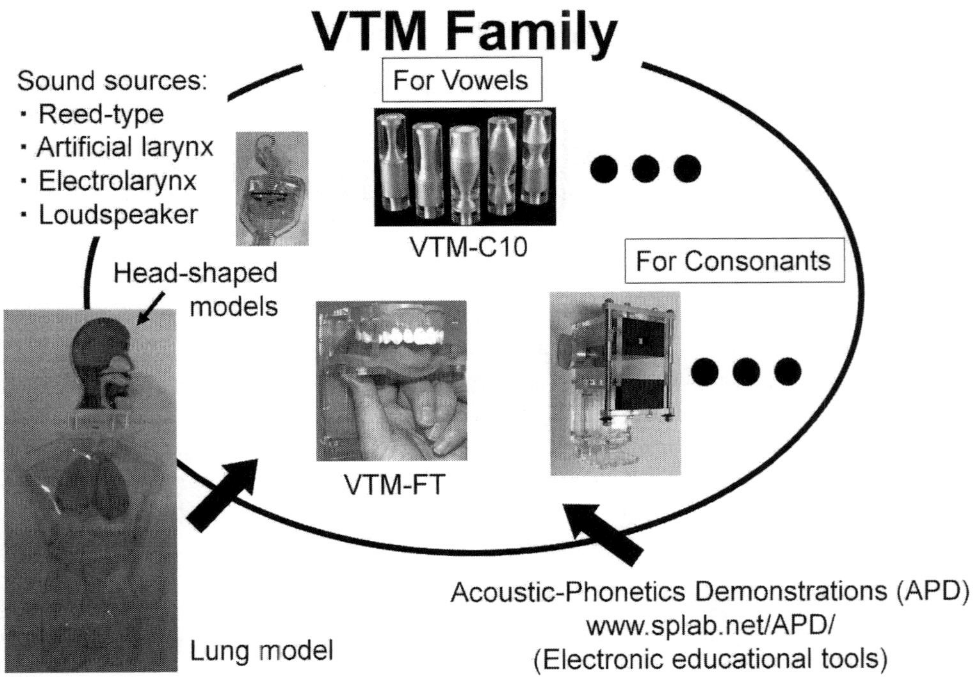

Figure 20.1 The VTM family, including a set of VTMs, sound sources, and computer- or web-based educational tools.

of the VTMs may be accessed at the following website: *Acoustic-Phonetics Demonstrations* www.splab.net/APD/

Sound sources

A sound source is needed to excite any vocal tract. An artificial larynx (Lebrun et al., 1973), which is used to simulate the glottal source in laryngectomy patients, is one of the sound sources that we often use, because it produces a reasonably clear vowel sound with our models. A whistle-type artificial larynx is available, including a reed-type (Lebrun et al., 1973; Riesz, 1930; Gardner and Harris, 1961). So far, different artificial larynxes were developed, such as Tapia's artificial larynx (the so-called "duck call" has a similar mechanism). Figure 20.2 (a) shows our reed-type sound source, SS-R30. In this case, a 0.1–0.2 mm thick plastic sheet is used. The plastic sheet is fixed on the curved support with a hole, so that the airflow sets the sheet into vibration. All of the above-mentioned sound sources produce reasonable glottal source sounds, which is important because the quality of the vowel production demonstration depends on the quality of the sound source. The spectrum of each of these sound sources is rich in harmonics and its envelope is smooth.

We also found that an electrolarynx, which is another type of artificial larynx, is useful for hands-on classroom demonstrations. First, students could touch their own throat and feel the vibration during phonation. They could also touch the top surface of the electrolarynx and feel a similar vibration. Then, with an electrolarynx, students were able to observe that the original buzz sound changes immediately to a humanlike vowel when the device is

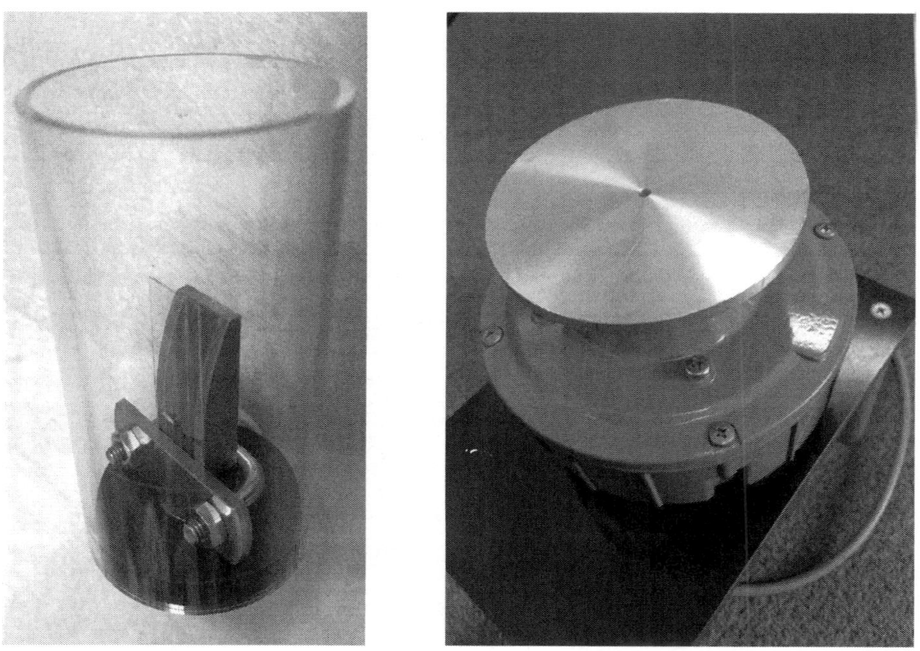

(a) (b)

Figure 20.2 (a) A reed-type sound source, SS-R30. (b) A driver unit of a horn speaker (TOA, TU-750).

gently pressed on the outside of the neck. This kind of demonstration can be done with an electrolarynx, but not with a whistle-type artificial larynx.

A driver unit of a horn speaker can be used as a transducer for producing an arbitrary sound. One can feed signals to the driver unit not only from an oscillator, but also from a computer by means of a digital/analog converter and amplifier, so that any arbitrary signal can be a source signal. To avoid unwanted coupling between the neck and the area behind the neck of the driver unit and achieve high impedance at the glottis end, Umeda and Teranishi (1966) filled the neck of their model with nails. We inserted a close-fitting metal cylindrical filler inside the neck, instead. As shown in Figure 20.2 (b), we can place the glottal end of the vocal-tract model on top of a thin metal plate, directly connected to the metal filling inside the neck. Ours has a hole in the center of the metal filling and plate with an area of 0.13 cm^2. If the area of the hole is small enough, high impedance at the glottal end is achieved. However, if the area is too small, the acoustic power coming from the hole becomes too weak. The diameter of 4 mm is a good compromise for the size of the hole.

The sound source for a driver unit could be virtually any signal. We typically use the following: an impulse train, triangular glottal pulse, white noise, an LPC residual signal or an acoustic signal recorded just outside a speaker's larynx during phonation. Another possibility is to use a model for the glottal waveform, such as Liljencrants-Fant (LF) glottal source model (Fant et al., 1985).

Lung model

Functionally, the lung model shows how we breathe and produce the airflow needed for making speech sounds. In our VTM family, the reed-type sound source requires airflow to produce sounds. For airflow, one may either blow into the sound source or use bellows/pumps. To imitate the human respiratory system with a simple device, we adopted a functional model of the lung and diaphragm (Arai, 2007). With this model, we can slowly pull on a knob attached to the "diaphragm" (a rubber membrane covering the bottom of the cavity) to inflate the "lungs" (two balloons). The balloons are connected to a Y-shaped tube simulating the trachea. Pulling down the diaphragm increases the volume of the thoracic cavity, thereby creating a negative pressure in the air inside the thoracic cavity. Air flows into the lungs to equalize the pressure inside the lungs with the atmospheric pressure, simulating inhalation. Pushing up on the diaphragm decreases the thoracic cavity volume, causing air to flow out of the lungs, simulating exhalation. By combining a whistle-/reed-type sound source with the lung model, a glottal sound is produced.

Models for vowels

People typically produce vowels using the vocal tract as a resonator by feeding a glottal sound into the vocal tract. To make different vowels, the shape of the vocal-tract configuration is critical, with the area function along the vocal-tract length determining vowel quality. In this sense, the issue of straight- vs. bent-tube is not crucial as long as the area function is consistent along the length of the tube. It is sometimes simple to show a straight model to see the change in the area function. However, with a straight model, it is a bit difficult to imagine where the vocal tract is located within one's head. Therefore, a bent-tube model has the advantage in demonstrating the location of the vocal tract. Also, if we want to demonstrate tongue movement within the vocaltract, we need a bent-tube model, as well.

Bent-tube models show the location and degree of constriction directly, because one can see the location of the tongue.

A model with many degrees of freedom is ideal for simulating human behavior. However, with too many degrees of freedom, it becomes difficult to demonstrate changes from one vowel to another. Therefore, we have developed several different types of models for specific applications and purposes.

A major set of the VTMs for vowels are shown in Figure 20.3. They are grouped into two categories; the bottom panel shows the straight-tube models, and the top panel shows the bent-tube models. The horizontal axis of this figure is the degree of freedom in terms of movement from static models with the null degree of freedom through dynamic models with moderate and high degrees of freedom. For example, VTM-N20 and VTM-T20 are the straight-tube and static models, with zero degrees of freedom. Because the vocal-tract configuration is fixed for each model, we need an entire set of models to cover all of the different vowels. However, these models have an advantage for quick demonstrations. For example, if one wants to make five vowels in a row, the fixed/static models are the most useful. VTM-HS has a bent vocaltract and a movable velum that acts as a valve between the pharyngeal and nasal cavities. Because the velum is the only moveable part, this model has a single degree of freedom. The vocal-tract configuration is again fixed for each vowel for VTM-HS. For VTM-P10 and VTM-UT, there are 10–20 degrees of freedom, because the area function of a vocal-tract configuration is simulated step-by-step with a 10 or 15 mm step width. With these models, different vowels can be made by changing the area function based on each configuration. Finally, VTM-FT is bent and made partially of a gel-type material, so that the vocal-tract configuration is flexible. Although one can dynamically change

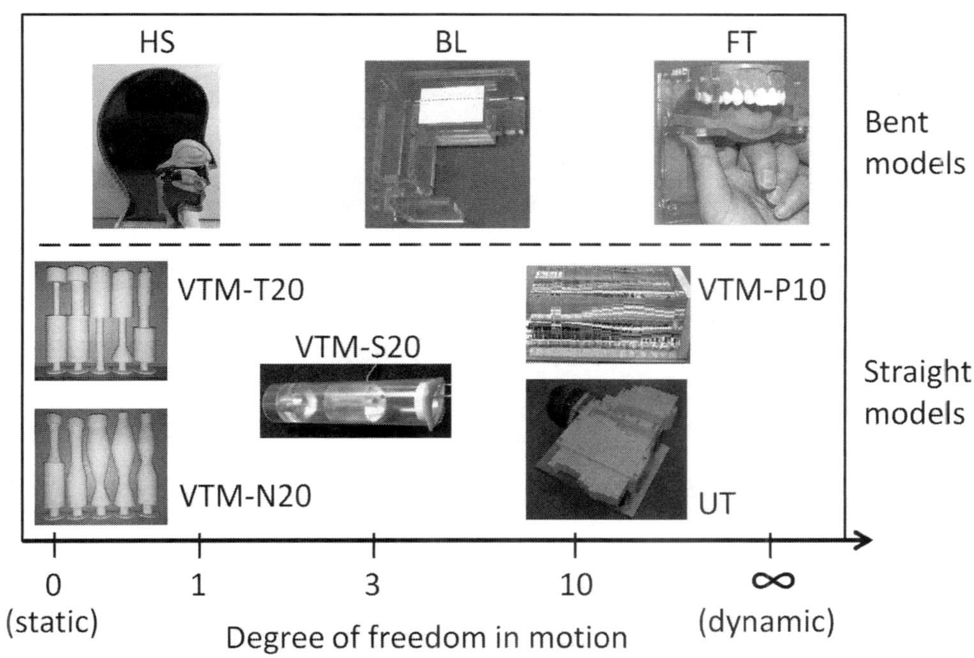

Figure 20.3 A major set of VTMs for vowels (see text for details).

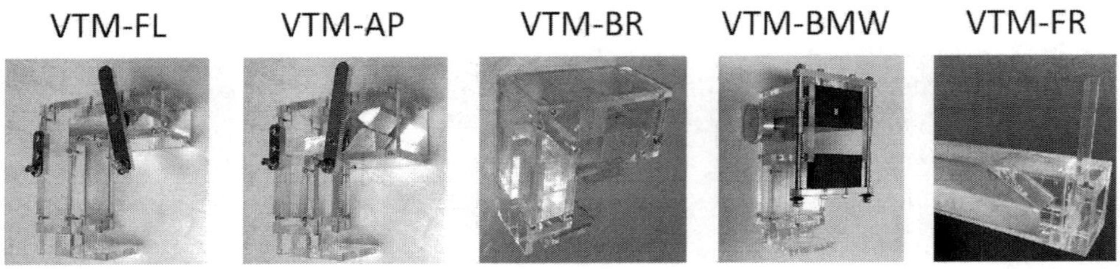

Figure. 20.4 A set of VTMs targeted for consonants (see text for details).

the vocal-tract configuration, a certain degree of knowledge and practice may be needed to successfully produce the target vowel.

Models for consonants

For pulmonic egressive sounds, consonants are articulated by completely or partially blocking the airstream from the lungs in the vocal tract. The way we articulate consonants is called "manner of articulation." For many languages, the manners of articulation include: stop, nasal, flap, fricative, affricate, trill, and approximant. With stop consonants, the airstream is completely blocked in the vocal tract. For nasal consonants, the airstream is completely blocked in the oral cavity, as with oral stops; however, the airstream passes through the nasal cavity due to the opening of the velopharyngeal port as the velum is lowered. Fricative consonants are articulated by letting the airstream pass through a narrow channel at a point of constriction in the vocal tract, producing a turbulent noise. For approximants, the constriction is wider than for fricatives, so there is no turbulence.

Thus, consonants are produced differently than vowels, and the manners of articulation are widely ranging. Although we articulate all of the vowels and consonants with our mouths, making a single physical model to produce all of these sounds is difficult. For simplicity, we provide a different model for a single consonant or a few consonants.

Figure 20.4 shows a set of VTMs targeted for different types of consonants. VTM-FL and VTM-AP are designed for making a flap sound and approximants (Arai, 2013b). VTM-BR is designed for bunched /r/ in English (Arai, 2014). VTM-BMW is a model for the sounds [b], [m], and [w] (Arai, 2016a). VTM-FR is a model for fricatives. Please see the following section of "Producing consonants" for more details.

Resonance of a uniform tube

In this section, we will examine what occurs when these models are given a pure tone source. More concretely, we will introduce pure tones of different frequencies into a uniform tube with a certain diameter and measure the output levels to see whether the levels show peaks depending on the input frequencies. The transfer function of the uniform tube is defined as the output levels relative to the input levels as a function of frequency. Finally, we will feed an impulse train into the uniform tube and observe the spectrum of an output signal showing harmonics with peaks in their spectral envelope.

Pure tone as an input signal

Figure 20.5 shows a tube with a uniform diameter of 28 mm and a length of 170 mm. When we input a sinusoidal acoustic wave from a loudspeaker (the driver unit of a horn speaker described in the previous section) with a metal attachment, as shown in this figure, a pure tone is produced through the tube. What happens when we vary the frequency of the sinusoidal wave from a low frequency to about 3 kHz? Figure 20.6 shows the output sound through the acoustic tube when we measure the output level relative to the input level of the sinusoid as its frequency varies. This figure shows that the output level fluctuates as the frequency increases. Specifically, the output-level curve has peaks at approximately 500 Hz, 1500 Hz, and 2500 Hz. These peaks are due to the resonance, and the peak frequencies are called resonance frequencies.

Thus, resonance is revealed when the input signal has matching frequency components. These resonance frequencies depend on the length of the tube, L, and resonance occurs when the sound wave inside the tube forms a standing wave. The lowest resonance frequency, f_{R1}, is $\frac{c}{4L}$, where c is the speed of sound (approximately 340 m/s). This is because the first standing wave occurs at one quarter of the wavelength of the sound. In this measurement, the tube length L was 170 mm (which is the average length of an adult male speaker); therefore, f_{R1} is going to be about 500 Hz. The consequent resonances occur at odd multiples of f_{R1}: $f_{R2} = \frac{3c}{4L} \cong 1500$ Hz, $f_{R3} = \frac{5c}{4L} \cong 2500$ Hz, and so on (in general, $f_{Rn} = \frac{(2n-1)c}{4L}$).

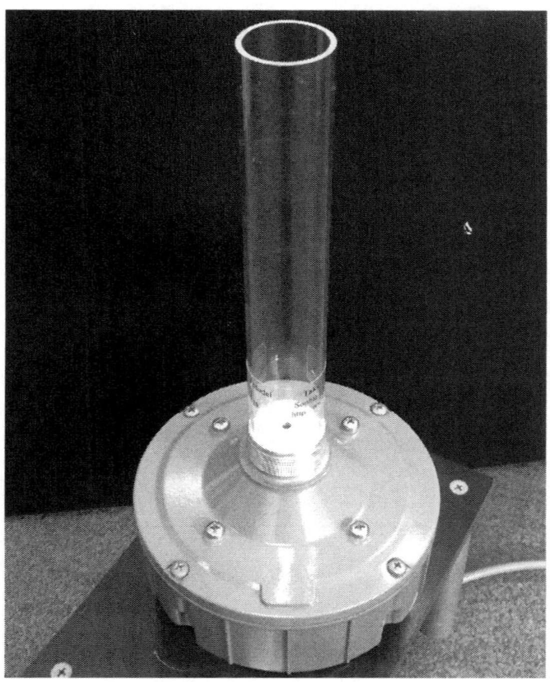

Figure 20.5 A uniform acoustic tube (inner diameter = 28 mm, length = 170 mm) placed on the top of the driver unit.

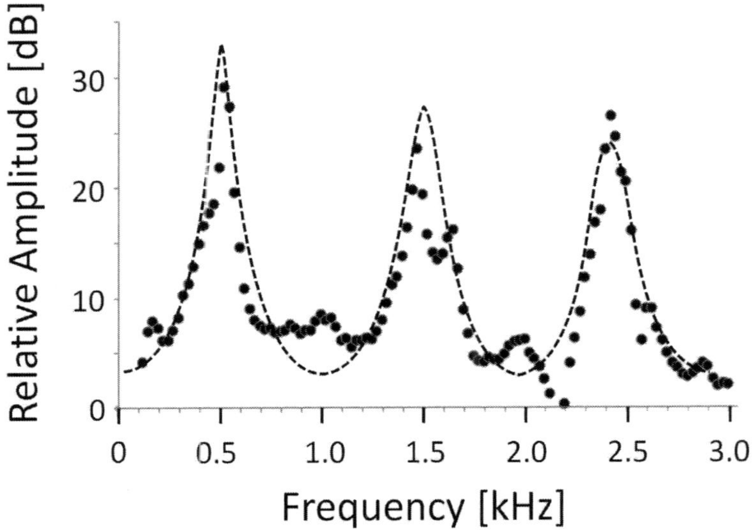

Figure 20.6 The output level relative to the input level in dB as a function of frequency. The dots denote the measured values every 25 Hz, while the dashed line shows a theoretical curve (Stevens, 1998). Note that the open-end correction was not accounted for, so that the frequencies of the peaks are slightly less than the theoretical values.

In Figure 20.5, the output end was open. However, if the output end is closed, the first standing wave occurs when the tube length is about half the wavelength of the sound: $f_{R1} = \frac{c}{2L}$. In this case, the consequent resonances occur at multiples of f_{R1}: $f_{Rn} = \frac{nc}{2L}$.

Impulse train as an input signal

Let us assume that we are going to input a combination of two sinusoids of 100 and 200 Hz. We already know what is going to happen when we input a single sinusoid from the previous measurement section on pure tones. According to the superposition principle, we can estimate the output signal when we combine input sinusoids of 100 and 200 Hz. The estimated output signal will be a combination of the two original output signals: the one obtained from the 100-Hz sinusoid and the other obtained from the 200-Hz sinusoid.

Next, let's assume we are going to input a combination of many sinusoids of multiples of 100 Hz. In this case, again, we can estimate the output signal as a combination of all the original output signals. Note that when we add sinusoids of multiples of 100 Hz with a certain phase condition, we will get an impulse train. In other words, we can say that the impulse train has a fundamental component at 100 Hz (fundamental frequency), and its multiples are called harmonics. (Later, we will see that a glottal source signal also has a similar spectrum, i.e., the harmonic structure, in the frequency domain.)

When we input the impulse train into the acoustic tube in Figure 20.5 instead of sinusoidal signals, the spectrum of the output signal looks like Figure 20.7, in which the impulses are repeated every $T = 10$ ms. Therefore, Figure 20.7 reveals the harmonic structure. In other words, there is the fundamental component at the fundamental frequency $f_0 = 1/T = 100$ Hz, and its harmonics are located at multiples of f_0. By comparing Figures 20.6 and 20.7, we can observe that the output signal with the impulse train input has the same spectral peaks as the

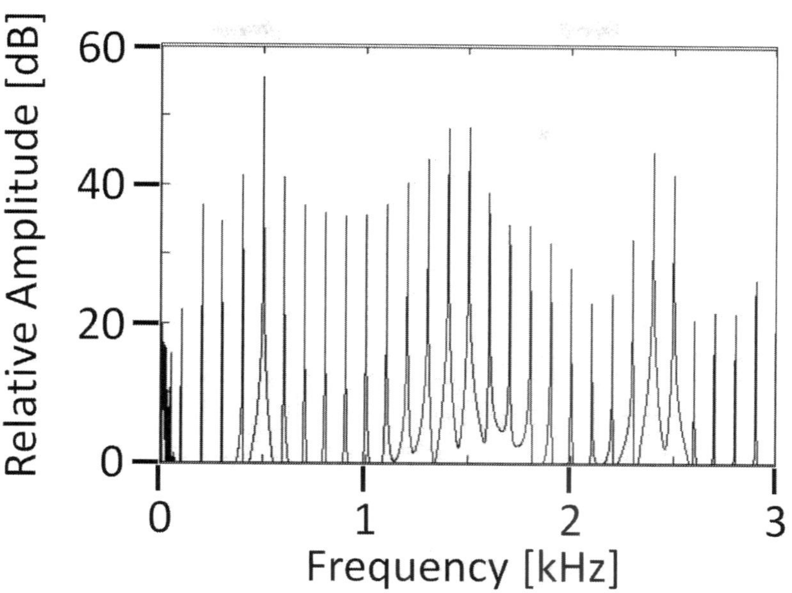

Figure 20.7 Spectrum of the output signal when the impulse train with f_0 = 100 Hz was fed into the uniform tube.

resonance curve in Figure 20.6. The uniform tube approximates the vocal-tract configuration of the neutral vowel, schwa ([ə] in the International Phonetic Alphabet, IPA). The spectral peaks are called "formants," and they are noted as F_1, F_2, F_3, and so on (although see Chapter 9 for discussion on different definitions of the formant). Note there is no guarantee that a formant frequency perfectly matches any frequencies of the harmonics.

Vocal-tract configuration of vowels

Figure 20.8 shows midsagittal cross-sections of the vocal-tract configuration for the five Japanese vowels (top), and their schematic straight models (bottom). The plots of this figure are adopted from Chiba and Kajiyama (1941–1942); they originally measured the configurations using a combination of x-ray photography, palatography, and laryngoscopic observation of the pharynx (Maekawa, 2002).

From this figure, one can note the following vowel features:

- /i/ has a narrow constriction in the front cavity, whereas the back cavity is relatively large
- /e/, as with vowel /i/, has a narrow constriction in the front cavity, but the degree of the constriction is less than that of vowel /i/
- /a/ is produced with lips (and front cavity) wide open, whereas there is a narrow constriction in the back cavity
- /o/, like /a/, has a narrow constriction in the back cavity, but the degree of lip opening is rather small
- /u/ has a narrow constriction in the middle of the vocal tract and the degree of lip opening is small

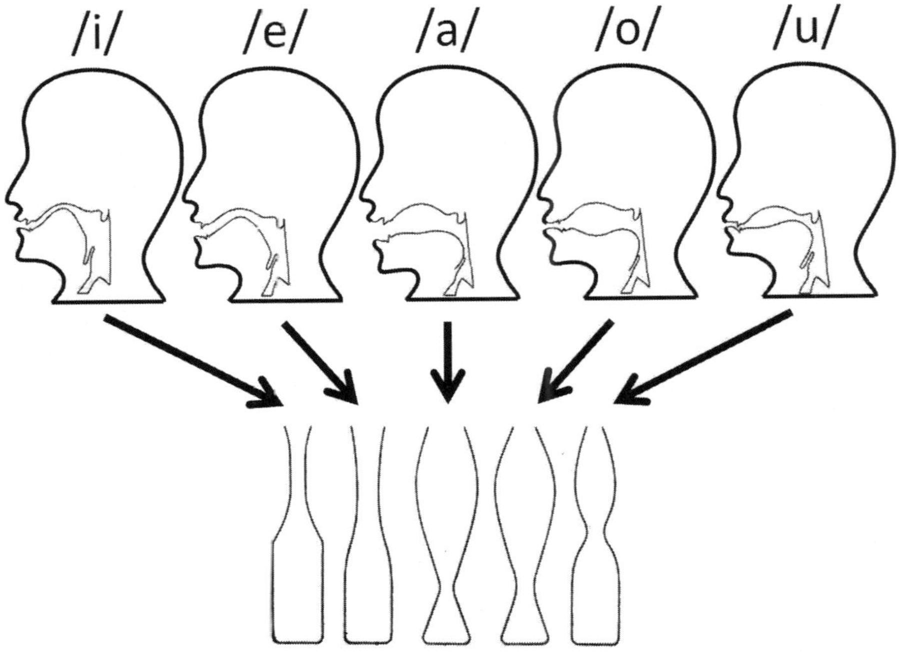

Figure 20.8 Midsagittal cross-sections of the vocal-tract configuration for the five Japanese vowels (top), and their schematic straight models (bottom).

Source: The plots are adopted from Chiba and Kajiyama (1941–1942).

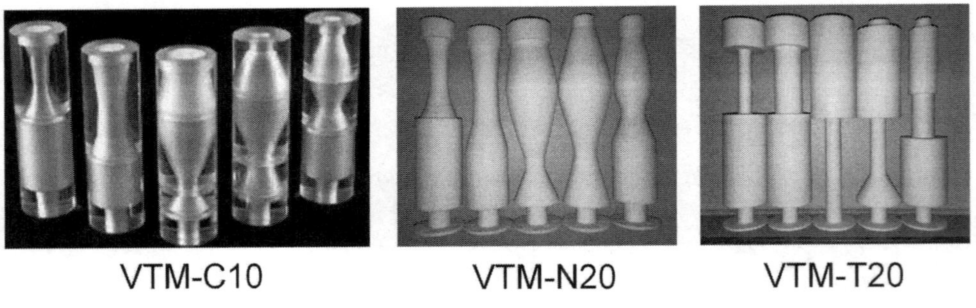

Figure 20.9 VTM-C10 (a) Precise reproduction based on Chiba and Kajiyama (1941–1942). VTM-N20 (b) The "outline" version of the VTM-C10. The interior area functions are the same as VTM-C10. VTM-T20 (c) A simplified version designed by connecting multiple uniform tubes with different diameters and lengths.

Chiba and Kajiyama (1941–1942) made vocal-tract models based on their measurements. By introducing a glottal sound into their models, they demonstrated that the vowel sounds produced by the models are close to their naturally produced counterparts. Arai (2001) replicated their models as shown in Figure 20.9 (a: VTM-C10, b: VTM-N20).

Figure 20.9 (c) shows a set of VTM-T20 for the five Japanese vowels. These models were obtained by simplifying the configurations of VTM-N20 and connecting several uniform tubes with different cross-sectional areas and lengths.

Source-filter theory of speech production

As discussed in Section 3, the output signal is the result of the combination of the sound source and the resonance characteristics of the acoustic tube. In general, speech sounds, especially vowel sounds, can be viewed as the linear combination of a sound source and the resonance characteristics of the vocal tract. In other words, one can model speech sounds as the response coming from a vocal-tract acting as a linear filter, where a sound source is fed into and filtered by the vocal tract. This kind of modeling by a linear system is called the source-filter theory of speech production. For vowels, the sound source is a glottal sound produced by vocal fold vibration (the phonation source). The basic concept of source-filter theory appears in Chiba and Kajiyama (1941–1942). Fant merged this concept with the filter in electrical circuit theory and formulated the "source-filter theory of vowel production" (Fant, 1960; Arai, 2004).

If the vocal-tract configuration is unchanged, the vocal-tract filter becomes a linear time-invariant (LTI) system, and an output signal $y(t)$ can be expressed by the convolution of an input signal $x(t)$ and the impulse response of the system $h(t)$, that is,

$$y(t) = h(t) * x(t),$$

where the asterisk denotes the convolution (top panel in Figure 20.10).

The equation above is expressed in the time domain, but it can also be expressed in the frequency domain as follows:

$$Y(\omega) = H(\omega)X(\omega),$$

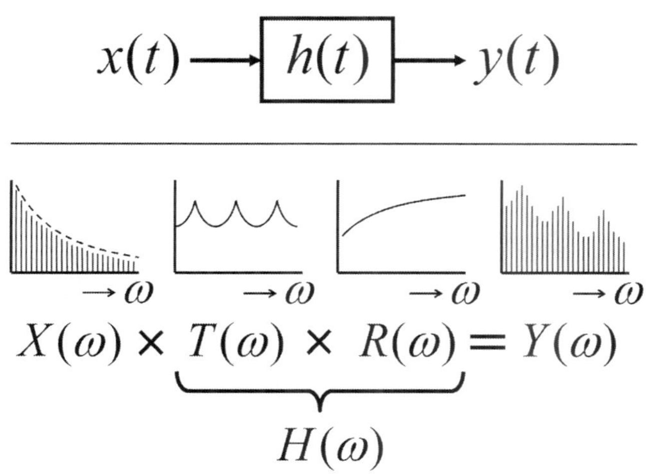

Figure 20.10 Top: Output signal y(t) of an LTI system can be expressed by the convolution of an input signal x(t) and the impulse response of the system h(t) in the time domain. Bottom: Speech spectrum Y (ω) is modeled as the product of the source spectrum X (ω), the transfer function of the vocal-tract filter T (ω), and the radiation characteristics from the mouth R (ω) in the frequency domain.

and this tells us the relation of each spectral representation. In other words, the speech spectrum $Y(\omega)$ is modeled as the product of the source spectrum $X(\omega)$ and the spectrum of the vocal-tract filter $H(\omega)$.

Strictly speaking, the spectrum of the vocal-tract filter $H(\omega)$ can be further viewed as the product of the vocal-tract transfer function $T(\omega)$ and the radiation characteristics from the mouth $R(\omega)$, that is,

$$Y(\omega) = \left[T(\omega)R(\omega)\right]X(\omega),$$

as shown in the bottom panel in Figure 20.10.

One can conduct a simple demonstration of the source-filter theory with our vocal-tract models in order to illustrate the respective contribution of sound source and vocal tract configuration to output sound. Let's say we have a sound source with a variable fundamental frequency, f_0, and two vocal-tract filters: one for /i/ and another for /a/. By combining the sound source with the model /i/, we obtain a vowel sound with the same f_0 contour as the sound source. Likewise, when one combines the sound source with the model /a/, one obtains a vowel sound with the same f_0 contour as the sound source. Figure 20.11 shows spectrograms of the output sounds of this demonstration. In both panels, one can observe a similar vertical movement of the harmonics, while the spectral peaks are steady and show different patterns depending on the vowel. This demonstrates that sound source mainly governs the fundamental frequency of the output sound, while vocal tract configuration mainly governs vowel quality.

For speech sounds, whether vowels or consonants, there are four sound sources: glottal (or phonation), aspiration, frication, and transient source, One of the sources or a combination of them becomes an input to the vocal-tract filter, and a vowel or a consonant can be

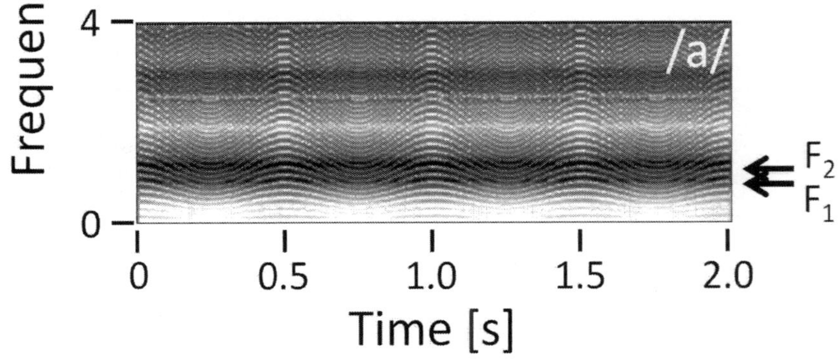

Figure 20.11 Spectrograms of the output sounds from the two vocal-tract models. The sound source is an impulse train with a variable fundamental frequency. Top panel: /i/. Bottom panel: /a/.

viewed as the response of such a filter. Thus, the source-filter theory can be expanded and applied not only to vowels but to any speech sound, including consonants (Stevens, 2005).

Talkers are able to more or less independently control phonation (source) with the larynx, and articulation (filter) with the vocal tract, and the source-filter theory is a good approximation of speech sounds. However, we have to remember this theory is only an approximation, and the actual process of speech production is nonlinear and time-variant. It is also true that there is an interaction between the source and the vocal-tract filter (see Section 310).

Sliding two-tube model

Figure 20.12 shows the sliding two-tube model (Arai, 2018), the S2T model, with a cross-sectional area of 100 or 1000 mm^2 and the total length of 170 mm (L in the figure). A cross-section of this model is either the main large square plus the small square (1000 mm^2) or the small square alone (100 mm^2). Because a 30 mm x 30 mm square bar can slide inside the main square pipe, the resulting acoustic tube consists of two connected, uniform tubes with different cross-sectional areas. Therefore, we call this model the sliding two-tube model. The lengths of the two tubes denote l_1 (the small square part) and l_2 (the large square part) hereafter.

To measure the resonances of this S2T model, we recorded output signals when with a 100-Hz impulse train input to the model. The sliding square bar was inserted from the left in Figure 20.12, and recordings were conducted at every 1-mm step. A flange with a diameter of 24 cm was attached at the open end of the tube. Figure 20.13 shows a two-dimensional representation of the concatenated output spectra, each having a duration of 100 ms, where the horizontal axis is the length of the back cavity, l_1. From this figure, one observes that the resonance frequencies vary depending on the position of the inserted sliding bar. For the S2T model, we can assume that the two uniform tubes are connected, and each has an open end. This assumption can be made because the gap of the cross-sectional areas between the two tubes is large enough, and this leads to the acoustic decoupling of the tubes. Therefore, we can think of two sets of resonances for the two tubes (cavities); $\frac{(2n-1)c}{4\ell_1}$ for the back cavity and $\frac{(2n-1)c}{4\ell_2}$ for the front cavity. Based on this approximation, the theoretical plots

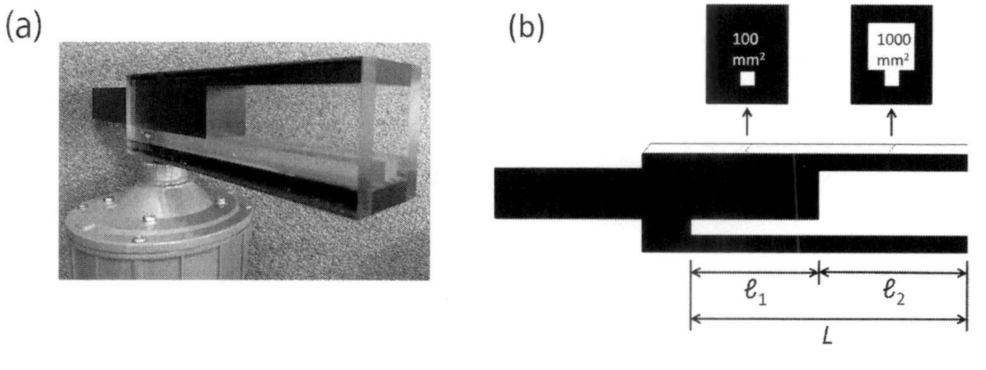

Figure 20.12 The sliding two-tube (S2T) model. (a) The model is connected to the driver unit and a small hole runs from the neck of the driver unit through the glottis end of the S2T model. (b) Schematic illustration of the midsagittal section of the model.

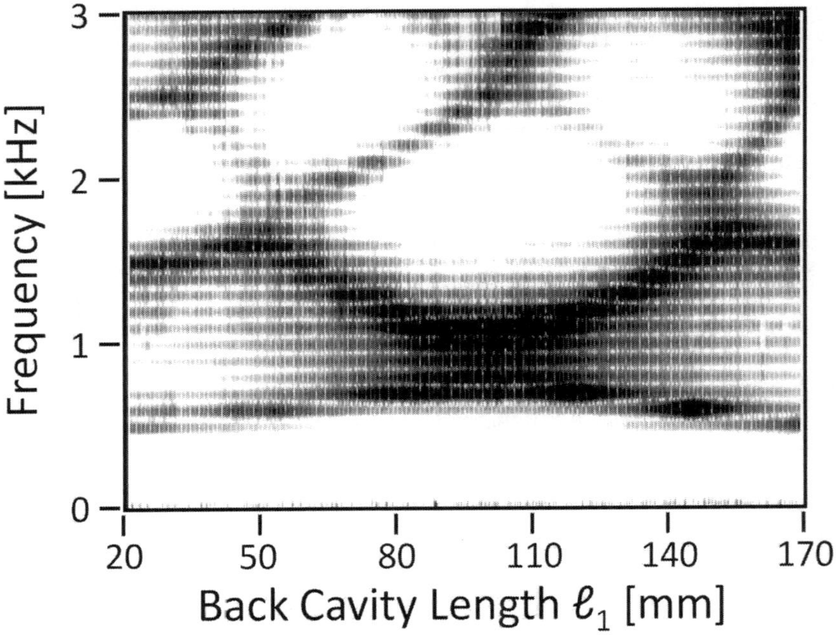

Figure 20.13 Two-dimensional representation of the output spectra (frequency vs. the back cavity length).

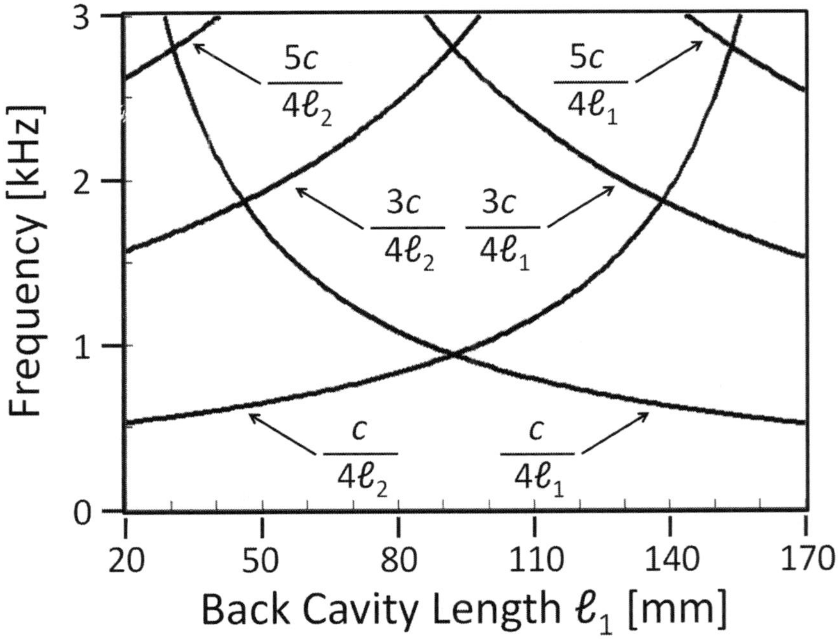

Figure 20.14 Underlying resonance curves of the S2T model as function of the back cavity length.

are shown in Figure 20.14. (An end correction of 0.82 r for the front cavity resonance with a flange was applied, where r is the effective radius of the mouth end.)

Notice that the underlying resonance curves intersect with each other in the middle of Figure 20.14. At the intersection, the systems avoid taking exactly the same resonance frequency (Stevens, 1998). As a result, the first and second formants show a plateau around l_1 = 90–100 mm. This stable region for F_1 and F_2 is less sensitive to the position of the articulators and shows an evidence of "the quantal theory of speech production" (Stevens, 1972, 1989). In fact, many languages use this region for the vowel /a/.

Sliding three-tube model

Working from the concept of the S2T model, we now turn to the sliding three-tube, or S3T, model, where three uniform tubes are connected to each other (Arai, 2006, 2012a). This model is based on the concept of Fant's three-tube model (Fant, 1960). Figure 20.15 is a schematic representation of the midsagittal cross-section of this model.

In Figure 20.15, the glottis end is on the left, and the lip end is on the right. The first tube is the leftmost one, with length l_1 and diameter D. The second tube is the middle one, with length l_2 and diameter d. The third tube is on the right, with length l_3 and diameter D. The total length of the three tubes is L (= $l_1 + l_2 + l_3$)

If the diameter d of the second tube is small enough compared to the diameter of the rest, that is, D, we can assume the tubes are acoustically decoupled and the resonance phenomena in the tubes can be treated independently. Thus, we can think in terms of three resonances in the lower frequencies. The first resonance is from the first tube. With this tube, both ends are considered closed, and the approximation of its first resonance frequency is given by $\frac{c}{2\ell}$. The second resonance is from the third tube. With this tube, one end is open, but the other end is closed, and the approximation of its first resonance frequency is given by $\frac{c}{4\ell_3}$. The third resonance is a Helmholtz resonance from a resonator formed by the first and second tubes. The resonance frequency is given by $\frac{c}{2\pi}\sqrt{\frac{A_2}{A\ell_1\ell_2}}$, where A and A_2 are the areas of circles with diameters D and d, respectively: $A = \frac{\pi}{4}D^2$ and $A_2 = \frac{\pi}{4}d^2$.

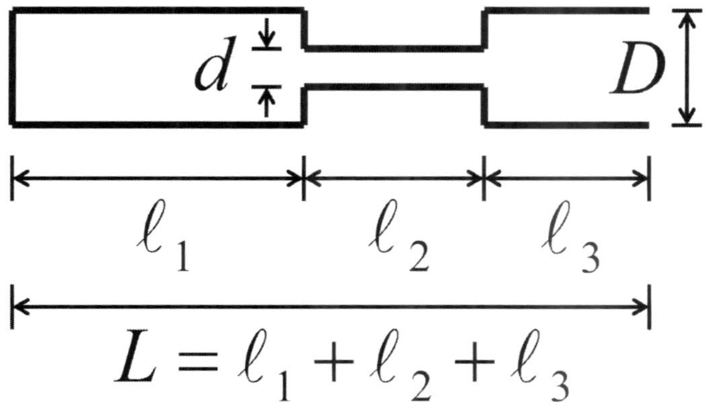

Figure 20.15 Schematic representation of the midsagittal cross-section of the S3T model.

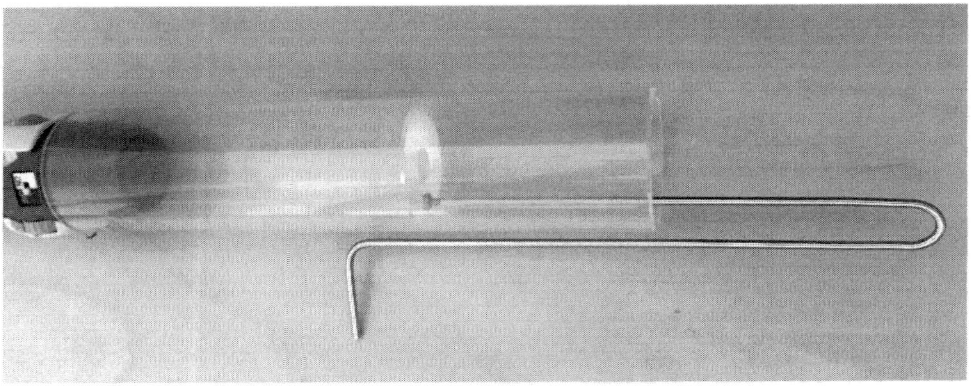

Figure 20.16 Sliding three-tube (S3T) model with an electrolarynx.

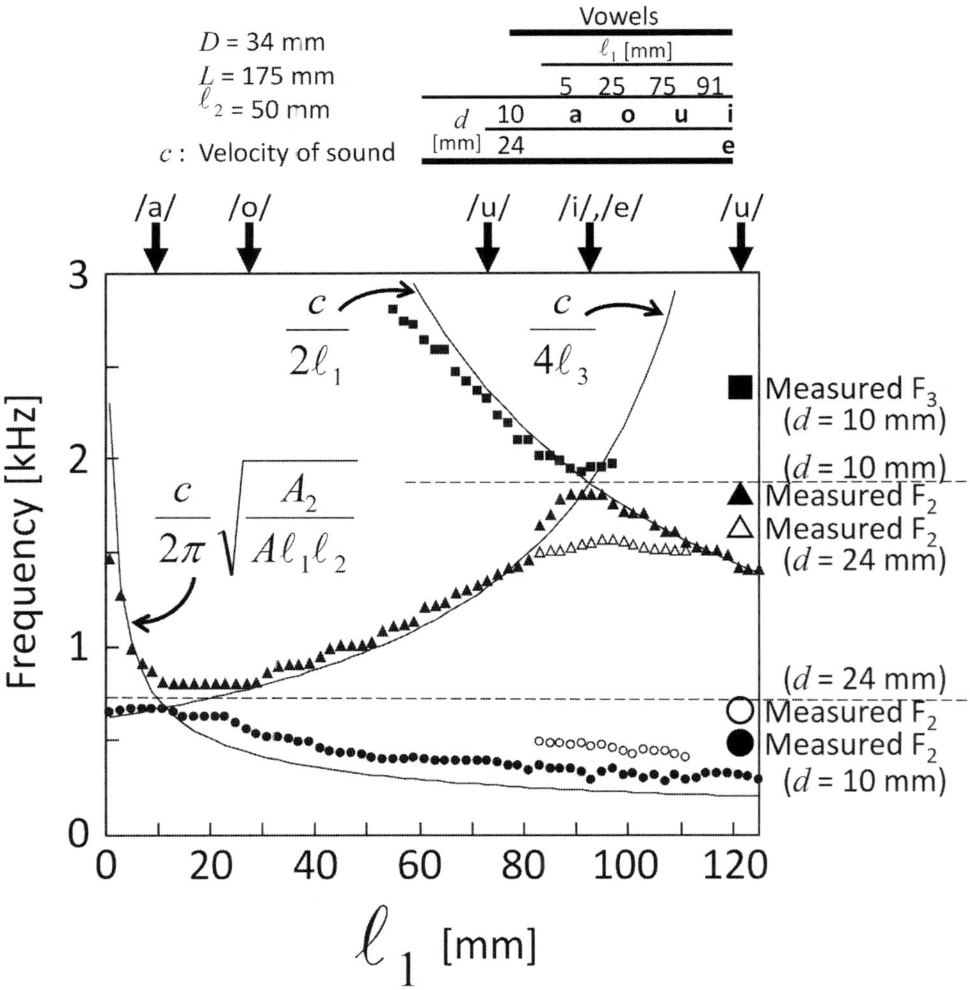

Figure 20.17 Measured formants and underlying resonance curves of the S3T model as function of the back cavity length (Arai, 2006, 2012a).

With this three-tube model, a wide range of vowels can be produced by appropriately defining the parameters. Figure 20.16 shows an example of the S3T model. In this model, there is an outer tube, with an inner diameter *D*, and an inner tube, with a hole having the diameter *d*. Because the inner tube slides back and forth inside the outer tube, the location of the constriction can change arbitrarily.

Arai (2006, 2012a) plotted the results of the actual measurements in terms of the spectral peak frequencies as well as the theoretical resonance curves by using the values listed in Figure 20.17, as a function of the length of the back cavity, l_1. The three resonance curves in this figure are obtained by the three formulas above by simple approximation. (An end correction of 0.82 *r* for the front cavity resonance with a flange was applied, where *r* is the radius of the mouth end.) The dots are the measured peak frequencies which correspond to the resonances.

From this plot, we can see that the vowels /a/ and /o/ are produced when the constriction is in the back, the /u/ is produced when the constriction is in the middle, and /i/ is produced when the constriction is in the front. The vowel /e/ is produced when the constriction is located at the same position as for /i/, but the diameter of the constriction *d* is larger.

Again, in Figure 20.17, we can observe that the underlying resonance curves intersect with each other. As a result, F_1 and F_2 show a plateau around l_1 = 10–20 mm for /a/, and F_2 and F_3 show a plateau around l_1 = 90–100 mm for /i/. These stable regions are less sensitive to the position of the articulators and show evidence of "the quantal theory of speech production" (Stevens, 1972, 1989).

Perturbation theory

As shown in Section 3, resonance occurs in a uniform tube, where one end is closed and the other end is open, when the resonance frequency is an odd-number multiple of the fundamental. Perturbation theory tells us whether each resonance frequency increases or decreases when a small change occurs in the diameter at a local region of the tube (Kent and Read, 2001). The top panels of Figure 20.18 show the volume velocity distribution of air particles inside the tube when the standing waves with the first resonance mode (R_1), the second resonance mode (R_2), and the third resonance mode (R_3) occur. In each panel, A_i and

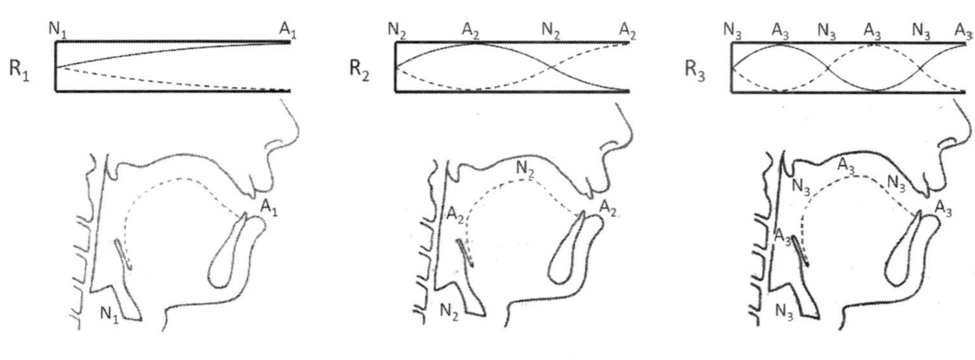

Figure 20.18 Top panels: The volume velocity distributions of inside the uniform tube when the standing waves with the first, second, and third resonance modes occur. Bottom panels: Corresponding uniform vocal-tract configurations.

Source: Adapted from Chiba and Kajiyama (1941–1942).

N_i denote volume velocity maximum (antinodes) and minimum (nodes), respectively. The bottom panels of the same figure show corresponding uniform vocal-tract configurations adapted from Chiba and Kajiyama (1941–1942).

According to perturbation theory, the resonance frequency of the particular resonance mode decreases when a constriction is located at an anti-node of that resonance mode; and the resonance frequency of the particular resonance mode increases when a constriction is located at a node of that resonance mode.

From these facts, we can derive the following (Kent and Read, 2001): (a) all resonance frequencies decrease when the lips are rounded, (b) the second resonance frequency decreases when a constriction occurs at the pharyngeal region because the second resonance mode has an anti-node in that region, and (c) the second resonance frequency increases when a constriction occurs at the palatal region because the second resonance mode has a node in that region. Thus, for vowel /i/, F_2 frequency is higher because there is a constriction in the palatal region. For vowel /a/, F_2 frequency is lower because there is a constriction in the pharyngeal region. For vowel /u/, F_1 and F_2 frequencies are both lower because there is a constriction at the lips.

To measure actual changes in the resonance frequencies, the following experiment was conducted using one of the mechanical models. A uniform tube, similar to the one in Section 33, was used as shown in Figure 20.19. While a ring-shape constriction was shifted

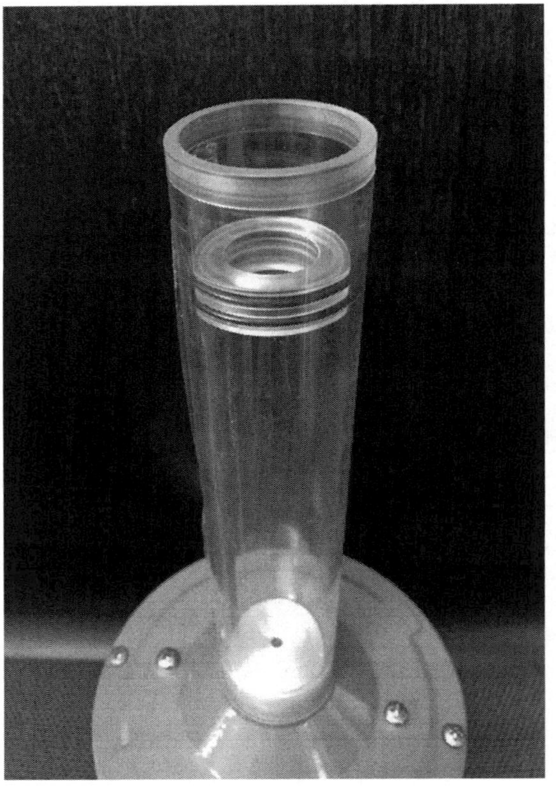

Figure 20.19 A uniform acoustic tube (inner diameter = 34 mm, length = 170 mm) placed on the top of the driver unit. There is a ring-shaped constriction (inner diameter = 28 mm, length = 10 mm) inside the tube, the position of which is movable.

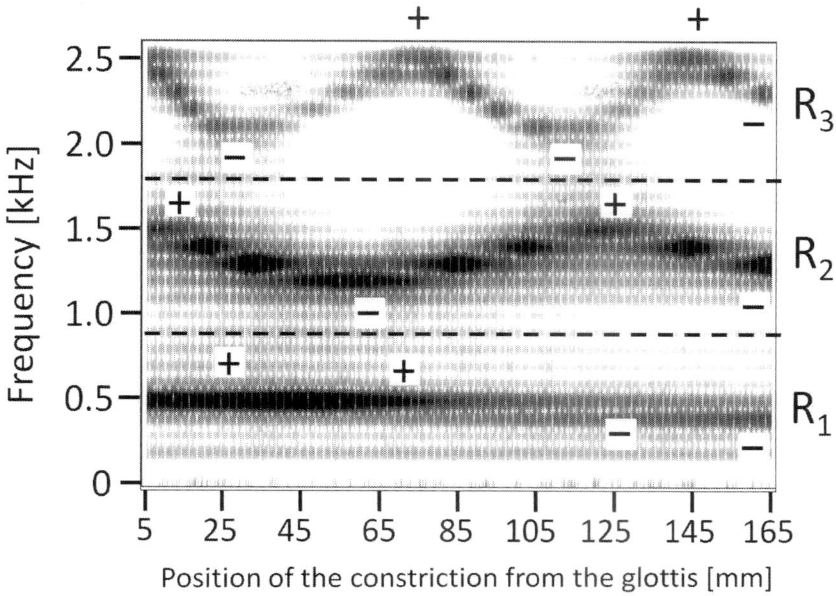

Figure 20.20 Two-dimensional representation of the output spectra as a function of the position of the constriction from the glottis.

from the glottis end through the lip end, the output sounds were recorded and analyzed by feeding a 100-Hz impulse train as an input signal. Figure 20.20 shows a two-dimensional representation of the output spectra as a function of the position of the constriction from the glottis. From this figure, each resonance frequency shifts up and down depending on the constriction position.

A general approach to perturbation theory is based on a theorem by Ehrenfest (1916). Perturbation theory tells us the relationships between vocal tract configurations and formant frequencies by examining the changes in the formant frequencies that occur as a result of small perturbations of the area function in some region along the length of the vocal tract (Stevens, 1998). In chapter XI of "The Vowel" by Chiba and Kajiyama (1941–1942), the researchers use their measurements to calculate the distribution of sound-pressure amplitude and velocity amplitude for the first two resonances for different vowel configurations. It is generally accepted that Chiba and Kajiyama showed the physical phenomenon of wave propagation in the vocal tract for the first time (Motoki, 2002). The relevance of their work was recognized some decades later, when Stevens used such plots to predict the acoustic effects of perturbations on vocal tract shape (Stevens, 2001). Figure 93 from "The Vowel" was cited by Fant and adopted by many subsequent monographs of acoustic phonetics, including recent ones (Maekawa, 2002).

Male vs. female and adults vs. children

The vocal tract lengthens as a baby grows. The average length of the vocal tracts varies between male and female, and the male vocal tract is longer than that of female on average (Stevens, 1998). Therefore, male formant frequencies are the lowest. Likewise, vocal folds grow as humans develop. The average fundamental frequency decreases as a child grows. However, an average male voice decreases drastically, while an average female voice decreases less. Even if the vowel distributions in terms of formants are overlapping among different types of speakers, humans correctly recognize vowels because they are able to normalize for speaker differences. Thus, it is worthwhile to examine and model the changes in vocal-tract length vs. fundamental frequencies, as these are two very salient speaker differences.

In Arai (2012b), the tube length of the S3T model was changed, and a perceptual experiment was conducted with four different lengths of the model (Figure 20.21). For this experiment, four different fundamental frequencies were also used, resulting in a 4x4 combination of stimuli (D = 34 mm and d = 10 mm). Participants were asked to judge the most likely speaker: an adult male, an adult female, an elementary-school child or a baby. As a result, listeners tended to identify the speaker as a female or child not only as f_0 increased, but also as L decreased. Figure 20.22 shows two-dimensional representations of the vowel spectra produced by each of the four S3T models (frequency vs. the length of the back cavity).

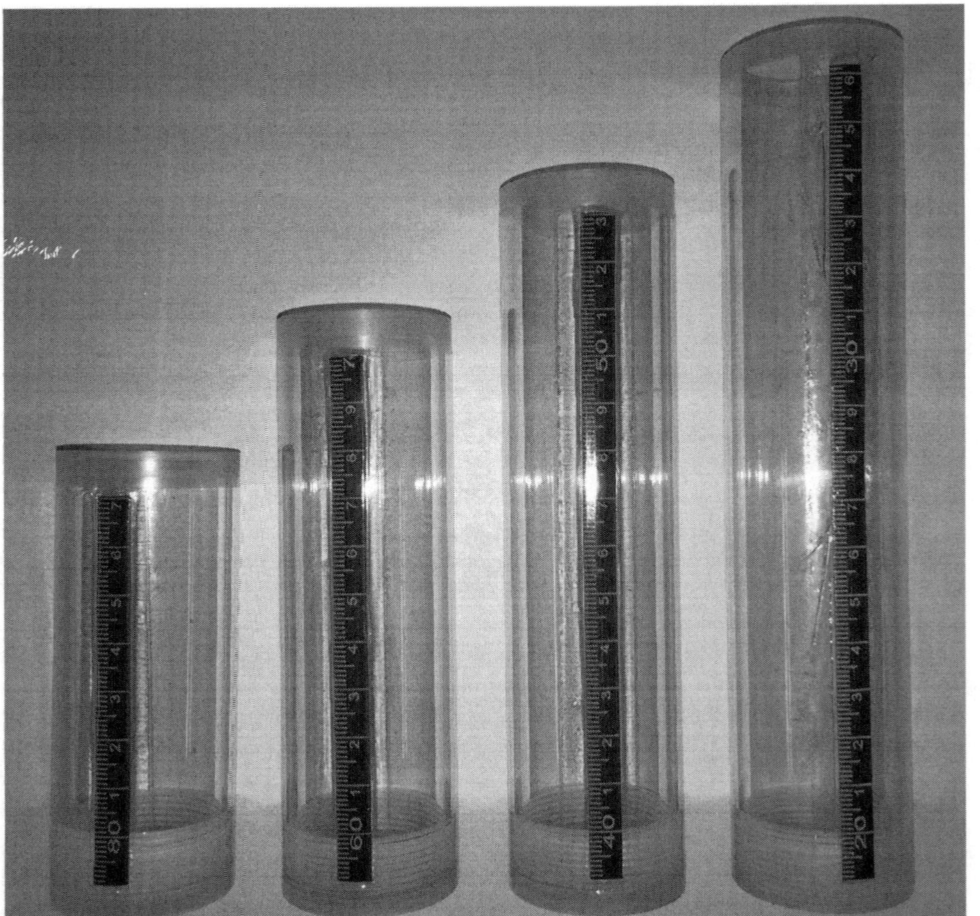

Figure 20.21 The four versions of the S3T model with the four different combinations of outer and inner cylinder lengths used in Arai (2012b).

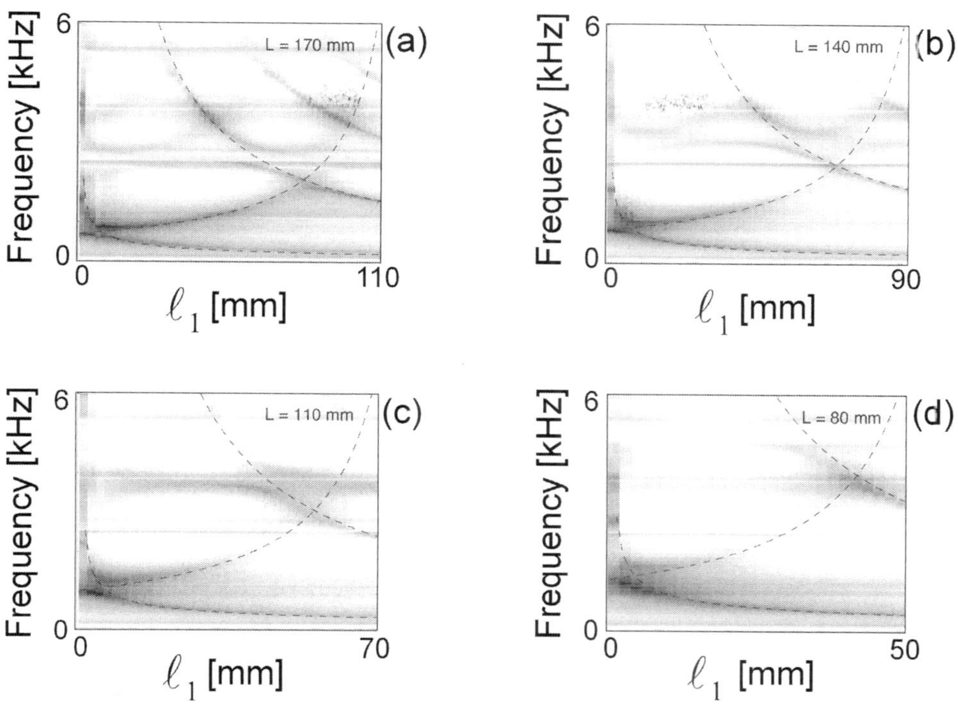

Figure 20.22 Two-dimensional representations of the vowel spectra produced by each of the four S3T models (frequency vs. the length of the back cavity). The horizontal axes are scaled. (a) L = 170 mm, (b) L = 140 mm, (c) L = 110 mm, and (d) L = 80 mm.

Source: Adopted from Arai (2012b).

As shown in Figure 20.22, as L decreased, the formant frequencies increased (the dashed lines show the three underlying resonance curves from Section 37). The same study also confirmed that good vowel quality was retained when the vocal-tract length and the fundamental frequency were inversely related.

Interaction between source and filter

In source-filter theory, we model speech sounds as a response of a linear filter. Nonlinear interaction between source and filter has been reported in several studies (e.g., Titze et al., 2008; Titze, 2008). Although the source-filter theory yields a good approximation in general, we also have to keep in mind that it is just an approximation, and it is possible to come across cases where such approximation is no longer valid.

The interaction phenomenon between source and filter is easily observed with physical models, especially when the fundamental frequency, f_0, and the first formant frequency, F_1, are close to each other. Figure 20.23 shows a spectrographic representation of an output sound with VTM-T20-u when f_0 decreases. Because the F_1 frequency is low (200–300 Hz) for /u/, this sound has a gap around the region where f_0 drops in that frequency range. In other words, a decreasing chirp sound fades out suddenly and comes back with a dropped pitch around the timing indicated the arrow in this figure.

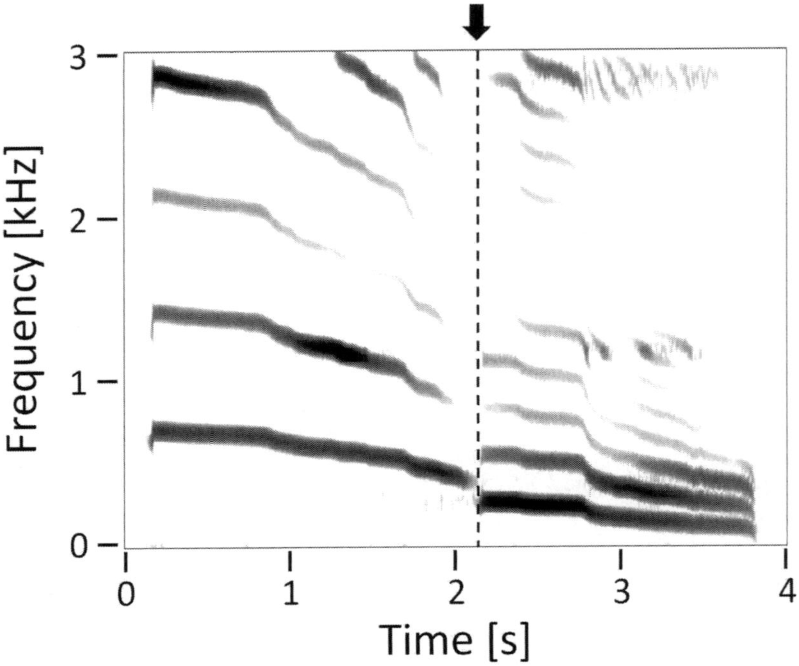

Figure 20.23 Spectrogram of an output sound with VTM-T20-u when f_0 decreases.

Nasalization

When we produce an "oral" vowel, the pharyngeal cavity only couples with the oral cavity. In other words, the velum is raised and the velopharyngeal port is closed. When we breathe naturally, however, the nasal cavity couples with the pharyngeal cavity, so that the air flows through nose. Therefore, the velum acts as a valve for velopharyngeal coupling. When we produce a vowel when the velum is open, the resulting sound is nasalized. In some languages, nasalization is phonemically contrastive (nasal vs. non-nasal vowels).

Figure 20.24 shows the head-shaped model (VTM-HS) for the vowel /a/ with the nasal cavity. This model has a moveable velum that can be used to simulate the effect of nasal coupling. In the following experiment (Arai and Budhiantho, 2015), we measured (a) the response of only the nasal cavity and (b) the response of the head-shaped /a/ model with various degrees of velopharyngeal opening. For the type (a) measurement, we prepared an independent model of the nasal cavity only, with exactly the same nasal cavity configuration as the one in Figure 20.24. With this model, the input hole was the position where the velopharyngeal port was originally located.

We measured the models using a multiple swept-sine signal fed to the driver unit (TOA, TU-750) of a horn speaker through a power amplifier (Onkyo, MA-500U). The swept-sine signal is a chirp tone, and its frequency increases or decreases as a function of time. Acoustic responses from the models were captured using the microphone attached to a sound level meter (Rion, NL-32). The microphone was positioned on an axis approximately 200 mm away at the height of the nostril of the models.

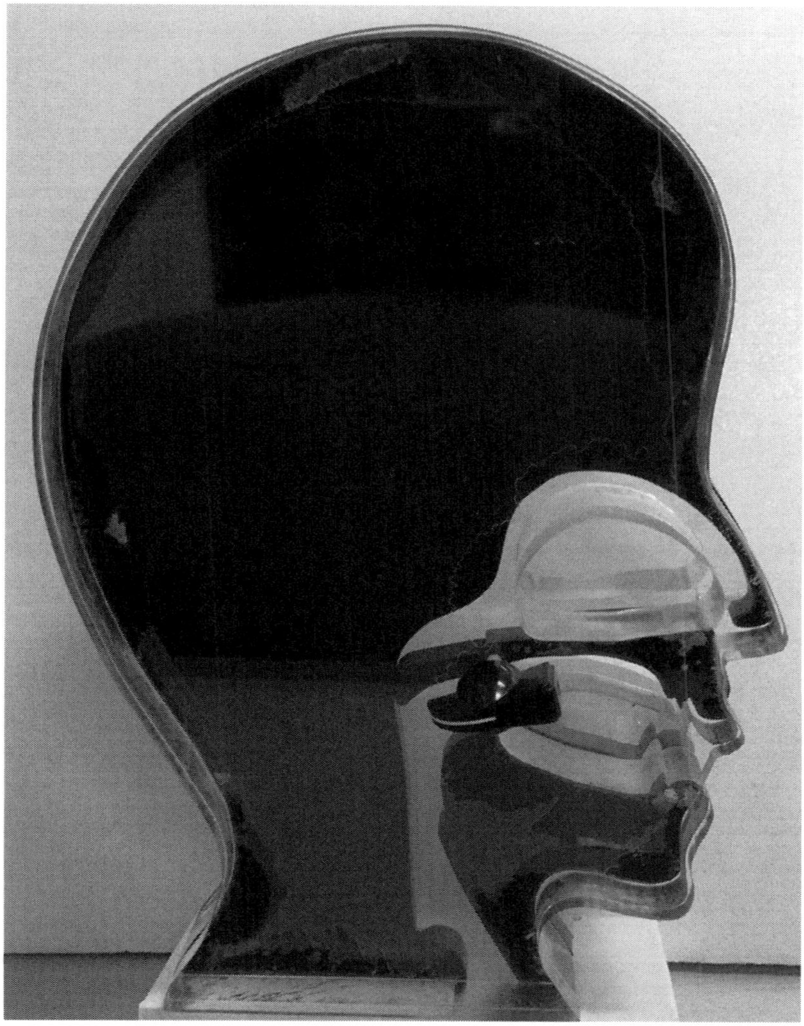

Figure 20.24 Head-shaped model (VTM-HS) of /a/ with the nasal cavity.

We used an external digital audio interface (Roland, UA-25EX) both to supply the excitation signal from the PC and to take the signal response from the microphone to the PC. A sampling frequency of 48 kHz and a 16-bit quantization were used in the signal processing of the measurements. The responses of the head-shaped /a/ model were measured from the closed velopharyngeal opening of 0° to a maximum opening of 40° in 10° increments.

From this measurement, the lowest resonance frequency of the nasal cavity model was approximately 482 Hz. Figure 20.25 shows the frequency responses of the head-shaped /a/ model as the velopharyngeal opening increases. The frequency responses in this figure reveal that (a) the F_1 frequency increases but its amplitude decreases, (b) the peak frequency around 500 Hz (nasal formant) increases, and its amplitude also increases, and (c) an anti-resonance dip (anti-formant) starts to appear around 800 Hz.

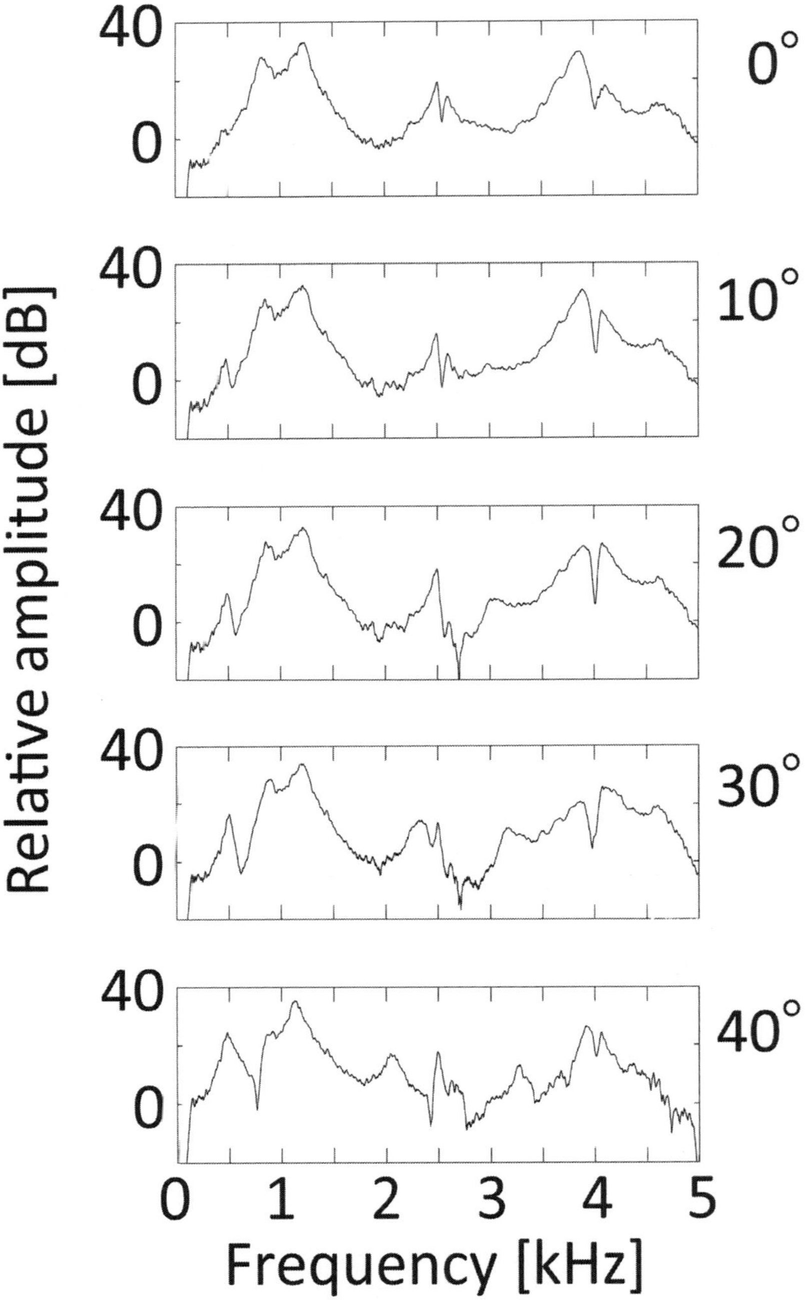

Figure 20.25 Frequency responses of the head-shaped /a/ model with increasing velopharyngeal opening from 0° to 40° in 10° increments (plotted by shifting 20 dB apart).

Producing consonants

As shown in Figure 20.4, the VTM family also has models for consonants. When the tongue is struck against the palate with a single muscle contraction, a flap or tap is produced. VTM-FL is designed for making a flap sound (Arai, 2013b). The front part of the tongue can rotate against the alveolar ridge. With this model, it is possible to produce a quick flapping tongue motion because the return motion of the lever for the rotation is boosted by a spring or rubber band.

VTM-AP (Arai, 2013b) is another model in which the tongue can rotate against the palate. It is designed for approximants, such as the alveolar lateral approximant (English /l/) and the retroflex approximant (English /r/). With this model, the length of the tongue is variable. If the tongue is extended, the tongue tip is made to touch the alveolar ridge by rotating the lever. Although there is contact between the tongue and alveolar ridge, there are still lateral pathways along both sides of the tongue. This simulates the alveolar lateral approximant. If the tongue is short, it does not touch the palate, which is how this model simulates alveolar/retroflex approximants.

Approximants are produced when the articulators come close together. When we produce an alveolar or retroflex approximant, such as English /r/, the tongue tip moves towards the alveolar ridge or the palate. However, the tongue tip does not touch anywhere. When we produce an alveolar lateral approximant, such as English "clear" /l/, the tongue tip touches and remains on the alveolar ridge. However, the sides of the tongue do not make contact with the articulators, so the airstream flows laterally along both sides of the tongue.

Another version of English /r/ is produced by bunching the tongue. Therefore, Arai (2014) developed another model for bunched /r/, or VTM-BR. This model consists of sliding blocks for the lips and tongue. The narrow constriction placed between 5 and 7 cm from the lips seems to be the key to producing bunched /r/. Bunched /r/ with lip rounding produce a clearer /r/ sound (enhancing gesture). Note that English /r/ is produced with the articulatory gesture of tongue root retraction (Zhou et al., 2008). In Arai (2013b) and Arai (2014), the tested sounds were /ra/ with a narrow pharyngeal cavity, where the tongue root was always retracted. It would be worthwhile to test this with a different vowel to see the contribution of the tongue root retraction. In any case, by using both VTM-AP and VTM-BR, we are able to produce the same English /r/ sound with different configurations of the vocal tract. This tells us that the mapping from a sound to a vocal-tract configuration is not a one-to-one mapping, but one-to-many.

Furthermore, the speed of articulators also gives us a different perceptual impression. In other words, for VTM-AP with the extended tongue, when we slowly move the tongue tip against the alveolar ridge and quickly release it back to resting position, it sounds more like a natural /l/ than when it moves back slowly. Also, when we quickly touch the tongue tip against the alveolar ridge it sounds more like a flap sound. This suggests that we can produce the same sounds with different configurations of the vocal tract but similar temporal changes.

Arai (2016a) developed another model for the sounds [b], [m], and [w] (VTM-BMW in Figure 20.4). This model is bent, and it has a nasal cavity. The elastic force of a spring or rubber band is again applied to boost the movement of the lower lip block to achieve more rapid movement. The difference between [b] and [m] is in the velopharyngeal port, which is closed for [b] and open for [m]. With this model, a slower manipulation of the lip block is needed for [w], while [b] and [m] require a faster movement. We can also demonstrate that close-open coordination of the lip and velopharyngeal gestures is important for [m].

We have also developed a fricative model, such as VTM-FR in Figure 20.4. With this model, one can blow air from the glottal end, and because of the constriction at the alveolar ridge, a jet stream comes out from a narrow hole, and it hits a half-closed thin plate simulating the teeth. As a result, a fricative sound, for example [s] in this case, can be produced. However, the sound quality is not yet as clear as a natural speech sound; fricative models will have to be improved in the future.

Although VTM-FT was originally designed for producing vowels, it can also produce consonants. This is possible because the tongue is made of a flexible material, and it mimics human speech production. VTM-FT and several other models in Figure 20.4 are designed for manual manipulation, but some readers might wonder whether it makes sense from a physiological point of view. To this question one might consider "Glove-Talk" proposed by Fels and Hinton (1993, 1997). With Glove-Talk, speech sounds were synthesized by physical movements of the hands mapped to a set of parameters for a formant synthesizer. In our previous study, we also discussed that the VTM-BR can be used for pronunciation training for second language learners (Arai, 2015).

Summary

In this chapter, a series of physical models of the vocal tract and speech articulatory organs were introduced, and basic theories and concepts in acoustic phonetics were reviewed. Some of the models are particularly suited for education, especially for explaining basic acoustic concepts in speech production, such as the source-filter theory and the relationship between vocal-tract configurations and vowel quality. Other models are helpful when second language learners want to differentiate between the vowels or consonants of their native language and those of another language, such as Japanese versus English vowels/consonants, or when they wish to master unfamiliar sounds from another language, such as the collection of /r/ sounds in English. For further information, readers might be interested in reading the following references and the APD website (www.splab.net/APD/).

Acknowledgments

This work was partially supported by JSPS KAKENHI Grant Numbers 18K02988, 15K00930, 24501063, 21500841, 19500758, 1750060 I would also like to thank members in Arai Laboratory and Phonetics Laboratory of Sophia University and Terri Lander for their support.

References

Arai, T 2001, 'The replication of Chiba and Kajiyama's mechanical models of the human vocal cavity', *Journal of the Phonetic Society of Japan*, 5(2), pp. 31–38.

Arai, T 2004, 'History of Chiba and Kajiyama and their influence in modern speech science', *Proceedings of From Sound to Sense*, MIT Press.

Arai, T 2006, 'Sliding three-tube model as a simple educational tool for vowel production', *Acoustical Science and Technology*, 27(6), pp. 384–388.

Arai, T 2007, 'Education system in acoustics of speech production using physical models of the human vocal tract', *Acoustical Science and Technology*, 28(3), pp. 190–201.

Arai, T 2012a, 'Education in acoustics and speech science using vocal-tract models', *The Journal of the Acoustical Society of America*, 131(3), pp. 2444–2454.

Arai, T 2012b, 'Vowels produced by sliding three-tube model with different lengths', *Proceedings of Interspeech*, Portland.
Arai, T 2013a, 'Mechanical models of the human vocal tract', *Acoustics Today*, 9(4), pp. 25–30.
Arai, T 2013b, 'Physical models of the vocal tract with a flapping tongue for flap and liquid sounds', *Proceedings of Interspeech*, pp. 2019–2202.
Arai, T 2014, 'Retroflex and bunched English /r/ with physical models of the human vocal tract', *Proceedings of Interspeech*, pp. 706–710.
Arai, T 2015, 'Hands-on tool producing front vowels for phonetic education: Aiming for pronunciation training with tactile sensation', *Proceedings of Interspeech*, pp. 1695–1699.
Arai, T 2016a, 'Mechanical production of [b], [m] and [w] using controlled labial and velopharyngeal gestures', *Proceedings of Interspeech*, pp. 1029–1103.
Arai, T 2016b, 'Vocal-tract models and their applications in education for intuitive understanding of speech production', *Acoustical Science and Technology*, 37(4), pp. 148–156.
Arai, T 2018, 'Sliding two-tube model for vowel production', *Proceedings of the Autumn Meeting, Acoustical Society of Japan*, pp. 805–806.
Arai T & Budhiantho M 2015, 'Education in acoustics of nasalized vowels using physical models of the human vocal tract with nasal cavity', *Proceedings of the Spring Meeting, Acoustical Society of Japan*, pp. 1291–1294.
Carré, R 2004, 'From an acoustic tube to speech production', *Speech Communication*, 42, pp. 227–240.
Chiba, T & Kajiyama, M 1941–1942, *The Vowel: Its Nature and Structure*, Kaiseikan, Tokyo.
Dang, J & Honda, K 1995, 'Acoustic effects of the pyriform fossa on vowel spectra', *Technical Report of IEICE*, SP95-10, pp. 1–6.
Denes, PB & Pinson EN 1993, *The Speech Chain: The Physics and Biology of Spoken Language*, 2nd edn, W. H. Freeman, New York, p. 199.
Dudley, H & Tarnoczy, TH 1950, 'The speaking machine of Wolfgang von Kempelen', *The Journal of the Acoustical Society of America*, 22, pp. 151–166.
Ehrenfest, P 1916, 'Adiabatische Invarianten und Quantentheorie', *Annalen der Physik*, 356, pp. 327–352 (Citation from Schroeder, MR 1976, *The Journal of the Acoustical Society of America*, 41, pp. 1002–1010.).
Espy-Wilson, CY, Boyce, SE, Jackson, M, Narayanan, S & Alwan, A 2000, 'Acoustic modeling of American English /r/', *The Journal of the Acoustical Society of America*, 108(1), pp. 343–356.
Fant, G 1960, *Acoustic Theory of Speech Production*, Mouton, The Hague, Netherlands.
Fant, G, Liljencrants, J & Lin, QG 1985, 'A four-parameter model of glottal flow', *STL-QPSR*, 2, pp. 1–1.
Fels, SS & Hinton, GE 1993, 'Glove-talk: A neural network interface between a data-glove and a speech synthesizer', *IEEE Transactions on Neural Networks*, 4, pp. 2–8.
Fels, SS & Hinton, GE 1997, 'Glove-talk II-A neural-network interface which maps gestures to parallel formant speech synthesizer controls', *IEEE Transactions on Neural Networks*, 9, pp. 205–212.
Flanagan, JL 1965, *Speech Analysis, Synthesis and Perception*, Springer-Verlag, Berlin.
Gardner, WH & Harris, HE 1961, 'Aids and devices for laryngectomees', *Archives of Otolaryngology*, 73, pp. 145–152.
Gick, B, Wilson, I & Derrick, D 2013, *Articulatory Phonetics*. Wiley-Blackwell, Malden, MA.
Gold, B & Morgan, N 2000, *Speech and Audio Signal Processing*, John Wiley & Sons, New York.
Honda, K, Takemoto, H, Kitamura, T, Fujita, S & Takano, S 2004, 'Exploring human speech production mechanisms by MRI', *IEICE Transactions on Information and Systems*, E87–D, 5, pp. 1050–1058.
Kent, RD & Read C 2001, *Acoustic Analysis of Speech*, Singular Publishing, San Diego, CA.
Korpiun, C 2015, 'Kratzenstein's vowel resonators-reflections on a revival', *Proceedings of International Workshop on the History of Speech Communication Research*, pp. 52–59.
Lebrun, Y, Lissens, D & Lissens-Doms, MC 1973, *The Artificial Larynx*, Swets & Zeitlinger, Amsterdam.
Lindsay, D 1997, 'Talking head', *American Heritage of Invention & Technology*, 13, pp. 56–56.

Maeda, S 1982, 'A digital simulation method of the vocal-tract system', *Speech Communication*, 1, pp. 199–229.

Maekawa, K 2002, 'From articulatory phonetics to the physics of speech: Contribution of Chiba and Kajiyama', *Acoustical Science and Technology*, 23(4), pp. 185–188.

Motoki, K 2002, 'Three-dimensional acoustic field in vocal-tract', *Acoustical Science and Technology*, 23(4), pp. 207–212.

Riches, M 2018, 'Martin Riches', http://martinriches.de/ (Last viewed May 5, 2018).

Riesz, RR 1930, 'Description and demonstration of an artificial larynx', *The Journal of the Acoustical Society of America*, 1(2A), pp. 273–279.

Stevens, KN 1972, 'The quantal nature of speech: Evidence from articulatory-acoustic data', in *Human Communication: A Unified View*, Denes, PB & David Jr, EE (eds), McGraw Hill, New York, pp. 51–66.

Stevens, KN 1989, 'On the quantal nature of speech', *Journal of Phonetics*, 17, pp. 3–46.

Stevens, KN 1998, *Acoustic Phonetics*, MIT Press, Cambridge, MA.

Stevens, KN 2001, 'The Chiba and Kajiyama book as a precursor to the acoustic theory of speech production', *Journal of the Phonetic Society of Japan*, 5(2), pp. 6–7.

Stevens, KN 2005, 'The acoustic/articulatory interface', *Acoustical Science and Technology*, 26(5), pp. 410–417.

Stevens, KN, Kasowski, S & Fant, CGM 1953, 'An electrical analog of the vocal tract', *The Journal of the Acoustical Society of America*, 25, pp. 734–742.

Story, BH 2005, 'A parametric model of the vocal tract area function for vowel and consonant simulation', *The Journal of the Acoustical Society of America*, 117, pp. 3231–3254.

Story, BH, Titze, IR & Hoffman, EA 1996, 'Vocal tract area functions from magnetic resonance imaging', *The Journal of the Acoustical Society of America*, 100, pp. 537–554.

Takemoto, H, Adachi, S, Kitamura, T, Mokhtari, P & Honda, K 2006, 'Acoustic roles of the laryngeal cavity in vocal tract resonance', *The Journal of the Acoustical Society of America*, 120, pp. 2228–2238.

Titze, IR 2008, 'Nonlinear source – filter coupling in phonation: Theory', *The Journal of the Acoustical Society of America*, 123(5), pp. 2733–2749.

Titze, IR, Riede, T & Popolo, P 2008, 'Nonlinear source – filter coupling in phonation: Vocal exercises', *The Journal of the Acoustical Society of America*, 123(4), pp. 1902–1915.

Trouvain, J & Brackhane, F 2011, 'Wolfgang von Kempelen's speaking machine as an instrument for demonstration and research', *Proceedings of International Congress of Phonetic Science*, pp. 164–167.

Umeda, N & Teranishi, R 1966, 'Phonemic feature and vocal feature: Synthesis of speech sounds, using an acoustic model of vocal tract', *Journal of Acoustical Society of Japan*, 22(4), pp. 195–120.

von Kempelen, W 1791, *Mechanismus der menschlichen Sprache und Beschreibung einer sprechenden Machine*, Degen, Wien.

Zhou, X, Espy-Wilson, CY, Boyce, S, Tiede, M, Holland, C & Choe, A 2008, 'A magnetic resonance imaging-based articulatory and acoustic study of "retroflex" and "bunched" American English /r/', *The Journal of the Acoustical Society of America*, 123(6), pp. 4466–4481.

21

Introduction to forensic voice comparison

Geoffrey Stewart Morrison and Ewald Enzinger

Introduction

In a court of law there is sometimes a dispute as to the identity of a speaker on an audio recording. For example, the prosecution contends that the speaker is the defendant, whereas the defense contends that the speaker is not the defendant. Other scenarios are possible; for instance, the issue could be whether the questioned speaker is a kidnap victim. The court may call on a forensic practitioner to compare the recording of the speaker of questioned identity with a recording of the speaker of known identity. The task of the forensic practitioner is to help the court decide whether the voices on the two recordings were produced by the same speaker or by different speakers.

The present chapter provides an introduction to *forensic voice comparison* (aka forensic speaker comparison, forensic speaker recognition, and forensic speaker identification). A general knowledge of phonetics is assumed, but previous knowledge of forensic inference and statistics is not. It is our hope that this chapter can provide phoneticians with a working sense of the challenges faced when conducting forensic voice comparison analyses for presentation in the courtroom. We also wish to address some current controversies concerning how such forensic voice comparison may be best implemented.

Forensic voice comparison is challenging because the quality of speech recordings in casework is often poor and there is often mismatch between the speaking style in and the recording conditions of the known- and questioned-speaker recordings. Recordings may contain only a few seconds of speech, they may include background noise of various sorts (e.g., babble, ventilation system noise, vehicle noise) at varying intensities, they may have been recorded in reverberant environments, they may have been recorded using microphones that are distant from the speaker of interest (e.g., covert microphones, telephone microphones picking up speakers other than the caller), they may have been transmitted through different transmission channels (e.g., landline telephone, mobile telephone, voice over internet protocol) that distort the signal, and they may have been saved in compressed formats (e.g., MP3) that also distort the signal. Mismatches in speaking style and recording conditions can make two recordings of the same speaker appear more different than if they were recorded under the same conditions. Mismatches in recording conditions can also mask or be mistaken for differences due to recordings actually being of different speakers. See Ajili (2017, ch. 3) for a review of the effects of speaker intrinsic and speaker extrinsic factors on the performance of automatic speaker recognition systems.

The present chapter is structured as follows:

- The first section below describes different approaches to extracting information from voice recordings
- The second section describes frameworks for making inferences based on that information
- The third section describes empirical validation
- The fourth section briefly discusses legal admissibility and case law in some common-law jurisdictions

The present chapter has some overlap with Morrison et al. (2018). The latter covers some topics in more detail and also covers other topics not included in the present chapter. The present chapter covers some material not included in the latter, including discussion of the UK framework and of legal admissibility in Canada.

Approaches to forensic voice comparison

We use the term *approaches* to refer to broadly different ways of extracting information from speech recordings. Historical and current practice in forensic voice comparison can be described in terms of four different approaches:

- auditory
- spectrographic
- acoustic-phonetic
- automatic

This section describes the different approaches, then presents information about their popularity. Many practitioners use combinations of approaches, e.g., auditory-spectrographic or auditory-acoustic-phonetic, but for simplicity we will describe each approach separately.

We will make a distinction between modes of practice in which the conclusion as to the strength of evidence is directly based on subjective judgment (subjective mode), and in which it is based on relevant data, quantitative measurements, and statistical models (statistical mode). Auditory and spectrographic approaches are intrinsically subjective, automatic approaches intrinsically statistical, and acoustic-phonetic approaches can be practiced in either a subjective or a statistical mode.

Auditory approaches

Auditory approaches, as the name implies, are based on listening. The practitioner listens to the known- and questioned-speaker recordings in search of similarities in speech properties that they would expect if the two recordings were produced by the same speaker but not if they were produced by different speakers, and in search of differences in speech properties that they would expect if the two recordings were produced by different speakers but not if they were produced by the same speaker. Properties that a practitioner attends to may include vocabulary choice, pronunciation of particular words and phrases, segmental pronunciation, intonation patterns, stress patterns, speaking rate, and voice source properties. Practitioners who have training in auditory phonetics can transcribe and describe segmental and suprasegmental properties, including attributing putative articulatory or physiological origins of what they perceive auditorily.

Some (perhaps most) practitioners listen only to the known- and questioned-speaker recordings, and rely on their training and experience to make judgments as to whether perceived differences are more likely to be due to same- or different-speaker origin. Some practitioners also listen to a set of *foil speakers*, i.e., speakers who sound broadly similar to the known and questioned speakers (including same sex, language spoken, and accent spoken), speaking in a similar speaking style and under similar recording conditions. One approach, known as *blind grouping* (see Cambier-Langeveld et al., 2014) is for one practitioner to prepare recordings of foil speakers, and present the known-speaker, questioned-speaker, and foil recordings to a second practitioner without telling the second practitioner the origin of each recording or how many speakers there are total. Each original recording may have been cut into a number of smaller recordings, and the recordings presented to the second practitioner are randomly labeled. The task of the second practitioner is to group the recordings by speaker. The correctness of grouping of foil speakers serves as a test of performance. Care must be taken so that the speaking style, linguistic content, or recording conditions of the known- and questioned-speaker recordings do not make them stand out relative to the foil recordings.

Descriptions of the auditory approach are provided in: Nolan (1997), Rose (2002), Nolan (2005), Jessen (2008), Hollien (2016), Hollien et al. (2016).

Spectrographic approaches

Practitioners of *spectrographic approaches* visually compare spectrograms of words or phrases that occur in both the known- and questioned-speaker recordings. Some protocols require the known speaker to be recorded saying the same phrases in the same speaking style as on the questioned-speaker recording. Practitioners look for similarities in the spectrograms that they would expect if the two recordings were produced by the same speaker but not if they were produced by different speakers, and for differences that they would expect if the two recordings were produced by different speakers but not if they were produced by the same speaker. Practitioners rely on their training and experience to make judgments as to whether differences they perceive between the known- and questioned-speaker spectrograms are more likely to be due to same- or different-speaker origin. Practitioners may attend to segmental and suprasegmental properties visible in the spectrograms, including fundamental frequency (f_0), formants, spectral tilt, word duration, and the effect of nasal anti-resonances (American Board of Recorded Evidence, 1999). Rather than documenting multiple visually perceptible properties, some practitioners use a Gestalt approach (Poza & Begault, 2005).

As with auditory approaches, some practitioners (perhaps most) only look at spectrograms from the known- and questioned-speaker recordings, but some also look at spectrograms from foil speakers (the latter is advocated in Gruber & Poza, 1995; Poza & Begault, 2005).

In the early 1970s, there was a debate about whether a visual only or a visual plus auditory approach was better. *Auditory-spectrographic approaches* (aka *aural-spectrographic approaches*) won out. Spectrographic/auditory-spectrographic approaches have also been called "voiceprint" or "voicegram" approaches. The term "voiceprint" has been criticized as suggesting a false analogy with fingerprint. Whereas fingerprints are images of friction ridge patterns which are relatively stable anatomical features, spectrograms are not images of anatomical features and the acoustic properties that are graphically represented in spectrograms are subject to considerable variation due to speaker behavior and recording conditions. In the 1960s and 1970s, unsubstantiated claims of near-perfect performance were made by some advocates of spectrographic approaches, and the term "voiceprint" fell into disrepute.

Descriptions of the spectrographic approach are provided in: Kersta (1962), Tosi (1979); and National Research Council (1979). There has been substantial controversy surrounding the use of the spectrographic approach. Reviews of the controversy around its use and admissibility are included in: Gruber and Poza (1995), Solan and Tiersma (2003), Meuwly (2003a, 2003b), Morrison (2014), and Morrison and Thompson (2017).

Acoustic-phonetic approaches

Practitioners of *acoustic-phonetic approaches* may examine many of the same acoustic properties that practitioners of auditory and spectrographic approaches examine via auditory or visual perception, but practitioners of acoustic-phonetic approaches make quantitative measurements of those acoustic properties. The most widely used acoustic-phonetic properties are fundamental frequency and formant frequencies, but quantitative measurements can also be made of voice onset time (VOT), fricative spectra, nasal spectra, voice source properties, speaking rate, etc. (Gold & French, 2011; French & Stevens, 2013). A common approach involves first finding and marking the beginning and end of realizations of particular phonemes or of major allophones of particular phonemes, for example, all tokens of /i/ or all tokens of /aɪ/ not adjacent to a nasal, lateral, rhotic, or labiovelar. Human-supervised formant measurements are then made using the same sort of signal-processing algorithms and procedures as are used in acoustic-phonetic research in general, e.g., linear predictive coding (LPC) plus a peak picking algorithm with the optimal number of LPC coefficients selected by the human supervisor. Measurements may be made at multiple points in time during the vowel to capture information about formant trajectories.

Since questioned-speaker recordings are often telephone recordings and traditional telephone systems have bandpasses of around 300 Hz – 3.4 kHz, first formant (F_1) frequencies close to 300 Hz (e.g., in [i] and [u]) are often distorted, and high frequency spectral information in bursts and fricatives (e.g., in [tʰ] and [s]) is often missing. Fundamental frequency is below the bandpass, but can be recovered from harmonic spacing. Practitioners of acoustic-phonetic approaches have to take such transmission-channel effects into account, especially when there is a mismatch in recording channel between the known- and questioned-speaker recordings. One solution is to not use certain measurements, such as measurements of F_1 in realizations of vowels with intrinsically low F_1; however, even in the middle of the bandpass, the codecs used in mobile telephone systems can distort formants. Zhang et al. (2013) reviewed previous research on the effects of telephone transmission on formants, and tested the effects of landline and mobile telephone transmission on the performance of forensic voice comparison systems.

Once they have made their measurements, some practitioners make tables or plots of the values, and use their training and experience to subjectively assess strength of evidence via examination of those tables or plots. For example, first versus second formant (F_1–F_2) values could be plotted for realizations of a particular vowel phoneme in both the known- and questioned-speaker recording, and the visual degree of overlap considered. Measurements made on recordings of foil speakers may also be plotted.

Other practitioners use their measurements as input to statistical models that calculate quantifications of strength of evidence. Some practitioners directly report the output of the statistical model as a strength of evidence statement, but others use it as input to a subjective judgment process, which may also include consideration of the results of other analyses such as an auditory analysis.

Descriptions of acoustic-phonetic approaches (non-statistical and statistical) are provided in: Nolan (1997), Rose (2002), Hollien (2002), Nolan (2005), Rose (2006), Jessen (2008), Rose (2013), Drygajlo et al. (2015), Rose (2017).

Automatic approaches

Human-supervised *automatic approaches* evolved from signal-processing engineering, and in particular speech processing. Automatic speaker recognition techniques developed for non-forensic applications have been adapted for forensic application. For most security applications the system has to be fully automatic and make a decision. For example, the system must decide to grant or deny a caller access to bank account information without intervention from a human member of staff. Also, the bank client will initially have been cooperative in enrolling sample recordings of their voice, and the bank client can also be asked to cooperate by calling from a quiet location and be asked to say particular words and phrases. In contrast, in forensic application:

- The questioned speaker is generally not cooperative
- The questioned speaker is not trying to be identified and they may not even be aware that they are being recorded
- The recording conditions and speaking styles are much more variable and the quality of the recordings often much poorer
- The output of the system is not a binary decision but a quantification of strength of evidence

Appropriate adaptation of automatic speaker recognition techniques to forensic problems is non-trivial. It requires human-supervised systems in which the practitioner carefully selects relevant data for training and testing so that the output of the system is a meaningful quantification of strength of evidence for the case. Inappropriate use of automatic systems is garbage in garbage out (GIGO).

Traditional automatic approaches do not explicitly exploit acoustic-phonetic, segmental, or suprasegmental information. Instead, they usually make spectral measurements at regular intervals, e.g., once every 10 ms within a 20 ms wide window. Such measurements are usually made throughout the recorded speech of the speaker of interest, and the results are pooled irrespective of whether they originated from vowels or consonants or realizations of particular phonemes. The most commonly made measurements are mel frequency cepstral coefficients (*MFCCs*, see Davis and Mermelstein, 1980). At each point in time, the MFCCs characterize the shape of the spectral envelope using a vector of around 14 numbers. *Deltas*, the rate of change of MFCC values over time, and *double deltas*, the rate of change of delta values over time, are usually appended to produce a vector of around 42 numbers (see Furui, 1986). The measurements made by automatic systems, and the derivatives of those measurements, are known as *features*.

The boundary between acoustic-phonetic and automatic approaches is, however, fuzzy. Some automatic approaches use phone recognizers from automatic speech recognition systems to model information related to specific phones or phone classes (e.g., vowels, fricatives, nasal consonants). See Ajili et al. (2016) for an exploration of the effect of excluding particular phone classes on the performance of an automatic forensic voice comparison system. Some systems automatically find voiced segments then automatically measure f_0 and formant frequency values at regular intervals throughout those voiced segments. The latter are called long-term formant (LTF) values (see for example Jessen et al., 2014). Some practitioners of acoustic-phonetic approaches mark realizations of particular phonemes, but then make MFCC measurements within those realizations. Using around 14 MFCC values provides more information about the spectrum than f_0 plus two or three formant values.

The measurements made in automatic approaches are invariably used as input to statistical models. The statistical modeling approaches used in forensic voice comparison (and automatic speaker recognition more broadly) have evolved over the last 20 years. An approach known as *GMM-UBM* (Gaussian mixture model–universal background model) was introduced around 2000 (Reynolds et al., 2000), and another approach known as *i-vector PLDA* (identity vector probabilistic linear discriminant analysis) was introduced around 2010 (Dehak et al., 2011; Prince and Elder, 2007). Current state of the art in automatic speaker recognition research makes use of *DNNs* (deep neural networks; e.g., Richardson et al., 2015), and these are beginning to be adopted for forensic application. GMM-UBM, i-vector PLDA, and DNN-based systems can be considered systems that output *scores*. Scores are similar to likelihood ratios (described in the "frameworks" section below) in that they take account of similarity and typicality, but their absolute values are not interpretable. This is not a problem in applications in which a decision is made by comparing a score value to a threshold, but is a problem when the purpose is to provide a strength of evidence statement to the court. *Calibration* can be used to convert scores to interpretable likelihood ratios. It was first used in forensic voice comparison around 2007. A standard statistical modeling approach for calibration is *logistic regression* (see: Pigeon et al., 2000; González-Rodríguez et al., 2007; Morrison, 2013).

A great deal of effort in automatic speaker recognition has focused on developing statistical techniques for dealing with mismatches in speaking styles and recording conditions between known- and questioned-speaker recordings (the statistical techniques are known as *mismatch compensation*, aka channel or session compensation). These techniques include *cepstral mean subtraction* (CMS, see Furui, 1981), *cepstral mean and variance normalization* (CMVN, see Tibrewala and Hermansky, 1997), *feature warping* (Pelecanos and Sridharan, 2001), and *linear discriminant analysis* (LDA). The first three are alternatives applied to features and the latter is usually applied to i-vectors. In automatic speaker recognition, LDA actually usually refers to the use of canonical linear discriminant functions for dimension reduction (see Klecka, 1980) prior to using a different probabilistic classification model.

Some practitioners directly report the output of the statistical model as a strength of evidence statement, but others use it as input to a subjective judgment process, which may also include consideration of the results of other analyses such as auditory and acoustic-phonetic analyses.

Descriptions of automatic approaches are provided in: Ramos Castro (2007), Becker (2012), Enzinger (2016), Marks (2017). For a review of approaches to automatic speaker recognition in general, see Hansen and Hasan (2015).

Popularity of different approaches

Gold and French (2011) published the results of a survey of practitioners working in a mixture of private, university, and law-enforcement or other government laboratories. In the reported results from 35 respondents:

- 2 (6%) used an auditory only approach
- Spectrographic approaches were not mentioned
- 25 (71%) used an auditory-acoustic-phonetic approach
- 1 (3%) used an acoustic-phonetic-only approach
- 7 (20%) used a human-supervised automatic approach

In 2016, INTERPOL published the results of a survey of speaker recognition capabilities of law-enforcement agencies in member countries (Morrison, Sahito et al., 2016). 44 respondents stated that their agency had speaker recognition capabilities. Of these, many reported using more than one approach, hence the following summary statistics add up to more than 44.

- 15 (25%) used an auditory approach
- 21 (34%) used a spectrographic or auditory-spectrographic approach
- 25 (41%) used an auditory-acoustic-phonetic (subjective) approach
- 15 (25%) used an acoustic-phonetic (statistical) approach
- 20 (33%) used a human-supervised automatic approach
- 9 (15%) used a fully automatic approach (Assumed to be for investigative rather than forensic application)

In the results of both surveys (auditory-)acoustic-phonetic approaches were the most popular, with human-supervised automatic approaches second or a close third. In the results of the INTERPOL survey (auditory-)spectrographic approaches were also popular. Auditory-only approaches were the least popular.

The two surveys were separated in time but also solicited responses from different groups, hence one cannot conclude that the differences between them are due to changes in practice.

Frameworks for evaluation of forensic evidence

In contrast to the term *approaches*, which we use to refer to different ways of extracting information from speech recordings, we use the term *frameworks* to refer to different ways of evaluating strength of evidence based on that information. Frameworks therefore refer to ways of reasoning or ways of drawing inferences. Historical and current practice can be described in terms of a number of different frameworks, including:

- Likelihood ratio
- Posterior probability
- Identification/exclusion/inconclusive
- The UK framework

We describe each of these frameworks below, and then give information about their popularity.

Frameworks are mutually exclusive of each other. Most frameworks can be used in a subjective or a statistical mode. In some frameworks strength of evidence can be expressed verbally or as a numeric value. To some extent, frameworks are independent of approaches, e.g., one could use either an acoustic-phonetic-statistical or an automatic approach in combination with either a posterior-probability or a likelihood-ratio framework. In practice, however, certain combinations are more common than others, e.g., a spectrographic approach combined with a verbal posterior-probability framework, an auditory-acoustic-phonetic approach combined with the UK framework, and an automatic approach combined with a numeric likelihood-ratio framework.

Likelihood-ratio framework

The likelihood ratio framework is considered the logically correct framework for the evaluation of forensic evidence by many forensic statisticians, forensic scientists, and legal scholars; see for example: Aitken et al. (2011), Willis et al. (2015), Drygajlo et al. (2015), Morrison, Kaye et al. (2017). General introductions to the likelihood ratio framework include: Aitken et al. (2010); Robertson et al. (2016), Balding and Steele (2015, chs. 1–3 and 11). Introductions in the context of forensic voice comparison include: Rose (2002), Morrison and Thompson (2017), Morrison et al. (2018).

Similarity is not enough

Just considering the degree of similarity of the voices on the known- and questioned-speaker recordings is not enough to quantify strength of evidence. Imagine that we measured the mean fundamental frequency of the voices on two recordings and found that they differed by 5 Hz. Would that indicate that the two recordings are of the same speaker? Would it indicate that it is highly probable that the two recordings are of the same speaker? You will probably answer "no" or "it depends." The two recorded voices are very similar on this metric, there is only a 5 Hz difference between them, but we have to consider whether that 5 Hz difference is more likely to occur because it really is the same speaker or more likely to occur by chance. How do we assess this? Our discussion below focuses on answering this question using *relevant data*, *quantitative measurements*, and *statistical models*.

Histogram models

Imagine that we have multiple recordings of the known speaker (N_k recordings total) and we measure the mean fundamental frequency in each recording. We will designate each of these values an x_{k_i} value, $i \in 1 \ldots N_k$. Let's begin with a simple statistical model based on the proportion of the x_{k_i} values that fall into 10 Hz wide ranges, e.g., what proportion of the x_{k_i} values are greater than 90 Hz and less than or equal to 100 Hz, what proportion are greater than 100 Hz and less than or equal to 110 Hz, etc. We can represent the results as a histogram as in Figure 21.1 (top panel darker rectangles).[1] We will draw the histogram such that the *area* of each rectangle represents the proportion of measurements falling within the range of x values which it covers. Since each rectangle represents a proportion of the whole, the sum of the areas of all of the rectangles must be 1. We can now use the histogram as a statistical model. We use the proportions as estimates of probability. We can use the model to estimate the probability that the mean fundamental frequency of a recording would have

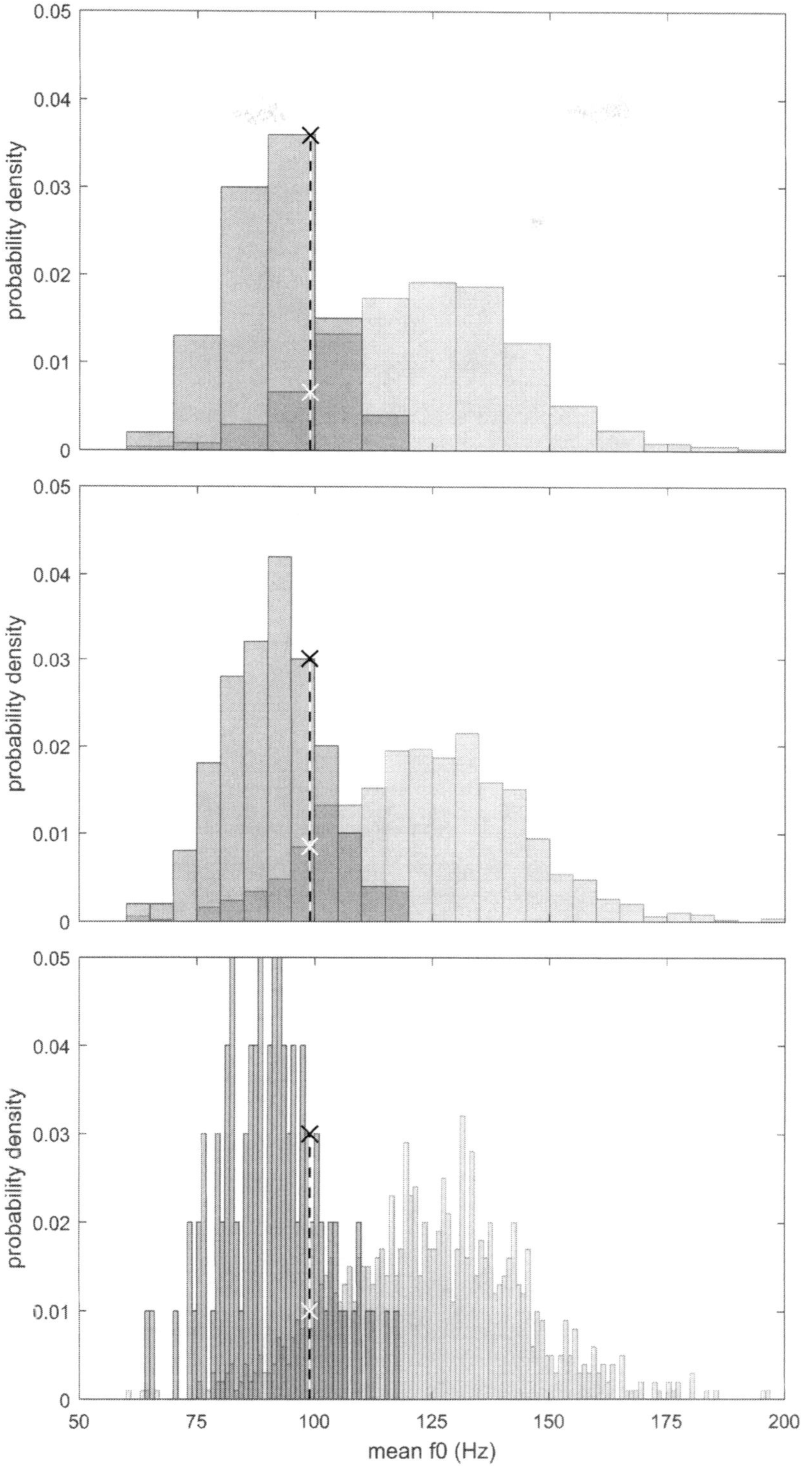

Figure 21.1 Histogram models for likelihood ratio calculation. The same data are modeled using histograms with different rectangle widths, i.e., from top to bottom: 10 Hz, 5 Hz, 1 Hz.

a value within a specified 10 Hz wide range if it were produced by the known speaker. Imagine that the mean fundamental frequency of the voice on the questioned-speaker recording, x_q, is 99 Hz. This falls in the range of greater than 90 Hz and less than or equal to 100 Hz. The area of the rectangle corresponding to this range, and hence the estimated probability of a value falling in this range if it were produced by the known speaker is 0.0360. This gives us a quantification of the *similarity* between the voice on the questioned-speaker recording and the known speaker's voice.

We also need to consider the probability of getting an x_q value of 99 Hz if the questioned speaker were not the known speaker but some other speaker selected at random from the relevant population. We will discuss the concept of relevant population in a later subsection. For now let us assume that the relevant population is adult males. We obtain recordings of a large number (N_r) of adult male speakers. This is a sample of the relevant population. For the recording of each speaker we measure the mean fundamental frequency, $x_{r_j}, j \in 1 \ldots N_r$. We then construct a histogram for these data in the same way as we did for the data from the known speaker. This is shown in Figure 21.1 (top panel lighter rectangles). We use the second histogram as our statistical model to estimate the probability that the x_q value would fall within the range greater than 90 Hz and less than or equal to 100 Hz if it came from a speaker selected at random from the relevant population. In this example, that value is 0.0066. This provides a quantification of the *typicality* of the voice on the questioned-speaker recording with respect to the relevant population.

We are now in a position to answer a question which has two parts:

- What is the probability of getting the measured property of the voice on the questioned-speaker recording if it came from the known speaker? (What is the degree of *similarity*?)

versus

- What is the probability of getting the measured property of the voice on the questioned-speaker recording if it came not from the known speaker but from a speaker selected at random from the relevant population? (What is the degree of *typicality*?)

If we divide the answer to the first part (the similarity part) by the answer to the second part (the typicality part), we get the ratio of the two, and we can say that we estimate that the probability of getting the measured property of the voice on the questioned-speaker recording is $0.0360/0.0066 = 5.45$ times higher if it came from the known speaker than if it came from some other speaker selected at random from the relevant population.

We can rephrase the two questions above as hypotheses:

- The measured property of the voice on the questioned-speaker recording (the evidence) came from the known speaker.

versus

- The measured property of the voice on the questioned-speaker recording (the evidence) came not from the known speaker but from a speaker selected at random from the relevant population.

For brevity, we will refer to these as the *same-speaker hypothesis* and *different-speaker hypothesis* respectively, and we will use the term *evidence* to refer to the measurement (or measurements) made on the questioned-speaker recording.

Note that using the model described above, we would have gotten the same result had x_q been any value between 90 and 100 Hz, but if the mean of the x_{k_i} were 90 Hz then perhaps the strength of evidence should be lower if x_q is toward the top of the 90–100 Hz range than if it is toward the bottom (further from the known-speaker mean rather than closer). We could address this by making the ranges of the rectangles in our histograms narrower. For example, in Figure 21.1, the middle and bottom panels have rectangles of widths 5 Hz and 1 Hz respectively. Using these histograms, the corresponding estimates of the probability of getting the measured property of the voice on the questioned-speaker recording if it came from the known speaker versus if it came from some other speaker selected at random from the relevant population are $0.0300/0.0084 = 3.57$ and $0.0300/0.0100 = 3.00$, respectively.

If we continue to make the widths of the rectangles narrower and narrower, however, we will eventually run into a problem. Because we are using proportions it does not matter exactly how many known-speaker recordings and how many relevant-population sample recordings we have, and we do not have to have the same number of each, but we do have to have a sufficient number of measurements in each rectangle for the proportions to be reasonable estimates of probability. Assuming we have a limited number of recordings that are a sample of the known speaker's speech, and a limited number of recordings which are a sample of the speech of speakers from the relevant population, as we make the rectangles narrower fewer and fewer x_{k_i} and x_{r_j} values will fall within each rectangle, and the quality of the estimate of the probability for each rectangle will deteriorate. At the extreme, most rectangles would have a zero count and some would have a count of one. The problem is already apparent in the bottom panel of Figure 21.1.

Parametric statistical models (Gaussian distributions)

A solution to the problem described at the end of the previous subsection is to use a parametric model. If we are willing to assume that the data have a Gaussian distribution (a normal distribution), then we can get relatively good parameter estimates (estimates of the mean and variance) using comparatively little data compared to the amount of data we would need to make a high resolution non-parametric histogram. We calculate the sample means $\hat{\mu}_k$ and $\hat{\mu}_r$ and sample variances $\hat{\sigma}_k^2$ and $\hat{\sigma}_r^2$ from the x_{k_i} and from the x_{r_j} values. This gives us the statistics (the parameter estimates) necessary to define the two Gaussian distribution models plotted in Figure 21.2: $y_k = f\left(x|\hat{\mu}_k, \hat{\sigma}_k^2\right)$ and $y_r = f\left(x|\hat{\mu}_r, \hat{\sigma}_r^2\right)$, where $f\left(x|\mu, \sigma^2\right)$ is the Gaussian probability density function (these were trained on the same simulated data used to train the histograms in Figure 21.1). Note that just as the total area of a histogram is 1, the area under the curve for each Gaussian distribution is 1. If we calculate the area under the curve within a range of values, e.g., greater than 90 Hz and less than or equal to 100 Hz, or greater than 98.5 Hz and less than or equal to 99.5 Hz, then we have an estimate of the probability of a value falling within that range. But if we pick an exact value, e.g., 99 Hz, then the width of that range is zero and the area is therefore zero. The y-axis value for the curve at an exact value is not zero, but the y value does not represent probability – it represents a quantity known as *probability density* or *likelihood*. At the value of the evidence, x_q, we assess the likelihood of the known-speaker model, $y_{q,k} = f\left(x_q|\hat{\mu}_k, \hat{\sigma}_k^2\right)$ (this quantifies similarity), and the likelihood of the relevant-population model, $y_{q,r} = f\left(x_q|\hat{\mu}_r, \hat{\sigma}_r^2\right)$ (this quantifies typicality), and we divide the former by the latter. The result is a *likelihood ratio*, which is a quantification of the strength of evidence. In this case we estimate that the likelihood of the evidence is $y_{q,k} / y_{q,r} = 0.0279 / 0.0089 = 3.12$ times higher if it came from the known speaker than if it came from some other speaker selected at random from the relevant population.[2]

Note that if we keep the degree of similarity the same, but reduce the degree of typicality, then the value of the likelihood ratio increases: see Figure 21.3 top left panel, in which $\hat{\mu}_r$ has been increased by 10 Hz relative to its value in Figure 21.2. The value of the likelihood ratio is 6.68.

Vice versa, if typicality increases the value of the likelihood ratio decreases: see Figure 21.3 top right panel, in which $\hat{\mu}_r$ has been decreased by 10 Hz relative to its value in Figure 21.2. The value of the likelihood ratio is 1.88.

Also, if we keep the degree of typicality the same, but the degree of similarity increases the value of the likelihood ratio increases: see Figure 21.3 bottom left panel, in which $\hat{\mu}_k$ has been increased by 10 Hz relative to its value in Figure 21.2. The value of the likelihood ratio is 4.12. In contrast, if similarity decreases the value of the likelihood ratio decreases: see Figure 21.3 bottom right panel, in which $\hat{\mu}_k$ has been decreased by 10 Hz relative to its value in Figure 21.2. The value of the likelihood ratio is 0.99.[3] The value of the likelihood ratio would also change if the value of x_q changed.

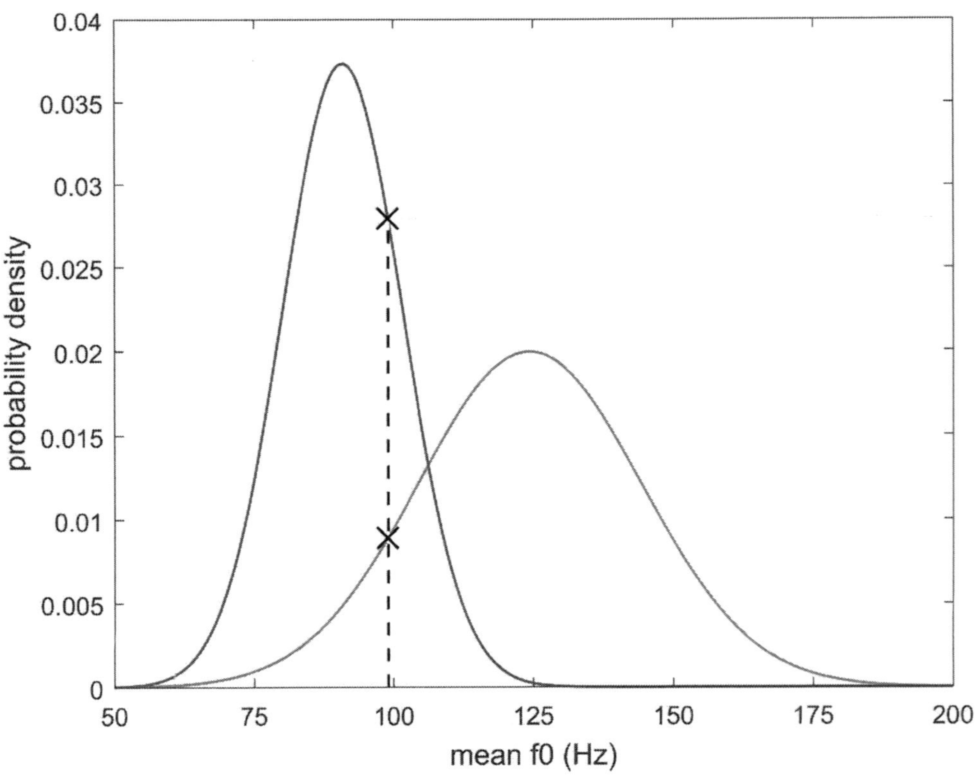

Figure 21.2 Gaussian distributions for likelihood ratio calculation. The distributions were fitted to the same data as represented by the histograms in Figure 21.1.

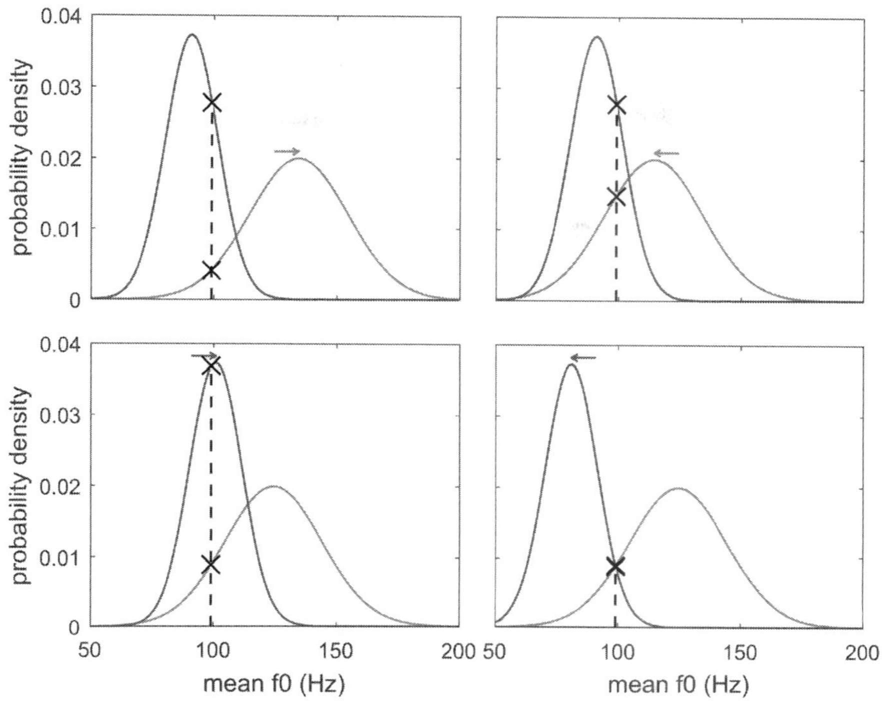

Figure 21.3 Gaussian distributions for likelihood ratio calculation. The distributions are shifted relative to Figure 21.2 in order to represent different degrees of typicality (top row) and different degrees of similarity (bottom row).

Statistical models are not restricted to univariate measurements and can be applied to multivariate measurements. In addition, statistical models are not restricted to Gaussian distributions, and much more complex distributions can be fitted. In both acoustic-phonetic statistical and automatic approaches, the data are usually multidimensional and have complex distributions. Multivariate Gaussian mixture models are used in both GMM-UBM and i-vector PLDA.

What does a likelihood ratio mean?

Likelihood ratios can have values that are > 1 or < 1. If the value of the likelihood ratio is > 1, then the evidence is more probable if the same-speaker hypothesis were true than if the different-speaker hypothesis were true. If the value of the likelihood ratio is < 1, then the evidence is more probable if the different-speaker hypothesis were true than if the same-speaker hypothesis were true. But, importantly, what matters is not just whether a likelihood ratio is > or < 1, but how far away it is from 1. The further the value from 1 the greater the strength of evidence.

What does the value of a likelihood ratio mean? From a normative perspective it is the amount by which the trier of fact (the judge or the jury depending on the legal system) should change their belief regarding the relative probabilities of the same- and different-speaker hypotheses.[4]

Before the trier of fact is presented with the forensic voice comparison testimony, they have some belief as to the relative probability that the speaker on the questioned recording will be the defendant versus that the speaker on the questioned recording will be some other speaker. A simplistic example assumes a crime committed on an island of 101 inhabitants. One of the islanders is the defendant and the trier of fact assumes that innocent until proven guilty implies that before considering any evidence the defendant is no more or less likely to be the questioned speaker than any other inhabitant of the island. The prior probability that the defendant is the questioned speaker is therefore 1/101 and the prior probability that someone else is the questioned speaker is 100/101 (1/101 for each inhabitant multiplied by the 100 inhabitants other than the defendant). The ratio of these is (1/101)/(100/101) = 1/100. The ratio of the prior probabilities is called the *prior odds*.

But the trier of fact may have already heard other evidence, and immediately prior to hearing the likelihood ratio from the forensic voice comparison their prior odds may no longer be 1/100. For example, if it is apparent that the voice on the questioned-speaker recording is male, and the defendant is male, and the trier of fact is told that 50% of the other inhabitants of the island are male, then the trier of fact's prior odds before hearing the forensic voice comparison testimony might be 1/50.

Irrespective of the actual value of the trier of fact's prior odds, normatively the trier of fact should update their belief according to the following formula (the *odds form of Bayes' Theorem*):

(1) $$\text{prior odds} \times \text{likelihood ratio} = \text{posterior odds}$$

$$\frac{p(H_s)}{p(H_d)} \times \frac{p(E|H_s)}{p(E|H_d)} = \frac{p(H_s|E)}{p(H_d|E)}$$

$$\frac{1}{100} \times 5 = \frac{5}{100} = \frac{1}{20}$$

$$\frac{1}{50} \times 5 = \frac{5}{50} = \frac{1}{10}$$

In which H_s stands for the same-speaker hypothesis, H_d for the different-speaker hypothesis, and E for the evidence. $p(E|H)$ reads as probability of evidence given hypothesis, and $p(H|E)$ reads as probability of hypothesis given evidence. After the trier of fact has heard the strength of evidence expressed as a likelihood ratio, the *posterior odds* are what their belief should be as to the relative probabilities that the defendant is the questioned speaker versus that someone else on the island is the questioned speaker.

Note that in the two examples at the bottom of Equation 1, the differences in the posterior odds are due to differences in the prior odds. The evidence is the same, the strength of evidence is the same, and the likelihood ratio calculated by the forensic practitioner is the same. Both examples use a likelihood ratio of 5. What the trier of fact should do with the likelihood ratio is the same, irrespective of what their prior odds are. A likelihood ratio has an unambiguous meaning. In the context of forensic voice comparison, it is the amount by which (in light of the evidence) the trier of fact should multiply their prior odds in order to update their belief about the relative probabilities of the same- versus the different-speaker hypotheses being true. With suitable changes in wording, an unambiguous definition of a likelihood ratio can be provided addressing strength of evidence questions in other branches of forensic science.

If the value of the likelihood ratio is > 1, the value of the posterior odds will be more than the value of the prior odds, and if the value of the likelihood ratio is < 1, the value of the posterior odds will be less than the value of the prior odds. In this sense, the likelihood ratio framework is symmetrical, it can lead to higher belief in the probability of the same-speaker hypothesis being true over the different-speaker hypothesis being true, or *vice versa*. Likelihood ratios < 1 are crammed into the range 0 to 1, whereas likelihood ratios > 1 are in the range 1 to infinity. A value < 1 can be inverted along with inversion of the hypotheses, e.g., $p(E|H_s)/p(E|H_d) = 0.001$ is equivalent to $p(E|H_d)/p(E|H_s) = 1000$, and, rather than use a fraction, it is easier to say the probability of the evidence is 1000 times greater if the different-speaker hypothesis were true than if the same-speaker hypothesis were true. For mathematical convenience, log likelihood ratios are often used, e.g., $\log_{10}(0.001) = -3$ and $\log_{10}(1000) = +3$. Likelihood ratios less than 1 convert to log likelihood ratios in the range minus infinity to 0, and likelihood ratios greater than 1 convert to log likelihood ratios in the range 0 to plus infinity. The log-odds version of Bayes' Theorem is additive rather than multiplicative:

(2) log prior odds + log likelihood ratio = log posterior odds

$$\log\left(\frac{p(H_s)}{p(H_d)}\right) + \log\left(\frac{p(E|H_s)}{p(E|H_d)}\right) = \log\left(\frac{p(H_s|E)}{p(H_d|E)}\right)$$

$$\log\big(p(H_s)\big) - \log\big(p(H_d)\big) + \log\big(p(E|H_s)\big) - \log\big(p(E|H_d)\big)$$
$$= \log\big(p(H_s|E)\big) - \log\big(p(H_d|E)\big)$$

Subjective likelihood ratios and verbal expression of likelihood ratios

Based on their training and experience, it should be intuitive for a phonetician that an f_0 of around 120 Hz is typical for an adult male. Thus, if the voices on the known- and questioned-speaker recordings both have values close to 120 Hz, this does not constitute strong evidence in support of the hypothesis that they were both produced by the same speaker rather than by different speakers. In contrast, an f_0 of 70 Hz is atypical. Thus if the voices on the known- and questioned-speaker recordings both have values close to 70 Hz, this does constitute strong evidence in support of the hypothesis that they were both produced by the same speaker rather than by different speakers. Without obtaining an explicit sample of the relevant population and without using a statistical model, it is therefore possible for a phonetician to subjectively assign values to a likelihood ratio. The phonetician could give subjective numeric estimates or could give a verbal expression, e.g., the evidence is much more probable if the same-speaker hypothesis were true than if the different-speaker hypothesis were true. Such statements would be consistent with the logic of the likelihood ratio framework.

The 2015 ENFSI guideline on evaluative reporting (Willis et al., 2015) includes examples of verbal expressions of likelihood ratios, such as shown in Table 21.1. Each expression is associated with a range of numeric likelihood ratio values. Terms such as "much more probable" and "far more probable" are, however, ambiguous. They may be interpreted differently by different people, and even differently by the same person in different contexts.[5]

Table 21.1 Examples of verbal expressions of likelihood ratios and corresponding ranges of numeric likelihood ratio values in the 2015 ENFSI guideline on evaluative reporting.

Verbal Expression			*Range of Values*
The forensic findings are	slightly more more appreciably more much more far more exceedingly more	probable given one proposition relative to the other.	2–10 10–100 100–1000 1000–10,000 10,000–1 million 1 million +

Relevant population

An important issue for calculating a likelihood ratio is: What is the *relevant population*? On listening to the questioned-speaker recording certain things are usually (but not always) obvious, including whether the speaker is male or female, what language they are speaking, and broadly what accent of that language they are speaking. If these are likely to be salient to the trier of fact and unlikely to be disputed by the prosecution or defense, then they can be used for defining the relevant population that the forensic practitioner will adopt. It is important that the forensic practitioner clearly communicate what relevant population they have adopted so that the judge at an admissibility hearing and/or the trier of fact at trial can decide whether it is appropriate, and so that the judge and/or trier of fact can understand what the calculated value of the likelihood ratio means – one cannot understand the answer if one does not understand the question.[6]

In addition, it is important to consider whether the sample is sufficiently representative of the specified relevant population. Part of this consideration is whether the sample is sufficiently large. Also to be considered is whether the sample is biased or is simply of some population other than the specified relevant population. For example, imagine that the questioned speaker and known speaker are adult males with f_0 values of approximately 120 Hz, and that the specified relevant population is adult males, but the sample used is actually a sample of adult females. The f_0 for the known and questioned speakers would be relatively atypical with respect to the distribution of f_0 values in the sample of female speakers. The calculated likelihood ratio value would therefore be large, but this value would be misleading because the question it actually answers involves typicality with respect to the wrong population. The actual question answered would be nonsensical: What is the probability of getting the f_0 of the male on the questioned-speaker recording if it were produced by the male known speaker, versus if it were produced by a female speaker?[7] What the forensic practitioner uses as a sample of the relevant population must be clearly communicated to the judge and/or trier of fact so that ultimately the judge and/or trier of fact can decide whether the sample is sufficiently representative of the relevant population.

Posterior-probability framework

Some practitioners express their conclusions as to strength of evidence as posterior probabilities. These could be generated using statistical models or could be subjectively assigned, and they could be expressed numerically or verbally. For example: "There is a 95% probability that the known speaker is the speaker on the questioned-speaker recording." Expressions of certainty are also posterior probability expressions, e.g., "I am 95% certain that it is the same speaker." The American Board of Recorded Evidence protocols for spectrographic approaches require the use of verbal expressions of posterior probability: "identification," "probable identification," "possible identification," "inconclusive," "possible exclusion," "probable exclusion," "exclusion" (American Board of Recorded Evidence, 1999).

The problem with expressing strength of evidence as a posterior probability is that logically in order to calculate a posterior probability one must consider two things: the likelihood ratio and the prior probability.[8] The forensic practitioner must therefore either use some arbitrary prior, or must assign a prior based on the other evidence in the case that the trier of fact has already heard.

Unless the trier of fact tells the forensic practitioner specific priors to use, the forensic practitioner cannot calculate the appropriate posterior probability. Given current legal practice around the world, it is extremely unlikely that the trier of fact would provide specific priors, and in some jurisdictions this is clearly impossible.

The task of the forensic practitioner is to assess the strength of evidence of the particular materials they have been asked to analyze, independent of any other evidence in the case. It is the task of the trier of fact to consider and combine all the evidence. It would be inappropriate for the forensic practitioner to consider the other evidence in the case. Even knowing about the other evidence could bias the forensic practitioner's conclusion. This would mean that the strength of evidence statement that the forensic practitioner presents to the trier of fact would not be (entirely) new independent information for the trier of fact, and the trier of fact would be in danger of double counting the same information. Cognitive bias is a problem of increasing concern in forensic science (see: Risinger et al., 2002; Saks et al., 2003; National Research Council, 2009; Found, 2015; Stoel et al., 2015; National Commission on Forensic Science, 2015; Edmond et al., 2017).

An arbitrary prior is problematic since if one practitioner used a high value for the prior and another practitioner used a low one, and otherwise acted the same, the difference in the priors would make the value of the first practitioner's posterior probability higher and that of the second lower, but this difference would have nothing to do with the materials they were asked to compare. If the value of the arbitrary prior were not revealed, then the reported posterior probability would be misleading. If the value of the arbitrary prior were revealed along with the value of the posterior, then the value of the likelihood ratio could be recovered, but it would have been much simpler just to present the value of the likelihood ratio in the first place.

It may be the case that practitioners who present posterior probabilities are not aware of the logical problems. Jackson (2009) discusses the problems with posterior probabilities and a range of other ways that have been used to express strength of evidence (see also Hicks, Buckleton et al., 2015)

Identification/exclusion/inconclusive framework

In an extreme version of the posterior probability framework, the practitioner only reports either "identification," i.e., 100% probability for same speaker, or "exclusion," i.e., 100% probability for different speaker, or declines to express an opinion "inconclusive." In making an "identification" or "exclusion" the forensic practitioner has made the decision as to same speaker or different speaker, which is properly a decision to be made by the trier of fact who also takes other evidence into consideration. Apart from the logical problems associated with a posterior probability framework in general, "identification" or "exclusion" leads to additional problems. Logically, a practitioner who makes an "identification" or an "exclusion" is claiming infallibility – if they acknowledged that they could be wrong then they could not be 100% certain. Also, logically, the practitioner is claiming that no other evidence in the case is relevant – the trier of fact weighs other evidence against the voice evidence, but a posterior probability of 1 equates to a posterior odds of infinity (which could only be obtained if the prior odds or the likelihood ratio were infinite), and no other evidence can have any counter effect against infinitely strong evidence. The trier of fact could, of course, decide to not believe the forensic practitioner.

President Obama's Council of Advisors on Science and Technology stated that forensic practitioners should not be allowed to claim 100% certainty (President's Council of Advisors on Science and Technology, 2016, p. 19).

UK framework

In 2007, a group of forensic voice comparison practitioners and researchers in the United Kingdom published a position statement that included a framework for evaluation of evidence (French and Harrison, 2007). This became known as the "UK framework." It was explicitly tied to auditory-acoustic-phonetic subjective approaches.

The framework has two stages: "consistency" and "distinctiveness." In the first stage, the practitioner makes a subjective judgment as to "whether the known and questioned samples are compatible, or consistent, with having been produced by the same speaker" (French & Harrison, 2007, p. 141). The choices are "consistent," "not consistent," or "no-decision." If the practitioner decides that the samples are "not consistent," the practitioner may state that they were spoken by different speakers and express their degree of confidence that this is so (this is a posterior probability). If the practitioner decides that the samples are "consistent," the practitioner then makes a subjective judgment as to whether the known- and questioned-speaker recordings fall into one of five levels of distinctiveness with respect to the relevant population: "exceptionally-distinctive," "highly-distinctive," "distinctive," "moderately-distinctive," or "not-distinctive."

Unlike the numerator and denominator of a likelihood ratio, "consistency" and "distinctiveness" are not measured on the same scale, and there are no explicit algorithms for assigning values to "consistency" or "distinctiveness." The latter are assigned "informally via the analyst's experience and general linguistic knowledge rather than formally and quantitatively" (French et al., 2010, p. 144). Also, the meaning of the conclusion is ambiguous, and there is no normatively correct way to combine it with the strength of other evidence.

The UK framework has been criticized in Rose and Morrison (2009) and Morrison (2009, 2010, 2014). In 2015, the lead authors of the UK position statement abandoned their framework (see French, 2017) in favor of the Association of Forensic Science Providers' standards (Association of Forensic Science Providers, 2009), which require the use of the likelihood ratio framework. French (2017) indicates that they have adopted the use of verbal expressions of likelihood ratios, with the level on the ordinal scale assigned on the basis of subjective judgment.

Popularity of different frameworks

In the Gold and French (2011) survey, the 35 respondents' use of different frameworks was reported as follows:

- 4 (11%) used numeric likelihood ratios
- 3 (9%) used verbal likelihood ratios

- 14 (40%) used posterior probabilities. It was suggested that most or all of these were verbal expressions of posterior probabilities
- 2 (6%) used identification/exclusion/inconclusive
- 11 (31%) used the UK framework
- 1 (3%) was reported as "other"

In the 2016 INTERPOL survey (Morrison, Sahito et al., 2017), of the 44 respondents who stated that their agency had speaker recognition capabilities, use of different frameworks was reported as follows:

- 10 (23%) used numeric likelihood ratios
- 9 (20%) used verbal likelihood ratios
- 3 (7%) used numeric posterior probabilities
- 4 (9%) used verbal posterior probabilities
- 22 (50%) used identification/exclusion/inconclusive
- 3 (7%) used the UK framework

Some respondents reported using more than one framework, or both a numeric and verbal variant, hence the preceding summary statistics add up to more than 44 (18, 41%, used numeric and/or verbal likelihood ratios).

Empirical validation

The only way to know how well a forensic comparison system works is to test it. US Federal Rule of Evidence 702 – *Daubert*[9] and England & Wales Criminal Practice Directions[10] Section 19A establish demonstration of scientific validity as a key requirement for admissibility. The following organizations also recommend or require empirical validation of forensic methodologies: National Research Council (2009); Forensic Science Regulator of England and Wales (2014, 2017), as part of accreditation; European Network of Forensic Science Institutes (Drygajlo et al., 2015), specifically for forensic voice comparison; President's Council of Advisors on Science and Technology (2016). Morrison (2014) reviewed calls going back to the 1960s for the validity and reliability of forensic voice comparison systems to be empirically validated under casework conditions.

President Obama's Council of Advisors on Science and Technology stated that:

> neither experience, nor judgment, nor good professional practices (such as certification programs and accreditation programs, standardized protocols, proficiency testing, and codes of ethics) can substitute for actual evidence of foundational validity and reliability. The frequency with which a particular pattern or set of features will be observed in different samples, which is an essential element in drawing conclusions, is not a matter of "judgment." It is an empirical matter for which only empirical evidence is relevant. Similarly, an expert's expression of *confidence* based on personal professional experience or expressions of *consensus* among practitioners about the accuracy of their field is no substitute for error rates estimated from relevant studies. For forensic feature-comparison methods, establishing foundational validity based on empirical evidence is thus a *sine qua non*. Nothing can substitute for it.[11]

Next, we describe empirical validation of forensic comparison systems within the likelihood ratio framework. A number of different metrics and graphics have been proposed for assessing and reporting the degree of validity and reliability of likelihood ratio systems (see: Morrison, 2011; Meuwly et al., 2017). Below, we describe the most popular metric (C_{llr}) and the most popular graphic (Tippett plot).

Black-box testing

Black-box testing is concerned with how well a system works, not with how it works. Black-box testing therefore treats all systems equally, irrespective of whether they are based on auditory, spectrographic, acoustic-phonetic, or automatic approaches.

The basic procedure for assessing validity using black-box testing is as follows. The tester presents the system with pairs of voice recordings. The tester knows whether each pair is a same-speaker pair or a different-speaker pair, but the system being tested must not know. For each pair, the system outputs a strength of evidence value. For simplicity, let us imagine a system that outputs "same-speaker" or "different-speaker" (this is an identification/exclusion framework). Table 21.2 shows the possible input and output combinations, and their correctness. If the answer is correct, the tester assigns it a penalty value of 0. If the answer is incorrect (a *miss* or a *false alarm*), the tester assigns it a penalty value of 1. After all the test pairs have been presented, the tester sums the penalty values and divides by the total number of pairs, i.e., calculates the mean penalty value. Usually, the proportion of misses for all same-speaker input and the proportion of false alarms for all different-speaker input are calculated, then the mean of those two proportions is calculated. The resulting value is called *classification error rate* (its inverse is *correct classification rate*).

Log likelihood ratio cost (C_{llr})

Classification error rate is not appropriate for assessing the validity of a system that outputs likelihood ratios. Classification error rate requires a same-speaker or different-speaker decision to be made, which logically requires deciding whether the value of a posterior probability exceeds a threshold or not. Also, even if one decided to use the neutral likelihood ratio value of 1 as a threshold, the further a likelihood ratio from 1 the greater the strength of evidence indicated. If, for example, the tester knew that the input was a different-speaker pair and the system returned a likelihood ratio of 1.1, that would be a

Table 21.2 List of input and output possibilities and corresponding correctness for a system which outputs either "same-speaker" or "different-speaker."

		output	
		same-speaker	different-speaker
input	same-speaker	✓ hit	× miss
	different-speaker	× false alarm	✓ correct rejection

false alarm and would attract a penalty value of 1. But if the system returned a likelihood ratio of 1000, that would also be a false alarm and also attract a penalty value of 1, even though a likelihood ratio of 1000 would be much more misleading to the trier of fact than a likelihood ratio of 1.1.

To perform empirical validation compatible with the likelihood ratio framework, instead of assigning penalty values of either 0 or 1 depending on a threshold, the procedure for calculating the *log likelihood ratio cost* (C_{llr}; see: Brümmer and du Preez, 2006; González-Rodríguez et al., 2007; Morrison, 2011) assigns a penalty value according to the magnitude of the likelihood ratio. The function for calculating C_{llr} is given in Equation 3:

$$(3)\quad C_{\text{llr}} = \frac{1}{2}\left(\frac{1}{N_s}\sum_i^{N_s}\log_2\left(1+\frac{1}{\Lambda_{s_i}}\right)+\frac{1}{N_d}\sum_j^{N_d}\log_2\left(1+\Lambda_{d_j}\right)\right)$$

Where Λ_s and Λ_d are likelihood ratio outputs corresponding to same- and different-speaker inputs respectively, and N_s and N_d are the number of same- and different-speaker inputs respectively. Figure 21.4 plots the penalty functions for likelihood ratio outputs corresponding to same- and different-speaker inputs, i.e., the functions within Equation 3's left and right summations respectively.

When the input is a same-speaker pair, large positive log likelihood ratios are good and are assigned low penalty values, small positive log likelihood ratios are not as

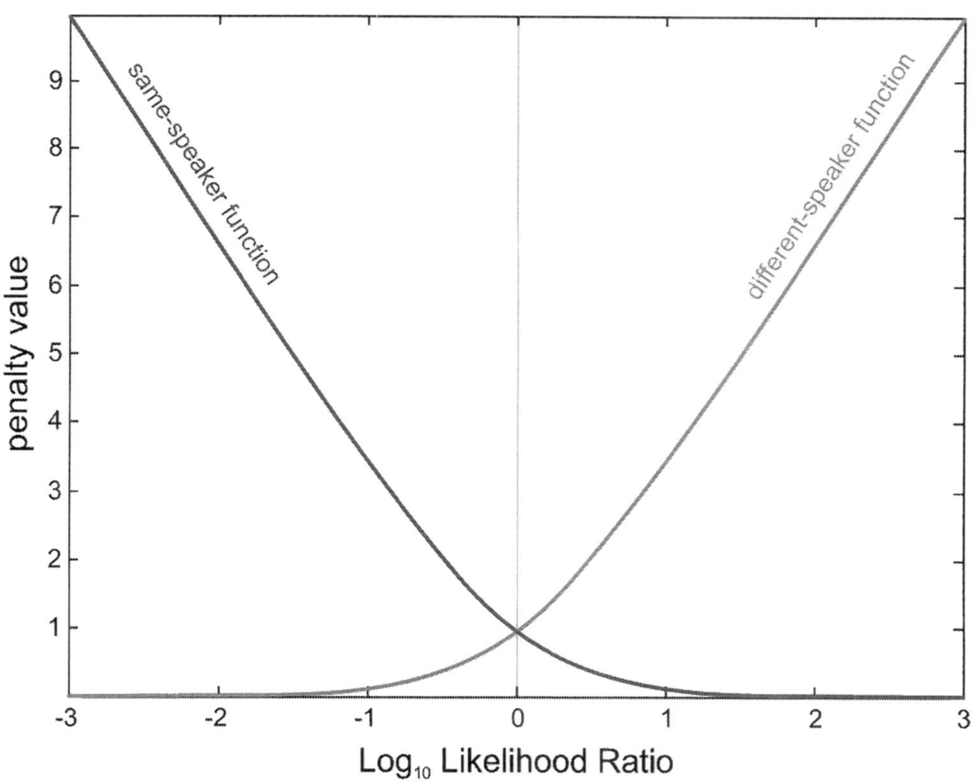

Figure 21.4 C_{llr} penalty functions.

good and are assigned higher penalty values, negative log likelihood ratios are bad and are assigned yet higher penalty values with higher penalty values for larger magnitude negative log likelihood ratios. *Mutatis mutandis* for when the input is a different-speaker pair.

The better the performance of the system, the lower the value of C_{llr}. A "perfect" system would always give infinite likelihood ratios when the input is same-speaker and always give likelihood ratios of zero when the input is different-speaker, and the value of C_{llr} would be 0. Perfect systems do not exist for non-trivial problems, so in practice C_{llr} will never reach 0. A system which always outputs a likelihood ratio of 1 irrespective of the input would provide no useful information to the trier of fact, and would have a C_{llr} value of 1. In practice, because systems are trained and tested on different data, C_{llr} values can be greater than 1. If a system has a C_{llr} value much greater than 1, then it is probably miscalibrated and better performance would be achieved if it were calibrated (see the subsection above on automatic approaches).

Tippett plots

The first step in drawing a *Tippett plot* (Meuwly, 2001) is the same as the first step in calculating C_{llr}: input same-speaker and different-speaker pairs to the system and get the corresponding output. The next step is to rank all the same-speaker results in ascending order, and all the different-speaker results in ascending order. Then the cumulative empirical distribution for each group of values is plotted. If, for example, there are $N_s = 100$ same-speaker outputs, Λ_s, the lowest ranked Λ_{s_i} $(i = 1)$ is plotted at its log likelihood ratio value on the x-axis and at its proportional rank on the y-axis, i.e., at $y = i/N_s = 1/100$. The second lowest ranked Λ_{s_i} $(i = 2)$ is plotted at $x = \Lambda_{s_2}$, $y = 2/100$, the third at $x = \Lambda_{s_3}$, $y = 3/100$, etc. The y values of the plotted points represent the proportion of likelihood ratios from same-speaker test pairs that have likelihood ratio values less than or equal to the value indicated on the x-axis. Conventionally, the points are joined by lines and no symbols are drawn at the actual point values. A similar procedure is used for the Λ_d values, but the y values of the plotted points represent the proportion of likelihood ratios from different-speaker test pairs that have likelihood ratio values greater than or equal to the value indicated on the x-axis.

Figure 21.5 shows two example Tippett plots based on artificial data created for illustrative purposes. The curve rising to the right represents the same-speaker results, and the curve rising to the left represents the different-speaker results. Learning to fully appreciate the information in Tippett plots may take some time, but at a basic level the further to the right and the shallower the slope of the same-speaker curve and the further to the left and the shallower the slope of the different-speaker curve the better the performance. A Tippett plot with fewer or less extreme values for misleading test output, i.e., same-speaker pairs resulting in negative log likelihood ratios and different-speaker pairs resulting in positive log likelihood ratios, generally indicates better performance even if the magnitudes of the log likelihood ratios pointing in the correct directions are less extreme. In Figure 21.5, the Tippett plot in the bottom panel represents a system with better performance than that in the top panel.

The C_{llr} values corresponding to the top and bottom panels in Figure 21.5 are 0.548 and 0.101 respectively. Tippett plots include all test results and therefore contain much more information than C_{llr}. C_{llr} is a single value summary metric, and is a many to one mapping – multiple different Tippett plots could correspond to the same C_{llr} value.

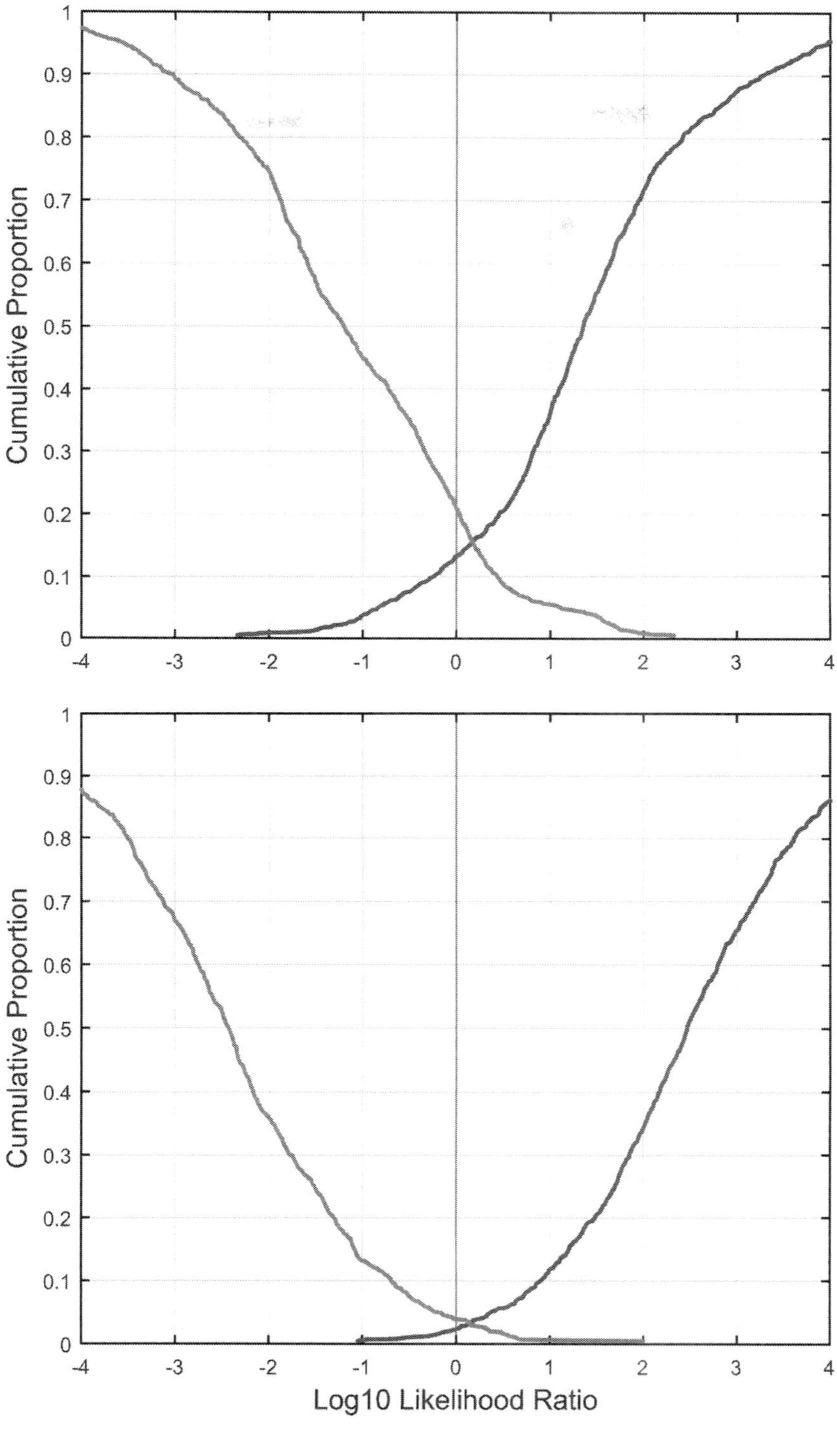

Figure 21.5 Example Tippett plots.

Appropriate test data

It is important to use test data that represent the relevant population and reflect the speaking styles and recording conditions for the case under investigation. Tests conducted using data that represent other populations and reflect other conditions may be highly misleading with respect to how well the forensic analysis system will perform when used in the case. A system that works well with studio quality audio recordings may work very poorly under casework conditions that include a mismatch between the known- and questioned-speaker recordings and poor quality recording conditions, e.g., due to background noise, reverberation, transmission through communication channels, and being saved in compressed formats. When putting together test pairs, one member of each pair must reflect the conditions of the known-speaker recording and the other must reflect the conditions of the questioned-speaker recording.

Whether the test data are sufficiently representative of the relevant population and sufficiently reflective of the speaking styles and recording conditions of the case is a judgment that will initially be made by the forensic practitioner, but the forensic practitioner must clearly communicate what they have done so that ultimately the appropriateness of their decision can be considered by the judge at an admissibility hearing and/or the trier of fact at trial.

It is important to test the system that is actually used to compare the known- and questioned-speaker recordings. For example, if an automatic system is used, but the output of the automatic system is used as input to a subjective judgment process which also includes consideration of the results of analyses based on other approaches, it is the output of the final subjective judgment process that must be empirically validated.

For admissibility, the judge first has to consider whether the test data were sufficiently representative of the relevant population and sufficiently reflective of the speaking styles and recording conditions of the case. If the judge decides that the data are sufficient, then the judge can consider whether the demonstrated degree of performance is sufficient to warrant the admission of testimony based on the forensic comparison system.

In addition, for systems based on statistical models, the test data must not be the same data as were used to train the statistical models. Training and testing on the same data gives misleadingly good results compared to when statistical models are tested on new data. In actual application, the known- and questioned-speaker recordings are new data. Therefore it is performance on new data that matters. Test data must therefore come from a completely separate sample of the relevant population, or a procedure known as cross-validation should be used to avoid training and testing on the same data.

Legal admissibility and case law

This section briefly discusses legal admissibility and case law in some common-law jurisdictions: United States (particularly Federal cases), Australia (particularly New South Wales), United Kingdom (particularly Northern Ireland and England and Wales), and Canada. We provide somewhat longer summaries of the Canadian cases because, unlike the cases from the other jurisdictions, they have not been previously described in an academic archival venue.

United States

In the United States, through the 1960s, 1970s, and 1980s, testimony based on spectrographic/auditory-spectrographic approaches was often proffered in court proceedings. Based on published rulings, the rate of admission appears to have been somewhat greater than the rate of exclusion. By the 1990s there had been a substantial decline in the number of cases in which it was proffered. In 2003 in *Angleton*,[12] in an admissibility hearing held under Federal Rule of Evidence (FRE) 702 and the criteria established by the Supreme Court in the 1993 case of *Daubert*,[13] the court ruled an auditory-spectrographic approach inadmissible. Among other criteria, FRE 702 – *Daubert* requires consideration of the empirically demonstrated level of performance of the forensic analysis system. The court found that demonstration of an adequate level of performance was lacking. Based on published rulings, no attempt to admit a spectrographic or auditory-spectrographic approach appears to have survived an FRE 702 – *Daubert* challenge since then.

In 2015 in *Ahmed*,[14] testimony was proffered which was in-part based on an automatic approach, but which was combined with auditory and acoustic-phonetic approaches to reach an ultimately subjective assessment of the strength of evidence. An FRE 702 – *Daubert* admissibility hearing was held, but before the judge ruled on the matter the case was resolved via a negotiated plea deal. Thus no decision on admissibility was issued in that case. During the hearing, questions were raised as to whether appropriate data had been used to train the automatic component of the system, whether the system had been empirically tested under conditions reflecting those of the case, and whether the subjective procedure for combining the output of the automatic component and the outputs of the subjective auditory and acoustic-phonetic components was influenced by cognitive bias.

For more detailed discussion of admissibility of forensic voice comparison testimony in the United States see Morrison and Thompson (2017).

Australia

In New South Wales in 1977 in *Gilmore*[15] the court ruled testimony based on an auditory-spectrographic approach admissible. The decision was based in part on the fact that such testimony had been ruled admissible by a number of courts in the United States in the early to mid-1970s. In a 2012 admissibility hearing in the New South Wales case of *Ly*,[16] the admissibility of testimony based on an auditory-spectrographic approach was challenged. Despite the change that had occurred in the US with respect to admissibility of auditory-spectrographic approaches, the court in *Ly* ruled that *Gilmore* was precedential and that the testimony was therefore admissible (for further discussion, see Enzinger and Morrison, 2017). In *Ly* the practitioner used a mixture of auditory, spectrographic, and acoustic-phonetic subjective approaches, with subjective judgment used to combine the results. We are aware of several other instances in which auditory-spectrographic-acoustic-phonetic-subjective or auditory-acoustic-phonetic-subjective analyses have been admitted in courts in several Australian jurisdictions.

In 2008 in *Hufnagl*,[17] testimony based on an acoustic-phonetic statistical approach was admitted (see Rose, 2013). In 2017, testimony based on an automatic approach was submitted in a New South Wales case, but the case was resolved by plea deal before going to trial (see Morrison, 2018b, in which questions are raised with respect to whether appropriate data were used for training and whether performance was empirically tested under conditions reflecting those of the case).

United Kingdom

There are rulings from Northern Ireland and from England and Wales specific to the admissibility of forensic voice comparison testimony. We are not aware of any such rulings from Scotland.

In Northern Ireland in the 2002 case of *O'Doherty*,[18] the appeal court ruled an auditory-only approach inadmissible, but auditory-acoustic-phonetic subjective approaches admissible. It was reported that most practitioners considered auditory-only approaches to be unreliable.

In England and Wales in 1991 in *Robb*,[19] the appeal court ruled an auditory-only approach admissible. In 2008 in *Flynn*,[20] the appeal court opined that *Robb* was still precedential and that courts in England and Wales should not follow the example set in Northern Ireland in *O'Doherty*. The opinion in *Flynn* was echoed in the 2015 appeal court ruling in *Slade*.[21]

The appeal court in *Slade* considered the admissibility of new evidence consisting of forensic voice comparison testimony based in-part on an automatic approach, but which was combined with an auditory-acoustic-phonetic subjective approach to reach an ultimately subjective assessment of the strength of evidence. Some empirical testing of the performance of the automatic component of the analysis was presented, but the court was not satisfied with the quantity and quality of the data used to train and test the automatic system. Nor was it satisfied with the empirically demonstrated level of performance of the system. Also note that what was tested was not the whole auditory-acoustic-phonetic-automatic plus combination-via-subjective-judgment system actually used to assess strength of evidence, but only the automatic component. What needs to be tested is the performance of the whole system, not just a component of the system (Forensic Science Regulator, 2014, §3.3.1–3.3.2). The appeal court ruled the testimony based in-part on the automatic analysis inadmissible. The ruling was specific to this instance, and did not preclude testimony based on an automatic approach being admissible in future cases. Ironically, testimony based on auditory-only and auditory-acoustic-phonetic subjective approaches had been admitted at trial despite the fact that they had not undergone any empirical testing (admissibility of these approaches does not appear to have been challenged at any point in the proceedings).

Shortly before the appeal in *Slade*, new Criminal Practice Directions on admissibility of expert evidence (CPD 19A) were introduced.[22] The CPD 19A admissibility criteria are similar to those of FRE 702 – *Daubert*. It is not clear whether they had any impact on the decision in *Slade*, but it may be that they will have an impact on future admissibility decisions. For more detailed discussion of admissibility of forensic voice comparison testimony in England and Wales and Northern Ireland see Morrison (2018a).[23]

Canada

In the 1998 labor arbitration case of *Ontario Hydro v Canadian Union of Public Employees*,[24] testimony was proffered from a university-based academic who taught applied linguistics, speech-language pathology, and phonetics and phonology, and who had conducted research in analysis of normal, pathological, and foreign-accented speech. He performed an auditory-only analysis. The Board of Arbitration considered a number of admissibility criteria identified in rulings made by courts of law. The Board found that the academic was not qualified as an expert in forensic voice comparison because he had no training or experience specifically in that field. The Board found that "his knowledge and experience as a phonetician are not sufficient for this purpose." The Board also found that "there is nothing to indicate that the method used by [the academic] to reach a conclusion regarding voice identification in this case has gained any acceptance and, based on the evidence, we find that it fails to meet a threshold test of reliability." The standards against which the Board compared the academic's auditory-only analysis were, however, those of organizations such as the American Board of Recorded Evidence (1999) which required auditory plus spectrographic analysis, and no mention was made of criticisms of the auditory-spectrographic approach (this case was prior to the US case of *Angleton*).

In 2018 in *R v Dunstan*[25] in a *Charter* Section 8 Application[26] the Ontario Superior Court of Justice considered forensic voice comparison testimony from three practitioners. For this judge-only hearing none of the testimony was ruled admissible or inadmissible *per se*, but in her ruling the judge commented on the appropriateness of the different methodologies used by the practitioners. The recording of interest was of a telephone call made to a police call center six years previously. The recording was noisy and had been saved in a lossy compressed format. The total duration of the speech of the speaker of questioned identity was approximately 10 seconds.

At trial, testimony had been presented by an audio engineer. He applied noise reduction to the questioned-speaker recording, then created multiple compilations in each of which the questioned-speaker recording was either non-synchronously intercalated/concatenated or synchronously mixed with a time-warped recording of either the known speaker, the practitioner, or a third speaker. The judge at the Section 8 hearing concluded that "The comparisons were not fair and reliable." Reasons included the following: Of several known-speaker recordings available, the particular known-speaker recordings used had been selected because they were the ones that sounded the most similar to the questioned speaker. The known-speaker recordings had been time-warped to make them more similar to the recording of the questioned speaker.

One of two practitioners to testify at the Section 8 hearing was a speech-language pathologist who conducted an auditory-acoustic-phonetic subjective analysis. The acoustic-phonetic component was based on acoustic measurements of jitter in vocal fold vibration. No data representative of a relevant population were used (a comparison was made with a recording of the practitioner's own voice), no empirical validation was conducted, and the practitioner's conclusion was reported as a subjective posterior probability. The judge concluded that the practitioner "was not an objective, unbiased witness. . . . He did not express, either in his report or in his testimony, an understanding of his duty to the court to be impartial, independent and unbiased." "[He] said that his task was to find similarities between the two voices, so he did not report dissimilarities that he observed." "[He] was unable to say what proportion of Canadian males have a jitter measurement of 7 per cent. . . . He did not give evidence from which it can be concluded that the nine test results he provided represent an empirically sound basis from which to draw inferences about voices in the forensic context."

The other practitioner to testify at the Section 8 hearing was the first author of the present chapter. He performed a human-supervised automatic analysis, which included a statistical procedure to reduce the likelihood of overstating the strength of evidence (Morrison and Poh, 2018), and a statistical procedure to take account of the six-year gap between the questioned- and known-speaker recordings even though the recordings available for training and testing were made only hours to days apart.[27] Steps were also taken to reduce the potential for cognitive bias, including that the practitioner did not listen to both the questioned- and known-speaker recordings, he listened to the questioned-speaker recording to prepare it for input into the automatic system but his assistant prepared the known-speaker recording. The automatic system was trained/optimized using multiple recordings of just over 100 speakers specially collected with the intention of representing the relevant population and reflecting the recording conditions in this case – male General Canadian English speakers made multiple mobile telephone calls to the same police call center using the same call recording system as had been used to record the questioned-speaker recording six years previously.

Empirical validation was conducted using the same recordings (cross-validation was used to avoid training and testing on the same data) and the validation results were reported. The questioned- and known-speaker recordings were then compared, and the likelihood ratio value output by the system was directly reported as the strength of evidence statement. The calculated likelihood ratio value was close to 1. In theory, a likelihood ratio value of 1 should have no effect on the trier of fact's belief as to the relative probabilities of the same- and different-speaker hypotheses, the posterior odds should be equal to the prior odds, but the practitioner was called to testify in order to contrast his methodology and result with the other practitioners' methodologies and their strong claims about the identity of the questioned speaker. The judge "accept[ed] that [the practitioner] is very well qualified in his field," but had reservations about his application of the human-supervised automatic approach: (a) "it is novel and must be carefully scrutinized"; (b) the questioned-speaker speech was only 10 seconds long;[28] (c) with respect to the statistical procedure used to compensate for the six-year time difference between the questioned- and known speaker recording, she was concerned that it had not been adequately validated;[29] and (d) with respect to the speakers intended to be representative of the relevant population, who were all police officers, she was concerned that police officers may speak differently from other speakers of General Canadian English.[30]

Conclusion

Although the case law and rulings on legal admissibility in common-law jurisdictions remain mixed, we believe that the future of forensic voice comparison lies in the use of human-supervised automatic approaches within the likelihood ratio framework, with empirical testing of system performance under casework conditions and direct reporting of the calculated likelihood ratio value. We argue that this is the most practical way to meet rigorous applications of legal admissibility criteria such as those of FRE 702 – *Daubert* and CPD 19A.

Systems in which the output is directly based on subjective judgment are not transparent, not replicable, and are highly susceptible to cognitive bias. Even if an explanation is given, there is no way to know whether it corresponds to what actually happened in the practitioner's mind or whether it is a *post hoc* rationalization. In contrast, systems based on relevant data, quantitative measurements, and statistical models are transparent and replicable. The procedures can be described in exact detail, and the data and software used can even be provided to another practitioner.

It should be noted that procedures based on relevant data, quantitative measurements, and statistical models do require subjective judgments, but these are judgments about relevant populations and relevant data which are far removed from the output of the system. The appropriateness of such judgments should be debated before the judge at an admissibility hearing and/or the trier of fact at trial. After these initial judgments, the remainder of the system is objective. Systems based on relevant data, quantitative measurements, and statistical models are therefore much more resistant to the potential influence of cognitive bias than are systems in which the output is directly based on subjective judgment.

In addition, procedures based directly on subjective judgment generally require considerable human time to perform each test trial. Thus they are practically difficult to test compared to an automatic procedure that can run thousands of test trials in seconds. If a subjective procedure were found to outperform an automatic procedure, it would be preferred, but performance would have to be empirically demonstrated under relevant conditions.

We prefer automatic approaches over acoustic-phonetic statistical approaches because we have found the former to outperform the latter, especially under forensically realistic conditions or conditions approaching forensically realistic conditions (see: Enzinger et al., 2012; Zhang et al., 2013; Zhang and Enzinger, 2013; Enzinger, 2014; Enzinger and Kasess, 2014; Jessen et al., 2014; Enzinger et al., 2016; Enzinger and Morrison, 2017).[31] We also prefer automatic approaches because acoustic-phonetic approaches generally require much greater investment of human time and therefore take longer and are more expensive.

In evaluation of strength of evidence for presentation in court, it would be inappropriate for a system to be fully automatic; it should be human-supervised. The forensic practitioner is responsible for determining an appropriate question to ask and selecting appropriate data and statistical models in order to answer that question. An automatic system is a tool, and inappropriate use of the tool will lead to inappropriate results. A potential danger of automatic systems is that they could be too easy to use, and therefore too easy to misuse. Appropriate training and knowledge is therefore essential.

Notes

1 All panels in Figure 21.1 were based on the same simulated data consisting of $N_k = 100$ recordings sampled from the simulated known speaker and $N_r = 1000$ recordings sampled from the simulated relevant population. The data were generated for illustrative purposes only and are not intended to accurately reflect real f_0 distributions.

2 Technically, when describing a likelihood ratio one should talk about *probability of evidence given hypotheses* if the data are discrete, but *likelihood of hypotheses given evidence* if the data are continuous. This, however, is confusing for non-statisticians, and our concern in a forensic or legal context is to avoid inducing the prosecutor's fallacy (Thompson and Schumann, 1987). We may therefore use phrases such as "likelihood of evidence given hypotheses" or "probability of evidence given hypotheses" rather than the technically correct "likelihood of hypotheses given evidence."

3 If increased similarity corresponds with increased typicality, however, then in some instances the value of the likelihood ratio could decrease as similarity increases.

4 This discussion is provided to explain the meaning of a likelihood ratio. It is not intended to instruct triers of fact as to how to reason on legal matters, nor to imply that triers of fact must assign numeric values to evidence which is not the result of a forensic analysis.

5 For more detailed criticism of verbal expressions and ordinal scales, see Marquis et al. (2016) and Morrison and Enzinger (2016). For a study of lay people's perception of various verbal and numeric expressions of strength of evidence, see Thompson et al. (2018).

6 Selection of the relevant population in the context of forensic voice comparison is discussed in Morrison et al. (2012), Gold and Hughes (2014), Hughes and Foulkes (2015), Hicks, Biedermann et al. (2015, 2017), Morrison et al. (2016, 2017), Hughes and Rhodes (2018).

7 We note, however, that it is not always obvious whether the questioned speaker is male or female and since the different-speaker hypothesis is that the questioned speaker is not the known speaker, the sex of the known speaker is not relevant for defining the relevant population. In such cases the relevant population could include speakers of both sexes, e.g., males plus females with low-pitched voices or females plus males with high-pitched voices.

8 For coherent odds: $o(H) = p(H) / p(\tilde{H})$, and $p(\tilde{H}) = 1 - p(H)$. $\tilde{H}$ means not *H*. Hence, via substitution and algebraic derivation, the formula to convert from posterior odds to posterior probability is: $p(H) = o(H) / (1 + o(H))$.

9 *William Daubert et al. v Merrell Dow Pharmaceuticals Inc.*, 509 US 579 (1993).

10 *Criminal Practice Directions* [2015] EWCA Crim 1567.

11 President's Council of Advisors on Science and Technology (2016) p. 6, emphasis in original.

12 *United States v Robert N. Angleton*, 269 F.Supp. 2nd 892 (S.D. Tex. 2003).
13 *William Daubert et al. v Merrell Dow Pharmaceuticals Inc.*, 509 US 579 (1993).
14 *United States v Ali Ahmed, Madhi Hashi, and Muhamed Yusuf*, No. 12–661 (E.D.N.Y.).
15 *R v Gilmore*, 1977, 2 NSWLR 935.
16 *R v Ly*, NSW District Court, 2010/295928 (note that this is a reference to an earlier hearing in the case).
17 *R v Hufnagl*, NSW District Court, 2008.
18 *R v O'Doherty* [2002] NICA 20 / [2003] 1 Cr App R 5.
19 *R v Robb* [1991] 93 Cr App R 161.
20 *R v Flynn and St John* [2008] EWCA Crim 970.
21 *R v Slade et al.* [2015] EWCA Crim 71.
22 *Criminal Practice Directions* [2015] EWCA Crim 1567.
23 For a history of forensic voice comparison in the UK from another perspective, see French (2017).
24 *Ontario Hydro v Canadian Union of Public Employees* [1998] OLAA No 691.
25 *R v Dunstan* [2018] ONSC 4153.
26 *Canadian Charter of Rights and Freedoms*, s 8, Part I of the Constitution Act, 1982, being Schedule B to the Canada Act 1982 (UK), 1982, c 11. Section 8 provides protection against unreasonable search and seizure.
27 This was developed specifically for use in this case building on research reported in Kelly and Hansen (2016).
28 This does not seem to have taken into account that the performance of the forensic voice comparison system was empirically validated under conditions reflecting those of the case under investigation, including the condition that questioned-speaker speech had a duration of 10 seconds. We would argue that a decision on whether to use the output of a system should be made on the basis of consideration of results of empirical testing of that system under conditions reflecting those of the case, rather than directly on what those conditions happen to be.
29 Published papers including descriptions of the data used to train the statistical procedure were submitted along with the original report, and the practitioner offered to provide a supplemental report he had prepared on the validation of the statistical procedure.
30 This was an argument advanced by the party who proposed the same-speaker hypothesis. We do not believe that this argument has any merit, but, even if it did, the same-speaker hypothesis they proposed was that the questioned speaker was a particular police officer. Hence there was no basis for their objection that the sample recordings were recordings of police officers and that typicality was therefore assessed with respect to male General Canadian English speakers who were police officers rather than with respect to male General Canadian English speakers in general.
31 These are primarily papers written by ourselves. Our backgrounds are in acoustic phonetics, and we thus had an interest in empirically assessing the performance of acoustic-phonetic-statistical approaches under casework conditions. Other than our work, there is very little published work in which acoustic-phonetic-statistical and automatic systems have both been empirically tested on the same test data under forensically realistic or close to forensically realistic conditions.

References

Aitken, C.G.G., Berger, C.E.H., Buckleton, J.S., Champod, C., Curran, J.M., Dawid, A.P., Evett, I.W., Gill, P., González-Rodríguez, J., Jackson, G., Kloosterman, A., Lovelock, T., Lucy, D., Margot, P., McKenna, L., Meuwly, D., Neumann, C., Nic Daéid, N., Nordgaard, A., Puch-Solis, R., Rasmusson, B., Redmayne, M., Roberts, P., Robertson, B., Roux, C., Sjerps, M.J., Taroni, F., Tjin-A-Tsoi, T., Vignaux, G.A., Willis, S.M. and Zadora, G. (2011). Expressing evaluative opinions: A position statement. *Science & Justice*, 51, 1–2. http://dx.doi.org/10.1016/j.scijus.2011.01.002

Aitken, C.G.G., Roberts, P. and Jackson, G. (2010). *Fundamentals of Probability and Statistical Evidence in Criminal Proceedings: Guidance for Judges, Lawyers, Forensic Scientists and Expert Witnesses*. London: Royal Statistical Society. Available at: http://bit.ly/1WnoXRx [Accessed 1 February 2017].

Ajili, M. (2017). *Reliability of Voice Comparison for Forensic Applications*. PhD. University of Avignon.

Ajili, M., Bonastre, J.F., Ben Kheder, W., Rossato, S. and Kahn, J. (2016). Phonetic content impact on forensic voice comparison. In *Proceedings of the 2016 IEEE Spoken Language Technology Workshop (SLT)*, pp. 201–217. http://dx.doi.org/10.1109/SLT.2016.7846267

American Board of Recorded Evidence. (1999). *Voice Comparison Standards*. Available at: www.tapeexpert.com/pdf/abrevoiceid.pdf [Accessed 1 February 2010].

Association of Forensic Science Providers. (2009). Standards for the formulation of evaluative forensic science expert opinion. *Science & Justice*, 49, 161–164. https://doi.org/10.1016/j.scijus.2009.07.004

Balding, D.J. and Steele, C. (2015). *Weight-of-Evidence for Forensic DNA Profiles*. 2nd ed. Chichester: Wiley-Blackwell. https://doi.org/10.1002/9781118814512

Becker, T. (2012). *Automatischer Forensischer Stimmenvergleich* [Automatic forensic voice comparison]. PhD. University of Trier.

Brümmer, N. and du Preez, J. (2006). Application independent evaluation of speaker detection. *Computer Speech and Language*, 20, 230–275. https://doi.org/10.1016/j.csl.2005.08.001

Cambier-Langeveld, T., van Rossum, M. and Vermeulen, J. (2014). Whose voice is that? Challenges in forensic phonetics. In van Heuven V. and Caspers, J., eds., *Above and Beyond the Segments: Experimental Linguistics and Phonetics*. Amsterdam: John Benjamins, pp. 14–27.

Davis, S. and Mermelstein, P. (1980). Comparison of parametric representations for monosyllabic word recognition in continuously spoken sentences. *IEEE Transactions on Acoustics, Speech, and Signal Processing*, 28(4), 357–366. https://doi.org/10.1109/TASSP.1980.1163420

Dehak, N., Kenny, P.J., Dehak, R., Dumouchel, P. and Ouellet, P. (2011). Front-end factor analysis for speaker verification. *IEEE Transactions on Acoustics, Speech, and Signal Processing*, 19(4), 788–798. https://doi.org/10.1109/TASL.2010.2064307

Drygajlo, A., Jessen, M., Gfroerer, S., Wagner, I., Vermeulen, J. and Niemi, T. (2015). *Methodological Guidelines for Best Practice in Forensic Semiautomatic and Automatic Speaker Recognition, Including Guidance on the Conduct of Proficiency Testing and Collaborative Exercises*. European Network of Forensic Science Institutes. Available at: http://enfsi.eu/wp-content/uploads/2016/09/guidelines_fasr_and_fsasr_0.pdf [Accessed 1 January 2018].

Edmond, G., Towler, A., Growns, B., Ribeiro, G., Found, B., White, D., Ballantyne, K., Searston, R.A., Thompson, M.B., Tangen, J.M., Kemp, R.I. and Martire, K. (2017). Thinking forensics: Cognitive science for forensic practitioners. *Science & Justice*, 57, 144–154. http://dx.doi.org/10.1016/j.scijus.2016.11.005

Enzinger, E. (2014). A first attempt at compensating for effects due to recording-condition mismatch in formant-trajectory-based forensic voice comparison. In *Proceedings of the 15th Australasian International Conference on Speech Science and Technology*. Australasian Speech Science and Technology Association, pp. 133–136 Available at: www.assta.org/sst/SST-14/6.A.%20FORENSICS%202/1.%20ENZINGER.pdf [Accessed 1 February 2017].

Enzinger, E. (2016). *Implementation of Forensic Voice Comparison Within the New Paradigm for the Evaluation of Forensic Evidence*. PhD. University of New South Wales. Available at: http://handle.unsw.edu.au/1959.4/55772 [Accessed 1 February 2017].

Enzinger, E. and Kasess, C.H. (2014). Bayesian vocal tract model estimates of nasal stops for speaker verification. In *Proceedings of the International Conference on Acoustics, Speech, and Signal Processing (ICASSP 2014)*, pp. 1685–1689. http://dx.doi.org/10.1109/ICASSP.2014.6853885

Enzinger, E. and Morrison, G.S. (2017). Empirical test of the performance of an acoustic-phonetic approach to forensic voice comparison under conditions similar to those of a real case. *Forensic Science International*, 277, 30–40. http://dx.doi.org/10.1016/j.forsciint.2017.05.007

Enzinger, E., Morrison, G.S. and Ochoa, F. (2016). A demonstration of the application of the new paradigm for the evaluation of forensic evidence under conditions reflecting those of a real forensic-voice-comparison case. *Science & Justice*, 56, 42–57. http://dx.doi.org/10.1016/j.scijus.2015.06.005

Enzinger, E., Zhang, C. and Morrison, G.S. (2012). Voice source features for forensic voice comparison – An evaluation of the Glottex® software package. In *Proceedings of Odyssey 2012: The Language and Speaker Recognition Workshop*, pp. 78–85. Available at: http://isca-speech.org/archive/odyssey_2012/od12_078.html [Accessed 1 February 2017] [Errata and addenda Available at: https://box.entn.at/pdfs/enzinger2012_odyssey_vsferradd.pdf Accessed 1 February 2017].

Forensic Science Regulator. (2014). *Guidance on Validation (FSR-G-201 Issue 1)*. Birmingham: Forensic Science Regulator. Available at: www.gov.uk/government/publications/forensic-science-providers-validation [Accessed 19 March 2017].

Forensic Science Regulator. (2017). *Codes of Practice and Conduct for Forensic Science Providers and Practitioners in the Criminal Justice System (Version 4.0)*. Birmingham: Forensic Science Regulator. Available at: www.gov.uk/government/publications/forensic-science-providers-codes-of-practice-and-conduct-2017 [Accessed 13 June 2018].

Found, B. (2015). Deciphering the human condition: The rise of cognitive forensics. *Australian Journal of Forensic Sciences*, 47, 386–401. http://dx.doi.org/10.1080/00450618.2014.965204

French, J.P. (2017). A developmental history of forensic speaker comparison in the UK. *English Phonetics*, 21, 271–286.

French, J.P. and Harrison, P. (2007). Position statement concerning use of impressionistic likelihood terms in forensic speaker comparison cases. *International Journal of Speech, Language and the Law*, 14, 137–144. https://doi.org/10.1558/ijsll.v14i1.137

French, J.P., Nolan, F., Foulkes, P., Harrison, P. and McDougall, K. (2010). The UK position statement on forensic speaker comparison: A rejoinder to Rose and Morrison. *International Journal of Speech, Language and the Law*, 17, 143–152. https://doi.org/10.1558/ijsll.v17i1.143

French, J.P. and Stevens, L. (2013). Forensic speech science. In Jones, M.J. and Knight, R.A., eds., *The Bloomsbury Companion to Phonetics*. London: Bloomsbury, pp. 183–197. http://dx.doi.org/10.5040/9781472541895.ch-012

Furui, S. (1981). Cepstral analysis technique for automatic speaker verification. *IEEE Transactions on Acoustics, Speech, and Signal Processing*, 29(2), 254–272. https://doi.org/10.1109/TASSP.1981.1163530

Furui, S. (1986). Speaker-independent isolated word recognition using dynamic features of speech spectrum. *IEEE Transactions on Acoustics, Speech, and Signal Processing*, 34, 52–59. https://doi.org/10.1109/TASSP.1986.1164788

Gold, E. and French, J.P. (2011). International practices in forensic speaker comparison. *International Journal of Speech, Language and the Law*, 18, 143–152. http://dx.doi.org/10.1558/ijsll.v18i2.293

Gold, E. and Hughes, V. (2014). Issues and opportunities: The application of the numerical likelihood ratio framework to forensic speaker comparison. *Science & Justice*, 54, 292–299. http://dx.doi.org/10.1016/j.scijus.2014.04.003

González-Rodríguez, J., Rose, P., Ramos, D., Toledano, D.T. and Ortega-García, J. (2007). Emulating DNA: Rigorous quantification of evidential weight in transparent and testable forensic speaker recognition. *IEEE Transactions on Audio, Speech, and Language Processing*, 15, 2104–2115. https://doi.org/10.1109/TASL.2007.902747

Gruber, J.S. and Poza, F. (1995). Voicegram Identification Evidence. *American Jurisprudence Trials*, 54. Westlaw.

Hansen, J.H.L. and Hasan, T. (2015). Speaker recognition by machines and humans: A tutorial review. *IEEE Signal Processing Magazine*, November 74–99. http://dx.doi.org/10.1109/MSP.2015.2462851

Hicks, T., Biedermann, A., de Koeijer, J.A., Taroni, F., Champod, C. and Evett, I.W. (2015). The importance of distinguishing information from evidence-observations when formulating propositions. *Science & Justice*, 55, 520–525. http://dx.doi.org/10.1016/j.scijus.2015.06.008

Hicks, T., Biedermann, A., de Koeijer, J.A., Taroni, F., Champod, C. and Evett, I.W. (2017). Reply to Morrison et al. (2016) Refining the relevant population in forensic voice comparison – A response to Hicks et alii (2015) The importance of distinguishing information from evidence/observations when formulating propositions. *Science & Justice*, 57, 401–402. http://dx.doi.org/10.1016/j.scijus.2017.04.005

Hicks, T., Buckleton, J.S., Bright, J.A. and Taylor, D. (2015). A Framework for interpreting evidence. In Buckleton, J.S., Bright, J.A. and Taylor, D., eds., *Forensic DNA Evidence Interpretation*. 2nd ed. Boca Raton, FL: CRC, pp. 37–86.

Hollien, H. (2002). *Forensic Voice Identification*. San Diego, CA: Academic Press.

Hollien, H. (2016). An approach to speaker identification. *Journal of Forensic Sciences*, 61, 334–344. http://dx.doi.org/10.1111/1556-4029.13034

Hollien, H., Didla, G., Harnsberger, J.D. and Hollien, K.A. (2016). The case for aural perceptual speaker identification. *Forensic Science International*, 269, 5–20. http://dx.doi.org/10.1016/j.forsciint.2016.08.007

Hughes, V. and Foulkes, P. (2015). The relevant population in forensic voice comparison: Effects of varying delimitations of social class and age. *Speech Communication*, 66, 218–230. http://dx.doi.org/10.1016/j.specom.2014.10.006

Hughes, V. and Rhodes, R. (2018). Questions, propositions and assessing different levels of evidence: Forensic voice comparison in practice. *Science & Justice*, 58, 250–257. https://doi.org/10.1016/j.scijus.2018.03.007

Jackson, G. (2009). Understanding forensic science opinions. In Fraser, J. and Williams, R., eds., *Handbook of Forensic Science*. Cullompton: Willan, pp. 419–445.

Jessen, M. (2008). Forensic phonetics. *Language and Linguistics Compass*, 2, 671–711. https://doi.org/10.1111/j.1749-818x.2008.00066.x

Jessen, M., Alexander, A. and Forth, O. (2014). Forensic voice comparisons in German with phonetic and automatic features using Vocalise software. In *Proceedings of the 54th Audio Engineering Society (AES) Forensics Conference*, Audio Engineering Society, pp. 28–35.

Kelly, F. and Hansen, J.H.L. (2016). Score-aging calibration for speaker verification. *IEEE/ACM Transactions on Audio, Speech, and Language Processing*, 24, 2414–2424. http://dx.doi.org/10.1109/TASLP.2016.2602542

Kersta, L.G. (1962). Voiceprint identification. *Nature*, 196, 1253–1257. https://doi.org/10.1038/1961253a0

Klecka, W.R. (1980). *Discriminant Analysis*. Beverly Hills, CA: Sage.

Marks, D.B. (2017). *A Framework for Performing Forensic and Investigatory Speaker Comparisons Using Automated Methods*. MSc. University of Colorado Denver.

Marquis, R., Biedermann, A., Cadola, L., Champod, C., Gueissaz, L., Massonnet, G., Mazzella, W.D., Taroni, F. and Hicks, T.N. (2016). Discussion on how to implement a verbal scale in a forensic laboratory: Benefits, pitfalls and suggestions to avoid misunderstandings. *Science & Justice*, 56, 364–370. http://dx.doi.org/10.1016/j.scijus.2016.05.009

Meuwly, D. (2001). *Reconnaissance de locuteurs en sciences forensiques: L'apport d'une approche automatique* [Speaker recognition in forensic science: The contribution of an automatic approach]. PhD. University of Lausanne.

Meuwly, D. (2003a). Le mythe de l'empreinte vocale I [The myth of voiceprinting I]. *Revue Internationale de Criminologie et Police Technique*, 56, 219–236.

Meuwly, D. (2003b). Le mythe de l'empreinte vocale II [The myth of voiceprinting II]. *Revue Internationale de Criminologie et Police Technique*, 56, 361–374.

Meuwly, D., Ramos, D. and Haraksim, R. (2017). A guideline for the validation of likelihood ratio methods used for forensic evidence evaluation. *Forensic Science International*, 276, 142–153. http://dx.doi.org/10.1016/j.forsciint.2016.03.048

Morrison, G.S. (2009). Forensic voice comparison and the paradigm shift. *Science & Justice*, 49, 298–308. https://doi.org/10.1016/j.scijus.2009.09.002

Morrison, G.S. (2010). Forensic voice comparison. In Freckelton, I. and Selby, H., eds., *Expert Evidence*. Sydney, Australia: Thomson Reuters, ch. 99.

Morrison, G.S. (2011). Measuring the validity and reliability of forensic likelihood-ratio systems. *Science & Justice*, 51, 91–98. http://dx.doi.org/10.1016/j.scijus.2011.03.002

Morrison, G.S. (2013). Tutorial on logistic-regression calibration and fusion: Converting a score to a likelihood ratio. *Australian Journal of Forensic Sciences*, 45, 173–197. http://dx.doi.org/10.1080/00450618.2012.733025

Morrison, G.S. (2014). Distinguishing between forensic science and forensic pseudoscience: Testing of validity and reliability, and approaches to forensic voice comparison. *Science & Justice*, 54, 245–256. http://dx.doi.org/10.1016/j.scijus.2013.07.004

Morrison, G.S. (2018a). Admissibility of forensic voice comparison testimony in England and Wales. *Criminal Law Review*, 1, 20–33.

Morrison, G.S. (2018b). The impact in forensic voice comparison of lack of calibration and of mismatched conditions between the known-speaker recording and the relevant-population sample recordings. *Forensic Science International*, 283, e1–e7. http://dx.doi.org/10.1016/j.forsciint.2017.12.024

Morrison, G.S. and Enzinger, E. (2016). What should a forensic practitioner's likelihood ratio be? *Science & Justice*, 56, 374–379. http://dx.doi.org/10.1016/j.scijus.2016.05.007

Morrison, G.S., Enzinger, E. and Zhang, C. (2016). Refining the relevant population in forensic voice comparison – A response to Hicks et alii (2015) The importance of distinguishing information from evidence/observations when formulating propositions. *Science & Justice*, 56, 492–497. http://dx.doi.org/10.1016/j.scijus.2016.07.002

Morrison, G.S., Enzinger, E. and Zhang, C. (2017). *Reply to Hicks et alii (2017) Reply to Morrison et alii (2016) Refining the Relevant Population in Forensic Voice Comparison – A Response to Hicks et alii (2015) The Importance of Distinguishing Information from Evidence/Observations When Formulating Propositions*. Available at: http://arxiv.org/abs/1704.07639

Morrison, G.S., Enzinger, E. and Zhang, C. (2018). Forensic speech science. In Freckelton, I. and Selby, H., eds., *Expert Evidence*. Sydney, Australia: Thomson Reuters, ch. 99.

Morrison, G.S., Kaye, D.H., Balding, D.J., Taylor, D., Dawid, P., Aitken, C.G.G., Gittelson, S., Zadora, G., Robertson, B., Willis, S.M., Pope, S., Neil, M., Martire, K.A., Hepler, A., Gill, R.D., Jamieson, A., de Zoete, J., Ostrum, R.B. and Caliebe, A. (2017). A comment on the PCAST report: Skip the "match"/"non-match" stage. *Forensic Science International*, 272, e7–e9. http://dx.doi.org/10.1016/j.forsciint.2016.10.018

Morrison, G.S., Ochoa, F. and Thiruvaran, T. (2012). Database selection for forensic voice comparison. In *Proceedings of Odyssey 2012: The Language and Speaker Recognition Workshop*. International Speech Communication Association, pp. 62–77.

Morrison, G.S. and Poh, N. (2018). Avoiding overstating the strength of forensic evidence: Shrunk likelihood ratios/Bayes factors. *Science & Justice*, 58, 200–218. http://dx.doi.org/10.1016/j.scijus.2017.12.005

Morrison, G.S., Sahito, F.H., Jardine, G., Djokic, D., Clavet, S., Berghs, S. and Goemans Dorny, C. (2017). INTERPOL survey of the use of speaker identification by law enforcement agencies. *Forensic Science International*, 263, 92–100. http://dx.doi.org/10.1016/j.forsciint.2016.03.044

Morrison, G.S. and Thompson, W.C. (2017). Assessing the admissibility of a new generation of forensic voice comparison testimony. *Columbia Science and Technology Law Review*, 18, 326–434.

National Commission on Forensic Science. (2015). *Ensuring That Forensic Analysis Is Based Upon Task-Relevant Information*. Available at: www.justice.gov/ncfs/file/818196/download [Accessed 1 January 2018].

National Research Council. (1979). *On the Theory and Practice of Voice Identification*. Washington, DC: National Academies Press.

National Research Council. (2009). *Strengthening Forensic Science in the United States: A Path Forward*. Washington, DC: National Academies Press.

Nolan, F. (1997). Speaker recognition and forensic phonetics. In Hardcastle, W.J. and Laver, J., eds., *The Handbook of Phonetic Sciences*. Oxford: Wiley-Blackwell, pp. 744–767.

Nolan, F. (2005). Forensic speaker identification and the phonetic description of voice quality. In Hardcastle, W.J. and Mackenzie Beck, J., eds., *A Figure of Speech: A Festschrift for John Laver*. Mahwah, NJ: Lawernce Erlbaum Associates, pp. 385–411.

Pelecanos, J. and Sridharan, S. (2001). Feature warping for robust speaker verification. In *Proceedings of Odyssey 2001: The Speaker Recognition Workshop*, International Speech Communication Association, pp. 213–218.

Pigeon, S., Druyts, P. and Verlinde, P. (2000). Applying logistic regression to the fusion of the NIST'99 1-speaker submissions. *Digital Signal Processing*, 10, 237–248. http://dx.doi.org/10.1006/dspr.1999.0358

Poza, F. and Begault, D.R. (2005). Voice identification and elimination using aural-spectrographic protocols. In *Proceedings of the Audio Engineering Society 26th International Conference: Audio Forensics in the Digital Age*, Audio Engineering Society, pp. 1–1.

President's Council of Advisors on Science and Technology. (2016). *Forensic Science in Criminal Courts: Ensuring Scientific Validity of Feature-Comparison Methods*. Available at: https://obamawhitehouse.archives.gov/administration/eop/ostp/pcast/docsreports/ [Accessed 6 February 2017].

Prince, S.J.D. and Elder, J.H. (2007). Probabilistic linear discriminant analysis for inferences about identity. In *Proceedings of the IEEE 11th International Conference on Computer Vision (ICCV)*, pp. 1–8. https://doi.org/10.1109/ICCV.2007.4409052

Ramos Castro, D. (2007). *Forensic Evaluation of the Evidence Using Automatic Speaker Recognition Systems*. PhD. Autonomous University of Madrid.

Reynolds, D.A., Quatieri, T.F. and Dunn, R.B. (2000). Speaker verification using adapted Gaussian mixture models. *Digital Signal Processing*, 10, 19–41. https://doi.org/10.1006/dspr.1999.0361

Richardson, F., Reynolds, D.A. and Dehak, N. (2015). Deep neural network approaches to speaker and language recognition. *IEEE Signal Processing Letters*, 22, 1671–1675. https://doi.org/10.1109/LSP.2015.2420092

Risinger, D.M., Saks, M.J., Thompson, W.C. and Rosenthal, R. (2002). The Daubert/Kumho implications of observer effects in forensic science: Hidden problems of expectation and suggestion. *California Law Review*, 90, 1–56. Available at: www.jstor.org/stable/3481305

Robertson, B., Vignaux, G.A. and Berger, C.E.H. (2016). *Interpreting Evidence: Evaluating Forensic Science in the Courtroom*. 2nd ed. Chichester, UK: Wiley. https://doi.org/10.1002/9781118492475

Rose, P. (2002). *Forensic Speaker Identification*. London: Taylor & Francis.

Rose, P. (2006). Technical forensic speaker recognition. *Computer Speech and Language*, 20, 159–191. https://doi.org/10.1016/j.csl.2005.07.003

Rose, P. (2013). Where the science ends and the law begins-likelihood ratio-based forensic voice comparison in a $150 million telephone fraud. *International Journal of Speech, Language and the Law*, 20, 227–324. http://dx.doi.org/10.1558/ijsll.v20i2.277

Rose, P. (2017). Likelihood ratio-based forensic voice comparison with higher level features: Research and reality. *Computer Speech & Language*, 45, 475–502. http://dx.doi.org/10.1016/j.csl.2017.03.003

Rose, P. and Morrison, G.S. (2009). A response to the UK position statement on forensic speaker comparison. *International Journal of Speech, Language and the Law*, 16, 139–163. http://dx.doi.org/10.1558/ijsll.v16i1.139

Saks, M.J., Risinger, D.M., Rosenthal, R. and Thompson, W.C. (2003). Context effects in forensic science: A review and application of the science of science to crime laboratory practice in the United States. *Science & Justice*, 43, 77–90. http://dx.doi.org/10.1016/S1355-0306(03)71747-X

Solan, L.M. and Tiersma, P.M. (2003). Hearing voices: Speaker identification in court. *Hastings Law Journal*, 54, 373–435.

Stoel, R.D., Berger, C.E.H., Kerkhoff, W., Mattijssen, E.J.A.T. and Dror, E.I. (2015). Minimizing contextual bias in forensic casework. In Strom, K.J. and Hickman, M.J., eds., *Forensic Science and the Administration of Justice: Critical Issues and Directions*. Thousand Oaks, CA: Sage, pp. 67–86. http://dx.doi.org/10.4135/9781483368740.n5

Thompson, W.C., Hofstein Grady, R., Lai, E. and Stern, H.S. (2018). Perceived strength of reporting statements about source conclusions. *Law, Probability and Risk*, 17, 133–155. http://dx.doi.org/10.1093/lpr/mgy012

Thompson W.C. and Schumann E.L. (1987). Interpretation of statistical evidence in criminal trials: The prosecutor's fallacy and the defense attorney's fallacy. *Law and Human Behavior*, 11, 167–187. http://dx.doi.org/ 10.1007/BF01044641

Tibrewala, S. and Hermansky, H. (1997). Multi-band and adaptation approaches to robust speech recognition. In *Proceedings of Eurospeech*, International Speech Communication Association, pp. 2619–2622.

Tosi, O. (1979). *Voice Identification: Theory and Legal Applications*. Baltimore, MD: University Park Press.

Willis, S.M., McKenna, L., McDermott, S., O'Donell, G., Barrett, A., Rasmusson, A., Nordgaard, A., Berger, C.E.H., Sjerps, M.J., Lucena-Molina, J.J., Zadora, G., Aitken, C.G.G., Lunt, L., Champod, C., Biedermann, A., Hicks, T.N. and Taroni, F. (2015). *ENFSI Guideline for Evaluative Reporting in Forensic Science*. European Network of Forensic Science Institutes. Available at: http://enfsi.eu/wp-content/uploads/2016/09/m1_guideline.pdf [Accessed 1 January 2018]

Zhang, C. and Enzinger, E. (2013). Fusion of multiple formant-trajectory- and fundamental-frequency-based forensic-voice-comparison systems: Chinese /ei1/, /ai2/, and /iau1/. In: In *Proceedings of the 21st International Congress on Acoustics (ICA), Proceedings of Meetings on Acoustics*, volume 19, paper 060044. Available at: http://dx.doi.org/10.1121/1.4798793

Zhang, C., Morrison, G.S., Enzinger, E. and Ochoa, F. (2013). Effects of telephone transmission on the performance of formant-trajectory-based forensic voice comparison – female voices. *Speech Communication*, 55, 796–813. Available at: http://dx.doi.org/10.1016/j.specom.2013.01.011

Index

Note: Page numbers in *italic* indicate a figure and page numbers in **bold** indicate a table on the corresponding page.